Complications in Surgery and Trauma

J. B. Lippincott Company
Philadelphia

London
Mexico City
New York
St. Louis
São Paulo
Sydney

Complications in Surgery and Trauma

Edited by
Lazar J. Greenfield, M.D.
Stuart McGuire Professor and
Chairman, Department of Surgery
Medical College of Virginia
Virginia Commonwealth University
Richmond, Virginia
67 Contributors

Foreword by
David C. Sabiston, Jr., M.D.
James B. Duke Professor of Surgery and
Chairman, Department of Surgery
Duke University Medical Center
Durham, North Carolina

Acquisitions Editor: John deCarville
Sponsoring Editor: Sanford J. Robinson
Manuscript Editor: Lee Henderson
Indexer: Sandra King
Art Director: Maria S. Karkucinski
Designer: Arlene Putterman
Production Supervisor: N. Carol Kerr
Production Assistant: S. M. Gassaway
Compositor: Ruttle, Shaw & Wetherill, Inc.
Printer/Binder: Halliday Lithograph

1 3 5 6 4 2

Library of Congress Cataloging in Publication Data
Main entry under title:
Complications in surgery and trauma.
Bibliography: p.
Includes index.
1. Surgery—Complications and sequelae. 2. Wounds and injuries—Complications and sequelae. I. Greenfield, Lazar J. [DNLM: 1. Intraoperative complications. 2. Wounds and injuries—Complications. WO 181 C737]
RD98.C66 1984 617′.01 83-9348
ISBN 0-397-50521-3

The authors and publisher have exerted every effort to ensure that drug selection and dosage set forth in this text are in accord with current recommendations and practice at the time of publication. However, in view of ongoing research, changes in government regulations, and the constant flow of information relating to drug therapy and drug reactions, the reader is urged to check the package insert for each drug for any change in indications and dosage and for added warnings and precautions. This is particularly important when the recommended agent is a new or infrequently employed drug.

To Sharon
and our families,
who forbear our commitment
to surgery

Contributors

Robert S. Adelaar, M.D.
Associate Professor of Surgery and Chief, Section of Hand and Sports Medicine, Medical College of Virginia, Richmond, Virginia

Aliasghar Aghdami, M.D.
Associate Professor of Anesthesiology, Medical College of Virginia, Richmond, Virginia

J. Wesley Alexander, M.D., Sc.D.
Professor of Surgery and Director, Transplantation Division, University of Cincinnati Medical Center; Director of Research, Shriners Burn Institute, Cincinnati Unit, Cincinnati, Ohio

Jeffrey S. Augenstein, M.D., Ph.D.
Assistant Professor of Surgery and Anesthesiology; Associate Director, Surgical Intensive Care Unit; and Director, Medical Information Systems Laboratory, University of Miami–Jackson Memorial Medical Center, Miami, Florida

Robert W. Barnes, M.D.
David Hume Professor of Surgery, Medical College of Virginia, Richmond, Virginia

Donald P. Becker, M.D.
Professor and Chairman, Division of Neurosurgery, Medical College of Virginia, Richmond, Virginia

Bruce Broecker, M.D.
Assistant Professor of Surgery, Medical College of Virginia, Richmond, Virginia

James W. Brooks, M.D.
Professor of Surgery, Medical College of Virginia, Richmond, Virginia

John A. Cardea, M.D.
Associate Professor and Chairman, Division of Orthopedic Surgery, Medical College of Virginia, Richmond, Virginia

Joseph M. Civetta, M.D.
Professor of Surgery, Anesthesiology, Medicine, and Pathology, University of Miami–Jackson Memorial Medical Center, Miami, Florida

I. Kelman Cohen, M.D.
Professor and Chairman, Division of Plastic and Reconstructive Surgery, Medical College of Virginia, Richmond, Virginia

Richard L. Corales, M.D.
Attending Surgeon, Southern Baptist Hospital, New Orleans, Louisiana

Kevin Ducey, M.D.
Assistant Professor of Surgery, Medical College of Virginia, Richmond, Virginia

Leo J. Dunn, M.D.
Professor and Chairman, Department of Obstetrics and Gynecology, Medical College of Virginia, Richmond, Virginia

Martin R. Eichelberger, M.D.
Assistant Professor of Surgery and Child Health, George Washington University; and Attending Surgeon, Children's Hospital National Medical Center, Washington, D.C.

Ronald C. Elkins, M.D.
Chief, Surgical Service, Veterans Administration Hospital, Oklahoma City, Oklahoma

Jack C. Fisher, M.D.
Professor and Head, Division of Plastic Surgery, University of California Medical Center, San Diego, California

David H. Frank, M.D.
Assistant Professor of Surgery, Division of Plastic Surgery, University of California Medical Center, San Diego, California

Mitchell H. Goldman, M.D.
Assistant Professor of Surgery, Medical College of Virginia, Richmond, Virginia

Cleon W. Goodwin, M.D., Lt. Col., M.C.
Chief, Surgical Study Branch, Department of the Army, Brooke Army Medical Center, Fort Sam Houston, Texas

Richard P. Greenberg, M.D., Ph.D.
Associate Professor of Neurosurgery, University of Arizona Health Science Center, Tucson, Arizona

Lazar J. Greenfield, M.D.
Stuart McGuire Professor and Chairman, Department of Surgery, Medical College of Virginia, Virginia Commonwealth University, Richmond, Virginia

Robert H. Hackler, M.D.
Associate Professor of Surgery, Medical College of Virginia, Richmond, Virginia

B. W. Haynes, Jr., M.D.
Professor of Surgery and Director, Burn Unit, Medical College of Virginia, Richmond, Virginia

Robert E. Hermann, M.D.
Chairman, Department of General Surgery, The Cleveland Clinic Foundation, Cleveland, Ohio

J. Shelton Horsley, III, M.D.
Professor of Surgery, Medical College of Virginia, Richmond, Virginia

Alan R. Hudson, M.D.
Professor and Chairman, Division of Neurosurgery, University of Toronto, Toronto, Ontario

W. Glenn Hurt, M.D.
Professor of Obstetrics and Gynecology, Medical College of Virginia, Richmond, Virginia

S. K. Kallar, M.D.
Assistant Professor of Anesthesiology, Medical College of Virginia, Richmond, Virginia

R. L. Keenan, M.D.
Professor and Chairman, Department of Anesthesiology, Medical College of Virginia, Richmond, Virginia

David G. Kline, M.D.
Professor and Chairman, Department of Neurosurgery, Louisiana State University Medical Center, New Orleans, Louisiana

Warren W. Koontz, Jr., M.D.
Professor and Chairman, Division of Urology, Medical College of Virginia, Richmond, Virginia

Donald S. Kornfeld, M.D.
Professor of Clinical Psychiatry, Columbia University College of Physicians and Surgeons; and Chief, Psychiatric Consultation and Liaison Service, Presbyterian Hospital, New York, New York

H. M. Lee, M.D.
Professor and Chairman, Division of Vascular and Transplantation Surgery, Medical College of Virginia, Richmond, Virginia

Paul R. Liebman, M.D.
Attending Surgeon, Good Samaritan Hospital and St. Mary's Hospital; and Director, Vascular Laboratories of the Palm Springs, West Palm Springs, Florida

James M. McGreevy, M.D.
Assistant Professor of Surgery, University of Utah College of Medicine, Salt Lake City, Utah

Hunter H. McGuire, Jr., M.D.
Professor of Surgery, Medical College of Virginia; and Chief, Surgical Service, McGuire Veterans Administration Hospital, Richmond, Virginia

James A. Majeski, M.D., Ph.D.
Assistant Professor of Surgery, Medical University of South Carolina, Charleston, South Carolina

Kimball I. Maull, M.D.
Professor and Chairman, Department of Surgery, University of Tennessee Health Sciences Center, Knoxville, Tennessee

C. Glen Mayhall, M.D.
Associate Professor of Medicine, Medical College of Virginia, Richmond, Virginia

G. Mendez–Picon, M.D.
Associate Professor of Surgery, Medical College of Virginia, Richmond, Virginia

Wyndell H. Merritt, M.D.
Associate Professor of Surgery, Medical College of Virginia, Richmond, Virginia

Michael R. Milano, M.D.
Assistant Clinical Professor of Psychiatry, Columbia University College of Physicians and Surgeons; and Liaison Psychiatrist, Surgical Service, Presbyterian Hospital, New York, New York

Frank G. Moody, M.D.
Professor and Chairman, Department of Surgery, University of Texas Health Sciences Center, Houston, Texas

David L. Nahrwold, M.D.
Loyal and Edith Davis Professor of Surgery; Chairman, Department of Surgery, Northwestern University Medical School; and Surgeon-in-Chief, Northwestern Memorial Hospital, Chicago, Illinois

H. H. Newsome, Jr., M.D.
Professor and Chairman, Division of General and Trauma Surgery, Medical College of Virginia, Richmond, Virginia

H. Newland Oldham, Jr., M.D.
Professor of Surgery, Duke University Medical Center, Durham, North Carolina

Mark B. Orringer, M.D.
Professor of Surgery, Section of Thoracic Surgery, University of Michigan Medical Center, Ann Arbor, Michigan

George A. Parker, M.D.
Assistant Professor of Surgery, Medical College of Virginia, Richmond, Virginia

Donald D. Price, Ph.D.
Associate Professor of Anesthesiology, Medical College of Virginia, Richmond, Virginia

Charles L. Puckett, M.D.
Associate Professor and Head, Department of Plastic and Reconstructive Surgery, University of Missouri Health Sciences Center, Columbia, Missouri

Judson G. Randolph, M.D.
Professor of Surgery and Child Health, George Washington University; and Surgeon-in-Chief, Children's Hospital National Medical Center, Washington, D.C.

Michael J. Rosner, M.D.
Associate Professor of Surgery (Neurosurgery), University of North Carolina, Chapel Hill, North Carolina

William R. Rout, M.D.
Assistant Professor of Surgery, Johns Hopkins University School of Medicine; and Assistant Chief of Surgery, Baltimore City Hospitals, Baltimore, Maryland

Arnold M. Salzberg, M.D.
Professor and Chairman, Division of Pediatric Surgery, Medical College of Virginia, Richmond, Virginia

Michael Scheflan, M.D.
Assistant Professor of Surgery, Medical College of Virginia, Richmond, Virginia

Seymour I. Schwartz, M.D.
Professor of Surgery, University of Rochester School of Medicine, Rochester, New York

David E. Sharp, M.D., Ph.D.
Assistant Professor, Department of Pathology, Medical College of Virginia, Richmond, Virginia

Donald Silver, M.D.
Professor and Chairman, Department of Surgery, University of Missouri Health Sciences Center, Columbia, Missouri

M. J. V. Smith, M.D., Ph.D.
Professor of Surgery, Medical College of Virginia, Richmond, Virginia

Harvey J. Sugerman, M.D.
Associate Professor of Surgery, Medical College of Virginia, Richmond, Virginia

John H. Texter, Jr., M.D.
Professor and Chairman, Division of Urology, Southern Illinois University School of Medicine, Springfield, Illinois

S. Dawson Theogaraj, M.D.
Professor, Division of Plastic and Reconstructive Surgery, Medical College of Virginia, Richmond, Virginia

Alexander J. Walt, M.B., Ch.B.
Penberthy Professor and Chairman, Department of Surgery, Wayne State University School of Medicine, Detroit, Michigan

Timothy Wolfgang, M.D.
Assistant Professor of Surgery, Medical College of Virginia, Richmond, Virginia

Harold F. Young, M.D.
Professor of Surgery, Medical College of Virginia, Richmond, Virginia

George D. Zuidema, M.D.
Surgeon-in-Chief, Johns Hopkins Hospital, Baltimore, Maryland

Foreword

Dr. Greenfield and his associates are to be highly commended for this superb text. The editor of this volume has covered a number of very important topics with an outstanding selection of contributors. Each is an authority in the field, and the range of complications discussed is both broad and thorough.

Despite many improvements in preoperative preparation, intraoperative surgical management, and postoperative care, complications continue, and for understandable reasons. Surgical procedures have become more complex in recent years, and those patients thought previously to be unsuitable candidates because of high risk have become operable as a result of numerous advances in surgery.

The editor of this outstanding volume is a well-recognized surgical scholar who has had a broad interest in both general and cardiothoracic surgery. His depth of knowledge in the pathophysiology of disease processes is well recognized and is brought sharply into focus in his editorship of this text. Those surgeons who follow the principles as recommended for the prevention and management of complications will provide their patients with a reduced incidence of morbidity and mortality. For these reasons it is easy to predict that this text will be a popular and widely read volume and will serve as a valuable reference for all those involved in the practice of surgery and the surgical specialties.

DAVID C. SABISTON, JR., M.D.

Preface

Just as advances across the field of medicine alter our approach to the primary management of surgical disorders, so should we continue to improve our ability to prevent, diagnose, and treat the complications that result from surgery and trauma. With this objective in mind I have attempted to provide a useful text of manageable size that addresses common complications across the broad field of surgery. The decision to include the surgical specialties of plastic, cardiothoracic, neurologic, genitourinary, gynecologic, and orthopaedic surgery was based on the principle that the patient benefits most from the continuity of care provided by a single surgical team that accepts overall responsibility.

The organization of *Complications in Surgery and Trauma* is based on the physiological-systems approach, beginning with surgical wounds and their complications. Since this is not a textbook of surgery, complications of breast surgery then become an appropriate topic for this section. However, this approach required compromises in some areas, such as in thermal burns, where the wound complications are separated from their systemic effects, which are included in the chapter on fluid loss and replacement. The remaining sections correspond to the recognized specialties, emphasizing the problems most likely to be encountered by the surgical resident or practicing surgeon. I have made the assumption that the reader will have enough familiarity with a given surgical disorder not to require an in-depth review of the basic anatomy or pathophysiology.

Even though the patient may understand the risk of complications after an elective surgical procedure, when a complication develops, his degree of disappointment and disability can result in a damaged relationship with the surgeon, sometimes to the point of a lawsuit. The management of the complication therefore deserves the same attention and documentation in the patient's record as did the original surgical problem. With this in mind the authors have called on their clinical experience to provide a review of the prophylaxis, diagnosis, and management of the complications of surgery and trauma in their respective specialties.

As hospitals find their own vulnerability increasing, they are most likely to request that surgeons establish methods of risk control. Such measures should include but not be limited to assurance of the continuity of follow-up care, occasional audits of selected procedures, and regular review of the deaths and complications that occur within the institution. Every surgeon should monitor the morbidity and mortality rates of his own patients, not only for medicolegal purposes but also to force himself to sharpen his skills and to be accurate in his predictions of outcome for his patients.

> Let us undertake, therefore, every one of us to fulfil
> the duties both of an observer and of an instructor.
> —R. Virchow, 1858

LAZAR J. GREENFIELD, M.D.

Acknowledgments

I am indebted to the many contributors who accepted the responsibility for adding this work to their many other obligations. I am particularly grateful to Judith McDevitt for her editorial assistance, to Donna Hensel and Rae Spivey for manuscript preparation and correspondence, to Sue Seif for her artwork, and to Sanford Robinson, Assistant Editor of Medical Books, and Lee Henderson, Manuscript Editor, J. B. Lippincott Company. The suggestions of Dr. Hunter H. McGuire, Jr., and Dr. H. H. Newsome, Jr., regarding organization and philosophy were most appropriate and very valuable.

Contents

Part One

Wounds in Surgery and Trauma

1 Complications of Wound Healing

I. Kelman Cohen

OVERVIEW—NORMAL WOUND HEALING

In order to prevent or correct complications of wound healing, one must have a clear concept of terms. This is particularly difficult because the term wound healing *is ambiguous and encompasses many distinct biologic phenomena. For example, local and systemic factors that affect hemostasis, cell function, and collagen metabolism will directly affect wound healing. Therefore, knowledge of the specific biologic processes involved is required if one is to diagnose and treat specific abnormalities of wound healing. We will briefly review the major wound-healing events that begin at the onset of injury and then consider complications that interfere with these events.*

BIOLOGIC EVENTS IN WOUND HEALING

Inflammation, the release of tissue fluids and the influx of cells and plasma into the wound, initiates and modulates the cascade of events leading to wound repair. Platelet and macrophage factors appear to regulate many aspects of fibroplasia.[4, 12, 14, 19] Lymphocytes and polymorphonuclear cells are probably involved in both fibroplasia and wound remodeling (collagen degradation).[21, 22]

Epithelialization includes the mitosis and migration of epithelial cells. These processes are essential for the healing of partial-thickness wounds, those in which the epithelium has been removed but in which a portion of the dermis (with epithelial islands) remains intact.

Contraction is the active phenomenon whereby a wound closes spontaneously. The same process occurs with injury to a hollow viscus such as the esophagus and results in stricture. The force causing wound contraction appears to be derived from a fibroblastlike cell, the myofibroblast, which contains cytoplasmic smooth muscle components. These contractile fibroblasts are thought to pull the wound margins together.[8, 16, 18]

Collagen metabolism includes the synthesis and deposition of collagen, which provides strength and integrity to the repaired wound.[3] Normally there is an equilibrium between collagen synthesis and degradation, and the result is a normal deposition of collagen. If insufficient collagen is synthesized or if there is excessive collagen degradation, there will be insufficient collagen deposition, which may result in diminished wound strength. Decreased collagen deposition and wound strength may also result from insufficient intermolecular and intramolecular crosslinking of the collagen molecule.

It is important to note that these four phenomena—inflammation, epithelialization, contraction, and collagen metabolism—occur in an ordered sequence, that they are interdependent, and that they may be altered by a variety of factors that can, and often do, ultimately lead to abnormal wound healing. Furthermore, there are different types of wounds that heal by different mechanisms, as well as different wound closure techniques that affect wound healing.

TYPES OF WOUNDS

Partial-thickness wounds are those in which most of the epithelium has been removed but part of the dermis remains with the epithelium in the sebaceous glands and hair follicles. Epithelial mitosis and migration (epithelialization) then resurfaces the dermis, resulting in a healed wound. Examples include abrasions, split-thickness skin-graft donor sites, and first- and second-degree burns.

Full-thickness wounds are those in which the entire skin is removed.

TYPES OF WOUND CLOSURE

Primary closure is defined as closure with sutures and tape within several hours after the wound was made. The primarily closed wound heals mainly by collagen deposition (synthesis, deposition, and crosslinking).

Delayed primary closure is defined as surgical closure from 24 hours to several days after injury. Indications for delayed primary closure are gross contamination with foreign materials or a significant contamination with bacteria, which would result in clinical infection and delayed healing.

Closure by secondary intention occurs when the open full-thickness wound is allowed to close by the normal biologic processes (epithelialization, contraction, and collagen deposition).

In addition to the *type* of wound and the *method* of wound closure, there are numerous other factors that influence healing. The most clinically significant of these are considered here.

Major Factors That Inhibit Normal Healing

NUTRITION

Starvation or protein depletion inhibits collagen synthesis and hence wound strength.[20] For example, ascorbate and molecular oxygen are required for the hydroxylation of proline on the nascent collagen chain. Ascorbate depletion or hypoxia results in the production of underhydroxylated collagen, which is rapidly degraded and therefore is not available for replacement in the injured site. Zinc depletion may result in insufficient collagen deposition and retardation of wound contraction.[2] Although the exact mechanism is unknown, there appears to be a greater influx of neutrophils and macrophages into the wounds of zinc-deficient animals. This abnormal influx of inflammatory cells inhibits normal wound healing. Moreover, it is also believed that zinc acts to stabilize inflammatory cell membranes and that zinc deficiency results in the spontaneous disruption of inflammatory cells, the release of increased amounts of degradative enzymes into the wound site, and the disruption of new tissue-matrix components deposited in the healing wound. Zinc may also perform a function in the transport of vitamin A, which is important in wound contraction.

PHARMACOLOGIC AGENTS

Corticosteroids are known to interfere specifically with several major wound-healing phenomena. For example, corticosteroids reduce collagen synthesis, increase collagen degradation, and inhibit epithelialization and wound contraction.[11, 15] However, vitamin A counteracts some of the deleterious effects of corticosteroids.[7] Following therapy with vitamin A, epithelialization and collagen synthesis return to normal. In open wounds, however, contraction remains inhibited. It would therefore seem advisable to treat patients who take corticosteroids with vitamin A before they undergo surgery. Observe caution in using large doses of vitamin A for a prolonged period because of the known complications of hypervitaminosis A. Moreover, transplant patients being treated with corticosteroids for immunosuppression could in theory have a rejection response from ingestion of vitamin A.

Colchicine, which is used commonly in the treatment of gout, could inhibit various wound-healing parameters in humans because it inhibits wound contraction and collagen secretion and enhances collagen degradation.[5, 9] However, the direct effects of colchicine on wound healing have not been studied in patients on pharmacologic dosages of the drug.

There is an additional group of drugs, the lathyrogens, that specifically inhibit collagen crosslinking and thereby disrupt the connective-tissue matrix in healing wounds. D-penicillamine (used in the treatment of Wilson's disease and homocystinuria) and isoniazid (used to treat tuberculosis) belong to this group. Curiously, the clinical significance of these drugs on wound healing in humans is unknown, but the surgeon should be aware of their potential effects. Patients receiving these agents could develop wound-healing problems related to decreased wound strength.

INFECTION

Gross bacterial contamination is a major cause of complications in wound healing.[6] Wounds closed in the presence of 1×10^5 bacteria per gram of tissue or greater will become infected and consequently will not heal, owing to the presence of excess inflammatory cells, bacterial toxins, and associated degradative enzymes. Moreover, the number of bacteria needed to produce infection may be less than 1×10^5 if host resistance is lowered. Although a wound may appear "clean" and "not infected," one should not rely on clinical judgment alone to decide the safe time for wound closure. Quantitative bacteriology (which can give immediate results with a slide-dilution technique as well as bacterial culture methods) should be performed whenever possible before wound closure. Clinically, however, one can make some calculated guesses about the degree of wound contamination. For example, in the noncontaminated wound, there should be no purulence; epithelial migration may be visible at the edge of the wound, and granulation tissue, if present, will be red and healthy looking. Furthermore, an allograft should "take" on a clean wound. One of the best ways to clean contaminated open wounds is with wet-to-dry fine-mesh gauze dressings. Several agents on the market are commonly used, but because of cost and their tendency to cause excessive tissue damage their use is unwarranted unless they are used very carefully. Pharmacology will never replace good manual wound care. Finally, there is clear evidence that the wound closed after a delay will soon be as strong as or stronger than a wound closed primarily.

GENETIC DEFECTS

There are certain genetic defects that may alter wound healing. For example, there are seven distinct types of Ehlers–Danlos syndrome. Some of these may be associated with fragile skin, lack of strength with subsequent disruption of skin wounds, spontaneous aneurysms in major vessels, and bleeding disorders. A careful history and physical examination should alert the surgeon to the possibility of these disorders in surgical patients. If any form of Ehlers–Danlos, Marfan's, or other genetic diseases of connective tissue is suspected on clinical grounds, biochemical confirmation may be very difficult because of the paucity of laboratories that can biochemically confirm the clinical diagnosis. Once a clinical diagnosis is made, great care should be exercised in wound closure, since there are no known methods to correct the metabolic errors.

FACTITIOUS WOUNDS

Although the true incidence of factitious wounds is unknown, it is probably much more common than one might suspect. The diagnosis is often very difficult to make. One should suspect a factitious wound in patients who have multiple scars or a history of wound-healing problems, or who are associated in some way with health care. Psychiatric consultation may help in the diagnosis of factitious wounding but will not provide a definitive diagnosis. Placing fluorescein on the open wound, dressing it, and then looking for fluorescence on the patient's digits with a Wood's lamp several hours later may provide evidence that the patient has manipulated the wound. When patients are confronted with the diagnosis, they will often be very angry and leave. Discovery does not appear to help the patient to seek treatment.

MALIGNANCY

Malignant neoplasms of the skin may be mistaken for nonhealing skin wounds. Melanoma and basal and squamous cell cancers have all been diagnosed as benign skin ulcers. Perhaps the most common diagnostic error is mistaking a Marjolin's ulcer for a simple ulcer in an old scar. All suspicious lesions deserve biopsy.

HEMATOMAS, SEROMAS, AND FOREIGN BODIES

Hematoma is a common surgical complication that can be avoided often by meticulous hemostasis at the time of surgery. Smooth awakening from anesthesia will also help to prevent the elevation of venous pressure associated with bucking. When there is any question about the adequacy of hemostasis, the wound should be drained. A Jackson–Pratt drainage system is recommended because it does not collapse and rarely gets obstructed.

Hematoma is detrimental to wound healing because it may become infected or fibrotic as healing progresses and can cause the death of an overlying flap, as clearly documented by Hillelson and colleagues.[10] The best treatment for most hematomas is surgical drainage under sterile conditions to prevent infection.

Foreign bodies such as tar and dirt located near the skin may require immediate removal, because once wound healing is complete, it may be impossible to remove the pigmented "tattoo." However, foreign bodies situated in deep tissues should not be treated unless the patient has symptoms. The most frequently ignored foreign bodies are tar and dirt that become embedded in the abraded skin after injury. It is therefore important to scrub the wound vigorously, a procedure that often requires a general anesthetic. Although harmful to cells it is sometimes necessary to use an organic solvent to remove tar and dirt. Failure to clean the wound thoroughly will result in a severe tattoo deformity.

Abnormal Surface Scarring

INCISIONS

Whenever possible, incisions should be placed in lines of minimal tension.[1] This will help prevent hypertrophic scarring. For example, the lines of minimal tension on the forehead are transverse, so a transverse incision should heal with a finer line than would a horizontal incision. If the surgeon is not sure of the lines of relaxation on the face, the patient should be asked to use his muscles of facial expression to show the wrinkle lines of relaxation. Lines of relaxation are generally transverse in the extremities and abdomen.

SCAR REVISIONS

The objective in scar revision should be to change the dimension of the scar to be in the line of relaxation. Z-plasty or W-plasty may be used for this purpose, as outlined by Borges.[1] The inexperienced surgeon will often create a deformity more noticeable than the original scar by doing a Z-plasty that does not fall into the lines of relaxation.

Perhaps the most common error in scar management is early revision. All scars are red and raised for several months after wounding. At least a year is required for the scar to mature with collagen remodeling and resolution of inflammation. Even scars that run at right angles to relaxation lines may mature in a manner that is satisfactory to the patient. In most circumstances early scar revision is inappropriate.

HYPERTROPHIC SCARS AND KELOIDS

Hypertrophic scars are raised and often red, but they are confined to the area of original wounding. They usually resolve very slowly (over 1 to 2 years) without surgical intervention. However, triamcinolone (40 mg/ml) injected directly into the scar every 6 weeks will often accelerate the process of scar regression. In contrast, keloids extend beyond the boundaries of the original wound and will not regress spontaneously.[17] In addition, they tend to recur after excisions. The surgeon often makes the mistake of excising keloids, only to have them recur even larger than they were before excision. Rarely is excision alone sufficient treatment to prevent recurrence. Again, intralesional triamcinolone will often result in marked regression.[13] Surgery may be useful to remove the large, bulky, disfiguring keloid, but postoperative intralesional triamcinolone must be used to prevent recurrence. Care must be taken in using this agent because skin atrophy and depigmentation may result. Although radiation therapy has been used for keloid treatment, a therapy that may promote the formation of skin malignancy in the future should be avoided.

Finally, one must be sure why the patient with keloid seeks medical attention. Many patients do not require excision because they are not troubled by appearance or functional loss. These patients simply want to get rid of the pain, burning, and itching that often accompany keloids. Both intralesional triamcinolone and diphenhydramine (Benadryl) tend to relieve these symptoms, thereby obviating the need for surgery. An antihistamine may be appropriate because of the high histamine content of these lesions.

MANAGEMENT OF DONOR SITES

Management of surgical donor sites is complicated by a multitude of rituals. The only known principle that is important is that epithelialization is enhanced with a moist dressing. Therefore, a hydrophobic dressing may be superior to a hydrophilic one. Although Scarlet Red will increase epithelial mitotic activity, there is no evidence that complete epithelialization of the wound will occur more rapidly with Scarlet Red or any other preparation. Some donor-site dressings are very expensive, and their manufacturers make claims that are unsubstantiated. The surgeon must be objective and cost accountable in selection.

Heat lamps are frequently used to dry out the donor site, but this method defies the known principle that the donor site should not be dry. In addition, patients have been burned by the heat or by direct contact with the lamp.

Donor-site dressings should not be wrapped with multiple layers of cotton gauze once the initial oozing of blood has ended (*i.e.*, 24 hours) since a single layer of gauze will suffice. If there is any evidence of purulence beneath the single-layered dressing, the dressing should be cut away and the wound drained. It is very rare to see gross infection in a well-attended donor site. The single-layer dressing covering the donor site should *never* be pulled off but should be allowed to separate. This separation will occur spontaneously as epithelium covers the surface of the donor site.

Complications of Surgical Technique

There are multiple complications of wound healing that can result from inappropriate surgical techniques. Although very obvious, it is important to remember that skin incisions should be made at right angles to the skin in all instances except for scalp incisions, which should be made obliquely to avoid damage to the hair follicles. Right-angle incision will allow even approximation of the dermis when the wound is closed.

Hemostasis should always be complete to avoid hematoma. Suction drainage should always be used if there is *any* question of bleeding.

The choice of suture material is one of the most frequently debated but least important issues. Permanent dark-colored sutures should not be placed in subcutaneous tissues of light-skinned patients because these sutures will be visible beneath the skin. "Dead space" should not be closed with sutures because this will increase the incidence of wound infection. To obtain optimal aesthetic healing, one should attempt to close the wound without tension. Biologically, sutures should be placed in the dermis because collagen gives the wound strength. These sutures should be placed to evert the edges of the skin. The only reason for skin sutures is to adjust the final positioning of the margins of the skin. Early removal of skin sutures will also prevent epithelial tracts from forming.

Crosshatch marks from sutures will always be avoided if the dermis is closed with minimal tension and the skin sutures are removed 3 to 5 days after placement. At that time, tapes can be placed across the wound for additional relief of tension. In many instances the wound can be closed with skin tapes instead of skin sutures. In fact, there are data to suggest that there is less infection and more rapid gain of tensile strength with tape closure.

Dog-ears may occur with wound closure and can be prevented by closing the wound with sutures that continually bisect the wound. If a dog-ear does occur, it can be corrected by simple ellipse or by lateral excision.

Improper debridement of abrasions is one of the most common problems in surgical technique. As mentioned previously, all foreign material such as tar and dirt must be excised from the wound. If this is not done, the foreign bodies will become intracellular and permanent in the wound.

Special Problems in Wound Healing

HERNIA

Groin hernia is a unique problem in wound healing. Clearly, recurrent groin hernia results from the surgeon's failure to obliterate the course of the hernia with collagenous tissues. The surgeon must always remember the biologic principle that *it is collagen that supplies tissues with strength and integrity*. If insufficient collagenous tissues are present, the surgeon must use free fascia lata or a tensor fascia lata myocutaneous flap to bring collagen of sufficient quality and quantity into the wound to obtain an adequate hernia repair. These principles are particularly apropos for the direct groin hernia, but the general principle applies to all types of hernia repair.

Biomaterials in Hernia Repair

Biomaterials should be used only if it is impossible to close the defect with autogenous material. For example, infection and ingrowth of bowel serosa in Marlex mesh is an extremely difficult problem to correct, whereas fascia lata can be used to close wounds without excessive morbidity.

HOLLOW VISCUS CONTRACTION

Any hollow viscus may undergo contraction after injury, and this contraction results in stenosis. For example, the process of contraction can occur in the esophagus, biliary tree, or urethra and can lead to stenosis or contracture in these areas. Although these specific complications are dealt with elsewhere in this text, it is important to recognize that these pathologic processes are the result of an abnormality in wound healing. Before they can be controlled, the surgical investigator must learn to control contraction. Preliminary evidence suggests that dilatation in conjunction with a collagen crosslink inhibitor may control this devastating process in a hollow viscus.

References

1. Borges AF: Elective Incisions and Scar Revision. Boston, Little, Brown & Co., 1973
2. Chvapil M: Zinc and other factors of the pharmacology of wound healing. In Hunt TK (ed): Wound Healing and Wound Infection. New York, Appleton–Century–Crofts, 1980
3. Cohen IK, McCoy BJ, Diegelmann RF: An update on wound healing. Ann Plast Surg 3:264, 1979
4. Diegelmann RF, Cohen IK, Kaplan AM: The role of macrophage in wound repair: A review. Plast Reconstr Surg 68:107, 1981
5. Diegelmann RF, Peterkofsky B: Inhibition of collagen secretion from bone and cultured fibroblasts by microtubular disruptive drugs. Proc Natl Acad Sci USA 69:892, 1972
6. Edlich RF, Thacken JG, Buchanan L et al: Modern concepts of treatment of traumatic wounds. Adv Surg 13:169, 1979
7. Ehrlich HP, Traver H, Hunt TK: Effects of vitamin A and glucocorticoids upon inflammation and collagen synthesis. Ann Surg 177:222, 1973
8. Gabbiani G: The role of contractile proteins in wound healing and fibrocontractive diseases. Methods Achiev Exp Pathol 9:187, 1979
9. Harris ED, Jr., Krane SM: Effects of colchicine on collagenase in cultures of rheumatoid synovium. Arthritis Rheum 14:669, 1971
10. Hillelson RL, Glowacki J, Healey NA et al: Microangiographic study of hematoma associated flap necrosis and salvage with isoxsuprine. Plast Reconstr Surg 66:528, 1980
11. Houck JC, Sharma VK, Patel YM et al: Induction of collagenolytic and proteolytic activities by anti-inflammatory drugs in the skin and fibroblast. Biochem Pharmacol 17:2081, 1968
12. Hunt TK: Wound Healing and Wound Infection. New York, Appleton–Century–Crofts, 1980
13. Ketchum LD, Cohen IK, Masters FW: Hyptertrophic scars and keloids. Plast Reconstr Surg 53:140, 1974

14. Leibovich SJ, Ross R: The role of the macrophage in wound repair : A study with hydrocortisone and antimacrophage serum. Am J Pathol 78:71, 1975
15. McCoy BJ, Diegelmann RF, Cohen IK: *In vitro* inhibition of cell growth, collagen synthesis and prolyl hydroxylase activity by triamcinolone acetonide. Proc Soc Exp Biol Med 163:216, 1980
16. Majno G, Gabbiani G, Hirschel BJ et al: Contraction of granulation tissue *in vitro:* Similarity to smooth muscle. Science 173:548, 1971
17. Peacock EE, Jr., Madden JW, Trier WC: Biologic basis for the treatment of keloids and hypertrophic scars. South Med J 63:755, 1970
18. Rudolph R, Guben S, Suzuki M et al: The life cycle of the myofibroblast. Surg Gynecol Obstet 145:389, 1977
19. Rutherford RB, Ross R: Platelet factors stimulate fibroblasts and smooth muscle cells quiescent in plasma serum to proliferate. J Cell Biol 69:196, 1976
20. Stein HD, Keiser HR: Collagen metabolism in granulating wounds. J Surg Res 11:277, 1971
21. Wahl LM, Wahl SM, Mergenhagen SE et al: Collagenase production by lymphokine-activated macrophages. Science 187:261, 1975
22. Wahl SM, Wahl LM, McCarthy JB: Lymphocyte-mediated activation of fibroblast proliferation and collagen production. J Immunol 121:942, 1978

2
Complications of Traumatic Wounds of the Face

S. Dawson Theogaraj

OVERVIEW

In their research on automotive crash injuries, a Cornell University group found that 72.1% of all victims of automobile crashes suffered facial trauma, and 8.7% had associated neck and cervical spine injuries (Fig. 2-1).[9] Automobile accidents account for 4 million injuries annually in the United States, and an equal number of accidents occur around the home. In contrast, industrial accidents are responsible for 2 million cases.

Acute Complications

AIRWAY COMPROMISE

Early oxygen debt may be heralded by restlessness and anxiety. If unrelieved, this will lead to cyanosis, stupor, and death. The airway may be obstructed by the tongue, by mucus, vomitus, or blood, or by fragments of bone and teeth. The person giving first aid should pull the tongue forward and promptly clear the obstructing material.[6,7] This is best accomplished manually. If the obstruction persists, an airway must be provided either by an endotracheal tube or by a formal tracheostomy.[10,29] However, when there is total airway obstruction, immediate cricothyroidotomy may be necessary (Fig. 2-2).

HEMORRHAGE

Bleeding from facial lacerations is usually from a superficial source, such as the facial or superficial temporal vessels. This type of bleeding is readily controlled by local pressure until the vessels can be ligated. However, in severe mid-facial injuries, repeated swallowing movements may be an early sign of concealed bleeding in the nasopharynx. If concealed bleeding is left uncontrolled, it could lead to shock. Such cases may require a postnasal pack to control the hemorrhage.

SHOCK

Shock is rarely caused by facial injuries alone, so it is wise to consider the possibility of associated injuries to the head, chest, or abdomen.[30] Meanwhile, establish an intravenous line and begin appropriate resuscitation measures with plasma expanders until crossmatched blood is available.[37] Ensuring a patent airway is mandatory, and administering oxygen is helpful. Provide adequate analgesia and keep the patient warm.

ASSOCIATED INJURIES

After the airway has been cleared and the hemorrhage and shock brought under control, the trauma team should carry out a thorough assessment for associated injuries.[22] The team should thoroughly check the status of the neuromuscular, gastrointestinal, and cardiopulmonary systems and assess for concealed hemorrhage from fractures of the pelvis or long bones.

Specific Considerations

TREATMENT OF SOFT TISSUE INJURIES

Most facial lacerations can be repaired with the patient under local anesthesia.[27,31] However, complicated lacerations such as those of the eyelids, facial nerve, and parotid duct warrant a general anesthetic for optimal repair.[7,35] Repairs of avulsion defects

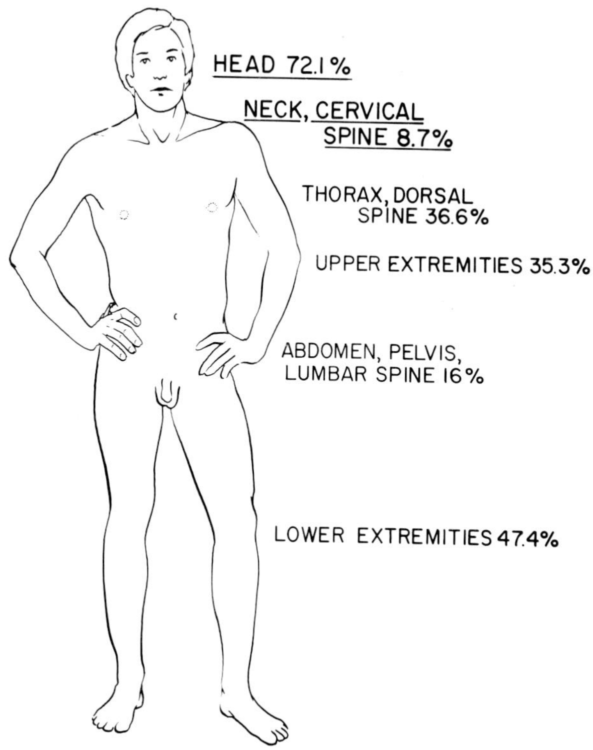

FIG. 2-1. Distribution of injuries from automobile accidents. (Data from Cornell University Automotive Crash Injury Research. The Injury-Producing Accident: A Primer of Facts and Figures. New York, Cornell University, August 1981)

also demand a more sophisticated environment than the emergency room.

Primary suture of lacerations, if carried out during the first 8 hours after injury—the "golden period"—do not need antibiotic coverage. With the advent of the powerful antibiotics available today (e.g., cephalosporins and semisynthetic penicillins) the golden period may be extended to 24 hours. Prior to closure, irrigate the wound copiously with saline. A technique that works very effectively is to fit a 35-ml syringe with a 19-gauge needle to deliver a fine stream of balanced salt solution (Ringer's lactate or 0.9% saline) into the wound.[11] This technique provides a jet of fluid that has far more cleansing force (7 psi) than that from an Asepto syringe. Then debride the wound edges judiciously. Closing the wound in layers with 5-0 chromic or Dexon in the dermis and 6-0 nylon for the skin completes the treatment.

Of the irrigation solutions available the most innocuous is 0.9% saline and Ringer's lactate. Bränemark and his colleagues have reported evidence of the cellular damage that results from various other solutions that may be used to cleanse wounds (Fig. 2-3).[2]

If a contaminated wound has a bacterial count of 10^5/g of tissue, surgical closure will result in frank infection.[12, 21] Although this is common knowledge, what is not commonly known is that buried sutures act as foreign bodies even in wounds with a low bacterial count (10^2/g of tissue). Elek and Conen reported that in the presence of a buried suture, introduction of 100 organisms (*Streptococcus pyogenes*) into volunteers created an abscess in every subject.[13] Without the suture it required 2 million organisms to produce a similar infection! Thus, wounds that are contaminated and those that are seen after the 24-hour limit must be treated expectantly.

The value of delayed closure of war wounds was reaffirmed by Heaton and his colleagues in the report of their experiences during the Vietnam war.[20] Their patients suffered an all-time low infection rate (2.58%) when treated in this fashion.

Edlich and his co-workers have proven the efficacy of delayed wound closure in all wounds that are judged to have a high risk of developing infection.[11, 12] Such wounds are treated with fine-mesh gauze dressings and reassessed after 4 days. If approximation of the wound edges is possible without tension, the use of skin tapes to bring the edges together will be successful in the majority of cases. If the tension is too great, consider using nylon or polypropylene monofilament sutures.

FIG. 2-2. Total airway obstruction is best relieved by a cricothyroidotomy, which can be performed more rapidly than a formal tracheostomy. The incision through the cricothyroid membrane is depicted here.

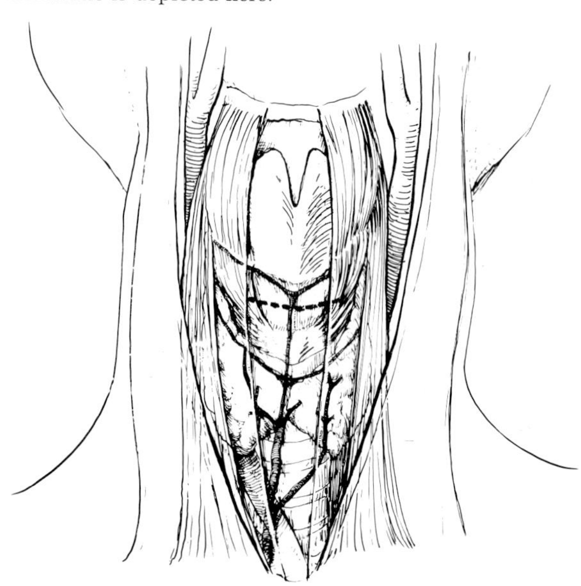

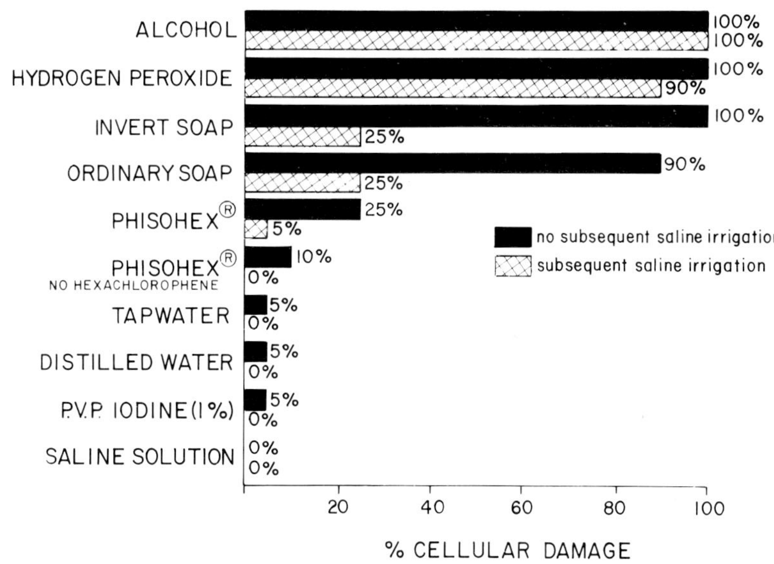

FIG. 2-3. Toxicity to cells of 10 common irrigating and cleansing solutions, based on the data of Bränemark and coworkers. Bränemark and his colleagues demonstrated in an experimental animal that alcohol and hydrogen peroxide are lethal to surface cells. Even organic iodine solutions (povidone-iodine [Betadine]) are mildly toxic. Saline and Ringer's lactate, however, are perfectly harmless to tissue. (Data from Bränemark PI, Albrektsson B, Lindstrom J et al: Local tissue effects of wound disinfectants. Acta Chir Scand [Suppl] 357:166, 1966)

INFECTION IN FACIAL WOUNDS

Because of the rich vascular supply of the scalp and face, infections in lacerations of these regions are very uncommon. Adequate débridement of wounds and copious irrigation prior to closure usually result in primary healing. However, infection in facial wounds can occur.

The proximity of the cavernous sinus and the danger of thrombosis prompt immediate hospitalization in cases of infected facial wounds. Institute bed rest, warm soaks, and intravenous antibiotic coverage with penicillin and nafcillin or penicillin and gentamicin immediately, and remove some of the sutures for drainage. Rapid control of the infection ensues following such aggressive therapy.

Types of Injuries

CONTUSIONS WITH OR WITHOUT HEMATOMA

A contusion, or bruise, is usually treated with ice-cold compresses, and prompt resolution can be expected. If a small hematoma forms, it may be treated expectantly. However, large clots should be evacuated through well-placed incisions. These are preferably made along lines of relaxed skin tension. For instance, if a hematoma of the cheek is to be evacuated, make the incision through the lower eyelid in one of the skin-crease lines. Milk the clot upward and evacuate it.[29] Then irrigate the cavity and allow it to heal spontaneously. If a hematoma is neglected, the periphery organizes and the center liquefies. Such collections may require repeated aspirations, and a depressed scar may be the final outcome.

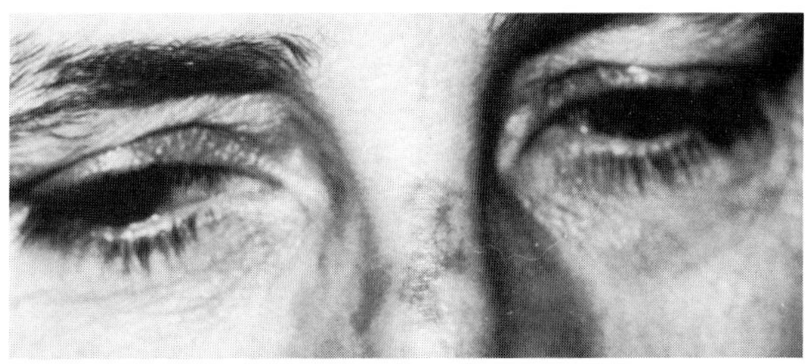

Fig. 2-4. An abrasion over the nose and cheek sustained 3 months earlier was not adequately treated. Rapid healing resulted in incorporation of gravel into the dermis, and a traumatic tattoo is the final outcome.

ABRASIONS

It is important in treating abrasions to avoid the occurrence of a traumatic tattoo (Fig. 2-4). Small particles of gravel, grease, or carbon may be ground into an abraded wound and, unless promptly removed, become incorporated into the layers of the skin. The epithelium regenerates over these particles, and permanent pigmentation of the skin occurs. Edlich and colleagues have shown conclusively that soil has infection-potentiating fractions (IPF) that carry a negative electric charge.[11] The basic (gentamicin) and amphoteric (tetracycline) antibiotics are inactivated by these particles.[11, 28] The acidic anti-

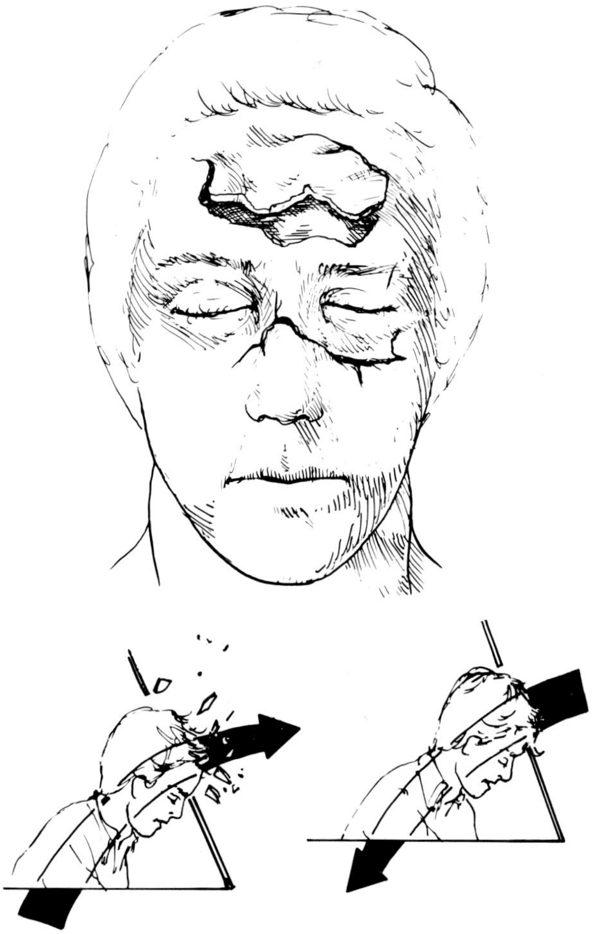

FIG. 2-5. The mechanism of sustaining an avulsion flap of the face. The automobile may stop suddenly during an accident, but the passenger continues to move forward, hitting his head against and shattering the windshield. When the body stops moving forward and slumps back, the forehead is scraped by the jagged glass and sustains a superiorly based avulsion flap.

biotics (cephalosporins and penicillins), on the other hand, are free to exert their antibacterial effects in wounds with IPF. Thus, prior to surgical treatment of wounds with ground-in dirt, it is logical to give an intravenous dose of one of the acidic antibiotics. The primary treatment of such abraded wounds is best carried out after adequate anesthesia (local or general) has been established. Either a sterile toothbrush or a scrub brush may be employed to cleanse the wound of all visible particles. If the particles are deeply imbedded, they may be picked out with a No. 11 blade. Ether or benzene may be needed to remove grease. Then dress the wound with Owens gauze or Xeroform gauze, leave it exposed, and allow it to dry. Prompt epithelialization occurs within 10 days.

AVULSION INJURIES

A typical windshield injury results in multiple avulsions of the forehead. These are extremely difficult to treat, and the prognosis is usually guarded. A dermabrasion (surgical planing) is often needed after several months. Such an injury in the black patient poses an even greater problem in management. Darkly pigmented skin cannot undergo dermabrasion, since any such additional insult results in deeper pigmentation of the whole area.

If the avulsion flap is small, it may be excised and the area closed primarily. If it is large but questionably viable, it is defatted and applied as a full-thickness skin graft.

Avulsion of parts of important features of the face, such as the nose, eyelid, or ear, constitutes a special problem. In such cases the avulsed piece is sewn back as a free composite graft in the hope of a "take." If the gamble succeeds, one may be able to avoid complicated reconstructive procedures.

TRAPDOOR LACERATIONS

The automobile passenger who hits his forehead on the dashboard usually has a large avulsion flap elevated from the region of the forehead (Fig. 2-5). Such a flap has an adequate blood supply and survives, but the scar that encircles two thirds of its circumference undergoes contracture and raises it in a biscuitlike elevation. After a waiting period of several months, it may be necessary to perform staged Z-plasties to redistribute the skin tension around the scar. These procedures are met with a moderate degree of success.

Injuries of Specific Sites

EAR

Lacerations of the ear usually heal without many problems. However, a healed scar may occasionally become a keloid.

Blunt trauma to the ear may result in an otohematoma (wrestler's ear, cauliflower ear). The injury raises the perichondrium off the cartilage, and the blood that collects in the dead space obliterates the various contours of the pinna, giving rise to a characteristic appearance. Prompt aspiration of the liquefied blood and a bolus tie-over dressing to hold the skin snug against the cartilage is the treatment of choice (Fig. 2-6). The dressing is removed in 7 to 10 days. If untreated, the hematoma stimulates fibrosis, and the cauliflower ear results.

In some avulsion injuries the ear may be hanging by a narrow pedicle. If a few key sutures are placed to reposition the pedicle, a significant portion of the ear usually survives (Fig. 2-7).

Missing parts of the ear, unless badly damaged, may be replaced as composite grafts. Occasionally, a large segment of ear may be torn off, in which case dermabrade the avulsed part and resuture it to the stump, then bury it in the retroauricular skin. This is the "pocket principle" of Mladick.[24] The ear is released from the pocket in a few days, and it usually survives. If this principle is neglected, the patient is left with a significant deformity.

PAROTID DUCT

Injuries to the parotid duct have a characteristic presentation. The surface anatomy of the duct is at the middle third of the line that extends from the tragus to the upper lip (Fig. 2-8). Any laceration that crosses

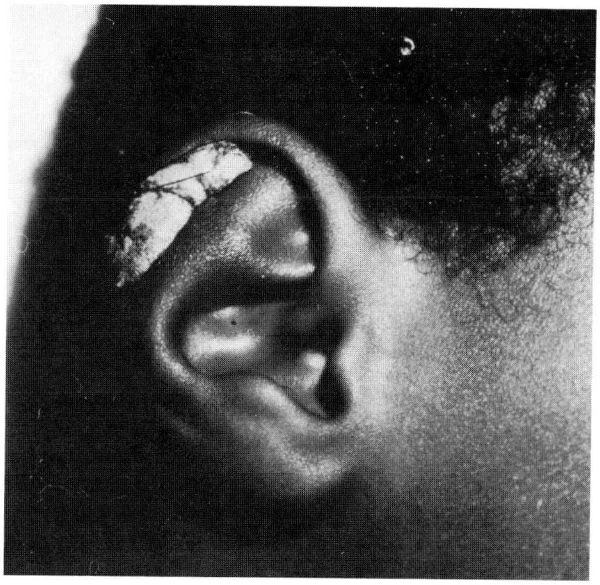

FIG. 2-6. After aspiration of the liquefied blood, a bolus tie-over dressing has been applied.

FIG. 2-7. (*A*) An automobile accident almost severed this ear. A few key sutures were placed initially. (*B*) Six months after the accident, the ear has almost entirely survived, despite some ischemic loss.

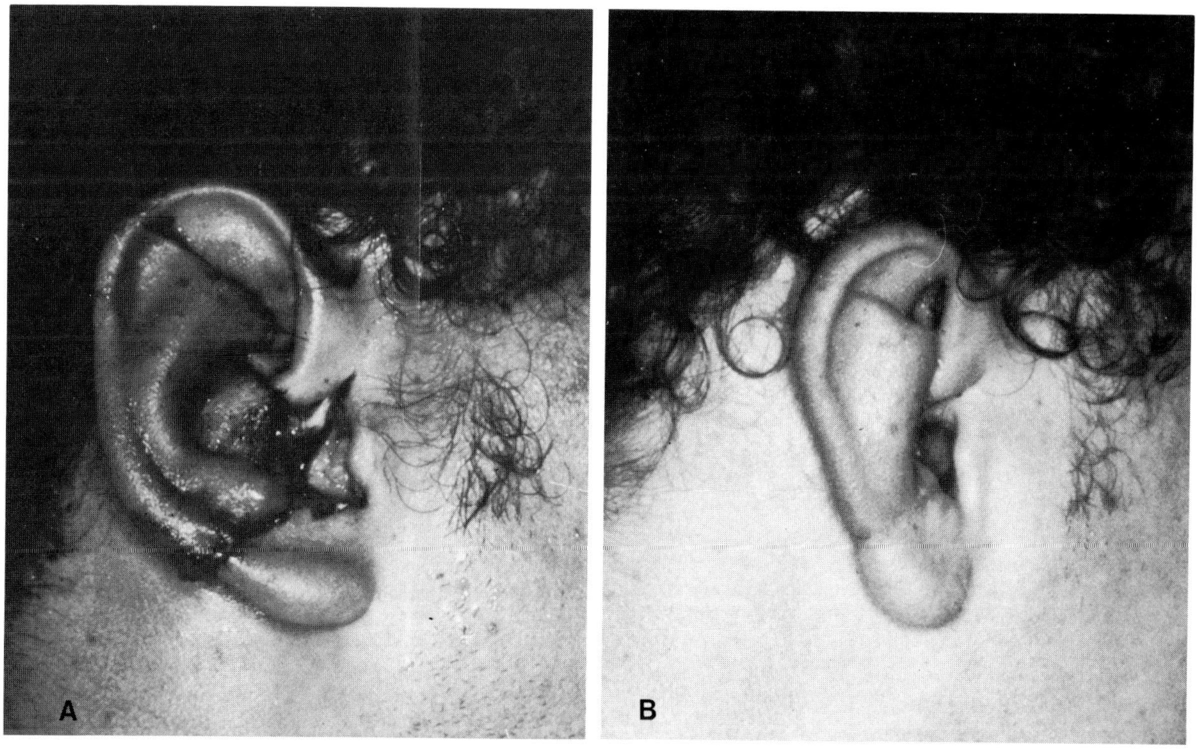

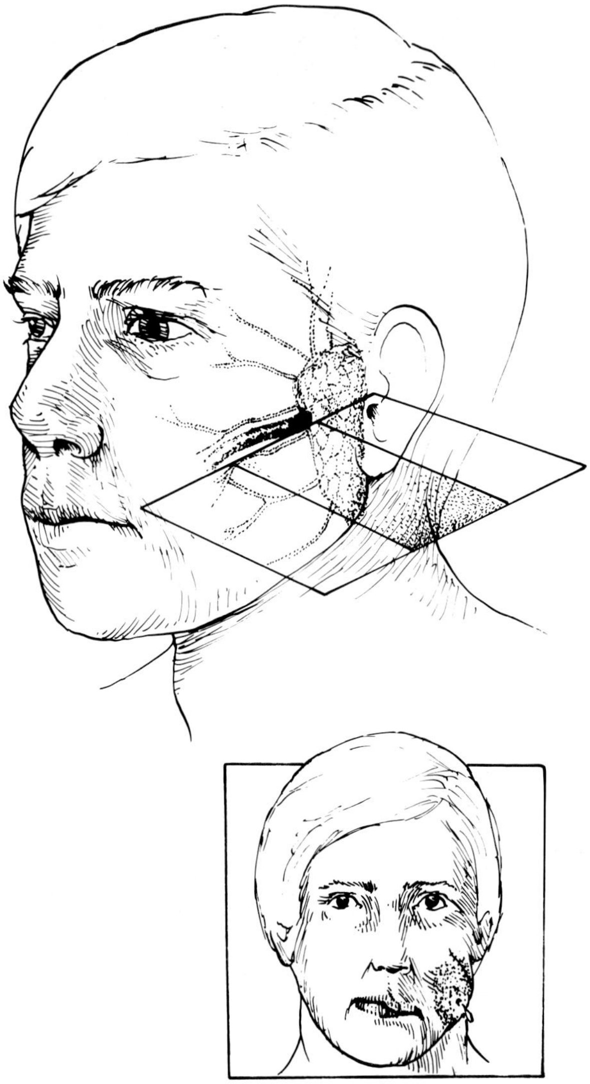

FIG. 2-8. The middle third of a line drawn from the tragus to the upper lip is the surface marking for the parotid duct. (*Inset*) Injury to the duct is often associated with damage to the buccal branch of the seventh nerve. If the injuries go undetected, the typical features of "parotid duct syndrome" result: The cheek swells up with saliva, and the upper lip droops from nerve injury.

this line is suspect. If the buccal branch of the facial nerve also is injured, resulting in a sagging upper lip, it is called the parotid duct syndrome.[8] The nerve should be repaired under magnification, and the parotid duct should be sutured over a polyethylene stent. The stent is left in place for 10 days. If Stensen's duct is left unrepaired, either an external fistula or a large collection of saliva in the cheek (sialocyst) may result. Early detection and prompt repair is therefore the treatment of choice.

FACIAL NERVE

The distal end of the cut facial nerve can be stimulated by faradic current for 48 to 72 hours after injury. Therefore, when the nerve is lacerated, prompt repair within this time is imperative (Fig. 2-9). By contrast, missile injuries of the nerve should be treated conservatively, since a large number of such injuries result in spontaneous recovery (Fig. 2-10).

EYELID

All eyelid injuries require a thorough assessment by an ophthalmologist to exclude intraocular damage. It is only after such an appraisal that the plastic surgeon should begin surgical repair. Injuries of the upper lid are more important because the cornea is more likely to suffer exposure if the lid is unrepaired. The Mustardé technique is the best type of lid repair to follow (Fig. 2-11).[25] If the levator palpebrae is lacerated, recognition and repair can prevent the occurrence of ptosis.

If the lacrimal canaliculus is damaged, the Worst pigtail probe method (Fig. 2-12) may be employed.[18] However, only 30% of patients with such an injury complain of excessive lacrimation if the duct is obstructed.

Medial canthal ligament rupture leads to a characteristic telecanthus, with a rounded intercanthal region and a shortened palpebral fissure (Fig. 2-13).[30] Prompt repair with wire sutures will prevent this deformity.

Injuries to the nasolacrimal ducts may eventually necessitate a dacryocystorhinostomy to restore lacrimal drainage. This operation opens the lacrimal sac into the nose.

Special Injuries

ANIMAL BITES

It is estimated that domestic animal bites in the United States occur 500,000 times each year.[1] Dog bites are the most common animal bites. In the "friendly dog syndrome," in which an unsuspecting child is allowed to crawl near a feeding dog, the animal snaps at the infant's face. The result is a trapdoor laceration of the cheek and an avulsion injury of the nose (Fig. 2-14).[29]

Because of the high bacterial content of the dog's saliva, rapid treatment of dog bites is imperative.

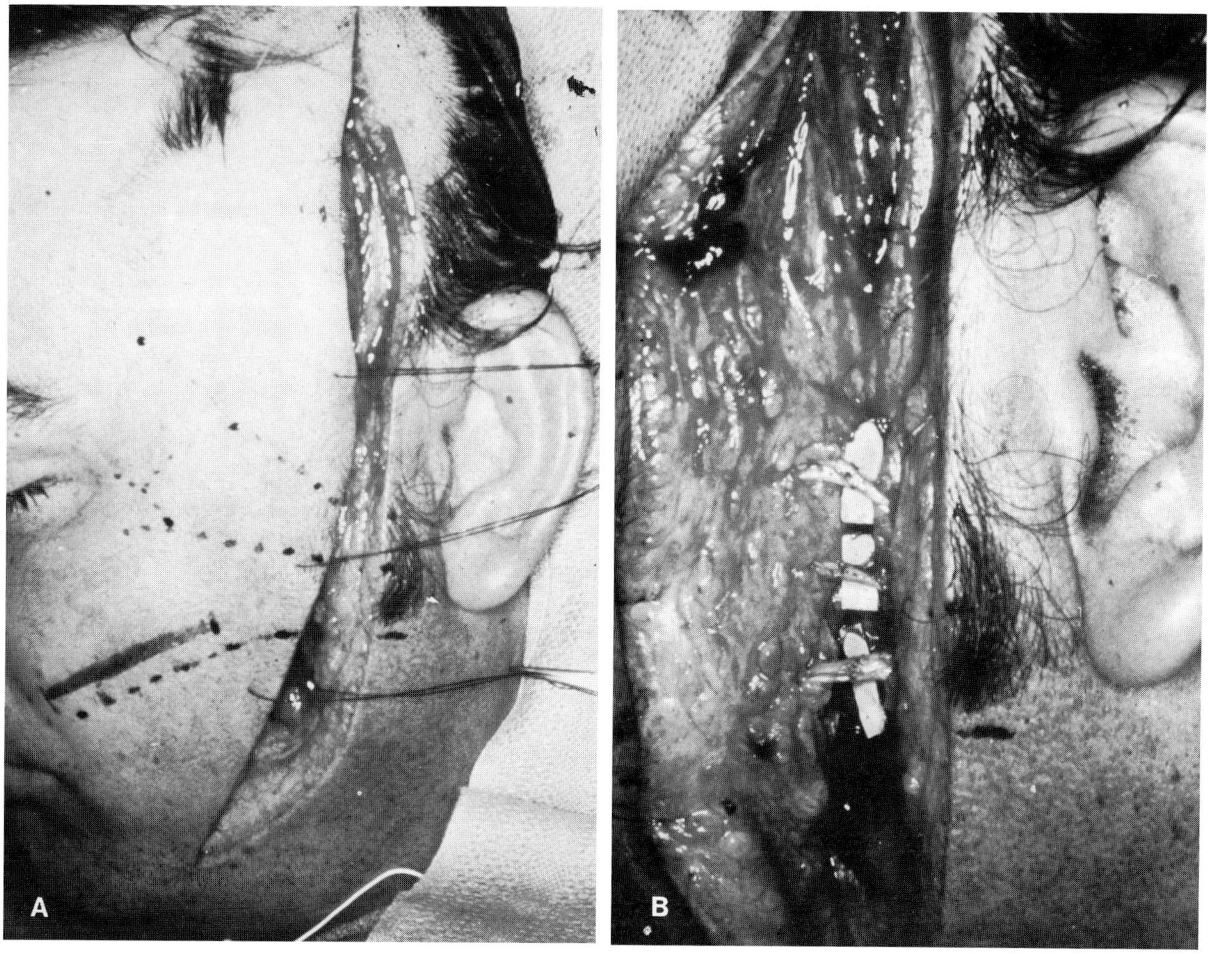

FIG. 2-9. (*A*) All of the peripheral branches of the facial nerve and the parotid duct have been lacerated by a knife. (*B*) An intraoperative picture shows that all divided structures have been repaired. Excellent recovery resulted.

Treatment, which should be provided within 6 hours of the injury, should include high-pressure saline (0.9%) irrigation, followed by thorough wound débridement.[11] Such aggressive management has helped to reduce the infection rate from 70% to 2% in some series.[4]

Fortunately, dog bites of the face are less likely to become infected (11%) than those of the hand (36%).[4] If infection becomes established within 24 hours, the most common pathogen found is *Pasteurella multocida*.[1] If infection sets in after 24 hours, the organisms are a mixed flora, with *Staphylococcus aureus* and *Streptococcus viridans* predominating.[1]

Penicillin is the antibiotic of choice for all of the common pathogens found. Certain strains of staphylococci may require the use of semisynthetic penicillins. In the presence of penicillin allergy, erythromycin is the recommended drug.

HUMAN BITES

Human bites are more serious than dog bites.[26, 34] The human mouth harbors a mixed flora of facultative species and obligatory anaerobes.[24] The predominant pathogens are *Staphylococcus aureus* and streptococci at the gram-positive end of the spectrum and *Bacteroides* strains from among the anaerobes.

The usual infective dose of bacteria for most soft tissue wounds is 10^5/g of tissue. The debris from the crevices between the teeth can contain as many as 10^{11} bacteria/g of tissue.[11] This is the same concentration of microbiota found in human feces. Human

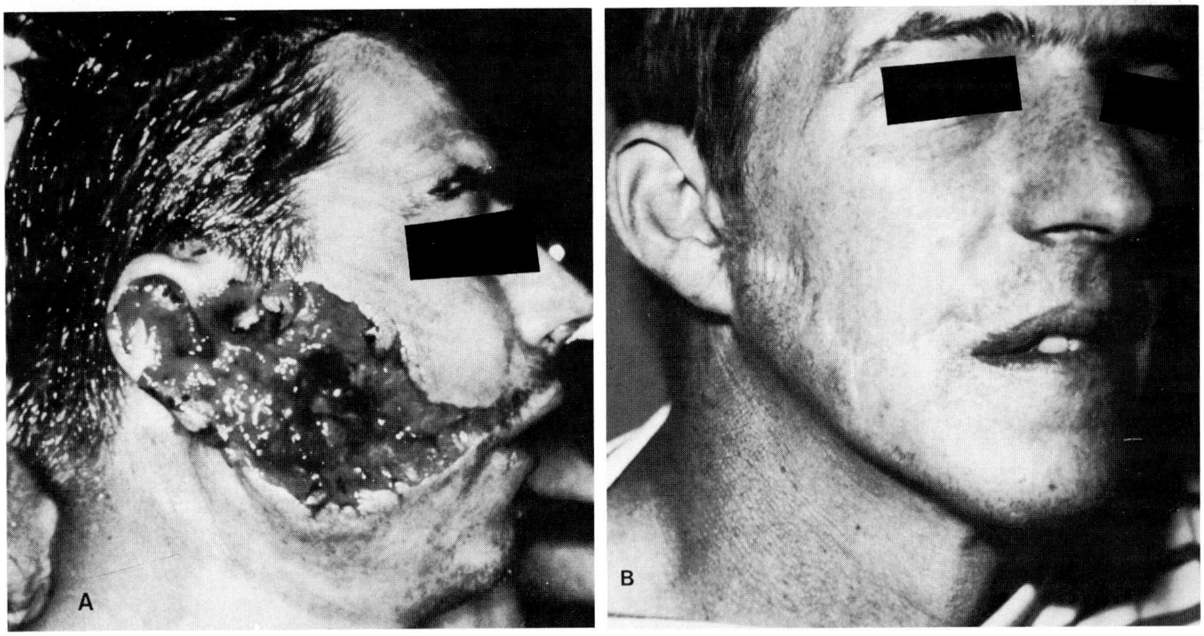

FIG. 2-10. (*A*) A self-inflicted gunshot injury to the right cheek caused by a handgun (the patient was left-handed). Notice the large area of missing cheek. (*B*) After scar revisions and no further reconstruction for the damaged facial nerve, spontaneous recovery of the majority of the branches occurred. A minimal droop of the upper lip was the only residual deformity.

FIG. 2-11. This superior method of lid repair (Mustardé) has become very popular. A key suture is placed at the gray line for alignment. The tarso-conjunctival layer is repaired by a continuous pullout suture of monofilament nylon. The superficial layers of the lid are then approximated.

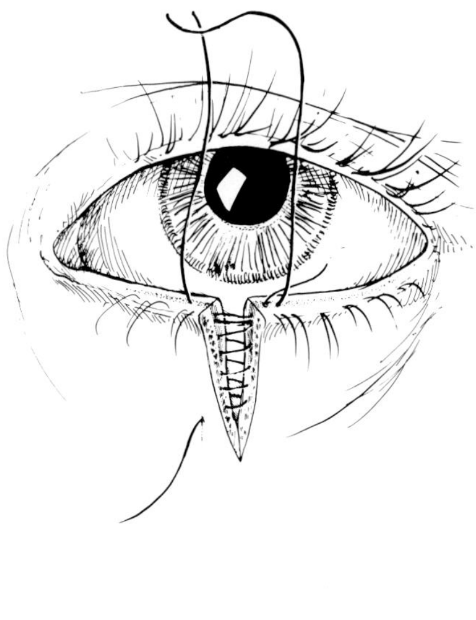

FIG. 2-12. The pigtail probe of Worst is introduced through the upper lacrimal punctum into the lower canaliculus. It is made to traverse the cut ends of the canaliculus and is then passed out through the lower punctum. A soft Silastic tube is then withdrawn, and this helps to stent the cut canaliculus. (*Inset*) The Silastic tube has been sutured to itself. The skin of the lid laceration has been approximated.

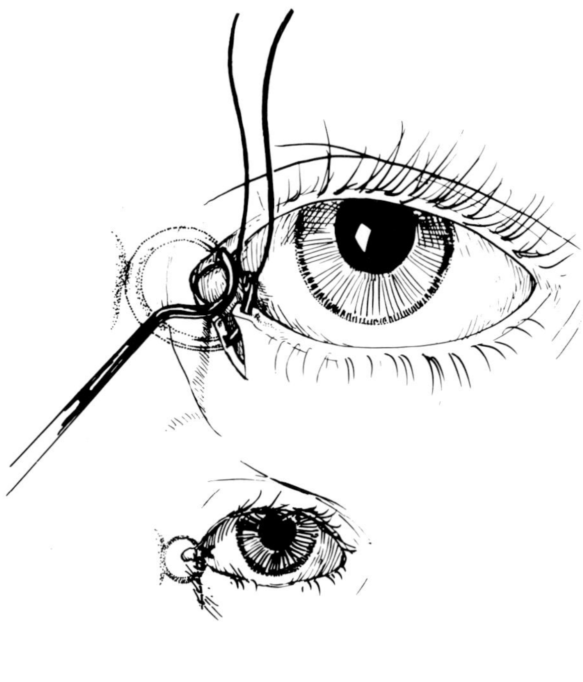

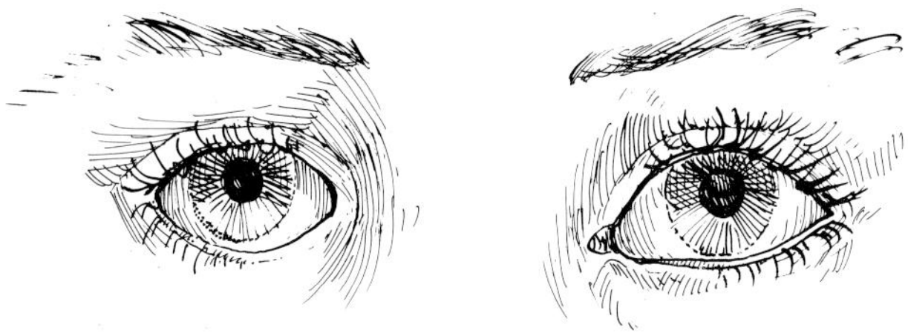

FIG. 2-13. A medial canthal disruption in the right eye following a nasoethmoidal injury. Notice the rounded contour of the canthus and the obscured lacrimal caruncle. The palpebral fissure is smaller transversely, and the medial canthus is farther away from the midline (telecanthus).

saliva has 10^8 bacteria/g of tissue. Thus, primary closure following a human bite is always contraindicated.

Treatment includes copious high-pressure irrigation and débridement of the wound, followed by wet-to-dry dressings for several days.[11] The antibiotic of choice is a combination of nafcillin and clindamicin given intravenously. This treatment plan is effective in preventing infection. Delayed closure is usually possible after a few days, and the nonsuture technique with skin tapes (Steristrips) is the preferred method.

GUNSHOT WOUNDS

The velocity of the missile is the prime determinant of tissue damage in gunshot wounds.[36] The kinetic energy expended is expressed in the formula

$$KE = \frac{M\,(V\ \text{entrance} - V\ \text{exit})^2}{2g}$$

where

KE = kinetic energy
M = mass of missile
V = velocity of missile
g = gravitational deceleration

Thus, missile injuries can be classified into three groups, according to muzzle velocity (Table 2-1).

The small-caliber, low-velocity missile (a .22 bullet from a handgun) is likely to cause minimal damage to structures, although occasionally an important structure such as the facial nerve may be hit. Suicide attempts using handguns result in wide local damage, since a larger-caliber bullet (.38 or .45) is usually used.[33] A right-handed person is likely to suffer injuries to the left cheek and maxilla (see Fig. 2-10, *A*).

Shotgun injuries in suicide attempts are unique.

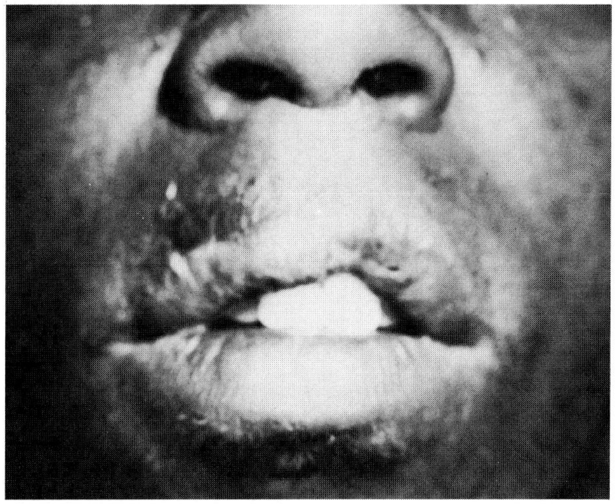

FIG. 2-14. A dog bite of the face in childhood has resulted in severe scarring of the upper lip with significant psychological sequelae in adolescence.

TABLE 2-1. CLASSIFICATION OF MISSILE INJURIES BY MUZZLE VELOCITY

Group	Type of Weapon	Muzzle Velocity
I	Shotgun	Low (<1000 ft/sec)
II	Handgun	Medium (<2000 ft/sec)
III	Rifle	High (>2000 ft/sec)

The pathogenesis is as follows: The gun butt rests on the floor and the barrel is placed under the chin. The barrel, which is approximately 30 inches long, tilts forward and to the left when the victim reaches down to pull the trigger.[17] Instead of blowing out the brains as intended, the shot blasts off the anterior mandible, maxilla, and nose. The frontal lobes and both eyes are often damaged. After this spur-of-the-moment event, the rest of the victim's life is spent undergoing reconstructive procedures to restore what has been lost (Fig. 2-15).[14] Emergency treatment includes a tracheostomy, along with other resuscitative measures.[17, 23] A frontal craniotomy is often needed, and soft tissue coverage is obtained with plastic surgical gymnastics.[17, 32] The underlying bone should be stabilized before soft tissue restoration is performed.

Multiple reconstructive efforts are required for the nasal deformity (bone grafts), mandible deformities, palatal defects (palatal flaps or obturators), and eyelid deformities (canthal ligament and other reconstructions). Rearrangement of the soft tissues by scar revisions is required many times.

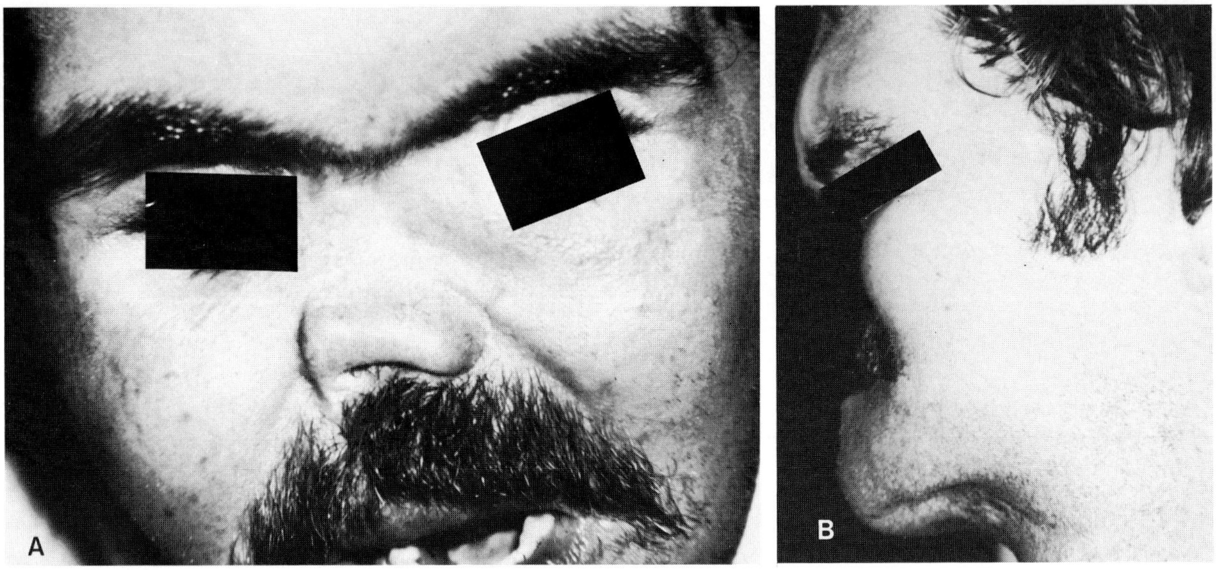

FIG. 2-15. Self-inflicted shotgun injuries resulted in severe trauma to the mandible, maxilla, nasal complex, and both orbits. The patient is completely blind. Notice the severe aesthetic and functional deformity in both the frontal (*A*) and profile (*B*) views.

CHAIN SAW INJURIES

"Man Versus Machine": such was the caption over a prize-winning exhibit at one medical meeting. The chain saw, held loosely, was shown to hit a knot on the limb of a tree. The sudden resistance encountered caused the saw to bounce up toward the face of the operator. The Consumer Product Hazard Index lists chain saws as the 67th most dangerous product of 367 product groups. In 1976 alone, 29,000 persons required emergency-room treatment for chain saw–related injuries.[19] The usual pattern of wounding is oblique, involves the left eye, and runs across the nose and onto the right cheek.

The injury devitalizes areas of tissue, fragments bones, and grinds in foreign material. Thus high-pressure irrigation, followed by wound debridement, is necessary prior to repair.[11] The injury to the eye is usually severe and the nasal injury results in loss of tissue. Surgical therapy is carried out by many specialists. The ophthalmic surgeon works to save the eye, and the plastic surgeon repairs the soft tissue injuries (Fig. 2-16). A neurosurgeon also should be involved if the posterior wall of the frontal sinus is fractured.

With the proliferation of these tools there is a great need for public-safety education. Appropriate clothing and gloves should be worn to avoid such mishaps, and it is essential to follow the correct operating procedures when using these power instruments. A thoughtful article by Graham and his colleagues provides valuable information on these preventive measures.[19]

Complications Following Bony Injuries of the Face

ORBIT

Blowout Fractures

The contents of the orbit at body temperature are essentially fluid. This is a very useful protective quality. Additionally, the human eye is surrounded by an elevated bony rim that takes the brunt of most injuries. However, any object that is smooth and larger than 5 cm in diameter (e.g., a tennis ball, a human fist) may hit the front of the orbit forcefully enough to cause severe damage. The essentially fluid contents are displaced inferiorly and medially, and a blowout injury of the thin bony walls results at these locations (Fig. 2-17).[8]

Under these conditions the eye appears sunken (enophthalmos) and may not be able to rotate up because the inferior rectus muscle is trapped below (Fig. 2-18). Such patients will have diplopia. Thus the presence of diplopia in an eyeball that does not rotate up raises the suspicion of the presence of a blowout fracture. Routine radiographs and tomograms are necessary to diagnose the extent of injury.

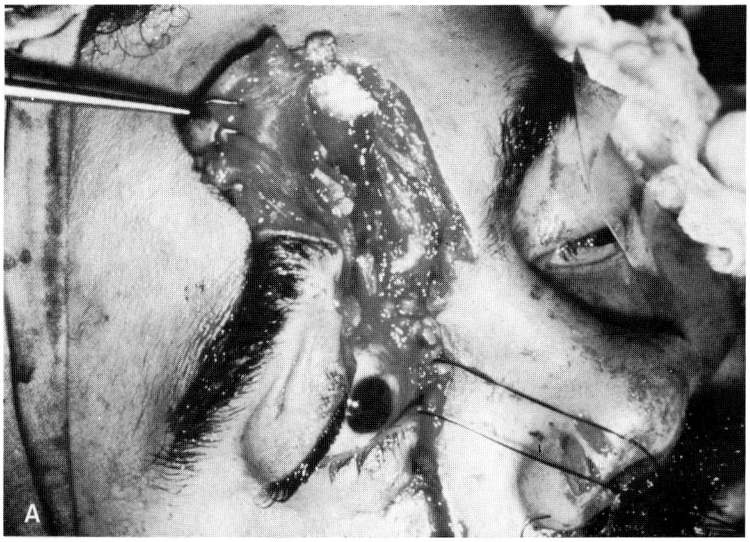

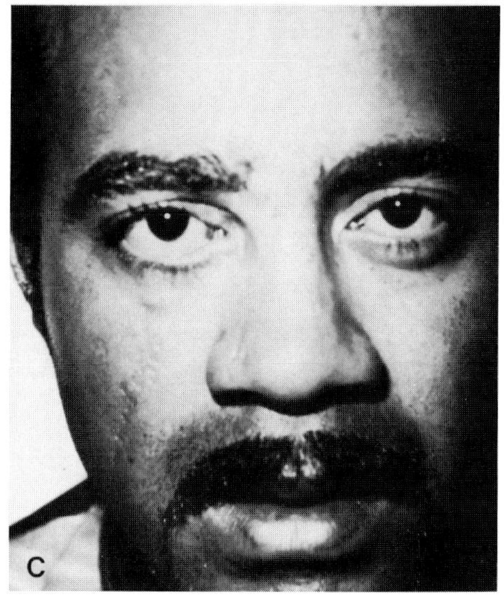

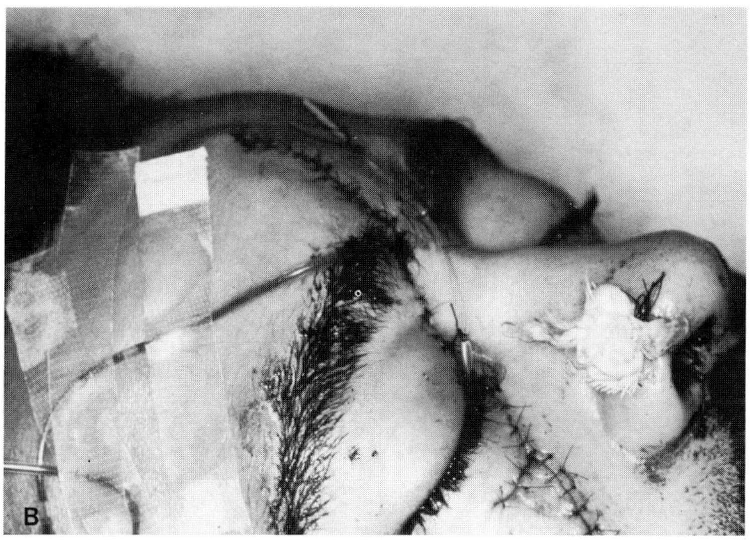

FIG. 2-16. (A) An ipsilateral injury from a chain saw to the frontal sinus, both lacrimal canaliculi, and the cheek. (B) The same patient after repair of all damaged structures, including the lacrimal apparatus by the Worst method (see Fig. 2-12). (C) The patient 1 year after the injury and after minor scar revisions.

A neuro-ophthalmologic evaluation is essential to rule out the possibility of damage to the cornea (abrasion), iris (traumatic iritis), lens (dislocation or cataracts), vitreous (hemorrhage), retina (detachment or tears), and eye muscles (hemorrhage or nerve palsies). The plastic surgeon is guided in his approach to the patient by the recommendations of specialists in these areas.

The surgical approach to the floor of the orbit is methodical (Fig. 2-19). If the floor is broken, a pack introduced into the maxillary antrum will hold up the fragments until they heal. If a piece of bone is missing, it may be replaced by a piece of Silastic or Supramid. Delayed treatment in these cases could result in permanent diplopia.

Malar Complex Fractures

The malar (zygomatic) bone forms the cheek prominence and a major part of the inferior and lateral walls of the orbit. An injury from the side (e.g., from a fist or dashboard) may push the bone downward, inward, and backward. The lateral canthal ligament will displace with it. The orbital floor fractures, the infraorbital nerve is damaged, and the maxillary antrum fills with blood.

Thus a typical case exhibits periorbital ecchymosis, downward displacement of the lateral canthus, flattening of the cheek, and diplopia (Fig. 2-20). Numbness of the cheek, nose, upper lip, and anterior teeth is usually present. Here again, a preoperative evaluation by an ophthalmologist is essential. Surgical reduction is through a lateral brow incision and an incision in the lower eyelid facilitates inspection of the floor of the orbit. Interosseous fixation at the junctions of the zygoma with the maxilla and frontal bone follows, and a good result is the usual outcome. If there has been a delay in management, however, the external deformity becomes permanent and is much more difficult to correct. Furthermore, late diplopia is almost impossible to correct surgically. The enophthalmos also may become permanent.

Superior Orbital Fissure Syndrome

Superior orbital fissure syndrome is a rare complication of malar fractures.[27] Bony impingement of important structures at the fissure causes a paralysis of the third, fourth, and sixth cranial nerves. Thus, the patient has ptosis of the upper lid (third nerve), dilatation of the pupil (third nerve), and an ophthalmoplegia (third, fourth, and sixth nerves). The fore-

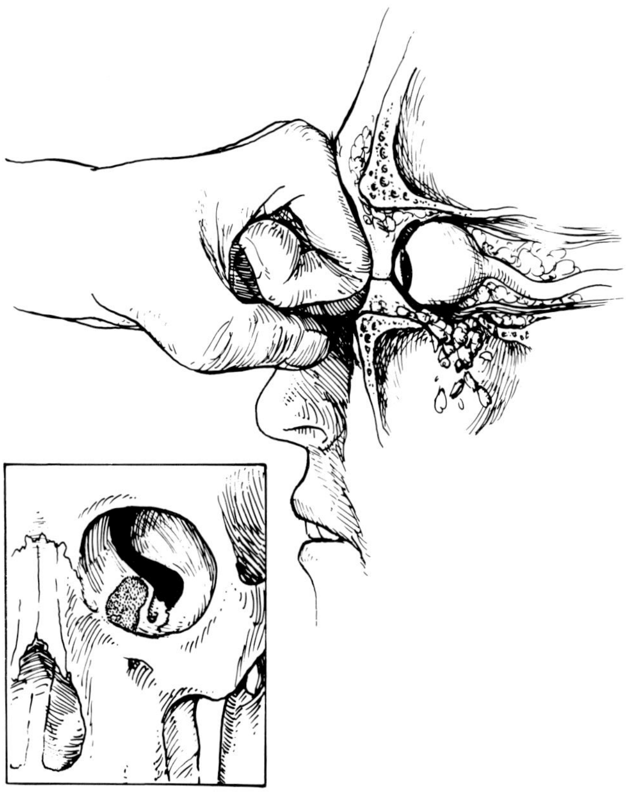

FIG. 2-17. The mechanism of a blowout fracture of the orbit. A human fist is shown hitting the front of the orbit, displacing the orbital contents backward. The floor, which is very thin inferiorly, "blows out" into the antrum. (*Inset*) The typical area of the fracture in the floor of the orbit (*shaded portion*).

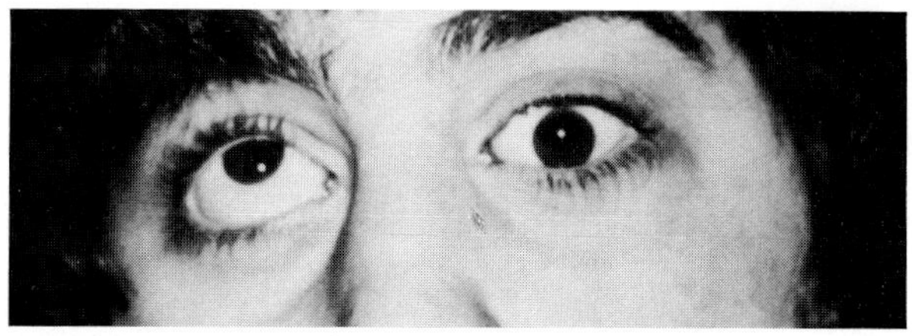

FIG. 2-18. Typical findings following a blowout fracture of the orbit. The normal eye rotates upward, but the eye with the inferior rectus muscle trapped in the defect is unable to do so, giving rise to diplopia and enophthalmos.

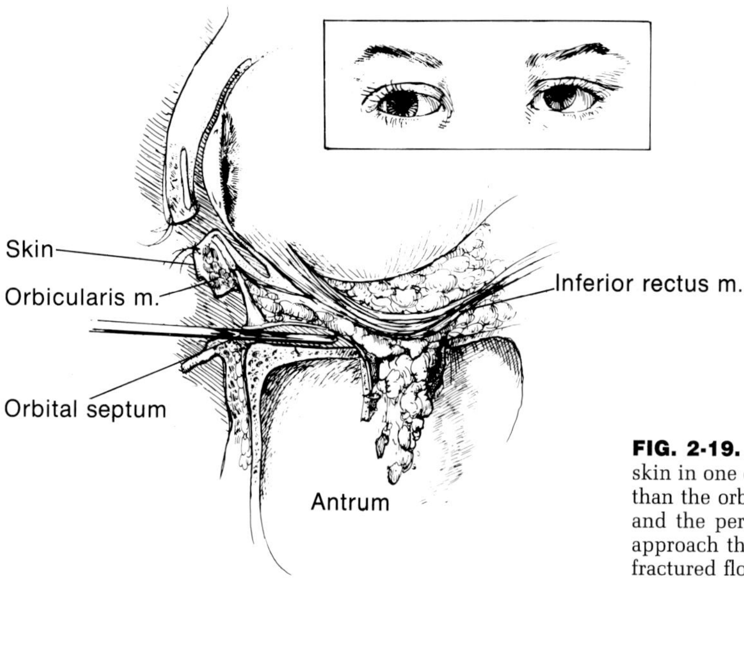

FIG. 2-19. The surgical approach to the orbital floor. The skin in one of the creases of the lid is incised at a higher level than the orbicularis muscle. The orbital septum is preserved, and the periosteum at the orbital rim is incised in order to approach the fracture site. (*Inset*) The right eye, which has a fractured floor, is unable to roll up and is entrapped.

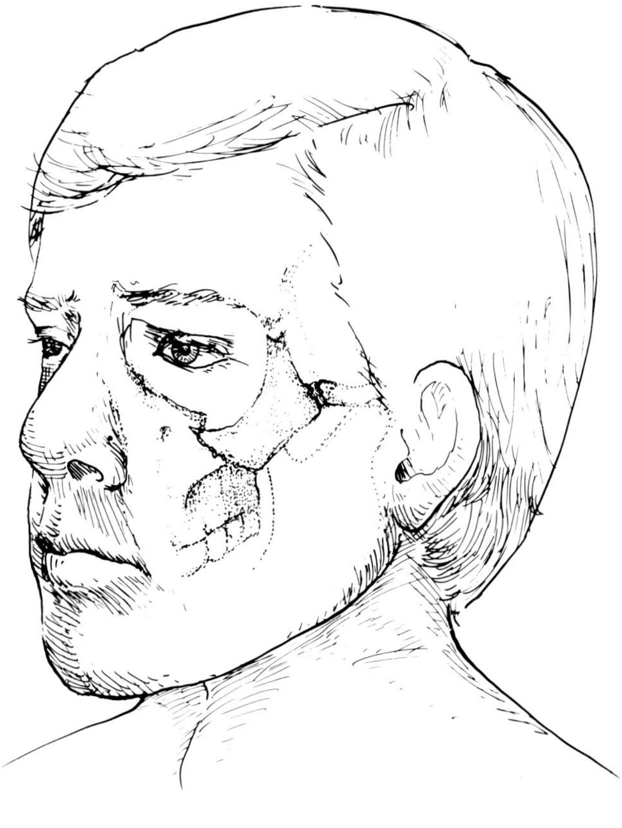

FIG. 2-20. A fracture with downward and medial displacement of the zygomatic bone. The lateral canthus becomes displaced downward, and the infraorbital nerve is often damaged. Numbness of the cheek is a common sequel.

head may be numb from paralysis of the fifth cranial nerve (ophthalmic division) (Fig. 2-21). Reduction of the malar fracture results in spontaneous recovery of eyeball movements. Decompression of the superior orbital fissure by the Kronlein technique has not been found to be necessary.

NOSE

Nasal Fractures

The usual type of deformity in a nasal fracture is either a lateral fracture dislocation or a depressed fracture of the nasal bones. If treated promptly, the aesthetic result is good. Reduction is achieved by

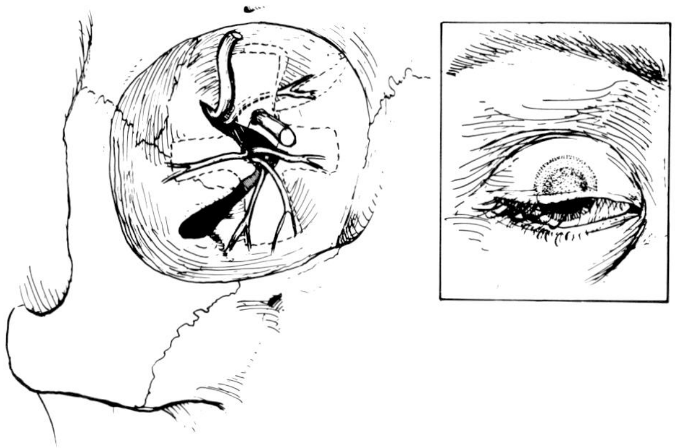

FIG. 2-21. The entry of the third through sixth cranial nerves through the superior orbital fissure. (*Inset*) The classic findings in superior orbital fissure syndrome: ptosis, mydriasis, and ophthalmoplegia.

FIG. 2-22. A septal hematoma is a rare complication of nasal injury. (*Left*) The blue black bulging of the septal mucoperichondrium must be drained promptly or a septal abscess is likely to result. (*Right*) The L-shaped incision used for drainage.

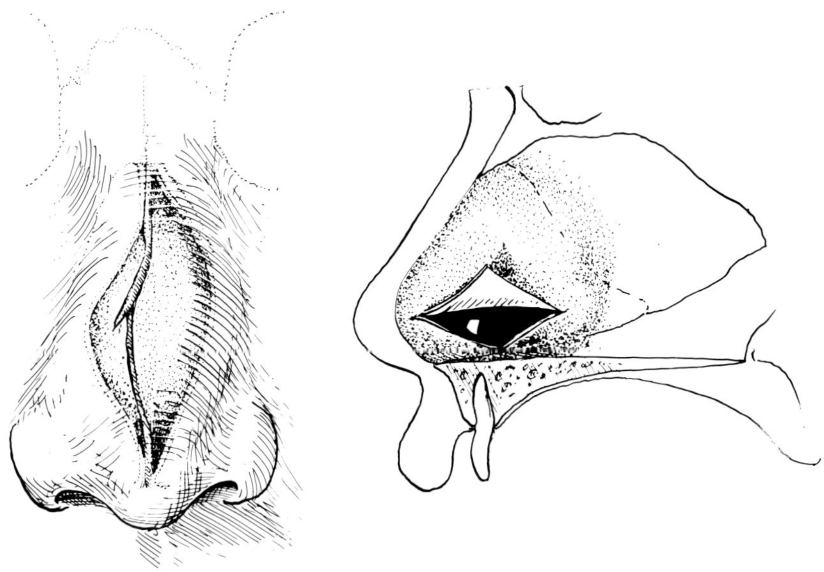

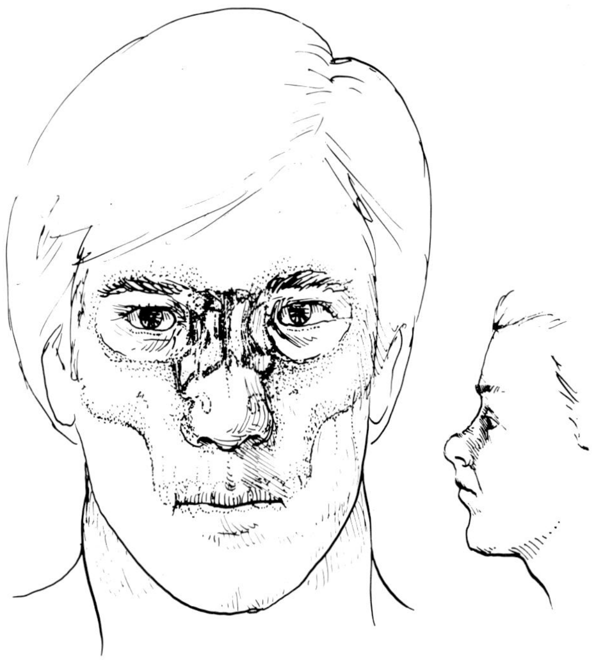

FIG. 2-23. In a classic nasoethmoidal fracture, the comminuted nasal bones are driven into the ethmoids between the orbits, causing traumatic telecanthus (increased distance between medial canthi) and leakage of cerebrospinal fluid through the cribriform plate. The *side view* shows the telescoped appearance of the nose, with tip tilting upward.

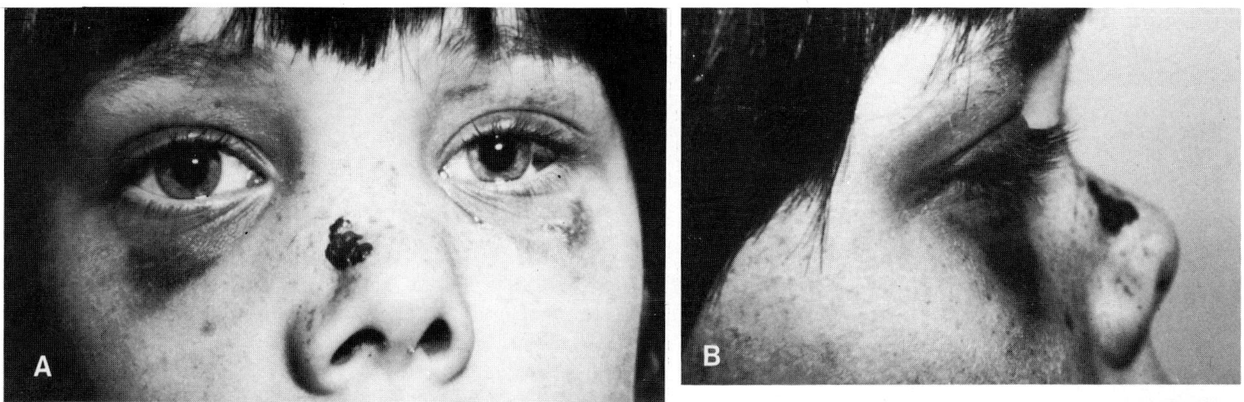

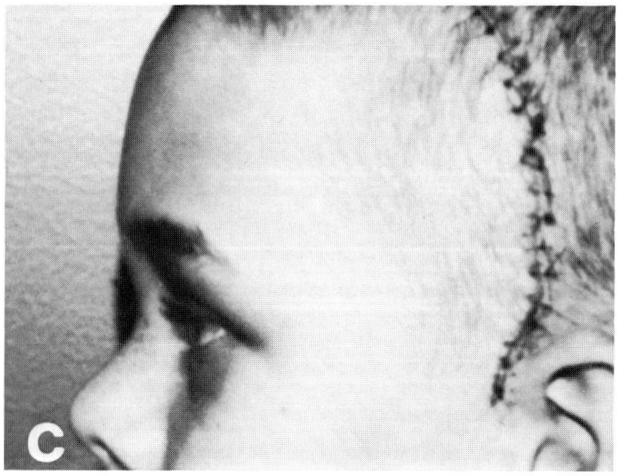

FIG. 2-24. (*A*) A severe frontal injury to the nasal pyramid has pushed in the nose between the orbits. (*B*) Notice the telescoping of the nose, with tip tilting upward. (C) The coronal approach to this region with complete reduction and internal fixation has resulted in excellent contour restoration of the nose.

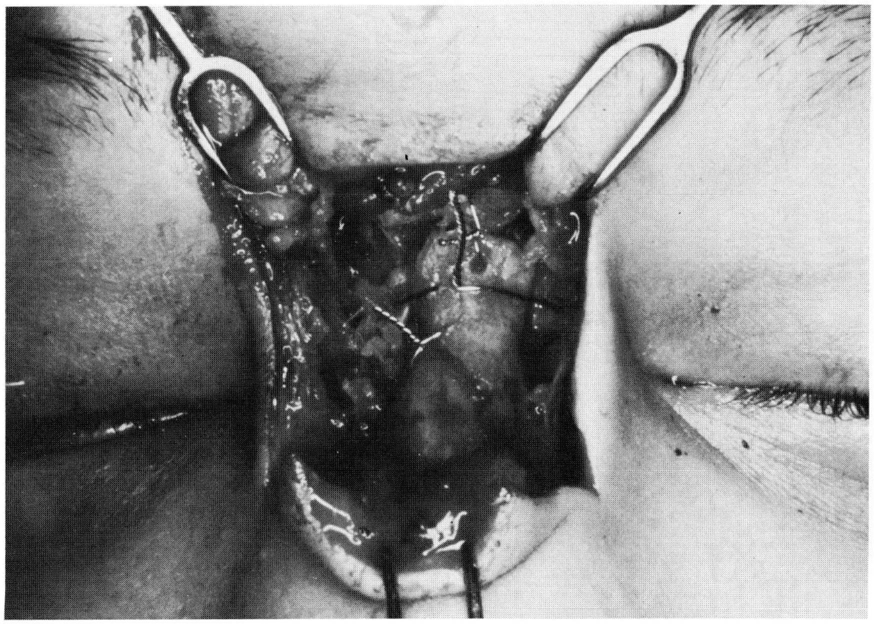

FIG. 2-25. A severe facial injury required the "open sky" approach to a comminuted nasoethmoidal fracture. Direct wiring is shown.

reversing the direction of force. If a septal hematoma is present, it should be recognized. Intranasal inspection in such a case would reveal a blue black bulging of the septal mucosa. This is usually bilateral, and obstruction of the airway is usually present. Prompt drainage by an L-shaped incision is the treatment of choice (Fig. 2-22). If the hematoma is neglected, either the septum thickens or a septal abscess develops. A septal abscess leads to a saddlenose deformity.

Fracture of the septal cartilage may initially appear to heal well. However, if the cartilage is broken on one side only, the internal stresses on the intact side may cause it to curve in a C or S fashion.[15, 16] These curves lead to a nasal deformity and intranasal obstruction, and a septorhinoplasty is usually needed to correct the deformities.

Nasoethmoidal Fractures

If a direct frontal force is severe and hits the nose squarely, it may drive the nose between the orbits, giving rise to the classic nasoethmoidal fracture (Fig. 2-23).[25, 29, 30] The ethmoidal sinuses crumple up on either side and the cribriform plate fractures, resulting in leakage of cerebrospinal fluid. A neurosurgical evaluation should be conducted, and prompt reduction of the depressed fracture may be accomplished in one of two ways, the direct method or the indirect method.

INDIRECT REPAIR. In the indirect method of repair, a coronal incision in the scalp allows exposure and repositioning of the fragments (Fig. 2-24).

DIRECT REPAIR—THE "OPEN SKY" APPROACH. An incision made on either side of the external nose exposes the frontal process of the maxilla.[8] Reduction of the bony fragments can then be carried out under direct vision. A wire suture passed in mattress fashion

FIG. 2-26. This patient, who sustained a nasoethmoidal fracture 9 years previously, had received inadequate treatment. Notice the severe flattening of the nose and the traumatic telecanthus.

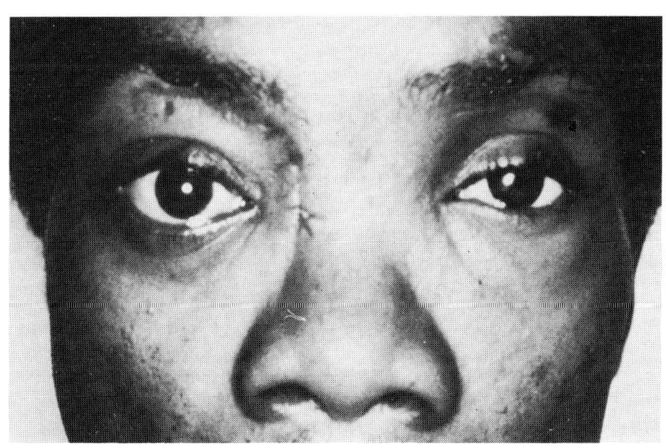

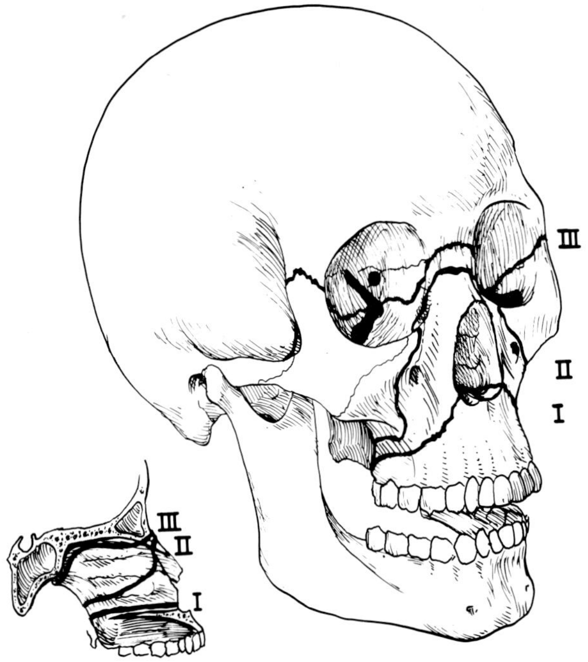

FIG. 2-27. The typical pattern of Le Fort fractures of the maxilla. Le Fort II and III fractures involve the orbit.

across the nose is tied over lead plates (Fig. 2-25). Such measures give pleasing results.

If nasoethmoidal fractures are neglected, severe deformities result (Fig. 2-26). Such malunited fractures require major craniofacial operations to restore functional and aesthetic balance to the face.

MULTIPLE FACIAL INJURIES

In a high-speed vehicular accident the victim may sustain a severe blow to the face that results in multiple fractures of the facial bones.[7, 8, 18] Commonly, the mandible, maxilla, and both zygomatic bones are broken. The usual kind of fracture through the maxilla (*i.e.*, the Le Fort II or III type) involves the orbit (Fig. 2-27). A tracheostomy early on in the management is almost mandatory. The surgical approach to these fractures is systematic from below upward. First reduce the mandible, if fractured, and apply an arch bar to the teeth. Next, reduce the maxilla and fix a similar arch bar to the teeth. Then bring the mandible and maxilla into a correct occlusal relationship with each other. Next, reduce the zygomatic fractures in the standard fashion and restore the orbital floor (Fig. 2-28). If there is a fracture of nose, reduce it next and employ appropriate packing and splinting techniques. A case illustrating the various steps in the management of these complicated injuries is demonstrated in Figure 2-29.

If treatment of these injuries is delayed beyond 4 weeks, the fractures become malunited. The permanent functional and aesthetic stigmata that remain are very difficult to correct. As pointed out by Dingman and Natvig, such severe deformities lead to alterations in the body image and are a prime cause of depression.[10] Often these patients are then forced to seek ongoing treatment at the hands of a competent psychiatrist. Early treatment of the facial injuries is the key to prevention of such sequelae.

FIG. 2-28. When multiple facial fractures are present, the sequence of reduction and internal fixation starts from below and proceeds upward. Illustrated here is open reduction and internal fixation of a mandibular fracture and the application of an arch bar to the teeth, together with reduction of the maxillary fracture and application of a similar arch bar. The teeth are then placed in occlusion. Open reduction of the bilateral zygomatic fractures and nasoethmoidal fractures completes the treatment. The upper jaw is slung to the frontal bone with wire (Adams slings) on each side in order to hold the maxilla suspended to the head.

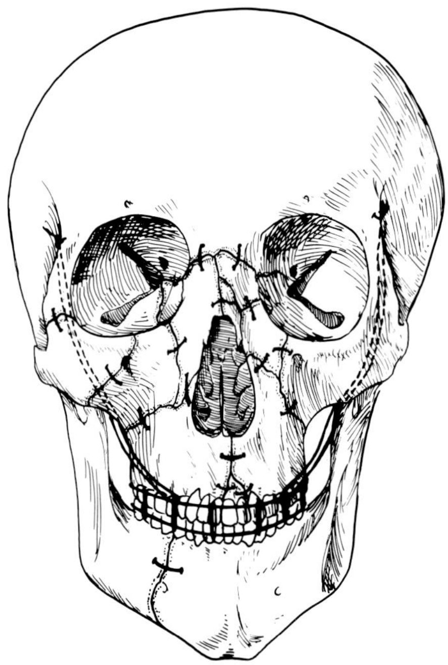

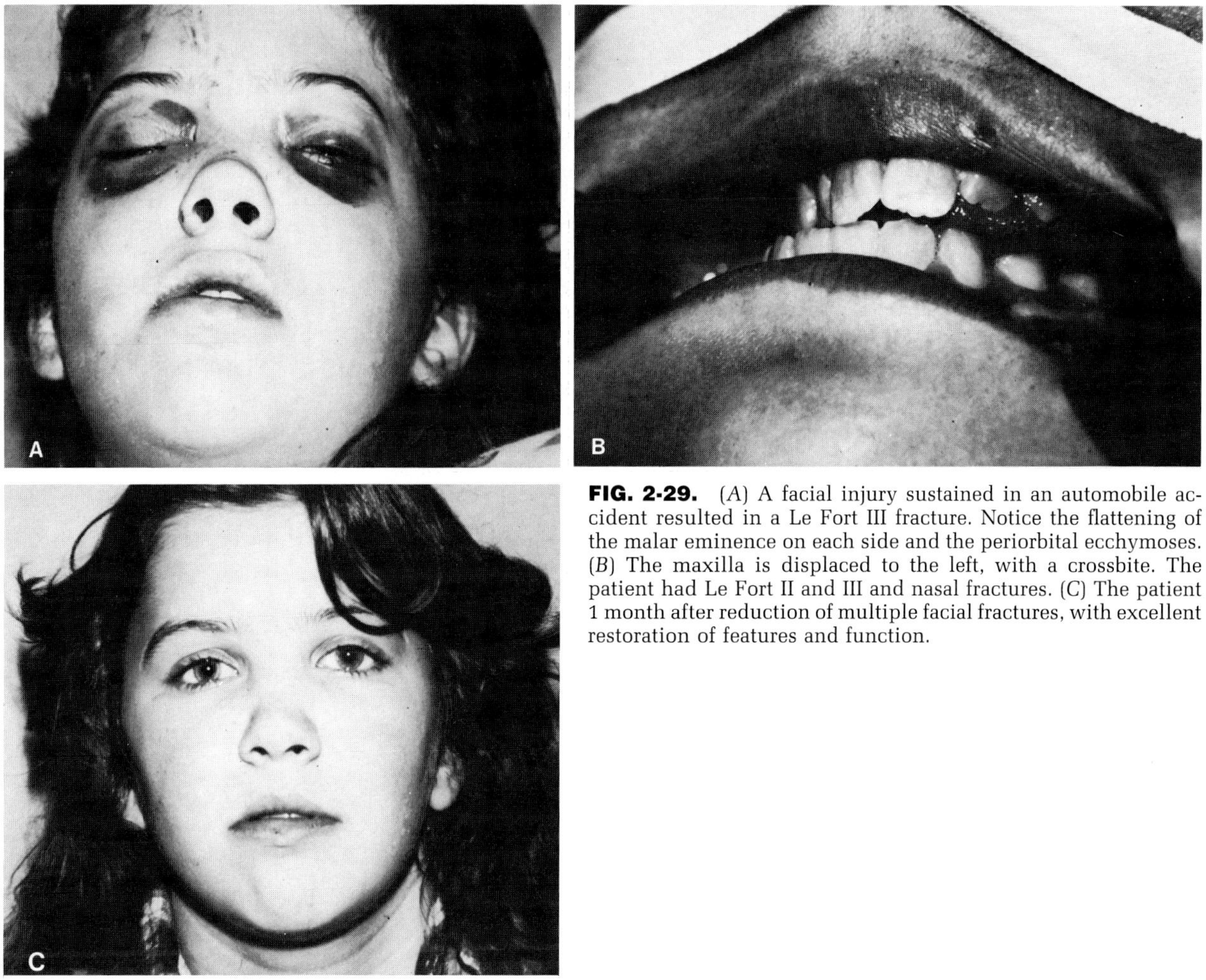

FIG. 2-29. (*A*) A facial injury sustained in an automobile accident resulted in a Le Fort III fracture. Notice the flattening of the malar eminence on each side and the periorbital ecchymoses. (*B*) The maxilla is displaced to the left, with a crossbite. The patient had Le Fort II and III and nasal fractures. (*C*) The patient 1 month after reduction of multiple facial fractures, with excellent restoration of features and function.

References

1. Aghababian RV, Conte JE, Jr: Mammalian bite wounds. Ann Emerg Med 9:79, 1980
2. Bränemark PI, Albrektsson B, Lindstrom J et al: Local tissue effects of wound disinfectants. Acta Chir Scand. [Suppl] 357:166, 1966
3. Callaham M: Treatment of common dog bites: Infection risk factors. J Am Coll Emerg Physicians 7:83, 1978
4. Callaham M: Prophylactic antibiotics in common dog bite wounds: A controlled study. Ann Emerg Med 9:410, 1980
5. Callaham M: Dog bite wounds. JAMA 244:2327, 1980
6. Constant E: Trauma to the face. In Schwartz GR, Safar, P, Stone JH et al (eds): Principles and Practice of Emergency Medicine. Philadelphia, WB Saunders, 1978
7. Converse JM: Surgical Treatment of Facial Injuries, 3rd ed. Baltimore, Williams & Wilkins, 1974
8. Converse JM: Reconstructive Plastic Surgery, 2nd ed. Philadelphia, WB Saunders, 1977
9. Cornell University Automotive Crash Injury Research. The Injury-Producing Accident: A Primer of Facts and Figures. New York, Cornell University, August 1961
10. Dingman RO, Natvig P: Surgery of Facial Fractures. Philadelphia, WB Saunders, 1964
11. Edlich RF, Thacker JG, Buchanan L et al: Modern concepts of treatment of traumatic wounds. Adv Surg 13:169, 1979
12. Edlich RF, Tsung MS, Rogers W et al: Studies in management of the contaminated wound. I. Technique of closure of such wounds with a note on a reproducible model. J Surg Res 8:585, 1968
13. Elek SD, Conen PE: The virulence of *Staphylococcus pyogenes* for man: A study of the problems of wound infection. Br J Exp Pathol 38:573, 1957
14. Finch DR, Dibbell DG: Immediate reconstruction of gunshot injuries to the face. J Trauma 19:965, 1979
15. Fry JH, Robertson WB: Interlocked stresses in human septal cartilage. Br J Plast Surg 19:392, 1967
16. Gibson T, Davis WB: The distortion of autogenous carti-

lage graft: Its cause and prevention. Br J Plast Surg 10:257, 1957
17. Goodstein WA, Stryker A, Weiner LJ: Primary treatment of shotgun injuries to the face. J Trauma 19:961, 1979
18. Grabb WC, Smith JW: Plastic Surgery, 3rd ed. Boston, Little, Brown & Co, 1973
19. Graham WP, Davis TS, Miller SH: Chain saw injuries. Am Fam Physician 16:89, 1977
20. Heaton LD, Hughes CW, Rosegay H et al: Military surgical practices of the U.S. Army in Vietnam. Curr Probl Surg, November 1966
21. Holl D, Rodeheaver GT, Edgerton MT et al: Potentiation of infection by suture closure of dead space. Am J Surg 127:716, 1974
22. Irby WB. Facial Trauma and Concomitant Problems: Evaluation and Treatment, 2nd ed. St Louis, CV Mosby, 1979
23. May M, West J, Heeneman H: Shotgun wounds of the head and neck. Arch Otolaryngol 98:37, 1973
24. Mladick RA, Horton CE, Adamson JE et al: Pocket principle: A new technique for reattachment of a severed ear part. Plast Reconstr Surg 48:219, 1971
25. Mustardé JC: Repair and Reconstruction in the Orbital Region. London, E & S Livingston, 1969
26. Peeples E, Boswick JA, Jr., Scott FA: Wounds of the hand contaminated by human or animal saliva. J Trauma 20:383, 1980
27. Pogrel MA: The superior orbital fissure syndrome: Report of a case. J Oral Surg 38:215, 1980
28. Roberts AM, Rye GD, Edgerton WT et al: Activity of antibiotics in contaminated wounds containing clay soil. Am J Surg 137:381, 1979
29. Schultz RC: Facial Injuries, 2nd ed. Chicago, Year Book Medical Publishers, 1977
30. Schultz RC (ed): Maxillofacial injuries from vehicular accidents. Clin Plast Surg, a, 2:80; b, 2:115, 1975
31. Schwartz GR, Safar P, Stone JH et al (eds): Principles and Practice of Emergency Medicine. Philadelphia, WB Saunders, 1978
32. Sherman RT, Parrish RA: Management of shotgun injuries: A review of 152 cases. J Trauma 3:76, 1963
33. Shuck LW, Orgel MG, Vogel AV: Self-inflicted gunshot wounds to the face: A review of 18 cases. J Trauma 20:370, 1980
34. Tomasetti BJ, Walker L, Gormley MB et al: Human bites of the face. J Oral Surg 37:565, 1979
35. Zaydon TJ, Brown JB: Early treatment of facial injuries. Philadelphia, Lea & Febiger, 1964
36. Zide MF, Epker BN: Short-range shotgun wounds to the face. J Oral Surg 37:319, 1979
37. Zook EG: The Primary Care of Facial Injuries. Acton, MA, Publishing Sciences Group, 1980

3 Complications of Wound Infections

James A. Majeski | J. Wesley Alexander

OVERVIEW

Wound infections following surgical procedures are major complications leading to significant morbidity and mortality, as well as contributing to increased health costs. Nearly half of all postoperative complications are wound complications, and among these, infections and dehiscence are the most common, affecting approximately 4% of all wounds. Surgical infections may be caused by endogenous organisms or by organisms acquired from exogenous sources, which sometimes include a traumatizing agent, the hospital environment, and medical personnel.

Bacteria enter many wounds without causing sepsis. The susceptibility to infection is determined by the involved tissue, by the virulence of the organism, and by the strength of the patient's natural host defense. Host defenses include local inflammation and leukocyte migration to the wound edge. Should there be a failure of local containment, regional lymph nodes are the next line of host defense. Beyond that the capacity of a normal reticuloendothelial system to clear bacteremia is impressive.

The risk of infection and its severity are increased by local and general factors that inhibit host defenses. Local factors that promote wound infection include the presence of extensive devitalized tissue, long surgical procedures, large incisions, poor surgical technique, a defective blood supply, and hematomas, seromas, and foreign bodies, which may include drainage tubes, indwelling catheters, and prostheses. General factors associated with a higher incidence of wound infections include old age and systemic diseases such as diabetes, malignancy, malnutrition, obesity, and atherosclerosis. Ancillary therapy such as that with broad-spectrum antibiotics that eliminate the competitive inhibition of the normal body flora on mucosal surfaces, steroids, cytotoxic agents, and immunosuppressive drugs have increased the hazards of infection.

Experimental data indicate that an inoculation of 10^6 or more viable staphylococci is required to produce a subcutaneous abscess in normal humans.[12] With acceptable aseptic technique, contamination of clean wounds with this large number of bacteria should be rare. However, surgical wounds are nearly always contaminated with a few microbes. Wound dead space and blood clots may predispose to growth of contaminating organisms. These areas become protected foci because of rapid loss of opsonizing activity from dead-space fluid and ineffective penetration of the coagulum by leukocytes and antimicrobial agents. Ischemia, even though transient, may favor bacterial growth in wounds contaminated with subinfective doses of bacteria.[19] Significant local factors that diminish host defense mechanisms at the time of operative contamination are the presence of foreign bodies and devitalized tissue in the wound.[23] When tied too tight, sutures used to approximate tissue lead to tissue necrosis and predispose to wound infection.[8] Skillful surgical technique that eliminates dead space, obtains hemostasis, and uses delicate tissue dissection with special care to prevent loss of the blood supply and eliminate tissue trauma results in the lowest incidence of surgical wound infections.

There is a strong correlation between deficiencies in immunologic and host defense mechanisms and protein–calorie malnutrition in humans.[1] Malnutrition results in a higher incidence of surgical infections. Estimates suggest that 20% to 30% of all surgical patients in industrialized nations have some element of malnutrition, and since malnutrition has been estimated to affect three fourths of the world's population, this percentage is unquestionably higher in many underdeveloped countries. Adequate nutritional support to meet the increased *metabolic demands of a major surgical procedure can decrease the incidence of morbidity and mortality from surgical infections. Thus, not only must preexisting nutritional disorders be corrected to return depressed host defenses to normal prior to surgery, but nutritional support also must be provided during times of infection or stress to maintain a functionally normal immunologic defense and to prevent abnormalities in this defense from developing.*[8]

Diagnosis

The cardinal signs of infection and inflammation have been known for centuries. Calor (heat) and rubor (redness) are the result of intense hyperemia. These signs are frequently found in infections of the skin itself. Tumor (swelling) is a result of accumulation of an inflammatory exudate. Dolor (pain) and functio laesa (disturbed function) are the most common signs of infection. These two features arise from multiple factors, which include the stimulation of sensory and motor nerve endings of the affected tissue. Additional nonspecific physical signs such as fever, tachycardia, and discoloration aid in the detection of an infection.

Diagnosis of surgical wound infections depends on a thorough awareness of the patient's history, a physical examination, laboratory data, and bacteriology information. Early and accurate diagnosis is of great importance in the control of surgical infections. Successful treatment depends on the employment of old and established surgical principles aided by the use of current antibiotic therapy.

With the presentation of a suspected wound infection in a postoperative patient, a relatively complete examination of the patient should be performed, along with a thorough review of the patient's history, postoperative course, and available laboratory data. Wound infections generally appear beginning at the fourth to the seventh postoperative day, but they may appear years after the surgical procedure, especially with implanted prosthetic devices. A majority of infections originate in the subcutaneous tissue, particularly in obese patients or diabetics.

The first sign of an infection usually is fever. An unexplained fever in a postoperative patient always requires inspection of the wound. Additional areas that must be examined are the lungs, for atelectasis, infiltrate, or pleural effusion; the heart, for a new murmur; the extremities, for intravenous sepsis or thrombophlebitis; the central lines placed for hyperalimentation, central venous pressure monitoring, or dialysis, or Swan–Ganz catheters, for positive culture; the central nervous system, for meningitis; and of course the abdomen, for subphrenic, subhepatic, or intrahepatic abscesses or for pelvic or interloop abscesses. All catheters, drainage tubes, feeding tubes, and endotracheal tubes are a possible source of infection or sepsis.

Laboratory data that may be of aid in the differential diagnosis are a complete blood count and urinalysis. Blood culture data may define the etiologic agent in a surgical infection and may occasionally help to determine the source and site of the infection. Current practice is to perform several cultures at frequent intervals and near the onset of chills or during the phase of ascending temperature. Chest and abdominal x-ray films frequently give important clinical clues in pulmonary infections or intra-abdominal abscesses. An x-ray film of the wound may occasionally lend important information toward the diagnosis of clostridial infection, necrotizing fasciitis, or retention of a foreign body.

The initial approach to an area of possible infection in a previous surgical incision is to obtain a sample of pus or exudate. Needle aspiration of the suspected abscess cavity, simple removal of several sutures with direct culture, and aspiration of the infected areas are all suitable methods. Microscopic examination of a smear of the material after Gram staining yields immediate information on the etiologic agent for the purpose of instituting appropriate antibiotic therapy. The material must also be cultured immediately with aerobic and anaerobic techniques. Material kept refrigerated or at room temperature and exposed to air frequently yields inconclusive or even false results, particularly when mixed infections are present.

Once the incision is found to be infected, open the area widely to allow free drainage. Carefully examine the underlying muscle and fascia if they are involved in the infection. Biopsy of the lesion is frequently an important diagnostic aid in establishing granulomatous infections and occasionally in establishing a systemic disease as the cause. After carefully examining the wound for any loculations or sinus tracts, debride it and irrigate the infected area. Establish dependent drainage when physically possible. Frequently an infected wound can be packed with an iodoform or simple gauze to ensure adequate drainage.

Primary treatment in a wound infection consists in widely opening the wound and establishing dependent drainage. The use of antibiotics is secondary and should not be substituted for incision and drainage. Systemic antibiotics are routinely employed to prevent the spread of bacteria, to decrease the incidence of complications, and to shorten convalescence. By contrast, antibiotic therapy is the major and primary method of treatment of cellulitis.

Other sources of postoperative fever can occur concurrently with a wound infection. The careful examination and diagnostic workup of an infection should rule out the presence of ancillary infectious problems. An algorithm presents the basic logical sequence of surgical decisions and workup for a wound infection (Fig. 3-1).

Prevention

There are several basic requirements for the establishment of a wound infection. First, bacteria must reach the incision in sufficient quantities to establish an infection.[12] Next, a nutrient supply must be available for bacterial growth. Old blood-clot or tissue-breakdown products are excellent nutrient sources for bacterial growth. Finally, unless the inoculum is very large, the patient's resistance must be systemically compromised or overcome in the local tissue environment. Frequent factors appear to be malnutrition, either acquired or inherited deficiencies of host defense or natural or acquired immunity, poor local blood supply, and systemic disease.

The prevention of wound infections is easily accomplished by adherence to the time-honored principles of surgery. Frequently, surgeons with experience gained during the pre-antibiotic era are the best practitioners and teachers of surgical technique. The use of strict aseptic technique can minimize bacterial contamination below the typical minimal infective dose of 10,000 bacteria. Elimination of devitalized tissue, complete débridement of traumatic wounds, and elimination of hematomas, seromas, and dead spaces with closed-catheter–suction drainage systems lead to a decreased incidence of surgical wound infections. A lengthy preoperative hospitalization increases the likelihood of colonization by pathogenic bacteria and may increase the likelihood of an operative wound infection.

Currently, we recommend a minimum of a 5-minute scrub with povidone-iodine or chlorhexidine gluconate by the surgeon. This scrub reduces bacterial counts on the hand to a level that persists throughout the surgical procedure. The same scrub should also be used for the operative site except in those few instances when contraindicated. Emerging concepts indicate that when hair is sparse the routine shaving of skin around the operative site may not be necessary. In a large, randomized prospective series at the University of Cincinnati Medical Center, removal of body hair by clipping on the morning of operation was shown to result in the lowest incidence of surgical wound infections. The use of disposable paper gowns designed to resist penetration by moisture may prove to decrease wound infections substantially.[16]

The advantages of laminar or unidirectional airflow systems to maintain clean air in the operating room and prevent wound infection appear more theoretical than practical. There are no data to indicate any significant benefit of these systems in decreasing the incidence of surgical wound infections. Ultraviolet irradiation of the air achieves an impressive 50% reduction in the number of airborne bacteria in the operating room, but unfortunately, this system fails to produce any clinically significant change in the overall infection rate of surgical wounds.[17, 18]

An emerging area of importance in the prevention of surgical wound infections is host defense and immunity. Certain systemic disease states can alter the complex interactions among lymphocytes, phagocytes, and humoral factors. A list of these states frequently seen by the surgeon includes malignant disease, extensive trauma, large burns, cirrhosis, inflammatory bowel diseases, old age, obesity, diabetes mellitus, uremia, and numerous chronic debilitating illnesses. Several important studies indicate that many of the abnormalities of host defense and immunity can be explained by protein malnutrition or deficiencies. Emerging principles indicate that major injury greatly increases metabolic expenditure, and this expenditure must be met with an increased nutritional caloric and protein intake.[6] Recommendations for nutritional therapy to prevent infection or supplement the treatment of infections are as follows:

Institute hyperalimentation in the postsurgical patient who will not be able to take oral nutrition for periods longer than 5 to 7 days.

In patients with preexisting malnutrition, correct the nutritional defects before performing any elective surgery.

Provide nutritional therapy for patients with severe infections that do not respond quickly to therapy.

Oral hyperalimentation is the preferred route of supplemental nutrition. Intravenous hyperalimentation should be reserved for those patients unable to take nourishment by the enteral route.

Hyperalimentation should ensure adequate caloric intake for the basal metabolic needs plus the estimated needs required by conditions associated with hypercatabolism, such as burn injury.

Vitamin supplementation for patients not previously vitamin deficient should be in the range of two to three times the recommended daily allowance, except for vitamin C, which should be given in doses of 500 mg to 1000 mg/day in adults.

Oral hyperalimentation programs usually contain enough trace metals to ensure against deficiencies, but trace metals must be added to intravenous regimens.[8]

FIG. 3-1. An algorithm outlining the steps in surgical wound evaluation.

Initial patient evaluation

- A. History and physical
  1. Temperature course (blood cultures for T ≥ 102)
  2. Operation
  3. Anesthesia
  4. Medications
  5. Lungs and heart
  6. Wound
  7. Abdomen
  8. Extremities
- B. Laboratory studies
  1. Complete blood count with differential
  2. Urinalysis → pyuria → Gram's stain culture → antibiotics
- C. Radiograph
  1. Chest
  2. Wound—if suspect
     - a. Clostridial infection
     - b. Necrotizing fasciitis
     - c. Retention of a foreign body

→

- A. Infected wound
  1. Usually 3–7 days after surgery
  2. Pain, tenderness, swelling, warmth, redness, pain on motion
     → a. Remove 2–3 sutures and probe with sterile swab OR b. Needle aspirate
     - Pus (note color, odor, and consistency) →
       1. Open wound wide
       2. Culture
          - a. aerobic
          - b. anaerobic
       3. Gram's stain
       4. Biopsy lesion → if suspect { a. Malignancy; b. Granulomatous disease }
       5. Irrigate
       6. Pack open with iodoform or gauze
       7. Institute appropriate antibiotics
     - No pus →
       1. Perform frequent repeat examinations
       2. Culture incision and Gram's stain
       3. Examine underlying fascia and muscle
  3. Crepitance → a. Gas gangrene; b. Necrotizing fasciitis } Surgery
- B. Noninfected wound → Repeat physical exam →
  - Lungs
    1. Atelactasis → Agressive pulmonary care
    2. Pneumonia
       - a. Bacterial
       - b. Aspiration

       } Gram's stain culture—antibiotics
    3. Pulmonary embolus → Scan—anticoagulants
  - Abdomen
    1. Subphrenic abscess
    2. Intrahepatic abscess
    3. Flank abscess
    4. Pelvic abscess
    5. Intraloop abscess

    } Localize by { a. Physical exam; b. Plain radiograph; c. ECHO; d. CT scan; e. Gallium isotope scan }

    (c–e) → Drain abscess { (1) Culture; (2) Antibiotics }
  - Extremity
    1. Infected IV site → Remove IV { a. Administer antibiotics; b. Occasionally must excise vein }
    2. Septic thrombophlebitis → a. Scan; b. Venogram { (1) Anticoagulants; (2) Blood cultures; (3) Antibiotics }
  - Negative physical exam
    1. Exclude drug allergy
    2. Perform random blood culture

    } a. Repeat exam in 24 hours; b. Change or stop antibiotics

Prophylactic Antibiotics in Surgery

In elective surgical patients, prophylactic antibiotics are often administered to treat contaminated wounds before contamination occurs. Unfortunately, the administration of antibiotic drugs is occasionally substituted for sound judgment and good surgical technique. With certain exceptions, prophylactic antibiotics should not be used in clean operative procedures that carry a minimal risk of sepsis, since patients undergoing clean-wound operations do not benefit from such systemic antibiotics. There are, however, a couple of currently acceptable indications for the use of prophylactic antibiotics. First, in clinical situations in which the incidence of infection has been shown to be significantly high, the use of prophylactic antibiotics to decrease wound morbidity, shorten the hospital stay, and decrease hospital costs is warranted. The only other indication is an operation the results of which would be uniformly disastrous if a postoperative infection were to occur.

Lists of clinical situations in which prophylactic antibiotics are usually recommended are available, but they can be summarized under several definite categories:

- Elective procedures opening contaminated areas such as the gastrointestinal, respiratory, or genitourinary systems
- Contaminated wounds or traumatic injuries in which the incidence of infection is high
- Surgery in a patient with a recent preexisting or current active infection
- Any surgical procedure in which a prosthesis is inserted or in which the patient is at exceptional risk

The antibiotic chosen should be effective against the organism expected to contaminate the operative field, a consideration often dictated by the anatomical site.[22]

Antibiotic therapy is ineffective in several situations. These include those clinical situations in which there is continued contamination and in which the antibiotic treatment is begun at the end of the surgical procedure. Prophylactic antibiotics also fail if the dosage is subtherapeutic or if the agent used has an inappropriate antibacterial spectrum. To be effective, prophylactic antibiotics must be started preoperatively, before bacterial contamination, and they must be present in the circulating blood—and most especially in the local tissues—at the time of contamination.[17, 18]

A new area of immunotherapy is emerging that has promise in the manipulation of immunologic responses to increase the patient's resistance to infection. Administration of one of the immunomodulators, levamisole, has led to reduced infection and improved survival in anergic surgical patients.[7, 15] Replacement therapy with plasma, γ-globulins, hyperimmune globulin, or granulocyte transfusions for isolated defects of the immune system may, in highly selected instances, be of significant value for the reduction of surgical infections.

Treatment of Established Wound Infections

Before the advent of antibiotic therapy, several principles of treating surgical wound infection were established, and these principles are still very applicable today. Frequently inspect the incision postoperatively for infection. Keep dressings dry and change them whenever they become moist or soiled. Early diagnosis is important, since current antibiotic therapy is more effective when started early in the course of a surgical infection.

Once an infection has established itself in the surgical incision, several procedures are employed to diminish the effect of the infection and to provide an effective means of recovery. Surgical intervention in a wound infection is based on the time-honored principle of incision and dependent drainage of localized collections of pus. Surgical drainage accomplishes several important tasks: bacteria are removed or substantially reduced in total numbers, toxins produced by bacteria are removed or decreased, and necrotic tissue is removed by débridement. Fluids collecting in wounds become progressively less able to support opsonization for phagocytosis and killing by neutrophils.[5] Débridement and drainage allow for fresh access to the infected area with phagocyte and bacteriocidal cells, antibiotic agents, and serum factors of host defense and immunity.

We occasionally irrigate an infected surgical incision with an antibiotic solution. Kanamycin or neomycin is the effective agent of choice in a concentration of 1g per 1 liter of normal saline. Despite reports of aminoglycoside-induced myoneural blockade and its resultant respiratory arrest, these complications are rare when the drugs are used judiciously in surgical wounds. Another irrigation solution that has been effective consists of 1 g of a cephalosporin in 1 liter of normal saline. The use of topical irrigation has been cited as a principal factor in the reduction of infection.[11, 21]

The choice of antibiotic therapy for a particular case depends on several factors. Initial therapy should be based on the results from Gram smears, clinical data, culture results, and sensitivity tests. When this information is not available, the choice of antimicrobial agent should be based on the type of infection and its location and clinical characteristics. It is most important to realize that the most common pathogens and their resistances vary from hospital to hospital, as well as within a particular hospital over time. An antibiotic regimen used successfully at a particular hospital may prove to be relatively ineffective in another hospital, and it may even prove ineffective at a later time in the same hospital.[2-4, 8, 9]

Treatment of Special Wound Infections

CELLULITIS

Cellulitis is one of the most common of infections seen by the surgeon during routine practice. The term *cellulitis* is frequently misused and should be limited to invasive nonsuppurative infection and inflammation of connective tissue with massive infiltration of neutrophils, typically seen on the extremities. Cellulitis usually arises from a surgical wound, an ulcer, or an area of gangrene. Although the responsible etiologic agents have been identified as any of a variety of aerobic and anaerobic bacteria, the most common agents are the hemolytic streptococci. Certain bacterial species (β-hemolytic streptococci) usually spread through tissue as extending cellulitis, but others (staphylococci) usually remain localized to form abscesses if they are not controlled. A moderate fever is usually present in either type. The area involved has widespread swelling, redness, and pain without a site of localization. Treatment consists in having the patient rest, elevating the infected area, applying warm packs, and instituting antibiotic therapy. Early therapy reduces the possibility of lymphatic or blood-borne spread and allows host resistance to function optimally with an increased blood supply and without the impediment of dependent edema. Penicillin is usually the drug of choice in non–hospital-acquired cellulitis. The infection usually begins to resolve within 48 hours of treatment. Because there are no localized areas of pus formation, drainage is indicated only to relieve pressure that may cause ischemia. Localized abscesses frequently have a surrounding area of cellulitis, in which case draining the abscess and instituting antibiotic therapy are essential parts of surgical treatment.

CLOSTRIDIAL INFECTIONS

Infections with anaerobic clostridia can result in three diseases of major consequence in surgery: clostridial cellulitis, gas gangrene or clostridial myositis, and tetanus.

Clostridial Cellulitis

Clostridial cellulitis is a severe septic anaerobic involvement of the subcutaneous and fascial tissue that is caused by one of the clostridia, most commonly *Clostridium perfringens*. Intact, healthy muscle is not usually invaded. The infection is characterized by a crepitant cellulitis that spreads in tissues rendered necrotic by ischemia, trauma, or bacterial activity. The cellulitis is characterized as a foul-smelling, seropurulent infection that spreads rapidly. Eventually, necrosis and sloughing of the areolar tissues, fascia, and skin may occur as a result of thrombosis of contiguous nutrient blood vessels. Mild pain about the area is characteristic. The symptoms associated with clostridial cellulitis are similar to those associated with clostridial myositis, but they occur to a lesser degree. The organisms multiply in the connective tissue spaces and may produce gas that escapes into the tissues. Gas is not present in the muscles in clostridial cellulitis.[26] Clostridial cellulitis generally has a gradual onset; the incubation period is 2 to 4 days. Systemic effects are usually mild, there is no profound toxemia, and there is rarely any skin discoloration or edema. Clostridial cellulitis seems to have its greatest incidence in diabetics.

Treatment should include extensive surgical decompression with elevation of skin flaps superficial to the fascia, as well as administration of systemic antibiotic agents in large doses, usually penicillin and tetracycline.[10]

Clostridial Myositis

Clostridial myositis, the most serious form of clostridial infection, primarily involves muscle and is characterized by rapid-spreading gangrene and profound toxemia. Gas gangrene is classically defined as a spreading clostridial myositis that rapidly progresses to myonecrosis.[9] The infection occurs in severe wounds of large muscle masses and is associated with delayed or inadequate surgical care and impaired blood supply. The chief etiologic agents are *C. perfringens, C. novyi, C. septicum,* and *C. sordellii*.[26] The average incubation period is 48 hours but can be as short as 6 hours. Pain is an early and very significant symptom. A rapid pulse with only mild elevations of temperature is common. Hypotension, renal failure, severe prostration, and jaundice with intravascular hemolysis then follow, with severe prostration and, ultimately, death. Crepitus, the classic sign, may occur late in the clinical course, but it may be absent if *C. novyi* is the causative organism.[8] Radiographic demonstration of tissue gas may lead to the diagnosis but is not by itself diagnostic. The most valuable diagnostic technique is Gram's staining of the exudate. The finding of large, gram-positive rods with few neutrophils is good evidence for an early diagnosis.[26] When present in tissues, *C. perfringens* does not contain spores. The other common toxigenic clostridia are frequently sporulated.[26] Rapid identification of *C. perfringens* can be made by inoculating a warmed exudate into a special milk medium that is then incubated anaerobically. Stormy fermentation in the medium and the presence of proliferating, nonmotile bacteria indicate the presence of *C. perfringens*. This test is helpful in the early diagnosis of some questionable cases of gas gangrene.[10]

Once bacterial growth is established and bacterial toxins accumulate, the invasion of uninjured tissue is promoted, and the anaerobic infection becomes established. The clostridial exotoxin is extremely potent and is among the most toxic poisons known to man. The most lethal component of the exotoxin is an α-portion containing a lecithinase that is responsible for hemolysis, tissue necrosis, and disruption of cell membranes, leading to capillary permeability.[26]

Early and adequate surgery is the only effective method of treating gas gangrene. Surgical treatment consists in extensive decompression of all involved muscle compartments by incision and fasciotomy, or in amputation of the part if irreversible gangrenous changes have developed in the extremity. Because of the frequently rapid spread of the infection, a 24-hour delay in surgery will frequently be fatal. Antibiotic therapy with penicillin and tetracycline has been most effective as an adjunct to operative treatment. Antitoxin therapy directed toward neutralizing these toxins has been ineffective in clinical practice. Hyperbaric oxygen therapy should be considered only as supportive therapy to surgery. Its effect is a direct oxygen-toxic action on the clostridial organism, and it inhibits the bacteria from producing an α-lecithinase toxin. However, it does not neutralize any toxin already present.[24]

Tetanus

Tetanus (lockjaw) is caused by an exotoxin released by the anaerobic bacteria *Clostridium tetani*. *C. tetani* is noninvasive, and a low oxygen tension is necessary for its growth. Tetanus commonly follows mild injuries because the routine protective measures employed in severe cases are occasionally omitted. The usual types of lesions leading to the development of tetanus are penetrating wounds or cuts due to splinters, thorns, or rusty nails, and even dirty soiled abrasions. As the bacteria grow in the tissue, a soluble toxin (tetanospasmin) is produced that acts on susceptible cells in the central nervous system and on neuromuscular end organs, causing local tonic contractions.[25] With the exception of botulinum toxin, this substance is the most powerful poison known.

The neurotoxin acts on four areas: the skeletal muscle motor end plate, the brain, the sympathetic nervous system, and the spinal cord. By inhibiting the release of acetylcholine from nerve terminals in certain muscles, the neurotoxin impairs neuromuscular transmission. This leads to dysfunction of polysynaptic reflexes, producing the unopposed contraction of muscles with the loss of antagonistic muscle function that is characteristic of tetanus.[25] At the onset of the illness, intermittent tetanic contractions of the muscles in the area of the wound are accompanied by headache, stiffness of the jaw muscles, and restlessness. Tonic spasm of the skeletal muscles with a generalized tetanus usually follows, along with the classic facial distortion, opisthotonos, and rigidity. Respiratory arrest often accompanies these seizures.

Usual laboratory studies are of little value in the diagnosis of tetanus, and examination of the spinal fluid reveals no abnormalities. The peripheral white blood cell count may be elevated or normal. Gram stains may show the characteristic gram-positive bacillus. Occasionally there is elevation of the creatinine phosphokinase level. The diagnosis of the disease is based primarily on a history of injury followed by the development of the characteristic symptoms.[20]

Even with current therapy the mortality rate for tetanus patients is approximately 30%. Prevention of clinical tetanus is more effective than treatment of the clinical disease. The successful treatment of generalized tetanus depends on early diagnosis, neutralization of the circulating toxin, and control of the systemic manifestations of the toxins. Careful sedation to control convulsive seizures is the most important symptomatic therapy.[25] The drug treatment of choice to control the seizures is a constant intravenous drip of a 0.05% to 0.1% solution of sodium pentothal.[9] Complete local excision and débridement of the tetanus infection should be performed as soon as possible.[9] The established disease is treated by administering human antitetanus globulin. Patients who have already received a full course of active toxoid immunization should receive full protection by a booster of tetanus toxoid at the time of injury. Injured patients who have not been immunized previously should be given tetanus immune globulins and immediately started on a program of active-toxoid immunization.[8] The patient with severe tetanus requires the use of muscle relaxants, sedation with a short-acting barbiturate, a careful balance of fluids and electrolytes, and elimination of visceral and external stimuli. A tracheostomy frequently is performed in severe cases or in those in which there is evidence of developing respiratory deterioration. Curare-like drugs may be of some benefit in controlling seizures. Antibiotic therapy is of no value in the treatment of established tetanus *per se*, but it should be given if there are associated or complicating infections such as bacterial pneumonitis.[25]

NECROTIZING FASCIITIS

Necrotizing fasciitis is a frequently lethal infection that occurs in elderly, debilitated, or diabetic patients. The infection is almost always diagnosed late in its course, a fact that accounts for its high incidence of lethal complications. The infection typically occurs in an ulcer or an injury to an extremity with an undermining fascial necrosis. The infective necrotic process can also involve the abdomen, perineum, and chest wall. The overlying skin frequently shows mild edema. The infectious agents are frequently streptococci or hemolytic staphylococci, but mixed infections are common. Antibiotic therapy alone is ineffective. The patient must be taken as soon as possible to the operating room, where the surgeon should follow two principles of surgical therapy: to excise all necrotic tissue and to provide wide surgical drainage. Perforating nutrient vessels to the skin and subcutaneous tissue can often be preserved by meticulous dissection.[13, 14]

Reconstruction is frequently much easier with skin preservation. As an initial antibiotic therapy in this infection, give penicillin plus an aminoglycoside, or clindamycin plus an aminoglycoside. Later, select more specific antibiotics according to the sensitivity patterns of the bacteria colonizing the wound.

Necrotizing fasciitis requires careful, aggressive therapy. Nutritional support, in addition to immediate surgery and antibiotic therapy, is considered essential to patient survival. Typical nutrient support measures for severe infections include two times the normal basal nutritional requirements with high-protein dietary supplements. The mortality from necrotizing fasciitis can be substantially reduced if these guidelines are followed closely.

References

1. Alexander JW: Nutrition and surgical infection. In Ballinger WF et al (eds): American College of Surgeons Manual of Surgical Nutrition. Philadelphia, WB Saunders, 1975
2. Alexander JW: Life-threatening sepsis. In Condon RE, De Cosse JJ (eds): Surgical Care: A Physiologic Approach to Surgical Problems. Philadelphia, Lea & Febiger, 1980
3. Alexander JW: Infection, host resistance and antimicrobial agents. In Dudrick SJ et al (eds): American College of Surgeons Manual of Preoperative and Postoperative Care, 3rd ed. Philadelphia, WB Saunders, 1981
4. Alexander JW (ed): Surgical infections. Surg Clin North Am 60, 1980
5. Alexander JW, Korelitz J, Alexander NS: Prevention of wound infections: A case for closed suction drainage to remove wound fluids deficient in opsonic proteins. Am J Surg 132:59, 1976
6. Alexander JW, McMillan BG, Stinnett JD et al: Beneficial effects of aggressive protein feeding in severely burned children. Ann Surg 192:505, 1980
7. Alexander JW, Stinnett JD: Immunotherapeutic approaches. In Simmons RL, Howard RJ (eds): Surgical Infection Diseases. New York, Appleton–Century–Crofts, 1981
8. Altemeier WA, Alexander JW: Surgical infections and choice of antibiotics. In Sabiston DC, Jr (ed): Christopher's Textbook of Surgery, 12th ed. Philadelphia, WB Saunders, 1981
9. Altemeier WA, Burke JF, Pruitt BA et al: Manual of Control of Infection in Surgical Patients. Philadelphia, JB Lippincott, 1976
10. Altemeier WA, Fullen WD: Prevention and treatment of gas gangrene. JAMA 217:806, 1971
11. Banowsky LH, Montie JE, Brown WE et al: Renal transplantation. III. Prevention of wound infections. Urology 4:656, 1974
12. Elek SD: Experimental staphylococcal infections in skin of man. Ann NY Acad Sci 65:85, 1956
13. Freeman HP, Oluwole SF, Ganepola GAP et al: Necrotizing fasciitis. Am J Surg 142:377, 1981
14. Kaiser RE, Cerra FB: Progressive necrotizing surgical infections—A unified approach. J Trauma 21:349, 1981
15. Meakins JL, Christou NV: Defects in host defense mechanisms. In Dick G (ed): Immunological Aspects of Infectious Diseases. Baltimore, University Park Press, 1979
16. Moylan JA, Kennedy BV: The importance of gown and drape barriers in the prevention of wound infection. Surg Gynecol Obstet 151:465, 1980
17. Polk HC: Prevention of surgical wound infection. Ann Intern Med 80:770, 1978
18. Polk HC: Operating room acquired infection: A review of pathogenesis. Am Surg 45:349, 1979
19. Polk HC, Fry O, Flint LM: Dissemination and causes of infection. Surg Clin North Am 56:817, 1976
20. Rothstein RJ, Barker FJ: Tetanus: Prevention and treatment. JAMA 240:675, 1978
21. Schweizer RT, Kountz SL, Belzer FO: Wound complications in recipients of renal transplants. Ann Surg 177:58, 1973
22. Stone HH, Hooper CA, Kolb LD et al: Antibiotic prophylaxis in gastric, biliary and colonic surgery. Ann Surg 184:443, 1976
23. Todd JC: Wound infection etiology, prevention and management. Surg Clin North Am 48:787, 1968
24. Van Unnik AJM: Inhibition of toxin production in *Clostridium perfringens in vitro* by hyperbaric oxygen. Antonie Van Leeuwenhoek 31:181, 1965
25. Weinstein L: Tetanus. N Engl J Med 289:1293, 1973
26. Weinstein L, Barza MA: Gas gangrene. N Engl J Med 289:1129, 1973

4 Complications of Skin Grafting

Michael Scheflan

OVERVIEW

For skin grafting to be successful, it must fulfill several criteria. The graft should ultimately fit in its recipient area as inconspicuously as possible and provide it with protective and aesthetic functions. The donor site should heal with little or minimally visible scarring. To achieve these goals, the potential complications of skin grafting must be prevented in several areas.[10] *These include donor-site complications, recipient-site complications, graft complications, and technical complications.*

Donor-Site Complications

The choice of a donor site depends on the type and size of graft needed. The choice of a graft, on the other hand, depends on the functions it is expected to perform and on the age of the patient. For example, full-thickness skin grafts (FTSGs) have a much better growing potential than split-thickness skin grafts (STSGs) and should therefore be used more commonly in children.

The secretory components of a skin graft that retain the characteristics of the graft are sweat and sebaceous glands. Sebaceous glands are transplanted intact in FTSGs and begin to function early and independently of the recipient bed. In STSGs they are injured and do not function. This results in a dry, scaly appearance of the graft.

Sweat glands, too, function more completely in FTSGs. Here, however, they are neurologically dependent on the recipient site, since sweating is regulated by the autonomic nervous system. Hair growth almost never occurs in STSGs but is frequently retained in FTSGs. Finally, although sensibility, which is patterned by the recipient site, returns faster in STSGs, it is much more complete in FTSGs.

FULL-THICKNESS SKIN GRAFTS

FTSGs contract less than partial-thickness skin grafts and provide excellent coverage for selected wounds of the face and the hand. Preferred donor sites for the face are the posterior auricular area and the supraclavicular area, which provide an excellent color and texture match for facial wounds. The donor sites for the hand and other areas are the lower abdomen, groin, inner thigh, and inferior gluteal fold.[4]

Since a full-thickness defect is created every time an FTSG is harvested, the scar that is produced must be linear and easy to conceal. To create such a scar, the donor defect must be closed without tension, and it must heal without infection or hematoma. The skin sutures should be removed within 5 days after surgery to prevent ugly hash marks. The scar should be placed in such a fashion that it will not be chronically irritated or traumatized by clothing, friction, skin folds, external appliances, and so forth. Although a secondary scar-revision procedure can usually improve an unacceptable donor-site scar, secondary surgery should not be required in the first place.

SPLIT-THICKNESS SKIN GRAFTS

STSGs are ideal methods of wound closure for coverage of the trunk and extremities when the defect cannot be closed primarily and when adequate subcutaneous fat and soft tissues are present to support the graft and protect the underlying structures.

Even though STSGs contract more than FTSGs and tend to hyperpigment and remain dry for longer periods, they provide an excellent, expeditious, simple measure for obtaining wound closure on most body surfaces. Thick STSGs contract less than thin STSGs.

The buttocks, lower abdomen, and upper thighs are the most common donor areas for STSGs. Whenever possible, an STSG is harvested within the "bikini" or "shorts" area so that donor-site scars, minimal as they may be, can easily be covered.

Although most partial-thickness donor sites heal within 10 days to several weeks and with minimal scarring, there is a long list of complications that may adversely affect wound reepithelialization and turn this seemingly simple process into a nightmare of disturbed and prolonged wound healing that may produce significant scarring. The most common of these problems are pain, delayed healing, and scarring.[11]

DONOR-SITE PAIN

The sensory nerve endings in the exposed dermis cause significant pain when irritated. Even the most gentle attempt to clean the wound or change the dressing can cause extreme pain and discomfort and may not be tolerated by the patient. Donor sites may be managed in the postoperative period by either the exposure method or the dressed-treatment method.

Exposure Method of Treatment

The donor site is left open and exposed to air immediately after surgery or the morning after. Since there are no dressings, there will be no dressing changes and, therefore, no pain. In reality, however, the exposed raw surface may still prove to be painful. Even the slightest airflow, underlying muscle contraction, or accidental friction from clothing or sheets may cause significant pain. The exposure method of treatment has proved to be practical in areas that do not lend themselves to simple and secure wound dressing (trunk, buttocks, upper thigh).

Dressed Method of Treatment

The donor site is dressed at the time of surgery and let practically alone for 10 days. By this time most wounds would have reepithelialized and permit painless removal of the dressing.

Donor-site dressings should never be forcefully pulled off (a common practice in the past—to prevent the dressing from "incorporating" into the patient). Not only is the procedure exquisitely painful, but it disrupts the thin and fragile epithelial film overlying the wound. Donor-site dressings that are "stuck" on the tenth postoperative day should be let alone for another 5 to 10 days and then gently soaked off.

Occlusive donor-site dressings not only reduce the postoperative pain, which is commonly more pronounced than that of the recipient site, but also protect the area from inadvertent trauma and help stop oozing in the immediate postoperative period. It is important, however, that occlusive dressings *not* be watertight and that serosanguineous drainage be absorbed by the dressing rather than being left to accumulate between the dressing and the raw surface. Secretions trapped underneath the dressing form a moist, warm, closed environment, an ideal medium for bacterial proliferation and infection.

TYPES OF DONOR-SITE DRESSINGS. Donor-site dressings include a variety of gauzes impregnated with an oily base and medicated to accelerate epithelialization, to reduce bacterial surface count, and to be as nonadherent to the wound as possible (Xeroform gauze, Betadine gauze, Scarlet Red gauze, and Vaseline gauze).[7] None has been conclusively shown to be superior or to shorten the period of wound healing, but they all remain popular because of their antiseptic and nonadhering properties.

STSG DONOR-SITE INFECTION

Although unusual, infection will, when it does occur, greatly delay the process of epithelialization and may convert a partial-thickness wound into a full-thickness defect.

When infection is recognized because of the incidence of increased pain, a foul-smelling discharge, a wet, purulent surface, blistering, epithelial breakdown, and inflammation that extends beyond the margin of the donor site, the dressing must promptly be removed. The wound should be cleaned with lukewarm saline, and wet-to-dry dressings should be applied several times daily. Systemic or topical antibiotics are usually unnecessary. This treatment should be continued until the area appears clean. From then on, the wound should be treated by the exposure method until it has completely reepithelialized.

INADVERTENT FULL-THICKNESS DONOR SITE

The inadvertent creation of a full-thickness donor site is a result of an error in technique in the operating room. A faulty or a poorly adjusted dermatome, a sudden change in the surface tension of the skin, or unequal skin traction by the operator and the assistant all may cause uneven or deeper-than-planned shaving of the skin.

When this complication is recognized, skin harvesting should immediately be stopped and the reason for the failure analyzed and corrected appropriately. If a full-thickness defect has already been created, it must be closed either by direct suturing of the defect or by thinning the graft and laying it back on the surface from which it came.

Infection and mechanical trauma also can convert partial-thickness defects into full-thickness ones. Fortunately, often only a portion of the wound

GUIDELINES FOR PREVENTING DONOR-SITE COMPLICATIONS

Appropriate choice of donor area: least visible, least subjected to chronic trauma

Meticulous preparation of the dermatome and the donor surface: preventing unintentional harvesting of FTSG

Protective dressing of the wound: reducing pain in the initial postoperative period

Protection of the wound if a dressing is not applied: using bed cradles to prevent mechanical trauma to the wound

Nontraumatic removal of the dressing not earlier than 10 days postoperatively: preventing tearing of wound epithelium

Lubrication and protection of the donor area for at least 4 months postoperatively: preventing scaling, itching, and mechanical trauma while wound strength is gradually increasing

becomes deeper, so it can usually heal by secondary intention (contraction and epithelialization). It is unusual for a skin graft to be required to close a large split-thickness donor site that has suffered this complication.

Recipient-Bed Complications

The wound that is about to receive a graft must be devoid of devitalized tissues, free of infection, and rich in blood supply. Careful preparation of the wound prior to surgery will prevent most of the complications related to the recipient bed.

PREPARATION OF THE WOUND

Débridement and Hemostasis

Begin wound débridement in the preoperative period at the patient's bedside. Excise all devitalized tissues sharply, in repeated sessions, without producing undue pain or excessive bleeding. Wet-to-dry dressings and occasionally collagenolytic enzymes and hydrophilic powders are useful. In the operating room, just prior to grafting, excise all involved tissues until clean and bleeding soft tissues are encountered, indicating a viable wound bed. All bleeding must now be meticulously arrested before the graft is laid onto the wound. Hematoma will prevent the graft from becoming vascularized and will invariably cause graft failure. Hemostasis may be obtained with the following measures:

Pressure (at least 5 to 7 minutes)

Electrocautery (producing as little burning in the wound as possible)

Topical thrombin, which will control capillary ooze within 30 seconds

Agents like oxidized cellulose (Oxycel, Surgicel) or absorbable gelatin sponge (Gelfoam) produce relatively avascular surfaces that will not support a graft and thus should not be used in hemostasis of the recipient-bed wound. Delaying grafting for 24 to 48 hours by applying gentle pressure with a sterile moist dressing to the wound is a time-honored method as well. The graft itself is kept folded in a moist sterile gauze in a sterile container and refrigerated at 4°C. Bedside application of the graft within 48 hours is then undertaken.

Controlling Bacteria

Although the recipient bed must be "clean," it is, nevertheless, contaminated with bacteria.[5] The mere presence of bacteria in the wound, however, is not necessarily detrimental to the ultimate outcome of the graft. It is rather the number and type of bacteria in the wound that will determine success or failure. The types of wound bacteria are determined by the following factors:

The individual resident flora of the skin

The proximity of the wound to body orifices

The patient's general nutritional condition

The patient's immunologic profile and competence

The presence of infections elsewhere in the body

Medications (antibiotics, antifungals, steroids, parenteral hyperalimentation)

Whether the patient has been hospitalized, and if so, for how long

The patient's personal hygiene

A wound that harbors a bacterial concentration of less than 10^5/g of tissue will usually accept a graft if it is otherwise devoid of devitalized tissues and is reasonably well vascularized.[8] It is the same number that defines the fine line between contamination and infection. Although all wounds are contaminated, infection occurs only in wounds whose local defense mechanisms are overwhelmed by either the large number of bacteria or the bacterial virulence.

A count of 10^5 bacteria/g of tissue is not a magic number. The actual quantity of bacteria that will cause invasive infection in a wound also depends on the rate of reproduction of the bacteria, as well as on the enzymatic factors that the bacteria elaborate, which facilitate invasion or produce excessive drainage. Some species of streptococci produce wound infection and, therefore, graft failure at much lower concentrations than 10^5/g. Whenever appropriate, submit wound biopsies for quantitative cultures to determine the actual number of bacteria in

GUIDELINES FOR PREVENTING RECIPIENT-BED COMPLICATIONS

Débridement of all devitalized tissues
Quantitative reduction of wound bacteria
Qualitative control of particularly virulent bacteria
Control of systemic illness
Reduction of edema
Shaving of hypertrophic chronic granulations
Avoiding grafting of surfaces that are better managed with a flap

the tissues. Wound biopsies are important because surface cultures do not accurately reflect the type of bacteria that exist deep in the wound. Systemic and topical antibiotics are useful adjuncts to repeated mechanical (excisional) preparation of the wound. Several agents are available as adjuncts to sharp excision in preparation for surgery.

Saline or povidone-iodine (Betadine) wet-to-dry gauze dressings are useful for fine surface débridement. Silver nitrate solution, silver sulfadiazine (Silvadene) and mafenide acetate (Sulfamylon) cream, acetic acid solution, and sodium hypochlorite (Dakin's) solutions are effective topical agents for controlling wound-surface bacteria.[9]

Debrisan, Travase, fibrinolysin (Elase), and similar preparations are helpful hydrophilic and enzymatic débriding agents in selected patients. No commercially available agent, however, takes the place of repeated sharp mechanical excision of the wound in preparation for surgery.

PROBLEM SURFACES

Bone and tendon will accept a skin graft if their periosteum and paratenon, respectively, have been preserved. Dried-out, denuded bone and tendon surfaces will not accept a skin graft. Since skin grafts do not provide adequate protective functions for bones or good gliding surface for tendons, they are, generally speaking, not suited for permanent, durable coverage of these surfaces, which are managed much better with a flap. Granulation tissues are made of endothelial capillary buds, fibroblasts, and bacteria, and they commonly accept skin grafts well. Chronic hypertrophied granulation tissues, however, are not good surfaces for grafting and must first be shaved down to a smooth, pink, bleeding bed prior to grafting.[3]

Chronically scarred edematous and indurated wounds are poor receiving beds for skin grafts. Wounds that belong in this category are frequently found in patients with the following conditions:

Peripheral vascular disease (ischemic soft tissues)
Radiation injury (obliterative vasculitis)
Varicosities (sustained venous hypertension or scarred, indurated, hyperpigmented soft tissues)
Diabetes mellitus (small vessel disease)
Sickle cell anemia (small vessel thrombosis)
Rheumatoid arthritis (autoimmune vasculitis)
Crohn's disease, ulcerative colitis, pyoderma gangrenosum

Complications Related to the Skin Graft Itself

GRAFTS THAT ARE TOO THIN OR TOO THICK

Harvesting grafts with a poorly adjusted or a malfunctioning dermatome may result in inadequate and damaged grafts. Very thin grafts harvested from very thick and highly keratinized skin may result in no living epidermal cells in the graft. On the other hand, a very thick graft that is placed on a poorly vascularized bed will fail before it has a chance to revascularize.[1]

Skin grafts that are improperly stored or stored for prolonged periods will not be successful. The viability of a skin graft wrapped in a moist gauze, dipped in saline, and kept in a sterile container at 4°C can be maintained for 10 days.[6] Liquid nitrogen tanks at −170°F can keep grafts viable for 6 months prior to grafting.[2] A skin graft harboring streptococci will fail in the immediate postoperative period, as will a skin graft that is excessively contused or traumatized.

Technical Reasons for Graft Failure

IMPROPER IMMOBILIZATION

All grafts should be gently compressed and secured to their recipient site. This compression is provided by a sterile soft dressing that is either circumferentially wrapped (extremities) or secured as a tieover dressing (trunk, head and neck). Many grafts are lost after the first dressing change because of the failure to replace accurately the protective and compressive dressing after the initial inspection of the graft. Occasionally, large grafts on large truncal surfaces (e.g., in large burn wounds) do not lend themselves to dressing application. These patients are best treated with the graft left exposed and frequently (every half hour) "rolled" by the nursing staff. Gentle rolling of the graft with cotton-tipped swabs expresses and absorbs the underlying accumulation of serosanguineous secretions. Grafts are sometimes placed upside down or on an epithelializing wound, conditions under which they cannot be expected to succeed.

Placing skin-grafted extremities in the dependent position is ill advised for at least 2 to 3 weeks postoperatively. Gradual ambulation is then permitted while the patient is wearing compressive stockings. A pressure garment is necessary on all skin-grafted extremities during ambulation for at least 3 months, while graft maturation is taking place.

References

1. Barker DE: Skin thickness in the human. Plast Reconstr Surg 7:115, 1951
2. Bondoc CC, Burke JF: Clinical experience with viable frozen human skin and frozen skin bank. Ann Surg 174:371, 1971
3. Eade GG: The relationship between granulation tissue, bacteria and skin grafts in burned patients. Plast Reconstr Surg 22:52, 1958
4. Kaplan I, Penn J: Grafting. In Goldwin RM (ed): The Unfavorable Result in Plastic Surgery. Boston, Little, Brown & Co, 1972
5. Krizek TJ, Robson MC: Biology of surgical infections. Curr Probl Surg 1, 1973
6. Ninneman JL, Fisher JC, Frank HA: Clinical skin banking: A simplified system for processing, storage and retrieval of human allografts. J Trauma 18:723, 1978
7. Peters WJ: Biological dressings in burns. Ann Plast Surg 4(2):133, 1980
8. Robson MC, Krizek TJ: Predicting skin graft survival. J Trauma 13:213, 1973
9. Robson MC, Samburg T, Krizek TJ: Quantitative comparison of biological dressings. J Surg Res 14:431, 1973
10. Robson MC, Krizek TJ: Biology of surgical infection. Curr Probl Surg 1, 1973
11. Rudolph R, Fischer JC, Ninneman JL (eds): Skin Grafting. Boston, Little, Brown & Co, 1979

5 Complications of Local Burn Wound Management

B. W. Haynes, Jr.

OVERVIEW

HEALING OF PARTIAL-THICKNESS BURNS

In partial-thickness burns the burning agent does not penetrate below the skin appendages, especially the sebaceous gland–hair follicle complex, which provide the source for epithelial regeneration. Partial-thickness burns characteristically blister as a result of separation of the epidermis from its subjacent dermis by a serous isotonic fluid, which contains approximately 3 g/dl of albumin.

The usual scald, or in some instances flame burn, damages approximately half of the dermis as a primary result of caloric transfer. Experimental studies have shown that approximately 3.9 calories/sq cm are required to produce partial-thickness injury.[3] Major factors in the injury potential of a given caloric input are duration of delivery, skin temperature, and blood flow, all of which are chiefly responsible for heat dissipation and can alter injury potential significantly. In this connection, data show that early cooling following injury diminishes the degree of injury and edema secondary to the caloric input. An apparent limiting factor is time after injury that cooling is applied. A delay of approximately 30 minutes in the application of cold makes the therapy ineffectual. Since marked vasospasm is commonly observed immediately after injury, this suggests that early caloric dissipation may have a significant role in minimizing injury. Thromboxane and prostaglandin E_1 also appear to play a role in advancing tissue destruction, since inhibitors minimize it.

Once a partial-thickness burn is sustained, two basic processes are initiated: the separation of devitalized dermis and the re-epithelialization from skin appendages over healthy dermis from which granulation tissue has formed. The separation process of the dermis is enzymatic, and the enzymes may be of body or bacterial origin. Known sources of body enzymes that produce proteolytic change in devitalized dermis have been found in two areas: (1) the leading edge of the epithelial growth and (2) mononuclear macrophages and, possibly, polymorphonuclear leukocytes. In the usual superficial partial-thickness injury, separation of the devitalized dermis may be observed by the fourth or fifth day and is often complete by 2 weeks. When such wounds are observed on a sequential basis, the island pattern of epithelial regeneration is readily visible and its effect on débriding surrounding dermis as the islands grow circumferentially is apparent (Fig. 5-1). Progress in wound healing can be readily observed and can be measured photographically. Islands join to form sheets, and wound healing is ordinarily complete at 14 days.

Deep dermal partial-thickness injury takes longer to heal since there are fewer island regenerative sources to accomplish the task. Such wounds may require 3 to 4 weeks to heal if good local wound care is provided. One surgical approach to managing deep dermal injury is instructive regarding wound healing. Tangential excision, as devised and practiced by Janzekovic, is a method for slicing off the devitalized dermis to a healthy layer that will accept a skin graft and heal promptly.[5] The studies of Jackson have characterized different zones of injury and clarified that if the surgeon slices to the zone of stasis, split-thickness grafts can be applied safely with the expectation of prompt growth and wound healing. Importantly, if the surgeon excises to this level and does not apply the graft, the wound then degenerates farther, often delaying healing by being converted to a full-thickness injury by secondary infection.

Certain abnormalities of partial-thickness wound healing may be observed at the clinical level. Each island of epithelialization begins as a small circular mound rising slightly above the dermal level. As the mound grows, it débrides the surrounding dermis around its circumference. Normally the pattern of growth changes from vertical to horizontal, progressing toward a juncture with its neighboring island and wound closure. One aberration of this pattern is continued vertical growth, so that the island rises phalluslike significantly above the dermal level (Fig. 5-2). Such a circumstance will eventually result in slough of the epithelium across the top of the phallus and a change in direction to the horizontal growth necessary for skin coverage.

Another abnormal pattern of partial-thickness wound healing occurring commonly on the dorsum of the hand is excess epithelial hyperplasia, in which the skin takes on a thickened appearance resembling scar hypertrophy. In reality, on microscopic section, this is pseudoepitheliomatous hyperplasia. Because itching is a common symptom and scratching results, small areas of injury with tiny clots appear, giving the wound a dotted melanomalike appearance (Fig. 5-3, *A*) The natural history of this variant is to regress slowly toward a more normal epithelial thickness, with the skin often becoming platelike and resembling the usual thin and atropic appearance of scar epithelium (Fig. 5-3, *B*).

FIG. 5-1. A partial thickness burn injury with islands of epithelial regeneration débriding devitalized dermis enzymatically in a circular manner as epithelial growth progresses.

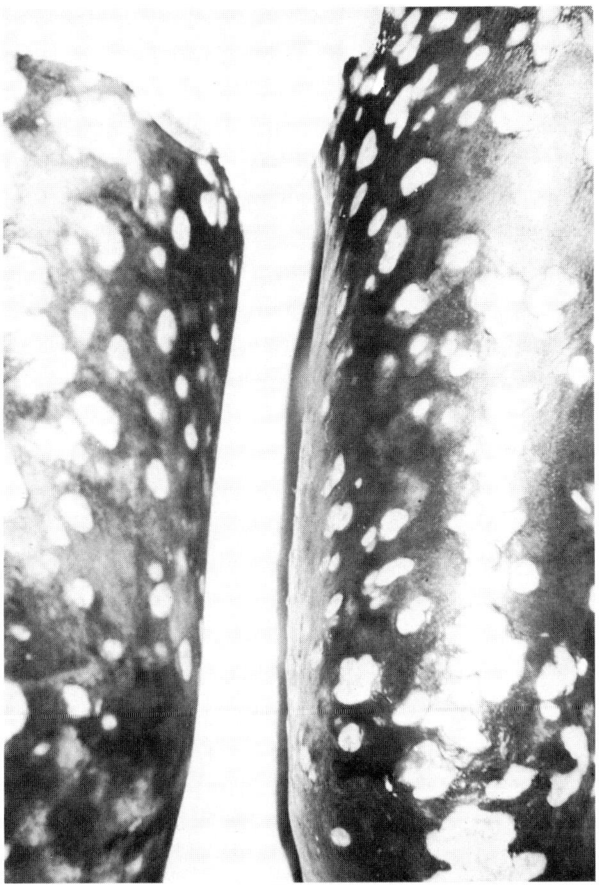

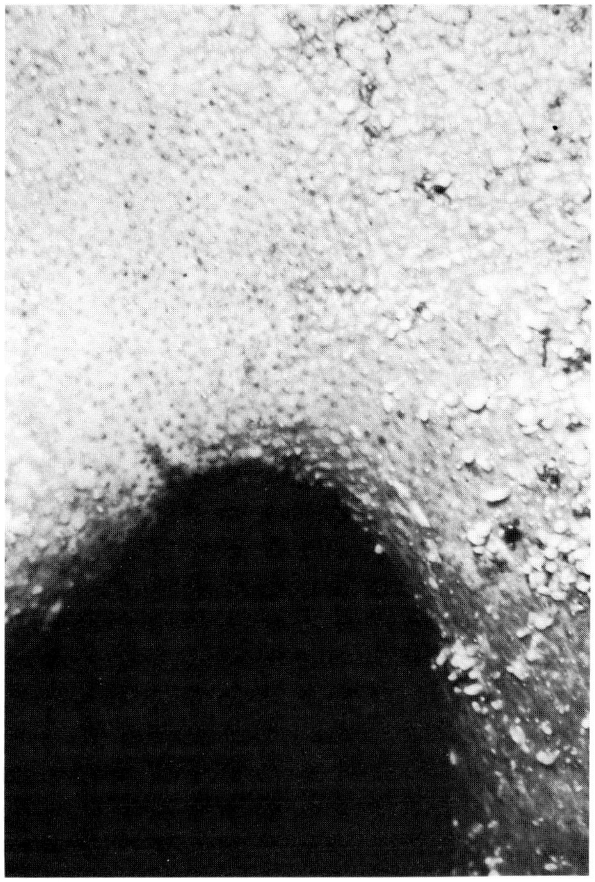

FIG. 5-2. An abnormality of epithelialization characterized by a phalluslike growth vertically above the dermal level. Healing occurs by sloughing of the tips and delayed horizontal growth. The island pattern of melanin deposition can also be seen at the center of the photograph.

The most significant variant observed in partial-thickness wound healing is epithelial arrest, which is characterized by cessation of epithelial growth in a wound that is relatively clean and free of dead tissue. It can occur at any age and often is seen in children who do not appear to have significant malnutrition. Factors that may contribute to this complication include topical therapy, sepsis, and vitamin and trace mineral deficiencies, particularly zinc

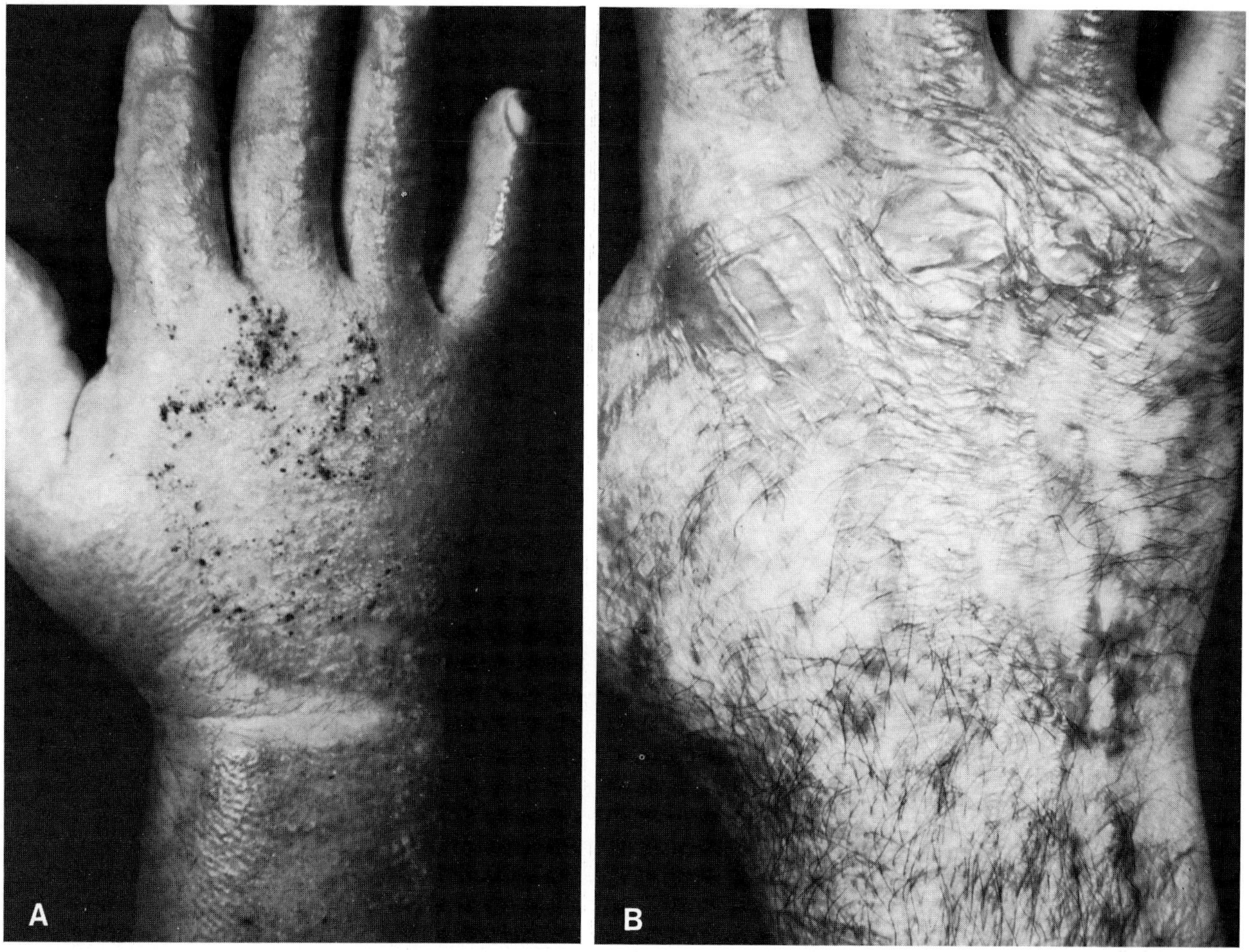

FIG. 5-3. (*A*) Pseudoepitheliomatous hyperplasia in a healed partial-thickness burn injury with a melanomalike appearance due to small blood clots secondary to scratching. (*B*) As the pseudoepitheliomatous hyperplasia matures and thins out, it takes on a platelike appearance.

deficiency. Deficiencies of vitamins A and B are of special significance.

HEALING OF FULL-THICKNESS BURNS

Full-thickness burns cause complete destruction of the dermis; this destruction includes the skin appendages, thus epithelial regeneration is not possible. After removal of the damaged tissue, skin grafting is necessary to achieve wound healing.

The first major step in wound healing is the removal of the devitalized tissue or eschar. As indicated, this is done enzymatically by body enzymes from mononuclear sources, but bacterial enzymatic débridement also plays a significant role. The common gram-negative organisms found on the burn wound, including *Pseudomonas aeruginosa*, have proteolytic enzyme systems, but the organism offering the best current débriding potential is *Bacillus subtilis*. The enzyme harvested from this particular organism is used clinically to foster separation of full-thickness injury. As the number of organisms increases in density in the wound, their débriding potential increases. However, their potential for producing sepsis of the burn wound increases as well. If the density of organisms does not exceed 10^5 organisms per gram of tissue, and the size of the burn injury is under 35% to 40%, débridement will progress satisfactorily without major septic complications. If the bacterial density of the organisms increases to 10^6 organisms per gram or more, and the size of the burn wound is significant, patient survival is threatened by overwhelming sepsis. Separation of full-thickness injury is well advanced by 2 to 3 weeks if assisted by good local wound care and surgical débridement of dead tissue. The development of a clean granulating wound 3 to 4 weeks post injury with an accompanying bacterial density of 10^4 organisms per gram of tissue permits expeditious skin grafting and wound healing with a high percentage of graft acceptance.

Effective split-thickness skin grafting converts an open, granulating wound to a healed, sterile wound in 1 to 3 days, with a resultant beneficial effect in general on the patient. Such grafts are remarkable in many ways in that they provide effective permanent skin cover that is durable and, when mature, soft and pliable. Although they have neither hair follicles nor sweat glands that are functional, the quality of the skin remains good, and, one of their most important characteristics is that they customarily will innervate, achieving sufficient sensory discrimination to protect the patient against injury and to function satisfactorily.

Wound contracture is a major force occurring in the granulating wound by the action of myofibrils, which cause a decrease in size of the wound by borrowing tissue from the surrounding normal skin. Although useful in wound closure, contracture may be detrimental to joint function if the tensions across the joint surface limit the range of movement. If wound contraction threatens a joint, it may be inhibited by range of motion exercises and its contractile effects may be prevented by early wound closure with grafting. Epithelialization at the edge of full-thickness injury has limited potential for wound healing. Such epithelium will grow approximately 1 cm beyond its edge.

THE CRITICAL ROLE OF OPTIMUM NUTRITION

It was first recognized that pronounced negative nitrogen balance followed major injury less than 50 years ago. Since that time, numerous nitrogen and caloric balance studies have demonstrated that burn injury is perhaps the most severe metabolic insult that humans can survive. It is only in recent years, however, that it has been possible to approach positive nitrogen balance and caloric balance in all severely burned patients. Optimum nutrition has had a positive effect on survival, but there are several problems associated with its delivery. It is likely that optimum nutrition improves the lagging host defense mechanisms that are commonly observed in the severely burned patient. Caloric requirements may be defined simply as follows:[2]

Adults
25 calories/kg/day
40 calories/percentage of burn/day
70-kg man, 50% burn = 3750 calories

Children (< 8 yr)
60 calories/kg/day
35 calories/percentage of burn/day
20-kg child, 50% burn = 2950 calories

The patient is encouraged to eat sufficient food containing the requisite number of calories. If he fails to eat this amount, an additional amount of liquid feedings containing 1 to 1.5 calories per milliliter is given him by gavage through a small inlying gastric or duodenal feeding tube. Because paralytic ileus is a common complication of major thermal injury, feedings may be inadequate to achieve the goal. If this is the case, the patient is alimented intravenously by a peripheral line if the need is small and by a central line if the need is large. By the combination of these delivery techniques, essentially every patient can obtain optimum nutrition regardless of the size of his injury.

The first important complication of alimentation is vomiting and aspiration in association with gavage and gastric atony. This event occurs more commonly later in the patient's course, when he is septic, seriously ill, and less reactive and when paralytic ileus has occurred. Diarrhea in association with tube feedings is best combatted by decreasing or stopping the osmotic load and re-establishing it more slowly.

The complications of hyperalimentation include those of catheter insertion, which in the peripheral line is usually thrombosis occurring within 4 to 8 days. Such thrombosis requires discontinuance of the catheter and change to another site. Insertion of a subclavian catheter for central-line hyperalimentation may be associated with pneumothorax, which will require catheter decompression of the pleural space. A postinsertion chest radiograph is a routine precaution. A more common complication of central-line insertion is the growth of organisms on the tip of the inlying catheter, which serves as a focus for bacteremia. Because the burn patient provides a large source for surface bacterial contamination of an indwelling catheter, the incidence of catheter-tip infection is high and various studies have reported culturable organisms on the tip of the catheter 3 to 5 days after its insertion. Furthermore, the severely burned patient may present with only burned areas through which a central line may be placed. In weighing the consequences of inadequate nutritional delivery against the risks of its administration, the overwhelming importance of optimum nutrition has led to the practice of changing the indwelling catheter every 2 to 3 days while hyperalimentation proceeds. This technique appears to reduce the risk of sepsis from the catheter while providing optimum nutrition.

Complications of Partial-Thickness Burns

INITIAL EVALUATION, CLEANSING, AND DÉBRIDEMENT

Evaluation of the burned patient must first emphasize maintenance or re-establishment of the airway, followed by appropriate fluid and electrolyte resuscitation.

In carrying out the initial therapy of the partial-thickness injury, it is important that all blisters greater than 1 inch be débrided and that the wound be cleansed appropriately with a bland detergent and saline solution. Although there are data to support the concept that the unruptured blister provides optimum conditions for epithelialization, the partially ruptured blister provides the opportunity for streptococcal or staphylococcal infection to occur, which is followed by delay in epithelialization.

Patients with partial-thickness burns of 15% of the body surface or more are generally candidates for hospitalization. After appropriate cleansing, the burns are well treated with the use of a topical antibacterial agent such as silver sulfadiazine (Silvadene) over the involved areas. Appropriate to such treatment is daily or twice-daily hydrotherapy, which assists in wound cleansing and removal of devitalized tissues and promotes epithelialization. Although there are data to show that the application of sulfonamide cream causes delay in epithelialization, silver sulfadiazine has many advantages, and this disadvantage does not appear to be a major problem.

Prophylaxis of wound infection is important, and it should be considered in the management of all hospitalized patients. Historically, in the burn patient β-hemolytic *Streptococcus* was the most common organism associated with septic death. With the control of β-hemolytic *Streptococcus* by penicillin, resistant hemolytic *Staphylococcus aureus* emerged as the most common cause of septic death, and it was not controlled until the advent of the semisynthetic penicillin, methicillin. At this point the septic picture again changed with the ascendency of the gram-negative organisms, especially *Pseudomonas aeruginosa*. If penicillin is given prophylactically for 5 days after injury, staphylococci and streptococci are cultured rarely on the burn wound. Discontinuance of prophylactically administered penicillin has resulted in a prompt increase in staphylococcal infection. A contribution to prophylaxis is made by commonly used topical agents that have staphylococcal coverage. The control of the pathogenic staphylococci followed by growth of opportunistic gram-negative organisms is less than ideal but does not cancel the advantage of using these topical agents. Third- and fourth-generation cephalosporins offer promise for control of specific gram-negative organisms on a level not yet attained. An imminent staphylococcal threat is reappearing in the form of a methicillin-resistant strain of hemolytic *Staphylococcus aureus*. To date the outbreaks have been sporadic.

As the patient progresses during the first 2 weeks of local treatment, hydrotherapy, and local débridement, cross infection complicating the recovery becomes a major concern. Cross infection in the burn wound occurs primarily as a result of personnel who may inadvertently transmit organisms from one patient to another. The opportunity for cross infection is provided during all contact with patients, such as during examinations, bed changing, wound treatment, or other care. The use of gloves and frequent hand washing between caring for patients are helpful.

The second area of opportunity for transfer of organisms occurs during hydrotherapy, which provides a central point of contact between patients, both in the transportation from bed to bath and in the treatment in the bath. Careful attention to isolation of each patient as he is handled is helpful, as is the use of individual plastic tank liners, which make each patient's bath bacteriologically separate from the previous patient. The wearing of elbow-length plastic gloves by personnel handling patients during the bath is also useful.

Autoinfection provides a major source of burn wound infection since organisms from the gastrointestinal tract contaminate the wound and may result in sepsis of the burn wound. Although intestinal antisepsis has been demonstrated to limit autoinfection, emergence of resistant strains such as staphylococci that cause enterocolitis has discouraged the use of this approach. On balance, effective topical therapy has been a more useful approach to the problem.

Wound hemorrhage is an occasional complication of wound débridement and is controlled by an appropriately placed suture ligature. Frequent observation of the patient following hydrotherapy and débridement is necessary to minimize this complication.

SURGICAL EXCISION AND GRAFTING

If the cleansing and débriding techniques described above are used, most partial-thickness wounds will heal in 3 weeks and be in a position to soften and mature into a satisfactory wound surface. Deep dermal injuries, however, take longer to separate, take longer to re-epithelialize, and are associated with an increased incidence of scar hypertrophy. The application of surgical excision and grafting of such wounds is a reasonable approach.

The use of tangential excision and grafting is a means of removing devitalized tissue and resurfacing the wound to secure early and prompt healing. The patient treated by this approach should be in good general condition, stabilized after his injury in terms of fluid and electrolyte balance. The surgeon must be familiar with excisional techniques. The tissue is excised in a slicing manner to the zone of stasis, which is recognized as a deep dermal layer that has a healthy bleeding base. Excision is followed by the application of either meshed or sheet grafts.

The first complication encountered in excision is hemorrhage, which may lead to significant blood transfusion requirements. It is controlled chiefly by the use of topical vasoconstrictor agents such as epinephrine in dilute concentrations, followed by the use of sheet or mesh grafts that are spread no more than 1.5 to 1 to permit egress of blood from capillary oozing.

Sheet grafts are preferred where hemostasis is excellent. Inadequate local hemostasis results in interference with graft take. The use of mesh grafting is of particular importance, since subgraft hematoma delays healing. However, sheet grafts give the best functional and cosmetic results, since small knobs of excess scar occur inevitably in the mesh area and cause a delay in wound healing. The choice of grafts may thus be a trade-off between the mesh graft, which causes more scar but less subgraft hemorrhage and good graft take, versus the sheet graft, which gives less scar, more subgraft hematoma, but good graft take, depending on hemorrhage control at the time of surgery.

Following hemorrhage control, the major complication that occurs is inadequate excision. Should dead tissue of significant amount be left in place, graft take suffers and the procedure results in secondary infection and undue prolongation of wound healing.

PRESERVATION OF RANGE OF MOTION IN INVOLVED JOINTS

A basic principle in the care of all burn injuries is preservation of range of motion in joints involved by the burn. Passive motion should be started on the first day of hospitalization and continued with supervised active therapy throughout the patient's stay. It is axiomatic that preservation of range of motion in involved joints means good function will result after wound healing. To the extent that this goal is not achieved, the quality of the result suffers. Even though range of motion exercises are painful, a high percentage of patients can be encouraged to progress toward full range of motion early in the course after injury and to maintain this throughout the wound-healing process. In the usual partial-thickness injury that heals in 3 weeks, a good functional result is to be expected.

THE PROBLEM OF SCAR HYPERTROPHY

Scar hypertrophy occurs primarily in patients with deep dermal partial-thickness injury and results from sepsis and delayed healing. The basic pathologic change is an inflammatory response that occurs in association with increased collagen deposition in an abnormal pattern. Such thickened hypervascular scars interfere with range of motion; they itch, burn, and are painful; and they constitute a major wound-healing problem following thermal injury. Prevention of this complication is of paramount importance; early wound closure helps to prevent it. In most instances, early skin grafting prevents the development of scar hypertrophy and results in a more cosmetically acceptable and functional wound. Tangential excision, described above, is a rational approach to the solution of the problem through early healing and thus the prevention of the complication.

Treatment of scar hypertrophy is generally supportive, with a view toward normal maturation of the wound, which will cause the process to resolve partially or completely. Compression bandages are used widely and may have some physical effect on scarring. They are particularly helpful in lower-extremity injuries, where they minimize edema and decrease itching. The use of lanolin-base creams provides some measure of relief from itching and from dryness of the skin. The use of topical steroids such as triamcinolone has only minimal effect, primarily because of the difficulty in getting the agent through the skin into the scar. Newer steroids that have the ability to penetrate skin may offer more relief for this problem. The oral administration of steroids is not effective and is not advised. Some patients with excessive scar hypertrophy, particularly involving the hands or critical joint areas, may benefit from excision and skin grafting.

Complications of Full-Thickness Burns

INITIAL EVALUATION, CLEANSING, AND DÉBRIDEMENT

A full-thickness injury customarily presents as an avascular wound without blister formation and is insensitive to pinprick. Many full-thickness flame burns will show signs of more intense heat damage, resulting in a translucent dermis with visible coagulated subdermal venous plexus, which is a hallmark of full-thickness flame burn.

It is crucial that patients with full-thickness burns should first have airway evaluation followed by initiation of adequate intravenous fluid and electrolyte resuscitation prior to therapy of the burn wound. The wound then should be cleansed with a mild detergent and saline solution and an evaluation made of the total amount of burn that the patient has suffered. The distribution and amount of partial versus full-thickness injury also must be assessed. Patients with full-thickness burns may be treated by the hydrotherapy-débridement technique on a day-to-day basis, followed by the development of a clean wound and skin grafting, or they may be treated by earlier surgical excision and grafting. Such a decision is ordinarily made after complete evaluation of the patient and his response to initial therapy so that a sound judgment may be made. Isolated areas of full-thickness injury are ideal for primary excision and grafting, although more recently there is a trend toward excising all deep dermal injury and third-degree injury as soon as is reasonable and practical, in a staged manner depending on the size of the burn and the condition of the patient.

PROPHYLAXIS OF WOUND INFECTION, INCLUDING TOPICAL THERAPY

The topical therapy of choice today in the prevention of wound infection in the full-thickness injury is the use of silver sulfadiazine. This agent is effective against the usual gram-negative organisms that colonize the burn wound, especially *Pseudomonas aeruginosa*. In addition, intravenous penicillin of the methicillin type is useful in preventing colonization of the wound by significant β-hemolytic streptococci or hemolytic *Staphylococcus aureus*. Such therapy is discontinued after 5 days while the topical therapy is continued.

PRINCIPLES OF WOUND CARE: HYDROTHERAPY AND DÉBRIDEMENT

The complications of hydrotherapy and débridement, that is, cross infection and hemorrhage, have been discussed in the section on partial-thickness burns and are similar in the full-thickness injury. Because of the depth of the wound, the incidence of hemorrhage is more frequent, and, therefore, requires surgical control more often. By the same token, the cross-infection problem is more severe since infection as a whole is more severe. As full-thickness injuries progress through their course, the risk of sepsis and septic shock increases. There is a close relationship between the size of the third-degree burn and mortality, and this appears to be based primarily on the risk of sepsis that is imposed by the full-thickness injury. As wound separation proceeds, it is tempting to excise large areas of full-thickness injury in an effort to control the septic problem. A complication of that approach is septic shock, and extensive excision must be approached with caution. Débridement generally is carried out on a day-to-day basis rather than on a full-scale basis in the operating room. Skin grafting is performed as soon as wounds become clean and granulating. Blood loss is a problem, and more frequent transfusions are required to correct actual losses as well as the losses secondary to the anemia of infection.

SURGICAL EXCISION AND GRAFTING

Surgical excision is adaptable to a full-thickness injury of circumscribed extent most readily and effectively. A prime example is a circumferential full-thickness injury of an extremity. Such wounds can be treated by excision in one operation under a tourniquet, which minimizes blood loss significantly. Since full-thickness injury commonly involves the subcutaneous tissue to a greater or lesser extent, it is a common experience that excision of the skin alone leads to a sloughing subcutaneous tissue, which markedly delays wound closure by grafting. One practical approach to the problem, which has been used extensively, is excision to the fascial level; it is simple and direct and can be closed readily by either primary or delayed primary skin grafting. Functional results without the subcutaneous tissue layer are satisfactory.

To accomplish primary grafting with sheet grafts after an extremity excision, excellent hemostasis is essential or subgraft hemorrhage may interfere with graft take. The use of mesh grafting may minimize this problem, or the use of sheet grafts following a period of delay (*i.e.*, 24 hours) to control the bleeding may be effective. Either approach will effectively avoid the problem of subgraft hemorrhage.

Surgical excision of the full-thickness injury has as its major advantage the early closure of the wound and avoidance of infection associated with the separation of the dead tissue. It also results in a shorter period of hospitalization. Although morbidity is decreased, evidence fails to show that it improves mortality over the hydrotherapy debridement regimen.

USE OF ALLOGRAFT AND OTHER SKINS

The use of allograft in the management of full-thickness injury is primarily of value in the clean excised or granulating wound that cannot be closed with autograft immediately. One application of allograft to such wounds provides prompt wound healing, freedom from infection, relief of pain, and decrease of fluid losses. Its basic effect is to provide primary wound healing that imitates the effect of autograft. When applied to a major wound, it has the ability to control wound infection and assist in making the patient's host defense mechanisms more effective. It is temporary, and a good take of allograft will reject in 4 to 6 weeks as a rule, using random donors.

The major complication in the use of allograft occurs when it is used as a debriding agent over a wound containing devitalized tissue. If it is applied and not changed frequently, it results in significant subgraft infection, even abscess formation, and an increase in sepsis. This sequence applies to all topical autograft substitutes.

Amnion has the ability to diminish bacterial growth in the clean granulating wound. It tends to dry readily and has a limited span of a few days' effectiveness. When compared with allograft, it may be more readily available but it is not as durable and as effective for the purpose. Pigskin has been used extensively as a débriding agent and as a substitute for autograft on a temporary basis. As a débriding agent, it is no more effective than ointment dressings and is much more expensive. As an agent for temporary wound closure it may diminish bacterial counts, but if it is allowed to become incorporated into granulation tissue it may require surgical excision for removal. A recent development of an artificial skin uses collagen from nonhuman sources fabricated into a sheet. When placed on the burn wound it is biodegraded and replaced by human collagen and permanent healing is achieved by a thin epidermal graft.[1] This technique may offer permanent wound closure for larger wounds with better utilization of available donor sites for epidermal grafts.

MANAGEMENT OF COMPLEX WOUNDS INVOLVING BONE, TENDON, AND CARTILAGE

Deep third-degree burn injuries involving bone, tendon, and cartilage pose special problems for the surgeon. The common areas that produce injuries to the bone are burns of the anterior surface of the tibia and the skull. In the past, such problems have been solved by either the transfer of pedicle flaps after developing clean bone and healthy surrounding tissue or by drilling small holes through the cortex, thus allowing granulation tissue to grow through and then to spread over the bone to resorb it and accept a split-thickness graft. Either of these methods is tedious and time consuming and requires long hospitalization.

The most effective way to solve problems of exposed bone is to close the surrounding wound with split-thickness grafts and then surgically remove sufficient cortex to provide bleeding Haversian canals. This bone will then accept a split-thickness graft and develop a secure surface that is durable and resistant to infection. Such grafts will heal readily if injured, and prolonged evaluation shows continued durability. Osteomyelitis, specifically, is not a problem.

Chondritis is a primary complication of third-degree burn of the ear. It may be prevented or minimized by good local wound care, emphasizing the use of topical therapy and local wound cleansing. The topical agent that is most effective is sulfamylon, because of its bacterial spectrum and its capability for effective penetration of the eschar. Burn wounds of the ear, even though they involve the cartilage and may result in loss of a part of the ear because of the full-thickness injury, may well heal without significant chondritis if good local wound care is provided. The onset of chondritis is recognizable because of increase in pain, increase in swelling, and the "wing" effect that occurs in comparison to the opposite uninjured ear. This complication is best treated early by the addition of intensive intravenous antibacterial therapy appropriate to the organism, which is commonly *Pseudomonas aeruginosa*. Gentamicin is used in doses to achieve good measured blood levels. If this approach does not correct the infection problem, it may be necessary to débride the wound and remove the cartilage in the involved area. If cartilagenous débridement is required, the ear loses its configuration and may shrink and scar significantly. Local injections of antibacterial agents are painful, difficult to achieve, and, in general, unrewarding.

Full-thickness injury involving tendon customarily results in loss of the tendon. In a few instances, if there is surrounding tissue that has good vascularity, a portion or all the tendon may become vascularized, in which case it may maintain sufficient viability and function for effective movement of the joint. For example, deep wounds about the anterior surface of the ankle may be managed conservatively with local débriding and wound cleansing, permitting separation of dead tissue with retention of one or more tendons. Even though several tendons may be sacrificed, the retention of one or two functional tendons may permit normal joint movement after grafting has healed the wound. This remaining tendon function would not be preserved if excision were carried out. Deep full-thickness burns of the hand also should be treated conservatively in the hope of preserving tendon function.

PRESERVATION OF RANGE OF MOTION IN INVOLVED JOINTS

In managing full-thickness injury about joints, the insistance on early and effective development of full range of motion is of paramount importance, even though the overlying tissues will require replacement. By using topical agents to maintain a soft full-thickness eschar, good range development is facilitated and good range of motion is possible whether the area is excised or is treated by hydrotherapy and day-to-day débridement to develop a clean wound and to allow subsequent grafting. When grafting is accomplished, splinting for a 5- to 8-day period is important in terms of facilitating graft take, but early range of motion exercises must be carried out thereafter and vigorously pursued to redevelopment of full range of motion. Deviation from these principles results in less effective functional results.

Pulmonary Complications

Inhalation injury is caused primarily by breathing smoke. Smoke is highly toxic to respiratory mucosa and often results promptly in glottic edema and obstruction. The passage of an endotracheal tube may be required soon after a major smoke inhalation injury. If the smoke inhalation is severe and continued, it may damage the mucosa of the tracheobronchial tree to the point where the formation of a tracheobronchial cast associated with sepsis, and sloughing of the mucosa may occur. This complication carries a high risk of mortality and will require tracheostomy and bronchoscopy to remove portions of the cast in order to facilitate gas exchange. Such serious injuries ordinarily result in long-term chronic pulmonary disease that is associated with hypoxia, shortness of breath, and severe pulmonary functional limitation.

The association of carboxyhemoglobin poisoning with smoke inhalation is significant, and the person often dies before the arrival of medical assistance. Patients with severe smoke inhalation who reach the hospital demonstrate carboxyhemoglobin levels up to 50%. Such levels are serious but can ordinarily be treated effectively by hyperventilation with enriched oxygen–air mixtures. Major brain damage may result, however, including severe optic degeneration.

Pneumonitis is a common complication of major full-thickness burn injury and may occur through bacteremic episodes infecting the lung or by inhalation of organisms. This complication is well treated by maintaining good tracheobronchial toilet, supporting pulmonary function by maintaining good gas exchange, and by selecting appropriate antibacterial therapy dependent on the organism cultured from the tracheobronchial tree. *Pseudomonas aeruginosa* is common and should be suspected until the identity of the pathogenic organism is confirmed. The use of appropriate intravenous gentamicin therapy achieving effective dosage levels is useful in controlling this complication.

Gastrointestinal Complications

Essentially all patients with major burns develop some degree of paralytic ileus as a result of the injury. Although the mechanism is not clear, it appears to be partly gastric atony and partly small intestinal distention. The main thrust of the complication is that it produces nausea and vomiting and limits food and fluid intake until the patient recovers, which ordinarily requires 2 or 3 days. Nasogastric suction is useful to minimize discomfort and vomiting. Once recovered, the patient may then have his food intake increased progressively to appropriate levels either by eating or by gastrointestinal gavage by way of a small tube. More serious paralytic ileus results when sepsis ensues. Prevention of or minimizing sepsis helps to lessen the risk of ileus as a complication and to preserve the gastrointestinal tract for its essential role of nutrition.

Curling's ulcer is ulceration of either the stomach or the duodenum, and it is associated with severe burn injury. Such lesions may occur in the first few days and be accompanied by hematemesis but rarely massive hemorrhage. Curling's ulcer and associated severe hemorrhage occurs later in the course and always in the presence of severe sepsis. The ulcers occur in the usual gastroduodenal areas that are associated with peptic ulcer disease, suggesting that there may be an acid relationship. Most Curling's ulcers are well controlled by methods that reduce gastric acidity. Cimetidine or alkali may be used to adjust the pH to a neutral range. Since Curling's ulcer occurs in children as well as adults, it is wise that both groups be treated prophylactically by antacid therapy, which is useful in preventing more serious complications of this disease. Curling's ulcer may perforate, in which case it is often a silent perforation occurring in a desperately sick and septic patient, usually in the second to third week after the injury. Since a patient with perforation may present with few abdominal complaints or signs, recognition may occur when free air under the diaphragm is observed on a chest film for pneumonitis. Surgical closure of the perforation is required, as is definitive surgical control of hemorrhage in those patients with excessive bleeding.

Renal Complications

Renal failure early in the course of treatment of burn patients who are healthy and without previous renal disease is due to inadequate volume replacement, resulting in shock and decreased renal blood flow plus increased hemoglobinuria and myoglobinuria. This circumstance results in acute tubular necrosis, which is a catastrophe for the burn patient. Modern therapy has essentially eliminated this complication in patients who have normal renal function at the time of injury and who receive adequate fluid therapy early enough after injury to prevent shock from occurring. The kidney that has a normal renal blood flow can clear hemoglobin and myoglobin through the distal tubule with little risk for acute tubular necrosis. The mortality risk in burn patients with acute tubular necrosis is high, but salvage of some by either hemodialysis or peritoneal dialysis can be accomplished. Since many burn patients require indwelling catheters for prolonged periods to measure urine volumes accurately, cystitis is a common, but rarely major, complication.

Reconstruction and Rehabilitation: Wound Maturation

In managing partial-thickness injuries, once the wound is healed, a prolonged follow-up is necessary while the wound progresses through its normal maturation to complete healing. The major complication is scar hypertrophy, and this may require a follow-up of 1 to 3 years or more in order to ensure that a cosmetic or functional problem that requires further surgical management does not result.

Major emphasis on active range of motion through exercise and strengthening is a most important aspect of the therapy. Failure to achieve full range of motion and strength is the major complication, and the services of trained physical therapists on a continuing outpatient basis are essential. In an effort to improve range of motion, the application of pressure over a thickened hypertrophied area is of benefit, and this may be done by the use of elastic bandages or by the use of more formal elastic stockings. Two types of splinting also may be useful. If there is a decrease in range, which is improved during the day but lost again during the night, an extension splint that maintains the joint in its fullest range should be worn at night. If the patient is unable to gain full range, for example in the finger joints, then functional splinting may be necessary, whereby rubber band traction is applied to the finger in order to improve range yet permit exercise against the stretching effect of the rubber band traction.

In all of these management problems, the complete cooperation, interest, and motivation of the patient is often the controlling factor in success. The extent that he can be induced to help himself often governs the quality of the result. If the patient, after intensive physical therapy, still maintains a significant joint contracture, then surgical revision of the scar may become necessary. In general, this is done approximately 1 year after injury, giving ample time for the more conservative methods to produce the desired result. Relief of contracture surgically is followed by skin grafting to replace the lost skin. Such procedures are generally effective in improving the range of motion.

References

1. Burke JF, Yannas IV, Quimby WC et al: Successful use of a physiologically acceptable artificial skin in the treatment of extensive burn injury. Ann Surg 194:413, 1981
2. Curreri P: Nutritional support of burn patients. World J Surg 2:215, 1978
3. Evans EI, Brooks JW, Schmidt FH et al: Flash burn studies on human volunteers. Surgery 37:280, 1955
4. Jackson D: Second thoughts on the burn wound. J Trauma 9:839, 1969
5. Janzekovic Z: The burn wound from the surgical point of view. J Trauma 15:42, 1975

6 Complications of Electrical Injury

David H. Frank | Jack C. Fisher

OVERVIEW

Electrical burns comprise only 3% of all burn injuries but account for over 15% of burn deaths.[11, 37] The greater proportion of fatal injuries as compared to fatalities caused by other forms of energy is due to the sudden and deep penetration of electrical current. In this chapter we will examine the more frequent complications associated with electrical injury and discuss their diagnosis, management, and prevention. Excellent review articles on this topic are available.[7, 21]

Electricity is a relatively safe and clean form of energy, but because of the pervasiveness of electrical technology in our society, the potential for injury is always at hand in our homes, our factories, and our hospitals. Although electrical energy became available as a commercial power source 30 years earlier, it was not until 1879 that the first electrocution was recorded in Lyons, France.[35] As the production of electrical energy increased during the first half of the 20th century, the mortality rate remained remarkably constant while the number of accidents increased (Fig. 6-1).[33] Since 1950, there has been a decrease in the frequency of electrical injury coincident with stricter regulation for electrical installation and safer appliances. Between 1960 and 1980 the per capita incidence of electrical injury has remained relatively constant.[37] In developing countries, the rapid introduction of electrical energy into rural areas continues to produce a sharp rise in the incidence of electrical burns worldwide.[32]

Each year in the United States and Canada, about 7 people per million population die from contact with electricity.[6] Over 200 utility company employees are killed annually, and another 100 to 600 deaths from lightning occur each year.[20, 35] The incidence of nonfatal electrical injuries is probably underestimated, since many are reported only as burn injury. During a 1-year period approximately 3500 injuries involving electrical appliances and extension cords were treated in emergency rooms in the United States, with 32% of these injuries involving children under 5 years of age.[38] Fortunately many of these injuries were relatively minor. However, even household current can produce instantaneous death, disability, or deformity.

ELECTROPHYSICS AND TISSUE DESTRUCTION

Electrical energy results in tissue destruction by its conversion to thermal energy (c = calories). This is most directly related to the amount of current flow (I = amperage) passing through the tissue and to the resistance (R = ohms) of the tissue as expressed by Joule's law:

$$c = I^2 \times R$$

(Heat equals the square of the amperage times the resistance.)

The amount of destruction produced by conversion of electrical to thermal energy is dependent on several factors. These include tissue resistance, type of current (alternating or direct), duration of exposure, area of contact, pathway of current flow, and number of amperes conducted. The relationship between amperage, voltage (V) and resistance is expressed by Ohm's Law:

$$V = R \times I$$

(Voltage equals the product of resistance times amperage.)

In the clinical situation where we wish to estimate or predict tissue damage, actual current flow and tissue resistance are rarely known or measured. And so it is helpful to rearrange the equation to read:

$$I = \frac{V}{R}$$

and use this in the Joule's law equation,

$$c = \frac{V^2}{R^2} \times R = \frac{V^2}{R}$$

With most accidents the voltage is usually known. Thus the current flow (and heat-related tissue damage) increases as the square of the voltage for a given tissue resistance.

Additional factors determining the extent of tissue damage are the duration of current flow and the volume of tissue through which the current is flowing. If the current can be distributed over a large area, the amount of tissue damage will be less severe than if it is concentrated to a single point. We apply this principle in our operating rooms where a large contact ground plate is used to disperse the exit of current, and the entrance of current at the pointed electrosurgical "knife" concentrates the resultant heat release to a local area of tissue destruction.

TYPES OF TISSUE INJURY

Four types of injury or tissue response may occur in association with electrical current: direct, conduction, arc, and flame.

Direct Electrical Injury

The effects of direct injury are usually seen with low voltages (less than 500 volts) and current flow. This is of greatest significance with 60-cycle alternating current. Tissue destruction may be minimal, but normal electrical phenomena within the body are interrupted with potentially lethal disruption of respiratory and cardiac rhythm. Nerve and muscle stimulation with alternating current produces a tetanizing effect on skeletal muscle. Contact with the current source may be prolonged as the victim is unable to let go. Similarly, small microcurrents of direct current can influence tissue growth, as demonstrated with the recent use of electrical induction of bone healing.[24]

Conduction Injury

With greater current flow associated with 500 volts and over, the conduction of electrical current through the body produces a significant release of thermal energy. This results in immediate coagulation and subsequent necrosis of tissue. In addition to the entrance and exit wounds there is often deep and hidden destruction. The resistance of various tissues within the body differs and partially explains the variable patterns of injury observed clinically. Listed in order of decreasing resistance are bone, cartilage, fat, tendon, skin, muscle, blood vessel, and nerve. Dry, clean skin is a relatively good insulator. However, in the presence of moisture, the skin becomes a better conductor. As current flow begins to coagulate the tissue, the skin resistance decreases and current flow increases further. This will continue until carbonization of the skin occurs and tissue resistance is again increased as moisture is driven out. Current flow eventually stops and external arcing may occur.[18]

Arc Burn

The third type of electrical injury is the arc burn produced by electrical current passing external to the body from the contact point to the ground. Since

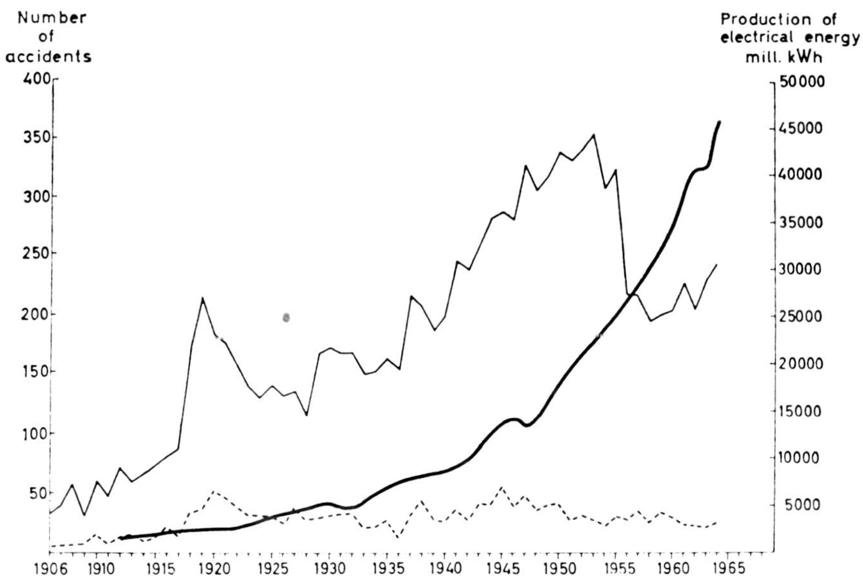

FIG. 6-1. The numbers of accidents and deaths from electricity are shown in relation to the production of electrical energy from 1906 through 1969. The heavy black line indicates the production of electrical energy; the lighter black line indicates the number of accidents related to electricity; the broken line indicates the number of deaths from electricity. (Skoog T: Electrical injuries. J Trauma 10:816, 1970. © 1970, The Williams & Wilkins Co., Baltimore)

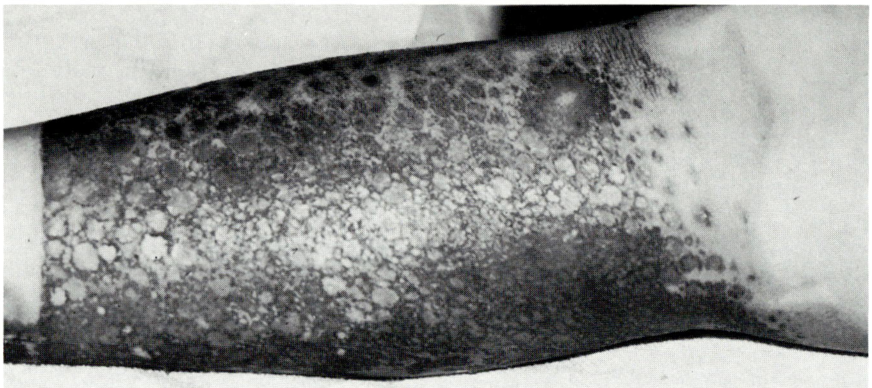

FIG. 6-2. The flowerlike appearance of lightning burns. (Courtesy of A.M. Kahn, M.D.)

TABLE 6-1. EARLY AND LATE COMPLICATIONS OF ELECTRICAL INJURY

Organ System	Early	Late
Central nervous	Coma, convulsions, hysteria, amnesia	Hysteria, psychosis, cataracts, hemiplegia
Neurovascular	Intense vasoconstriction, paralysis, hypesthesia	Neuritis, neuralgia
Skin	Second- and third-degree burns	Scar contracture, Marjolin ulcer
Cardiorespiratory	Acute myocardial injury, arrhythmias, apnea	Normal electrocardiogram
Musculoskeletal	Muscle necrosis, fractures	Fibrosis and tissue loss
Gastrointestinal	Gastric dilation, nausea, vomiting	Stress ulcers
Renal	Myoglobinuria, acute tubular necrosis	Normal function

the current is passing through the air, ionized particles are produced and extreme temperatures as high as 2500°C may be produced. Usually associated with high-tension current, arcing initially starts at approximately one inch per 20,000 volts in normal air. This distance is lengthened with increased humidity, and once the arc is established it may be drawn out to greater distances. The extent of damage may be extreme because of these high temperatures, and tissues and even bone may be physically melted.

Flame Injury

Often associated with electrical injuries are direct flame burns produced by electrical sparks igniting clothing and surrounding flammable materials. These burns may be extensive and deep because the dazed victim is unable to move away from the flames.

Lightning Injury

The damage resulting from being struck by lightning is the result of the combined effect of one or more of the four types of electrical injury. Lightning is a direct current discharge of static electricity between the clouds and the earth that lasts between 1/100 and 1/1000 of a second and involves a current between 12,000 and 200,000 amperes.[2] A person struck by lightning is often hurled several feet either by the effect of violent muscular contractions or the repelling of intense positive and negative charges.[26]

The direct electrical effect of the lightning may produce immediate disruption of the central nervous system with apnea or cardiac arrythmias. Immediate, and if necessary prolonged, respiratory and circulatory support frequently is rewarded by complete recovery.[28] While conduction injury may occur with deep wounds of entrance and exit similar to that caused by other high voltage current, this is unusual with lightning victims. Instead, a characteristic, usually superficial skin burn occurs, probably as the result of arcing of the current over the wet skin. The typical spidery arborescent patterns (Fig. 6-2), called lightning prints or keraunographic markings, may heal spontaneously within days.[2, 20] Grafting is usually not needed unless there are associated flame burns. Intense vasoconstriction leading to white, pulseless extremities may occur with lightning injury. This lesion usually responds to fluid therapy with low-molecular-weight dextran. Fasciotomies are not routinely required.[2] The early and late complications of lightning injury are included with other types of electrical injury in Table 6-1. The treatment of lightning injury may be summarized as follows:

1. Provide early, prolonged cardiopulmonary resuscitation and treat arrhythmias.
2. Institute fluid therapy (low-molecular-weight dextran, osmotic diuresis)

3. Provide tetanus prophylaxis.
4. Administer topical antibacterials and perform grafting for thermal and electrical burns.
5. Continue observation and treatment of late sequelae.

Recognize that musculoskeletal, gastrointestinal, and renal complications may occur with lightning injury but are more frequently associated with high-voltage alternating-current conduction injury.

Complications of Electrical Injury

ACUTE COMPLICATIONS

The acute complications of electrical injury (coma, apnea, ventricular fibrillation, paralysis), which are produced by direct electrical disturbance without tissue destruction have been described under lightning injuries. Their diagnosis and management are discussed elsewhere in this book. Associated injuries such as closed head injury, fractures, and blunt abdominal trauma may occur and must be systematically evaluated. Tetanic muscle contractions with alternating current may result in fractures independent of falls. Palpation and, where appropriate, radiographic evaluation of the bony skeleton are indicated even when it is known that the victim has not fallen.

ONGOING COMPLICATIONS

The intermediate and ongoing complications of electrical injury are the result of actual tissue damage produced by conduction and arcing of the electrical current. It is the extensive and often hidden tissue damage that leads to the fluid shifts, renal failure, compartment syndromes, muscle and nerve necrosis, and infection that result in the vast majority of deformity and in-hospital deaths from electrical accidents. The challenge to the trauma surgeon is to anticipate, recognize, and treat these complications early and vigorously.

Shock and Renal Failure

Fluid resuscitation and protection of renal function requires much larger volumes of fluid than would be calculated from the visible surface area of the burn. The typical flame burn is a surface phenomenon, while the electrical burn injury is more analogous to a crush injury with deep muscle damage. This produces large fluid shifts or "third space" fluid sequestration and vascular collapse. Shock will occur unless large volumes of fluid are administered rapidly. Initially, a noncolloid fluid such as Ringer's lactate is given through a large-bore venous catheter. The goal is to maintain adequate perfusion as monitored by stable vital signs and a urine output greater than 75 ml/hr. The release of myoglobin from damaged muscle may result in acute tubular necrosis unless a large, continuous flow of urine is maintained to remove the toxic material. The use of osmotic diuretics and alkalinization of the urine may be helpful. Underresuscitation is the most frequent cause of renal failure and is the result of underestimating the extent of tissue damage.[5] In contradistinction to surface burns, early destruction of red blood cells may require the use of transfusions within the first few hours after electrical injury.[6]

Compartment Syndromes

Another type of complication of electrical injury is the development of compartment syndromes. As injured muscles swell and fill the various anatomical compartments of the upper and lower extremities, uninjured vessels and nerves are compressed resulting in distal ischemia and nerve injury. This must be distinguished clinically from the immediate vasoconstriction and neuropraxis seen following lightning injuries. If, early following injury, the physician has the benefit of an initial examination showing adequate circulation and sensation and should repeat examination demonstrate progressive loss of function, pain, and impaired circulation, then increased compartment pressure must be suspected. If the compression is allowed to go untreated, permanent fibrosis and nerve dysfunction greater than the original injury may occur. Elevation and frequent monitoring of the involved extremity are necessary to prevent and detect this disabling complication. Observation of capillary refill in the nail bed and sensory tests are useful clinically. However, these should be supplemented by use of Doppler detection of distal pulses, and if peripheral flow is decreasing or the patient develops symptoms of pain, then direct measurement of compartment pressure with wick devices can be employed.[15, 23] In the presence of increased pressure, appropriate fasciotomies must be performed and may need to be supplemented with surface escharotomies of burned skin to relieve fully the pressure on the vessels and nerves. The wick pressure measurements are helpful in confirming complete release of the compartment.

Necrosis and Infection

Necrosis of muscle and nerve tissue and subsequent infection are the most critical complications of electrical injury. The surgeon's challenge is to remove the damaged tissue from the wound before infection and sepsis occur. There are two approaches to this problem: (1) immediate excision and reconstruction or (2) stepwise daily débridement.

The most direct method is to excise the wound completely back to normal tissue and effect immediate reconstruction by primary closure (with skin grafts or flaps if necessary). This has its widest application in small injuries in nonessential tissue away from vital structures. Proponents of this type of approach emphasize the decreased risk of infection because the necrotic tissue is removed early in the first few days after injury.

Because it is difficult to determine the extent of injury, various techniques may be used to evaluate the extent of necrotic tissue. Preoperative arteriograms will help demonstrate the extent of small vessel damage, since nonperfusion of muscle is an indication of nonviability. Muscle damage was previously thought to be progressive. However, recent evaluation of these injuries indicates that actual progression probably does not occur.[18] Because of irregularities in resistance of various tissues, skip areas of injury within muscle groups may occur, leaving areas of viable and nonviable muscle interspersed. Large vessels may remain patent initially, although damaged, and lead to underestimation of the extent of injury. The intimal damage in these initially patent vessels will lead to thrombosis. Arteriographic study of the smaller intermuscular arterioles demonstrates no progession on subsequent arteriograms and correlates directly with the initial extent of damage.[17] During surgery, contractility is one of the better tests of muscle viability. Frozen-section histology may also be helpful.[27]

For practical purposes, the soft tissues of the body can be considered to have a relatively uniform resistance during high-voltage injury. Once the initial skin resistance is bridged, the electric current takes the shortest path of least resistance to the exit point. The high electrical resistance of bone limits current flow and subsequent heat production and correlates with the rarity of full-thickness bone injury. Clinically observed cortical bone death and subsequent sequestra with delayed healing are probably due to periosteal injury. The temperature can become extremely high at the superficial bony cortex and partially explains the clinical finding of deep muscle damage adjacent to bone with uninjured overlying superficial muscle.[31] Current flows best along the neurovascular structures, which are commonly adjacent to bone.

An alternative approach to the early, radical excision of the injury is a more conservative stepwise removal of nonviable tissue. This minimizes excision of potentially viable and useful tissue in areas such as the hand and face where structure and function are important. An obvious risk with this approach is secondary bacterial infection and sepsis before the necrotic tissue is removed. Further excision and systemic antibiotics will usually result in control of the infection unless massive injury and involvement of vital organs preclude complete excision (Fig. 6-3). In order for this conservative approach to be effective and still prevent infection, daily inspection of the wound with frequent excision of all clearly dead material must be performed. Topical antibacterials such as mafenide acetate (Sulfamylon) and daily hydrotherapy are employed to help reduce the bacterial load within the tissues. Mafenide acetate is the topical agent of choice in electrical injury because of its greater penetration into necrotic tissue.[19] Quantitative bacterial cultures by biopsy of the wound are done three times per

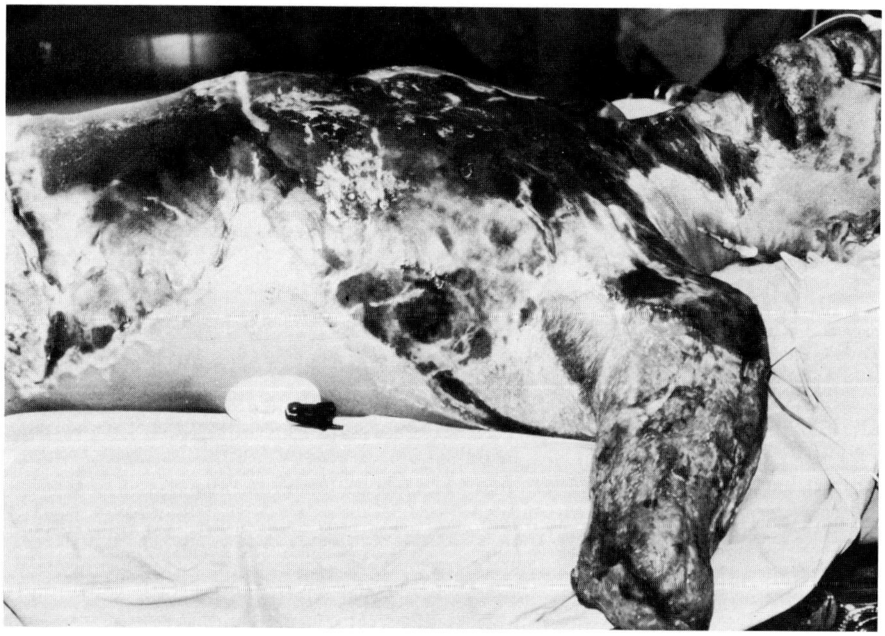

FIG. 6-3. Despite amputation of both arms and legs following extensive electrical burns, severe intra-abdominal injury resulted in this patient's death.

week to monitor bacterial proliferation and warn of impending sepsis.[29]

Because of the large extent of avascular necrotic tissue, there is always a risk of tetanus or clostridial myositis. Anaerobic or enteric organisms may also produce "gas" gangrene, requiring vigorous excision and sometimes amputation to salvage the patient. Systemic antibiotics and tetanus prophylaxis are necessary for the management of these patients. However, surgical debridement remains the most important therapeutic maneuver.

As potentially viable tissue is exposed by this stepwise debridement, it must be protected until the wound can be closed and reconstructed. Initial protection of the exposed wound with moist saline dressings will prevent dehydration. After the necrotic tissue has been completely removed, biologic dressings can be applied.[22]

Hidden Abdominal Injury

Hidden abdominal injury is a more severe and less easily detectable complication of tissue damage. With severe electrical injury, tissue destruction of the abdominal viscera may be present, leading to delayed perforation and sepsis. In the presence of overlying superficial burns the detection of these intra-abdominal injuries can be most difficult and perplexing. Mucosal hemorrhage, pancreatic necrosis, and necrosis and perforation of the gallbladder and bile duct have been reported.[40] Gastrointestinal bleeding, either as the result of direct injury or secondary stress (Curling's) ulcers, may occur.[9] A high index of suspicion and consideration of early abdominal exploration may be indicated in patients with otherwise salvageable injuries.

LATE COMPLICATIONS

Late sequelae of electrical injury may interfere with the eventual reconstruction and rehabilitation of these patients (see Table 6-1). Impairment of extremity function may occur from a combination of initial tissue destruction and subsequent progressive muscle fibrosis. In addition, initial nerve loss and delayed-onset nerve dysfunction at both the peripheral and spinal cord level may occur. Specific and serial evaluation of nerve and muscle function should be measured and recorded. When segmental injury can be demonstrated or anatomically suspected from previous excisional treatment, tendon grafts and transfers and nerve grafting may result in useful function and sensation. Other late complications include cataracts, contractures, bone sequestra, convulsions and other neurologic sequelae.[1, 9, 34] Psychosocial maladjustment is not unusual in posttraumatic patients, and particularly in those with severe burn injury. With the more severe injuries, return of patients to gainful employment is infrequent due to both physical and emotional reasons.

The frequency of early and late complications of electrical injury is quite variable. The known incidence of electrical injury sequelae either as percent of patients with a given complication or as percent of all complications listed by the authors of recently published studies is cited in Table 6-2.

TABLE 6-2. COMPLICATIONS OF ELECTRICAL INJURY

Type of Complication	Percentage of Occurrence						
Amputation	28	35	31	45		44	
Cardiac	20	25	12				
Renal	9	10	25			4	
Neurologic				12			
Central	7	55	45		9	7	
Peripheral	7	15	22		49	13	
Infection or sepsis	4		32	45	33	16	
Cataracts	6		2		27	9	1
Gastrointestinal hemorrhage			15		13		
Cholelithiasis					13		
Fractures		5	7	8	11	7	
No. of patients	46	20	65	80	45	45	141
No. of complications	114	29	118	90	64	55	
Data reported as % of patients (P) or of complications (C)	C	P	P	P	P	P	P
Reference	34	16	11	32	9	30	33
Year	1977	1971	1969	1978	1970	1978	1970

Electrical Burns of the Mouth

Oral burns in children are one of the most common types of electrical injury. While precise incidence figures are not available, we see at least an equal if not greater number of these, as compared with the more serious conduction type of injury. This injury typically occurs in toddlers who are learning to explore their world. However, we have seen it in older children using their teeth to pull extension cords apart, and in one series 20% were over age 5 and 5% were over age 10.[36]

The injury frequently occurs at the oral commissure (Fig. 6-4), producing a deep, leathery eschar with a surrounding area of white vasoconstricted skin. These wounds are remarkably painless. Because the injury is due to an arc of electric current between two electrically active conductors in close proximity (aided by the moisture in the mouth) there is severe local damage with minimal systemic effects. Electrical conduction may occur locally, but

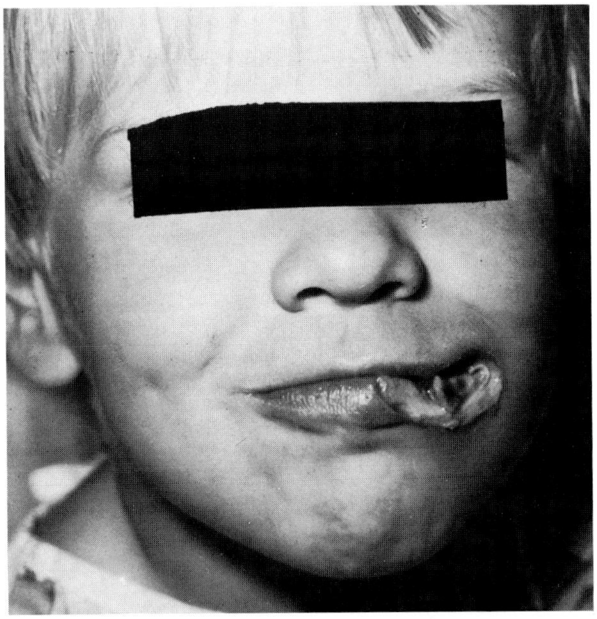

FIG. 6-4. Typical appearance of an electrical burn injury of the commissure in a 5-year-old boy on the day following injury.

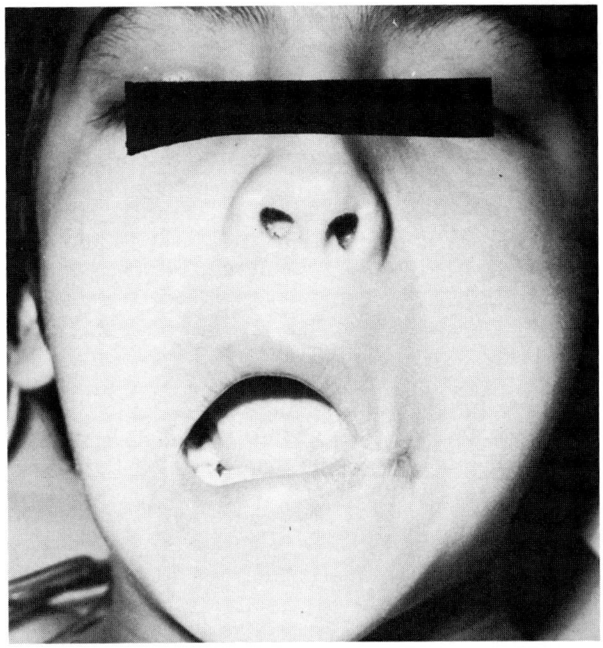

FIG. 6-5. If the wound is left to granulate and contract, microstomia frequently develops.

FIG. 6-6. (*A*) An external oral expander in place on the same boy as in Figure 6-4. (*B*) The same boy 2 months after the injury without reconstructive surgery.

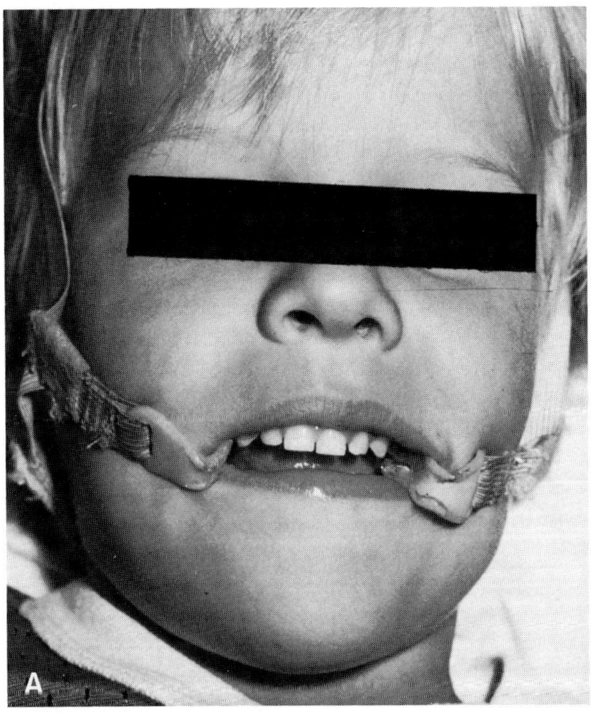

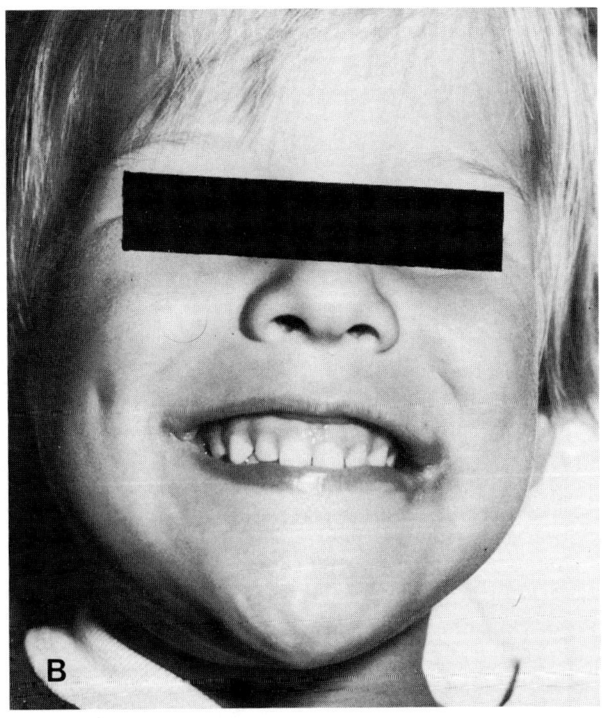

disruption of cardiac, respiratory, or neurologic function is extremely rare.[13] In the past these children were frequently hospitalized immediately following injury. Now we are selective and admit the child only if the local wound interferes with eating or secondarily bleeds or becomes infected. Part of our decision is based on the ability of the parents to care for the wound and cope with an injured child. The parents frequently need more support than the child.

The wound begins to swell after a few hours and develops a small rim of inflammation. Tetanus prophylaxis is checked and systemic antibiotics (oral penicillin) are given for a few days, although these have not been shown to be effective.[12] Topical antibiotic ointment may be applied to soften the eschar and help the parent clean the wound. After 7 to 10 days the eschar begins to separate. At this stage, conservative débridement may be employed for deeper wounds, which are more likely to involve the labial artery, but surgery is not routinely needed. In one series, less than 10% of patients managed without surgical excision developed bleeding or infection.[36] Early resection of the wound and immediate reconstruction has not proved advantageous and may lead to complications of tight lips and altered bone growth.[25]

The eschar-free open wound at the oral commissure initially results in drooling, owing to incompetence of the orbicularis muscle. As the wound granulates and contracts, the typical microstomia deformity occurs (Fig. 6-5) and is ready for reconstruction when the scar softens.[47] Over the past several years we have not waited for contracture to develop and are inserting an external oral expander starting early after the eschar separates (Fig. 6-6, *A*). If the expander is used the final deformity at 3 to 6 months after injury is often minimal and frequently requires little or no reconstructive surgery (Fig. 6-6, *B*).

Prevention of Electrical Injury

As in most forms of traumatic injury, prevention is always preferable to treatment. The electric utilities and heavy industry maintain training and safety inspection programs both for humanitarian and economic reasons. More stringent product liability codes are also an economic incentive to produce safer appliances. However, the human element remains the weakest safety link. The momentary forgetfulness in the tired lineman or the intentional misuse of altered wiring leads to disaster. Awareness of the problem and common-sense application of simple rules for electrical safety will prevent most electrical accidents. There are two areas in which physicians can have the greatest impact on prevention: in the home environment of the patients and in hospitals and operating rooms.

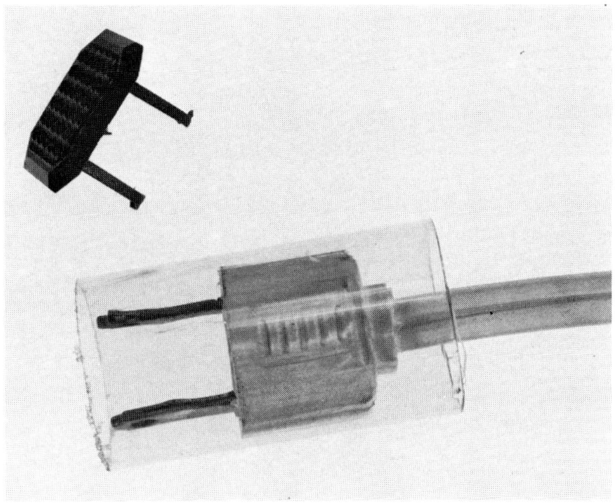

FIG. 6-7. The clear plastic cuff protects the prongs of the male plug while still allowing it to be plugged into the socket of an extension cord. The plastic plug fits into a female socket and prevents insertion of metal objects. This device is readily available at many hardware stores.

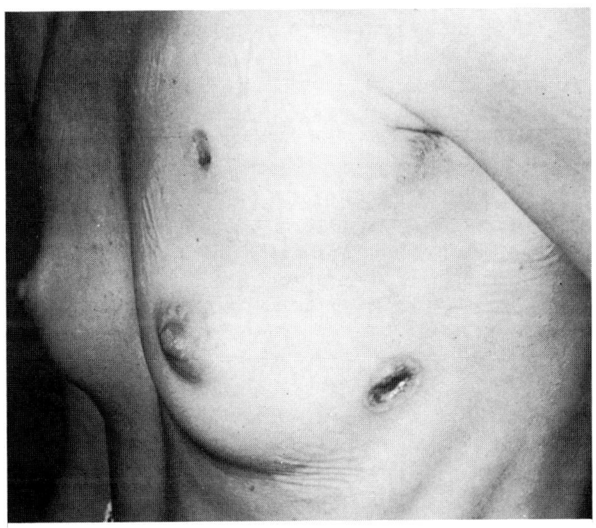

FIG. 6-8. Inadequate contact of the grounding plate allowed the electrocautery current to exit through the leads of an electrocardiograph and produce these burns.

The parents of every child treated should be advised and instructed to inspect their homes for safety. In addition to the usual cautions against medicine, cleaning products, and poisons, they should be questioned about protective covers for electrical outlets and plugs (Fig. 6-7).[10] Extension cords (the most frequent cause of injury in children) should be

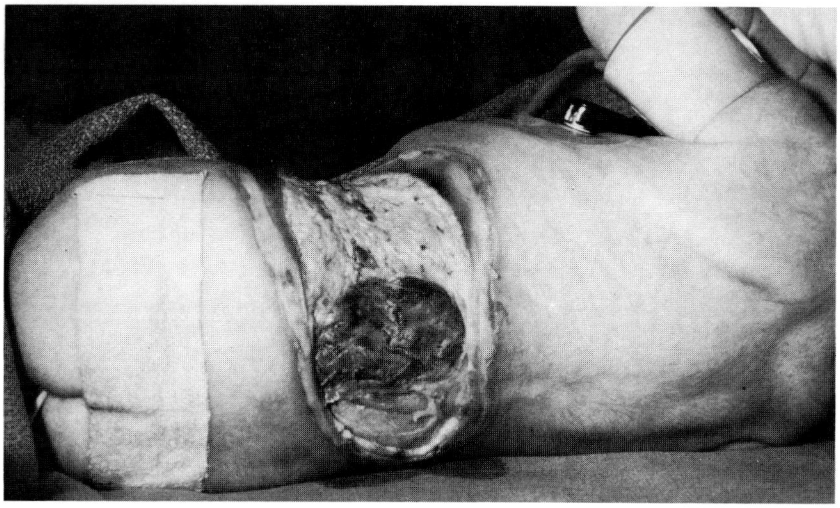

FIG. 6-9. Following uneventful cranial surgery, an extensive burn was discovered at the site of the ground plate. The wound is shown here 1 week following injury after two excisions of eschar.

securely fastened to the wall or hidden behind furniture. Better yet, avoid their use. Electric heaters and toys should be carefully inspected; specifically, one must look for exposed or accessible wires and contacts. Common-sense avoidance of electrical appliances such as radios and hair dryers near bathtubs and pools would save countless lives each year.

The other area where physicians must exhibit more safety consciousness is in hospitals and offices. If small children visit the office, then the same safety rules should be followed there as in the home. We also need to be more aware of the electrical monitoring devices we use. Although many now have safety circuits and disconnect alarms, none is foolproof.[3] Electrocardiographic monitoring leads are frequent offenders (Fig. 6-8).

In the operating room radiofrequency electric currents are intentionally used to cut and coagulate tissue. The biophysics of electrosurgery current is beyond the scope of this chapter but is reviewed elsewhere.[14] The principal concern in the operating room is that the circuit from the electrosurgical unit to the patient and back to the unit is not interrupted; otherwise current will flow in unpredictable pathways. Depending on the type of unit, the specific instructions for grounding or *not grounding* the patient and machine must be strictly adhered to. The patient contact plate must be firmly applied in an area away from bony prominences, excess hair, scars, metal prostheses, or cardiac monitors. The adequacy of the conducting gel or paste should be confirmed. During surgery, care should be taken to prevent fluids from accumulating near the plate, and if the patient is turned, the plate must be rechecked. If progressively increasing or excessive power settings are required for the active electrode to be effective, then the entire machine, conductive plate, and circuit should be rechecked. Even when all safeguards are followed and everything seems to be working well, occasional severe accidents will occur (Fig. 6-9)[8, 39]

References

1. Adam AL, Klein M: Electrical cataract: Notes on a case and a review of the literature. Br J Ophthalmol 29:169, 1945
2. Apfelberg DB, Masters FW, Robinson DW: Pathophysiology and treatment of lightning injuries. J Trauma 14:453, 1974
3. Arbeit SR, Parker B, Rubin IL: Controlling the electrocution hazard in the hospital. JAMA 220:1581, 1972
4. Argamaso RV, Strauch B, Lewin ML et al: Lip commissuroplasty after electrical burns. Chir Plastica 3:27, 1975
5. Artz CP: Electrical injury simulates crush injury. Surg Gynecol Obstet 125:1316, 1967
6. Artz CP: Changing concepts of electrical injury. Am J Surg 128:600, 1974
7. Artz CP: Electrical injury. In Artz CP, Moncrief JA, Pruitt BA (eds): Burns: A Team Approach. Philadelphia, WB Saunders, 1979
8. Battig CG: Electrosurgical burn injuries and their prevention. JAMA 204:91, 1968
9. Baxter CR: Present concepts in the management of major electrical injury. Surg Clin North Am 50:1401, 1970
10. Crikelair GF, Dhaliwal AS: The cause and prevention of electrical burns of the mouth in children: A protective cuff. Plast Reconstr Surg 58:206, 1976
11. DiVincenti FC, Moncrief JA, Pruitt BA: Electrical injuries: A review of 65 cases. J Trauma 9:497, 1969
12. Durtschi MB, Orgain C, Counts GW et al: A prospective study of prophylactic penicillin in acutely burned hospitalized patients. J Trauma 22:11, 1982
13. Frank DH: Special categories of thermal injury: Evaluation and management. Topics of Emergency Medicine 3:45, 1981

14. Glover JL, Bendick PJ, Link WJ: The use of thermal knives in surgery: Electrosurgery, lasers, plasma scalpel. Curr Prob Surg 15:1, 1978
15. Hargens AR, Romine JS, Sipe JC et al: Peripheral nerve-conduction block by high muscle-compartment pressure. J Bone Joint Surg [Am] 61:192, 1979
16. Hartford CE, Ziffren SE: Electrical injury. J Trauma 11:331, 1971
17. Hunt JL, McManus WF, Haney WP et al: Vascular lesions in acute electric injuries. J Trauma 14:461, 1974
18. Hunt JL, Mason AD, Masterson TS et al: The pathophysiology of acute electric injuries. J Trauma 16:335, 1976
19. Hunt JL, Sato RM, Baxter CR: Acute electric burns. Arch Surg 115:434, 1980
20. McCrady-Kahn VL, Kahn AM: Lightning burns. West J Med 134:215, 1981
21. Masters FW, Robinson DW, Ketchum LD: Management of electrical burns. In Lynch JB, Lewis SR (eds): Symposium on the Treatment of Burns. St. Louis, CV Mosby Co., 1973
22. Mills W, Switzer WE, Moncrief JA: Electrical injuries. JAMA 195:852, 1966
23. Mubarak SJ, Owens CA, Hargens AR et al: Acute compartment syndromes: Diagnosis and treatment with the aid of the wick catheter. J Bone Joint Surg [Am] 60:1091, 1978
24. Paterson DC, Lewis GN, Cass CA: Treatment of delayed union and nonunion with an implanted direct current stimulator. Clin Orthop Rel Res 148:117, 1980
25. Pitts W, Pickrell K, Quinn G et al: Electrical burns of lips and mouth in infants and children. Plast Reconstr Surg 44:471, 1969
26. Pritchard EAB: Changes in the CNS due to electrocution. Lancet 1:1163, 1934
27. Quinly WC, Burke JF, Trelstad RF et al: The use of microscopy as a guide to primary excision of high-tension electrical burns. J Trauma 18:423, 1978
28. Robinson DW: Discussion following Apfelberg DB, Masters FW, Robinson DW et al: Pathophysiology and treatment of lightning injuries. J Trauma 14:472, 1974
29. Robson MC: Bacterial control in the burn wound. Clin Plast Surg 6:515, 1979
30. Rouse RG, Dimick AR: The treatment of electrical injury compared to burn injury: A review of pathophysiology and comparison of patient management protocols. J Trauma 18:43, 1978
31. Sances AS, Myklebust JB, Larson SJ et al: Experimental electrical injury studies. J Trauma 21:589, 1981
32. Sinha JK, Khanna NN, Tripathi FM et al: Electrical burns: A review of 80 cases. Burns 4:261, 1978
33. Skoog T: Electrical injuries. J Trauma 10:816, 1970
34. Solen L, Fischer RP, Strate RG: The natural history of electrical injury. J Trauma 17:487, 1977
35. Sturim HS: The treatment of electrical burns. Surg Gynecol Obstet 128:129, 1969
36. Su CT, Manson PN, Hoopes JE: Electrical burns of the oral commissure: Treatment results and principles of reconstruction. Ann Plast Surg 5:251, 1979
37. U.S. Bureau of the Census: Statistical Abstract of the United States: 1980, 101st ed. Washington, DC, 1980
38. U.S. Consumer Product Safety Commission: Appliance cords and extension cords. National Electronic Injury Surveillance System News, Vol 3, No. 4, December 1974/January 1975
39. Wald AS, Mazzia VDB, Spencer FC: Accidental burns. JAMA 217:916, 1971
40. Wray RC: Electrical injuries in care of the thermally injured patient. In Zuidema, Rutherford, Ballinger (eds): The Management of Trauma, Philadelphia, WB Saunders, 1979

7 Complications of Ionizing Irradiation

Jack C. Fisher | David H. Frank

OVERVIEW

The focus of this chapter is on tissue injury as it affects the practice of a surgeon, and not just the reconstructive surgeon but also the urologist, the gynecologist, the gastrointestinal surgeon, the orthopaedist—in other words, all who must commit their technical skills and clinical judgment to the unpredictable healing response that follows administration of ionizing irradiation. It does not comprehensively detail all of the complications that might follow the use of radiation therapy for malignant disease. It has been written for surgeons by surgeons rather than by radiobiologists or radiation oncologists.

SURGEON VERSUS RADIATION ONCOLOGIST

Controlled administration of ionizing irradiation continues to be an integral part of the treatment spectrum for malignant disease. This fact will likely remain valid until a specific cure is found for cancer. During the past several decades, the relative risks and benefits of surgical excision *versus* radiation therapy for malignancy have been debated. Chemotherapeutic agents are a more recent development, and physicians who use them seem willing to combine drugs with the other two major methods of treatment. Surgeons and radiologists also have been willing to combine their efforts, but an appropriate sequence of therapy has not been resolved. "Radiation is most effective when tissue oxygenation has not been interrupted by the surgeon's knife," says one camp. "Wound healing is uncertain and options for surgical reconstruction are limited following irradiation," says the other. Indeed, surgeons prefer surgery because that is what they do best, and radiation oncologists prefer irradiation because it is the only form of therapy at their disposal. Coordinated management of the cancer patient therefore requires a panel of consultants or else someone with broader and more objective understanding of both the risks and the benefits of each component of therapy. Perhaps this explains in part the derivation of the tumor board and of the newer subspecialties of medical and surgical oncology.

Meanwhile, the polarization of the surgeon and radiologist has unfortunately precluded anticipation of certain inevitable consequences of radiation. This chapter points out that certain patterns of radiation injury are quite predictable and are an expected consequence of effective irradiation. Well-planned reconstructive surgery, by anticipation of tissue injury, may prevent some of the complications that can follow radiation therapy.

DOMINANCE OF RADIATION AS A MODE OF THERAPY

Surgery has been the principal choice for treatment of breast and gastrointestinal malignancies, but radiation therapy predominates for cancer affecting the head, neck, and pelvic regions. Surgical loss of a breast or of a segment of the gut can be tolerated more readily than can surgical alteration of the orofacial or laryngeal anatomy, and there is significant fear of lost urogenital function. Furthermore, radiation therapy does have a curative advantage for advanced prostatic or uterine malignancies.

But think for a moment of the potential for morbidity in the following regions where radiation therapy is dominant:

- The face, where ultraviolet sunlight may already have served as a carcinogenic influence
- The oral cavity, with its secreting glands and mucosal surfaces
- The teeth, fighting for stability and health in an environment high in dietary sucrose
- The pelvic viscera, where there are soft disten-

sible mucosal surfaces, subclinical forms of chronic intestinal irritation, bladder trigones in contact with intermittently contaminated fluid media

Aging hip joints, already prone to arthritic change even in the absence of ionizing irradiation

Radiation therapy morbidity can be predicted from our knowledge of the sensitivity of specialized tissues within likely treatment fields. In this chapter we define some of the radiation morbidity factors that might influence success or failure following cancer treatment.

EPIDEMIOLOGY OF RADIATION INJURY

The demography and epidemiology of cancer as a disease are well studied. We are fully informed of the geographic and genetic patterns of malignancy, the relative incidence and prevalence of the many primary forms of cancer, and the environmental factors that contribute to the origin of certain neoplasms. But we are not yet capable of determining the outcome of a particular form of therapy such as irradiation except in terms of survival.

The traditional index for success in cancer therapy is survival. The principal measure of failure is death resulting from recurrence or uncontrolled spread of disease. Survival experience is organized according to the tumor, nodes, and metastases (TNM) staging system, which is based upon morphologic criteria. But TNM staging overlooks the ways a host might respond to a particular malignant disease. Although the TNM system encourages use of survival data as the principal measure of treatment effectiveness, it discourages use of such morbidity parameters as chronic pain or disability.

Consider, for example, use of ionizing irradiation for pelvic malignancy. It is estimated that more than 85% of women with cancer of the uterus are treated by radiation therapy. In the case of endometrial carcinoma and late-stage cervical carcinoma, this practice appears justified by the curative advantage of x-ray over surgery. However, in the case of Stage I and Stage IIA cervical cancer, there is no survival advantage from radiation. And yet, most women so affected choose x-ray therapy! Avoidance of a surgical operation seems preferable, at least at the moment of decision. But what is the long-term outcome of that decision?

The precise answer to the question is that we still do not know. We are not yet in the habit of examining the long-term sequelae of a particular therapeutic decision in light of significant morbidity rather than of survival. We are willing to accept an 88% survival for either form of treatment but overlook the high incidence of postradiation dyspareunia.

Our point is that the long-term outcome of any cancer treatment must be examined, paying as much attention to morbidity as to mortality. But before learning what we do know about specific radiation sequelae, it is necessary to review some basic facts about ionizing irradiation and about mechanisms of tissue injury following exposure to radiation sources.

What is Ionizing Radiation?

Radiation can be a general term that refers to heat or to light, and it can be a specific term that refers to the electromagnetic spectrum. This discussion considers the latter, a continuous array of energy bundles known as *photons*. Photons are propagated by wave motion and categorized according to wave length and frequency (Fig. 7-1).

Microwaves and radiowaves have very long wavelengths, but their frequency is low. Cosmic, gamma, and x-rays exhibit short wavelengths and very high frequencies. In between are ultraviolet, visible light, and infrared rays. All wavelengths of the electromagnetic spectrum travel at the speed of light (186,282 miles/sec), but the penetrating power of a given wavelength varies considerably (Fig. 7-2). Those with short wavelengths and high frequency (gamma, x-rays) carry sufficient energy to produce ionization of the organic and inorganic materials that absorb them. Ionizing radiation is a very specific term that refers to high-energy radiation sources, high enough to inflict physical damage by producing ions (atoms or molecules with electric charge). We have already learned one source of ionization by radiation—the high energy end of the electromagnetic spectrum. There is a second source: namely, particulate radiation.

Particulate radiation means movement of discrete atomic particles. Particulate radiation may be generated two ways:

Directly by accelerating electrons, protons, or other particles in either a cyclotron or a linear accelerator

Indirectly through decay of naturally occurring or artificially produced radioactive substances

Particulate radiation is categorized according to the kind of particle involved. Biologically important are the alpha and beta particles, protons, neutrons, deuterons, and mesons. Alpha particles are identical to helium nuclei. Beta particles are high-speed electrons with extremely small mass. Unlike electromagnetic radiation, particulate radiation does not travel at a uniform velocity.

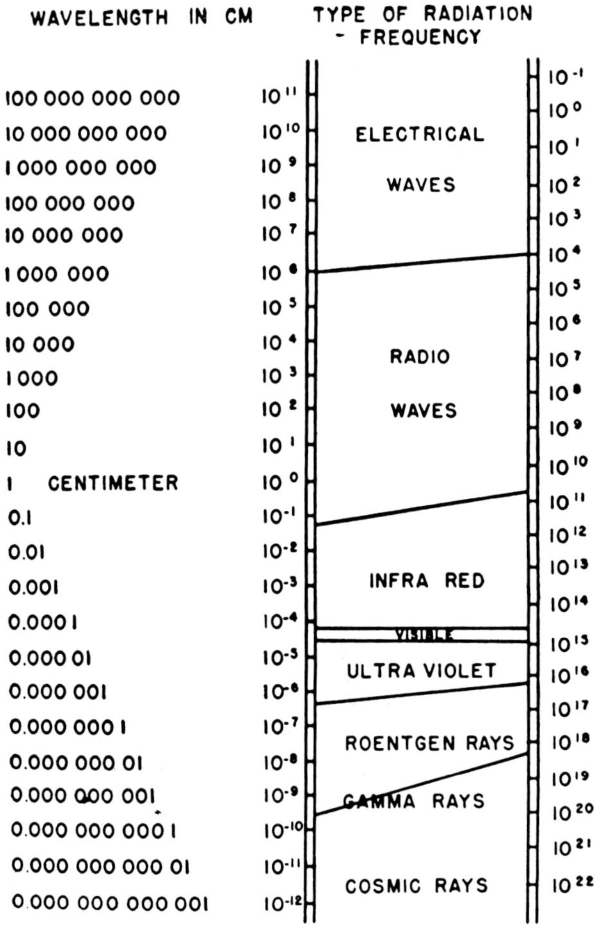

FIG. 7-1. The electromagnetic spectrum. Penetration energy is inversely related to wavelength but directly related to frequency. Gamma wavelengths are short, but the frequency of these waves is high. Radio wavelengths are long, their frequency low. (Berdjis C: Pathology of Irradiation, p 2. Baltimore, Williams & Wilkins, 1971. © 1971, The Williams & Wilkins Co., Baltimore)

Ionizing radiation is often called *high energy* because its units are far greater than the binding requirements of valence electrons within atoms. Molecular binding energies are on the order of 5 to 10 electron volts, whereas x-rays and gamma rays generate 1 million electron volts (MEV) of energy. Atomic particles are stronger, in the range of 1 to 10 million electron volts (MEV). There is no essential physical difference between gamma and x-rays. Historically, the term *x-ray* was applied to high-energy radiation emitted from radioactive substances. Today, little distinction is maintained.

In summary, think of two principal kinds of ionizing radiation: (1) particulate (alpha, beta, etc.) and (2) electromagnetic (x-ray, gamma ray). These are the energy forms capable of irreversibly damaging live tissue.

Biologic Effects of Radiation

CELL INJURY

Ionizing radiation can produce both direct and indirect effects in a biologic system.[1, 10] Direct cellular damage has been explained by the "hit" or "target" theory, whereas indirect effects include secondary ionization of cell water with concurrent liberation of free radicals. Ionizing injury can lead to cell death or to partial repair, depending on the cell component affected by the energy.

The target theory predicts that a cell unit will react adversely following a minimum number of "hits" or energy-absorption events. The number of cells inactivated by a given high-energy exposure event is directly proportional to the density of cells present. Direct effects of radiation appear at random along the pathways traveled by ionizing particles. The frequency of "hits" is related directly to size of the sensitive cellular structure or molecule.

Indirect effects of ionizing energy involve chemical sequelae of intracellular ionization. Free ionized molecules are uncommon in biology except as the result of ionizing irradiation. Intact or fragmented molecules, once ionized, become highly reactive, and they may enter into reactions that yield unstable secondary products known as *free radicals*. Secondary effects are not completely understood, but free radicals are known to be strong oxidizing and reducing agents. They can react with water to form toxic peroxides or they can form crosslinkages with critical macromolecules like DNA and RNA. They can even attach themselves to cell membranes, thereby blocking certain surface-attachment functions.

Which structures within a cell are most sensitive to ionization energy? This question is not easily answered since the sum of direct and indirect effects can inactivate an entire cell or may partially damage more than one cell component. A reduction in cell reproductive potential constitutes one of the most important effects of radiation because of the genetic importance of the DNA molecule. Following exposure, any cell may become pyknotic, undergo lysis, or otherwise display evidence of death. Adjacent cells remain viable but lose reproductive capacity. Irradiated cells may also replicate without physical separation, resulting in the formation of multinucleated cells so characteristic of radiation injury.

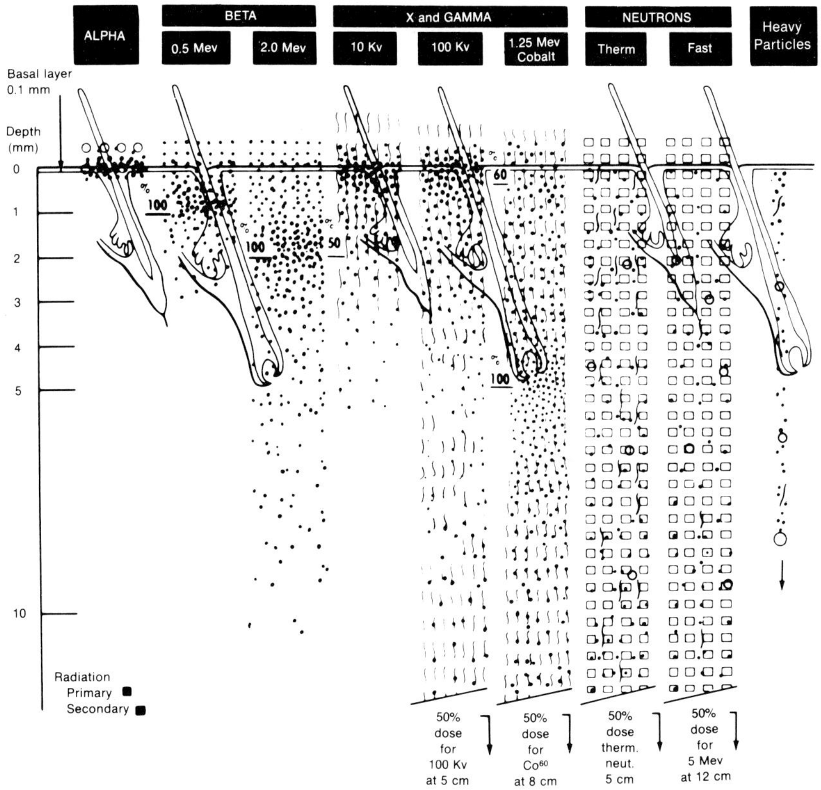

FIG. 7-2. Penetration of tissue, in this case skin, is variable among electromagnetic and particulate sources of ionizing radiation. (Berdjis C: Pathology of Irradiation, p 147. Baltimore, Williams & Wilkins, 1971. © 1971, The Williams & Wilkins Co., Baltimore)

Several factors influence the response of cells exposed to ionizing radiation:

- The character of the radiation, e.g., total dose administered
- The level of energy to be absorbed and the radiation source involved
- Chemical factors, such as ambient oxygenation, which can significantly influence the cellular effect (oxygen potentiates ionization)
- Biologic factors such as the relationship between radiation exposure and the reproductive cycle

In 1906, Bergonie and Tribondeau observed that "x-rays are more effective on cells which have greater reproductive activity." This principle was confirmed by the observation that tumor cells were more readily injured by irradiation than were normal cells.

TISSUE VASCULARITY

Clinical evidence of a tissue response to irradiation can be acute or chronic. Vascular changes are observed soon after irradiation of both normal and neoplastic tissues, despite the fact that endothelial cells are not especially radiosensitive. Vascular dilatation is responsible for the erythema that follows irradiation. Vacuolization of the endothelium and focal necrosis of the vessel wall come later when repair should be well underway. Several months after exposure, permanent degenerative abnormalities will include subintimal hyaline sclerosis, endothelial proliferation, diminished capillary proliferation, and ectasia of the vessels that remain.

Plastic surgeons have been fond of attributing most of the wound complications from radiation they treat to the vascular deficits adjacent to the wound. There is no abundance of granulation tissue within an indolent radiation ulcer. The most carefully designed flaps often fail if their base is adjacent to a site of prior radiation injury.

However, surgeons who deal with chronic radiation wounds also know that bleeding is vigorous near a radiated wound. Furthermore, intravenous fluorescein administration can be done during surgery to confirm flap viability. And it is known that in time, a few radiation wounds will yield granulation tissue and accept skin grafts.

Although vascular damage cannot therefore be discounted altogether, it is possible that we have overemphasized blood vessel injury and overlooked

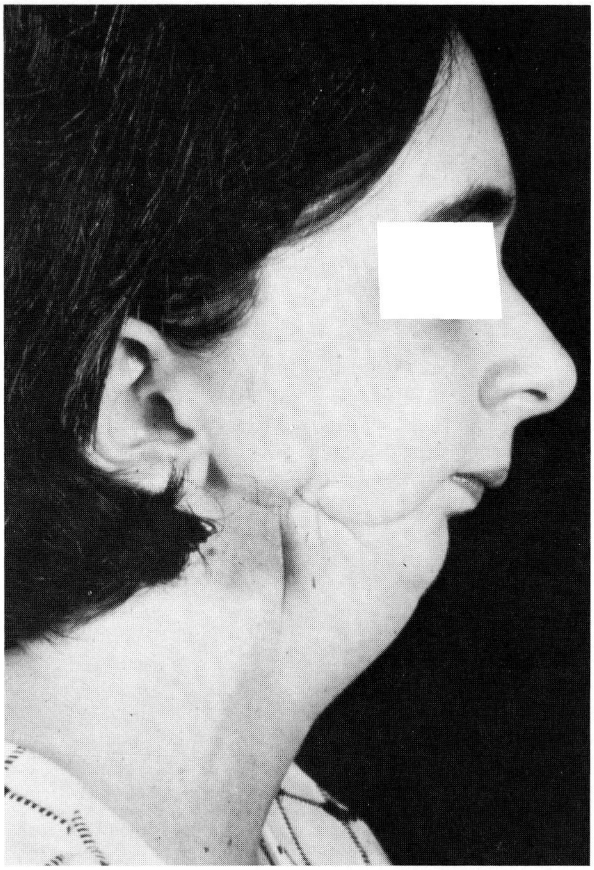

FIG. 7-3. A patient who was facially crippled during infancy because of a decision to irradiate a benign cystic hygroma and thus "avoid surgery." This congenital vascular lesion is known to involute spontaneously. The effects of the radiation included mandibular hypoplasia, dental agenesis, and chronic skin atrophy.

other mechanisms for tissue breakdown and incomplete healing.

CHRONIC ATROPHY

Atrophy is an appropriate term to describe what clinicians see when they look at a chronic radiation wound (Fig. 7-3). Wound biologists are aware that healing is a continuous process. There is constant turnover of collagen within a healed primarily closed wound or within a skin grafted surface wound. The continuous nature of this process is shown by ascorbic-acid-deficient animals, which cannot heal wounds and cannot maintain tensile strength of prior wounds.

Collagen is a product of fibroblast proliferation operating under the stimulus of substances liberated by macrophages. The origin of fibroblasts is local, that is, from the immediate zone of wound repair. One can therefore speculate that local fibroblast damage is the basis for nonregeneration of a radiated tissue surface. Evidence of chronic injury may be immediate, or it might be delayed several years, depending upon the density of cell death. Radiation wounds are indeed confounding in that they can appear many years after exposure.

GENETIC EFFECT

Ionizing radiation is known to be a potent mutagen. Radiation-induced mutations may involve somatic cells, in that case only the irradiated patient will be affected; or they may involve germinal cells, in that case, genetic offspring may suffer adverse consequences.

Two kinds of genetic change are seen following radiation exposure; the point mutation and the chromosomal aberration. The first of these involves small alterations in DNA sequencing not detectable by chromosome karyotyping. The second follows direct injury to an entire chromosome, which is detectable by karyotype analysis. Not all chromosomal aberrations are permanent. A fractured chromosome may rejoin without residual injury, but it may also join another chromosome or fail to heal altogether.

CARCINOGENIC EFFECTS

The carcinogenic effects of ionizing radiation have been recognized for the greater part of this century, first appearing only a very few years after Roentgen's rays were first used clinically. Early radiation workers, unaware of the cumulative effect of radiation injury and of the need for protection, soon developed basal and epidermoid malignancies of the skin of their hands.

Other clinical evidence for the association of malignant transformation and radiation exposure included the plight of the radium-dial painters, who tipped their brushes with the lips before applying radium-containing paint to watch dials. Bone sarcoma and other visceral malignancies appeared 10 and 20 years later.

These specific events are dramatic and widely retold. Less apparent are the malignancies that develop 20 and 30 years after curative therapeutic irradiation. Bone sarcomas of the pelvis may follow early-stage cervical carcinoma. There is no good long-term epidemiologic survey of carcinogenesis following radiation therapy, but the accumulation of isolated case reports suggests a greater clinical problem than we have been willing to admit.

Regardless of what is and is not known about radiation carcinogenesis, the following generalizations seem appropriate:

All forms of ionizing radiation are carcinogenic.
Multiple doses are more tumorigenic than is a single dose of identical magnitude.
Tumors of almost any type may be induced by irradiation.
The incidence of some malignancies (e.g., of hematopoietic tissues) is increased by very small amounts of radiation exposure.

Clinicians must recognize that a decision to use irradiation to control one malignancy might, in time, lead to development of another.

ACUTE RADIATION SICKNESS

While a thorough discussion of the acute radiation syndrome is not appropriate here, a brief account of its primary manifestations provides an understanding of the systemic biologic effects of radiation. There are three recognized phases:

1. A prodromal phase, characterized by nausea, apathy, and vomiting, lasting 12 to 24 hours
2. An asymptomatic interval, corresponding to the time required for development of specific organ-system deficiencies
3. The principal phase of illness, including hematologic, gastrointestinal, and central nervous manifestations

The death rate is extremely high. The effectiveness of newer treatment advances such as bone-marrow transplantation has not yet been determined because acute radiation sickness is, fortunately, rare.

Regional Specificity of Injury

SKIN

Historically, skin damage provided the earliest clinical evidence of the biologic destructiveness of ionizing radiation. Prior to 1950, ionizing radiation was characteristically lethal to the skin because tissue penetration was limited. In fact, the germinal layers of the skin absorbed nearly all of the energy. Later, when more potent sources were introduced, surgeons and patients were told that skin sparing would result in fewer complications. Perhaps this has been true, but significant injury to the skin commonly follows therapy with high-speed particulate irradiation.[8, 12] Much of that damage is self-limited to the period immediately following therapy, but some injury is permanent and progressive.

Early changes include erythema, epilation, bleb formation, ulcer formation, and hyperpigmentation. Chronic changes include epidermal atrophy, hyperkeratosis, telangiectasis, susceptibility to injury, and very poor healing potential. And there is a genuine potential for development of skin malignancies!

Today, the appearance of multiple skin malignancies in someone aged under 50 years may often be the result of adolescent exposure to therapeutic irradiation, administered for acne or other benign dermatoses. In one surgeon's experience, 10% to 20% of all women who seek surgical excision of a basal cell carcinoma provide a history of radiation exposure. But this incidence cannot be determined without careful interrogation of all patients with skin cancer. Cutaneous malignancy was at one time an occupational hazard for those working in radiation facilities, but modern safeguards have largely eliminated this problem. Neither do we see skin cancer among those treated for head and neck malignancy, perhaps because cancer of this region occurs at an older age and outcomes of treatment are neither favorable nor prolonged.

A chronic radiation ulcer may undergo malignant degeneration just as any chronic wound may. Carcinoma has been described that arose in an old burn scar, but a foundation of x-ray–damaged integument is a more likely site for neoplasia. Biopsy therefore becomes a clinical mandate for surgeons who accept responsibility for managing these difficult wounds.

HEAD AND NECK

The primary sites for cancer of the head and neck region are heterogeneous, as are the many tissues susceptible to injury. Rapidly multiplying mucosal cells are perhaps the most vulnerable, and one can therefore expect some diminution of salivary function in every patient treated with radiation. Studies of parotid-gland function after radiation therapy show cessation of function when lesions of the oral cavity or nasopharynx are irradiated. As much as 30% of glandular function can be interrupted following x-ray treatment of supraglottic or laryngeal malignancies. Most studies of salivary function have been carried out within 6 months of treatment, but functional loss can be progressive after longer intervals. As little as 500 R delivered to the entire area of the parotid gland virtually eliminates salivary flow from that organ. Therefore, we can assume that the late progression of dry mouth symptoms is related to scatter effect among the multitude of small accessory salivary glands distributed throughout the oropharyngeal region.

Dry mouth is not a casual aftermath of cancer treatment. Taste and dental hygiene are closely related to salivary function. Postirradiated patients with oral cavity cancer often select radiation, the form of treatment least threatening to their sense of well-being. Following treatment, those with aftereffects such as dryness of mouth will, when asked, express a different opinion about surgery, particularly when recurrence leads to a subsequent decision for surgical excision.

The teeth, when present, are in a precarious state, bathed in an environment rich in bacteria and worsened by our dependence on refined sugars. Therefore, patients with oral carcinoma are likely to have unstable dentition long before ionizing radiation is introduced. In the past, extraction of carious teeth was recommended before beginning radiation therapy. This was not a wise policy. The frequency of "dry sockets" (failure to granulate and close an alveolus) was very high, presumably because radiation held in check the proliferative capacity of the microvasculature. Chronic bone exposure soon led to mandibular pain and progressive necrosis.

Nowadays, restorative dentistry is the prudent choice for all who will undergo radiation therapy for head and neck malignancy. It should be instituted soon after admission, even before the workup is completed. Dental restorations take time. Outpatient care may be necessary; dental care must be completed before the patient begins radiation.

Surgery for head and neck malignancy often involves elevation of skin flaps used for reconstruction of a wound defect. The viability of these flaps and of primary wound healing depend upon a functioning microvasculature as well as upon the proliferative capacity of fibroblasts and capillary endothelium. Whenever flaps die or mucosal suture lines break down, development of pharyngeal fistulae or exposure of major vessels in the neck can lead to complications if not permanent disability. Furthermore, combined-therapy protocols that predispose to patient complications, particularly when irradiation precedes surgery, are currently popular.

Nutrition is recognized as an essential requirement for postoperative recovery, but the combination of salivary atrophy, loss of dental stability, and the presence of an orocutaneous fistula can mean surgical malnutrition. It is little wonder then that surgical approaches to head and neck malignancy have fallen into disfavor, a "Catch-22" since concomitant ionizing radiation often contributes to the problem.

Whenever longevity permits follow-up long after application of radiation to the head and neck region, secondary malignant degeneration becomes a genuine threat. This was learned initially from those who developed thyroid cancer many years after x-ray treatment for such benign conditions as thymic or tonsillar enlargement.

Even megavoltage radiation administered for potentially curable cancers like retinoblastoma or an early oral cavity lesion may in time (10 yr–20 yr) lead to a secondary malignancy. These are often sarcomas of osteogenic or fibrous origin.[7] It is extremely difficult to calculate the frequency of these late malignant sequelae. Most observers assume that these neomalignancies are rare and isolated events, while others suggest that the likelihood is far from remote, given sufficient time following cure.

CHEST WALL

Chronic radiation-induced defects of the anterior chest wall should diminish significantly in the next decade, but their prevalence remains unchanged according to many reconstructive surgeons. Temporary fascination with combined therapy for treatment of breast carcinomas has left many thousands of women disabled. The wide surgical field of the mastectomy, flaps of variable thickness and durability, and occasional wound complications have led to chronic tissue breakdown when irradiation followed surgery.

The least of these injuries involves instability of the integument and exposure of devascularized cartilage, often with concomitant pain but always associated with chronic odor and drainage. There is little tendency toward spontaneous healing despite modest dimensions of the ulcerative site. The worst of these injuries involve the full thickness of the thoracic cage together with underlying viscera. Following removal of necrotic ribs, cartilage, and connective tissue, the heart and great vessels may be observed at the base of an awesome cavity, a sight sufficient to strike fear in the hearts of patients, family, and surgeon alike.

The results of clinical surveys administered by the National Surgical Adjuvant Breast Project have demonstrated no advantage in survival or longevity when irradiation was added to surgical management for breast carcinoma. Only the frequency of local recurrence was affected, but the price—disability—was considered by most medical and surgical oncologists not to be worth the temporary gain, a gain that represents only a change in the pattern of recurrence, not a drop in overall recurrence rate. In the future the use of postmastectomy irradiation will be less frequent.

Rehabilitation in the form of breast reconstruction of the mastectomy patient will also become more feasible. Reconstructive procedures are not impossible in an irradiated field, but they are more challenging for reasons already defined.

PELVIS

The principal indication for pelvic irradiation is uterine cancer, one of the most common of malignancies that affect women. End-result data show a clear advantage for those with corpus lesions and those with Stage III and IV cervical carcinoma who are given irradiation instead of or in addition to surgery. But for those with earlier stages of malignant disease, there is no demonstrable advantage to radiation other than freedom from having to endure a surgical procedure. Preliminary studies at the University of California/San Diego indicate that the long-term sequelae of a decision for radiation therapy may be more frequent than was formerly believed.

Immediate postirradiation complications (*i.e.*, those appearing within 1 to 6 months of treatment) have been recorded by many observers. These include fistulae, cystitis, and proctitis. But far less commonly evaluated are the sexual functions, bladder and intestinal function, and various forms of musculoskeletal disability. It is after all not a part of our usual cancer follow-up protocols to arrange for interviews yielding full disclosure of altered sexual habits. Yet the incidence of painful intercourse following irradiation has been estimated to be as high as 75%.

Appropriate decisions for management of highly curable, early-stage malignancies must await a better understanding of the late aftereffects of megavoltage therapy. Successful skin-sparing techniques will still leave their effects on the femoral head, the bladder trigone, and the intestinal tract. Ionizing irradiation can tip the balance from asymptomatic to permanently symptomatic pelvic disease, a price worth paying for increased survival, but not a price to be asked of those who would be just as effectively cured by surgery.

GASTROINTESTINAL TRACT

The evolution of radiation-induced injury to mucosal surfaces is similar to that seen in skin but takes place at a faster rate. Gastritis, enteritis, and colitis are an integral part of the acute radiation syndrome because of the rapidity with which our intestinal lining replaces itself.

Delayed sequelae of gastrointestinal (GI) exposure to ionizing radiation deserves mention independent of our consideration of the pelvis, even though the most serious injuries are often the late result of irradiation administered for pelvic malignancy.[4, 9, 13] Chronic inflammation leading to stricture and obstruction or to ulceration and hemorrhage can be permanently disabling because the GI surgeon cannot easily isolate the very worst segments of injury from a surrounding environment of radiation damage. Successful anastomosis of bowel is heavily dependent on the vascular requirements for successful healing. Abdominal surgeons are therefore as handicapped as reconstructive surgeons when they attempt surgery in the absence of necessary biologic responses to the wound. Furthermore they are dealing with an organ system the integrity of which is necessary for continued life.

DeCosse has reviewed a series of 100 consecutive x-ray–induced injuries to the GI tract.[4] Nearly all patients had been treated for malignant disease although there were three whose radiation had been administered for chronic infection many years before. DeCosse established a 12% incidence of significant GI complications over a 15-year period following treatment for carcinoma of the uterine cervix. He is to be commended because few observers have taken the time to measure the overall long-term effects of irradiation on a specific organ system. Those effects include rectal stricture, rectovaginal fistula, chronic ileitis, and, in one instance, a new rectal malignancy.

The long-term outcome of this series of patients is worthy of comment. After 5 years, one third were alive and two thirds were dead. Death was attributed to cancer in 28 cases. Nearly as many (25) died as a result of complications of the GI system or nearby tissues. In other words, the treatment was nearly as serious as the disease!

What are the contributing causes of radiation injury to the gut? In other words, why doesn't everyone develop bowel sequelae after pelvic irradiation? DeCosse and associates compared their series with a matched population treated for carcinoma of the cervix who did not develop GI injury. Prior hysterectomy increased the likelihood of bowel injury after x-ray, but prior pelvic inflammatory disease did not. Concurrent hypertension seemed to have an influence on induction of intestinal injury after x-ray treatment. Age, race, or weight were not factors that influenced frequency of bowel damage.

The rectum appears to be the most frequently injured segment of the alimentary tract, not just because of the pelvic focus of the beam, but also because this is where the heavily contaminated fecal stream becomes concentrated and causes chronic inflammation even without ionizing irradiation. Ulcers may lead to fibrosis, scarring, and, in time, stenosis. Loss of integrity of the delicate linings that separate the rectum from the vagina results in fistulas (29 in this limited series of 100 patients).

Chronic ileitis is another frequent pattern of disease. These patients endure prolonged bouts of chronic abdominal pain, and the dilemma is whether to attempt resection in advance of obstruction or to wait until an abdominal emergency mandates surgical intervention. Most surgeons are not seeking reasons to enter the peritoneal cavity in order to avert tragedy, because in the presence of radiation injury, disaster is often the result. On the other hand, no surgeon likes to wait until perforation or obstruction has already taken place. The environment adjacent to these events is even less capable of responding—in the form of a walled-off abscess, something that requires all of the normal, nonradiated body's capacity for repair.

And so GI radiation injury carries many disadvantages that outweigh its benefits. Reconstructive surgeons who deal with surface defects have learned that waiting does not lead to a more opportune time or more favorable circumstances for the surgical solution. Should GI surgeons carefully examine their problems in the same terms?

CARDIOVASCULAR, NEUROLOGIC, AND MUSCULOSKELETAL INJURY

No specialized tissue or organ system is resistant to the effects of ionizing energy. We have already considered the possible effects of x-ray on small vessels. There is evidence that large-caliber vessels can be involved, as can such critical medium-sized vessels as the coronary arteries. Stenoses and aneurysms of large named arteries have been described in association with high-energy irradiation, but without a complete explanation derived from our traditional understanding of the pathogenesis of atherosclerotic disease. Angina pectoris in a young woman followed heavy administration of x-ray to the mediastinum for Hodgkin's disease. Indeed, rather typical histologic changes compatible with atherosclerosis may follow the sort of injury to a vessel wall described earlier in this chapter (see Tissue Vascularity).[5]

All connective tissues can show effects of ionization injury, but consider briefly bone and cartilage, generally thought to be the most durable and least cellular of our many tissues. The skeleton is not resistant to the effects of radiation, particularly when growth is incomplete or when we require of our joints and limbs the highest performance during athletic or recreational endeavors.

Indeed, our joints tell us very quickly after irradiation that their range of tolerance has become limited. When cortical bone, most dense among our tissues, becomes damaged sufficiently to cause symptoms, pain is one of the most troublesome and least controllable characteristics. "Radium jaw" is not easily managed for patient comfort, short of surgical resection. Development of connective tissue or bone sarcomas is an event no longer rare.[2, 14] Once again epidemiologic assessments of frequency are difficult to find, but case reports and clinical series are a regular feature of orthopaedic journals. Often a young woman treated for early-stage cervical cancer and subsequently cured may return years later with aseptic femoral head necrosis or an osteogenic sarcoma.

The axial and peripheral nervous systems may bear permanent ionizing injury just as the brain can. Necrosis and transverse myelitis of the spinal cord can lead to permanent and irreversible paralysis. Opinions vary over whether this is a direct neurogenic effect or the result of vascular thrombosis. Cranial nerves and brachial nerve neuropathy have also been described whenever heavy doses of energy are directed at these important neural structures. Recovery from ionizing injury to nerves and nerve sheaths is rare. Chronic wounds may then develop more easily within the radiation portal as a derivative of the paralysis that follows radiation neuropathy. Rarely has the patient been warned or prepared for the development of these events.

Principles of Reconstruction for the Radiation Defect

Radiation wounds most frequently requiring surgical reconstruction are surface defects, the end result of chronic atrophy. Because the integument overlying a radiation field has failed to regenerate itself, the surgeon cannot expect to benefit from all of the advantages he has at his disposal when he makes an elective incision or repairs a traumatic wound. Dealing surgically with a radiation defect has been likened to practicing surgery in the absence of a wound-repair system.

Based upon our understanding of what is happening (or not happening) at a cellular level in the radiation wound, we can assemble a reasonable list of principles applicable to the treatment of most radiation wounds:[1, 3, 6, 11]

1. *The most compelling indication for surgery is often pain.* We have not yet begun to predict or anticipate radiation injury, and so most of the wounds we see are late wounds. Pain is ordinarily the most common reason for reconstruction of a radiation wound. It can be an intense, unremitting pain similar in character to that experienced by the patient with sickle cell disease or hypertensive leg ulcers. The source of pain is not well understood, but the presence of pain and its severity will assure a cooperative and devoted patient throughout the course of reconstruction. The patient's desire is to be relieved of pain, although the surgical steps necessary to achieve that goal will at times seem forbidding.
2. *Confirm all suspicions of recurrent cancer with biopsy.* The disorganized character of the typical radiation wound will lead some to conclude that recurrent cancer is present. More often than not, this assumption is false. In fact, it is safe to say that cancer

does not exist in the wound until a biopsy proves that it does. Remember also that the cancer patient may believe that a radiation defect represents cancer recurrence until his physician tells him otherwise. Biopsies are therefore important, whether positive or negative. Even if recurrent malignancy is found, the presence of pain can justify a noncurative excision and wound closure, particularly if it can be accomplished in one surgical step.

3. *Tell the patient that the course ahead is difficult.* Before embarking on any surgical adventure, the patient must be fully informed of the challenge. He must be told that complications (*i.e.*, delayed wound healing) are the rule rather than the exception. A wise reconstructive surgeon prepares his patient to expect slow progress. Radiation injuries are brought under control in months and years, not in days or weeks.
4. *Immediate reconstruction of the excised defect may prevent progressive necrosis.* The inevitable presence of necrosis in a radiation ulcer would ordinarily call for débridement in advance of surgical closure. But isolated débridement is *not* a useful maneuver. Even if a bleeding base can be found beneath the necrosis, this surface is only viable to the extent that granulation tissue will form. And so we must limit ourselves to preliminary removal of only the worst necrosis and defer actual wound excision until we can at the same time cover the wound with a flap.
5. *The area of radiation damage is always larger than you think.* Clinical evaluation of the radiation wound must take into account the diffuse nature of ionizing radiation. The ulcer has definable borders, and although the surrounding zone of partial cutaneous injury is visible to the trained observer, the greater zone of microscopic injury lies beneath normal-appearing skin and its fragility is not known until flaps are designed and elevated.
6. *Skin grafting is not to be relied upon!* Because surgeons cannot depend on the usual wound-repair processes, skin grafting is not a technique on which to depend except to cover residual zones after flap loss when granulation has at long last appeared. Skin grafting should not be part of an initial operative plan except as immediate cover for a distant flap-donor site.
7. *Don't depend on traditional flaps either!* The random pattern flap is not a good choice for repair of radiation defects, particularly when it is taken from a zone immediately adjacent to the problem (Fig. 7-4). The subdermal vascular plexus is probably injured. The so-called scatter effect of the initial radiation exposure is usually more extensive than the quality of overlying skin would seem to indicate.
8. *Consider arterial flaps, but cautiously.* The arterial flap is a better choice except that the tips of these flaps are also dependent on the subdermal vascular plexus for part of their survival. Therefore, select no flap from a site anywhere near the radiation defect!
9. *Insist on a "permanent pedicle flap."* More distant flaps would be applicable to the problem save for one critical limitation: flaps must not only bring their own blood supply but must also carry a permanent blood supply, an observation first made by J. Barrett Brown many decades ago. Flaps cannot be "jumped" or secondarily transferred into a radiation wound. To repeat: flaps covering radiation wounds must carry their own blood supply, and that supply must be permanent, not temporary.
10. *Myocutaneous flaps have potential, but are not complication free.* The myocutaneous flap has great advantage for service as a cover of radiation wounds. But in our hands, its use is not without likelihood of complication. The abundant blood supply of the muscle is just what the doctor ordered for the indolent radiation wound. The skin island supplied by the muscle will be durable if it comes from a site well outside the radiated zone. But if the wound is not adequately excised, the vascularly enriched myocutaneous flap will fail to adhere to the wound surface, a problem we have witnessed more than once.
11. *Microvascular free flaps require adequate recipient vessels.* The microvascular free flap has potential but unproven benefit. The limiting feature, of course, is adequacy of the recipient vessels. We suspect that sources like the latissimus dorsi flap will be more useful than is the more precarious groin flap.
12. *The omentum may be the best source of all.* The omentum is a rich and valuable source for cover of many deep and extensive radiation defects. It may be transferred directly, or it may be transferred by microvascular anastomosis. Skin grafts are fully applicable in this case, for they are applied to a viable surface rich in vascularity (Fig. 7-5).

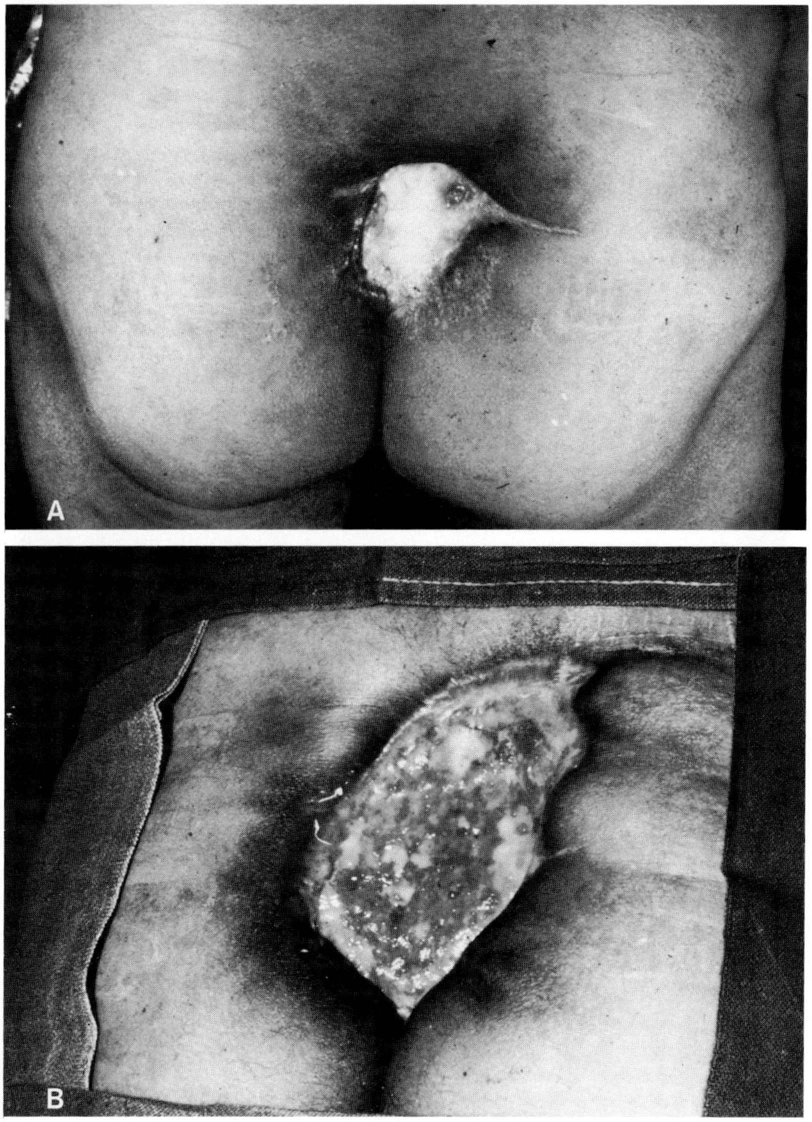

FIG. 7-4. (*A*) A sacral ulcer following pelvic irradiation for prostatic cancer, surrounded by apparently healthy skin. (*B*) Following wound excision and rotation of a random-pattern buttock flap of standard dimension, the distal half of the flap failed to survive. Months after surgery, débridement and local wound care led to the eventual formation of a granulation-tissue base. Pain remained a persistent feature of this unsuccessfully treated radiation injury.

13. *Conservative management is sometimes the best choice.* For some unfortunate patients, there may be no good reconstructive answers, or else rapid progression of their disease precludes a surgical solution. Conservative management of a chronic radiation wound is not easy, particularly if pain is a dominant feature.

    Conservative débridement, good hygiene, and a simplified dressing routine are the hallmarks of pragmatic care. Use of agents to limit bacterial proliferation is also important. The topical antibacterials of burn care (mafenide, sulfadiazine) have been used. We also recommend a classical remedy, balsam of Peru. It is hyperosmolar, keeps bacterial growth to a minimum, changes a bad wound odor to a favorable one, and one dressing change per day seems sufficient. Terminal care and convalescent home referral are facilitated by use of a simplified wound regimen such as this.
14. *Provide emotional support.* Finally, something can be said about sustaining a patient's mood throughout the interval of care for a radiation wound. Time and funds are spent in great amounts. The patient's spirit can be destroyed by pain and recurrent un-

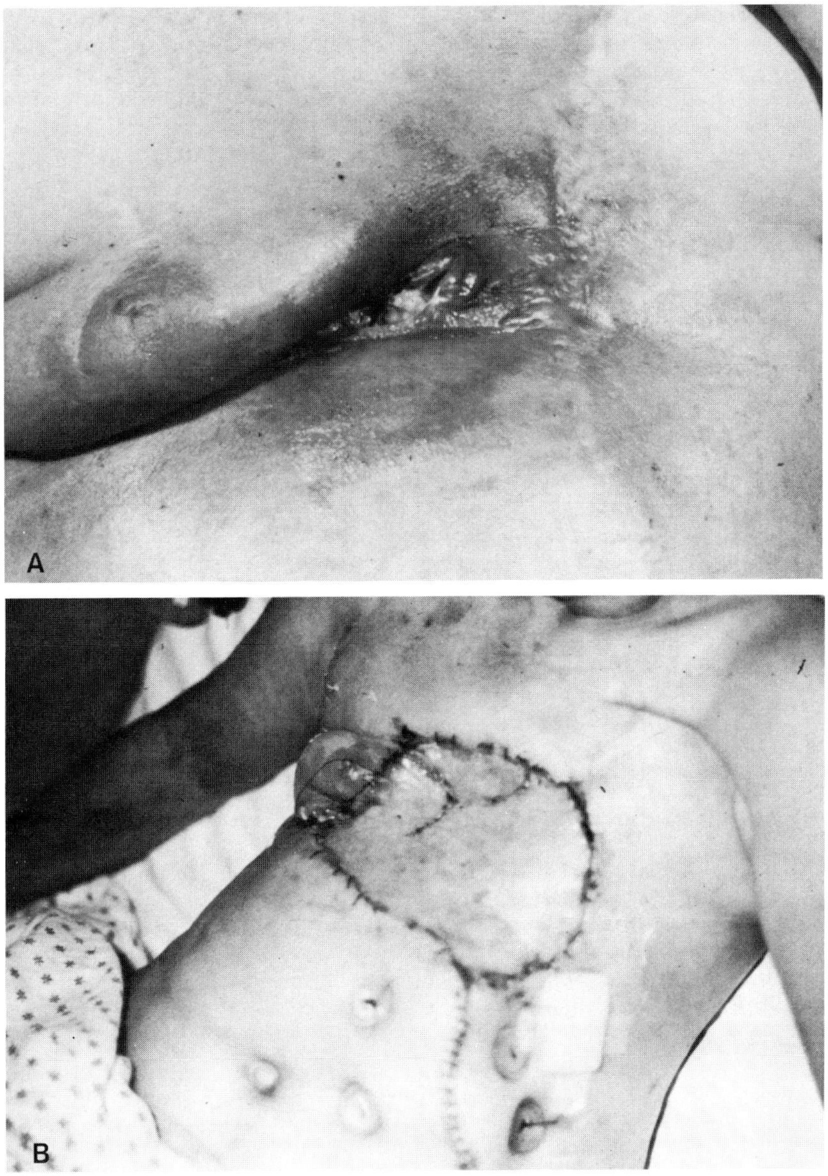

FIG. 7-5. (*A*) A close-up view of a midline sternal ulceration medial to an old mastectomy scar on the patient's left breast and on her distorted right breast. Pulmonary metastases are present. The principal indication for surgery is unrelenting pain. (*B*) The patient immediately following wide resection, including the sternum, ribs, pericardium, and pleura. Cancer was left at the base of the wound. The defect was filled with omental flap and covered with a split skin graft. Relief from pain was immediate. After surgery, the patient resumed her principal avocation, playing golf, and was alive, pain-free, and disease-stable 1 year later.

certainty about surgery. It is almost inevitable that the patient will question the wisdom and skill of those who administer the radiation. Careless comments by surgeons and their less experienced housestaff when they view the aftereffects of radiation can reinforce the patient's anger.

We find that these negative comments help no one and may provoke counterproductive medicolegal activity. We prefer supportive words when discussing the causes of the problem. Radiation was after all selected for treatment of a serious disease, cancer, and powerful forms of treatment cannot always be controlled when they are applied to the difficult challenge. When cure has been the result of treatment, these complications should be viewed by the patient as a side-effect that accompanies cure. Meanwhile, let us in the medical profession work hard to control all forms of cancer therapy as well as to fit the appropriate mode of cure to the appropriate disease. Gilbert and Sullivan would suggest that we "let the punishment fit the crime."

The Surgeon's Role in Prevention of Radiation Injury

As surgeons, we can favorably influence the frequency of complications following therapeutic irradiation:

1. We can discourage the use of ionizing irradiation for benign disease, a practice that remains commonplace in our sophisticated medical society despite countless reports of tragic outcomes, often malignant, many years later. It is not prudent to advocate ionizing radiation for shrinking congenital hemangiomata, for preventing keloid scar formation, or even for inhibiting certain benign cutaneous disorders. There is no evidence to support these notions.
2. As surgeons who are aware of reconstructive methods for repair of certain radiation wounds, we should anticipate tissue destruction and provide alternative surface closure well in advance of breakdown, necrosis, vascular erosion, bone exposure, or pain. Chronic unrelenting pain is the single most characteristic feature of a radiation wound. All too often, denial is the physician's defense as sequelae of radiation become progressively apparent. A false assumption that malignant disease has returned and that the patient has little time left can lead to months of misery. Our first duty is to control pain, and nowhere is this a more compelling mandate than for the victim of a radiation wound, *whether or not recurrent cancer is present.*
3. Our participation on tumor boards and other multiple-disciplinary teams provides an opportunity to assess carefully the long-term as well as short-term sequelae of our treatment choices, both surgical and nonsurgical.
4. Finally, as physicians committed to seeking a scientifically valid basis for the practice of medicine, we can demand of our investigators and of our editors that reports of success following cancer treatment include valid measurements of the long-term outcomes for each form of therapy, including measurement of quality as well as length of life.

In a significant passage from Solzhenitsyn's *Cancer Ward,* a patient reflects on the wisdom of accepting his physician's recommendation of x-ray therapy for a neoplasm of unproven nature that later turns out to be self-limiting. He says: ". . . In short, I would not care to pay too great a price for the hope of being able to live at some time in the distant future."

References

1. Anderson RE: Radiation injury. Chap 8. In Anderson WAD: Pathology, 7th ed. St Louis, CV Mosby, 1977
2. Arlen M et al: Radiation induced sarcoma of bone. Cancer 28:1087–1099, 1971
3. Brown JB, McDowell F, Fryer MP: Surgical treatment of radiation burns. Surg Gynecol Obstet 88:609–622, 1949
4. DeCosse JJ et al: The natural history and management of radiation induced injury to the gastrointestinal tract. Ann Surg 170:369, 1969
5. Hayward RH: Arteriosclerosis induced by radiation. Surg Clin North Am 52:359–366, 1972
6. Krizek T: Difficult wounds: Radiation wounds. Clin Plast Surg 6:541–543, 1979
7. Mahmoud NA: Radiation-induced fibrosarcoma of the head and neck. J Laryngol Otol 94:231–242, 1980
8. Malkinson FD, Keane JT: Radiobiology of the skin: Review of some effects on epidermis and hair. J Invest Dermatol 77:133–138, 1981
9. Palmer JA, Bush RS: Radiation injury to the bowel associated with the treatment of carcinoma of the cervix. Surg 80:458–464, 1976
10. Platzman RL: What is ionizing radiation? Sci Am 201:74–83, 1959
11. Rudolph R: Complications of surgery for radiotherapy skin damage. Plast Reconstr Surg (in press)
12. Rudolph R et al: The ultrastructure and etiology of chronic radiotherapy damage in human skin. Ann Plast Surg (in press)
13. Stuart M et al: Irradiation injuries of the large intestine. Dis Colon Rectum 23:94–97, 1980
14. Weatherby RP et al: Postradiation sarcoma of bone. Mayo Clin Proc 56:294–306, 1981

8
Complications of Flap Surgery

Michael Scheflan

OVERVIEW

While skin grafts are a simple, time-honored surgical modality for wound closure, they are frequently inadequate. Flap surgery is indicated when there are

Little or poorly vascularized bed that will not support a graft (bare bone and tendons, irradiated tissues)
Vital structures exposed in the wound (nerves, blood vessels, bone, intestines, mediastinum, etc.) that will not be adequately protected by a graft
A weight-bearing, pressure, and friction zone centered in the wound with inadequate subcutaneous tissues to which a skin graft will not provide protection, padding, and durability
Certain conspicuous exposed areas (face) where skin grafting may not achieve an adequate aesthetic result
Large amounts of composite tissues that have been lost (trauma, infection, ablative surgery, etc.), and tissue that carries its own blood supply must be "brought in" to reconstruct the function and appearance of the area (breast, abdomen, and chest wall)

Complications of flap surgery may arise in the recipient site, the donor area, and the flap itself. Complications related to the first two are similar to those described in Chapter 4, Complications of Skin Grafting.

Complications related to the flap itself are in general inadequate blood supply, tension, hematoma, and infection, as well as specific complications unique to each individual flap.

A large and ever-growing variety of flaps are available for soft tissue transfer. This chapter presents the essential principles of flap surgery and the most likely complications.

For ease of discussion flaps are divided into three categories: (1) skin and fat flaps, (2) skin and muscle flaps (musculocutaneous), and (3) free flaps (microvascular transplantation of tissues).

Skin and Fat Flaps

Inadequate blood supply and tension are the major foes of flap surgery in general and of skin and fat flaps in particular. Very few skin and fat flaps receive their blood supply directly from an underlying subcutaneous artery (dorsalis pedis flap, deltoid flap, groin flap, etc.—commonly used in free microvascular tissue transfer). More often, a skin flap has segmental perforators in its base (deltopectoral flap), but most commonly the skin and fat flap receives its vascularity from the subdermal plexus in a random fashion.[5] Most random flaps must maintain a width-to-length ratio of approximately 1:3 in order to predict adequate circulation to the flap's tip reliably. In reality, however, the length of a skin and fat flap is dependent on the local perfusion pressure. Flaps created under equal conditions of blood supply and pressure flow will survive to the same length regardless of width.[9]

Design of skin and fat flaps must, therefore, be particularly precise so that the flap can easily be rotated to cover a defect, be sutured without tension, and have its vascularity maintained at the same time. While this is true for all flaps, skin and fat flaps are particularly vulnerable to reduced circulation and tension. Swelling of the flap invariably follows its transfer and contributes to increased tension and reduced circulation. This must be considered when the flap is designed.

The secondary donor defect created by the transfer of a flap may require skin grafting unless the flap is so designed that it gradually "borrows" tissue from the donor site, usually spherically, so that the secondary donor defect may be closed primarily.

Transposition and rotational random skin and fat flaps are commonly used to close moderately small defects that cannot be approximated and closed directly.

Skin and Muscle Flaps

Muscle and musculocutaneous flaps have revolutionized the art and science of soft tissue transfer.[6] Most larger reconstructions are better managed with musculocutaneous flaps because of the more direct and predictable blood supply and since larger amounts of soft tissues can be reliably transferred this way.[4]

Accurate mapping and definition of reliable and versatile musculocutaneous units has, on the one hand, enormously diversified the surgical options of reconstructive plastic surgery and, on the other hand, created a new generation of related complications.[2, 14]

Although the detailed knowledge of anatomy and anatomical variations of muscles, their function, and blood and nerve supply has afforded great and bold leaps in soft tissue and bone reconstruction, this renaissance of often heroic surgery is not without its problems.

Problems in Musculocutaneous Flaps

ANATOMY

As much as anatomical expertise is the *sine qua non* for muscle flap surgery—so is the recognition of anatomic variability. Since the pivot point around which to rotate a flap is its neurovascular pedicle, the surgeon must be prepared at the time of surgery to learn that the major pedicle is lower or higher than expected or absent altogether (as in the case of the gracilis muscle that occasionally has no major dominant axial pedicle from the deep femoral artery and relies upon segmental perforators from the superficial femoral artery).

PHYSIOLOGY

Muscles that are nondispensible should in general not be sacrificed for soft tissue coverage even though they may be ideal choices according to their blood supply and proximity to the defect. Examples include biceps humerus for shoulder coverage, flexor carpi ulnaris for elbow coverage, and rectus femoris for thigh coverage.

Utilizing muscle and musculocutaneous territories while still preserving their function is a developing art that is discussed below for individual musculocutaneous flaps.[8] Examples include pectoralis major for dehisced median sternotomy wound coverage, posterior trapezius for head and neck coverage, and "reverse" latissimus for posterior trunk coverage.

DESIGNING AND ELEVATING A MUSCULOCUTANEOUS FLAP

Although the vascularity of musculocutaneous flaps is more predictable and these flaps carry large amounts of soft tissues reliably, they should be carefully designed so that the skin portion completely overlies muscle (with notable exceptions where skin and fat extensions are documented to be safe), the flap is large enough to resurface the wound without tension, and the pivot point is underestimated so that there is no direct pull on the isolated vascular pedicle. Flap elevation should proceed with caution in the correct intermuscular or subfacial plane. Minor pedicles should not be transected until the presence and location of the major dominant pedicle to the flap has been verified. The skin island should be secured to the underlying muscle with interrupted sutures to prevent its shearing during elevation, tunneling, and transfer. In many instances, the vascular pedicle must not be isolated or skeletonized even though its location is verified. Often the flap may be so fashioned that the secondary defect can be closed primarily rather than skin grafted, although doing so should not, in any way, add tension to the closure of the primary defect.

TRANSFERRING AND INSETTING THE FLAP

Avoiding traction on and avoiding kinking of the vascular pedicle are essential. Even though it is not routinely skeletonized or isolated, the pedicle may undergo severe spasm from rough handling of the flap, undue tension upon transfer, or postoperative swelling. If the skin territory of a musculocutaneous flap is designed as an island, the arc of rotation will be augmented and formation of a dog-ear will be prevented. This, however, increases the risk of vascular torsion and of putting the pedicle under tension.

Island musculocutaneous flaps isolated on their neurovascular pedicle, like any other flap, undergo immediate postoperative swelling that peaks in about 48 hours. This must be borne in mind when tunneling a flap. Swelling inside an inadequately large tunnel will obstruct blood flow to the tissues and lead to ischemic necrosis of the flap. Tunneling should be avoided whenever possible.

Representative Complications of Musculocutaneous Flaps

HEAD AND NECK AND CHEST WALL AREA

PECTORALIS MAJOR MUSCULOCUTANEOUS FLAP is a thick, fan-shaped muscle with a dual blood supply. The dominant axial pedicle is the thoracoacromial vessels, and the minor segmental blood supply is from the internal thoracic pedicle. This unit is particularly useful for reconstruction of the head and neck area after ablative surgery for cancer and for chest-wall reconstruction after traumatic, neoplastic surgical, or infectious processes.

The muscle may be rotated on either blood supply to cover a variety of defects. When designed as a "turnover flap" for closure of median sternotomy defects, the muscle is halved at the midclavicular line. The medial portion is turned over and based on the internal thoracic pedicles to obliterate the defect, while the lateral portion is sutured down to the chest wall. Since the neurovascular bundle to this lateral portion remains intact, pectoralis major adduction function is preserved.

Complications of the pectoralis major flap are usually related to its bulkiness (it is pulled down by gravity from the head and neck area), the inconsistent viability of the skin island if positioned below the inferior distal aspect of the muscle, and finally seroma, hematoma, or infection of the donor area, which are uncommon.

LATISSIMUS DORSI MUSCULOCUTANEOUS FLAP is the mirror image of the pectoralis major muscle. It, too, has a dual blood supply.[1] The dominant pedicle is the thoracodorsal vessels. The minor segmental blood supply comes from paraspinal perforators. This flap represents one of the safest and most reliable musculocutaneous territories, and it is particularly useful for reconstruction of the breast, chest wall, posterior trunk, upper arm, head and neck, and as free-flap transfer.

In some extended axillary dissections for breast cancer, the thoracodorsal pedicle is ligated. This results in atrophy of the muscle. Although the latissimus muscle can still be utilized (based on "reverse" flow from a branch to the serratus anterior), the transfer is less reliable. For posterior midline coverage (meningomyelocele, dehisced laminectomy wounds, etc.), a portion of the muscle may be distally based on the paraspinal perforators and transposed to close the posterior midline defect—while preserving the main neurovascular bundle and longitudinal continuity of the muscle fibers, thereby preserving function.[11]

Complications from this flap include inadvertent damage to the pedicle; tight tunneling, which will lead to ischemia; and accidental shearing of the skin island, all of which are very uncommon. Seroma accumulation in the back is the most common complication of this flap and is easily managed with needle aspiration and pressure. Few patients will complain of a slightly winging or "clicking" scapula.

TRAPEZIUS MUSCULOCUTANEOUS FLAP. Based on its blood supply from either the occipital artery or the transverse cervical artery, the trapezius is a versatile unit for reconstruction of the ipsilateral neck, the auriculotemporal area, and the posterior base of the neck.[7]

If the transverse portion of the muscle is used as a flap, the spinal accessory nerve must be sacrificed to allow an adequate arc of rotation. This will obviously result in a shoulder drop, which is sometimes unavoidable but should be discussed with the patient.

The posterior descending portion of the muscle between the spinous processes and the scapula can be included in a flap that will have a similar arc of rotation but will preserve shoulder function.

A complication of using the trapezius muscle flap stems from attempts to extend the cutaneous territory inferiorly so that the tip of the flap will reach past the anterior midline of the neck. This will often result in tip necrosis.

ABDOMINAL WALL

RECTUS ABDOMINIS MUSCLE AND MUSCULOCUTANEOUS FLAP. Based on the superior and inferior deep epigastric systems, the rectus abdominis flap is particularly useful for reconstruction of the abdominal wall, the chest wall, and the breast.[12]

Complications from this flap result from failure to repair the remaining anterior rectus sheath, particularly below the arcuate line where there is no posterior sheath. This will lead to an abdominal wall hernia.

BUTTOCKS

GLUTEUS MAXIMUS MUSCULOCUTANEOUS FLAP. The superior and inferior gluteal arteries vascularize the superior and inferior aspects of the muscle and its overlying skin. This bulky and reliable unit is commonly used for reconstruction of the sacral, ischial, and trochanteric areas.[13]

Being a strong extensor of the hip, the entire muscle should not be sacrificed on either side in ambulatory patients. Half the muscle, however, may be used on each side as a musculocutaneous flap without interfering with function. Complications from this flap are uncommon. However, when dissecting around the inferior gluteal pedicle in the sciatic foramen, the sciatic nerve is at risk and should be located in all patients. Because of the great vascularity of this bulky muscle and the lack of a clear surgical plane between it and the gluteus medius, a raw surface created when elevating the flap must be thoroughly drained to prevent hematoma.

THIGH

TENSOR FASCIA LATA MUSCULOCUTANEOUS FLAP. Based on the lateral femoral circumflex artery, the tensor fascia lata flap may include the entire iliotibial tract for soft tissue transposition. This is a subfacial flap that includes the overlying skin and is particularly useful for closure of trochanteric pressure sores, groin wounds, reconstructing the abdominal wall, and in free-tissue transplantation. A block of posterior superior iliac crest may be included in the origin of the muscle to reconstruct bony defects.

Complications from this versatile and reliable flap occur in the most distal thin portion of the flap, which cannot provide adequate padding to bony prominences.[10] Distal necrosis also often occurs when the flap is stretched to resurface the ischium or sacrum.

GRACILIS MUSCULOCUTANEOUS FLAP. Based on a proximal pedicle from the medial circumflex femoral artery, a branch of the profunda femoris artery, the gracilis flap is one of the most difficult musculocutaneous units.

It is a narrow and flat muscle in the medial thigh, and its cutaneous territory must be accurately defined prior to elevation of the flap. This is accomplished by identifying the tendon in the distal medial thigh and putting the unit under stretch. The flap is useful for reconstructing the perineum, vagina, penis, perianal area, and in free-tissue transplantation. Several distal segmental perforators are present from the superficial femoral artery. The exact hemodynamic contribution of each pedicle is variable, although the major proximal pedicle will usually support the flap. Complications from this flap result because the skin that overlies the distal third of the muscle cannot predictably and reliably be carried with the unit.[3] The entire overlying skin portion must be sutured down to the muscle since it may be easily sheared from its blood supply.

LOWER LEG

GASTROCNEMIUS MUSCULOCUTANEOUS FLAP. Based on sural branches of the popliteal artery, either the medial or the lateral head of the gastrox may be transposed to resurface defects in the upper third of the tibia and the knee area. While elevating the flap, it is easy to dissect in the wrong plane above the muscle and thereby devascularize the overlying skin. Should this occur, the flap must be restored to its original position. It can be re-elevated in the proper plane 3 weeks later.

The posterior tibial and perineal neurovascular bundles are protected by the underlying soleus muscle and are not disturbed if dissection is carried out in the correct plane. A distal subfascial extension of the flap may reliably be elevated beyond the muscle and transferred with the flap.

Complications of Microvascular Tissue Transplantation (Free Flaps)

A surgeon may resort to "free" transfer of tissue when options such as skin grafts or local flaps are inadequate or have been exhausted. Also, when highly "differentiated" tissues are required (*i.e.*, reconstruction of the cervical esophagus, mandible and overlying skin, neurosensory heel pad, etc.), free flaps are often chosen as the mode of reconstruction.

Although complications from donor and recipient sites are similar to those from grafts and flaps, the intra-abdominal complications—for instance, following free transfer of the jejunum to reconstruct the esophagus—may be severe. Independent clinical use of this surgical modality is just beginning, so that there has been relatively little experience with it, and no complications of this nature have yet been reported.

Although success rates of around 95% are currently reported, failure or complication of free flaps often means complete loss of the transplanted tissue. The most common complication of free tissue transplantation is anastomotic failure. Mechanical occlusion of the vessels causes gradual cessation of arterial inflow (white flap) or venous outflow obstruction (blue flap).

Increased sophistication in postoperative monitoring of free-flap circulation using transcutaneous PO_2 sensors, sensitive temperature electrodes, and microflow meters will inevitably lead to early detection of flow obstruction, early re-exploration, and revision of the microvascular anastomosis. All of these will improve the salvage rate.

The factors that contribute to successful microvascular surgery are the following:

Degree of surgical precision practiced
Size of the vessel
Rate and nature of blood flow
Tension
Use of anticoagulant and antithrombotic medications

As more experience is gained in this exciting and versatile microsurgical modality, clear indications, guidelines, and limitations are being defined. The development of technical expertise will be accompanied by development of our ability pharmacologically to manipulate the microcirculation to our advantage. This progress and our ability to monitor more accurately the postoperative course of free flaps will undoubtedly lead to a decreased complication rate and increased success of free microvascular tissue transplantation.

References

1. Bostwick T, Scheflan M: The latissimus dorsi musculocutaneous flap—a one stage breast reconstruction. Clin Plast Lung 7(4):71, 1980
2. Grabb WC, Cherry GW, Phil D et al: A prospective study of complications in 120 consecutive flaps in humans. Plast Surg Forum IV:22, 1981
3. Heckler FR: Gracilis muscle and musculocutaneous flaps. Clin Plast Lung 7(1):27, 1980
4. McCraw JB, Vasconez LO: Musculocutaneous flaps: Priciples. Clin Plast Surg 7(1):9, 1980
5. McGregor IA: Flaps. In Goldwin RM (ed): The Unfavorable Results in Plastic Surgery—Avoidance and Treatment. Boston, Little, Brown & Co, 1972
6. Mathes SJ, Alpert BS: Advances in muscle and musculocutaneous flaps. Clin Plast Lung 7(1):15, 1980
7. Mathes SJ, Nahai F (eds): Clinical Atlas of Muscle and Musculocutaneous Flaps. St Louis, CV Mosby, 1979
8. Mathes SJ, Nahai F (eds): Clinical Applications of Muscle and Musculocutaneous Flaps. St Louis, CV Mosby, 1982
9. Milton SH: The survival of experimental pedicled skin flaps—the fallacy of the length : width ratio. Br J Surg 52:502, 1970
10. Scheflan M: The tensor fascia lata—Variations on a theme. Plast Reconstr Surg 68(1):59, 1981
11. Scheflan M: Letter: The distally based ("reverse") latissimus dorsi myocutaneous flap. Ann Plast Surg 8(3): 267, 1982
12. Scheflan M, Hartrampf CR, Black PW: Breast reconstruction with a transverse abdominal island flap. Plast Reconstr Surg 69:85, 1982
13. Scheflan M, Nahai F, Bostwick T III: Gluteus maximus island musculocutaneous flap for closure of sacral and ischial pressure wounds. Plast Reconstr Surg 68:533, 1981
14. Vasconez LO, McCraw JB, Hall EJ: Complications of musculocutaneous flaps. Clin Plast Lung 7(1):123, 1980

9 Complications of Breast Surgery

J. Shelton Horsley, III

OVERVIEW

The principal reason for removing a mass in the breast is the suspicion of cancer. Fortunately, only 20% to 25% prove to be carcinoma. However, the American Cancer Society estimated that in 1982 112,900 new patients in the United States would be diagnosed with this disease.[1] *Because there has been a significant increase in the number of augmentation and reduction mammoplasties, as well as of breast reconstructions, surgical procedures on the female breast account for a significant number of operations in the United States each year.*

The incidence of breast cancer in the male is rare, approximately 1 for every 100 cases in the female. The same complications, however, would be applicable.

Preoperative Preparation

DIAGNOSIS

There are several ways to diagnose a mass in the breast, but they all require microscopic study of tissue or cells. The most commonly used method is incisional or excisional biopsy. Needle-tissue biopsy is becoming more frequent, as is needle-aspiration cytology. The most disastrous complication in the diagnostic procedure would be the incorrect diagnosis because of inadequate tissue. Whenever there is the suspicion of cancer, the entire mass must be submitted to histologic study before the lesion can be pronounced benign.

Another increasingly important complication is failure to excise the suspicious nonpalpable lesion found only on xeromammography. A localization technique utilizing xeromammography or mammography of the excised specimen is mandatory to confirm that the lesion has been removed.[1]

Whenever a mass, whether it is an occult or a palpable lesion, is removed for a total excisional biopsy, the surgeon should not incise any closer to the chest wall than is necessary to remove the lesion completely. If the pectoralis major fascia is not transgressed and the lesion is not in close proximity to the muscle, this muscle may be preserved in the subsequent definitive surgical procedure if the diagnosis is cancer.

SELECTION OF THERAPY

The clinical staging of breast cancer is made on physical examination with utilization of x-ray and bone scans, where appropriate, and less commonly liver and brain scans. The most significant complication would be to deny the patient appropriate primary therapy on the basis of a false-positive finding on one of these studies. Such a finding on bone scan would be a solitary area of increased uptake that might be the result of trauma or arthritis. If there is any question, confirmatory findings on radiograph or, better yet, microscopic tissue diagnosis should always be obtained.

There are several options available to the patient with potentially curable breast cancer.[11] Both surgical resection and radiation therapy are suitable for local therapy.[9, 14] The addition of chemotherapy or endocrine therapy depends on the histology of the axillary nodes and the determination of the estrogen-receptor status of the cancer.[16] All of these factors are vital for determination of therapy for the patient with either potentially curable or proven metastatic breast cancer.

It is beyond the objective of this chapter to discuss the various therapeutic options available to the patient. The surgeon should make his recommendations for therapy to the patient so that she understands the plan. There is considerable publicity about therapy for breast cancer, and some patients have many questions. The surgeon should answer her questions clearly and support the reasons behind his choice. If a second opinion is requested, cooperation is important. A well-informed patient, who has had her questions suitably answered, is in a much better frame of mind to start her therapy.

If the patient is a candidate for some type of clinical trial, the protocol should be carefully explained in detail and informed consent obtained.[15] The surgeon should have the patient seen prior to the initiation of definitive treatment by all physicians and allied health personnel, such as radiation oncologist, anesthesiologist, and rehabilitation workers, who participate in her therapy. The surgeon should make every effort to minimize misunderstanding and apprehension and maximize support. The patient's family should be included in these discussions when appropriate.

Operative Complications

INCISION

The incision should give the best exposure for the particular surgical procedure to be employed. If a small lesion is to be excised, a curving skin incision in Langer's lines directly over the mass gives adequate exposure and affords good healing and a satisfactory cosmetic result. Whenever possible, incisions in the circumareolar and inframammary areas should be utilized because they heal with minimal deformity. If a segmental resection of breast tissue is planned, a curving transverse incision in the upper half of the breast but a radial incision in the lower half is recommended. Meticulous hemostasis, primary closure without attempting to reapproximate breast tissue, and no drainage but only a pressure dressing for 24 hours give the best aesthetic result.

Whenever a mastectomy is peformed, a transverse incision provides excellent exposure, good healing, minimal restriction of shoulder and arm motion, and a most acceptable appearance. Incisions into the axilla are to be avoided because they lead to restriction of motion. The common practice of extending the vertical incision outside the brassiere strap line laterally over the shoulder is painful and ugly and restricts motion. Moreover, it offers nothing more than an unnecessary burden to the patient.

A 4-cm to 5-cm margin of grossly normal skin around the tumor should be included with the mastectomy specimen to avoid leaving behind cancer cells. The primary considerations for the incision are adequate exposure and a satisfactory border around the tumor; secondarily, the incision should be functional and cosmetic.

PREPARATION OF FLAPS

The thin superficial fascial level (4 mm–6 mm) is the proper thickness for the skin flaps. Too often these are thick at the margin and thin at the base, which leads to necrosis and slough. The surgeon will notice a minimal loss of blood if he is in the proper plane of dissection. During the surgical procedure, the flaps should be treated gently and not allowed to become dry.

AXILLARY DISSECTION

Adequate exposure is essential to the performance of a satisfactory dissection of the adipose tissue and lymph nodes of the axilla. In a standard radical mastectomy, with removal of both the pectoralis major and minor muscles, the exposure is excellent. When the pectoralis major muscle is preserved, the pectoralis minor removed, and the arm mobilized, the exposure is quite satisfactory and a thorough dissection of the axillary contents equal to that of a radical mastectomy can be accomplished. Failure to divide the pectoralis minor muscle and to mobilize the arm restricts the dissection to the lower and mid portions of the axilla while the upper third remains intact.

The most frequent complications in this area are hemorrhage from transection of one of the many branches of the axillary vein or artery. Although the main vessels can be injured, this is rare, but the branches are susceptible to injury. The brachial plexus is easily identified. No dissection should be undertaken in this area since there are no lymph nodes and surgical manipulation will only increase the possibility of injury or postoperative pain. The surgeon must be careful not to place the brachial plexus on undue or prolonged stretch by manipulation of the arm to obtain better exposure, particularly with modified radical mastectomy.

The two principal nerves vulnerable to injury are the thoracodorsal (lateral), motor to the latissimus dorsi muscle, and the long thoracic (medial) to the serratus anterior muscle (Fig. 9-1).[6] With the former, the entire thoracodorsal neurovascular bundle should be preserved because the latissimus dorsi muscle may play a vital function in eventual breast reconstruction. Damage of the long thoracic nerve leaves a severe deformity, winged scapula.

If the pectoralis major muscle is preserved, as in a modified radical mastectomy, the pectoral nerves should be preserved for motor function.[13] Frequently, the lateral pectoral nerve will be sacrificed when the pectoralis minor muscle is removed because their courses are so intimately involved (Fig. 9-2). Preservation of the medial pectoral nerve results in satisfactory function. Once the nerve has been divided, atrophy of the muscle will occur and

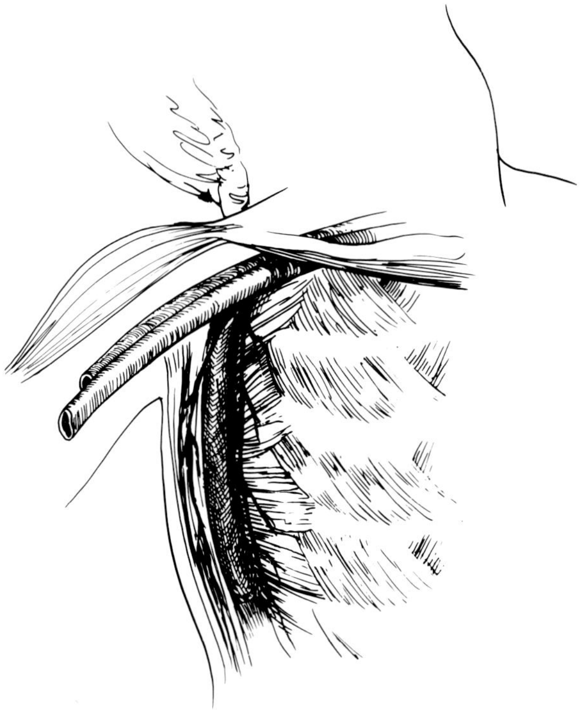

FIG. 9-1. The two principal nerves vulnerable to injury during axillary dissection: (*lateral*) the thoracodorsal nerve, motor to the latissimus dorsi muscle, and (*medial*) the long thoracic nerve, motor to the serratus anterior muscle.

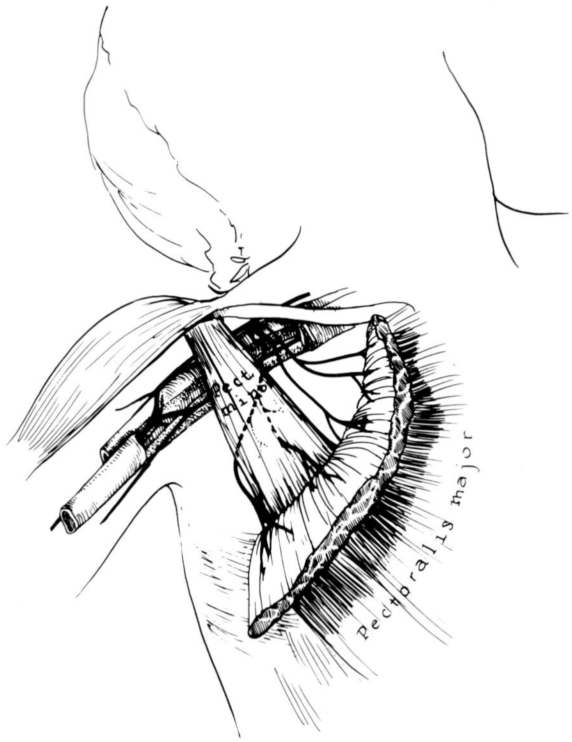

FIG. 9-2. Course of the lateral pectoral nerve.

the muscle becomes unsuitable for prosthesis coverage in breast reconstruction. If the nerve is only traumatized, return of function can be expected within several weeks to several months.

SURGICAL SPECIMEN

Once the specimen has been removed—whether by lumpectomy, segmental resection, or mastectomy alone or with axillary contents and with or without pectoral muscles—an adequate sample of the cancer (a minimum of 250 mg, preferably more) should be cleared of fat and breast tissue. It should be placed promptly in a sterile container on ice and quickly frozen in liquid nitrogen for storage for the determination of estrogen and progesterone receptor activity. The longer the devitalized cancer remains at room temperature, the less accurate are the results. Storage should not exceed 3 weeks before analysis is performed. Receptor activity is vital in determining subsequent therapy, either adjuvant to the primary treatment or therapeutic for metastatic disease, which may become apparent later.

In obtaining cancer tissue for the receptor determinations, adequate tissue should be preserved for the surgical pathologist. The entire specimen is appropriately labeled and sent to the pathology department for microscopic study.

WOUND CLOSURE

The wound should be inspected carefully for hemostasis and to be sure sponges or instruments do not remain under a flap or in the axilla. If the tumor is small and only locally removed, reconstruction of the breast tissue with several interrupted sutures may be helpful for hemostasis. Primary closure without drainage using a well-fitted compression dressing for the entire breast gives a most satisfactory result.

When a mastectomy of any type is performed and skin over the mass removed, the possibility of skin grafting must be considered. Although most of the time (70%) the closure is primary, the surgeon should always prepare an appropriate donor site for the split-thickness skin graft. I have utilized the anterior lateral thigh of the contralateral leg, which is prepared at the time of preparation of the breast for the mastectomy. This avoids the unnecessary problems and hazards of having to prepare a donor site at the completion of the mastectomy. The opposite thigh has been used so that the patient can more easily hold the hospital gown away from the donor site with her uninvolved hand and arm when getting in and out of bed and walking (a patient's suggestion). Primary closure of the mastectomy wound with minimal tension is preferred. Whenever the tension is great or the defect of such magnitude that primary closure is impossible, a split-thickness skin graft should be utilized.

Primary closure is usually done with multiple interrupted subcutaneous absorbable sutures and nonabsorbable sutures or staples for the skin. Steri-strips also give an excellent result, avoiding suture marks. If the closure requires a skin graft, the wound edges should be secured to the underlying pectoral muscle or chest wall and then the graft placed over the defect. The graft can be either left open or closed with a bolus type of dressing, depending on the preference of the surgeon. Attention to details of proper thickness of the graft, 0.0014 inch to 0.0018 inch, and meticulous placement should lead to 100% take!

With the increasing utilization of transverse incisions, a problem with the closure posteriorly often arises in obese patients. Often a sizable mound of tissue, "dog-ear," is created. It may annoy the patient considerably after healing has taken place. Rubbing against the patient's arm may be a source of chronic irritation. This can easily be modified at the time of closure if the surgeon performs appropriate excision. A slight upswing of the posterior lateral portion of the transverse incision facilitates the ease of a myocutaneous flap if breast reconstruction of this type is done later.

WOUND DRAINAGE

Drainage after simple excision of a breast mass or a segmental mastectomy is not necessary. For the patient who has had a mastectomy with or without an axillary dissection, suction drainage is beneficial to remove the serosanguineous fluid that accumulates over such an extensively denuded and traumatized area. The principal sites are the pectoralis major muscle (modified radical mastectomy) or chest wall proper (radical mastectomy) and the axilla. This requires two separate drains which should be attached to gentle suction. They should be properly placed in the wound and can be easily held there with a loosely placed absorbable suture about the drain tied to the underlying pectoral muscle or chest wall. To avoid inadvertent removal and ensure an airtight seal, the stab wound through which the drain is placed should be sutured snugly about the drain and the long ends of the suture tied securely about the drain. If the drain is silicone, indentation by the suture is easily accomplished. If it is a firm plastic, placing a rubber band or a small piece of Penrose drain between the drain and the suture increases the friction and holds more stably. The drains are brought out of separate stab wounds in the lower portion of a transverse incision or on either side of a vertical incision in a medial and lateral location for convenience of handling and comfort for the patient.

A covering dressing of the wound and the entire area of dissection is applied with gentle pressure for the first 24 hours. The wound is then re-dressed on the first postoperative day to check for hematoma. If the wound is satisfactory, a light dressing over the wound edge is applied for an additional 48 hours. After 72 hours, the wound edges should be sufficiently adherent and no dressing needed. However, some patients are apprehensive about an exposed incision, and there is no harm in keeping a light superficial dressing in place.

The sites where the drainage tubes exit through the skin should always have a dressing and should be dressed every 24 hours with a local bactericidal ointment, such as povidone-iodine (Betadine), reapplied about the drain as it passes through the skin.

The drains are all attached to a gentle portable suction apparatus, which is pinned to the patient's hospital clothes. These suction drains remove the fluid beneath the skin flaps so that the flaps become adherent to the underlying tissues. Once the drainage stops and the flaps are adherent to the muscle or chest wall, the mission of the drains has been accomplished and they should be removed. All drains are foreign bodies and will create fluid drainage by their presence in the body. The drains can usually be removed in 3 to 5 days.

Complications of the drains are inadvertent removal and premature plugging. Attention to details during the placement of drains and repeated careful observation of the wound can prevent these problems. Once plugged, drains usually require removal or replacement. Attempts to irrigate are not only unsuccessful but hazardous as a source of infection of the wound.

Postoperative Complications

HEMORRHAGE

Hemorrhage as a complication may be heralded by a sudden drop in the patient's blood pressure with tachycardia. It is not unusual to underestimate the blood loss during the surgical procedure, so this should be promptly checked with an evaluation of measured blood loss and fluid replacement during the operation. An increase in bloody drainage or a bulging wound may be a telltale sign of hemorrhage. The wound should be inspected immediately. If a hematoma is present, the patient should be returned promptly to the operating room, the incision opened, the hematoma evacuated, and all bleeding points meticulously controlled. The wound is then closed with drainage as previously described and the results are uniformly good with no increased morbidity.

DRAINAGE

The persistence of serosanguineous or serous drainage after the completion of the surgical procedure can lead to delayed healing of the wound flaps. As long as the drainage catheters are removing the fluid and the flaps are adherent to the underlying tissue, the wound will heal. The most troublesome problem is recurrence of serous fluid collections after the drains have been removed. Fortunately, this recurrence usually responds to intermittent aspirations several days apart. If aspirations fail and the seroma persists, reinstitution of catheter drainage with or without suction is necessary, but this is infrequent. At the same time, the patient should be requested to restrict her shoulder and arm activity on the involved side.

PULMONARY COMPLICATIONS

The most frequently encountered pulmonary complication postoperatively is atelectasis. This will respond promptly to deep breathing, coughing, and chest physiotherapy. Formerly, bulky pressure dressings, some circumferential about the entire thorax, were employed and restricted full expansion of the thoracic cavity and occasionally caused loss of viability of skin flaps.

Infrequently a pneumothorax will occur, particularly with a radical mastectomy or an extended radical mastectomy with internal mammary node dissection. The most common cause is when a hemostat perforates the pleura during an attempt to clamp a perforating vessel coming through the intercostal muscle. All hemostatic instruments should be placed parallel to the chest wall to avoid this problem. Any suspicion of pneumothorax should lead to a portable chest x-ray to confirm the diagnosis. Treatment consists in prompt placement of a high anterior chest drainage tube connected to underwater seal suction to re-expand the lung fully. This will promptly correct the problem, and the tube can usually be removed within 2 to 3 days.

INFECTION

Infection is a most serious complication. It can lead to skin edge necrosis and lymphedema of the arm. Fortunately, it is infrequent. Most patients who undergo any type of excisional breast surgery do not warrant prophylactic antibiotics.

The prompt recognition of infection and treatment with appropriate antibiotics and adequate drainage, if there is an abscess, will be successful. The surgeon should not hesitate to open the wound widely if there is purulent material present. Cultures should be taken and antibiotics chosen on the basis of this information.

WOUND HEALING

One of the most common complications of mastectomy is poor wound healing with necrosis of the skin edges.[2, 5, 17] This is most often the result of using an uneven skin flap sutured primarily under too much tension in an effort to avoid skin grafting. Wide undermining of skin flaps will help avoid tension. A small area of skin loss will adequately heal by secondary intention with proper débridement and wound care. However, a large area may require split-thickness skin grafting, after appropriate débridement and preparation of a good vascular base to receive the graft. Skin loss may delay the use of an external prosthesis and inhibit shoulder and arm motion.

SHOULDER AND ARM MOTION

An avoidable complication is limitation of shoulder and arm motion. So much emphasis has been placed on this phase of rehabilitation that sometimes therapy is too vigorous too soon after the surgical resection. Patients who have had extensive mastectomies requiring a skin graft to cover the resulting defect should not start active shoulder and arm exercises as soon as the patient whose wound is closed primarily. Although our patients are seen preoperatively and postoperatively by a member of our Breast Rehabilitation Team, active motion is started on an individualized basis, usually after the drains have been removed. A recent study done at the National Cancer Institute showed a most satisfactory range of motion being obtained in patients whose active motion exercises were delayed up to 7 days after surgical resection.[12] Every effort should be made to get complete return to preoperative range of motion (ROM) but not at the expense of seroma formation and delayed wound healing.

The maintenance of good motion requires the attention of both the patient and her physician. An appropriate exercise program should become a part of the daily routine until the wound is completely healed and the functional ROM desired has been obtained, usually in 3 to 4 months. However, some patients may need a lifetime commitment to such a program of exercise.

LYMPHEDEMA

Lymphedema is the most common chronic complication involving the arm following radical mastectomy.[7] Initially, this may present as a slight transitory edema that usually disappears with restoration of function and activity of the arm. However, in about 10% of patients, edema can persist, resulting in a genuine disability. The causes of lymphedema are many, including surgical techniques, infection, and radiation. Venous obstruction, autonomic nervous system reflex spasm, and obesity also have been suggested as etiologic factors. Certainly the best evidence supports an insufficiency of lymphatics draining the arm as the result of removal and obstruction. The more extensive resections with skin grafting and radiation have a higher incidence of this problem. The surgical procedures that do not include axillary dissection, or only limited lower axillary dissection, without radiation of the axilla, rarely have this complication.

Restoration of shoulder and arm motion greatly enhances lymphatic drainage, but elevation, motion, and compression can be used to treat the problem. Infection is to be avoided as it will lead to further lymphatic obstruction, thus creating a vicious cycle. At the first sign of cellulitis, appropriate antibiotics, usually penicillin, should be started.

For all patients having a mastectomy of any type, any trauma to the affected arm, such as needle sticks for obtaining blood or administering drugs or application of blood pressure cuff, should be avoided. Patients are also cautioned to be especially careful in case of any injuries, such as thorn pricks, splinters, or blisters, and to wear protective gloves when working in the garden. All rehabilitative programs stress exercises and motion to recover shoulder and arm motion and avoid the development of edema.

The most devastating complication of lymphedema of the arm is lymphangiosarcoma, which fortunately is rare.[18] It presents in a chronically lymphedematous upper extremity on the average of 10 years or longer after radical mastectomy. Typically, it appears as a blue, red, or purple, well defined, mildly tender cutaneous nodule with satellite lesions that will coalesce to form a large, ulcerated, hemorrhagic mass. This is a highly malignant tumor that spreads rapidly. If it is localized to the extremity, the most effective treatment is amputation, usually an interscapulo-thoracic resection. The outlook is poor.

ADJUVANT THERAPY

Adjuvant therapy refers to treatment in addition to the primary treatment of the breast cancer. The most frequently employed adjuvant therapeutic measures are radiation therapy, combination chemotherapy, and endocrine therapy. It is most important for the patient to be well informed and understand the rationale for such a treatment plan. Because the overall prognosis is sufficiently good in women whose axillary nodes are free of metastases on microscopic examination, there are no indications for adjuvant therapy in this group at present.

Radiation therapy is being utilized more frequently in the primary treatment of breast cancer to conserve breast tissue. It is less often used as adjuvant to primary surgical resection since, similar to surgery, it is local therapy. The local skin changes are minimal, but lymphedema of the arm is more common after radiation.

Combination chemotherapy attacks the problem of systemic spread of breast cancer. In a consensus report from the National Cancer Institute in August 1980, it was recommended that combination chemotherapy be given following primary surgical therapy (radical or modified radical mastectomy) in premenopausal women with axillary node metastases.[16] Postmenopausal women should receive it only as part of a clinical trial until it can be shown to be beneficial for this group. The morbidity may be significant depending on the drug combinations. Side-effects include nausea and vomiting, alopecia, stomatitis, and bone marrow depression.[3] Since most regimens are given for 1 or 2 years, the quality of life is definitely disturbed. Close observation of the patient to adjust her dosages according to signs, symptoms, and laboratory blood studies is mandatory. The patient also needs much psychological support during this time. The physician must be knowledgeable about these drugs and explain and re-explain to the patient the various effects she will experience.

Endocrine therapy is principally the use of the antiestrogen, tamoxifen, as an adjuvant in estrogen receptor positive (ER+) breast cancers with axillary node metastases. The side-effects of this drug are minimal.

The entire field of adjuvant therapy is currently being explored.[20] All therapeutic modalities have the potential to cause adverse side-effects so the physician must inform his patients of these possibilities and be able to treat them effectively.

REHABILITATION

Recently, increased emphasis has been placed on the rehabilitation of the patient who has undergone mastectomy for cancer of the breast.[8, 21] No group of people has contributed more to understanding this rehabilitation than have the volunteers of the American Cancer Society's Reach to Recovery Program.[19]

These women have had a mastectomy and been selected and trained for these activities. It is a free service of the American Cancer Society available, with the approval of the patient's surgeon, to any woman who has had breast cancer surgery. These volunteers usually see the patient in the hospital and help start her physical and psychological recovery. They are knowledgeable about various breast prostheses—where to purchase one and be properly fitted.

The surgeon should make the patient aware of the possibilities of reconstructive surgery of the breast. Although approximately 75% of patients following mastectomy will decide to use only a prosthesis, those who desire reconstruction should be referred to a suitable plastic surgeon.

Despite all of the supportive groups for the patient who has undergone therapy for breast cancer, her primary physician, most often a surgeon, is the one to whom she looks for support and answers to her questions.[10] The patient should be aware that she will be followed for the rest of her life. It would be a most unfortunate complication if the patient was "lost to follow-up," or did not have a physician to whom she could turn for advice and support. The physician unwilling to make such a commitment should not treat the woman with cancer of the breast.

References

1. American Cancer Society: Cancer Facts and Figures, 1982, p 10. New York, 1981
2. Budd DC, Cochran RC, Sturtz DL, Fouty WJ Jr: Surgical morbidity after mastectomy operations. Am J Surg 135:218–220, 1978
3. Costanza ME: Sounding board: the problem of breast cancer prophylaxis. N Engl J Med 293(21):1095–1098, 1975
4. Egan JF, Sayler CB, Goodman MJ: A technique for localizing occult breast lesions. Ca-A Cancer Journal for Clinicians 26(1):32–37, 1976
5. Feigenberg Z, Zer M, Dintsman M: Comparison of postoperative complications following radical and modified radical mastectomy. World J Surg 1(2):207–211, 1977
6. Feller I, Woodburne RT: The long thoracic and thoracodorsal nerves in radical mastectomy. Surg Gynecol Obstet 107:789–791, 1958
7. Grabois M: Rehabilitation of the postmastectomy patient with lymphedema. Ca-A Cancer Journal for Clinicians 26(2):75–79, 1976
8. Healey JE Jr: Role of rehabilitation medicine in the care of the patient with breast cancer. Cancer 28(6):1666–1671, 1971
9. Hellman S, Harris JR, Levene MB: Radiation therapy of early carcinoma of the breast without mastectomy. Cancer 46(4):988–994, 1980
10. Holland JC, Mastrovito R: Psychologic adaptation to breast cancer. Cancer 46(4):1045–1052, 1980
11. Lazaro EJ, Rush BF Jr, Swaminathan AP: Changing attitudes in the management of cancer of the breast. Surgery 84(4):441–447, 1978
12. Lotze MT, Duncan MA, Gerber LH et al: Early versus delayed shoulder motion following axillary dissection: A randomized prospective study. Ann Surg 193(3):288–295, 1981
13. Moosman DA: Anatomy of the pectoral nerves and their preservation in modified mastectomy. Am J Surg 139:883–886, 1980
14. Moxley JH III, Allegra JC, Henney J, Muggia F: Treatment of primary breast cancer: Summary of the National Institutes of Health consensus development conference. JAMA 244(8):797–800, 1980
15. Muss HB, White DR, Michielutte R et al: Written informed consent in patients with breast cancer. Cancer 43(4):1549–1556, 1979
16. The NIH Consensus-Development Panel: Special report, NIH consensus-development statement, adjuvant chemotherapy of breast cancer. N Engl J Med 303(14):831–832, 1980
17. Say CC, Donegan W: A biostatistical evaluation of complications from mastectomy. Surg Gynecol Obstet 138:370–376, 1974
18. Schreiber H, Barry FM, Russell WC et al: Stewart-Treves syndrome, a lethal complication of postmastectomy lymphedema and regional immune deficiency. Arch Surg 114:82–85, 1979
19. Timothy FE: The reach to recovery program in America and Europe. Cancer 46(4):1059–1060, 1980
20. Weiss RB, Henney JE, DeVita VT Jr: Multimodal treatment of primary breast carcinoma, analysis of accomplishments and problem areas. Am J Med 70:844–851, 1981
21. Winick L, Robbins GF: The postmastectomy rehabilitation group program: Structure, procedure and population demography. Am J Surg 132:599–602, 1976

10 Complications of Breast Reconstruction Following Mastectomy

I. Kelman Cohen | Michael Scheflan

OVERVIEW

Although only approximately 20% of all women who have undergone mastectomy later undergo breast reconstruction, the percentage is increasing steadily. As reconstructive efforts are standardized, simplified, and improved, the procedure may be accomplished in one stage, and the results become increasingly attractive. Reconstruction of the female breast following mastectomy presents a formidable challenge but is, nevertheless, commonly performed in reconstructive surgical practice.

Each patient considered for breast reconstruction presents a unique problem, and patient selection must be based on patient goals, body image, tumor biology, and general mental and physical health. Thoughtful discussions between the extirpative and the reconstructive surgeons will often expand the understanding and insight of both and lead to better patient care.

We believe that reconstruction should be discussed with almost all patients who undergo mastectomy. Psychologically, this provides the patient with realistic optimism *that her breast can be restored and may avoid the depression, anger, and anxiety which are reported so commonly in mastectomy patients.*[11] *Furthermore, knowing that their breasts may be reconstructed soon after the mastectomy, women may face breast cancer with less fear of the physical, psychological, and sexual deformity.*

CRITERIA FOR PATIENT SELECTION AND BIOLOGY OF TUMOR

If each patient is considered with depth and sensitivity, disease staging should have no bearing on the ultimate decision for or against reconstruction. The prospect of an enhanced quality of life as a result of the restoration of body image may make reconstruction extremely worthwhile to the patient with a limited life expectancy, while, on the other hand, a patient informed of limited prognosis may reject reconstruction.

CHEMOTHERAPY

Although normal hematologic parameters, serum proteins, and so on, should be present at the time of reconstruction, chemotherapy *per se* is not a contraindication to reconstruction.[10] The therapeutic index of surgery should be of utmost importance in decision making.

TIMING OF THE RECONSTRUCTION

Although some authors have reported immediate reconstruction at the time of tumor removal, the increased tension of the implant on the chest wall skin flaps may cause flap necrosis and implant extrusion. If immediate reconstruction is performed, it should be limited to patients with small lesions and clinically normal axillary nodes. Some argue that the patient who has never experienced breast removal may be more critical of reconstructive efforts than is the patient who has lived for a while with the deformity that resulted from her mastectomy. This argument is self-serving and unwarranted. The psychologic benefits of primary rather than delayed reconstruction are unpublished. When these data are available, they may be helpful in deciding which patients should be selected for immediate reconstruction. At present, immediate reconstruction may be performed on patients with small primary lesions and clinically negative axillary nodes when adequate skin is present and the patient is eager for immediate reconstruction. Of course, this places the reconstuctive surgeon on "standby" call for potential reconstruction and may present awkward timing problems.

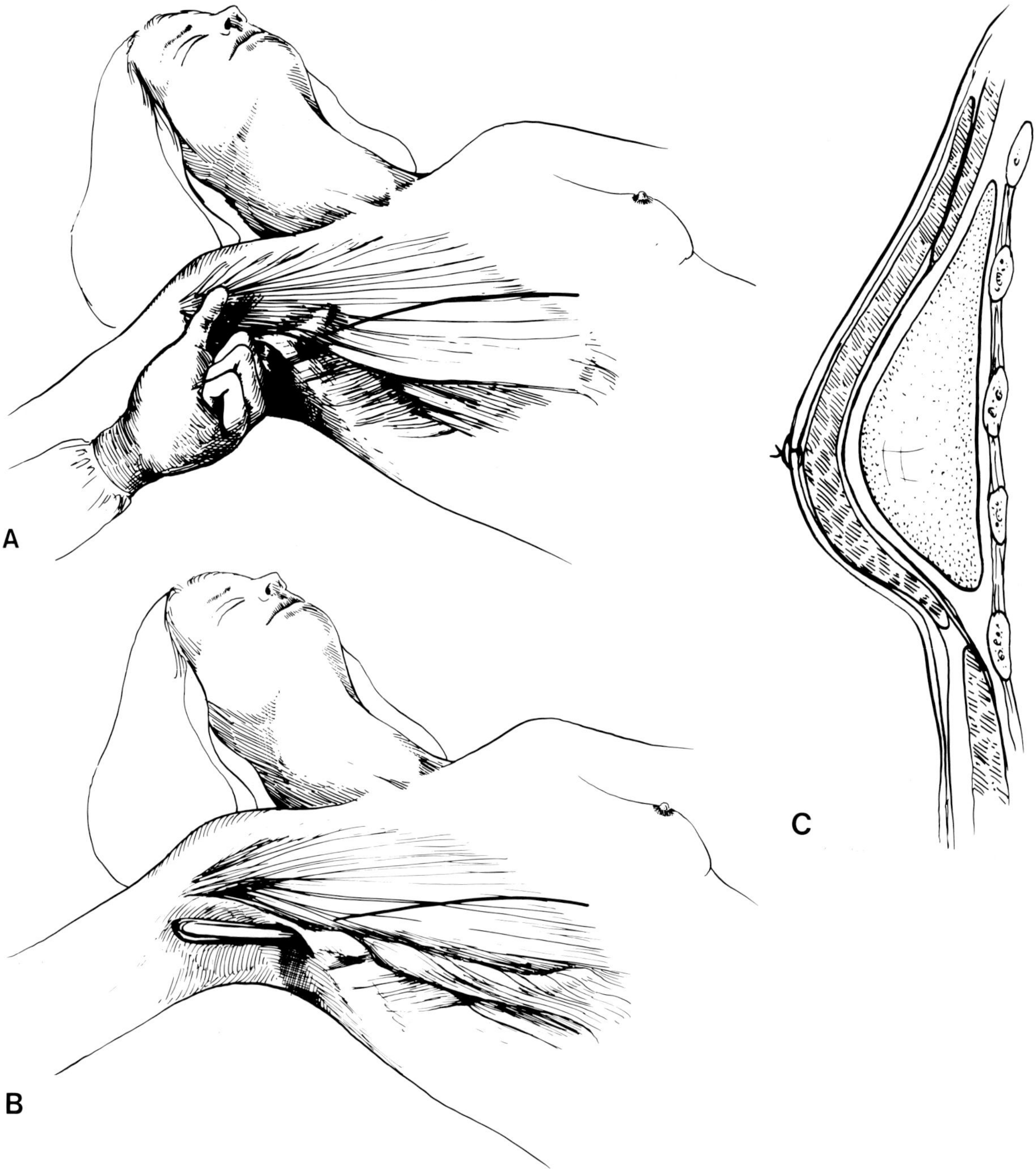

FIG. 10-1. Subpectoral breast reconstruction following modified radical mastectomy when an adequate amount of skin and muscle are present to accommodate an implant. The subpectoral pocket is created through a small incision in the axilla or through the old mastectomy scar. First by finger dissection (*A*) and then with a large uterine dilator (*B*), a large pocket is created, extending the dissection to create a symmetrical inframammary fold. (*C*) The lateral view demonstrates the subpectoral position of the breast implant.

In general, reconstruction should be performed when the incisional scar is matured and the chest wall skin is soft and pliable. This is usually at least 3 months from the time of mastectomy. Reconstruction before scar maturity may cause excessive firmness to the reconstructed breast.

Problems in Selection of Ablative Operative Procedures

DENERVATED PECTORALIS MAJOR

When possible, for most general surgeons modified radical mastectomy has become the choice ablative procedure for breast cancer. However, some general surgeons denervate the pectoralis major during modified radical mastectomy. It then becomes a thin, atrophic muscle that will not provide adequate soft tissue bulk suitable for prosthesis coverage.[8] As a result, replacement with the latissimus dorsi muscle or an abdominal flap becomes necessary in order to create a soft, natural-appearing breast. Denervation of the pectoralis major can be avoided by preservation of the medial and lateral pectoral nerves and by *never* dividing the pectoralis major muscle.

MASTECTOMY SCAR

Oblique or vertical scars extending to the axilla detract from the aesthetic result that can be achieved with reconstruction. The scar is difficult to hide in bathing suits and low-cut dresses. A transverse incision with a gentle upward curve laterally is the best for reconstructive purposes. This allows placement of a subpectoral implant through the lateral portion of the mastectomy incision without an additional incision (Fig. 10-1). All too often, the incision is designed without regard to postoperative aesthetics. This is inexcusable.

THE LATISSIMUS DORSI MYOCUTANEOUS FLAP

The latissimus dorsi myocutaneous flap is frequently used for breast reconstruction following mastectomy.[2] Based on its major pedicle, the thoracodorsal artery and vein, the muscle and an ellipse of overlying skin can be rotated from a pivot point in the axilla to resurface the anterior chest wall and replace the missing skin and muscle that were removed at the time of mastectomy.[1] One must carefully plan the position of the skin island so that it will be rotated easily to its new position on the anterior chest to replace the missing skin where it is needed and also so that the underlying latissimus muscle will be located in the proper position for maximal resurfacing of the chest wall and subclavicular, and axillary deformities. When indicated, the humeral origin of the latissimus must be detached and transferred anteriorly for correction of the missing lateral pectoral fold. We prefer to ignore the old mastectomy scar in most cases, placing the skin island at the inframammary fold and extending it laterally along the normal breast contour (Fig. 10-2).[9]

Placement of the skin island by opening the old mastectomy scar is acceptable as well in the appropriate patient.

Complications of Reconstructive Procedures

PROSTHESIS PLACEMENT

The implant *must* be placed under muscle in order to attain breast softness. Moreover, subcutaneous placement is more likely to cause skin necrosis and should *never* be done. If functional muscle is absent, muscle such as the latissimus dorsi should be brought into the defect to cover the prosthesis or a transverse abdominal island flap used that allows for breast reconstruction without a prosthesis.

The inframammary fold must be marked carefully with the patient in the upright position. The inferior margin of the pocket should extend about 2 cm below this fold. It is preferable to place the implant too low than too high. If the implant is found to be too low in the early postoperative period, it can usually be corrected by supporting the implant with tape in the desired position. If the implant is placed too high, only surgery can correct the deformity. In addition, lateral dissection of the pocket must be carefully controlled so the implant will fall to the side the same as the unoperated breast. Failure to perform lateral dissection properly (beneath the serratus muscle when a flap is not used) can result in severe deformity because the implant is either too anterior or too lateral.Superior dissection should extend to the clavicle and medially to the sternum.

FAILURE TO USE A FLAP

If the pectoralis major muscle is absent, denervated, or partially resected, a muscle flap must be used to cover the implant. If additional skin is required, a myocutaneous flap must be used to achieve the best results. Failure to cover the implant with muscle and provide tension-free skin closure will produce a poor aesthetic result. Of course, there are borderline cases in which skin deficiency is questionable. Frequently, however, most patients are best treated with a latissimus dorsi myocutaneous flap or a transverse abdominal island flap.

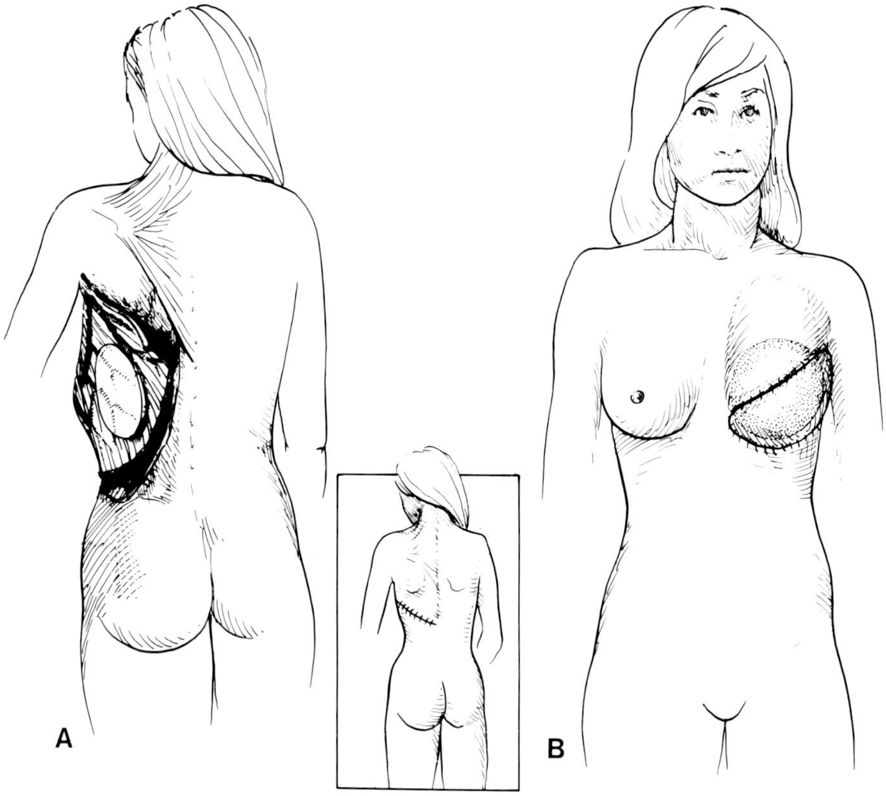

FIG. 10-2. (*A*) A large segment of the latissimus dorsi muscle is elevated with an island of overlying skin. Based on its major axial blood supply from the thoracodorsal pedicle high in the axilla, the flap is rotated anteriorly. The muscle will simulate the missing pectoralis major, and the skin island replaces the skin that was removed at the time of the mastectomy. The skin is placed in the inframammary fold to give the breast a natural appearance (*A, inset; B*).

PLACEMENT OF MYOCUTANEOUS FLAP

The mastectomy breast scar may be ignored in most patients and the myocutaneous flap placed in the inframammary fold extending up laterally. This minimizes the visible scar if the patient is wearing a low-cut dress and provides the forward projection where it is needed. Designing the skin island with a lazy S curvature may enhance the breast contour.

FAILURE OF LATISSIMUS DORSI MYOCUTANEOUS FLAP

Uncommonly, necrosis of this reliable flap may occur. If the tunnel from the posterior to the anterior chest is not made wide enough, there will be excessive pressure on the pedicle when the usual postoperative swelling occurs within the flap. This will result in venous or arterial occlusion and lead to irreversible soft tissue ischemia. Excessive twisting of the pedicle or tension on the flap when it is placed on the anterior chest wall could also result in flap necrosis. If the thoracodorsal artery was sacrificed at the time of mastectomy, the reconstructive surgeon must be careful to preserve the feeder branch between the serratus anterior and latissimus dorsi muscles, for this branch becomes the dominant arterial supply to the latissimus when the thoracodorsal pedicle has been divided.[7] If the motor nerve has also been cut, muscle atrophy will develop and the reliability of the flap is markedly reduced. Of course, severance of the thoracodorsal pedicle at the time of reconstruction will almost inevitably result in flap death. Care must even be taken in later procedures in which one wishes to divide the thoracodorsal pedicle. It should always be clamped first, atraumatically, and the viability of the skin island assessed.

PROSTHESIS FAILURE

All breast prostheses on the market today are made of silicone, and all produce some degree of foreign-body reaction. If this is severe, then capsular contraction will occur, which results in unnatural breast firmness and an external spherical deformity of the breast. The silicone elastomer envelope may disrupt, leaking silicone gel or saline, depending on the filler used within the implant. Although rare, silicone gel extruded from the damaged implant may form a foreign-body giant cell or granulomatous reaction. For these reasons, we prefer to use a double-lumen implant wherein both chambers are filled with saline at the time of surgery.* Because of the small volume

*American Heyer Schulte Company, Goleta, CA

in the outer chamber, outer chamber failure would not cause a noticeable difference in breast size. Only failure of both chambers would require replacement. Moreover, fluid leakage of saline would be innocuous in contrast to silicone gel leakage, which could form local granuloma or migrate some distance. Silicone migration or granuloma formation could also be confused with recurrent breast carcinoma. Frequently, the surgeon may cause implant failure by damaging the implant upon insertion. Closure of muscle around the implant may result in implant damage when the point or back end of the needle scratches across the surface of the silicone elastomer shell. Therefore, deep sutures should be preplaced prior to implant insertion and tied down after implant insertion.

IMPROPER IMPLANT SIZE

To avoid asymmetry, one should attempt to match the volume of the opposite breast unless the opposite breast is excessively large. Several measuring devices are available to give a rough guide to implant size. Test implants of various sizes are also available to be used at surgery as a guide to selecting the proper implant. It is always wise to err on the large side because it is easier to make the implant smaller than to increase the size of the pocket. This is because replacement with a larger implant will require additional dissection to enlarge the pocket. Moreover, if the implant is reduced in size at a second stage, the reconstructed breast will often develop a slight ptotic look, which may at times improve the match with the normal breast.

NIPPLE–AREOLAR RECONSTRUCTION

Nipple–areolar banking in the groin at the time of mastectomy used to be a popular procedure. However, the technique is to be condemned today because nipple–areolar placement in the groin may seed cancer in this area. Breast cancers have about a 25% periareolar involvement.[6,12] Moreover, "banked nipples" often become hypopigmented and are unsuitable for transfer to the reconstructed breast. The reconstructive surgeon can create a more aesthetic areolar complex using full-thickness skin grafts from the pigmented area of the upper inner thigh. The donor site can be closed primarily, and the areolar color match is usually excellent. The nipple is reconstructed by sharing the opposite nipple. If ptosis correction is done on the opposite breast, areolar sharing may also be done. The corkscrew-sharing procedure described by Cronin and colleagues is mentioned only to be condemned. It results in a bizarre corkscrewlike areola.[3]

Nipple–areolar reconstruction should usually be delayed for 2 months to 6 months following creation of the breast mound to avoid malposition of the nipple–areolar complex. No matter how carefully one places the nipple–areolar complex at the time of the primary procedure, the breast will change shape over several months and "settle" so that the nipple-areolar complex that looks perfect at surgery may appear in a very abnormal position several months later.

SURGICAL ALTERNATIVES IN BREAST RECONSTRUCTION

Alternative flaps can be used (1) when the patient does not want an internal prosthesis and desires reconstruction with autogenous tissue; (2) when large amounts of skin and fat are required; or (3) when one does not wish to turn the patient during surgery. Repositioning is required when a latissimus dorsi musculocutaneous flap is used for reconstruction. The most promising flap for breast reconstruction without an implant is the transverse abdominal island flap based on one superior epigastric pedicle. This flap allows for total breast reconstruction without the use of a prosthesis. The operation first described by Hartrampf, Scheflan, and Black opens new vistas for breast reconstruction.[5] A large transverse abdominal ellipse, which is commonly removed at the time of abdominoplasty, may be used with the entire rectus muscle on one side based on one superior epigastric pedicle (Fig. 10-3). This new flap will reconstruct the entire breast without use of a prosthesis. The resulting donor scar is in a highly desirable suprapubic location; the breast is reconstructed with autogenous tissues; and the patient receives an additional benefit of the abdominal lipectomy, which further enhances her body image. Abdominal hernia would appear to be the major complication of this procedure, especially below the arcuate line. Therefore, enough anterior rectus fascia must be left to allow for careful closure of the anterior rectus sheath.

Free flaps of latissimus dorsi, omentum, and buttock have been utilized for breast reconstruction but should be used only under very unusual circumstances.[4] The other alternatives described are safer and often can be completed in less time by most surgeons.

INFECTION AND HEMATOMA

Infection requires removal of the implant, in most instances, waiting several months until healing is complete, and then reinsertion of another implant. Although the data are inconclusive, perioperative antibiotics may decrease the incidence of infection with breast reconstruction.

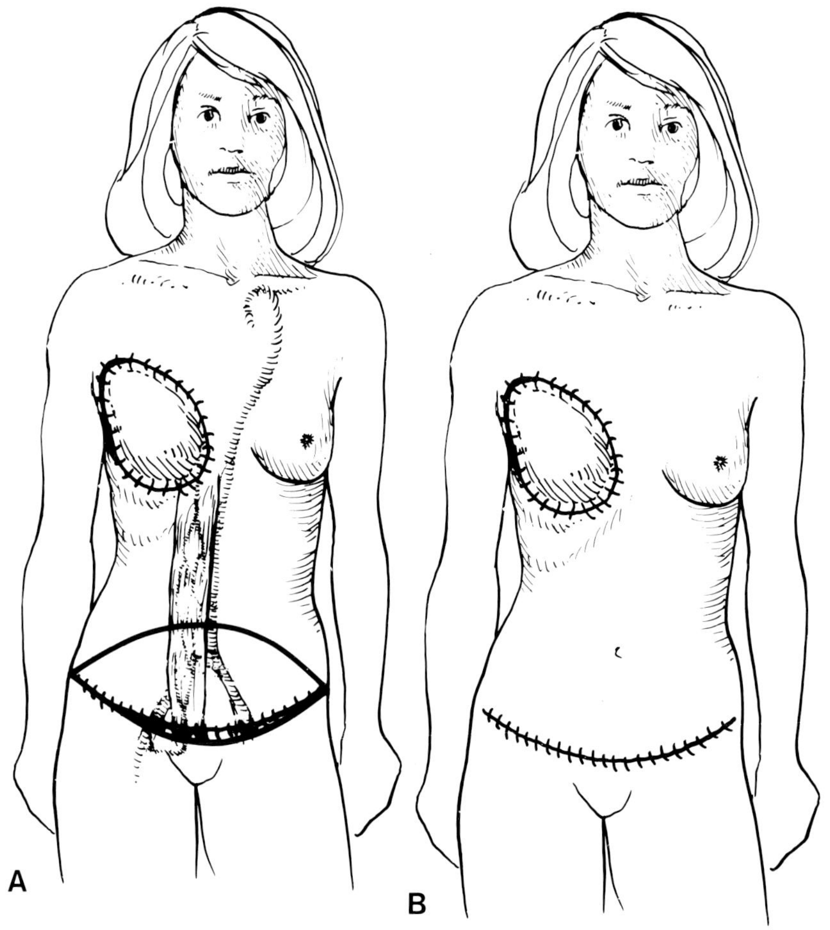

FIG. 10-3. (*A*) Based on one rectus abdominis muscle and its underlying pedicle, the superior deep epigastric vessels, a large ellipse of skin and fat is tunneled under the abdominal apron and brought up to the chest wall, where it is reshaped to look like a breast (*B*). The anterior rectus sheath is carefully repaired to prevent abdominal hernia, particularly below the arcuate line, where no posterior rectus sheath exists.

Hematoma formation underneath the reconstructed breast is quite rare. Whenever present, however, the incidence of unnatural hardening of the breast is high even after appropriate expeditious drainage.

References

1. Bostwick J III, Scheflan M: The latissimus dorsi flap—a one-stage breast reconstruction. Clin Plast Surg 7:A, 1980
2. Bostwick J III, Vasconez LO, Jurkiewicz MJ: Breast reconstruction of the radical mastectomy. Plast Reconstr Surg 61:685, 1978
3. Cronin TD, Cronin DE: Nipple areola reconstruction. In Gant JD and Vasconez LO (eds): Post-Mastectomy Reconstruction. Baltimore, Williams & Wilkins, 1981
4. Gant JD, Serafin D, Buncke H Jr: Free flap reconstruction of the breast. In Gant JD and Vasconez LO (eds): Post-Mastectomy Reconstruction. Baltimore, Williams & Wilkins, 1981
5. Hartrampf CR, Scheflan M, Black PW: Breast reconstruction with a transverse abdominal island flap. Plast Reconstr Surg 69:216, 1982
6. Lagios MD et al: A guide to the frequency of nipple involvement in breast cancer. Am J Surg 138(1):135, 1979
7. Maxwell GP, Manson PN, Hoopes JE: Experience with thirteen latissimus dorsi myocutaneous free flaps. Plast Reconstr Surg 64:1, 1979
8. Moosman DA: Anatomy of pectoral nerves and their preservation in modified mastectomy. Am J Surg 139(6):883, 1980
9. Ruetschi MS, LeWinn LR, Chaglassian FA: Variation of latissimus dorsi design for post-mastectomy reconstruction. Ann Plast Surg 6(3), 1981
10. Shamberger RC, Devereux DF, Murray FB: The effect of chemotherapeutic agents on wound healing. International Chemotherapeutic Agents in Surgical Oncology 4:15, 1981
11. Silverman JJ, Cohen IK: Psychological aspects of breast cancer and reconstructive surgery. Va Med Monthly 106:140, 1971
12. Smith J, Payne SW, Carney AJ: Involvement of the nipple and areola in carcinoma of the breast. Surg Gynecol Obstet 143(4):546, 1976

11
Complications of Lymphadenectomy and Lymphedema

Charles L. Puckett | Donald Silver

OVERVIEW

The complications of lymphadenectomy may be grouped into two general areas: those related to the surgical wound and the occasional problem of resultant lymphedema.

Wound Complications

TREATMENT FAILURE

A potential complication of any surgical effort is the failure of that procedure to accomplish its goal. The goals for regional lymphadenectomy (in the neck, axillary, or groin) are both diagnostic (staging) and therapeutic (ablation). The presence of residual tumor in the wound after lymphadenectomy obviously represents a therapeutic failure but may have adequately served the staging goal.

> Lymphography may offer information about the status of lymph nodes prior to and following surgery. The size and number of lymph nodes in the different areas vary, especially in the pelvic and lumbar areas, and from patient to patient. As it is very difficult to interpret defects in the lymph nodes from a single x-ray, anterior–posterior, lateral, and right and left oblique views are recommended to delineate filling defects, replacement, or enlargement of lymph nodes. The poppyseed oil disappears slowly from noninflamed lymph nodes, with 70% still being visualized at 1 year and 12% at 2 years after injection, so that postoperative or intraoperative x-ray film can indicate the thoroughness of a lymphadenectomy.[5]

SKIN SLOUGH

The majority of wound complications are related to skin slough. Late hemorrhage and infection often result from this problem. A major cause of skin slough, assuming gentle surgical technique, is preoperative irradiation. Skin loss, while uncommon following axillary lymphadenectomy, still occasionally occurs in radical neck surgery and is a frequent problem after groin lymphadenectomy. Skin slough in each of these regional locations is particularly dangerous because major vessels (carotid, axillary, femoral arteries) may be exposed.

DIAGNOSIS. The early diagnosis of a skin slough may be difficult. Eventually, however, the slough will be manifest as a necrotic and blackening eschar. The diagnosis can be established earlier by the intravenous injection of fluorescein dye (Fig. 11-1). Fluorescein staining under a Wood's lamp 20 minutes after injection closely correlates with adequate perfusion and thus tissue viability. The failure to "stain" a suspicious area is virtually synonymous with evolving flap loss. Intraoperative diagnosis may allow excision of the ischemic area and selection of an alternative closure technique (such as a flap). It will, at least, signal the need for some protective mechanism for the vessels (e.g., a muscle flap placed over the artery).

TREATMENT of later-evolving skin sloughs will be dictated largely by the occurrence of major vessel exposure. Small or nonstrategically located sloughs may be allowed to granulate and heal by secondary intention; or they may be closed with a skin graft. Larger sloughs with vessel exposure should be treated by débridement and flap coverage. Fortunately, a plethora of flaps are available as a result of the recent widespread interest in the various myocutaneous flaps. In the neck, trapezius, latissimus dorsi, and pectoralis major flaps are used most often. The deltopectoral flap is an old standard and reliable choice, as well. Although we have not observed significant axillary skin flap sloughs, the latissimus

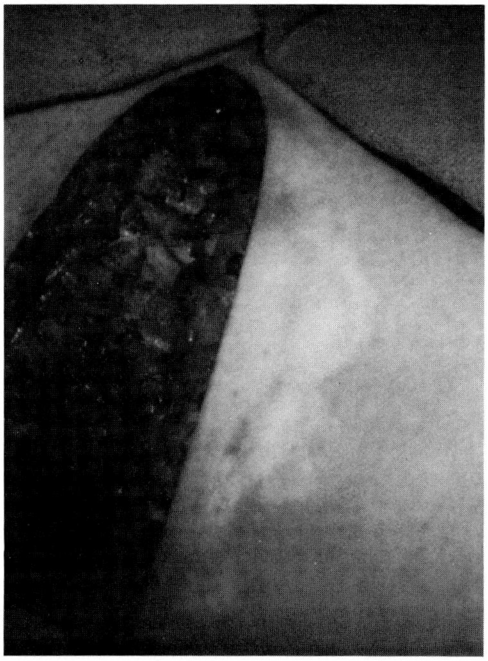

FIG. 11-1. This groin wound was photographed with blue and orange filters 20 minutes after injection with fluorescein dye. The right margin of the wound, which appears blue, represents a failure of fluorescein staining, which would appear yellow. A persistent lack of staining (in the absence of vasoconstrictors) indicates impending necrosis. This part of the wound should be excised primarily.

dorsi flap is an adjacent good choice should necrosis occur. A number of muscles and myocutaneous flaps are available to resurface the groin. These include the sartorius, gracilis, rectus femoris, and the very ample tensor fascia lata flaps. One of these choices should be available in almost any case. In the rare instance that one of these is not, a "free flap" may be considered (see Chap. 8).

PREVENTION. Obviously, the prevention of a complication is preferable to correcting one successfully. Skin slough appears to be related to (1) inappropriate or poorly designed incisions, (2) excessive thinning of the flaps (thus injuring the subdermal plexus), and (3) the preoperative use of large doses of radiation. The use of the modified McFee incision for a radical neck dissection and the avoidance of preoperative radiation have virtually eliminated skin slough following radical lymphadenectomy in the neck. Institutions and surgeons that continue to use preoperative irradiation report a significantly higher incidence of skin flap loss.[26] In the groin, the use of a more vertical incision and the avoidance of a long, thin inferior–lateral flap have decreased the occurrence of skin slough. The intraoperative use of fluorescein dye to identify ischemic areas has also enabled immediate correction and thus avoidance of late skin-slough problems.

NERVE INJURY

Nerve injury is, fortunately, not frequently associated with lymphadenectomy in any of the three regions. In the axilla, the annoying anesthesia associated with sacrifice of the intercostobrachiocutaneous nerve is an occasional complaint, but a major motor or sensory deficit in the arm is rare. In the groin, major nerve damage is unusual, presumably owing in part to the fact that the femoral nerve has a diffuse structure and composite injury would be less likely. Hypoesthesia is an occasional mild complaint but is rarely of consequence.

Potential nerve injuries in the neck are many and varied. Probably the most common one of major concern is *phrenic nerve injury* with unilateral diaphragmatic paralysis. The diagnosis is often not made until several days postoperatively when a chest film reveals an elevated and paralyzed hemidiaphragm. Treatment usually consists of careful observation to be certain that pulmonary mechanics and toilet are progressing satisfactorily. Only in the patient with a minimal respiratory reserve is there likely to be a significant problem. Obviously, in the pulmonary cripple, decompensation may ensue and may necessitate tracheostomy and respirator assistance. Preventive techniques include careful anatomic dissection with particular care being exercised when the cervical cutaneous branches are transected. At this point, with traction on the specimen, the phrenic nerve can be tented and attached to the neck-dissection specimen. Careful identification of these cervical cutaneous branches can help avoid injury.

The nerve stimulator is also useful in identifying nerves during the dissection in order to prevent their injury. Fortunately, injury of the lingual, glossopharyngeal, vagus, and hypoglossal nerves is uncommon since they are easily identified.

Injury to the spinal accessory nerve is often a planned part of the lymphadenectomy procedure. The major disability subsequently is related to loss of shoulder girdle support by the trapezius muscle. Patients often complain of a chronic ache in the shoulder region. A variety of muscle transfers using muscles such as the levator scapulae offer a degree of improvement of this disability, but some discomfort is likely to persist. Prevention of this problem is offered by the various modified neck-dissection procedures that preserve the spinal accessory nerve or, at least, the branch to the trapezius. If one chooses to save the spinal accessory nerve, magnification can aid in the dissection. In selected cases, this preservation of the nerve apparently does not compromise the therapeutic potential of the procedure.

HEMORRHAGE

EARLY HEMORRHAGE. The potential for immediate or early postoperative hemorrhage is ubiquitous to all surgical procedures. Hemorrhage and hematoma are usually heralded by swelling at the operative site. If drains are in place, rapid passage of blood through the drains may be evident. Significant hemorrhage is treated in the operating room by control of the bleeding vessel. Prevention of postoperative hemorrhage is mandated by meticulous hemostasis at the time of surgery. Closing an oozing or wet surgical wound is an invitation to disaster. Although sealed suction-drainage systems will not prevent major hemorrhage, some protection against the occurrence of hematoma may be offered by pulling the flaps down snugly and preventing the accumulation of fluid.

LATE HEMORRHAGE is often related to wound problems, particularly skin slough with secondary exposure of large vessels. The most dreaded complication of radical lymphadenectomy procedures is a late major arterial bleeding as a result of vessel exposure. Mortality related to carotid "blow out" is very high, and only heroic efforts with rapid return to the operating room can offer an opportunity for salvage. From the diagnostic standpoint, any late bleeding from a lymphadenectomy site should be considered serious and should prompt a careful evaluation of the wound. When significant late bleeding does occur, direct application of pressure will usually control the bleeding but in the neck may do so at the expense of cerebral circulation. Exposure of the proximal and distal healthy vessel with careful ligation away from the wound is necessary. Rarely is vascular bypass feasible or required. Unfortunately, even with control of the vessel, the neurologic sequelae of carotid ligation may be devastating. Obviously, the best management of this situation is prevention, and the best assurance against late carotid hemorrhage is a healthy wound with hearty skin flaps covering the vessels. The incidence of carotid blow out is quite low in series not employing preoperative irradiation, versus those that do.[26] Fortunately, axillary artery blow out is extremely rare, and the femoral artery seems to have more resistance to this problem than does the carotid.

INFECTION

Infection is another complication indigenous to all surgical procedures. If there is a sealed wound, wound infection is usually indicated by erythema, swelling, and fluctuance. Culture and smear are indicated for accurate diagnosis. Treatment of the infection requires proper wound toilet and the replacement of unhealthy tissues with healthy ones. Débridement, frequent dressing changes, and then later coverage with a flap (particularly a myocutaneous one) will usually allow a satisfactory result. Treatment of an abscess is the same as in any other area of the body. Antibiotic coverage is often indicated, but rarely is a sophisticated antibiotic duel necessary. In general, healthy wounds do not become infected even when there is some degree of contamination. It is worth emphasizing that most infections are usually secondary problems following skin slough. Careful and gentle surgical technique with the avoidance of strangulated wads of tissue that have been ligated or cauterized will help prevent these problems. Preoperative irradiation is another factor predisposing the patient to the development of infection.[1]

LYMPH FISTULA

A problem unique to radical lymphadenectomy procedures is the occurrence of a lymph leak with either fistula or lymphocele. This problem probably occurs with equal frequency in the neck, axilla, and groin. Usually, it is self limiting and, if it is not accompanied by infection, will generally resolve without permanent problem. Lymphocele is usually diagnosed from the observation of swelling or lymph accumulation under the flaps. As long as there is no erythema or temperature elevation, one should not feel great urgency about treating this problem. However, unless the fluid is evacuated, the flaps will not adhere to the wound and a more chronic problem may ensue. The lymph accumulation usually responds to needle aspiration on one or several occasions. This should be done using careful sterile technique to avoid the introduction of organisms. Occasionally the recurrence of fluid requires catheter drainage.

If a skin slough is associated, a more chronic problem can develop from fistula formation, but even here the problem usually resolves with time. Since the etiology of lymph fistula is probably related to the transection of lymphatics without ligature (and the failure to appreciate this at the time of surgery), prevention is best accomplished by careful technique with meticulous identification and control of lymphatics. Although lymph has most of the proteins and other substances necessary for coagulation, their amounts are reduced and coagulation is inefficient. Therefore, the electric cautery is probably not a satisfactory method to control lymph leak from transected lymphatics. The problem of lymph fistula is somewhat more troublesome in the left neck than in the right because of the presence of the thoracic duct and its tributaries. Closed suction-seal drainage with a strong negative pressure may help prevent this problem by assisting in the early adherence of the skin flaps to the wound.

SCAR

Problems related to the scar include contracture and hypertrophy. Fortunately, both of these problems are usually not of major concern. Occasionally an axillary scar contracture will be functionally significant, but this is rare (as it is also in the neck and the groin). Problems with scar are more frequently of aesthetic than of functional concern. Especially in women the scars in the neck and those of the radical mastectomy may be difficult to conceal. Revision of these scars and possibly a Z-plasty, other flap, or a graft may be indicated. Careful tissue handling and healthy wounds will prevent many of the scar problems. The use of the modified McFee incision in the neck usually offers good scars without significant contracture or hypertrophy. The avoidance of longitudinal scars in the axilla at right angles to the axillary fold will usually prevent problems here. Interestingly, the safest incision (vertical) for groin dissection is also one that should lend itself most likely to contracture. However, this has not been a frequent problem.

AESTHETIC PROBLEMS from lymphadenectomy are often related to the disfiguring scars, particularly in the case of radical mastectomy. However, other problems can occur. In the thin neck, the removal of the sternocleidomastoid is especially noticeable. Although some muscle transfers have been offered as a correction of this deformity, very little realistic improvement can be offered. The aesthetic disadvantage of radical mastectomy is obvious. Fortunately, very excellent reconstructive measures are currently available. This will not be dealt with in this chapter, but the latissimus dorsi myocutaneous flap has virtually revolutionized breast reconstruction (see Chap. 10). The resection of the pectoralis major muscle leaves an awkward hollow below the shoulder that is very difficult to correct secondarily. Modified radical mastectomy procedures with the preservation of the pectoralis major muscle have prevented this problem. Also, the use of transverse incisions and the avoidance of the upper extent of the scar being visible have improved aesthetic results. One of the most significant aesthetic problems that can follow lymphadenectomy occurs when there is development of lymphedema.

Lymphedema

PATHOPHYSIOLOGY

Chronic obstructive lymphedema secondary to lymphadenectomy is a frequently disabling, often confusing, and consistently incurable disorder. Why one patient develops secondary lymphedema following lymphadenectomy and another does not is an unanswered question. However, if one considers the variable severity of lymphedema to be a reflection of the degree of lymphatic obstruction, some answers are suggested. An explanation offered for the different age at onset of the various primary lymphedemas has been that they represent degrees of the same disability. The more severe the lymphatic abnormality, the earlier the lymphedema would be manifest (as in congenital types). A lesser degree of lymphatic abnormality may become manifest later in life or after infection or trauma further reduces the lymphatic channels to a disabling level. It is believed by some that the patients who develop obstructive lymphedema following lymphadenectomy were marginally compensated before surgery. Perhaps their number of lymphatic channels was congenitally deficient, compared to the norm, but was functioning adequately until surgical ablation reduced this number below the critical level. There seems no better explanation for why the same operation performed in a similar manner results in lymphedema in only a few cases. Furthermore, the occurrence of lymphedema does not seem directly related to the vigor with which lymphatic ablation is accomplished. Irradiation also increases the incidence, presumably by destroying more lymphatics.

The function of the lymphatics appears to be the removal of macromolecules from the interstitial space. The failure to do this adequately results in anoncotic disadvantage with resultant edema. Strangely, certain areas of the body, such as the brain, do not have lymphatics and yet seem to accomplish the functions of this system in some other equally satisfactory manner.

ANATOMY

Larger lymphatics are visible to the naked eye, and some, such as the thoracic duct, are quite striking in size. Because lymph is colorless, all lymphatics are more difficult to see than blood vessels. Lymphatics have delicate unidirectional valves that, together with muscular contraction, aid in the propulsion of lymph. Peripheral lymphatics have been observed to pulsate weakly, and these pulsations may also contribute to lymph flow. The lymphatic end point is the central venous circulation. The failure to return lymph from an area usually results in swelling. If this persists beyond 6 months, it is considered to be permanent lymphedema. The lymphatics in obstructive lymphedema are usually dilated and have incompetent valves; thus unidirectional flow is lost.

DIAGNOSIS

The diagnosis of obstructive or secondary lymphedema can usually be made by clinical evaluation. In the arm following axillary dissection, there are not

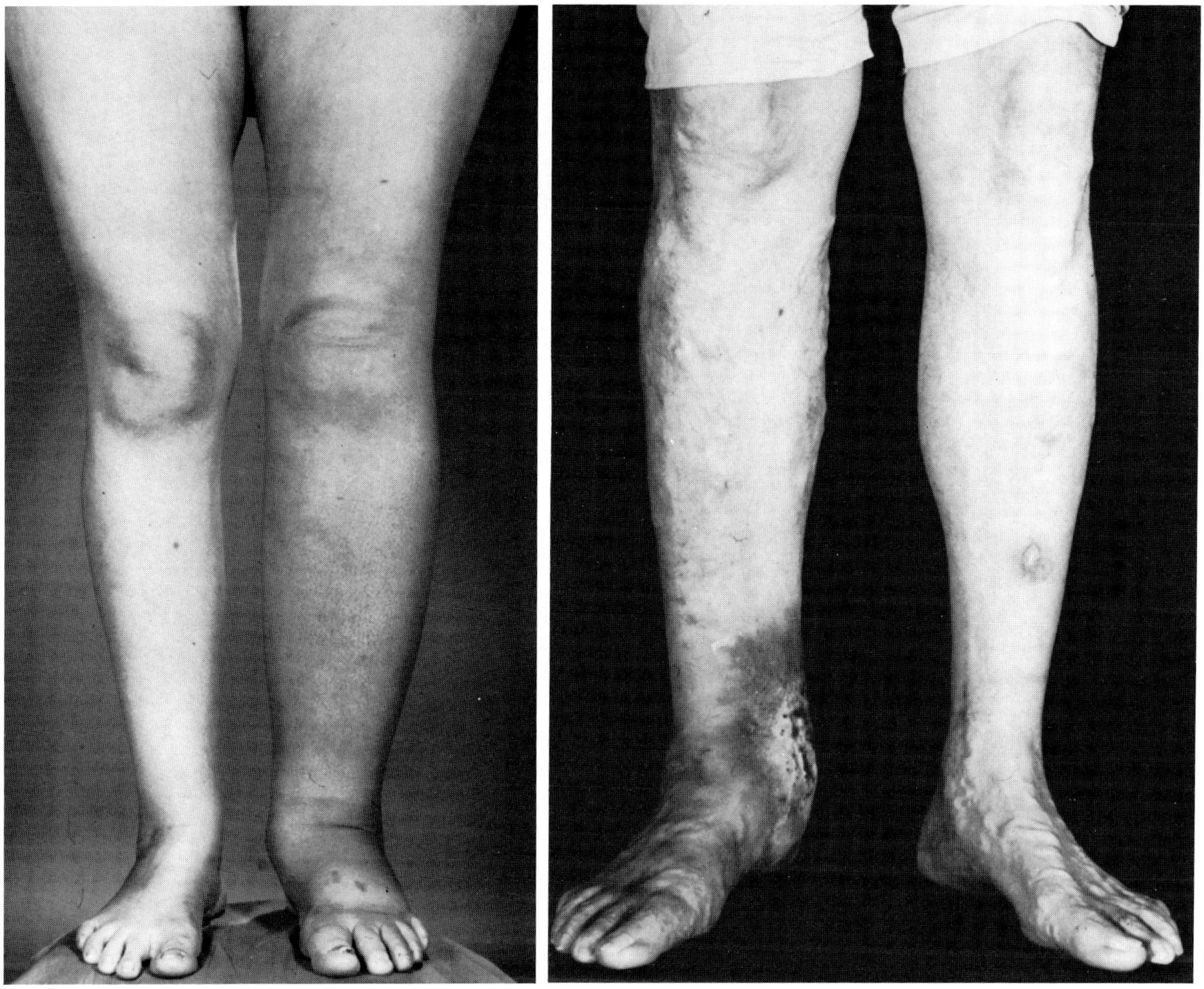

A B

FIG. 11-2. (*A*) A patient with lymphedema of the left leg. Note that there is no pigmentation and that the digits are slightly swollen (see Table 1). (*B*) A patient with postphlebitic venous insufficiency. Note the pigmentation and varicosities and the ulceration over the medial malleolus (see Table 1).

TABLE 11-1. DIFFERENTIATION OF LYMPHEDEMA FROM VENOUS INSUFFICIENCY

	Pigmentation	Swollen Digits	Ulceration	Verrucae	Infection
Lymphedema	No	Yes	Rare	Common	Lymphangitis frequently
Venous insufficiency	Usual	Rare	Often	No	Rare (unless ulceration)

many plausible alternative explanations for chronic swelling. In the lower extremity following inguinal lymphadenectomy there is only one significant rivaling diagnosis, venous insufficiency. For the most part, these disorders can be accurately differentiated by clinical signs. However, occasionally more sophisticated measures such as venography or lymphography may be necessary. Rarely, the two problems may coexist and complicate diagnosis and therapy (Fig. 11-2). Table 11-1 provides a handy checklist to differentiate lymphedema from venous insufficiency.

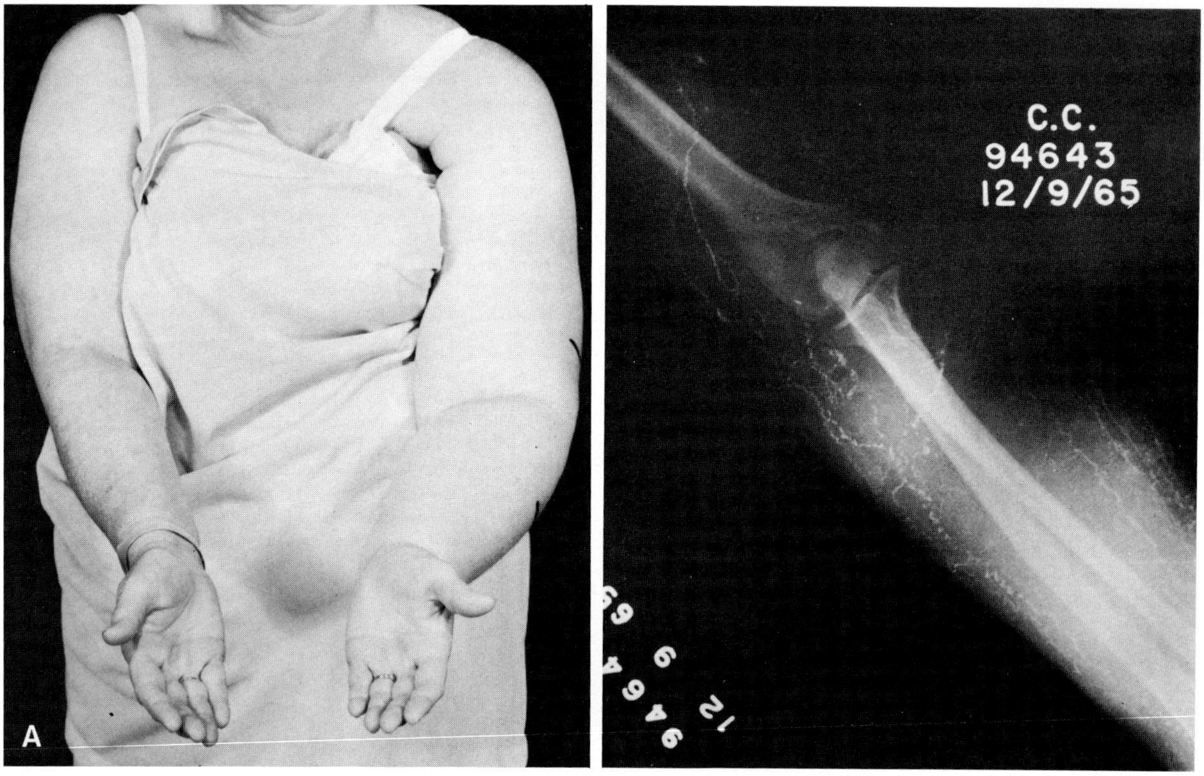

FIG. 11-3. (*A*) A patient with postmastectomy lymphedema of the left upper extremity. (*B*) A lymphogram of the patient shows dilated, tortuous lymphatics, indicative of retarded flow.

Obviously, systemic causes of edema (such as cardiac and renal) must be differentiated, but the history of lymphadenectomy and the unilateral nature of the swelling will usually eliminate these considerations. With the exception of venous insufficiency, diagnosis is usually not difficult.

Lymphography

Only within the past 30 years has clinical investigation of the lymphatic system utilized vital dyes to visualize surface lymphatics and iodinated oils to visualize radiographically deeper lymphatics and lymph nodes. Properly performed lymphography provides information about the functional status of the lymphatics of the extremities and thus helps with the classification of lymphedema. The lymphograms help establish whether the patient has hypoplastic (87%), aplastic (5%), or hyperplastic (8%) types of primary lymphedema or secondary lymphedema (Fig. 11-3).[12] Lymphography also is very useful in detecting primary and secondary tumors in peripheral, retroperitoneal, and other lymph nodes.

The method of lymphography popularized by Kinmonth has become the standard for lymphography.[10]

VITAL DYES. The patent blue used by Kinmonth, a 10% solution, is usually tolerated by most patients. We mix 0.5 ml of 10% patent blue with 1.5 ml of 1% lidocaine in order to reduce the discomfort of the dye injections. Koehler noted only 57 cases of sensitivity to the vital dyes during 32,000 lymphograms reported by 70 investigators.[13] Our experience parallels that of Kinmonth, with no significant complications from the dye.[12] Only small amounts of the dye are required, with the usual injection being 0.1 ml or 0.2 ml in each web space of the foot (Fig. 11-4). If larger amounts of dye are injected or if the patient is an infant, the urine may assume a bluish discoloration, much to the consternation of the nursing and anesthesia staff, unless they are forewarned.

CONTRAST MATERIAL. Iodinated poppy-seed oil is the contrast material most often used to visualize the lymphatic trunks and nodes. This oil is quite viscous and requires mechanical injectors to maintain a constant flow at pressures that should not rupture the lymphatics or cause extravasation of the contrast material. The minimum amount required to visualize the lymphatics is determined with serial radiographs but should not exceed 7 ml per lower extremity in adults (with 3 ml–4 ml per extremity being the rule). The contrast is usually injected at about 1 ml per 8 to 10 minutes.

COMPLICATIONS. Complications have been encountered from the vital dyes, the iodinated oils, the rate of the injection, and the interpretation of the lymphograms. Koehler noted only 40 patients who were sive infusion of the poppy-seed oil may result in too 32,000 lymphograms reviewed, while Kinmonth had only 2 patients who were sensitive to the "iodine in the preparation."[12, 13] A rapid infusion or an excessive infusion of the poppy-seed oil may result in too large a volume of the contrast reaching the lungs, with obstruction of pulmonary arterioles and adverse effects upon the patient's cardiopulmonary physiology. Koehler noted 81 pulmonary infarcts, 10 cases of pulmonary edema, 13 cases of pneumonia, and 10 cases of hemoptysis in the patients undergoing the 32,000 lymphograms.[13] Thus, the contrast should be given with care to patients with compromised pulmonary function. Frequent radiographs should be obtained during the infusion of the contrast material to be certain that the infusion is into a lymphatic rather than a vein. If an intravenous infusion occurs, the patient is at increased risk for pulmonary problems. Koehler also noted 24 cases of fever, 4 lymph fistulas, and 9 cases of cerebral dysfunction. In addition, 18 deaths occurred 3 hours to 21 days after the lymphograms.[13] Complications have been infrequent in our patients, and we have not observed aggravation of the lymphedema or infection.

Secondary Problems

FUNCTIONAL DISABILITY. The patient with a lymphedematous extremity will have functional disability directly proportionate to the degree of lymphedema. Mild cases offer little more than a cosmetic consideration. Extreme cases, however, may render the extremity functionless by virtue of the excessive weight and the mechanical disadvantage inhibiting movement of muscles and joints.

SKIN ULCERATION. Fortunately, skin ulceration is a rare occurrence in lymphedema, unlike its frequency in venous insufficiency. When ulceration occurs, however, the risk of infection in the form of lymphangitis seems more prevalent and potentially more dangerous. Therefore, impending or early skin breakdown should be meticulously cared for to prevent a full-thickness skin loss.

LYMPHANGITIS is a frequent problem in the patient with lymphedema. The portal of entry for the bacteria may occasionally be obvious, as with an ulceration or a specific injury, but often there is no specific cause. The risk of infection is much greater in lymphedematous extremities, perhaps owing to an immunologic disadvantage existent in the limb. Furthermore, each bout of lymphangitis probably pro-

FIG. 11-4. (*A*) Patent Blue dye injection in normal feet. Note the diffuse pattern, with little staining of the toes. (*B*) Patent Blue dye injected into the lymphedematous foot. Note the patchy pattern on the dorsum of the foot, indicating dilated lymphatics, and the dermal backflow into the toes.

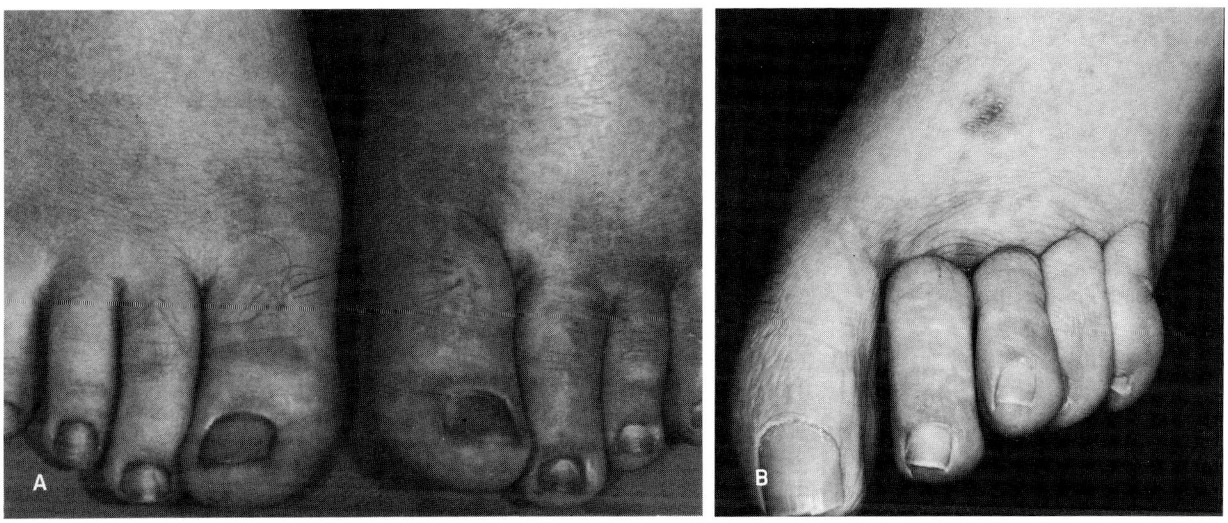

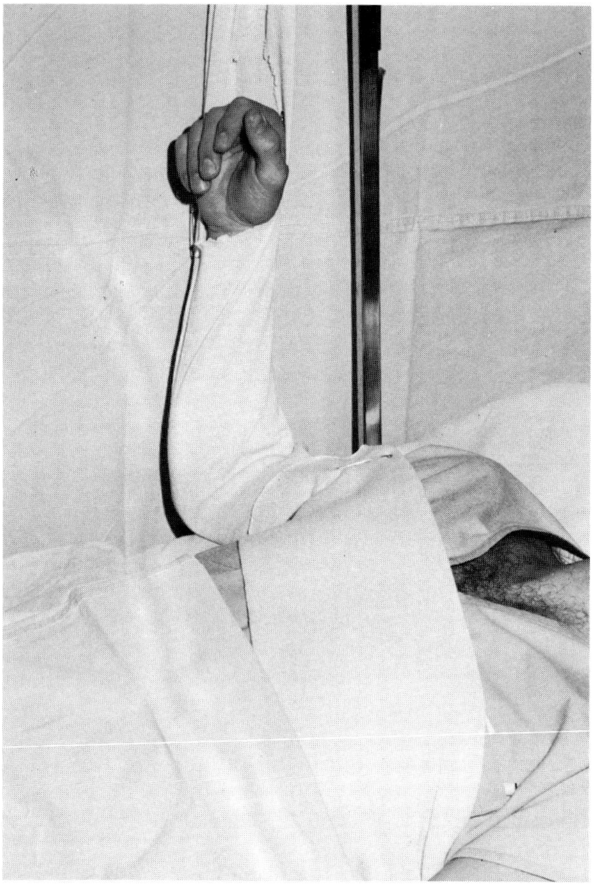

FIG. 11-5. The proper method of arm elevation. Pillow elevation alone is difficult to maintain with any movement by the patient. The stockinette, however, supports the arm resting on the bed or a pillow.

duces additional fibrosis and further loss of lymphatic channels. This compounds the problem and contributes to the potential for aggravation of the lymphedema. Lymphangitis should be treated vigorously at the first sign. Hospital admission with bed rest, extremity elevation, and intravenous antibiotics are usually rapidly successful in correcting these bouts of infection. Fortunately, pathogens are usually common varieties of streptococci and staphylococci and respond readily to traditional antibiotics such as penicillin.

VERUCCOUS CHANGES. The verrucae that occur, usually on the toes, in the more advanced stages of lymphedema are difficult to treat. Their presence is presumably related to an immunologic alteration that persists as long as the lymphedema does. Salicylic acid, podophyllin, and other wart remedies may help with individual troublesome lesions. However, success is often contingent upon relief or improvement in the degree of lymphedema.

HYGIENE. With severe lymphedema in which there is infolding of the skin at the joints and excessive skin stretching, hygiene may become difficult. Intertrigo may precipitate episodes of lymphangitis. Meticulous care of the skin should be encouraged along with the use of protective clothing and appropriate drying agents to prevent maceration.

TREATMENT

Medical Therapy

The treatment of the lymphedema patient should be considered predominately a nonsurgical effort. At present there is no surgical method consistently capable of eradicating this disorder, nor is there any medication yet available to alleviate the edema reliably. A major goal should be the education of the patient to an understanding of the disease. Once this is accomplished, the intelligent and well-intentioned patient can use common sense to live with the disorder, limiting its progression and the degree of disability as much as is possible.[11]

GRAVITATIONAL DRAINAGE. The patient must be taught the advantages of gravitational drainage of the extremity. This may require explaining with diagrams how the affected limb must be above the level of the heart for a significant period of time each day. The patient must understand that failure to improve the swelling indicates that the period of elevation is inadequate or that something else is wrong. Rarely is placement of the limb on a pillow adequate for a night's sleep. With lower-extremity edema, drainage can best be accomplished by elevating the entire foot of the bed with 8- to 10-inch blocks. The arm can be elevated efficiently by suspending it in a stockinette sling (Fig. 11-5).

ELASTIC SUPPORT. The patient should be educated in the use of elastic support. What is best is one of the heavy-gauge elastic-support garments specifically tailored for the individual (Jobst). The dangers of constriction with wrinkling must be pointed out. Elastic-bandage wrapping can be taught and may be used as a short-term adjunct to elevation and the stockings. It must be demonstrated that wrapping must be from distal to proximal parts of the extremity to avoid a tourniquet effect. Furthermore, the extremity should be wrapped in its entirety rather than a short segment of it, which might also act as a tourniquet.

PROGNOSIS AND RELATED TREATMENT. Gravitational drainage and elastic support in concert are the foundation of the conservative management of lymphedema. The patient who understands them and is diligent in their applications will usually be successful in controlling his lymphedema. The patient who does not can expect a progressive and deteriorating course.

Other adjunctive measures include meticulous hygiene to decrease the likelihood of surface infection and lymphangitis. The patient's weight must be controlled, as must other systemic conditions that predispose the patient to peripheral edema and thus increase the load on an already compromised system. In addition, lymphangitis should be treated promptly. In Europe considerable interest has evolved in the use of benzopyrones for the control of lymphedema.[4] Several series have reported encouraging results. The benzopyrones seem to work by lysing proteins and enhancing phagocytosis.

Lymphedema patients are often a neglected group. Many times they are shuttled from one physician to another, perhaps because of professional lack of interest or understanding of the problem. Consequently, many patients arrive for care at a rather advanced stage of lymphedema. Other patients will have a progressive, deteriorating course even with good medical management. For these patients, surgery may become necessary.

Surgery

Conceptually, the surgical approach to the treatment of lymphedema follows one of two courses. One method is an attempt to ablate the lymphedematous tissue, and the other is an attempt to augment lymph flow from the lymphedematous area.

ABLATIVE TREATMENT. In the ablative techniques, the edematous subcutaneous tissue is excised. The wound is then covered by either skin grafts or flaps. Coverage of the wound with skin grafts is known as the *Charles procedure*.[2] In this operation, all skin and subcutaneous tissues are removed down to and including the fascia of the muscles of the extremity. Skin grafts are then harvested either from another area of the body or occasionally from the removed skin of the edematous leg. (There are both proponents and opponents of this approach, some feeling that it predisposes the patient to a later development of verrucae.) Aesthetic results following this procedure are usually wretched, but amazing functional improvement may accompany the removal of an enormous amount of edematous tissue. Recurrence seems related to the adequacy of tissue removal. The durability of the skin grafts directly applied to muscle is often less than optimal, and later revisions are frequent.

Excision of the subcutaneous tissue and replacement with skin flaps is often (erroneously) referred to as the *Kondoleon procedure;* it is also known (more correctly) as the *Sistrunk* or *Homans* procedure.[9, 14, 23] It has been most extensively described and reported in recent years by Miller and can appropriately be referred to as the *Miller procedure*.[16, 17] Cases treated successfully in this manner have far superior aesthetic results to those accomplished by the Charles procedure. However, the very thin skin flaps are treacherous, and flap loss is not uncommon. Massively swollen legs are sometimes difficult to treat in this manner. Usually two, and occasionally three or more, operative procedures are necessary. The medial (or lateral) side of the leg can be approached first with the elevation of anterior and posterior skin flaps followed by the removal of the subcutaneous tissue to the level of the muscle. The flaps are trimmed to remove redundancy and closed with suction drainage. Results reported with this method have been quite good.

AUGMENT LYMPH FLOW. The procedures to augment lymph flow fall into one of three categories: to develop communications between the superficial and the deep systems, to secure alternative drainage, or to establish lymphovenous anastomosis.

ESTABLISH COMMUNICATIONS BETWEEN SYSTEMS. Because of the suspected competence and adequacy of the deep lymphatic system, various attempts have been made to establish communications between the inadequate superficial system and the normal deep system. In 1912, Kondoleon described an attempt to do this by creating a fascial window.[14] In the 1960s, Thompson introduced his buried-dermal-flap operation, which was intended to establish communications from the dermal lymphatics to the deep system.[24, 25] He extensively reported on this operation with good early results in 92% of his cases. Kinmonth has endorsed this operation as his procedure of choice, but other authors have been unable to produce consistently good results with it.[3] Many have believed that the main value of the procedure derives from its ablative potential and that no genuine communication between superficial and deep lymphatics can be established.

SECURE ALTERNATIVE DRAINAGE. A second approach to the augmentation of lymph flow is to provide some alternative mechanism of lymph drainage from the lymphedematous area. Handley described the subcutaneous "wick" principle in 1908.[8] However, the procedure fell into disuse for many years. More recently, our experience with subcutaneous nylon or Teflon "wicks" would suggest that they can provide significant short-term edema relief.[22] Eventually, longer follow-up study reveals a return to the original level of edema, but subcutaneous wicks have been suggested for use when short-term benefit would be appropriate. The use of skin flaps to bridge areas of lymphatic obstruction was originally advocated by Gillies but has failed to produce consistent improvement.[6] Goldsmith's transfer of omentum into the chronic lymphedema extremity initially held promise, but the most recent report showed a rather unexciting long-term success rate and an inordinate incidence of significant serious complications.[7]

ESTABLISH LYMPHOVENOUS ANASTOMOSES. The third approach to the augmentation of lymph flow has been the establishment of lymphatic-to-venous anastomoses. Conceptually, this is based on a sound physiologic principle since lymph is ultimately returned to the venous circulation. Laine and Howard first reported experimental lymphaticovenous anastomoses in 1963.[15] However, these studies were done on normal dogs. In the late 1960s, there was some enthusiasm for lymphnodovenous anastomoses (a macroscopic procedure).[20] However, long-term patency was only occasionally demonstrated. O'Brien has been the major proponent of the clinical use of direct microlymphaticovenous anastomoses.[19] In his most recent report, 35 patients had had such anastomoses, but a number of the patients had had ancillary ablative procedures, as well.[18] An approximate 44% improvement rate was reported, although there is no documentation of lymphovenous anastomotic patency. Our experience with lymphovenous anastomoses in lymphedematous dogs demonstrated that while anastomoses are patent, significant improvement in the edema can be expected.[21] However, long-term patency of the anastomoses was not demonstrated and was presumed to be, in part, related to an alteration in tissue compliance with decrease in the lymphatic pressure. Currently, we are pessimistic about the long-term potential of lymphovenous anastomoses. However, additional cautious trials seem warranted on an experimental basis, and final judgment must be reserved.

In summary, the surgical approach to the treatment of lymphedema should be considered adjunctive when a medical regimen fails. Also the success of any surgical procedure mandates the continuation of all medical methods, as well. To date, none of the procedures described can be considered curative. Probably the one offering the most consistent long-term improvement would be Miller's modification. If some mechanism can be discovered for maintaining lymphovenous anastomotic patency, then the microsurgical approach to this unfortunate disease may assume a significant role.

Horizons in the treatment of lymphedema include ongoing research directed at more effective therapeutic modalities and at a better understanding of the disease. Only by a precise understanding of the pathophysiology can innovative ideas for therapeutic measures be conceived. Ongoing and future research interest in our laboratories should be concerned with additional approaches to the augmentation of the lymph-flow system.

LYMPHANGIOSARCOMA

Lymphangiosarcoma is fortunately a very rare sequel to lymphedema. It is more common in obstructive lymphedema and seems particularly likely to occur in the upper extremity in the patient with marked postmastectomy lymphedema. Therapy is generally inadequate and usually only palliative. Some opportunity for cure is offered by radical amputation.

References

1. Ariyan SA, Marfuggi RA, Harder G, Goodie MM: An experimental model to determine the effects of adjuvant therapy on the incidence of postoperative wound infection: I. Evaluating preoperative radiation therapy. Plast Reconstr Surg 65:328, 1980
2. Charles RH: Elephantiasis scroti. In Latham A and English TC (eds): A System of Treatment, vol 3. London, Churchill, 1912
3. Chilvers AS, Kinmonth JB: Operations for lymphoedema of lower limbs. J Cardiovasc Surg (Torino) 16:115, 1975
4. Clodius L, Pillar NB: Conservative therapy for postmastectomy lymphedema. Chirurgia Plastica 4:193, 1978
5. Fabian CE, Nudelman EJ, Abrams HL: Postlymphangiogram film as an indicator of tumor activity in lymphoma. Invest Radiol 1:386, 1966
6. Gillies H, Frazer FR: Treatment of lymphoedema by plastic operation. Br Med J 1:96, 1935
7. Goldsmith HS: Long term evaluation of omental transposition for chronic lymphedema. Ann Surg 180:847, 1974
8. Handley WS: Lymphangioplasty: A new method for the relief of the brawny arm of breast cancer and for similar conditions of lymphatic oedema. Lancet 1:783, 1908
9. Homans J: The treatment of elephantiasis of the legs. N Engl J Med 215:1099, 1936
10. Kinmonth JB: Lymphangiography in clinical surgery and particularly in the treatment of lymphoedema. Ann R Coll Surg Engl 15:300, 1954
11. Kinmonth JB: Conservative Treatment of Lymphoedema. In Kinmonth JB (ed): The Lymphatics, p 314. Baltimore, Williams & Wilkins, 1972
12. Kinmonth JB: Methods of Lymphography. In Kinmonth JB (ed): The Lymphatics, pp 1–19. Baltimore, Williams & Wilkins, 1972
13. Koehler P: Complications of Lymphography. In Mayall, Witte (eds): Progress in Lymphology, p. 209. New York, Plenum Press, 1977
14. Kondoleon E: Die operative behandlung der elephantiastischen odeme. Zentralbl Chir 39:1022, 1912
15. Laine JB, Howard JM: Experimental lymphatico-venous anastomosis. Surgical Forum 14:111, 1963
16. Miller TA: A surgical approach to lymphedema. Am J Surg 134;191, 1977

17. Miller TA: Surgical management of lymphedema of the extremity. Ann Plast Surg 1:184, 1978
18. O'Brien BM, Shafiroff BB: Microlymphaticovenous and resectional surgery in obstructive lymphedema. World J Surg 3:3, 1979
19. O'Brien BM, Sykes PJ, Threlfall GN, Browning FSC: Microlymphaticovenous anastomoses for obstructive lymphedema. Plast Reconstr Surg 60:197, 1977
20. Politowski M, Bartkowski S, Dynowski J: Treatment of lymphedema of the limbs by lymphatico-venous fistula. Surgery 66:639, 1969
21. Puckett CL, Jacobs GR, Hurvitz JS, Silver D: Evaluation of lymphovenous anastomoses in obstructive lymphedema. Plast Reconstr Surg 66:116, 1980
22. Silver D, Puckett CL: Lymphangioplasty: A ten year evaluation. Surgery 80:748, 1976
23. Sistrunk WE: Further experiences with the Kondoleon operation of elephantiasis. JAMA 71:800, 1918
24. Thompson N: The surgical treatment of chronic lymphoedema of extremities. Surg Clin North Am 47:445, 1967
25. Thompson N: Buried dermal flap operation for chronic lymphedema of the extremities. Plast Reconstr Surg 45:541, 1970
26. Vandenbrouck C, Sancho H, Le Fur R et al: Results of a randomized clinical trial of preoperative irradiation versus postoperative in treatment of tumors of the hypopharynx. Cancer 39:1445, 1977

Suggested Reading

Kinmonth JB (ed): The Lymphatics. Baltimore, Williams & Wilkins, 1972

Clodius L (ed): Lymphedema. Stuttgart, Georg Thieme Publishers, 1977

Part Two

Systemic Complications and Trauma

12
Complications of Acute Fluid Loss and Replacement

Cleon W. Goodwin

OVERVIEW

Acute nonhemorrhagic fluid loss characterizes the majority of surgical disorders, and the extent of fluid loss may be greater than that of hemorrhage and produce consequences just as dire. Hemorrhage represents loss of both red cells and plasma from the intravascular space, and its clinical manifestations present almost entirely as hemodynamic instability. The clinical picture of acute massive fluid loss, such as that which follows large thermal injury, emerges slightly less rapidly than that of hemorrhage, but intravascular volume deficits can be as profound. Hemodynamic instability characterizes the clinical presentation and determines the eventual outcome. Shock can rapidly ensue, as in hemorrhage, and fluid therapy must be instituted expeditiously. Fluid losses of less rapid onset (e.g., with gastrointestinal fistulas) allow compensatory mechanisms partially to alleviate the plasma volume deficits. Hemodynamic instability is less a feature of the clinical presentation until losses are long-standing, and disorders of tissue hydration and electrolyte concentration dominate the clinical presentation. An understanding of the forces governing fluid distribution and electrolyte concentration (primarily, water and sodium) allows the assessment of acute fluid loss, the choice of the appropriate fluid therapy, and the treatment of the underlying disorders.

Physiologic Basis of Body Fluid Distribution

FLUID COMPARTMENTS AND COMPOSITION

Total body water (TBW) constitutes approximately 45% to 60% of body weight, depending on sex, age, and extent of body fat (Table 12-1). Males have proportionately more TBW than do females because females have more body fat, which is essentially water free. Overall, TBW constitutes a rather constant 70% of the fat-free body mass and is partitioned into the extracellular fluid (ECF) and the intracellular fluid compartments, which have unique electrolyte compositions (Tables 12-2). The functional ECF, which is of primary importance in understanding the effects of acute fluid loss, consists of the plasma, interstitial fluid, and lymph. These subcompartments are in functional equilibrium and rapidly exchange with one another. The total ECF constitutes approximately 21% of the body weight of a young male. The transcellular fluid volume (secretions of organs, etc.) and inaccessible bone water slowly exchange

TABLE 12-1. APPROXIMATE VALUES FOR TOTAL BODY WATER OF NORMAL SUBJECTS*

Age	TBW (Percentage of Body Weight)
0–6 mo	75
1/2–14 yr	65
15–55 yr	50–60
56+ yr	45–50

* Proportions are greater in adult males than in adult females.

TABLE 12-2. BODY WATER DISTRIBUTION OF NORMAL 70-kg MALE

	Body Weight (%)	BW (%)	Liters
Plasma volume	4.5	7.5	3
Blood volume	8.2	12	5
Functional extracellular volume	21	35	14.5
Total intracellular water	33	55	32
TBW	60	100	42

Plasma

Cations (153 mEq/L)		Anions (153 mEq/L)	
Na	142	Cl	102
		HCO_3	26
		SO_4	1
K	4	HPO_4	2
Ca	5	Organic acids	6
Mg	2	Protein	16

Interstitial fluid

Cations (149 mEq/L)		Anions (149 mEq/L)	
Na	145	Cl	113
		HCO_3	31
		SO_4	1
K	4	HPO_4	2
		Protein	2

Intracellular fluid

Cations (195 mEq/L)		Anions (180+ mEq/L)	
K	156	HPO_4	95
		SO_4	20
		HCO_3	10
Na	10	Protein	55
Ca	3		
Mg	26		

FIG. 12-1. Electrolyte composition and concentration in the three major body-fluid compartments.

with other extracellular subdivisions, are not detected by ECF tracers, and do not participate in fluid derangements during acute fluid loss.

Sodium and chloride are the major cations and anions of the ECF (Fig. 12-1). The average adult contains approximately 3700 mEq of sodium ion. Eighty-five percent of the exchangeable sodium resides in the ECF, with the remaining 15% of exchangeable sodium in the cells. Most of the nonexchangeable sodium (25% of the total) is in the crystalline matrix of bone. The body content of chloride is approximately 2100 mEq and distributes with sodium in the ECF. Potassium in the extracellular fluid is quite low. Calcium is 35% to 45% bound to protein, while 5% to 15% is complexed to anions. Protein and lipids form solids that add 7% to the serum volume, and the true concentrations of electrolytes in serum water can be calculated by dividing the measured value by 0.93. If these solids are abnormally increased, as by hyperlipidemia associated with pancreatitis, diabetic ketoacidosis, or infusions of fat emulsions, spuriously low plasma electrolyte concentrations may be obtained. Intracellular fluid volume cannot be determined directly and is calculated indirectly as the difference between the TBW and the ECF, both of which can be measured by tracer techniques. The intracellular fluid constitutes 33% of adult body weight, or approximately 55% of total body water, and is the largest fluid space in the body. Potassium is the dominant cation, and 90% of the total body content of 3600 mEq is intracellular; magnesium is the other major cation. Phosphate, sulfate, and protein are the major intracellular anions.

MAINTENANCE OF WATER AND ELECTROLYTE DISTRIBUTION

The capillary bed is the major filtering surface for water and most solutes. The surface is quite large, 6300 m^2 in adults, and is highly permeable to water. Fluid balance is maintained by capillary hydrostatic pressure and osmotic force. The balance between hydrostatic and osmotic (including oncotic) pressures is modified in individual vascular beds by known anatomical differences and by sudden changes in capillary and tissue fluid composition. Water moves along osmotic gradients across membranes by diffusion (slow) and by bulk flow through pores. Imbalances of fluid distribution between the vascular space and the tissue manifest as edema or dehydration.

Hydrostatic pressure arises from the force generated by cardiac contraction and is transferred along the vascular tree to the capillaries. Intravascular pressure falls from a mean of 95 torr in the major arteries to less than 30 torr in the capillary bed, where fluid exchange occurs. The net pressure gradient across the endothelial wall at the arterial end of the capillary bed is sufficient to drive water and solute into the interstitial space. This process is reversed at the venous end of the capillary bed according to the classical mechanism described by Starling (Fig. 12-2), so that the net transfer of fluid secondary to hydrostatic pressure under normal conditions is small.[32]

Osmotic pressure is generated when solute is asymmetrically partitioned by a membrane that is permeable to water but not to the solute. Water flows

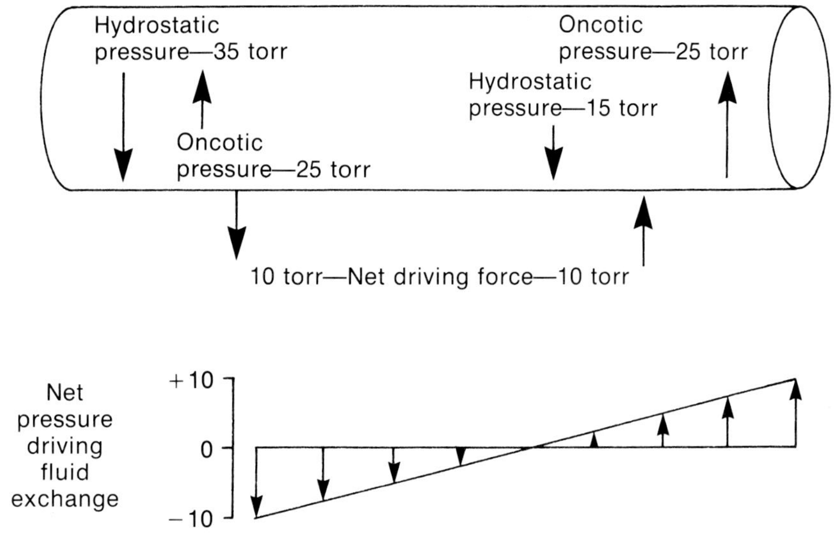

FIG. 12-2. The classic representation of the Starling forces governing water equilibrium between the capillary and tissue. The *lower panel* illustrates graphically the net driving pressure along the capillary. Recent studies indicate that these pressures are lower than originally proposed by Starling and that other factors, including tissue hydrostatic and oncotic forces, influence the net balance of fluid distribution.

from the side of lower solute concentrations to the side of higher concentration until the hydrostatic pressure equals the osmotic pressure. The forces generated by osmotic pressure can be quite large: a change in osmotic pressure of 6 mOsm across a perfect semipermeable membrane approximates mean arterial pressure. In reality, cell membranes are not perfectly semipermeable, and solutes pass through them with varying facility. Such solutes produce much less than ideal osmotic pressure.

Sodium salts account for 90% of osmotically active solutes in the ECF. Sodium is freely dissociated from its anions, which are also osmotically active. Potassium, glucose, and urea contribute minor extracellular osmotic effects under normal conditions. Glucose, in particular, is restricted in large part to the ECF and exerts an osmotic force that increases net water movement into the extracellular space (which by itself will dilute the sodium concentration) when glucose concentration increases. Urea moves freely between the extracellular and intracellular compartments, so that no redistribution of water occurs with changing urea concentrations. The osmolality generated by these solutes in plasma can be calculated by the following equation:

$$\text{Plasma osmolality} = 2\ \text{Na(mEq/L)} + \text{K(mEq/L)} + \text{BUN(mg/dl)}/2.8 + \text{blood glucose (mg/dl)}/18$$

In the capillary bed, plasma ions pass easily into the interstitial space; therefore, the osmotic gradient between the plasma volume and interstitial space is relatively small. Plasma proteins, on the other hand, do not freely pass through the capillary endothelium, and this asymmetry of distribution contributes the major osmotic force preventing loss of fluid from the plasma volume into the interstitial space. This osmotic force, generated largely by albumin, is called the *oncotic pressure*. The proteins also influence electrolyte concentrations in the various fluid compartments. Proteins at pH 7.4 have a net negative charge and behave as anions. The restriction of the anionic form of proteins to one side of a membrane causes an asymmetry of electrolyte concentrations between the plasma and interstitial fluid, which is called the *Gibbs-Donnan equilibrium*. On the side of the membrane with the negative impermeant ion (plasma protein), the concentration of diffusible cations (sodium) is greater than on the opposite side. To maintain charge balance, the concentration of diffusible anion (chloride) is less in plasma than in the interstitial fluid. Furthermore, the total number of diffusible ions will also be greater on the side containing the impermeant anion (see Fig. 12-1). Thus, the major differences between the plasma and interstitial fluid are the much higher concentration of anionic protein and slightly higher total quantity of ions in the plasma. The protein gradient between the plasma volume and interstitial space is maintained by the constant pumping of interstitial fluid, including its protein, into the lymphatic circulation. In contrast, the capillary membrane retards flow of protein into the interstitial space. A complex nonlinear relationship exists between the volume capacities of the plasma space and the interstitial fluid space. With normal water balance, the size of the interstitial volume will change two- to threefold for a given change in blood volume. Above a critical level of blood volume, fluid will leak more rapidly into the interstitial space, which will increase its size up to 50-fold for a given increment in blood volume. With a decrease in blood volume, the same relationships hold in the opposite direction. In a sense, the interstitial space behaves as a buffer or reservoir for the intravascular space during periods of fluid loss, while large fluid infusions are in part stored in the interstitial tissues, with eventual edema formation.

Intracellular volume is maintained by mechanisms similar to those responsible for maintaining fluid and electrolyte distributions between the plasma and interstitial fluid. Cells contain large quantities of anionic protein, which generate a Gibbs-Donnan equilibrium relative to the extracellular space. Because of its higher protein content, the concentration of diffusible ions is increased relative to the extracellular fluid. Cells do not swell, however, because sodium is pumped out of the cell by energy requiring active transport mechanisms. A potential difference is generated as a consequence of the active extrusion of sodium, with the inside of the cell negatively charged. Potassium moves into the cell in response to the electrical gradient, while chloride remains in the ECF with sodium. The extracellular and intracellular spaces are in osmotic equilibrium, since water moves rapidly across membranes to dissipate any osmotic gradients. Although measured concentrations of intracellular ions are greater than extracellular values, a proportion of the former are bound to protein and are not osmotically active.

REGULATION OF INTRAVASCULAR VOLUME AND BALANCE OF SODIUM AND WATER

Maintenance of intravascular volume during rapid fluid loss is regulated by a feedback system involving blood volume, arterial pressure, renal perfusion, and urine output. In addition, a number of hormonal mechanisms influence control of vascular volume but are much more important in regulating extracellular electrolyte concentration. In essence, a decrease in intravascular volume causes a decrease in mean arterial pressure, which in turn causes a decrease in the glomerular filtration rate directly and indirectly by activating peripheral baroreceptors. The decrease in glomerular filtration results in a fall in urine output. In addition, volume receptors believed to be located in the atria and in the major vessels may also contribute to this control. With restoration of blood volume, the process is reversed. This simplified mechanism provides a basic schema on which the effects of acute fluid loss and response to therapy can be assessed.

Restitution of plasma volume at the microvascular level can be separated into two phases.[12] Initially, arterial hypotension results in sympathetically mediated arteriolar vasoconstriction. The ensuing decrease in capillary pressure allows movement of protein-free fluid from the interstitium into the capillaries. This initial shift of fluid allows restitution of 20% to 50% of lost intravascular volume. At the end of this phase, interstitial tissue pressure is reduced and its fluid is hypo-osmolar. Both of these factors now promote movement of fluid from cells into the extracellular space, leading to a further restitution of plasma volume. These compensatory changes partially restore hemodynamic stability, and complete restitution of fluid volume occurs only after replacement of lost fluid. Fluid losses of a lesser nature and occurring over a longer period of time elicit a wider range of compensatory mechanisms, which govern not only the metabolism of sodium and water, but also that of potassium, hydrogen ion, and other electrolytes.

Total body sodium content closely reflects intravascular volume and is determined by renal mechanisms. If sodium intake increases (whether enteral or parenteral), sodium excretion rises, and almost half of the excess is excreted within 24 hours. Sodium loading increases the glomerular filtration rate and decreases the proximal tubular reabsorption of sodium. Decrease in body sodium content is interpreted as a decrease in extracellular volume, and sodium reabsorption is accelerated by the kidney. While extracellular volume is controlled primarily by the kidneys, the concentration of sodium is determined primarily by antidiuretic hormone (ADH) and thirst acting by way of hypothalamic osmoreceptors. Sodium concentration is determined by ADH and water balance, not by total body sodium content. A less than 2% increase in the normal plasma osmolality of 280 to 300 mOsm/kg water will elicit release of ADH, which increases renal reabsorption of water and restoration of normal osmolality. If sodium is loaded, ADH will increase water reabsorption and decrease urine output until osmolality is restored to normal, at which point urinary output will return to levels equal to intake. Total body water content will be at a higher plateau (ADH escape). A sodium load results in an expanded extracellular volume, not hypernatremia, and water content is adjusted to maintain normal sodium and, hence, osmolal concentration. To compensate for this relative hypervolemia, sodium is lost in the urine and water is unloaded.

Aldosterone also causes increased tubular reabsorption of sodium in the distal nephron, but this action is overshadowed by the influence of the glomerular filtration rate and proximal tubular reabsorption, which are predominantly under hemodynamic control by the microcirculation. Instead, aldosterone primarily regulates postassium concentration by promoting tubular reabsorption of this cation, an effect that is at least tenfold more potent that its similar action on sodium.[16]

Acute Resuscitation

Acute ECF volume deficit with rapid internal translocations of sodium and water and minimal loss of red cells is the most common major fluid management problem seen by the surgeon and requires rapid resuscitation to restore and maintain hemodynamic stability. Almost without exception, the fluid lost is isotonic with respect to sodium and water, and resuscitation should be carried out with a similar fluid. Fluid is lost from the entire extracellular space, including the plasma compartment, the contribution of which is proportional to the total volume of ECF lost. Although the displaced fluid may be lost entirely from the body, such as by vomiting, it more often shifts into an injured tissue or a body cavity. Such sequestered fluid is nonfunctional in that it cannot participate in the normal physiologic mechanisms that maintain the integrity of the functional ECF compartment. The rate of plasma volume reduction parallels the rate of isotonic fluid loss even in the face of profound hypotension. The increased concentrations of plasma proteins do not maintain intravascular volume in the presence of extracellular sodium and water deficits. The importance of sodium is illustrated by its potency in the restoring of intravascular volume. Plasma volume increases approximately 75 ml for each 1000 ml of water administered and 1150 ml for each 1000 mEq of sodium given. Sodium depletion of 4 to 8 mEq/kg body weight is associated with an intravascular volume deficit of 10% to 20% and presents clinically as profound hypotension, oligemia, decreased glomerular filtration rate, and elevated blood urea concentrations. A 10% to 20% blood volume deficit following hemorrhage produces only minimal symptoms of hypovolemia. In contrast, treatment of severely burned patients with balanced electrolyte solutions restores hemodynamic stability, urine output, and mental function in the face of existing plasma volume deficits. Clearly, sodium itself has a uniquely beneficial effect and is of major importance in determining physiologic response to acute fluid loss and to subsequent therapy. With acute fluid loss, there is insufficient time for fluid to shift from the intracellular compartment to compensate for the ECF deficits, and restoration of cardiovascular stability must be accomplished by exogenous administration of fluid and electrolytes.

CLINICAL SETTING AND ASSESSMENT

A variety of surgical diseases may cause massive acute fluid loss and are described in detail below. The causes and magnitude of the deficits are often invisible and difficult to assess, and the diagnosis of acute depletion of the ECF is made almost entirely on clinical grounds. The history and physical examination are of paramount importance not only in diagnosing the underlying surgical disease but also in assessing the resuscitation therapy required to restore hemodynamic stability. Swelling of injured areas (burns, fractured femur), contained fluid (ascites), or empty spaces (empty hemithorax following pneumonectomy) indicate locations of lost fluid. Weakness and mental confusion may indicate poor perfusion and hypovolemia. Assessment of external injury, as in burned patients, allows rough measurement of fluid deficits that exist at the time of initial evaluation and that can be expected to continue for a period of time. An accurate indication of the time of onset of the disease causing massive fluid losses is extremely important.

Cardiovascular instability is the predominant clinical manifestation of rapid ECF loss and reflects primarily the plasma volume deficit. The deficit in the remainder of the ECF is largely unmeasurable by clinical methods. Hemodynamic instability associated with total ECF loss represents a much larger fluid deficit than do similar signs associated with pure blood volume loss. Since very little fluid is transposed from the intracellular space following acute fluid loss, normal tissues do not show signs of shrinkage for hours, and assessment of skin turgor, ocular tension, and other indices of tissue hydration will not reflect fluid deficits. Weight decrease attending acute fluid loss may provide some indication of fluid deficits, but if fluid is transported from the extracellular space to a physiologically nonfunctional reservoir, very little weight reduction occurs. Since fluid therapy is often instituted while acute fluid losses continue, serial weight determinations usually document weight gain, not weight loss, during resuscitation. Changes in plasma electrolyte concentrations are uncommon during the acute phase of fluid loss. The hematocrit often becomes elevated with depletion of the plasma volume and can serve as a rough guide to the extent of plasma volume contraction. However, during restitution of fluid volume, change in the hematocrit often does not parallel the restoration of cardiovascular stability.

Assessment of blood pressure, pulse rate, and urinary output is the cornerstone for assessing intravascular volume. In most cases of acute fluid depletion associated with surgical diseases, a urinary catheter should be inserted into the bladder so that urinary output can be accurately monitored. Additional information is obtained by measuring cardiac filling pressures with a right atrial or wedged pulmonary artery catheter. The latter more accurately reflects intravascular volume and can also be used to measure cardiac output. Tachycardia, hypotension, and oliguria indicate hypovolemia and dictate timely fluid replacement. Severe intravascular volume deficits accompany ECF losses exceeding the equivalent of 8 mEq/kg of sodium (5 L in a 70-kg patient) and are often associated with pulse rate over 150 beats/minute, mean arterial pressure less than 40 torr, impalpable peripheral pulses, and anuria. Without fluid restitution, death may rapidly ensue, especially if fluid losses continue. Loss of consciousness associated with fluid loss is a dire sign and confirms severe deficits. With rapid fluid loss of such extent to produce these conditions, measurement of venous pressure is not needed, and therapy should not be delayed to confirm the obvious.

GOALS OF RESUSCITATION

The goal of acute resuscitation is to restore intravascular volume and hemodynamic stability as quickly as possible without producing fluid overload. Since the ECF loss is essentially isotonic with respect to plasma, a fluid of similar composition must be used to replace any ECF deficit. Severe fluid deficits associated with shock may be replaced with such fluid at rates initially up to 2000 ml/hour. The quantity and speed with which fluid is administered is determined by the patient's response to therapy. After approximately one third to one half of the intravascular volume deficit has been replaced, improvement will be reflected by rising blood pressure and urinary output and falling pulse rate. At this point, the rate of fluid administration can be decreased, and attainment of a urinary output of 30 to 50 ml/hour in adults (and 1 ml/kg in children weighing less than 30 kg) indicates that prior intravascular deficits have been nearly restored and that additional therapy should be directed toward replacing continued loss and the persisting extravascular tissue deficits.

The rapid administration of isotonic solutions may transiently expand the intravascular volume faster than repletion of the extravascular space, so that vital signs are restored and adequate urinary output may be obtained in the presence of severe depletion of the total ECF space. Overzealous fluid administration in this case may result in fluid overload with pulmonary edema and congestive heart failure, and monitoring of central venous or pulmonary artery wedge pressure is particularly useful in guiding fluid therapy. It is important to emphasize that the early response to therapy (first 3 to 6 hours) does not predict long-term fluid requirements since part of the rapidly administered fluid may be lost into the extravascular tissues. Once the patient's vital signs have stabilized, any remaining deficits should be replaced more slowly and attention directed toward more definitive treatment of the underlying disease.

AVAILABLE FLUIDS

The choice of fluids to replace any volume deficit is determined by the quantity and composition of fluid lost. Acute isotonic depletion of ECF should be replaced with a fluid of similar composition. Such a fluid is similar to plasma and is effective as a plasma-volume expander. The optimal electrolyte composition and the efficacy of including protein as an oncotic agent are subject to a debate that is beginning to be resolved. In more protracted fluid losses with associated electrolyte abnormalities, an isotonic fluid is used initially to restore plasma volume and cardiovascular stability, and the subsequent fluid regimen is dictated by any residual fluid deficit and electrolyte disturbance.

Crystalloids

BALANCED ELECTROLYTE SOLUTIONS. The prototypic balanced electrolyte solution is lactated Ringer's solution. Its electrolyte composition closely approximates that of the ECF and includes 130 mEq sodium, 109 mEq chloride, 28 mEq lactate, and small amounts of potassium and calcium (Table 12-3). Lactate serves as an alkalinizing agent after its conversion to bicarbonate by the liver. A potential disadvantage of lactated Ringer's solution is its hypo-osmolality with respect to sodium, and each liter furnishes 100 ml to 150 ml of free water. Other polyionic solutions are available in which the lactate has been replaced by acetate, gluconate, or citrate as the bicarbonate precursors. Although the pH of lactated Ringer's solution is approximately 6.5 to 6.7, and is further decreased by the addition of glucose, titratable acidity is quite small. Although liver dysfunction theoretically may impair conversion of lacate to bicarbonate and promote buildup of blood lactate levels, such a potential drawback is not observed clinically, even during treatment of patients with profound shock and poor organ perfusion. Lactated Ringer's solution is particularly effective for replacing a variety of gastrointestinal losses and is the most commonly employed fluid to rectify preexisting plasma and associated ECF volume deficits.

ISOTONIC SODIUM CHLORIDE. Isotonic sodium chloride contains 154 mEq each of sodium and chloride. Its main disadvantage is its high chloride content, compared to a normal plasma concentration of 103 mEq/

TABLE 12-3. ION COMPOSITION OF COMMONLY USED ELECTROLYTE SOLUTIONS IN mEq/L

Solution	*pH*	Na^+	K^+	Ca^+	Cl^-	HCO_3^-* Precursor	mOsm
Lactated or acetated Ringer's	6.7	130	4	3	109	28	280
0.9 sodium chloride	6.1	154			154		308
1/6 M sodium lactate	6.9	167				167	334
5% sodium bicarbonate	7.8	595				595	1190
3% sodium chloride	6.0	513				513	1026

* HCO_3^- equivalent as bicarbonate, lactate, gluconate, citrate, etc.

L. The extra chloride must be excreted by the kidney, which acts quite slowly. As a result, isotonic sodium chloride dilutes other electrolytes, including the bicarbonate buffer base, and produces a dilutional acidosis.[13] This solution is useful when chloride losses exceed sodium losses, as with nasogastric suction and when metabolic alkalosis is present.

HYPERTONIC SODIUM SOLUTIONS. Solutions containing sodium in concentrations of 175 to 300 mEq/L have been utilized for resuscitation of thermally injured patients. They have no demonstrated superiority over balanced electrolyte solutions. The theoretical advantage of a smaller administered fluid volume is often negated, especially at higher concentrations, by the development of severe hypernatremia and the necessity of vigorous treatment with additional free water. Molar sodium lactate or 3% to 5% sodium chloride is used to correct symptomatic hyponatremia, but none of these solutions has any place in acute volume replacement. The chloride salt is used if alkalosis is present, and the lactate salt if acidosis is present. Hypertonic solutions must be administered into a high flow vein.

DEXTROSE IN WATER. Dextrose in water is available in concentrations between 2.5% and 70%. Glucose furnishes energy at 3.4 kcal/g and is metabolized to carbon dioxide and water. Thus, such solutions are essentially electrolyte-free water and, as such, are poor volume expanders. The administered water rapidly distributes in the TBW, with only about 7.5% remaining in the intravascular space (red cells and plasma). Dextrose solutions are indicated primarily as a source of calories and of free water in hyperosmolal states.

Synthetic Colloids

DEXTRANS. Dextrans are glucose polymers produced by bacterial enzymatic action on sucrose. Following fractionation and purification, two preparations with potential clinical usefulness for volume replacement are available. Low molecular weight dextran (LMWD) has an average size of 40,000 daltons (range 10,000–90,000 daltons). Each gram of this dextran theoretically exerts a colloid oncotic effect equivalent to 25 ml of plasma. Thus, 500 ml of a 10% solution will draw approximately 750 ml of additional fluid from the extravascular tissues into the plasma compartment (provided no fluid deficit exists in the tissues). Since the glomerular filtration threshold for dextrans is approximately 50,000 daltons, LMWD is of limited usefulness as a plasma volume expander, with over 50% of the administered dose excreted in the urine within 3 hours.[3] An osmotic diuresis ensues following LMWD administration, with urine concentrations exceeding 40 g/L; as a consequence, urine output may prove unreliable as a clinical guide to fluid administration. A number of rheologic and anticoagulant effects purported to improve microcirculatory flow have been attributed to LMWD, but controlled studies demonstrating improved tissue perfusion and restoration of function are lacking. A number of adverse reactions, including urticaria, chills, fever, nausea, and anaphylaxis, have been reported. Particularly worrisome are reports of acute renal failure precipitated by LMWD administered to hypovolemic oliguric patients, in whom this dextran apparently precipitates in the renal tubule.[9] Abnormal bleeding occasionally occurs with doses exceeding 1000 ml/day. LMWD interferes with the crossmatching of blood and some laboratory determination of glucose, bilirubin, and protein concentrations. LMWD can be administered in doses up to 20 ml/kg/day and is available as 10% solutions in either 0.9% saline or 5% glucose in water.

Medium molecular weight dextran (MMWD) has a mean molecular weight of 75,000 daltons (range 25,000–200,000 daltons). In contrast to LMWD, whose plasma volume effect lasts approximately 90 minutes, that effect of MMWD lasts over 4 hours. Only 40% of this larger dextran is lost in the urine in 12 hours, and it produces a minimal osmotic diuretic effect. MMWD is used primarily as a plasma volume expander and an antithrombotic agent. MMWD is a relatively poor agent for restoring large ECF deficits, and, in fact, its volume expansion effect depends on intact ECF volume. MMWD has no beneficial effect on the microcirculation and, in fact, promotes platelet aggregation and rouleaux formation. Adverse reactions are similar to those of LMWD, and MMWD should not be used in patients with congestive heart failure, coagulopathies, and acute renal failure. MMWD is available as a 6% solution in 0.9% saline. Its recommended dosage of 20 ml/kg in 6 to 12 hours limits its usefulness in replacing large plasma volume deficits such as those that occur with large thermal injuries.

HYDROXYETHYL STARCH. Hydroxyethyl starch (HES) is made from starch amylopectin, which is modified by adding hydroxyethyl groups in ether linkages to its glucose moieties. This chemical modification prevents alpha amylase from rapidly degrading the amylopectin. The average molecular weight of HES is 450,000 daltons (range 10,000–1,000,000 daltons). Since HES is a compact, brushlike molecule, its oncotic properties more closely resemble those of the MMWD, which is a more linear molecule. The plasma volume expansion effect of HES and its plasma-disappearance kinetics are quite similar to those of MMWD, but it is less immunologically reactive and causes fewer sensitivity reactions than does MMWD. HES is available as a 6% solution in 0.9% saline. Dosage is limited to 1.2 g/kg/day or approximately 1000 ml for adults.

Blood and Blood Products

WHOLE BLOOD. Whole blood is the preferred fluid replacement for major intravascular volume deficits arising from blood loss. With acute nonhemorrhagic fluid loss and accompanying depletion of the ECF, the need for red cell replacement becomes increasingly unimportant, and when hemoconcentration has occurred, administration of blood may produce detrimental effects by impeding microvascular flow. Rather, when planning fluid repletion following acute fluid loss, red cells are administered in amounts sufficient to maintain the hematocrit between 30% and 35%. Used in this context, whole blood (or packed cells) contributes only a small proportion of fluid therapy of rapid ECF depletion. The disadvantages of whole blood administration and the place of component therapy are discussed in greater detail in Chapter 15.

ALBUMIN. Albumin provides approximately 80% of the colloid osmotic pressure of plasma. Exogenously administered albumin is regarded as the best available plasma volume expander since it is identical to the natural component most responsible for maintaining fluid equilibrium between the vessels and the tissue. However, it is expensive and relatively scarce and occasionally causes hyperpyrexic reactions. It is obtained from heat-treated pooled plasma and does not transmit hepatitis. Albumin is a transport protein for hormones, vitamins, drugs, fatty acids, and trace elements, and its ability to bind these agents renders many of them less toxic. Albumin is supplied as 5% and 25% solutions. The protein content of the 5% albumin solution resembles that of normal plasma, and this preparation acts to expand plasma volume on a milliliter for milliliter basis. Twenty-five percent albumin solution is hyperoncotic and theoretically adds three to four times its volume to the intravascular space. However, this effect is blunted, if not absent, in patients with large ECF deficits, which may be accentuated by hyperoncotic albumin. If this fluid shift is relied upon in such patients, resuscitation will be underestimated, and loss of albumin into injured tissues may compound the plasma volume deficit by causing a shift of intravascular water into the tissues.[15] If albumin is to be utilized during fluid restitution, no more should be administered than is required to maintain the plasma albumin concentration around 2.5 g/dl. This concentration produces an oncotic pressure of approximately 20 torr, an optimal level for maintaining circulating blood volume. Albumin is suspended in 0.9% saline and is nonviscous and easy to infuse. It is stable for 3 years at room temperature and for 10 years when refrigerated.

PLASMA PROTEIN FRACTION (PPF) is composed of 4.4% albumin and 0.6% globulin. It is slightly hypotonic, with sodium and chloride concentrations of 112 and 50 mEq/L, respectively. PPF is prepared by pasteurization of ethanol-precipitated pooled plasma. The anti-gamma and anti-beta globulins are removed, so PPF can be given to patients of any blood type. PPF is used as a plasma-volume expander (effective up to 48 hours) and to replace protein losses. It is less expensive than albumin and can be mixed with glucose and electrolytes, but not with amino acids. PPF can be given at rates exceeding 1000 ml/hour to patients in shock. Intractable hypotension occasionally follows administration of PPF and has been attributed to its acetate content and to retained pre-kallikrein factors. New preparations are apparently free of this complication.

CRYSTALLOID *VS* COLLOID

The necessity of large volumes of electrolyte-containing fluid to correct fluid deficits associated with acute injury and inflammation became evident with the realization that such deficits were associated with losses not only from the intravascular compartment but also from the functional ECF.[29, 30] The inclusion of colloid, whether as plasma proteins or as synthetic colloid, is widely practiced in the belief that such products produce more effective resuscitation. The increasing sophistication of hemodynamic monitoring techniques has allowed detailed physiologic studies that, for the most part, have defined the optimal properties of resuscitation solutions.

Early studies demonstrated an apparent superiority of colloid-containing solutions in restoring hemodynamic stability. When equal volumes of colloid and crystalloid were administered to hypovolemic animals, colloid solutions produced a more prompt and sustained rise in cardiac output.[4] When indices of adequate intravascular fluid volume, such as urinary output or venous filling pressures, served as the guide to fluid administration, colloid and crystalloid solutions were equally effective in restoring cardiac output and hemodynamic stability.[31, 35] To achieve comparable hemodynamic effects, larger volumes of crystalloid solutions must be administered, usually between two and four times the equivalent volume of colloid solutions. As a result, patients resuscitated with crystalloid solutions gain more weight, develop more peripheral edema, and have a lower plasma oncotic pressure than do similar patients resuscitated with colloid-containing electrolyte solutions. The postulated benefit of colloid solutions derives from the maintenance of plasma oncotic pressure and the minimization of peripheral edema and, by inference, of organ edema, especially of the kidney and lung. However, plasma oncotic pressure does not correlate with pulmonary extravascular water and restoration of large fluid deficits.[19, 34] No early superiority in minimizing water content or maintaining function of the uninjured lung can be demonstrated for either type of solution.[14, 20] Renal tubular function may be better maintained in patients resuscitated with crystalloid solutions, and after the immediate resuscitation phase, increased lung water, respiratory failure, and renal dysfunction are associated with the administration of large quantities of colloid solutions.[15, 21, 31, 35] Weight gain and peripheral edema do not indicate overexpansion of the intravascular volume or compromised organ function. In almost all cases of severe nonhemorrhagic fluid depletion, major deficits of the interstitial and intracellular compartments coexist with the more clinically obvious intravascular volume depletion. Failure to restore extracellular deficits concomitantly may cause organ dysfunction later in the patient's clinical course. Although colloid solutions and blood primarily replace intravascular deficits, crystalloid solutions more rapidly and more completely replenish all of these compartments and are the preferred fluid for acute resuscitation.

Occasionally, cardiovascular instability and poor tissue perfusion persist in spite of large infusions of crystalloid solutions. Such patients may respond to a single infusion of a colloid with restoration of vital signs and urinary output to normal levels. This unusual situation occurs most often when resuscitation is delayed and volume deficits are pronounced. Resuscitation with colloid solutions may also be indicated in patients in whom lung injury is associated with acute fluid loss.[25] When hemorrhage is a major feature of acute fluid loss, blood replacement is always indicated.

CLINICAL CONDITIONS

Major Burns

Cutaneous thermal injury of sufficient intensity and duration produces coagulation necrosis and cell death in the involved tissues. As a consequence, capillary permeability is increased in the burned skin, and the barrier to water vapor is lost. In burns exceeding 25% of the total body surface, additional intravascular fluid may be lost into unburned tissue.[2] Initially, lymph flow from the burned area is increased, but later the lymphatic circulation ceases as lymphatic channels become blocked with coagulated protein, and tissue pressure rises owing to accumulation of extravasated fluid. The net effect of this increased capillary permeability is loss of isotonic fluid from the plasma compartment into the surrounding tissue and massive edema formation, the severity of which depends on extent and depth of injury.

As plasma volume decreases, cardiac output, blood pressure, and urinary output fall, while hematocrit and plasma protein concentration rise. Severe hypovolemic shock and acidosis ensue if the patient remains untreated. The loss of plasma volume is too rapid and too massive in patients with large burns to allow partial correction of the intravascular volume deficit by shift of fluid from the interstitial and intracellular compartments. With resuscitation, the initial depression in cardiac output is reversed, while plasma and blood volume continue to decrease (Fig. 12-3). Cardiac output usually returns to normal by 18 to 24 hours after the injury, and it is a better initial guide to fluid therapy than are plasma and blood volume measurements. Although the net change in plasma volume is dependent upon the amount of infused resuscitation fluid, the rate of plasma volume loss is relatively unaffected by fluid therapy during the first 24 hours following thermal injury.[24] During the second day after the burn, capillary permeability returns to normal, and a net shift of fluid occurs from the extravascular tissues into the plasma compartment. Crystalloid infusion now has a remedial effect on plasma volume. Plasma volume is not restored to normal levels by fluid infusions until 24 to 48 hours after the burn,

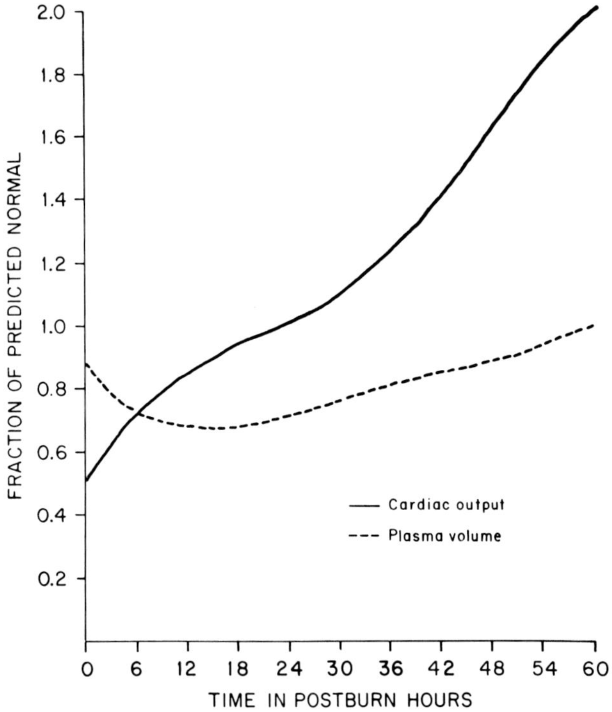

FIG. 12-3. Changes in cardiac output and plasma volume during resuscitation following burn injury. Cardiac output increases more rapidly in response to fluid infusion than does plasma volume. When plasma volume has returned to preinjury levels (at 60 hours postburn), cardiac output is at supranormal levels, where it remains until the wound has healed or been grafted.

when cardiac output has risen to supranormal values typical of the early postinjury hypermetabolic response.

To replace the large volumes of isotonic fluid lost into the injured tissues, balanced electrolyte solutions (lactated Ringer's solution) produce satisfactory results in most patients with large burns. The fluid requirements during the first 24 hours following injury can be estimated by the formula 2 ml/kg body weight/percent body surface burn for adults. Children require approximately 50% greater volume of fluid because of their higher surface area to body mass ratio.

Current Formulas for Estimating Resuscitation Fluid Requirements

First 24 hours

Adult, lactated Ringer's solution, 2 ml/kg body weight/percent body surface burn

Child, lactated Ringer's solution, 3 ml/kg body weight/percent body surface burn

Infusion rate adjusted according to patient response

Second 24 hours

Electrolyte-free water to maintain urinary output

Colloid-containing fluid equivalent to 0.3 ml to 0.5 ml plasma/kg body weight/percent burn

The calculations are based on the full extent of the burn. Approximately one half of the resuscitation requirements is administered over the first 8 hours after the burn and the remainder over the following 16 hours. The lactated Ringer's solution should be dextrose free; otherwise, profound hyperglycemia may occur. Larger volumes of fluid may be required by patients with high-voltage electrical injury, inhalation injury, and delayed resuscitation. Formulas for estimating the resuscitation fluid requirements serve only as initial guidelines, and the actual amount administered should be determined by the patient's physiologic response. Blind adherence to any formula will lead to inappropriate resuscitation of many patients.

The addition of colloid to balanced electrolyte solutions is advocated by some for resuscitation of burned patients. However, colloid administered during the first 24 hours following thermal injury appears to be lost rapidly from the circulation, and its presence does not influence the overall beneficial hemodynamic effects of crystalloid infusions.[6, 22] Because 1 mEq of sodium exerts the same effect as approximately 13 ml of salt-free fluid volume in restoring cardiac output, hypertonic saline solutions (250 mEq/L) have been used to decrease resuscitation volume requirements and the intensity of postinjury peripheral edema. The principal limitation of such solutions is the development of hypernatremia, which induces oliguria and renal dysfunction when serum sodium concentrations exceed 165 mEq/L.[28]

The adequacy of resuscitation and the rate of fluid infusion are guided by the patient's physiologic response to therapy. Animal studies defining the distribution of blood flow following thermal injury indicate that the kidney is the most poorly perfused organ following plasma volume depletion.[4] In contrast, when renal function is adequate, other major organs usually are being satisfactorily perfused, and urinary output is the most reliable and readily accessible index of effective resuscitation. In adults, fluid is administered at a rate to produce urine flow of 30 to 60 ml/hour. In children under 30 kg body weight, 1 ml/kg body weight/hour reflects adequate resuscitation. Patients with high-voltage injury may have hemochromogens in the urine, reflecting deep muscle necrosis. To prevent precipitation of these toxic agents in the renal tubule, urinary output should be increased to 100 ml/hour until the urine has cleared. If the patient does not respond to an increase in infusion rate, 12.5 g of mannitol should be added to each liter of lactated Ringer's solution. Diuretics are rarely indicated in other circumstances, and a low urinary output during the first 48 hours following the burn almost always reflects inadequate resuscitation, decreased renal blood flow, and impending acute renal failure. The proper treatment is increased fluid infusion, not diuretic administration.

The pulse rate is also a useful guide to resuscitation. With adequate fluid administration, pulse rate ranges between 100 and 125 beats/minute in healthy adults. Rates exceeding 140 beats/minute are usually related to hypovolemia and are accompanied by oliguria. Elderly patients may maintain pulse rates considerably below 100 beats/minute, and such a response usually reflects their limited cardiovascular reserve and attendant high mortality. Blood pressure measurements are notoriously inaccurate because of the edema often present in burned extremities. Approximate cuff pressures can be obtained with the aid of an ultrasonic flow probe placed over the artery, but if accurate blood pressures are required, an arterial cannula should be inserted and advanced into the central circulation. However, invasive monitoring by either arterial or venous routes is seldom required in most burned patients and is avoided because of the high incidence of infection associated with intravascular cannulas in burned patients. Invasive monitoring of intravascular pressures is most helpful in elderly patients, those with inhalation injury, and patients who do not respond to reasonable quantities of crystalloid infusions.

Peripheral pulses should be assessed continuously in patients with circumferential third-degree extremity burns. Edema accumulating beneath the unyielding eschar can cause a rise in tissue pressure that may exceed arterial pressure and result in necrosis of the extremity. A clinically compromised circulation is suggested by impaired capillary refilling in unburned distal tissue, neurologic deficits, and deep muscle pain and is confirmed by the absence of pulses on ultrasonic examination. Escharotomies can be carried out at the bedside without the need of anesthesia. Occasionally, escharotomy does not restore pulsatile blood flow in the adequately resuscitated patient, and fasciotomy is indicated. Following escharotomy (and fasciotomy), the patient will often demonstrate a rather sudden increase in fluid requirements.

Acute Intestinal Obstruction

Mechanical intestinal obstruction is caused by a physical barrier to the normal progression of intestinal contents (as opposed to ileus, a motility disorder). With simple obstruction, the bowel lumen is compromised, but the blood supply remains intact. Because large quantities of water are absorbed by the small intestine, small bowel obstruction is associated with large translocations of fluid. In addition to the accumulation of fluid and gas from above the obstruction, the distended small bowel begins to secrete more and absorb less fluid. Furthermore, the bowel wall itself becomes edematous and in advanced cases leaks a transudate fluid into the peritoneal cavity.[27] This sequestered fluid is approximately isotonic and is derived from the extracellular compartments. With continued distension, the small bowel may partially decompress by vomiting. With increasing intestinal distension, ECF deficit increases, and severe hypovolemia, renal failure, and shock ensue.

When both the gut lumen and associated vascular supply are compromised, as occurs with a volvulus, large quantities of fluid and eventually blood are lost into the compromised gut segment. The mucosal barrier is disrupted and bacteria spill into the peritoneal cavity with profound consequences. In a closed loop obstruction, in which the obstructed bowel segment is unable to decompress proximally, continued intestinal secretion progressively increases intraluminal pressure until it exceeds venous pressure, at which point tissue perfusion is compromised and bowel wall necrosis occurs. Many of the signs and symptoms of simple mechanical intestinal obstruction are absent initially, and significant ECF deficits and hypovolemia do not appear until bowel necrosis and peritonitis occur.

The physiologic effects of colon obstruction are usually less dramatic than those of small-bowel obstruction. Since fluid and electrolyte flux through the colon is relatively small, associated derangements are less severe and slower to develop. Except for volvulus, the colon rarely strangulates. The nonstrangulated colon progressively distends above the site of obstruction. If the ileocecal valve is incompetent, the colon partially decompresses into the small intestine. If it is competent, a closed loop obstruction is produced, and rupture may occur, usually at the cecum.

The treatment principles of bowel obstruction are fluid resuscitation, decompression of the bowel, and timely surgical intervention. With simple mechanical intestinal obstruction of short duration, salt and water deficits are usually not severe, and adequate resuscitation can be accomplished with a balanced electrolyte solution within a few hours. If the obstruction has been untreated for more than 24 hours, profound hypovolemia is associated with large ECF deficits and major electrolyte derangements. Such patients may require 6 to 24 hours of fluid therapy before surgery (if intestinal strangulation has not occurred). The hematocrit is a rough guide to the contraction of plasma volume and ECF loss; a hematocrit of 55% reflects approximately a 40% loss of extracellular fluid volume, which is most effectively replaced by a balanced electrolyte solution. Antibiotics are administered if bowel integrity is in doubt. Intestinal intubation is usually employed to decompress the gut as a prelude to resuscitation and prompt surgery. Replacement of external drainage must be considered in planning fluid therapy. With volume repletion and relief of obstruction, mobilization of sequestered fluid may cause a sudden massive diuresis, and the patient must be carefully monitored to detect early signs of vascular overload.

Peritonitis

Peritonitis occurs as an inflammatory response to chemical or bacterial injury to the peritoneal membranes. If this response is acute and generalized, large volumes of isotonic fluid are rapidly lost into the injured tissue. With the initial insult, the peritoneal membranes become hyperemic and lose large quantities of low protein fluid transudate into the peritoneal cavity. Later, the protein and fibrin content of the extravasated fluid increases, and the high protein concentration may play a role in sequestering fluid in the peritoneal cavity. The response of the bowel following the onset of peritonitis contributes to the ECF deficit. The initial hypermotility is rapidly followed by adynamic ileus, with the accumulation of large quantities of air and fluid in the bowel lumen. Secondary bacterial contamination accentuates the fluid deficits. If peritonitis arises from a perforated viscus, additional fluid losses from the viscus occur, and the electrolyte disturbances are influenced by the ion content of the viscus fluid. The signs and symptoms are those of an acute abdomen and severe hypovolemia. Since the primary hemodynamic defect is caused by ECF deficit and loss of plasma volume, an isotonic crystalloid solution should be employed to replace these losses.

Pancreatitis

Rapid fluid loss associated with acute pancreatitis arises from dysfunction of the gastrointestinal tract and from the inflammatory process itself. Patients are often nauseated and may vomit large quantities of fluid. As the disease progresses, ileus often develops with additional loss of ECF. However, the major sequestration of fluid occurs into tissues injured by the corrosive pancreatic exudate. This exudate spreads diffusely in the peritoneal cavity and may dissect into the thorax and retroperitoneal areas, inducing a massive inflammatory response. Severe hypovolemia and shock rapidly ensue. The volume deficit is corrected by isotonic crystalloid solutions, and up to 20 L in 24 hours may be required to resuscitate patients with acute pancreatitis. If significant hemorrhage is associated with pancreatitis, blood replacement is also indicated. Traumatic injury to the pancreas and rupture of a pancreatic pseudocyst can produce severe peritonitis and acute fluid loss, and prompt resuscitation with a balanced electrolyte solution is required prior to surgical intervention.

Fluid Replacement and Electrolyte Disturbances

Unlike acute fluid loss, which causes volume deficits primarily in the extracellular compartments, prolonged fluid loss is associated not only with serious fluid deficiencies in all body compartments but also with severe electrolyte disturbances and acid–base derangements. Subsequent therapy must be directed toward the concurrent correction of these disorders. The sequence in which these disorders are evaluated and treated is important in restoring hemodynamic stability and minimizing complications of therapy.

WATER AND SODIUM DISORDERS

Sodium and water remain the primary determinants of volume adequacy, and isolated disturbances of sodium or water metabolism are uncommon in patients with surgical diseases. Primary sodium excess is usually a manifestation of other diseases such as congestive heart failure and prompts retention of water and edema formation. Primary sodium deficit is nearly always accompanied by water depletion manifested clinically as extracellular volume deficit. Isolated water excess and deficit produce hyponatremia and hypernatremia, respectively. External losses or internal shifts of fluid are most commonly associated with surgical diseases and present as signs and symptoms of volume depletion with or without changes in plasma sodium concentration. Less often, and usually as a result of inappropriate therapy, abnormalities of sodium concentration occur without major fluid deficits.

Plasma sodium concentration is an index of the relative proportions of sodium and water not only in the ECF but also in the TBW and thus reflects the relation of total body solutes to TBW. Following any change in sodium or TBW, water redistributes in body compartments to produce a plasma sodium concentration that would occur if sodium had been distributed in the TBW, thus maintaining equal tonicity in all fluid spaces. Therefore, any corrections in sodium or water balance can be calculated from TBW and plasma sodium concentration:

$$TBW_D \times Na_D + Na_{balance} = TBW_P \times Na_P$$

where D is the desired concentration and P is the pathologic concentration. TBW can be estimated from body weight. This formula is utilized most often to calculate sodium deficit, but it can be utilized in any case of sodium or water imbalance. When water deficit or excess is being calculated, sodium balance is usually assumed to be zero.

Volume Depletion

Volume depletion almost always implies combined water and sodium deficits (see chart on this page). Most surgical diseases are associated with either isotonic or hypertonic dehydration. Volume depletion in which sodium loss is greater than water loss is rare in surgical patients and occurs most frequently in patients with altered renal function. If volume depletion is large, signs and symptoms of intravascular volume deficit and cardiovascular instability assume major importance. When water is lost in excess of sodium, shock does not occur until death is imminent. Blood pressure and urinary output are normal or slightly below normal, while the pulse is bounding until shortly before shock ensues. The degree of illness is roughly proportional to the rise in plasma sodium concentration. Loss of large quantities of sodium-containing fluid (e.g., small bowel obstruction) in conjunction with the intake of electrolyte-free water (a common management error) will produce symptoms of acute hyponatremia, but the major clinical manifestation of this condition will be hypovolemia. The severity of the associated hypovolemia is proportional to the sodium deficit. The hematocrit is often elevated, since the plasma volume is decreased. Fluid therapy is determined by the clinical condition of the patient, and the presence of clinically evident hypovolemia dictates parenteral therapy with a balanced electrolyte or physiologic saline solution until cardiovascular stability is reestablished. When laboratory data become available, fluid composition may require alteration.

Hyponatremia

Hyponatremia occurs in the presence of excess water relative to sodium content. Most episodes of hyponatremia result from defective urinary dilution involving three basic mechanisms, any one of which may pertain to surgical patients. First, ADH secretion may be inappropriately high in spite of ECF hypotonicity (ADH concentrations should be undetectible in such situations). Second, as a result of decreased glomerular filtration rate or increased proximal tubular reabsorption in the hypovolemic patient, insufficient sodium reaches the diluting sites in the ascending limb of Henle's loop and distal convoluted tubule; subsequently, water also begins to be reabsorbed into the circulation, producing hyponatremia and urine that is hypotonic relative to plasma (in spite of the absence of ADH). Finally, defective sodium reabsorption and excessive water permeability in the nephron may occur in conditions unrelated to ADH secretion; osmotic diuretics operate by this mechanism.

DISORDERS OF SODIUM AND WATER METABOLISM

COMBINED SODIUM AND WATER DEPLETION (VOLUME DEPLETION)

Extrarenal

Skin—sweating, burns
Gastrointestinal—fistulas, suction, diarrhea, vomiting
Sequestration—peritonitis, third-space losses with inflammation

Renal Losses

Renal diseases—recovery phase of acute tubular necrosis
Osmotic diuretics
Adrenal insufficiency

HYPONATREMIA

Sodium and water depletion—volume depletion
Adrenal insufficiency
Primary dilutional—usually iatrogenic water excess
Inappropriate secretion of ADH
Sick cell syndrome
Osmotic diuresis—glucose, mannitol
Spurious—hyperlipidemia, hyperproteinemia
Sodium retention and edema—congestive heart failure

HYPERNATREMIA

Extrarenal water losses—sweat, burns, lungs
Renal losses—osmotic diuresis, diabetes insipidus
Adrenal cortical hypersecretion
Excessive solute loading—excessive sodium intake, total parenteral nutrition

Several causes of hyponatremia are of importance in surgical patients requiring fluid therapy (Table 12-4). Hyponatremia associated with prolonged ECF depletion operates by renal and ADH mechanisms: with the latter, the maintenance of ECF volume takes precedence over the demands for normal tonicity. The severity of the accompanying hypovolemia is proportional to the true sodium deficit. The accompanying hyponatremia is rarely of clinical importance. Dilutional hyponatremia occurs as a frequent postoperative complication, when excessive sodium-free fluids have been administered to replace previous fluid losses. Such treatment fails to restore blood volume but results in hyponatremia, and excessive ADH secretion impairs the ability to excrete excess free water. The diagnosis of dilutional hyponatremia is often suggested by history, especially in patients receiving electrolyte-free fluids. Total body sodium content is rarely deficient and often is elevated. Consequently, ECF is usually expanded; vital signs are well maintained; and edema

TABLE 12-4. CLINICAL FEATURES OF ACUTE SODIUM IMBALANCES

System	Hyponatremia		Hypernatremia	
Cardiovascular	Minimal change unless cerebral edema present		Tachycardia, hypotension with large intravascular volume deficit	
Renal	Oliguria or anuria		Oliguria or anuria	
Metabolic	None or slightly hypometabolic and hypothermic		Fever	
CNS	*Moderate* Muscle twitching Hyperactive deep tendon reflexes	*Severe* Coma Seizures Loss of reflexes	*Moderate* Lethargic Restlessness Weakness Confusion	*Severe* Delirium Coma Seizures
Tissue	Edema, salivation, increased gastrointestinal secretions (nasogastric tube aspirates, diarrhea)		Dry mucous membranes, poor skin turgor, flushed skin, beefy tongue	

is frequently present. Prolonged hyperglycemia causes a redistribution of TBW, restoring osmotic equilibrium but producing hyponatremia. As a consequence, plasma sodium decreases 1.6 mEq/L for every 100 mg/dl increase in glucose concentration above normal.

The incidence and severity of clinical symptoms of hyponatremia are related to the rate of onset as well as the magnitude of the decline in plasma sodium concentration (see Table 12-4). In chronic conditions, patients are rarely symptomatic until plasma sodium concentration falls below 115 mEq/L. Treatment of hyponatremia is dictated by the patient's clinical condition. Hemodynamically significant volume deficits should be corrected expeditiously using a physiologic saline solution. However, since most patients are both fluid and sodium overloaded, simple fluid restriction is usually an effective and safe treatment in the absence of neurologic symptoms (if sodium decreases slowly, raise slowly). If central nervous system dysfunction occurs, the use of hypertonic saline (3% or 5%) increases survival.[1] Any underlying systemic disease causing hyponatremia should be treated.

Hypernatremia

Hypernatremia develops when water is deficient in relation to sodium content and can occur under conditions of true sodium excess or major water deficit. All body fluids are hypertonic. An increased sodium concentration normally stimulates thirst with subsequent fluid intake, so this disorder is usually seen in infants or critically ill obtunded patients who cannot regulate their water intake. Most patients with hypernatremia have lost salt-poor fluids; two thirds of this water deficit is derived from the intracellular compartment, so ECF deficits become manifest clinically only when water deficits are massive. Hypernatremia usually arises from insufficient replacement of hypotonic fluid losses, especially sweat and insensible losses (see Table 12-4). Less often, hypernatremia is caused by renal excretion of inappropriately dilute fluid in patients with diabetes insipidus and solute diuresis. With pure water deficit, signs of volume depletion are minimal; with mixed sodium and water deficit, signs of intravascular volume deficit may be evident. Primary sodium excess is usually iatrogenic and follows excessive use of hypertonic sodium solutions or prolonged administration of physiologic saline solutions. Under normal conditions, the renal response to physiologic saline infusion is urine containing 180 to 260 mEq/L of sodium. Thus, the normal kidney can "distill" sodium-containing solutions to some degree. However, this ability to eliminate sodium may be impaired in injured or postoperative patients.

Most symptoms (see Table 12-4) reflect intracellular water deficits, and with severe hypernatremia (plasma sodium greater than 165 mEq/L), the patient is critically ill. Central nervous system dysfunction and hypotension due to intravascular volume depletion are the major clinical manifestations. Children are particularly sensitive to increasing plasma sodium concentrations. Hyperglycemia by itself induces hyponatremia; the associated presence of hypernatremia indicates severe depletion of TBW following osmotic diuresis. Hypertonicity impairs insulin release and tissue glucose uptake, and hyperglycemia is resistant to treatment until volume deficits are replenished and normal tonicity restored.

Balanced electrolyte solutions should be given until volume deficits are corrected and cardiovascular stability restored. The speed with which these fluids are administered is dictated by the patient's initial condition, but balanced electrolyte solutions can be employed rapidly, if necessary, to correct severe hypovolemia. Once the patient has stabilized, tonicity should be very slowly restored to normal over a period of 24 to 48 hours. The rapid administration of hypotonic fluids is extremely dangerous because sodium-free water will shift rapidly into the intracellular space and produce tissue edema, especially in the brain. Insulin administration will drive glucose into the cells, and water will follow along osmotic gradients, increasing cell swelling. Hyperglycemia often corrects by itself when water deficits are replaced, and insulin should be used in small doses only in later stages of treatment when plasma sodium concentrations are approaching normal levels. Water requirements can be calculated from body weight (as a reflection of TBW) and plasma sodium concentration.

POTASSIUM AND ACID–BASE DISTURBANCES

Hypokalemia and Hyperkalemia

Moderate hypokalemia causes weakness and hyperreflexia. Severe deficits can produce areflexia, ileus, and psychosis. Electrocardiographic abnormalities become evident when plasma potassium concentrations fall below 2.5 mEq/L and present as lengthened Q–T interval, depressed ST segment, and U waves. Hyperkalemia is the more dangerous condition, with cardiac conduction defects occurring when plasma potassium concentrations exceed 7 mEq/L. At lesser degrees of hyperkalemia, peaked T waves and depressed ST segment changes are evident on the electrocardiogram. The effects of hyperkalemia on cardiac conduction are amplified if hypocalcemia, hyponatremia, or acidosis is also present. Although plasma concentrations of potassium bear no direct relation to total body content of that ion, careful regulation of the plasma concentration is of paramount importance because of potential cardiac effects.

Hyperkalemia may be treated by cation exchange resins, calcium, sodium bicarbonate, and glucose, alone or in combination. Hypokalemia is treated by potassium replacement. Several guidelines will aid planning of potassium therapy:[7]

1. For every change in *p*H of 0.1 units, potassium concentration changes in the opposite direction approximately 0.6 mEq/L.
2. In metabolic alkalosis with paradoxical aciduria (urine *p*H = 6), the potassium deficit in adults is at least 400 mEq.
3. If the plasma potassium concentration is less than 3.0 mEq/L, an infusion of 200 to 400 mEq is needed to raise plasma concentration by 1 mEq/L.
4. If plasma potassium is between 3.0 and 4.5 mEq/L, 100 to 200 mEq will raise the concentration by 1 mEq/L.

Before potassium is administered, plasma concentration and renal function must be assessed. When severe potassium losses occur (burned patients may lose up to 600 mEq/day), infusions of up to 40 mEq/hour may be required. If infusion rates of potassium must exceed 120 mEq/day or 20 mEq/hour, the patient should be monitored by electrocardiography and by measurement of plasma concentrations after every 50 to 100 mEq is administered. Potassium chloride is the optimal drug if plasma concentrations of chloride are also reduced. Potassium acid phosphate (KH_2PO_4) corrects any accompanying hypophosphatemia, and potassium acetate is an effective alkalinizing agent if acidosis is present. Basic potassium phosphate (K_2HPO_4) accentuates urinary loss of potassium and is seldom used. Potassium-containing solutions should be thoroughly mixed, since concentrated potassium preparations will layer out in fluid containers, causing a dangerously concentrated bolus to be infused into the patient. Normal daily intake of potassium is 50 to 90 mEq.

Acid–Base Disturbances

The primary disorders of acid–base equilibrium are respiratory and metabolic acidosis and alkalosis. Each of these disturbances stimulates a compensatory response that tends to restore *p*H toward normal. Full compensation of a simple disorder never occurs and when full compensation or an overshoot is seen, more than one primary disturbance is present. The *p*H is determined by the ratio of HCO_3^- to H_2CO_3, and the conventional Henderson–Hasselbach equation $pH = pK' + \log\frac{HCO_3^-}{H_2CO_3}$ can be thought of as $CNS = 6.1 + \log\frac{\text{kidney}}{\text{lung}}$, reflecting the interaction of these three organs. Respiratory disorders begin with an abnormal PCO_2 and metabolic disorders with an abnormal HCO_3^-. Obtaining an accurate history yields valuable clues to the underlying causes of acid–base disturbance. Essential laboratory studies include measurement of arterial blood gases,

BUN, blood sugar, potassium, anion gap, and blood cultures.

RESPIRATORY ACIDOSIS. Systemic *p*H decreases as a consequence of carbon dioxide retention arising from decreased pulmonary blood flow, shunting, depressed respiratory drive, or increased carbon dioxide production. Therapy is directed toward increasing the minute ventilation to eliminate excess carbon dioxide, and in most critically ill patients, this is most effectively accomplished by mechanical ventilation.

RESPIRATORY ALKALOSIS is due to hyperventilation and hypocarbia in response to anxiety, hypoxia, hypermetabolism, sepsis, or excessive mechanical ventilation. Treatment is directed toward correction of the underlying disorder eliciting this ventilatory response. Large urinary losses of potassium are associated with respiratory alkalosis and are treated with potassium replacement.

METABOLIC ACIDOSIS is caused by abnormal losses of bicarbonate (diarrhea, fistulas, renal tubular acidosis), increased endogenous acid production (ketoacidosis, lactic acidosis), impaired renal acid excretion (renal tubular acidosis), or excessive intake of acid. A number of these causes are a consequence of fluid therapy. Earlier preparations of hyperalimentation solutions contained amino acids as their hydrochloride salts, which on ionization resulted in a large acid load and metabolic acidosis. Current use of acetate salts of amino acids has avoided this potential source of acidosis. Metabolism of cystine and methionine results in a net production of hydrogen ion, and preformulated solutions with high concentrations of these amino acids should be avoided in patients prone to the development of acidosis. Most intravenous solutions have low *p*H, but their titratable acidity is quite low. Large infusions of isotonic saline frequently result in hyperchloremic acidosis. The excessive administration of chloride (in relation to plasma concentration) dilutes the other major anion, bicarbonate, causing its renal wasting. In contrast to the widening of the anion gap (normal: 8–12 mEq/L) with acid accumulation, the anion gap remains normal with bicarbonate loss.

The physiologic effects of severe acidosis are depressed myocardial contractility, decreased sensitivity of peripheral vasculature to catecholamines and bronchodilators, increased susceptibility to arrhythmias and acute renal failure, and finally shock. The underlying disorder producing acidosis must be identified and treated appropriately. Treatment of the acidosis should proceed expeditiously but only at a rate sufficient to establish a reversal of the acidifying process. Rapid correction of severe metabolic acidosis, particularly with bicarbonate, may cause a further decline in *p*H of the cerebrospinal fluid, producing increased obtundation and convulsions.[23] Rapid correction of acidosis is accompanied by a large shift of potassium into cells, and the resulting hypokalemia requires vigorous potassium supplementation. If hypocalcemia accompanies metabolic acidosis, correction of the acidosis may precipitate tetany. The Q–T interval on the electrocardiogram should be monitored during alkali therapy, and hypocalcemia treated with separate infusions of calcium salts.

Sodium bicarbonate is the preferred agent for the treatment of metabolic acidosis. Since the bicarbonate space is distributed in approximately 50% of the TBW, the bicarbonate deficit can be estimated by the expression

$$(HCO_3{}^-{}_D - HCO_3{}^-{}_P) \times 0.5\ TBW = HCO_3{}^- \text{ deficit}$$

where D is the desired concentration and P is the pathologic concentration. One half of this deficit should be administered over 2 to 4 hours, following which, the acid–base balance is reassessed and subsequent dosages determined. No attempt should be made to reverse the acidosis fully; successful treatment of the underlying disease usually results in eventual total correction. Chronic metabolic acidosis should be treated more slowly than the acute form. Lactated Ringer's solution with moderate amounts of added sodium bicarbonate (45 mEq/L) is an effective modality, especially in surgical patients with large losses of bicarbonate-containing fluid. Potassium acetate is an effective alkalinizing agent if acidosis is not severe and hypokalemia is also present.

METABOLIC ALKALOSIS. Causes of metabolic alkalosis fall into two general categories: depletion of body stores of sodium and chloride and, hence, extracellular fluid volume, and excessive loss of potassium and hydrogen ion while preserving near normal sodium, chloride, and water composition. Most cases of metabolic alkalosis are associated with ECF depletion following loss of large quantities of gastric acid, diuretic therapy, diarrhea, and rapid correction of hypercarbia. Urinary chloride concentrations are less than 10 mEq/L. Volume contraction increases tubular reabsorption of bicarbonate, producing alkalosis. Treatment with isotonic sodium chloride restores ECF volume and restores *p*H to normal. Potassium deficits are usually small, and treatment with potassium chloride supplements replenishes both the potassium and chloride deficits.

Alkalosis following excessive losses of potassium and hydrogen ion is associated with prolonged steroid therapy, excessive alkali regimens (e.g., stress ulcer prophylaxis), and occasionally prolonged gastric drainage with less than optimal electrolyte replacement. Urinary chloride concentrations under these conditions exceed 20 mEq/L. Since in most cases ECF depletion is minimal, the alkalosis responds poorly to sodium chloride administration. Potassium chloride is usually necessary to restore body stores and normal plasma concentrations. Acidosis persisting after reestablishing adequate fluid volume and replacing potassium deficits may require the use of acidifying agents. *L*-arginine monohydrochloride, when given intravenously, gives rise to equimolar quantities of hydrochloric acid; the arginine is metabolized, and its nitrogen is excreted as urea. It is available as a 10% solution with an osmolarity of 950 mOSm/L and a chloride content of 47.5 mEq/dl, and must be infused into a high flow vein. More recently, solutions of hydrochloric acid have been demonstrated to be efficacious in treating resistant cases of metabolic alkalosis. A 0.1 to 0.2 molar solution (100–200 mEq/L) is infused over 6 to 24 hours into a high flow vein.[7] To estimate the amount of hydrochloric acid required, the chloride deficit is calculated as

$$(Cl_D - Cl_P) \times 0.2 \text{ TBW}$$

where D and P are the desired and pathologic concentrations. One half of this estimated deficit is administered over the first 24 hours. As with metabolic acidosis, no attempt should be made to achieve rapid and total correction.

CLINICAL EVALUATION

The diagnosis of fluid balance disturbances associated with protracted body fluid losses is more difficult and subtle than that which occurs with massive deficits of rapid onset and is based primarily on the history and physical examination. Such information can define the character of the fluid–electrolyte disorder, the underlying cause, the magnitude of deficits or excesses, and the rates of continuing fluid losses. Only then can rational fluid therapy be instituted. It is important to know that a fluid deficit and not an excess is present so that initial treatment can be begun expeditiously. Better definition of subsequent therapy is determined by the patient's initial response. Laboratory data, which are rarely available immediately, allow precise quantification of electrolyte disturbances and facilitate fine tuning of initial therapy. Careful questioning can define external losses or internal translocations. The amount, duration, and character of vomitus, diarrhea, and fistulous drainage indicates the magnitude of fluid loss and potential electrolyte disturbances. Documentation of weight loss allows quite precise definition of external fluid losses. More difficult to measure is fluid lost into injured or inflamed tissues. Although this fluid remains within the body, it is unavailable to the normal body fluid compartments.

Findings on physical examination provide additional information about the underlying disease and the magnitude of fluid deficits. Dehydration is not evident until approximately 6% to 10% of TBW has been lost. Signs of tissue dehydration—decreased ocular tension, decreased skin turgor, dry and shrunken mucous membranes—do not appear until 6 to 24 hours following large water losses. Abdominal examination is particularly important. The shape of the abdomen can suggest underlying diseases. Hernias should be searched for not only in the inguinal area but in all other locations of natural abdominal wall weakness. Tenderness, rigidity, and absence of bowel sounds denote intra-abdominal inflammation. Examination of the rectum allows further assessment of the abdominal and pelvic contents.

Sodium content of the extracellular compartment is the prime determinant of cardiovascular stability during episodes of prolonged fluid loss. Dehydration in the absence of significant sodium losses has only a moderate effect on intravascular volume. Plasma volume decreases by 7.5% of the total of sodium-free fluid lost. In contrast, if the lost fluid is isotonic, plasma volume falls by 25% of the total volume lost. A sodium deficit of 2.5 to 4.0 mEq/kg results in a modest fluid deficit and is characterized by mild weakness and a urinary output of less than 40 ml/hour in the adult. With sodium deficits of 4 to 8 mEq/kg, the patient feels extremely weak and exhibits orthostatic hypotension. Urinary output ranges between 10 and 20 ml/hour, and the pulse pressure is decreased. Sodium deficits greater than 8 mEq/L produce profound shock.

PRIORITIES AND ASSESSMENT OF FLUID REPLACEMENT

Fluid replacement following long-standing fluid losses is often a more complex process than acute resuscitation following rapidly occurring massive fluid losses. As with most other disturbances of body homeostasis, the time required for correction should reflect the duration of the disorder. Thus, protracted untreated fluid deficits require a relatively long period of time to restore physiologic balance safely. An orderly approach to the diagnosis of the existing pathophysiology suggests the appropriate therapeutic sequence.

1. *Restore fluid volume.* Initially, hemodynamic stability is reestablished by restoring plasma volume. This phase of treatment must be accomplished rapidly to prevent acidosis and organ dysfunction. A balanced electrolyte solution (lactated Ringer's) is rapidly infused until adequate circulation and urinary output are reestablished. Up to 40 ml/kg can be infused with relative safety over 30 to 45 minutes if the patient is continuously reassessed.

Once cardiovascular stability is attained, the remaining ECF deficit is replenished over 4 to 8 hours, using urinary output as a guide to infusion rate. Thereafter, any remaining deficits and ongoing losses are assessed by clinical and laboratory assessment.

2. *Restore normal osmolality.* After restitution of plasma volume and cardiovascular stability by balanced electrolyte or isotonic solutions, fluid composition (particularly with respect to sodium) is altered to correct existing hyponatremia or hypernatremia. Fluid loss in most surgical patients is associated with either isotonic or free water volume deficits, and, at this stage, hypotonic sodium solutions are often indicated. Hyperglycemia is usually associated with dehydration and is treated with small doses of insulin after fluid replacement.
3. *Correct hydrogen ion disturbance.* Acidosis associated with large fluid deficits will usually resolve without the need for alkali therapy when fluid volume is replaced. Severe or persisting metabolic acidosis is safely treated by giving a portion of the sodium in the replacement solution as an alkali instead of chloride salt. Specific forms of treatment are discussed above.
4. *Replace intracellular ions.* The primary ion of concern is potassium.
5. *Correct other biochemical abnormalities.* Hypocalcemia frequently occurs following fluid replacement in dehydrated patients, and acidosis will accentuate the effects of hypocalcemia. Disorders of other ionic species (magnesium, phosphate, etc.) are guided by laboratory data.

Assessment of fluid replacement is best accomplished by the use of a flowchart on which intake, output, body weight, and vital signs are recorded. Intake totals should reflect measurement of volume and content not only of fluid administered by oral and intravenous routes but also that by enema and enteral tubes. Output totals should include urine, stool, vomitus, and all tube drainage. The net balance of intake and output records may grossly underestimate insensible fluid losses, especially in hypermetabolic, critically ill patients, and at least daily measurements of body weight are necessary to detect these discrepancies. Continuous monitoring of blood pressure, pulse rate, respiratory rate, and urinary output facilitates the recognition of trends which may suggest increasing fluid deficits and provide sufficient data for guiding therapy. Monitoring the central venous or wedged pulmonary arterial pressure reflects intravascular volume but provides no information about TBW and, therefore, is of limited value in gauging repletion of the chronically dehydrated patient. Frequent measurements of body weight, on the other hand, are quite efficacious. Patients receiving no caloric intake will lose 0.2 to 0.5 kg/day, and stable or increasing weight under these circumstances reflects a net increase in body water. The best guide to fluid therapy is continuous assessment of the patient's response to initial attempts at correcting suspected deficits. Maintenance requirements must be added to calculated deficits, and fluid therapy will alter continuing losses. Hypertonic and occasionally isotonic saline infusions may amplify renal and extrarenal sodium and water losses even while intravascular volume deficits persist and before fluid balance has occurred.

CLINICAL CONDITIONS

Complex water and electrolyte disorders accompany prolonged fluid loss associated with a variety of surgical diseases. Fluid can be lost to the external environment (vomiting, diarrhea, fistulous drainage) or to physiologically nonfunctional diseased tissue (peritonitis, burns). Such losses are usually isotonic in early stages, but with continuing chronicity, plasma sodium concentration decreases, especially if the patient attempts to rehydrate himself by drinking water. Potassium and hydrogen ion deficiencies frequently occur in advanced stages of chronic fluid loss.

Burns After the Resuscitative Phase

Approximately 24 hours following burn injury, when resuscitation with balanced electrolyte solutions is essentially complete, the goals of fluid therapy shift to replacement of continued losses and maintenance of hemodynamic stability. Capillary integrity returns to normal at this time, and the circulation will now retain protein in the intravascular compartment. Existing plasma volume deficits should be replaced with colloid-containing solutions equivalent to plasma in a dosage of 0.3 to 0.5 ml/kg body weight/percent body surface burn. Additional colloid usually need not be administered after the second day following the burn, and adequate plasma protein concentrations are best maintained by vigorous nutritional support. Unless severe blood loss accompanies thermal injury, blood transfusion is not indicated in the early treatment of burned patients. The hematocrit immediately following thermal injury is elevated, usually exceeding 60% to 70%, in spite of a 10% to 15% loss of red cell mass soon after severe injury.[33] Even with adequate resuscitation and continued fluid replacement, the hematocrit does not return to normal until the fourth or fifth day following the burn. Thereafter, blood is administered to maintain the hematocrit between 30% and 35%.

Beginning on the second day after the burn, electrolyte-free water is administered to facilitate excretion of the massive sodium load received during resuscitation and to prevent excessive water loss by evaporation. Thermal injury destroys the water vapor barrier of skin, and the burn becomes a free water surface that permits unimpeded evaporative loss. Such losses can be huge, up to 6 to 10 L/day, depending on the extent of the patient's hypermetabolic response and on his immediate environment. Evaporative loss in ml/hour can be estimated by multiplying the sum of 25 plus the percent body surface burn by the patient's body surface area; this calculation approximates the lower range of evaporative loss. The rate of fluid infusion is regulated to maintain normal serum osmolal and sodium concentrations and to allow a controlled reduction of the fluid sequestered in injured tissues. An adequately resuscitated patient with a large thermal injury will gain 15% to 20% of his preburn weight by the end of the first day following the burn. Subsequent fluid therapy is directed toward returning to preinjury weight by days 7 to 10 after the burn. A urinary output of at least 40 to 50 ml/hour is required to assure normal renal function and excretion of solute loads. By calculating expected evaporative loss and desired urinary output, a rough estimate of fluid requirements can be obtained. Although volume requirements are considerably lower than those needed for resuscitation, requirements nevertheless range from 4 to 6 L/day. Not infrequently, in patients whose catabolic response results in a large urinary solute load, a brisk diuresis may ensue as early as the second day after injury and the administration of sodium-free water (D_5W) must be increased to control weight loss and to prevent dehydration.

Hyponatremia is especially common in children but occurs at all ages as a result of excessive administration of free water. Total body content of exchangeable sodium is massively increased after resuscitation (up to 4000 mEq positive sodium balance), and remains so for up to 3 weeks after injury. Hence, the proper treatment of hyponatremia in most patients is restriction of water intake, not sodium administration. Rarely, sodium loss through the eschar, normally quite low, may be large when silver nitrate dressings are employed for wound protection. Sodium replacement in this situation may have to be used early. Hyponatremia producing neurologic symptoms requires the use of hypertonic saline. Hypernatremia almost always results from underestimation of evaporative water loss and subsequent severe water deficits. Appropriate therapy is to increase free water administration. Episodes of hypovolemia associated with deterioration of vital signs at any point following resuscitation should be treated first with a balanced electrolyte solution to restore cardiovascular stability; afterward, any abnormality of sodium concentration can be corrected by manipulating free water therapy as dictated by body weight and by sodium and osmolal concentration.

Potassium is not administered in the first 48 hours. The potassium in balanced electrolyte solutions and that released by injured tissues is sufficient to maintain normal serum concentrations at this time, and exogenous administration may result in dangerous hyperkalemia. By the third day after the burn, potassium loss in the urine begins to rise and may exceed 600 mEq/day. Topical treatment with silver nitrate accentuates potassium loss through the burn, while use of topical mafenide acetate (Sulfamylon) increases urinary losses.[37] Potassium supplements are administered to maintain plasma concentrations between 3.5 and 4.0 mEq/L. Glucose, which was omitted from resuscitation solutions to prevent hyperglycemia, is included in replacement solutions, usually beginning with 5% dextrose solutions. In patients with large burns, intensive nutritional support, with its attendant high osmolar loads, is delayed until the end of the first week after injury when the major fluid shifts are nearly complete.

Perioperative Fluid Therapy

Perioperative fluid management is directed toward replacing existing fluid deficits and correcting any electrolyte imbalances. Injuries produce "third space" losses which are replaced with isotonic solutions. Gastrointestinal losses are replaced as indicated by their volume and content. Frequently unrecognized causes of preoperative fluid deficits are the use of extended bowel preparations and long periods of no fluid intake prior to operation. Chronically ill, hypermetabolic patients whose operations are scheduled near the end of the day may lose 2 L to 3 L, appear stable, but develop profound shock with the induction of anesthesia.

Intraoperative fluid management involves replacing both ongoing blood loss and third space losses into injured tissues. The latter deficit may greatly exceed blood loss, especially with intra-abdominal procedures requiring extensive tissue dissection. ECF deficits should be replaced as they occur to minimize the hormonal changes induced by hypovolemia. Balanced electrolyte solutions, 500 to 1000 ml/hour, effectively maintain tissue hydration and organ perfusion.

Postoperative fluid therapy should correct any existing volume deficits immediately and replace ongoing losses for the remainder of the patient's course. ECF losses may continue for several days after operation and are assessed by following intake and output balances, vital signs, changes in mental status, and body weight. Insensible losses are usually 750 to 1000 ml/day but may be higher in hypermetabolic patients; they are replaced with 5% dextrose in water. External drainage and internal sequestration of fluid are replaced with crystalloid solutions. Urinary output of 1000 to 1500 ml/day is required to excrete solutes generated by tissue catabolism. Fluid retention tends to occur postoperatively, especially if water in excess of sodium has been administered. However, this proposed ADH effect may, in fact, represent an intravascular volume deficit as a result of underreplaced blood loss or sequestration in the wound or injury sites. In such cases, isotonic solutions are required as dictated by vital signs and urinary output. Postoperatively, the fasting state leads to breakdown of protein, glycogen, and fat, releasing large quantities of endogenous water and leading to hyponatremia. After the first postoperative day, high urinary volumes may reflect not only continued high intake but also mobilization of sequestered fluids. In the latter case, fluid infusion rate should not be increased to match output but rather the patient's fluid balance should be allowed to fall slowly to his preinjury state. No potassium is given during the first 24 hours following surgery unless a large preoperative deficit existed beforehand. Thereafter, potassium administration is guided by plasma measurements.

Vomiting

Vomiting is usually caused by a visceral disorder, either within or adjacent to the gastrointestinal tract. Vomiting causes depletion of hydrochloric acid and ECF, leading to dehydration and alkalosis as the primary disturbances, and more than 2 L/day can be lost. Hypokalemia and hypocalcemia develop with prolonged fluid loss. Hypochloremic alkalosis is the major acid–base imbalance if the fluid is mainly gastric in origin. If vomiting empties the upper small intestine, losses of sodium, potassium, and water are often larger, but the added loss of bicarbonate minimizes the acid–base derangement. With progressive loss of gastric fluid, plasma bicarbonate and *p*H increase, and urine *p*H initially exceeds 7.0, with loss of bicarbonate in the urine as a compensatory mechanism. However, the obligatory loss of sodium with bicarbonate in the urine soon limits the loss of the bicarbonate since severe total body sodium deficits and associated volume depletion cause the kidney to preserve volume (sodium) at the expense of acid–base balance.[10] The appearance of a paradoxical aciduria at this stage denotes severe ECF deficits. Fluid therapy is based on measurements of volume of vomitus and electrolyte content of serum and vomitus.

Diarrhea

Diarrhea is a manifestation of many underlying diseases and presents as increased frequency and water content of stools. It almost always results from impaired absorption or excessive secretion of solutes, usually sodium, but also others (sugars, magnesium, etc.). Water follows passively along osmotic gradients. The fluid lost is most often isotonic with ECF and may reach 2 to 8 L/day with ulcerative colitis and over 11 L/day with pseudomembranous enterocolitis. Loss of sodium, bicarbonate, chloride, and water leads to dehydration, acidosis, and shock. Hyponatremia may be accentuated by concomitant oral intake of water. Osmotic diarrheas (enteral feedings, lactase deficiency) produce large non–sodium-containing fluid losses and hypernatremic dehydration, which is aggravated if sodium replacement is excessive. Losses of sodium approach 1500 mEq/day and are directly related to the volume of diarrhea. Maximal potassium losses are less severe, up to 150 to 200 mEq/day, and with increasing fluid loss, potassium concentration in diarrhea declines.[11] Therefore, potassium depletion is unusual except in longstanding diarrhea and that associated with islet cell tumors and villous adenomas. Sodium, potassium, and chloride in the stool should be measured: if the sum of stool sodium and potassium concentrations exceeds the sum of stool chloride and plasma bicarbonate concentration, bicarbonate is being lost in the stool and severe acidosis will develop. Balanced electrolyte solutions provide adequate volume replacement. The exact volume and electrolyte content, as always, are guided by assessing stool and plasma electrolytes, volume of diarrhea, and the patient's response to therapy.

Gastrointestinal Fistulas

External fistulas are abnormal communications between bowel and skin, while internal fistulas connect the bowel and another hollow viscus. Fistulas can occur spontaneously or as a result of a surgical procedure. Major physiologic derangements arise from loss of absorptive surface, either by resection or by bypassing large segments of the gastrointestinal tract. Subsequent bacterial colonization of a bowel segment may amplify the fluid–electrolyte disorders. Bacteria deconjugate and dehydroxylate bile acids, which precipitate in the colon and lead to fat malabsorption and steatorrhea. Most physiologically significant fistulas are external and are caused by peptic ulcer disease, cancer, inflammatory bowel disease, trauma, and postoperative anastomotic leaks. Their metabolic consequences depend on their location in the gastrointestinal tract (Table 12-5).

GASTRIC, DUODENAL, AND JEJUNAL FISTULAS. Approximately 8 L of fluid traverse the intact gastrointestinal tract each day, and fistulas in these locations result in large losses of fluid, up to 5 L/day.[8] The lost fluid is isotonic, and rapid dehydration and shock ensue if fluid replacement is delayed. The anion lost depends on the site of the fistula: gastric fistulas cause

TABLE 12-5. ELECTROLYTE CONTENT OF BODY FLUIDS (RANGE)

Fluid	Na^+	K^+	Cl^-	HCO_3^-
Plasma	135–150	3.5–5.0	98–106	22–30
Gastric juice	30–90	4.3–12	52–124	0
Bile	120–170	3–12	80–120	30–40
Pancreatic juice	113–153	2.6–7.4	54–95	70–110
Small bowel	72–158	3.5–6.8	70–127	20–40
Ileum	90–140	6–30	82–125	25–30
Fecal	50–116	11–28	35–70	15–30

alkalosis, while those in the duodenum tend to produce acidosis. Jejunal fistulas are rare, produce low volumes of neutral pH fluid, and usually do not disturb acid–base equilibrium. Losses are replaced by isotonic solutions.

BILIARY AND PANCREATIC FISTULAS. Biliary fistulas primarily cause depletion of sodium, chloride, and water. Volumes are relatively small, less than 500 ml/day, although T-tube drainage (which, in effect, is a fistula) occasionally reaches 1000 to 2000 ml/day. Although pancreatic fistulas do not usually drain the entire pancreas, they can still produce large volumes (over 2000 ml/day) of bicarbonate-rich fluid. Acidosis readily develops, and the fistulas are very slow to heal because of the action of pancreatic enzymes on abdominal wall. Complete gastrointestinal tract rest and total parenteral nutrition facilitate spontaneous closure of these chronic fistulas.

ILEAL AND COLONIC FISTULAS. Fistulas in the ileum and colon by themselves rarely cause fluid–electrolyte problems. If they are a consequence of generalized bowel disease (e.g., regional enteritis), the fistulas may produce copious drainage, which is primarily an isotonic exudative fluid. Such losses are replaced with isotonic fluids.

ILEOSTOMY. According to the basic definitions, an ileostomy is a true fistula. Most chronic ileostomies are well tolerated. A new ileostomy may require a period of adjustment during which intravenous fluids are needed. Large losses of sodium and water occur during this time, up to 1 L of fluid containing over 100 mEq/L of sodium daily, and, if prolonged, severe dehydration and hypovolemia ensue. Associated magnesium loss can be severe. With time, the small intestine is able to adapt with increased fluid absorption. Partial obstruction of previously well functioning ileostomy stoma may produce catastrophic fluid loss. Massive diarrhea, up to 11 L/day, causes hypovolemia and shock. Fluid deficits are replaced with isotonic solutions, and the stoma must be surgically revised.

INTERNAL FISTULAS. Symptoms arise from a decrease in absorptive surface and bacterial overgrowth in the bypassed segment. *Gastrocolic fistula* is the most common example of this type and is usually a consequence of cancer or peptic ulcer disease. If the pylorus is unobstructed, gastric contents usually continue their normal course through the bowel. Symptoms such as diarrhea usually arise from contamination of the upper gastrointestinal tract by fecal bacteria. After fluid deficits are replaced, surgical intervention is indicated in most cases. *Short bowel syndrome* is, in essence, an internal fistula resulting in decreased intestinal absorptive surface. It follows massive resection for mesenteric vascular disease, regional enteritis, and midgut volvulus in children. Although 12 inches of upper small bowel may support life, less than 50 inches of small bowel causes typical symptoms which reflect the lack of adequate absorptive surface. Hypermotility, rapid transit of nutrients, decreased bile acid pool, and bacterial colonization impair digestion and cause massive diarrhea. Persistent diarrhea causes acidosis and hyperkalemia. Following rehydration, bowel rest and total parenteral nutrition reduce stool losses. During this interval small meals of low osmolality are begun in an attempt to allow the bowel to adapt its absorptive capacities. Success is more common with longer bowel segments, but relapses associated with massive stools occur frequently.

Ileus

Ileus is a functional, nonmechanical obstruction of the bowel resulting from neural inhibition of coordinated motor activity of the bowel wall. It is usually caused by intra-abdominal inflammation but also results from occlusive vascular disease of the bowel, distant sepsis, drugs, thoracic trauma, and electrolyte imbalance. Pseudo-obstruction of the colon is a visceral neuropathy similar to ileus, occurs most frequently in the elderly, and is often a manifestation of diabetes mellitus, progressive systemic sclerosis, and vascular disease. The most common cause of ileus is intra-abdominal surgery. Bowel motility usually returns in the small intestine within 24 hours, in the stomach within 24 to 48 hours, and in the colon within 3 to 5 days.

The underlying disease causing the ileus usually determines the clinical presentation and dictates treatment. Postoperative ileus lasting longer than 5 days should prompt investigations for anemia, sepsis, excessive drug therapy, and electrolyte imbalance, which, if present, should be corrected. Fluid lost into the atonic bowel is isotonic with respect to plasma and losses of 3 L to 4 L are not uncommon. In long-standing cases, severe hypovolemia associated with plasma volume deficits up to 50% have been identified.[10] Therapy consists of volume repletion with a balanced electrolyte solution, intestinal intubation, and treatment of the underlying cause.

Intestinal Bypass

Although intestinal bypass procedures for the treatment of obesity have declined in popularity in recent years, the many patients who have had the operation continue to require medical supervision. The purpose of the operation is to produce weight loss by inducing controlled malabsorption. With resumption of oral feedings postoperatively, massive diarrhea of up to 6 L/day ensues until gut adaptation takes place. However, the degree and duration of this adaptation is unpredictable, and diarrhea continues to persist 1 year postoperatively in 25% of patients.[26] The direct introduction of bile acids into the colon initiates severe fluid–electrolyte disturbances associated with intestinal bypass procedures. Bile acids block colonic absorption and may stimulate secretion of sodium and water, promoting ECF losses. Colonic bacteria metabolize bile acids to their hydroxy-analogues, which are potent cathartics. In addition, since ileal reabsorption is bypassed, the total bile acid pool soon is depleted, impairing fat digestion in the proximal small bowel and resulting in steatorrhea.

Potassium depletion is the most common electrolyte disorder following intestinal bypass procedures. All patients undergoing this operation should be treated chronically with potassium supplements, but severe hypokalemia frequently occurs in spite of this precaution. Fecal losses are accentuated to three to four times normal rates during episodes of severe volume depletion, possibly by an effect of increased aldosterone concentrations on the colonic mucosa. Chloride losses do not parallel sodium losses in diarrhea, and hyperchloremic acidosis usually accompanies significant volume depletion. The acidosis readily responds to the inclusion of alkali (bicarbonate) in the fluid replacement regimen. Calcium depletion is caused by diarrhea, steatorrhea, vitamin D deficiency, and increased urinary excretion. Since magnesium is absorbed throughout the small bowel, bypass results in increased losses and depressed serum concentrations. Both respond to mineral supplementation.

Bacterial overgrowth of the excluded bowel segment causes a bypass enteropathy, which presents as bloating, anorexia, nausea and vomiting, weight loss, and rectal burning. Unpredictable episodes of explosive diarrhea and severe dehydration occur when the excluded intestinal segment periodically evacuates its contents. Bypass enteropathy causes the most severe fluid–electrolyte derangement and is the most common cause for readmission of bypassed patients to the hospital. Opiates are of no benefit since they increase stasis and promote bacterial overgrowth. Bacterial suppression with a broad-spectrum antibiotic and replacement of diarrheal fluid losses with a balanced electrolyte solution are the primary forms of treatment. Large exudative protein losses in the stool may reach 17 g/day, and total parenteral nutrition may be required to maintain nutritional balance during episodes of massive diarrhea.

Tubes in the Digestive Tract

Tubes for the drainage of digestive secretions are utilized in practically all locations in the gastrointestinal tract. It is important to remember that these tubes are, in effect, external fistulas and can cause any of the fluid–electrolyte disorders described for fistulas. The precise derangement depends on the anatomical location of the tube. The most common management error is underreplacement of tube drainage both in volume and in electrolyte content. Accurate intake and output records and measurement of the electrolyte content of drainage aliquots allow timely replacement of tube losses. Fluid replacement of tube drainage should be integrated into considerations of the patient's total fluid needs. Blind volume-for-volume replacement of tube drainage may lead to overhydration, increased digestive secretions, and an increasing cycle of chasing fluid losses. The stomach, in particular, can act like a "third kidney," producing up to 5 L/day with constant nasogastric suction when fluid replacement is overzealous.[36] These complications can be avoided by titrating fluid replacement to maintain stable vital signs, body weight, and acceptable urinary outputs (50–60 ml/hour).

References

1. Arieff AI, Llach F, Massry SG: Neurological manifestations and morbidity of hyponatremia: Correlation with brain water and electrolytes. Medicine 55:121-9, 1976
2. Arturson G: Pathophysiological aspects of the burn syndrome. Acta Chir Scand 274:1-135, 1961
3. Arturson C, Cranath K, Thoren L, Wallenius G. The renal

excretion of low molecular weight dextran. Acta Chir Scand 127:543-51, 1964
4. Asch MJ, Feldman RJ, Walker HL et al: Systemic and pulmonary hemodynamic changes accompanying thermal injury. Ann Surg 178:218–21, 1973
5. Asch MJ, Mason AD Jr, Pruitt BA Jr: Regional blood flow in the burned unanesthetized dog. Surgical Forum 22:55,1971
6. Baxter CR: Fluid volume and electrolyte changes of the early postburn period. Clin Plast Surg 1:693-709, 1974
7. Burnell JM, Villamil MF, Uyeno BT, Scribner BH: The effect in humans of extracellular pH change on the relationship between serum potassium concentration and intracellular potassium. J Clin Invest 35:935-9, 1956
8. Edmunds LH Jr, Williams GM, Welch CE: External fistulas arising from the gastro-intestinal tract. Ann Surg 152:445-71, 1960
9. Feest TG: Low molecular weight dextran: A continuing cause of acute renal failure. Br Med J 2:1300, 1976
10. Fine J, Fuchs F, Gendel S: Changes in plasma volume due to decompression of the distended small intestine. Arch Surg 40:710-16, 1940
11. Fordtran JS, Dietschy JM: Water and electrolyte movement in the intestine. Gastroenterology 50:263-85, 1966
12. Gann DS: Endocrine and metabolic responses to injury. In Jeffers JD, Boynton SD, Leap B (eds): Principles of Surgery, pp 1-63. New York, McGraw–Hill, 1979
13. Garella S, Chang BS, Kahn SI: Dilution acidosis and contraction alkalosis: Review of a concept. Kidney Int 8:279-83, 1975
14. Goodwin CW, Mason AD Jr, Pruitt BA Jr: Colloid and crystalloid resuscitation have same effect on lung water after thermal injury. Surgical Forum 32:294-7, 1981
15. Goodwin CW, Long JW, Mason AD Jr, Pruitt BA Jr: Paradoxical effect of hyperoncotic albumin in acutely burned children. J Trauma 21:63-5, 1981
16. Guyton AC, Taylor AE, Granger HJ: Synthesis of the total system for control of body fluid volumes. In (eds): Circulatory Physiology II: Dynamics and Control of the Body Fluids, pp 316-29. Philadelphia, WB Saunders, 1975
17. Harken AH, Gabel RA, Fencl V, Moore FD: Hydrochloric acid in the correction of metabolic alkalosis. Arch Surg 110:819-21, 1975
18. Kassirer JP, Schwartz WB: The response of normal man to selective depletion of hydrochloric acid. Am J Med 40:10-18, 1966
19. Lam V, Goodwin CW Jr, Treat RC et al: Does pulmonary extravascular water vary with colloid oncotic pressure after burn injury? Am Rev Respir Dis 119 (Suppl 1): 139, 1979
20. Lowe RJ, Moss GS, Jilek J, Levine HD: Crystalloid versus colloid in the etiology of pulmonary failure after trauma–A randomized trial in man. Crit Care Med 7:107-12, 1979
21. Moss GS, Siegel DC, Cochin A, Fresquez V: Effects of saline and colloid solutions on pulmonary function in hemorrhagic shock. Surg Gynecol Obstet 133:53-8, 1971
22. Moylan JA, Mason AD Jr, Rogers PW, Walker HL: Postburn shock: A critical evaluation of resuscitation. J Trauma 13:354-8, 1973
23. Posner JB, Plum F: Spinal-fluid pH and neurologic symptoms in systemic acidosis. N Engl J Med 277:605-13, 1967
24. Pruitt BA Jr, Mason AD Jr, Moncrief JA: Hemodynamic change in the early postburn patient: The influence of fluid administration and of a vasodilator (Hydralazine). J Trauma 11:36-46, 1971
25. Richardson JD, Franz JL, Grover FL, Trinkle JK: Pulmonary contusion and hemorrhage-crystalloid versus colloid replacement. J Surg Res 16:330-336, 1974
26. Salmon PA: The results of small intestine bypass operations for the treatment of obesity. Surg Gynecol Obstet 132:965-79, 1971
27. Shields R: The absorption and secretion of fluid and electrolytes by the obstructed bowel. Br J Surg 52:774-9, 1965
28. Shimazaki S, Yoshioka T, Tanaka N et al: Body fluid changes during hypertonic lactated saline solution therapy for burn shock. J Trauma 17:38-43, 1977
29. Shires T, Coln D, Carrico J, Lightfoot S: Fluid therapy in hemorrhagic shock. Arch Surg 88:688-93, 1964
30. Shires T, Williams J, Brown F: Acute change in extracellular fluids associated with major surgical procedures. Ann Surg 154:803-10, 1961
31. Siegel DC, Cochin A, Geocaris T, Moss GS: Effects of saline and colloid resuscitation on renal function. Ann Surg 177:51-7, 1972
32. Starling EH: On the absorption of fluids from the connective tissue spaces. J Physiol (Lond) 19:312-26, 1953
33. Topley E, Jackson MG, Cason JS, Davies JW: Assessment of red cell loss in the first two days after severe burns. Ann Surg 155:581-90, 1962
34. Tranbaugh RF, Lewis FR, Christensen JM, Ealings VB: Lung water changes after thermal injury. Ann Surg 192:479-88, 1980
35. Virgilio RW, Rice CL, Smith DE et al: Crystalloid vs colloid resuscitation: Is one better? Surgery 85:129-39, 1979
36. Wangensteen OW, Paine JR: Treatment of acute intestinal obstruction by suction with the duodenal tube. JAMA 101:1532-8, 1933
37. White MG, Asch MJ: Acid–base effects of topical mafenide acetate in the burned patient. N Engl J Med 284:1281-6, 1971

13 Complications of Hypovolemic Shock

Lazar J. Greenfield

OVERVIEW

Shock is a recognized and readily diagnosed complication of trauma but may be less obvious in the surgical patient during an elective procedure or postoperatively where hypotension may not be seen. This happens because the definition of shock includes any state of imbalance between the metabolic needs of the tissues and the available oxygenated blood supply, leading to impaired cellular function.

Under the usual circumstances of a sudden reduction in blood volume of 30% to 40%, the adrenergic response produces sweating, hyperventilation, tachycardia to compensate for the reduced stroke volume, and peripheral vasoconstriction. Organ function is affected adversely, as demonstrated by a urine output reduced to less than 25 ml/hour and progressive metabolic acidosis. The cellular response is to shift to anaerobic glycolysis in an effort to maintain availability of high-energy phosphate, but the cost of this inefficient conversion is high, resulting in the production of pyruvate and lactate. If the shock state is uncorrected, there is increased platelet aggregation, increased capillary permeability, and eventual organ failure, which becomes lethal when pump action deteriorates in heart failure. With proper expeditious management, normal hemodynamics are readily restored (Table 13-1).

TABLE 13-1. GUIDELINES FOR NORMAL HEMODYNAMIC MEASUREMENTS

Determination	Normal Adult Range
Central venous pressure	5–10 cm H_2O
Pulmonary arterial pressure	23–30/8–10 torr
Pulmonary wedge pressure	8–10 torr
Systemic arterial pressure	120/80 torr
Cardiac index	3.0–4.5 L/min/M^2
Heart rate	70–80/min
Hematocrit	37–45%

Differential Diagnosis

The patient who demonstrates inadequate circulation may be suffering from one of several treatable problems. First and foremost is hypovolemia, which may be secondary to exogenous fluid losses or due to hemorrhage or diarrhea. The deficit may be more subtle, however, as with internal hemorrhage, anaphylaxis, or in the presence of a pheochromocytoma.

If the volume status of the patient is adequate, as demonstrated by filling pressure of the left ventricle (pulmonary capillary wedge pressure, PCWP) in the range of 10 to 15 torr, or shown less reliably by rising central venous pressure to a fluid challenge, then the heart may be at fault. In this type of cardiogenic shock, the PCW will usually exceed 15 torr. Other causes that must be excluded include mechanical problems such as cardiac tamponade, ball valve thrombus in the heart, dissecting aneurysm, and pulmonary thromboembolism. There are also the blood-volume-distributive disorders in which venous capacitance may be increased as in early sepsis, neurogenic shock, barbiturate intoxication, and other low-vascular-resistance problems that should be treated as functional hypovolemia. Further discussion of cardiogenic shock and related entities in the differential diagnosis as listed above can be found in the chapters that discuss those topics.

Complications of Treatment

The most serious complication of hypovolemic shock treatment occurs when the need for additional volume replacement is not recognized and a vasopressor agent is administered. This sequence in the face of physiologic vasoconstriction compounds the tissue damage and worsens the degree of acidosis. Further efforts to reverse the acidosis with sodium bicarbonate are unsuccessful and may contribute to the deterioration by added hyperosmolarity and central nervous system irritability. With further ischemic injury to the capillary network, the resultant increased permeability may make any subsequent attempts at volume repletion unsuccessful.

MILITARY ANTI-SHOCK TROUSERS

Advances in training of paramedical personnel have made it possible to initiate treatment of shock at the scene of an accident by use of the military anti-shock trouser (MAST) suit, which redistributes blood from the lower half of the body into the central circulation and increases arterial resistance. It is estimated that 0.6 L to 2 L of blood can thus be autotransfused to improve perfusion of the critical organs. In addition, the MAST suit provides tamponade of underlying bleeding vessels, both arterial and venous, at suit pressures as low as 15 to 50 torr.[9] The lowest possible pressure required to control the bleeding is preferred since pressures that exceed systemic levels have been associated experimentally with the development of metabolic acidosis.[7] This complication is difficult to dissociate from the metabolic acidosis produced by shock alone, but it would seem advisable to utilize sodium bicarbonate administration at the time of deflation of the suit if there is evidence of acidosis. Other complications such as compromised ventilation depend on the patient's ability to raise his respiratory rate in compensation for the reduced lung volume produced by restricted diaphragmatic movement. The patient with a head injury is most vulnerable to the development of this type of respiratory acidosis. Limb loss has also been reported as a complication of use of the MAST suit.[6] The suit is contraindicated in the presence of an acute myocardial infarction since it produces a significant added afterload for the left ventricle.[1]

FLUID RESUSCITATION

The type of fluid used for correction of hypovelemia continues to be controversial, although there is much less enthusiasm for colloid solutions currently than in the recent past when electrolyte solutions were felt to be contributory to the development of interstitial pulmonary edema. The concern that the use of Ringer's lactate solution might worsen any preexisting lactic acidosis proved to be unfounded in clinical studies that compared its effects to those of normal saline.[4] Since the distribution of electrolyte solutions used for resuscitation must include the extravascular space, some degree of overhydration must result from this type of resuscitation, which requires ratios of 3:1 to 4:1 above the actual volume lost. In an effort to minimize this effect,

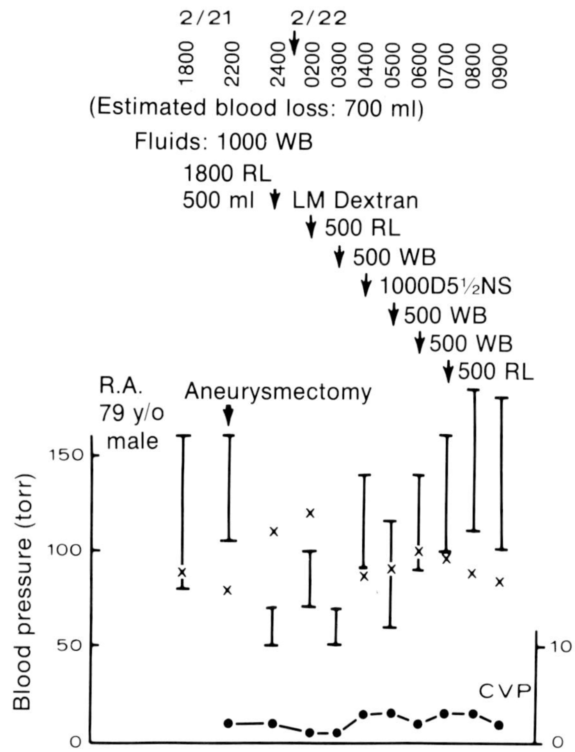

FIG. 13-1. Systemic blood pressure and heart rate (*X*) in a 79-year-old man who underwent emergency aneurysmectomy with an estimated blood loss of 700 ml. Immediately after surgery, he showed hypotension and tachycardia with a low central venous pressure (*CVP*), which was improved only after transfusion of an additional 1500 ml of whole blood (*WB*) and 2000 ml of lactated Ringer's solution (*RL*).

Jelenko and colleagues have suggested the use of a regimen of hypertonic, albuminated fluid on demand (HALFD), which limits fluid administration based on mean arterial pressure.[3] Although their experience has been favorable, it must be confirmed through other work. Since it has not been possible to demonstrate significant superiority of colloid over electrolyte solutions, the electrolyte solutions are preferred because of their practical advantages of ease of storage and cost, which is one tenth the cost of colloid resuscitation.

Both under- and overestimations of fluid volumes required for resuscitation may prove disastrous for the patient (Fig. 13-1). It has been customary to use the central venous pressure (CVP) as a guide to the adequacy of volume repletion; this is appropriate when its limitations are recognized. The normal limits of CVP are considered to be from 2 cm to 10 cm H_2O, assuming that the catheter is positioned correctly within the thorax and the zero reference point is at the level of the right atrium (Fig. 13-2). It is also essential to exclude treatable causes of abnormal elevation of pressure such as pneumothorax or cardiac tamponade. In hypovolemic shock, the CVP will be very low or negative, encouraging further fluid administration. As volume is restored, the CVP tends to rise, but there is no absolute end point that assures adequacy of repletion or that protects against overload. There is also a poor correlation between CVP levels and overall fluid requirements for resuscitation.[10]

If the patient still shows signs of inadequate perfusion once the CVP is within normal range, a bolus trial of fluid infusion may provide useful information. This consists of rapid infusion of 200 ml crystalloid over a 10-minute period to assess the CVP response. If there is no increase, then additional fluid can usually be administered, but if the CVP rises 2 cm or more, then additional fluid may be harmful. In these circumstances as well as in any patient whose cardiopulmonary status makes the CVP unreliable, such as in patients with chronic lung or heart disease, a pulmonary arterial (Swan–Ganz) catheter should be introduced to allow measurement of the PCWP as a more accurate reflection of the preload for the left ventricle. The catheter traverses the right heart to enter the pulmonary artery, and its progress can be followed by a pressure tracing (Fig. 13-3). Catheter position should be confirmed by chest films. Further verification of its position can be obtained by aspiration of fully oxgenated blood from the catheter.

Errors of catheter positioning may lead to incorrect assessment, and particular caution is required for patients on positive pressure ventilation with end-expiratory pressure (PEEP). If the catheter tip is above the level of the left atrium, the pressure reading may reflect alveolar rather than atrial pressure. Consequently, it is advisable to disconnect the PEEP during the pressure measurement and to reposition the catheter if the readings do not match the clinical picture. It may also be very difficult to obtain readings from the patient with dyspnea and wide swings in intrathoracic pressure. A pressure tracing with markings that identify expiration may be useful in this instance of an unstable baseline.

Other complications of balloon–catheter use include balloon rupture with air embolism, arrhythmias, sepsis, and pulmonary infarction or hemorrhage. These are fortunately rare and usually can be prevented by limiting catheter placement to 72 hours and minimizing periods of balloon inflation.

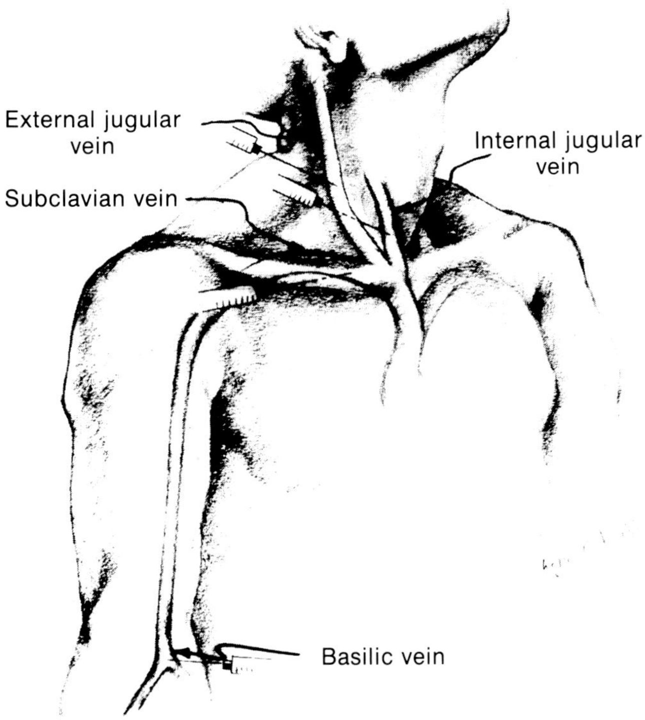

FIG. 13-2. Routes of access for measuring CVP. Catheters can be directed percutaneously into the superior vena cava from any of the veins shown.

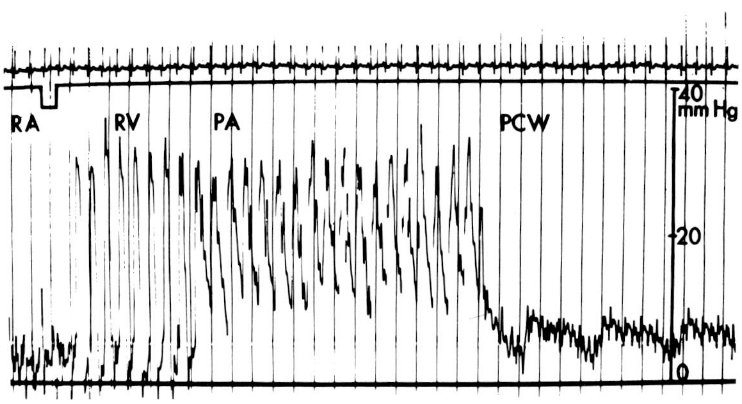

FIG. 13-3. A sequential pressure tracing obtained from the passage of a balloon-tipped (Swan–Ganz) catheter. Entry from the right atrium (*RA*) into the right ventricle (*RV*) is marked by an increase in systolic pressure; entry into the pulmonary artery (*PA*) is marked by a diastolic pressure increase. As the catheter proceeds to the pulmonary capillary wedge (*PCW*) position, the pressure falls, a reflection of left atrial pressure alone.

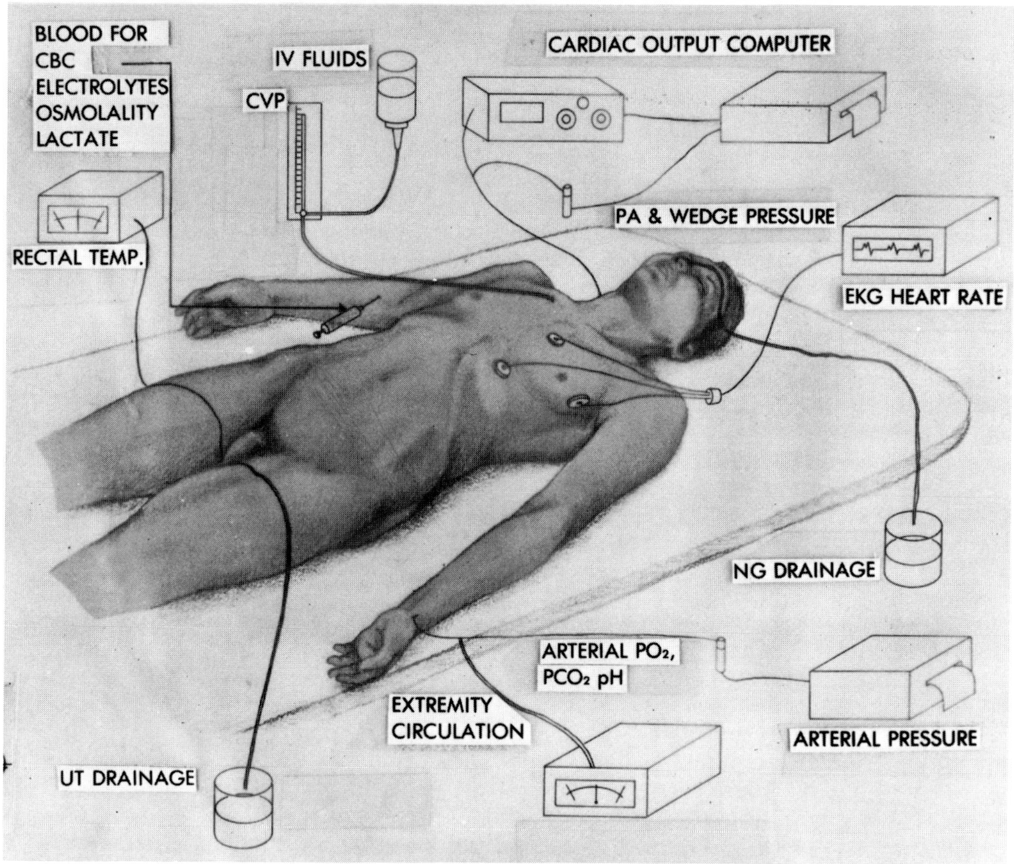

FIG. 13-4. A comprehensive approach to the patient in shock permits rapid assessment of his response to therapy. Although some of the hemodynamic determinations are less commonly available, they should be added whenever possible to permit evaluation of drug and fluid responses.

The Swan–Ganz catheter can also be used for cardiac-output determinations if a thermistor bead is attached. This indicator-dilution method registers the temperature change when a bolus of cold saline is injected. A computer calculates the area under the resulting curve for the direct reading of cardiac output. When cardiac output is high, a large curve is generated and there is little error in the method. When cardiac output is low, however, the curve is smaller and more difficult to analyze, making the temperature gradient critical. It is also advisable to use a computer that analyzes most of the curve rather than estimating the projected downslope to avoid the recirculation error. The balloon catheter's position in the pulmonary artery also allows sampling of the mixed venous oxygen tension ($P\bar{v}O_2$). Normally, this is in the range of 40 torr and falls to 30 torr and below during hypovolemic shock. A rising value shows improved circulation and usually parallels increasing cardiac output. The finding of an abnormally high $P\bar{v}O_2$ of 45 torr or more shows a narrow A–V difference and usually reflects the hyperdynamic state associated with sepsis.

The Swan–Ganz catheter has many advantages that outweigh its risks, provided that customary precautions are observed. These should include electrical isolation since the catheter is also a conductor that can allow random currents to produce arrhythmias. Comprehensive sequential measurements of the functions identified in Figure 13-4 provide optimal data for assessment of the response to treatment.

CARDIAC FAILURE

In noncardiogenic shock, the heart can be considered to be an innocent bystander that persists in valiant attempts to preserve the circulation until it too is overcome by acidosis and underperfusion. The adrenergic response that is fueled by catecholamines serves to increase myocardial oxygen demands at a time when oxygen supply is impaired. This imbalance leads to deterioration of myocardial function and eventual irreversible cardiac failure. The deterioration of myocardial performance during its global ischemia is a function of limited coronary flow redistributed away from the subendocardium, which decreases contractile force and the compliance of the ventricles. One can also find "zonal lesions" that consist of focal destruction of contractile elements.[5] These lesions can be prevented by beta-adrenergic blockade and therefore may be due to inotropic stimulation. There is also some evidence that a polypeptide from the splanchnic circulation may depress myocardial function, although this seems to be a late manifestation of splanchnic ischemia. The presence of acidosis also results in the release of lysosomal enzymes and the activation of the kinin system, which increases vascular permeability and reduces vascular tone. These effects further compromise venous return and arterial pressure, perpetrating the vicious cycle that leads to progressive cardiac depression.

The diagnosis of cardiac depression should be confirmed by the finding of an elevated PCWP in excess of 15 torr. This finding assures the adequacy of volume repletion, although additional volume may be required for improved cardiac output. Since this pressure is at the threshold of pulmonary edema, however, it is advisable to measure cardiac output by thermodilution before additional volume is administered. Although pharmacologic afterload reduction has been used successfully in the therapy of cardiogenic shock, its role in noncardiogenic shock is unknown. It would have some theoretical value in the face of very elevated systemic vascular resistance and low cardiac output, such as the late stages of septic and hypovolemic shock. However, since elevated vascular resistance is the result of hypovolemic shock and not a cause, volume repletion should be able to reverse the vasoconstriction. The agent that allows the most flexible control is nitroprusside, which acts to reduce preload by venodilation and increase ejection fraction by reducing impedance.

Under most circumstances of myocardial depression in late shock, an inotropic agent such as dopamine or dobutamine should be used. If higher doses of dopamine are required, its alpha vasoconstrictive effects may be ameliorated by adding nitroprusside. This combination often works effectively to improve the output of even a severely depressed heart and it has been better in our experience than dobutamine, which is a pure beta agonist, or any other inotropic agent. Although intra-aortic balloon counterpulsation has been used effectively in cardiogenic shock, it remains to be seen whether it can provide any improvement in the heart failure of late hypovolemic shock.

METABOLIC COMPLICATIONS

The combined effects of gluconeogenesis, glycogen breakdown, and impaired insulin production lead to hyperglycemia during the early stages of shock. In the later stages, especially in septic shock, hypoglycemia tends to develop, and hypertonic glucose has been shown to improve hemodynamics and rates of survival.[2] Insulin levels remain elevated for prolonged periods after resuscitation, and similarly elevated glucagon levels may be seen. The effects of glucagon are now recognized to be more widespread than those of its primary role of sustaining glucose levels since it is also a potent splanchnic vasodilator. The increased thrombocytosis and platelet adhesiveness after hemorrhage contribute further to the capillary stasis that produces cellular hypoxemia.

At the cellular level, there is decreased ability to remove metabolites, including potassium, which seep out of injured cells. The anaerobic production of lactate provides one measure of the severity of injury and seems to correlate with the mortality rate. Initially, most patients in the early stages of shock have levels of 1 mM to 2 mM of lactate with a low mortality rate. With progression, however, the lactate level increases and the mortality rate approaches 100% when the lactate level reaches 8 mM/L. Serial measurements can be useful indicators of the adequacy of resuscitation. The mortality rate also increases with multiple organ dysfunction, representing the most lethal complications of shock.

RENAL FAILURE

The most sensitive cells in the kidney to ischemia are the tubular lining cells. The development of acute tubular necrosis is perhaps the most common serious complication of shock and the most dangerous for the older patient who rarely survives this complication. The relationship to the duration of shock is variable, but without the protection of hypothermia, warm ischemic injury becomes apparent after 20 to 30 minutes of hypotension. The injury may initially be manifested as polyuria but more commonly is heralded by oliguria and failure of concentration of the urine. When oliguria persists after volume restoration, a trial of diuretic administration is indicated before a diagnosis of renal failure can be made. Once the diagnosis is confirmed, the treatment includes fluid restriction and the measures outlined in Chapter 56.

HEPATIC FAILURE

The consequences of hepatic cell ischemia, in addition to deranged glucose metabolism, include deficits in the factors responsible for coagulation. The coagulopathy is aggravated by multiple transfusions, excessive consumption of clotting factors, and hypothermia. Treatment consists of the administration of fresh frozen plasma and other specific factors identified by coagulation assays.

GASTRIC MUCOSA

The loss of the protective properties of the gastric mucosa following shock makes it vulnerable to the back diffusion of H^+ ions. The injury produces the characteristic stress ulceration and hemorrhage. Although cimetidine was originally thought capable of protecting against such ulceration, it is now recognized that the optimal protection is provided by regular *p*H monitoring of gastric juice and administration of alkaline buffers to maintain the *p*H at 5 or above.

IMMUNE RESISTANCE

The immune defenses of the patient can be compromised by all forms of shock. After multiple transfusions, the reticuloendothelial system can become overloaded with debris that may also originate from capillary stasis. Opsonization is affected adversely by the loss of fibrin for hemostasis and from reduced fibronectin ($\alpha 2$ glycoprotein). There are variable effects on the T- and B-cell subpopulations of lymphocytes and on neutrophils, all of which render the patient more susceptible to secondary infection. Preliminary studies suggest that the opsonic defect in septic shock can be corrected by infusion of cryoprecipitate to restore the fibronectin.[8]

PULMONARY FAILURE

The association between shock and respiratory failure is well established, but the pathophysiology remains controversial. This subject is treated separately in Chapter 22.

References

1. Gaffney FA, Thal ER, Taylor WF et al: Hemodynamic effects of medical anti-shock trousers (MAST garment). J Trauma 21:931, 1981
2. Hinshaw LB: The role of glucose in endotoxin shock. Circ Shock 3:1, 1973
3. Jelenko C III, Williams JB, Wheeler ML et al: Studies in shock and resuscitation: I. Use of a hypertonic albumin-containing fluid demand regimen (HALFD) in resuscitation. Crit Care Med 7:157, 1979
4. Lowery BD, Cloutier CT, Carey LC: Electrolyte solutions in resuscitation in human hemorrhagic shock. Surg Gynecol Obstet 133:273, 1971
5. Martin AM Jr, Hackel DB, Jurtz SM: The ultrastructure of zonal lesions of the myocardium in hemorrhagic shock. Am J Pathol 44:127, 1964
6. Maull KI, Capehart JE, Cardea JA, Haynes BW: Limb loss following military anti-shock trousers (MAST) application. J Trauma 21:60, 1981
7. Ransom KJ, McSwain NE: Metabolic acidosis with pneumatic trousers in hypovolemic dogs. J Am Coll Emerg Phys 8:184, 1979
8. Scovill WA, Saba TM, Blumenstock FA et al: Opsonic 2 surface binding glycoprotein therapy during sepsis. Ann Surg 188:521, 1978
9. Wangensteen SL, Ludewig RM, Co JM, Lynck JN: The effect of external counterpressure on arterial bleeding. Surgery 64:922, 1968
10. Wilson RF, Sarver E, Birks R: Central venous pressure and blood volume determinations in clinical shock. Surg Gynecol Obstet 132:631, 1971

14 Complications of Septic Shock

Harvey J. Sugerman

OVERVIEW—PATHOPHYSIOLOGY

Septic shock is a profound fall in arterial blood pressure that is usually accompanied by a shaking chill, temperature spike, and tachypnea associated with a bacterial or fungal infection. Although most definitions of shock include a fall in blood pressure with inadequate perfusion of vital organs, there is often normal, or even excessive, peripheral perfusion in septic shock. Although septic shock is usually thought to arise from a bacteremia, the syndrome may also occur, in the absence of bacteria in the bloodstream, from the absorption of toxic products of bacteria (i.e., endotoxin) or from the release of vasoactive substances as a result of the interaction of bacteria or endotoxin with infected tissues, white blood cells, or platelets. The mortality of septic shock is related to the underlying disease. Patients who have overwhelming infection or a marked neutropenia secondary to chemotherapy have a dismal prognosis. In contrast, patients who have a transient bacteremia from infusion of a contaminated parenteral solution or urinary-tract manipulation have an excellent prognosis if appropriately treated.[80] A clearer understanding of the pathophysiology of septic shock has evolved over the past 20 years. However, some patients remain refractory to treatment, a fact that emphasizes the deficiencies in our knowledge and the need for the development of additional therapeutic interventions.

MacLean initially demonstrated that patients in septic shock suffer from a diffuse peripheral vasodilatation with a marked increase in their intravascular capacitance so that they are relatively hypovolemic.[67] Although blood-volume measurements were normal, his patients required a significant increase in volume loading to maintain cardiac output and renal function and to prevent metabolic acidosis (Fig. 14-1). It was concluded that they suffered from a diminished "effective blood volume."[68]

Patients in hyperdynamic shock are usually plethoric with warm extremities, often called "warm" shock. The marked decrease in systemic vascular resistance, associated with a marked increase in cardiac output and a narrow arteriovenous oxygen-content difference (as noted by several groups of investigators in the 1960s) was initially presumed to be secondary to the opening of systemic arteriovenous shunts.[3,14,18,100] Subsequent studies using radioactive Xenon muscle washout or radioactive microspheres showed diffuse vasodilatation and the opening of normally closed or "resting" capillary beds rather than arteriovenous shunts.[8,32] Although the majority of patients in septic shock are hyperdynamic, approximately 25% have a reduced cardiac index and elevated systemic vascular resistance, producing "hypodynamic" or "cold" shock.[68]

The pathophysiology of the hyperdynamic low resistance state is still not clearly understood. There is probably a release of vasoactive substances from the interaction of bacteria or endotoxin with infected tissues, blood vessels, white blood cells, and platelets.[44] The substances that have been incriminated include serotonin, endorphins, prostaglandins, histamine, bradykinin, anaphylaxatoxin released from complement activation, and possibly angiotensin.[16,23,33,45,54,92,108] It is probable that most of these substances are involved, working in concert to produce the hemodynamic effects seen. Septic shock is probably the result of normal body defense mechanisms that are out of control. The classical signs of infection (i.e., calor, rubor, tumor, and dolor) are secondary to the release of powerful vasoactive substances such as histamine, serotonin, and prostaglandins that increase capillary permeability and permit the diapedesis of white cells and platelets into infected tissues. Chemotoxins attract the formed elements of the blood to the bacteria, where they undergo phagocytosis and killing with the intracellular, controlled release of extremely toxic substances such as superoxide, phospholipase, lysozyme, nucleotidase, and cathepsin. Should these powerful defenses get out of control, they could produce septic shock and multiple systemic organ failure, which are common fatal sequelae of overwhelming infection. This would include the acute respiratory distress syndrome, acute renal failure, disseminated intravascular coagulation, liver failure, myocardial depression, and coma.

Evidence that platelets and leukocytes are intimately involved in the pathophysiology of septic shock and its sequela is beginning to accrue. Severely septic patients frequently become thrombocytopenic, which may be the most valuable indicator of severe sepsis in the infant.[17, 20] *Direct platelet-bacterial and platelet-endotoxin interactions have been noted in* vitro.[25, 40] *A canine peritonitis model studied in our laboratory was associated with a marked thrombocytopenia that was proportional to the severity of infection. This was unassociated with fibrinogen or complement consumption.*[104] *When a focus of infection was placed in the canine hind limb, Indium-111 platelets were noted to go to the site of infection (Fig. 14-2). Complement activation produces white cell and, perhaps, platelet aggregation, which may be responsible for the development of the acute respiratory distress syndrome (ARDS) associated with septicemia.*[42] *Platelets contain large quantities of vasoactive substances such as thromboxane A_2, serotonin, and histamine. Platelets may react with bacteria to release these vasoactive substances, which markedly decrease peripheral vascular resistance and increase capillary permeability in all tissues of the body. Severely septic patients can become extremely edematous with a diffuse capillary leak refractory to volume expansion.*

Endotoxin has been implicated as the primary culprit in the etiology of gram-negative septic shock. Gram-positive bacteremias, however, can produce an identical shock syndrome.[55] *Endotoxin is a complex lipopolysaccharide found only in the cell wall of gram-negative organisms.*[83] *Intravenous Escherichia coli endotoxin will produce a fatal, hypodynamic shock with a low cardiac output and high systemic vascular resistance in dogs.*[60] *It will poison mitochondria and produce ARDS when infused into sheep.*[4, 75] *Platelet incubation inactivates endotoxin, and enhanced tolerance to Pseudomonas bacteremia has been noted following immunization with antiserum to E. coli endotoxin.*[24, 115] *Since there are many different endotoxins from many strains of bac-*

FIG. 14-1. Effective blood volume, that volume that restored arterial blood pressure, urine output, and tissue perfusion, exceeded the normal blood volume for each of these patients in septic shock. (MacLean LD, Duff JJ, Scott HM et al: Treatment of shock in man based on hemodynamic diagnosis. Surg Gynecol Obstet 120:1, 1965. By permission of SURGERY, GYNECOLOGY & OBSTETRICS)

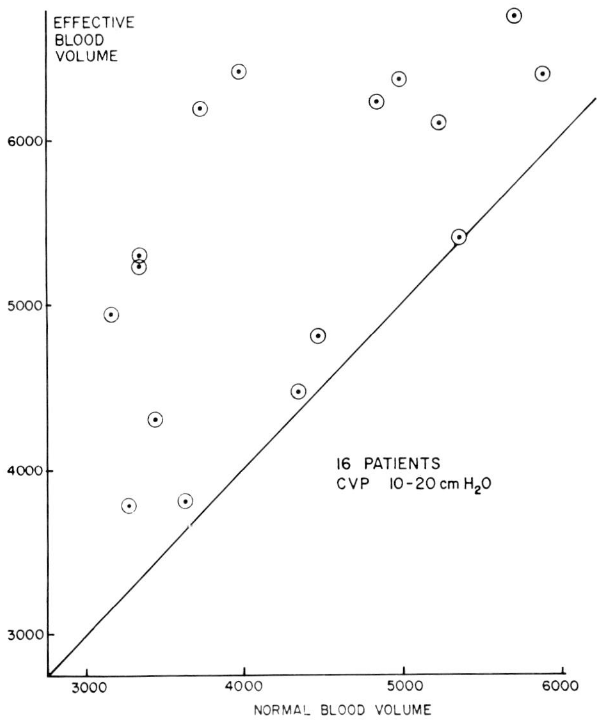

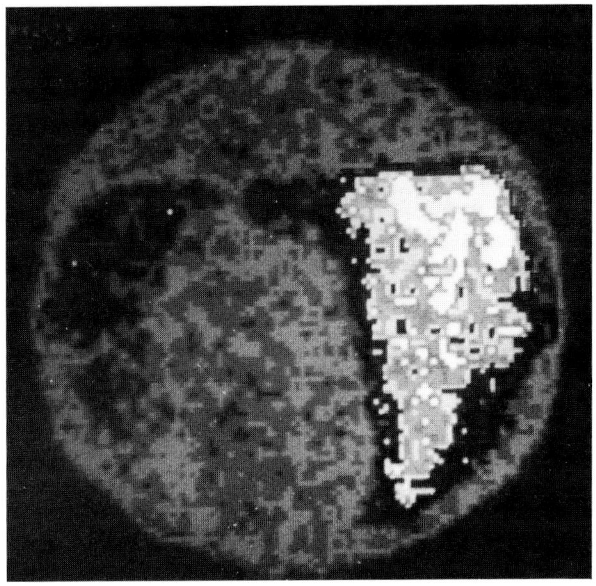

FIG. 14-2. Uptake of ^{111}In platelets at 24 hours in a focus of infection in a canine hind-limb preparation. (Reproduced with permission from Sugerman HJ, Peyton JWR, Greenfield LJ: Gram-negative sepsis. In Ravitch MM et al (eds): Current Problems in Surgery 18:405, 1981. Copyright © 1981 by Year Book Medical Publishers, Inc., Chicago)

teria, the degree of immunologic protection afforded by immunization with a single strain remains to be shown.

Diagnosis

The diagnosis of septic shock is often quite easy but may be deceptively difficult (Table 14-1). The earliest sign is usually a marked tachypnea and hyperpnea or "Kussmaul-like" breathing in the absence of ketoacidosis.[68] This is thought to be due to stimulation of the respiratory center by endotoxin or one of the vasoactive substances already mentioned. It may also be a result of microembolism of aggregates of platelets, leukocytes, and bacteria. A shaking chill often precedes a temperature spike prior to the fall in blood pressure. Occasionally, a paradoxical hypothermia occurs. The fundamental feature of septic shock is the marked fall in blood pressure. This is usually associated with warm, well-perfused extremities, so-called warm shock.[67] Central venous (CVP) and pulmonary capillary wedge (PCWP) pressures are usually low. Approximately 25% of patients, however, have cold or hypodynamic shock.[67] This usually occurs at the end stage of septic shock but can be seen early, especially in the presence of a severe volume deficit. Cardiac output in this circumstance would be reduced, and the arteriovenous oxygen-content difference wide. The oxygen consumption in both hyperdynamic and hypodynamic patients may be normal or somewhat elevated. Urine output is usually low in septic shock, but occasionally patients will present with an inappropriate polyuria.[89] The patient is often quite confused and may even be combative. Blood cultures, documenting the presence of a bacteremia, require several days to grow. The limulus assay is quite sensitive for the presence of endotoxin but is nonspecific.[57] Lactic acidemia may be present but is nonspecifically elevated in any shock state.

TABLE 14-1. DIAGNOSIS OF SEPTIC SHOCK

Shaking chill
Tachypnea
Spiking temperature (usual), hypothermia (rare)
Hypotension with warm toes (75%), cold toes (25%)
Low CVP or PCWP (usual)
High cardiac output (75%), low cardiac output (25%)
Elevated mixed venous oxygen tension (usual)
Oliguria (usual), polyuria (often)
Hyperglycemia (early), hypoglycemia (late)
+ limulus test
+ blood cultures (late)

TABLE 14-2. TREATMENT OF SEPTIC SHOCK

Blood culture
Broad spectrum antibiotics: aminoglycoside + ampicillin + clindamycin or metronidazole or chloramphenicol
Volume expansion: monitor CVP or PCWP and urine output
Vasoactive drugs if necessary: dopamine, digitalization, ? nitroprusside (if cardiac output low)
Intubation, mechanical ventilation, high F_IO_2, PEEP as needed
Physiologic dose of corticosteroid
Possible pharmacologic dose corticosteroid (30 mg/kg methylprednisolone)
Drain pus

Treatment

PRIMARY THERAPEUTIC MODALITIES

Appropriate blood, urine, sputum, and central-catheter cultures should be obtained and the patient begun on broad-spectrum antibiotics. These should include an aminoglycoside such as gentamicin or, if gentamicin resistance is considered, amikacin. Anaerobic coverage should be obtained with clindamycin, chloramphenicol, or metronidazole. In addition, ampicillin should be given to cover *Streptococcus faecalis*. Amphotericin may be required if candidemia is suspected. Once specific sensitivities are obtained, the appropriate antibiotic can be administered.

Following appropriate cultures and the administration of broad-spectrum antibiotics, the most important therapeutic intervention is to correct the deficit in "effective intravascular volume," as initially suggested by MacLean (Table 14-2).[68] Measurement of central venous pressure (CVP) was initially the guide for volume replacement and may still be useful. It is most important to follow not only the absolute level of CVP but its response to a fluid challenge.[111] It has been shown that the CVP may not be related to the PCWP in severely ill, septic, or traumatized patients, as shown in Figure 14-3.[12] By measurement of the PCWP, the use of the Swan–Ganz catheter provides more accurate information as to the status of left ventricular filling. In addition, one can measure cardiac output, using the thermodilution technique, and mixed venous oxygen tension. The PCWP measurement can occasionally be misleading, especially if the patient is receiving mechanical ventilation with positive end-expiratory pressure (PEEP).[35] Evidence is mounting that volume expansion, ARDS, and PEEP therapy all can lead to an excessive right ventricular end-diastolic volume with a shift of the interventricular septum to the left, impairment of left ventricular function, and a depressed cardiac output.[7, 73, 98] Right ventricular volume and contractility have been measured by Burke and colleagues using a modified Swan–Ganz catheter where the proximal opening is ad-

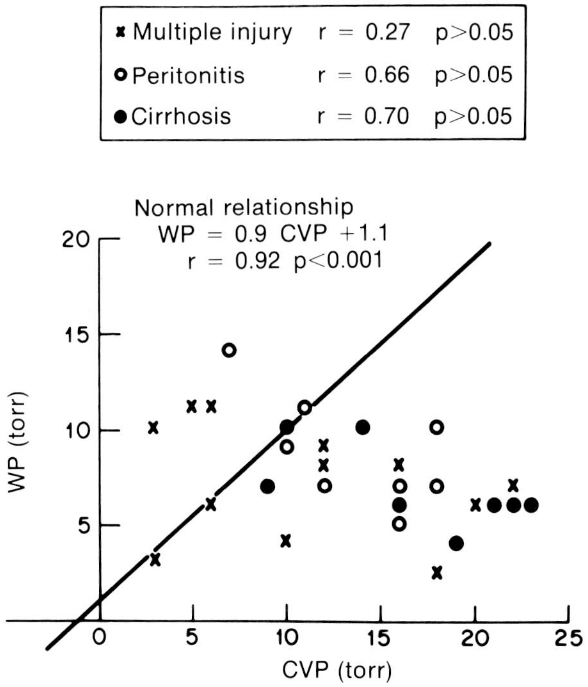

FIG. 14-3. Relationship of central venous pressure (*CVP*) and pulmonary capillary wedge pressure (*WP*) in normal patients and those with severe multi-system injury, decompensated cirrhosis, or peritonitis. Notice the regression line indicating the normal relationship between CVP and WP: $p < 0.001$ indicates a significant relationship. The relationship for values obtained in these three disease states was not significant. Wide scattering of points is evident. (Civetta JM, Gabel JC: Flow-directed pulmonary artery catheterization in surgical patients: Indications and modifications of technique. Ann Surg 176:753, 1972)

vanced from the superior vena cava to the right ventricle.[73] This may improve the usefulness of the Swan–Ganz catheter. Gated gamma camera scintigraphic measurement of both right and left ventricular chamber size as well as ejection fractions in response to a volume challenge may provide further physiologic information but is unlikely to be applicable on a broad clinical scale.[7]

In an earlier study from our laboratory, volume expansion alone was able to correct hypotension and oliguria in almost 50% of patients in septic shock.[105] It previously was our policy to raise the PCWP to 15 torr to provide maximum left ventricular function according to the Frank–Starling curve. There is evidence, however, that an increased pulmonary microvascular permeability secondary to sepsis is associated with an increased rate of protein and fluid leak following volume expansion (Fig. 14-4).[4] Under these conditions it may be more appropriate to expand volume to a PCWP of 10 torr or less. The choice of solutions for volume expansion is controversial. The data suggest that excessive use of colloid is not only expensive but offers no advantage over crystalloid solutions in the prevention of hypoxemia. and, furthermore, may possibly lead to even greater pulmonary damage.[64, 78, 100] Therefore, unless the patient has a markedly reduced serum albumin, we would elect to expand volume primarily with lactated Ringer's solution.

If the patient remains hypotensive and oliguric following volume expansion, vasoactive drug support is needed. Most investigators believe that the patient should receive digitalis.[68, 100] In the early 1970s, isoproterenol was used for inotropic support; however, in recent years dopamine has been shown to be more effective with less risk of arrhythmia.[113] At low doses (4–8 mcq/kg/minute), dopamine is primarily a beta-inotropic agent. High doses of dopamine (> 10 mcg/kg/minute) produce an "alpha-effect" with peripheral vasoconstriction. In either case, dopamine increases renal blood flow and glomerular filtration rate with an increased urinary output.[112] A more recent vasoactive drug, dobutamine, has been recommended because its action is limited to increasing myocardial inotropic activity.[34] It too offers less risk of cardiac arrhythmias. No studies that compare dobutamine to dopamine have been published. In early 1970, our laboratory showed that patients who are in high-output, hyperdynamic shock, will frequently respond to an alpha agent

FIG. 14-4. Compared to control animals, there is a marked increase in lung lymph flow following left atrial pressure elevation in sheep with endotoxin- and *Pseudomonas*-induced microvascular lung injury. (Brigham KL, Bowers RE, Haynes J: Increased sheep lung vascular permeability caused by *Escherichia coli* endotoxin. Circ Res 45:292, 1979, by permission of the American Heart Association, Inc.)

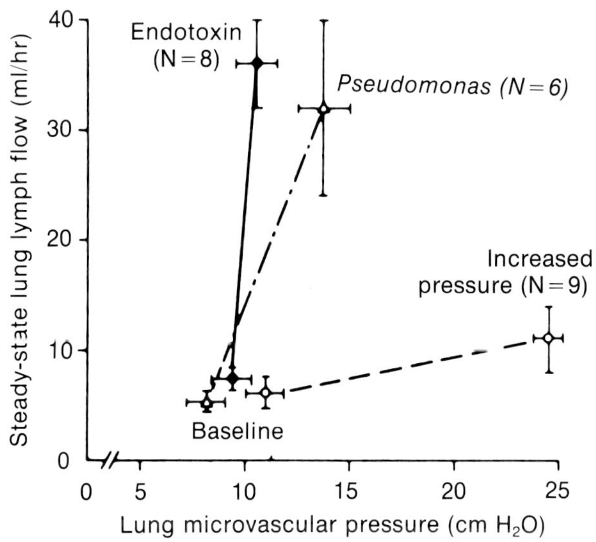

such as metaraminol.[105] These patients received high-dose metaraminol infusion; 12 to 19 hyperdynamic patients, refractory to isoproterenol, responded with a fall in cardiac output and a significant rise in urinary output with correction of their lacticacidemia.[105] Dopamine acts primarily as a "beta-agent" at low doses and as an "alpha-agent" at high doses so that it can be used initially to provide inotropic support and, if this is unsuccessful in a hyperdynamic patient, then an increased rate of infusion can be used to provide an "alpha-effect," which would mimic the action of metaraminol. This would not be possible with dobutamine.

If the patient is in hypodynamic shock with a low cardiac output, a high-peripheral vascular resistance, and a wide arteriovenous oxygen-content difference, then the primary effort must be directed toward improving cardiac inotropic activity. Again, digoxin should be used and a low-dose dopamine infusion begun. If the patient fails to respond to these maneuvers, one should consider afterload reduction with a nitroprusside infusion at 10 to 15 mcg/minute.[34] Some have suggested the application of nitroglycerine paste, but cutaneous absorption in a patient with cold shock is probably limited and would be more difficult to control than would an intravenous infusion.[9]

One of the most important aspects of managing a patient in septic shock is to remove or drain the source of infection. Should it be necessary to operate, the patient should be taken to the operating room as soon as hemodynamic stabilization can be achieved. It is rarely necessary to operate on a patient while he is in shock.

ADJUNCTIVE AGENTS

A number of other agents have been proposed for the treatment of septic shock. Pharmacologic doses of corticosteroids (30 mg/kg every 4 hours, methylprednisolone, or 4 mg/kg every 4 hours, dexamethasone) have been recommended for the management of septic shock since the studies by Lillehei in the early 1960s using a canine endotoxin model.[59] This model was subsequently found to represent an overwhelming insult, with the development of immediate hypodynamic (*i.e.*, low cardiac output, high resistance) shock. Use of a vasoconstrictor in the presence of a pathologically elevated peripheral vascular resistance led to rapid tachyphylaxis and death.[13] Lillehei and colleagues initially proposed the use of corticosteroids for their vasodilating properties.[59] They found that pharmacologic doses of corticosteroids produced a significant increase in survival in the canine endotoxic shock model. It has subsequently been suggested that steroids may work by stabilizing lysosomal membranes, improving mitochondrial function, or, more recently, preventing leukocyte agglutination.[13, 42, 74] There is only one randomized, prospective clinical study evaluating the efficacy of pharmacologic doses of corticosteroids in the treatment of septicemic shock. In this study Schumer found a significantly reduced mortality in patients so treated.[97] Another group of nonrandomized patients was also included in this study. In the discussion of this article, Baue questioned the ability to run a randomized and nonrandomized study at the same time on such a large volume of septic shock patients.[97]

The timing of the administration of corticosteroids is an additional cause for concern. The majority of patients who die have recurrent septic episodes. Steroids are known to suppress the immunologic response and mask the signs of sepsis.[50, 90] Hinshaw and colleagues have shown that pharmacologic doses of steroids administered to baboons prior to an *E. coli* bacteremic challenge significantly increased the rates of survival if the animals were also treated with gentamicin sulfate.[48] Nevertheless, the clear efficacy of corticosteroids in the treatment of patients in septic shock is still unproven. The greatest potential danger from their use is that the physician might neglect other, more important interventions, such as volume expansion and vasoactive amines. A physiologic dose of corticosteroid (*i.e.*, 100 mg hydrocortisone) should be given in the case of the rare possibility that the patient may have adrenal insufficiency.

More recently, data are beginning to show that blockade of prostaglandin synthesis or infusion of prostacyclin (PGI_2) may be beneficial in reducing the mortality of endotoxic shock in experimental animals.[33] Reynolds and colleagues found that septic shock was associated with endorphin or enkephalin release and that the narcotic antagonist, naloxone, reduced mortality in an endotoxic model.[92] Hess and colleagues have postulated that angiotensin activation may be responsible for the myocardial depression that is seen in late septic shock and that angiotensin blockade may be of value.[45] Lefer and colleagues have attributed this reduced cardiac function in sepsis to a myocardial depressant factor, or MDF.[56] Others have found a beneficial effect of ATP-$MgCl_2$ in the survival of shocked rats.[10]

Sepsis and Multisystem Organ Failure

It is now uncommon for a patient to die in intractable septic shock. Septic shock and infection, however, are the most common causes of multisystem organ failure, which carries a high morbidity and mortality and markedly increases the cost of medical

TABLE 14-3. MULTISYSTEM ORGAN FAILURE IN SEPSIS

Organ	Problem	Treatment/ Prevention
Lung	ARDS	Mechanical ventilation/PEEP
	↓ V/Q	↑ tidal volume
	Pneumonia	Antibiotics/good side down
	Excessive CO_2	↑ % fat to ↓ RQ
Kidney	Oliguric ARF	Early diagnosis, TPN with possible essential AA
	Nonoliguric ARF	+/− dialysis, TPN with standard AA solutions.
Liver	Cholestatic jaundice	r/o extrahepatic obstruction
		"Tincture of time"
		↑ % fat in TPN or d/c TPN
	Coma	Possible BCAA
	Hypoglycemia	Hypertonic glucose infusion (usually preterminal)
Gut	Stress bleeding	TPN + gastric acid neutralization
	Acalculous cholecystitis	Cholecystectomy
	Pseudomembranous colitis	Vancomycin
Heart	Myocardial failure	Possible afterload reduction (nitroprusside)
Coagulation	Thrombocytopenia	"Tincture of time"
	DIC	Heparin (rarely needed)
CNS	Nonketotic hyperglycemic coma	Insulin—slowly
	Obtundation of sepsis	Possible BCAA

care.[27, 37] Every organ in the body is at risk for failure in severe sepsis (Table 14-3).

THE EFFECT OF SEPSIS ON THE LUNG

The lungs are the human organ most susceptible to injury in septicemia and septic shock.[6, 15] The syndrome is known as the *acute respiratory distress syndrome*, or ARDS (see also Chap. 22). ARDS results from pulmonary microvascular injury with an increased pulmonary capillary membrane leak to protein.[94, 101] The increased interstitial fluid and protein pass along the alveolar walls to the peribronchiolar lymphatics where the fluid is returned to the vascular system. The pulmonary lymphatics are able to increase flow by a factor of 10.[94] When the lymphatic system is overwhelmed, there is a sudden leakage of fluid with a high protein content into the alveoli.[94] The increased swelling of the alveolar ductules may lead to decreased alveolar air flow. When the alveoli become flooded, there is either an inhibition or washout of surfactant with subsequent alveolar collapse. The perfusion of unventilated alveoli produces a ventilation–perfusion (V/Q) mismatch with arterial hypoxemia that may be refractory to increasing the inspired oxygen concentration (F_IO_2). In addition, a septic patient may suffer from V/Q mismatch without permeability edema when an extremely high cardiac output increases flow to poorly ventilated, dependent areas of the lung (zone III of West.)[99]

Etiology

The cause of the pulmonary capillary membrane injury is not yet fully understood. Hammerschmidt and colleagues have presented studies that suggest that bacteria or bacterial endotoxins activate the complement cascade that then produces granulocyte aggregation.[42] Disruption of these agglutinated leukocytes, with the release of toxic intracellar enzymes, produces capillary membrane injury. It is also possible that endotoxin or bacteria may react directly with the pulmonary capillary membrane. Furthermore, the release of autacoids such as histamine, serotonin, and prostaglandins may be responsible for the increase in pulmonary capillary membrane permeability. Platelet aggregation has also been incriminated in the pathogenesis of ARDS.[95, 96] Furthermore, experimental ARDS produced by administration of the fibrinogen degradation product, fragment D, was prevented by antiplatelet-serum-induced thrombocytopenia.[71]

Diagnosis

ARDS can be diagnosed when a patient becomes progressively hypoxemic (PaO_2<60 torr) despite increasing concentrations of inspired oxygen (Table 14-4). ARDS can be present even if the chest x-ray film is normal, but a diffuse infiltrate in both lung fields without evidence of cardiomegaly on chest film is usually required to be certain of the diagnosis. There may be bilateral rales on auscultation, but signs of congestive heart failure such as distended

TABLE 14-4. DIAGNOSIS OF ARDS

Tachypnea, air hunger
Hypoxemia without hypercarbia
Normal PCWP (<15 torr)
Diffuse infiltrate on chest radiograph (may be delayed finding)
Minimal ↑ PaO_2 with ↑ F_IO_2
Rapid ↑ PaO_2 with PEEP

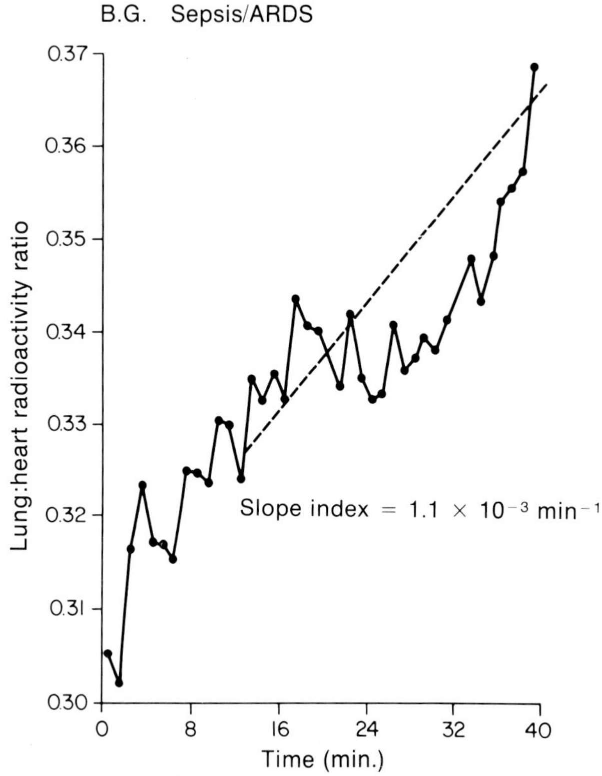

FIG. 14-5. A steep slope of injury was noted with portable computerized gamma scintillation camera measurements of the leak of ^{99m}Tc human serum albumin into the lung 8 hours following the onset of septic-induced ARDS in a patient with suppurative cholangitis. (Reproduced with permission from Sugerman HJ, Peyton JWR, Greenfield LJ: Gram-negative sepsis. In Ravitch MM et al (eds): Current Problems in Surgery 18:405, 1981. Copyright © 1981 by Year Book Medical Publishers, Inc., Chicago)

neck veins or a diastolic gallop are absent. Patients with ARDS have an alveolar-arterial oxygen tension difference on 100% F_IO_2 of greater than 300 torr with more than 20% right-to-left shunt.[101] The arterial $PaCO_2$ is either normal or reduced, since the CO_2-hemoglobin dissociation curve is linear, permitting almost complete removal of CO_2 from ventilated alveoli. Swan–Ganz right-heart catheterization will reveal a PCWP less than 15 torr. There may be an increased pulmonary vascular resistance and a wide pulmonary artery end-diastolic pressure to PCWP gradient. The differentiation between V/Q mismatch secondary to ARDS versus that due to an increased flow to zone III of the lung can be made by determining the response to increasing the tidal volume. This improves ventilation to zone III and minimizes a flow-induced V/Q mismatch with an improved PaO_2.[99] ARDS requires the institution of PEEP before a large rise in PaO_2 is seen.[101]

More accurate techniques for the detection and measurement of the severity of ARDS are needed, but many of the newer approaches are problematical. The double-isotopic indicator dilution technique for the measurement of extravascular lung water, developed by Chinard and Enns, is influenced by actual extravascular lung water as well as by changes in pulmonary vascular recruitment.[11] Thus, a patient with a high cardiac output would have an increased pulmonary blood flow, which would erroneously indicate an increased extravascular lung water in the absence of pulmonary edema.[72] The thermal-cardiogreen double-indicator dilution technique may overcome this problem because of the much more rapid distribution of the heat indicator.[85] Nevertheless, it is unproven whether this technique is also affected by changes in pulmonary vascular recruitment. Our laboratory has recently developed a computerized gamma camera scintigraphic technique for the detection and quantitative analysis of a pulmonary capillary membrane leak to protein.[107] In this method, ^{99m}Tc-tagged human serum albumin (Tc-HSA) is administered intravenously and the lungs and heart defined scintigraphically. The computer-constructed lung:heart radioactivity ratio is constant unless there is a pulmonary capillary protein leak, which reveals a rising ratio with time that we have called the "slope of injury." We have since applied this technique in a number of patients with ARDS secondary to sepsis. A slope of injury which persisted in some for several days was noted in these patients (Fig. 14-5). This method should permit us to evaluate the effectiveness of various therapeutic agents.

Treatment

The cornerstone in the treatment of ARDS is mechanical ventilation with a volume ventilator. Many of these patients have rigid lungs with poor compliance and cannot be adequately ventilated with a pressure-regulated ventilator. Although occasional patients may be managed without intubation by using continuous, positive airway pressure (CPAP), the safest and most effective technique is intubation and the use of continuous PEEP and high tidal volumes (800 ml –1000 ml).[28] Occasionally, an end-inspiratory hold may be helpful.[22] Since high-dose inspired oxygen is toxic, leading to the development of absorption atelectasis and, with prolonged use, to superoxide damage to pulmonary alveolar cells, every attempt should be made to use 0.6 F_IO_2 or less.[79, 84]

A rapid PEEP titration can be undertaken. In this procedure, the cardiac output or the mixed venous oxygen tension ($P\bar{v}O_2$) is measured with PEEP raised by 5-cm H_2O increments at 10-minute intervals up to 20 cm H_2O. The goal is the amount of PEEP that can maintain a PaO_2 above 60 torr with

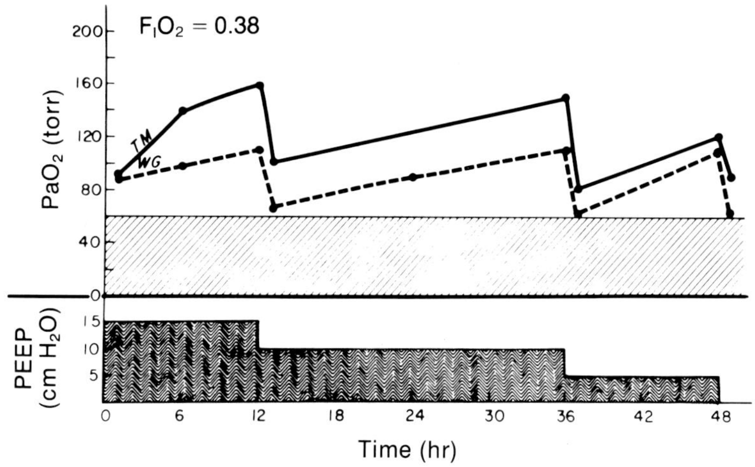

FIG. 14-6. Progressive improvement in arterial oxygen tension (PaO_2) in two patients with septic-induced ARDS. The PaO_2 could be maintained above 60 torr with 0.38 fraction inspired oxygen (F_IO_2) only when 15 cm H_2O positive end-expiratory pressure (*PEEP*) was used. Over 48 hours the steady increase in PaO_2 permitted a progressive reduction and eventual cessation of PEEP. (Sugerman HJ et al: Continuous positive end-expiratory pressure ventilation (PEEP) for the treatment of diffuse interstitial edema. J Trauma 12:263, 1972. © 1981, The Williams & Wilkins Co., Baltimore)

an F_IO_2 of 0.6 or less without interfering with cardiac output, as measured directly or as reflected by a decreased $P\bar{v}O_2$. Should the cardiac output fall, it may be necessary to expand intravascular volume to counteract the effect of PEEP on venous return.[88] When a patient is being treated with PEEP, PCWP measurements must be interpreted carefully. The increased ventilatory pressures can be transmitted to the pulmonary capillaries that are being measured if PEEP reduces flow to that zone of the lung.[65] Some patients require extremely high levels of PEEP, or "super-PEEP" in order to achieve adequate oxygenation. This can be facilitated by the use of intermittent, mandatory ventilation (IMV) so that the average mean airway pressure is reduced by the negative inspiratory force of the patient.[52]

In general, the sicker the patient is, the stiffer is the lung and the lower is the pulmonary compliance; hence, a greater amount of PEEP can be tolerated, since the higher airway pressures are dissipated and not transmitted to the venous system.[106] The effect of PEEP is quite rapid and usually reaches a maximum within 15 to 20 minutes. The use of PEEP for pulmonary injury is analogous to the use of a cast for a fracture. It, in effect, splints the lung and permits it to heal itself. In general, the level of PEEP can gradually be reduced over several days if no additional insult to the lungs occurs (Fig. 14-6). The danger of barotrauma must be considered when PEEP is used since a tension pneumothorax can develop rapidly.

Although several reports have recommended the use of pharmacologic doses of corticosteroids, none have proved their effectiveness in controlled, randomized, prospective trials. Hammerschmidt and colleagues noted that 30 mg/kg methylprednisolone will inhibit leukocyte aggregation induced by complement activation, which may prevent pulmonary capillary membrane injury.[42] Studies by Brigham and colleagues using the Staub sheep model have shown, however, that corticosteroids are only efficacious if given prior to endotoxin or *Pseudomonas* injection.[5]

Additional Pulmonary Problems

In addition to ARDS and V/Q mismatch, septic patients with ARDS are at high risk for the development of bilateral bronchial pneumonia.[1] The large amount of proteinaceous fluid that accumulates in ARDS is a rich culture medium that can be readily inoculated with bacteria from a mechanical ventilator or an indwelling endotracheal tube. Furthermore, these patients are quite debilitated with a decreased cough reflex and depressed ciliary activity and have difficulty mobilizing pulmonary secretions. They are dependent on the nursing staff for pulmonary toilet. With indwelling Swan–Ganz catheters and arterial lines, it is difficult to turn these patients. This increases the danger of fluid accumulation in the dependent regions of the lung with secondary bacterial invasion and overgrowth. In addition, septic patients are extremely catabolic. Even under the best of circumstances with vigorous total parenteral nutrition (TPN), it may be very difficult to achieve a positive nitrogen balance. They are also likely to have impaired respiratory muscle function, which impedes their ability to mobilize secretions and to be weaned from the ventilator. The catabolic energy state can also interfere with immunologic protection and leukocyte function, which increases their risk for pneumonia. Finally, septic, comatose patients are at risk for aspiration pneumonitis. At postmortem examination, these patients frequently have hepatization of their lungs. Should a unilateral pneumonia be present, the patient should be kept as much as possible with the good side down to increase flow to the well ventilated side.[91]

RENAL INSUFFICIENCY

It is probably less common for patients in septic shock to develop oliguric acute renal failure (ARF) than it is for patients with hypovolemic shock. This may be related to the fact that the majority of patients in septic shock have an elevated cardiac output with a low peripheral vascular resistance and continue to perfuse their kidneys while being hypotensive. Indeed, many patients with severe sepsis have an inappropriate polyuria that relates to an increased renal blood flow.[66] Radioactive Xenon washout studies showed a normal distribution of intrarenal blood flow in three such patients.[21] The greatest cause of oliguric ARF in septic patients is a nephrotoxic aminoglycoside antibiotic.[47] The toxicity of these drugs may be enhanced when they are used in combination with the cephalosporins.[31]

The development of ARF markedly increases the mortality rate of critically ill patients. It is still estimated, despite the advances in nephrology, that ARF carries a 50% mortality.[70] The presence of ARF complicates efforts with parenteral nutrition and the ability to provide adequate calories for the hypercatabolic septic patient.

The diagnosis of ARF is made in the presence of a progressively rising level of BUN and creatinine and a urinary sodium more than 40 mEq/L. This is to be differentiated from the hepatorenal syndrome in which the urinary sodium is less than 10 mEq/L. The pathogenesis of ARF is still unknown. These patients should be managed with early and frequent hemodialysis since the catabolic state of an extremely septic patient causes an accelerated production of urea as well as of other metabolites and can rapidly produce dangerous levels of hyperkalemia. Data suggest improved survival rates after early dialysis.[19] Should hyperkalemia become life-threatening, the patient should be treated prior to dialysis with intravenous regular insulin (10 units) and 250 ml, 50% glucose, to facilitate intracellular potassium movement, with electrocardiographic monitoring. A calcium infusion should be instituted to counteract the effect of an elevated serum potassium on the heart, but it is contraindicated in the digitalized patient.[81] Kayexalate enemas should also be given but are much slower to work.

The hypercatabolic, oliguric septic patient should be nourished with low volumes of highly concentrated dextrose solutions (47%). Recent studies have suggested that there is no advantage to the administration of essential amino acids (Nephramine) over standard amino acid solutions in the patient with ARF.[27,77] Intravenous mannitol or high-dose intravenous furosemide (100 mg–200 mg) have been suggested as useful in either preventing or treating early acute renal failure but neither has been proven efficacious.[58] Nonoliguric ARF is more frequently present as a result of nephrotoxic drugs. It carries a lower mortality rate than does oliguric ARF. These patients require less frequent dialysis for control of uremia or hyperkalemia, and TPN is much easier to manage since fluid restriction is not required.

LIVER ABNORMALITIES

The most common hepatic abnormality seen in gram-negative sepsis is cholestatic jaundice associated with a rise in bilirubin and alkaline phosphatase and minimal elevation of serum glutamic-oxaloacetic acid transferase (SGOT), serum glutamic-pyruvate transferase (SGPT), and lactic acid dehydrogenase (LDH).[82] The bilirubin can reach levels greater than 20 mg/dl from this cause. Furthermore, acute fatty infiltration of the liver associated with TPN can also produce a cholestatic picture.[39] Differential diagnosis between extrahepatic and intrahepatic obstructive jaundice can now be made easily with ultrasonography. An experienced radiologist can determine extrahepatic ductal dilatation of more than 5 days' duration with above 95% accuracy.[116] More invasive studies, such as percutaneous transhepatic cholangiography (PTC) or endoscopic retrograde cholangiopancreatography (ERCP), are usually unnecessary. With resolution of the septic condition, the cholestatic jaundice of sepsis will spontaneously resolve. Cholestatic jaundice from hyperalimentation will respond to either cessation of TPN or the use of an intravenous fat emulsion to provide a greater proportion of the caloric load.[39] Occasionally, a patient with overwhelming sepsis and septic shock will develop a marked increase in levels of SGOT and SGPT as well as LDH. We have seen values in the thousands in such patients with complete recovery. A large portion of the SGOT might be derived from muscle ischemia and the LDH from red-cell hemolysis.

With overwhelming infection, the liver may be unable to convert amino acids or lactate into glucose, resulting in the development of a fulminant, refractory hypoglycemia.[30] This is almost always a preterminal event. Although infrequently seen clinically, severe hypoglycemia is a common observation following experimental endotoxic shock, which suggests a severe injury to liver cells associated with endotoxemia.[30] The study of liver mitochondria following endotoxemia in rats has demonstrated several metabolic derangements.[76] This probably represents the ultimate, irreversible injury associated with septic shock with irreparable damage to the cell.

There is little information on the treatment of the metabolic aspects of liver insufficiency in sepsis. Massive infusions of glucose are not effective in the patient who develops fulminant hypoglycemia. Research laboratories are now working to tailor parenteral feeding solutions to fill the specialized metabolic needs of septic patients. Use of the branch chain amino acids (valine, leucine, and isoleucine) is being studied.[36]

EFFECT ON COAGULATION

Severe thrombocytopenia frequently develops in severe gram-negative infection. Pediatricians use this as a sensitive indicator of infection in infants in whom the other usual signs of sepsis (level of temperature, white count, and hyperpnea) may be absent.[20] Thrombocytopenia was initially thought to be invariably associated with disseminated intravascular coagulation (DIC).[17] However, a diagnosis of DIC requires a prolongation of the prothrombin time (PT) and the partial thromboplastin time (PTT), a decrease in serum fibrinogen to less than 100 mg/dl (normal being >160 mg/dl), and a rise in fibrin degradation products (FDPs) to above 40 mg/dl. Using these criteria, a number of studies have shown that thrombocytopenia in sepsis is rarely associated with DIC.[38, 93] This has also been our experience. A canine septic peritonitis model, developed in our laboratory, was found to produce a marked thrombocytopenia with an increased serum fibrinogen level without complement consumption.[104] The degree of thrombocytopenia was proportional to the severity of the illness (Fig. 14-7). Several *in vitro* studies have shown that platelets react directly with bacteria as well as with endotoxin.[24, 25, 40] It has been suggested that platelet lysis induced by endotoxin and bacteria may be responsible for the release of the high levels of autacoids (histamine and serotonin) responsible for the shock state.[23] Furthermore, activated platelets may go to pulmonary capillaries and produce ARDS.[42] When a focus of infection was placed in the canine hind limb, ^{111}In platelets went to the site of infection (see Fig. 14-2). This confirmed our hypothesis that platelets travel to the site of infection.

Although the vast majority of patients with thrombocytopenia do not develop DIC, this complication is occasionally seen, probably owing to bacteremia or endotoxemia with intravascular activation of platelets. Systemic heparinization has been recommended to abort the process.[26] The use of heparin in a critically ill patient, which itself has the potential of aggravating bleeding in the presence of thrombocytopenia, should be restricted to patients who have clinically significant bleeding and DIC documented according to the previously enumerated criteria.

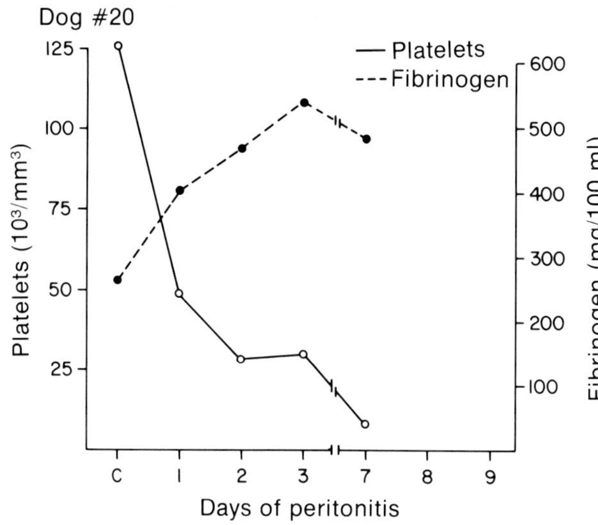

FIG. 14-7. A rapid fall in platelets without fibrinogen consumption found in experimental canine peritonitis. (Reproduced with permission from Sugerman HJ, Peyton JWR, Greenfield LJ: Gram-negative sepsis. In Ravitch MM et al (eds): Current Problems in Surgery 18:405, 1981. Copyright © 1981 by Year Book Medical Publishers, Inc., Chicago)

EFFECT ON CENTRAL NERVOUS SYSTEM

Severely septic patients are at risk for developing an encephalopathy. This may be due, in part, to the inability of the liver to metabolize the aromatic and sulfur-containing amino acids as well as to the production of false neurotransmitters, such as octopamine.[35] Cerebral dysfunction in sepsis might also result from the direct effect of bacteria or endotoxin or to the indirect effect of the release of powerful autacoids associated with sepsis. Also, hypophosphatemia may lead to cerebral dysfunction, and massive fluid shifts seen in septic patients may produce cerebral edema with coma.[63] Of greater danger and clinical importance is the nonketotic hyperglycemic coma that can occur with TPN in septic patients with impaired glucose metabolism.[69] It carries a 40% to 60% mortality. These causes of cerebral dysfunction can be prevented if the patient is carefully monitored. The development of hyperglycemia in a septic patient can be quite rapid and precede clinical evidence of sepsis (see Fig. 17-5).

EFFECT ON THE HEART

Impaired myocardial function is also seen in severe sepsis. Approximately 25% of patients in septic shock have a low cardiac output, high-resistance shock. Furthermore, many patients who die in septic shock pass from a hyperdynamic (high cardiac output, low-resistance) state to a hypodynamic phase preterminally. Lefer and colleagues have proposed the release of a myocardial depressant factor (MDF) in severe sepsis.[56] Hess and colleagues have suggested that this may be related to excessive angiotensin release.[45] They have also shown that endotoxin is quite damaging to myocardial sarcoplasmic reticulum.[46] In late septic shock there is an excessive production of lactic acid and organic anions which cannot be metabolized in a failing liver. This large metabolic anion gap produces a profound metabolic acidosis that further impedes myocardial contractility. All of these circumstances lead to a stiff, dilated ventricular chamber with a decreased myocardial function on the Starling curve. This can be diagnosed by following the PCWP response to volume loading. Decreased cardiac function should be treated with inotropic agents such as dopamine, dobutamine, or digitalis.[61, 68, 112] A nitroprusside infusion will reduce both preload and afterload and usually increase cardiac output.[34] When a patient reaches the stage of hypodynamic septic shock, the prognosis is quite guarded.[68]

EFFECT ON THE GUT

Although the human gastrointestinal system appears to be more resistant to shock than in other species, stress bleeding from gastritis is a major complication in a severely ill patient. The incidence of stress ulceration appears to be diminishing, though possibly as a result of improved care of multiple system organ failure in critically ill patients. These patients appear to have a breakdown of the gastric mucosal barrier with a back diffusion of hydrogen ion.[53] It is essential that stressed patients be protected from their own acid by continuous infusions of antacids through a nasogastric tube or have acid production reduced with intravenous cimetidine.[41, 43] Gastric pH should be regularly monitored.[102] The dose of cimetidine may have to be increased to maintain gastric acid neutrality. Two recent studies have shown that antacid infusions were more effective than is cimetidine in preventing bleeding.[87, 103] Also, large doses of cimetidine may induce mental confusion.[114]

In addition, vigorous TPN may play a major role in the reduction of stress bleeding in patients in intensive-care units. Gastric mucosa undergoes continuous regeneration. In the presence of protein-calorie malnutrition, this intestinal mucosal restoration may be impeded with loss of the gastric mucosal barrier and increased acid back diffusion. A recent primate study has confirmed an increased incidence of aspirin-induced gastric erosions in nutritionally depleted monkeys, which could be prevented by the use of TPN.[49]

Septic patients on multiple-dose antibiotics are also at risk for the development of pseudomembranous colitis.[51] This appears to be secondary to colonic overgrowth of *Clostridium difficile* with the release of a toxin that damages the colonic mucosa. Treatment of this condition demands discontinuance of the antibiotics as well as the administration of oral vancomycin to eliminate the clostridia.[51]

Acalculous cholecystitis is another intestinal condition seen in septic patients.[62] This may be related to decreased gallbladder contractility in patients who are critically ill as well as to bile stasis in a gallbladder that is not stimulated to contract as a result of TPN administration.[86] It may be extremely difficult to diagnose in a sick, septic patient so that the physician should maintain a high index of suspicion. Emergency cholecystectomy may be necessary. Low-flow shock may also produce intestinal necrosis or pancreatitis, but there is little evidence that pancreatitis is an expected consequence of gram-negative sepsis.[2, 110]

References

1. Ashbaugh DG, Petty TL: Sepsis complicating the acute respiratory distress syndrome. Surg Gynecol Obstet 135:865, 1972
2. Boley SJ, Sprayregan S, Siegelman SS, Veith FJ: Initial results from an aggressive roentgenological and surgical approach to acute mesenteric ischemia. Surgery 82:848, 1977
3. Border JR, Gallo E, Schenk WG: Systemic arteriovenous shunts in patients under severe stress: A common cause of high output cardiac failure? Surgery 60:225, 1966
4. Brigham KL, Bowers RE, Haynes J: Increased sheep lung vascular permeability caused by *Escherichia coli* endotoxin. Circ Res 45:292, 1979
5. Brigham KL, Bower RE, McKeen CR: Methylprednisolone prevention of increased lung vascular permeability following endotoxemia in sheep. J Clin Invest 67:1103, 1981
6. Burke JF, Pontoppidan H, Welch CE: High output respiratory failure. An important cause of death ascribed to peritonitis or ileus. Ann Surg 158:581, 1963
7. Calvin JE, Driedger AA, Sibbald WJ: The hemodynamic effect of rapid fluid infusion in critically ill patients. Surgery 90:61, 1981
8. Carroll G, Snyder J: Peripheral anatomic systemic venous shunting high cardiac output septic shock. Crit Care Med 8:230(A), 1980
9. Cerra FB, Hassett J, Siegel JH: Vasodilator therapy in clinical sepsis with low output syndrome. J Surg Res 25:180, 1978
10. Chaudry IH, Sayeed MM, Baue AF: Effects of adenosine triphosphate—magnesium chloride administration in shock. Surgery 75:220, 1974
11. Chinard FP, Enns T: Transcapillary pulmonary exchange of water in the dog. Am J Physiol 178:197, 1954
12. Civetta JM, Gabel JC: Flow directed pulmonary artery catheterization in surgical patients: Indications and modifications of technique. Ann Surg 176:753, 1972
13. Clermont HG, Williams JS, Adams JT: Steroid effect on the release of the lysosomal enzyme acid phosphatase in shock. Ann Surg 179:917, 1974
14. Clowes CHA, Vucinic M, Weidner MG: Circulatory and

metabolic alterations associated with survival or death in peritonitis. Clinical analysis of 25 patients. Ann Surg 163:866, 1966
15. Clowes GHA Jr, Zuschneid W, Turner M et al: Observations on the pathogenesis of the pneumonitis associated with severe infection in other parts of the body. Ann Surg 167:630, 1968
16. Cochrane CG, Muller–Eberhard HJ: The derivation of two distinct anaphylatoxin activities from the third and fifth components of human complement. J Exp Med 127:371, 1968
17. Cohen P, Gardner FH: Thrombocytopenia as a laboratory sign and complication of gram-negative bacteremic infection. Arch Intern Med 117:113, 1966
18. Cohn JD, Greenspan M, Goldstein CR et al: Arteriovenous shunting in high cardiac output shock syndromes. Surg Gynecol Obstet 127:282, 1968
19. Conger JD: A controlled evaluation of prophylactic dialysis in posttraumatic acute renal failure. J Trauma 15:1056, 1975
20. Corrigan JJ: Thrombocytopenia: A laboratory sign of septicemia in infants and children. J Pediatr 85:219, 1974
21. Cortez A, Zito J, Lucas CE, Gerrick SJ: Mechanisms of inappropriate polyuria in septic patients. Arch Surg 112:471, 1977
22. Dammann JF, McAslan TC, Maffeo CJ: Optimal flow pattern for mechanical ventilation of the lungs. 2. The effects of a sine wave versus square wave flow pattern with and without an end-inspiratory pause on patients. Crit Care Med 6:293, 1978
23. David RB, Meeker WR, McQuarrie DG: Immediate effects of intravenous endotoxin on serotonin concentrations and blood platelets. Circ Res 8:234, 1960
24. DesPrez RM, Bryant RE: Effects of bacterial endotoxin on rabbit platelets. IV. The divalent ion requirement of endotoxin-induced and immunologically-induced platelet injury. J Exp Med 124:971, 1966
25. DesPrez RM, Horowitz HI, Hook EW: Effects of bacterial endotoxin on rabbit platelets. I. Platelet aggregation and release of platelet factors in vitro. J Exp Med 114:857, 1961
26. Deykin D: Clinical challenges of disseminated intravascular coagulation. N Engl J Med 283:636, 1970
27. Eiseman B, Beart R, Norton L: Multiple organ failure. Surg Gynecol Obstet 144:323, 1977
28. Falke KJ, Pontoppidan H, Kumar A et al: Ventilation with end-expiratory pressure in acute lung disease. J Clin Invest 51:2315, 1972
29. Feinstein EI, Blumenkratz MJ, Healy M et al: Clinical and metabolic responses to parenteral nutrition in acute renal failure. A controlled double-blind study. Medicine 60:124, 1981
30. Filkins JP: Phases of glucose dyshomeostasis in endotoxicosis. Circ Shock 5:347, 1978
31. Fillastre JP, Laumonier R, Humbert G et al: Acute renal failure associated with combined gentamicin and cephalothin therapy. Br Med J 52:396, 1973
32. Finley RJ, Duff JH, Holliday RL et al: Capillary muscle blood flow in human sepsis. Surgery 78:87, 1975
33. Fletcher JR, Ramwell PW: The effects of prostacyclin (PGI_2) on endotoxin shock and endotoxin-induced platelet aggregation in dogs. Circ Shock 7:299, 1980
34. Forrester JS, DaLuz PL, Chatterjee K: Peripheral vasodilators in low cardiac output states. Surg Clin North Am 55:531, 1975
35. Freund H, Atamian S, Holroyde J, Fischer JE: Plasma amino acids as predictors of the severity and outcome of sepsis. Ann Surg 190:571, 1979
36. Freund HR, Ryan JA, Fischer JE: Amino acid derangements in patients with sepsis. Treatment with branched chain amino acid rich infusions. Ann Surg 188:423, 1978
37. Fry DE, Pearlstein L, Fulton RL, Polk HC: Multiple system organ failure. The role of uncontrolled infection. Arch Surg 115:136, 1980
38. Garcia–Barreno P, Balibrea JL, Aparicio P: Blood coagulation changes in shock. Surg Gynecol Obstet 6:147, 1978
39. Grant JP, Cox CE, Kleinman LM et al: Serum hepatic enzyme and bilirubin elevations during parenteral nutrition. Surg Gynecol Obstet 145:573, 1977
40. Guckian JC: Coagulopathy in experimental sepsis with streptococcus pneumoniae in rabbits: Effect of drug therapy and splenectomy. J Infect Dis 134:150, 1976
41. Halloran LG, Zfass AM, Gayle WE et al: Prevention of acute gastrointestinal complications after severe head injury: A controlled trial of cimetidine prophylaxis. Am J Surg 139:44, 1980
42. Hammerschmidt DE, White JG, Craddock PR, Jacob HS: Corticosteroids inhibit complement-induced granulocyte aggregation. A possible mechanism for their efficacy in shock states. J Clin Invest 63:798, 1979
43. Hastings PR, Skillman JJ, Bushnell LS, Silen W: Antacid titration in the prevention of acute gastrointestinal bleeding: A controlled randomized trial in 100 critically ill patients. N Engl J Med 298:1041, 1978
44. Herrneck AS, Thal AP: Mechanism for the high circulatory requirements in sepsis and septic shock. Ann Surg 170:677, 1969
45. Hess ML, Hastillo A, Greenfield LJ: Spectrum of cardiovascular function during gram negative sepsis. Prog Cardiovasc Dis 23:279, 1981
46. Hess ML, Soulsby ME, Davis JA, Briggs FN: The influence of venous return on cardiac mechanical and sarcoplasmic reticulum function during endotoxemia. Circ Shock 4:143, 1977
47. Hewitt WL: Gentamicin: toxicity in perspective. Postgrad Med J 50:(S)55, 1974
48. Hinshaw LB, Archer LT, Beller–Todd BK et al: Survival of primates in LD_{100} septic shock following steroid/antibiotic therapy. J Surg Res 28:151, 1980
49. Hobbs CL, Mullen JL, Buzby GP et al: The effects of nutrition on aspirin-induced mucosal ulceration in primates. Surgery 86:49, 1979
50. Howes EL, Plotz LM, Blunt JW, Ragan C: Retardation of wound healing by cortisone. Surgery 28:177, 1950
51. Keighley MRB: Antibiotic-associated pseudomembranous colitis—pathogenesis and management. Drugs 20:49, 1980
52. Kirby RR, Downs JB, Civetta JM et al: High level positive end-expiratory pressure (PEEP) in acute respiratory insufficiency. Chest 67:156, 1975
53. Kivilaakso E, Silen W: Pathogenesis of experimental gastric-mucosal injury. N Engl J Med 30:364, 1979
54. Kobold EE, Lucas R, Thal AP: Chemical mediators in clinical septic shock. Surg Forum 14:16, 1963
55. Kwaan HM, Weil MH: Differences in the mechanisms of shock caused by bacterial infections. Surg Gynecol Obstet 128:37, 1969
56. Lefer AM, Martin J: Origin of myocardial depressant factor in shock. Am J Physiol 218:1423, 1970
57. Levin J, Poore TE, Zauber NP, Oser RS: Detection of endotoxin in the blood of patients with sepsis due to gram-negative bacteria. N Engl J Med 283:1313, 1970

58. Levinsky NG, Bernhard DB, Johnston PA: Enhancement of recovery of acute renal failure: Effects of mannitol and diuretics. In Brenner BM, Stein JH (eds): Acute Renal Failure, pp 163–179. New York, Churchill Livingstone, 1980
59. Lillehei RC, Longerbeam JK, Bloch JH: Physiology and therapy of bacteremic shock. Experimental and clinical observations. Am J Cardiol 12:599, 1963
60. Lillehei RC, MacLean LD: Physiological approach to the successful treatment of irreversible endotoxin shock in the experimental animal. Arch Surg 78:464, 1959
61. Loeb HS, Khan M, Saudye A, Gunnar RM: Acute hemodynamic effects of dobutamine and isoproterenol in patients with low output cardiac failure. Cir Shock 3:57, 1976
62. Long TN, Heimbach DM, Carrico CJ: Acalculous cholecystitis in critically ill patients. Am J Surg 136:31, 1978
63. Lotz M, Zisman E, Bartter FC: Evidence for a phosphate depletion syndrome in man. N Engl J Med 278:409, 1968
64. Lowe RJ, Moss GS, Jilek J et al: Crystalloid versus colloid in the etiology of pulmonary failure after trauma—A randomized trial in man. Surgery 81:676, 1977
65. Lozman J, Powers SR Jr, Older T et al: Correlation of pulmonary wedge and left atrial pressures: A study in the patient receiving positive end-expiratory pressure ventilation. Arch Surg 109:270, 1974
66. Lucas CE, Rector FE, Werner M, Rosenberg IK: Altered renal homeostasis with acute sepsis. Clinical significance. Arch Surg 106:444, 1973
67. MacLean LD, Duff JH, Scott HM, Peretz DI: Treatment of shock in man based on hemodynamic diagnosis. Surg Gynecol Obstet 120:1, 1965
68. MacLean LD, Mulligan WG, McLean APH, Duff JH: Patterns of septic shock in man—A detailed study of 56 patients. Ann Surg 166:543, 1967
69. McCurdy DK: Hyperosmolar hyperglycemic nonketotic diabetic coma. Med Clin North Am 54:683, 1970
70. McMurray SD, Luft FC, Maxwell DR et al: Prevailing patterns and predictor variables in patients with acute tubular necrosis. Arch Intern Med 138:950, 1978
71. Manwaring D, Curreri PW: Platelet mediation of fragment D-induced respiratory distress syndrome. Surg Forum 31:242, 1980
72. Marshall BE, Teichner RL, Kallos T et al: Effects of posture and exercise on the pulmonary extravascular water volume in man. J Appl Physiol 31:375, 1971
73. Martyn JAJ, Snider MT, Farago LF, Burke JF: Thermodilution right ventricular volume: A novel and better predictor of volume replacement in acute thermal injury. J Trauma 21:619, 1981
74. Mela L, Hinshaw LB, Archer LT et al: Protection against brain metabolic failure by antibiotic glucocorticoid treatment. Fed Proc 38:1262(A), 1979
75. Mela L, Miller LD, Bacalzo LV et al: Role of intracellular variation of lysosomal enzyme activity and oxygen tension in mitochondrial impairment in endotoxemia and hemorrhage in the rat. Ann Surg 178:727, 1973
76. Mela L, Miller LD, Diaco JF, Sugerman HJ: Effect of E. coli endotoxin on mitochondrial energy-linked functions. Surgery 68:541, 1970
77. Mirtallo JM, Schneider PJ, Mavko K et al: A comparison of essential and general amino acid infusions in the nutritional support of patients with compromised renal function. JPEN 6:109, 1982
78. Moss GS, DasGupta TK, Brinkman R et al: Changes in lung ultrastructure following heterologous and homologous serum albumin infusions in the treatment of hemorrhagic shock. Ann Surg 189:236, 1979
79. Nash G, Blennerhassett JB, Pontoppidan H: Pulmonary lesions associated with oxygen therapy and artificial ventilation. N Engl J Med 276:368, 1967
80. Neely WA, Berry DW, Rushton FW, Hardy JD: Septic shock: Clinical, physiological and pathological survey of 244 patients. Ann Surg 173:657, 1971
81. Ng RC, Suki WN: Treatment of acute renal failure. In Brenner BM, Stein JH (eds): Acute Renal Failure, pp 229–273. New York, Churchill Livingstone, 1980
82. Norton L, Moore G, Eiseman B: Liver failure in the postoperative patient: The role of sepsis and immunologic deficiency. Surgery 78:6, 1975
83. Nowotny A: Molecular aspects of endotoxic reactions. Bacteriol Rev 33:72, 1969
84. Oliven A, Abinader E, Berzstein S: Influence of varying inspired oxygen tensions on the pulmonary venous admixture (shunt) of mechanically ventilated patients. Crit Care Med 8:99, 1980
85. Oppenheimer L, Elings VB, Lewis FR: Thermal-dye lung water measurements: Effects of edema and embolization. J Surg Res 26:504, 1979
86. Peterson SR, Sheldon GF: Acute acalculous cholecystitis: A complication of hyperalimentation. Am J Surg 138:814, 1979
87. Priebe HJ, Skillman JJ, Bushnell LS et al: Antacid versus cimetidine in preventing acute gastrointestinal bleeding. A randomized trial in 75 critically ill patients. N Engl J Med 302:426, 1980
88. Qvist J, Pontoppidan H, Wilson RS et al: Hemodynamic responses to mechanical ventilation with PEEP: The effect of hypervolemia. Anesthesiology 42:45, 1972
89. Rector F, Goyal S, Rosenberg IK, Lucas CE: Sepsis: A mechanism for vasodilatation in the kidney. Ann Surg 178:222, 1973
90. ReMine SG, McIllrath DC: Bowel perforation in steroid-treated patients. Ann Surg 192:581, 1980
91. Remolina C, Khan AV, Santiago TV, Edelman NH: Positional hypoxemia in unilateral lung disease. N Engl J Med 304:523, 1981
92. Reynolds DG, Gull NJ, Vargish T et al: Blockade of opiate receptors with naloxone improves survival and cardiac performance in canine endotoxic shock. Circ Shock 7:39, 1980
93. Riedler GF, Staub PW, Frick PG: Thrombocytopenia in septicemia. A clinical study for the evaluation of its incidence and diagnostic value. Helv Med Acta 36:23, 1971
94. Robin ED, Cross CE, Zelis R: Pulmonary edema. N Engl J Med 288:239, 1973
95. Saldeen T: The microembolism syndrome. Microvasc Res 11:227, 1976
96. Schneider RC, Zapol WM, Carvalho AC: Platelet consumption and sequestration in severe acute respiratory failure. Am Rev Respir Dis 122:445, 1980
97. Schumer W: Steroids in the treatment of clinical septic shock. Ann Surg 184:333, 1976
98. Sibbald WJ, Anderson RR, Reid B et al: Alveolar capillary permeability in human septic ARDS: Effect of high dose corticosteroid therapy. Chest 79:133, 1981
99. Siegel JH, Giovannini I, Coleman B: Ventilation: perfusion maldistribution secondary to the hyperdynamic cardiovascular state as the major cause of increased pulmonary shunting in human sepsis. J Trauma 19:432, 1979

100. Siegel JH, Greenspan M, DelGuercio LRM: Abnormal vascular tone, defective oxygen transport and myocardial failure in human septic shock. Ann Surg 165:504, 1967
101. Staub NC: Pulmonary edema. Physiol Rev 54:678, 1974
102. Stothert JC Jr, Dellinger EP, Simonowitz DA, Schilling JA: Gastric pH monitoring as a prognostic indicator for the prophylaxis of stress ulceration in the critically ill. Am J Surg 140:761, 1980
103. Stothert JC, Simonowitz DA, Dellinger EP et al: Randomized prospective evaluation of cimetidine and antacid control of gastric pH in the critically ill. Ann Surg 192:169, 1980
104. Sugerman HJ, Austin GL, Qureshi CD et al: Thrombocytopenia in progressive lethal canine peritonitis. Surg Gynecol Obstet (in press)
105. Sugerman HJ, Diaco JF, Pollock TW, Miller LD: Physiologic management of septicemic shock in man. Surg Forum 22:3, 1971
106. Sugerman HJ, Olofsson KB, Pollock TW et al: Continuous positive end-expiratory pressure ventilation (PEEP) for the treatment of diffuse interstitial pulmonary edema. J Trauma 12:263, 1972
107. Sugerman HJ, Strash AM, Hirsch JI, Greenfield LJ: Sensitivity of scintigraphy for detection of pulmonary capillary albumin leak in canine oleic acid ARDS. J Trauma 21:520, 1981
108. Thal AP, Sardesai VM: Shock and the circulating polypeptides. Am J Surg 110:308, 1965
109. Virgilio RW, Smith DE, Zarins CK: Balanced electrolyte solutions: Experimental and clinical studies. Crit Care Med 7:98, 1979
110. Warshaw AL, O'Hara PJ: Susceptibility of the pancreas to ischemic injury in shock. Ann Surg 188:197, 1978
111. Wilson RF, Sarver E, Birks R: Central venous pressure and blood volume determinations in clinical shock. Surg Gynecol Obstet 132:631, 1971
112. Wilson RF, Sibbald WJ, Jaanimagi JL: Hemodynamic effects of dopamine in critically ill septic patients. J Surg Res 20:163, 1976
113. Winslow EJ, Loeb HS, Rahimtoloa SH et al: Hemodynamic studies and results of therapy in 50 patients with bacteremic shock. Am J Med 54:421, 1973
114. Wood CA, Isaacson ML, Hibbs MS: Cimetidine and mental confusion. JAMA 239:2550, 1978
115. Ziegler EJ, McCutchan JA, Douglas H, Braudie AI: Prevention of lethal Pseudomonas bacteremia with epimerosa-deficient *E. coli* antiserum. Trans Assoc Am Physicians 38:101, 1975
116. Zusmer NR, Harwood SR, Pevsner NH et al: Gray scale ultrasonography and rose bengal scintigraphy in the evaluation of the patient with jaundice. Surg Gynecol Obstet 147:321, 1978

15
Complications of Blood and Blood-Product Transfusion

David E. Sharp

OVERVIEW

The decision to transfuse blood should be made only after consideration of the potential risks (Table 15-1) versus the expected benefits. Although transplant surgeons are aware that blood is an immunogenic tissue, they often tend to consider blood as an innocuous life-supporting fluid that can be given freely with few adverse consequences. In reality, however, up to 5% of carefully monitored transfusions are followed by untoward reactions.[2, 24] These range from transient chills or fever, which frequently go unreported, to the fulminant acute hemolytic transfusion reaction or the later development of acute viral hepatitis and its sequelae.

The hemolytic reaction is the most feared immediate complication of transfusion, but today it is relatively rare, occurring only once in 17,000 transfusions.[33, 36] When grouped with all other types of red-cell incompatibility, the incidence of complications is somewhat higher, occurring in 1% of transfusions; however, few deaths now result from such incompatibilities owing to improved surveillance and detection and vigorous treatment.[20] In my view the most serious risk of blood transfusion therapy today is the delayed morbidity and mortality associated with hepatitis.[1, 8, 15, 40] Hepatitis with jaundice occurs in a half to 1% of all blood recipients, and death occurs in 1 of every 3000 to 5000 of these cases.[8, 16, 24, 28]

From this chapter the surgeon should be able to identify the early stages of reactions associated with blood transfusion, to determine their probable cause, and to begin appropriate treatment. Late complications, particularly hepatitis, are also considered. Finally, the identification of high-risk patients

TABLE 15-1. MAJOR COMPLICATIONS OF BLOOD TRANSFUSION AND THEIR CAUSES

Complication	Most Common Cause	Less Common Cause	Rare Cause
Hepatitis	Non-A, non-B agent(s)	Hepatitis B virus	Cytomegalovirus, Epstein-Barr virus
Febrile transfusion reaction	Leukocyte antigens	Platelet antigens	Passive infusion of antibodies to platelet or leukocyte antigens, bacterial or pyrogen contamination
Allergic transfusion reaction	Plasma proteins	Platelet or leukocyte antigen	Albumin, plasma expanders
Acute hemolytic transfusion reaction	Clerical error	Laboratory error	Passive infusion of antibodies to recipient erythrocytes
Delayed hemolytic transfusion reaction	Anamnestic antibody response (secondary)	Primary antibody response	Bacterial contamination
Circulatory overload	Whole blood	Plasma or other colloid	Red blood cells
Isoimmunization	RBC antigens	WBC antigens	Plasma proteins Platelet antigens

and situations are discussed with a view to preventing or minimizing the likely complications.

HISTORICAL BACKGROUND

The first attempt at transfusion therapy was recorded in 1667, when animal blood was used, and as a result the patient died. Transfusions were then banned until the 1800s, when arm-to-arm transfusions using random donors without crossmatching were recorded with variable results.[41] (It is interesting to remember that bloodletting by the surgeon was a common therapeutic procedure in that era.) Blood groups were first identified in 1901, but the first anticoagulant was not developed until 1915. World War II greatly expanded the use of whole blood from Group O donors (universal donors) and of plasma, which were vital in saving lives, and, in 1943, the first anticoagulant that allowed the storage of blood was developed. During the 1950s and early 1960s, refrigerated centrifuges and the use of satellite plastic bags permitted component separation in a closed system and eliminated the risk of contamination that the use of glass bottles had carried. Today the blood bank can provide blood and its components in so many forms that transfusion therapy can be individualized.[6, 7, 12, 14, 22–24, 29, 30, 34, 37]

ROLE OF COMPONENT THERAPY

The indications and contraindications for the most significant blood products are listed in Table 15-2. Other commercially available derivatives of blood, including albumin, Factor VIII and IX concentrates, immune serum globulins, hyperimmune globulins, and RhoGAM have been reviewed elsewhere.[6, 7, 18]

Blood often seems to follow a cyclic course from its donation to its eventual use. Despite the value of whole blood for use in massive hemorrhage, the prevailing practice is for blood banks to immediately separate blood into its components to allow the best possible storage for each and to ensure the most efficient utilization. Those who order blood often reconstitute whole blood by combining packed red cells with fresh frozen plasma. This practice increases the risk of hepatitis exposure, since the components usually come from different donors. An example would be the use of fresh frozen plasma to reconstitute packed red cells into "whole" blood to provide additional volume expansion. If the patient in fact is not in need of coagulation-factor replacement, this therapy exposes him to the risk of hepatitis, which would not accompany the use of crystalloid or albumin instead of fresh frozen plasma.[17, 19, 31, 43]

Although the trend is toward component therapy, fresh whole blood is still the best product to transfuse in some specific situations, for example in trauma when there is rapid blood loss. The major advantage of fresh whole blood is that it both replaces volume and improves oxygen-carrying capacity at once and also limits the exposure to fewer donors and hence limits the exposure to hepatitis. Some coagulation factors and platelets are not effectively replaced, however, because in order to conserve inventory, blood banks preferentially supply

TABLE 15-2. INDICATIONS AND CONTRAINDICATIONS FOR THE USE OF WHOLE BLOOD AND ITS COMPONENTS

Blood Product	Major Indications	Major Contraindications
Whole blood	Acute blood loss	Chronic anemia Anemia responsive to proper medication
Packed red blood cells	Symptomatic anemia	Anemia responsive to proper medication
Washed red blood cells	Symptomatic anemia Febrile reactions to packed red blood cells	Anemia responsive to proper medication
Frozen red blood cells	Symptomatic anemia Red blood cell incompatibilities	Anemia responsive to proper medication
Platelet concentrate	Thrombocytopenia	Presence of antiplatelet antibodies
Fresh frozen plasma	Hypovolemia Deficiency of labile coagulation factors	Need for high potency coagulation factors
Cryoprecipitate	Hemophilia A von Willebrand's disease Hypofibrinogenemia	Need for high-potency coagulation factors

their oldest units and substitute packed red cells when whole blood is unavailable. Because of logistical and supply problems, whole blood and fresh blood have limited availability for use in indicated situations.

Pathophysiology

PYROGENIC REACTIONS

Although in the past pyrogenic reactions were due to infusion of blood products contaminated from either bacteria or bacterial products, most fever-producing reactions today are immunologic in origin.[3–5, 11, 12, 25, 26, 32, 38] Fever, often with chills, occurs during or shortly after blood-product transfusion; the patient is usually multiparous or has had multiple previous transfusions. More severe symptoms such as nausea, vomiting, headache, chest pain, and back pain may occur if transfusions are continued after the initial symptoms appear.[35] In elderly and severely debilitated patients, hypotension may result from severe reactions, and the patient may die.

Immunologic reactions, usually between leukocyte antigens and IgG antibodies already produced in susceptible multiparous or multitransfused patients, lead to damage of the involved leukocytes, especially granulocytes but also lymphocytes to a lesser extent, and release of pyrogens. Plasma products that contain preformed antibodies may react with the leukocytes of the recipient in a similar manner. Less frequently, the pyrogenic reactions are due to immunologic reactions involving platelet or plasma antigens. The severity of the pyrogenic reaction is related directly to the quantity of infused antigens and the titer of circulating antibodies.

ALLERGIC REACTIONS

Allergic immunologic-transfusion reaction results from the infusion of antigen, usually a plasma protein, to which the individual previously has formed an antibody. Less common, the transfused blood product contains a preformed antibody that reacts with antigens within the recipient plasma or with plasma antigens present in additional transfused blood products. The plasma protein most frequently implicated is IgA, although many other plasma protein antigens, such as Gm determinant on the heavy chains and V determinant on light chains, have been identified as the cause of allergic reactions. The most susceptible patient lacks IgA in his serum and forms high titers of class-specific antibodies, although most persons who are IgA-deficient produce only low titers of anti-IgA antibodies of limited specificity.

When the soluble antigen is infused into a presensitized patient, it may form soluble antigen–antibody complexes with specific IgG antibodies, or it may bind to specific IgE antibodies fixed to the surface of mast cells. The soluble antigen–antibody complexes may activate the early components of complement with release of C_3a and C_5a. The binding of antigen to IgE on the mast cell, and also C_3a and C_5a themselves, cause the degranulation of mast cells with release of histamine and serotonin, producing urticaria and pruritis.

ANAPHYLACTIC REACTION

The most severe form of allergic reaction is the anaphylactic reaction, which is associated with dyspnea, hypotension, and flushing of the skin. This rare reaction is usually triggered by infusion of blood products containing IgA into a recipient with high titers of IgG anti-IgA antibody. The anti-IgA antibody may be class specific or of limited specificity. The circulating IgA anti-IgA complexes fix complement and release large amounts of C_3a and C_5a fragments. In addition, mast-cell-histamine release occurs, and bradykinin may be generated from plasma kininogens. Hypotension results from the widespread rapid vasodilatation caused by these vasoactive amines. Bronchial smooth muscle constriction and laryngeal edema lead to dyspnea and hypoxia.

HEMOLYTIC TRANSFUSION REACTION

The hemolytic transfusion reaction is basically similar to other immunologically mediated transfusion reactions. This reaction may be due to either infusion of incompatible red blood cells or infusion of incompatible plasma, but the most severe reactions occur with the former. The local manifestations of the reaction, such as burning pain at the site of infusion or along the vein, are due to the activation of the early complement components with liberation of C_3a and C_5a. The hemoglobin released from the lysed cells and the stroma of the lysed compatible erythrocytes have little, if any, effect. The activation of Hageman factor by antibodies attached to the red cell antigens then triggers the coagulation cascade and also activates the kininogen system. Although significant intravascular coagulation is rare, the combined effects of the C_3a and C_5a fragments and bradykinin formation lead to profound systemic vasodilatation and hypotension. Some microcirculatory beds, especially in the kidney, heart, and lungs, may have considerable arteriolar vasoconstriction—producing dyspnea, chest tightness, angina, and flank pain.

Differential Diagnosis and the Role of Laboratory Tests

The first concern in evaluating a possible blood transfusion reaction is to recognize the early manifestations of a potentially life-threatening complication such as anaphylactic or endotoxic shock or acute red cell hemolysis. These complications may be accompanied by apparently insignificant signs and symptoms rather than by those more commonly attributed to the reaction. For example, anxiety, transient chills, or a slight temperature elevation may be associated with the hemolytic reaction rather than the flank pain, pain at the site of infusion, hypotension, or generalized bleeding traditionally associated with intravascular hemolysis. Therefore, even minimal signs and symptoms should be evaluated promptly and appropriate laboratory tests performed so that the blood transfusion can be terminated and appropriate management started.

The first step in evaluating any transfusion reaction is a clerical check of all identifying information on the unit of blood, laboratory slips, and the patient's arm. Next, the most critical laboratory tests, those that can quickly provide evidence to support or rule out a possibly lethal transfusion reaction, should be performed.

1. Examination for hemolysis of a clotted or anticoagulated blood sample drawn at the time of the suspected reaction may provide the earliest evidence of a hemolytic transfusion reaction. Visually detectable hemolysis produced by the destruction of as little as 10 ml to 20 ml of blood may be apparent in the blood sample at the bedside, but the blood sample should be centrifuged and the plasma or serum compared to a suitable pretransfusion sample from the patient in order to ascertain the presence of hemolysis. The presence of hemolysis does not confirm immunologic destruction, however, since physical agents may have produced the hemolysis. At the same time, a direct antiglobulin test or direct Coombs' test can provide evidence of an immunologic process within minutes. A positive direct Coombs' test on the patient's blood sample following transfusion that succeeds a sequence of negative Coombs' tests on previous blood samples strongly supports the presence of red blood cell incompatibility. False-positive direct Coombs' tests not infrequently are associated with long-term Aldomet or other drug therapy. That possibility should be considered before accepting the Coombs' test as definitively indicating red cell antigen incompatibility. False-negative Coombs' tests result from the complete destruction of the incompatible red blood cells, which not uncommonly occurs in ABO-incompatible transfusions. Rarely, the direct Coombs' test is negative when the class of offending antibody is not IgG, but IgA instead.
2. If the clerical check has uncovered an error or if the reaction sample from after the transfusion results in a direct positive Coombs' test, the cross matches should be repeated for both pre- and post-transfusion blood samples.
3. When these clerical checks and laboratory tests fail to define the cause of the suspected transfusion reaction, the presence of bacterial contamination of the blood or blood products should be determined. This examination can be done quickly by Gram staining a dried smear of blood or, even better, of supernatant plasma from the unit of blood or blood product. The presence of bacteria should be presumptive evidence of contamination; however, units containing clostridia or significant cryophilic organisms may be found rarely.
4. Examination of the urine for hemoglobinuria may be useful in documenting the presence of significant hemolysis, but this is usually delayed because filtration of hemoglobin occurs only after the plasma haptoglobin is saturated (about 100 mg hemoglobin/dl of plasma) and the level of free hemoglobin exceeds about 150 mg/dl.
5. Determinations of plasma hemoglobin and haptoglobin levels by quantitative means require additional time and testing facilities and usually are not useful initial studies. In addition, both levels may be elevated or depressed as a result of the patient's state of nutrition, the presence of acute inflammation, and the effects of recent blood transfusions. Serum bilirubin levels reach their maximum some 5 hours to 7 hours following acute hemolysis. Most often they provide evidence supporting hemolysis, although there are many other intrahepatic and extrahepatic causes for hyperbilirubinemia.

Treatment

Most complications from blood transfusions can be readily divided into two categories. The first type is the immediate transfusion reaction that occurs during or shortly after the end of the transfusion. Included in this category are febrile, allergic, anaphylactic, and acute hemolytic reactions. The second

TABLE 15-3. INITIAL MANAGEMENT OF BLOOD TRANSFUSION REACTIONS

Type of Reaction	Manifestation	Usual Cause	Management
Febrile reaction	Fever, chills	Leukocyte or platelet antigen incompatibility; rarely, bacterial contamination of blood	Stop infusion, treat with antipyretics, rule out bacterial contamination, treat with broad-spectrum antibiotics if contamination is suspected
Allergic reaction	Urticaria; pruritis; rarely, anaphylactic shock	Plasma protein incompatibility	Slow or stop infusion, treat with antihistamines
Anaphylactic reaction	Hypotension, bronchospasm	Immunoglobulin (IgA) incompatibility	Stop infusion, use epinephrine and corticosteroids if necessary
Acute hemolytic reaction	Shock, hemoglobinuria, diffuse bleeding	ABO-incompatible red blood cells, occasionally due to other blood group antigen incompatibility	Stop infusion, maintain high urine output with mannitol, fluids, and furosemide; consider heparin if bleeding is due to disseminated intravascular coagulation
Lysis of compatible blood	Hemoglobinuria, hemoglobinemia	Physical damage due to improper infusion or storage technique	Stop infusion, observe for additional signs
Circulatory overload	Labored respirations	Excessive infusion of plasma or whole blood	Slow or stop infusion, use diuretics, digitalis, and phlebotomy if necessary

type of reaction, the delayed transfusion reaction, generally occurs days to months after the transfusion. Other reactions such as circulatory overload and reaction to hemolyzed compatible red cells that may occur several hours after the end of the transfusion are included in this discussion of immediate reactions. The initial treatment of immediate blood transfusion reactions is outlined in Table 15-3.

IMMEDIATE TRANSFUSION REACTIONS

The most common transfusion-related complication, the febrile reaction, is due most frequently to infusion of leukocyte antigens and, less frequently, to infusion of platelet antigens into a susceptible recipient with corresponding preformed antileukocyte or antiplatelet antibodies (see Table 15-1). When the infusion is stopped early in the course of the reaction, antipyretic agents alone may be sufficient to alleviate the signs and symptoms.

Second in frequency to the febrile reaction is the allergic reaction, which is due largely to infused plasma proteins and leukocyte or platelet antigens reacting with corresponding antibodies in the recipient. The allergic transfusion reaction, usually manifest by pruritus or urticaria, may resolve quickly when the patient is given antihistamines orally or intravenously. After a short period of observation of symptom resolution, the blood transfusion can be resumed safely.

If the early symptoms are accompanied by or replaced with additional signs and symptoms, the transfusion should be terminated and the reaction should be presumed to be febrile or hemolytic. If no other manifestations of a transfusion reaction occur and there is no evidence of red cell incompatibility (such as visual detection of hemoglobinemia or a positive direct antiglobulin test), then bacterial contamination of the unit should be ruled out by examination of a Gram-stained smear. When there is no evidence of bacteria, antipyretic agents should be given. If bacteria are found on the smear, broad-spectrum antibiotics should be started.

Anaphylactic Reaction

An anaphylactic reaction commonly occurs after the infusion of a relatively small amount of blood product, perhaps only a few milliliters, but it may not progress if the infusion is stopped immediately. However, severe bronchospasm and profound hypotension may occur and require the immediate institution of appropriate therapy, including the administration of epinephrine or corticosteroids. In the anesthetized or comatose patient, the early phases of the reaction may be obscured and the precise etiology of the reaction may be complicated by consideration of factors such as the adverse effects of anesthetic agents or occult hemorrhage.

Anaphylactic shock associated with significant mortality may occur with blood products that contain IgA, other plasma proteins, or any soluble or cell-bound antigen in a susceptible individual with corresponding antibodies whose infusion is not closely monitored. Early treatment with intravenous epinephrine usually reverses the shock, although corticosteroids may be needed to prevent continuing sequelae.

Acute Hemolytic Reaction

The acute hemolytic reaction most commonly occurs when ABO-incompatible blood is transfused following a clerical mistake or misidentification of the intended recipient or the source of the initial pretransfusion blood sample. In the conscious patient, the reaction usually produces sufficient signs and symptoms so that the transfusion is stopped.[21, 42]

If shock accompanied by bleeding or hematuria are the presenting symptoms, an acute hemolytic reaction is likely and should be confirmed by visual inspection of the plasma for hemoglobin and laboratory testing for a positive direct antiglobulin test. In addition, by rechecking the clerical work and visually identifying once again the blood type of the recipient, any discrepancy between the ABO groups of the donor and recipient blood will become apparent. When the volume of infused blood is less than 200 ml of packed cells, serious sequelae such as renal failure and disseminated intravascular coagulation (DIC) rarely occur. In contrast, large amounts of incompatible blood may be transfused into an unconscious or anesthetized patient, resulting in shock or diffuse bleeding as initial evidence of a reaction. If this happens, initial therapy is to maintain renal function because irreversible renal failure leads to death 50% of the time. Kidney function should be monitored closely, and mannitol and fluids should be used to maintain urine output at greater than 100 ml per hour. Early heparinization and replacement of depleted clotting factors are advocated as the best management of DIC, once the initiating cause is eliminated or corrected.

Acute hemolysis is more frequently associated with minor blood group incompatibility, and the sequelae are usually less severe than those outlined above; however, renal failure occurs in a small percentage of cases and again is associated with greater mortality rates than are the reactions not complicated by renal failure.[10, 13] Immunologically mediated hemolysis may occur when products with plasma containing a high titer of blood cell antibody are infused into a susceptible recipient.

Lysis of Compatible Blood

If the only manifestation of a reaction is hematuria, red blood cell lysis may have occurred through a nonimmune mechanism. This form of lysis occurs when the red blood cells are subjected to osmotic injury, thermal injury (such as excessive heating or freezing), or physical injury (such as the effects of high-shear forces when blood is forced under pressure through a small-gauge needle).

The lysis of compatible blood caused by nonimmune mechanisms is generally asymptomatic in adults, but the associated hyperkalemia may lead to fatalities in neonates and susceptible adults. Visual examination of the tubing from the bag and of the bag of blood itself usually will establish the presence of hemolysis. However, the precise cause may be obscure and require retracing the route the unit of blood took within and outside the blood bank up to the time of discovery of hemolysis.

Circulatory Overload

Circulatory system overloading, signaled by labored respirations, occurs when blood, especially whole blood or plasma, is infused in too large a quantity or at too fast a rate. It can often be prevented by carefully monitoring the patient and the rate of transfusion and by the use of packed red cell products. Elderly and neonatal patients are most sensitive to rapid volume shifts and constitute the largest groups in whom this condition commonly develops. Also, patients with impaired cardiac function require more careful monitoring to prevent circulatory overloading during blood transfusions.

In the most severe instances of circulatory overload, oxygen may be required to prevent hypoxemia, and phlebotomy will most rapidly reduce the cardiac and respiratory decompensation. In less severe cases, simply decreasing the rate of infusion or stopping the transfusion altogether will allow equilibration of the circulatory system. Diuretic and digitalis therapy may provide benefit to patients who have continued signs and symptoms of hypervolemia with cardiac and respiratory embarrassment.

DELAYED HEMOLYTIC REACTIONS

Delayed hemolytic transfusion reactions are more subtle in presentation and frequently are undetected, the symptoms being dismissed as the expected consequence of surgery and hospitalization.[9, 27] Although delayed hemolytic transfusion reactions are generally less serious than are acute hemolytic transfusion reactions, renal failure is an occasional consequence and may lead to death in critically ill patients. The treatment usually is to improve renal function, although additional transfusions may be urgently needed to treat continued severe anemia in patients with red cell antibodies that elude identification.

Posttransfusion Hepatitis

Transfusion-associated hepatitis has been a focus of concern for several decades and has led to improved detection of infectious blood products, yet it remains

TABLE 15-4. TRANSMISSION OF HEPATITIS FROM BLOOD PRODUCTS

Product	Source	Risk
Factor IX concentrate	Pooled plasma, multiple donors	High
Factor VIII concentrate	Pooled plasma, multiple donors	Increased
Cryoprecipitate	Single donor	Present
Plasma, fresh frozen, or liquid	Single donor	Present
Red blood cells or whole blood	Single donor	Present
Red blood cells, washed	Single donor	Present
Red blood cells, frozen, deglycerolized	Single donor	Low
Platelets or granulocytes	Single donor	Present
Plasma protein fraction or albumin	Pooled plasma multiple donors	None
Hyperimmune gamma globulin	Pooled plasma multiple donors	None

a frequent and serious complication. Improved screening and the elimination of paid donors have significantly reduced the occurrence of hepatitis due to hepatitis B virus; however, the incidence of non-A, non-B hepatitis has increased.

All blood products containing plasma are potentially infective, especially pooled plasma products such as Factor IX concentrate (Table 15-4). The plasma derivatives—albumin and plasma protein fraction—are effectively sterilized during preparation and are not associated with hepatitis transmission. Frozen blood products, although extensively washed to remove cryoprotective agents such as glycerol, are still infectious owing to a remaining minute amount of plasma.

Other Infectious Agents

Other infectious agents such as malarial parasites and bacterial organisms such as spirochetes are increasingly uncommon contaminants in blood. Since spirochetes survive only a few days in blood maintained at 1°C to 6°C, cryophilic bacteria such as clostridia and bacteroid species are more commonly cultured from infrequently contaminated units of blood.

Prevention of Transfusion Complications

Improvements in the science of blood banking during the last 40 years have reduced the risks of morbidity and mortality associated with blood transfusion. Proper identification of blood samples and blood recipients greatly reduces the risk of an ABO-incompatible acute hemolytic transfusion reaction, the most feared complication. Strict adherence to proper indications for transfusion with elimination of unnecessary transfusions, the anticipation of complications, and constant vigilance for the early manifestations of reactions will lead to increased safety. In addition, the improved identification of patients at increased risk of complications, such as multiparous or previously transfused patients, will further decrease the risk of a hemolytic transfusion reaction.

The use of autologous transfusions provides the patient with the best possible blood, his own, and eliminates virtually all risk of disease transmission. Although contamination at the time of collection or during storage is possible, modern collection techniques and methods of storage render this unlikely. Misidentification of the intended recipient remains a potential hazard, and nonimmune hemolysis may result from improper handling and infusion, but in practice transfusion reactions are virtually eliminated when proper care is taken.

Blood-conservation techniques include such practices as preoperative and intraoperative blood removal from the patient, autotransfusion during surgery, and hemodilution.[39] These techniques allow surgery for trauma and open-heart procedures, which usually require many transfusions, to be performed safely with minimal use of homologous blood. The recently developed techniques of automated filtration, centrifugation, and washing of large volumes of shed blood allow autotransfusion when blood loss is massive. However, contamination of blood in the wound and inadequate anticoagulation of the shed blood remain significant problems. Hemodilution and reinfusion of oxygenator blood are used extensively in open-heart surgery employing cardiopulmonary bypass with membrane oxygenators. When the patient refuses blood transfusion on religious grounds, these forms of autotransfusion are acceptable and are widely employed.

Many groups are investigating improved methods of screening primarily for non-A non-B hepatitis in order to exclude blood donors capable of transmitting disease. Donors with elevation of liver enzyme levels of SGPT (ALT) are most likely to be infectious for non-A non-B, but this criterion will eliminate many noninfectious donors and not detect many infectious donors. The elimination of non-A non-B hepatitis as a hazard after blood transfusion still awaits the discovery of the specific antigens and antibodies analogous to hepatitis B virus. Vaccines to hepatitis viruses offer protection to those at high risk of exposure to hepatitis.

Further improvement of blood infusion results from the improved filtration of blood, which removes not only particulate debris but also platelets and leukocytes. When sufficient amounts of platelets and leukocytes are removed, even patients with preformed antiplatelet and antileukocyte antibodies have significantly fewer febrile transfusion reactions. In fact, the initial sensitization to foreign platelet and leukocyte antigens may be prevented by future improvements in filtration, although this has not yet been achieved.

Multiparous and previously transfused patients are known to be at increased risk of a transfusion reaction. Although they may develop delayed transfusion reactions, these patients should be monitored more closely for signs of an acute transfusion reaction. In the future, a blood recipient's ability to form antibodies to blood cells may be determined by immunologic testing prior to elective blood transfusions. Patients who may develop antibodies will be candidates for selective transfusion of blood products from HLA-matched donors or donors whose red blood cell antigens closely correspond to the recipient's.

References

1. Aach RD, Kahn RA: Post-tranfusion hepatitis: Current perspectives. Ann Intern Med 92:539–546, 1980
2. Baker RJ, Moinichen SL, Nyhus LM: Transfusion reaction: A reappraisal of surgical incidence and significance. Ann Surg 169(5):684–693, 1969
3. Barton JC: Nonhemolytic, noninfectious transfusion reactions. Semin Hematol 18(2):95–121, 1981
4. Bashir H: Adverse reactions due to leucocyte and platelet antibodies. Anaesth Intensive Care 8(2):132–138, 1980
5. Beal RW: Quality control and transfusion reactions. Anaesth Intensive Care 8(2):172–177, 1980
6. Blajchman MA, Shepherd FA, Perrault RA: Clinical use of blood, blood components and blood products. Can Med Assoc J 121:33–42, 1979
7. Collins JA: Use of blood and blood components. In Kinney JM, Bendixen HH, Powers SR Jr (eds): Manual Of Surgical Intensive Care, Chap 10, pp 121–142. Philadelphia, W.B. Saunders, 1977
8. Conrad ME: Diseases transmissible by blood transfusion: Viral hepatitis and other infectious disorders. Semin Hematol 18(2):122–146, 1981
9. Croucher BEE: Differential diagnosis of delayed transfusion reaction. In A Seminar on Laboratory Management of Hemolysis, Chap 8, pp 151–160. Washington, DC, American Association of Blood Banks, 1979
10. Goldfinger D: Acute hemolytic transfusion reactions—A fresh look at pathogenesis and considerations regarding therapy. Transfusion 17(2):85–98, 1977
11. Goldfinger D: Adverse reactions to blood transfusion. In A Seminar on Laboratory Management of Hemolysis, Chap 14, pp 137–154. Washington, DC, American Association of Blood Banks, 1979
12. Greenwalt TJ: Blood banking. Surg Clin North Am 58(5):1095–1100, 1978
13. Greenwalt TJ: Pathogenesis and management of hemolytic transfusion reactions. Semin Hematol 18(2):84–94, 1981
14. Harden PA: Blood transfusion in particular clinical situations. Anaesth Intensive Care 8(2):162–167, 1980
15. Holland PV, Alter HJ: Non-A, Non-B viral hepatitis. Hum Pathol 12:1114–1122, 1981
16. Honig CL, Bove JR: Transfusion-associated fatalities: Review of Bureau of Biologics Reports, 1976–1978. Transfusion 20(6):653–661, 1980
17. Isbister JP, Fisher MM: Adverse effects of plasma volume expanders. Anaesth Intensive Care 8(2):145–151, 1980
18. Isbister JP, Scurr RD: Blood transfusion therapy: Components, indications, complications and controversies. Anaesth Intensive Care 6(4):297–309, 1978
19. Kahn RA, Staggs SD, Miller WV, Ellis FR: Use of plasma products with whole blood and packed RBC's. JAMA 242(19):2087–2090, 1979
20. Kay AB: Some complications associated with the administration of blood and blood products. Clin Haematol 5(1):165–181, 1976
21. Klarkowski DB: The serological investigation of red cell incompatible transfusion reactions. Anaesth Intensive Care 8(2):120–124, 1980
22. Lundsgaard–Hansen P: Component therapy of surgical hemorrhage: Red cell concentrates, colloids and crystalloids. Bibl Haematologica 46:147–169, 1980
23. Lundsgaard–Hansen P, Koch St. Lindt R et al: Influence of a blood component program on postoperative complication rates. Vox Sang 41:193–200, 1981
24. McKittrick JE: Bank autologous blood in elective surgery. Am J Surg 128:137–142, 1974
25. McLeod BC: Immunologic factors in reactions to blood transfusions. Heart Lung 9(4):675–681, 1980
26. Miller WV: Adverse effects of blood transfusion. In Rutman RC, Miller WV (eds): Transfusion Therapy. Principles and Procedures, Chap 22. Rockville, Maryland, Aspens Systems Corporation, 1982
27. Moore SB, Taswell HF, Pineda AA, Sonnenberg CL: Delayed hemolytic transfusion reactions. Am J Clin Pathol 74(1):94–97, 1980
28. Myhre BA: Fatalities from blood transfusion. JAMA 244(12):1333–1335, 1980
29. Ness PM: Blood Banking. Clin Lab Med 1(1):67–76, 1981
30. Newland PE, Pastoriza–Pinol J, McMillan J et al: Maximal conservation and minimal useage of blood products in open heart surgery. Anaesth Intensive Care 8(2):178–182, 1980
31. Olinger GN, Werner PH, Bonchek LI, Boerboom LE: Vasodilator effects of the sodium acetate in pooled protein fraction. Ann Surg 190(3):305–311, 1979
32. Perkins HA, Payne R, Ferguson J, Wood M: Nonhemolytic febrile transfusion reactions. Vox Sang 11:578—600, 1966
33. Pineda AA, Brzica SM, Taswell HF: Hemolytic transfusion

reaction. Recent experience in a large blood bank. Mayo Clin Proc 53:378–390, 1978
34. Rice CL, Moss GS: Blood and blood substitutes: Current practice. Adv Surg 13:93–114, 1979
35. Rush B, Lee NLY: Clinical presentation of nonhemolytic transfusion reactions. Anaesth Intensive Care 8(2):125–131, 1980
36. Schmidt PJ: The mortality from incompatible transfusion. In Sandler SG, Jamieson GA (eds): Immunobiology of the Erythrocyte, pp 251–261. New York, Allen R. Liss, 1980
37. Silver H: Clinical aspects of autologous transfusion. Conn Med 43(4):201–205, 1979
38. Snyder EL: Non-infectious and non-immunologic complications of blood transfusion. Conn Med 43(4):206–211, 1979
39. Utley JR, Moores WY, Stephens DB: Blood conservation techniques. Ann Thorac Surg 31(5):482–490, 1981
40. Wallace J: Blood transfusion and transmissible disease. Clin Haematol 5(1):183–200, 1976
41. Walsh RJ: Adverse reactions to blood transfusion. Introduction—Historical overview. Anaesth Intensive Care 8(2):112–114, 1980
42. Webster BH: Clinical presentation of haemolytic transfusion reactions. Anaesth Intensive Care 8(2):115–119, 1980
43. Wells JV, King MA: Adverse reactions to human plasma proteins. Anaesth Intensive Care 8(2):139–144, 1980

16
Complications of Coagulopathy and Splenectomy

Donald Silver

OVERVIEW

Most of the bleeding that occurs after trauma or during or after major surgery is mechanical; that is, the bleeding can be controlled with appropriately placed pressure, clamps, ligatures, and so forth. Bleeding from coagulopathies—nonmechanical bleeding—although occurring infrequently, may contribute substantially to the morbidity and mortality of surgery or trauma.[13] *This chapter defines the various coagulopathies and offers methods for preventing, recognizing, and managing them. The complications following splenectomy are also discussed.*

Coagulopathies

Most of the coagulopathies encountered in surgical or trauma patients are related to the surgery or the trauma and its management. A few patients with hemostatic mechanisms that were previously *clinically* intact may exhibit a coagulopathy during or after surgery or trauma because they have congenitally deficient or abnormal coagulation factors or platelets that become manifest during the time of active bleeding. Thus, most coagulopathies encountered by the surgeons are acquired, and a few are congenital; all are difficult to recognize and may be made worse by inappropriate therapy.

It should be remembered that inherited or acquired abnormalities of blood vessels may be associated with bleeding, mainly from mucous membranes or into the skin, usually in association with trauma. Some of the conditions associated with vascular bleeding include amyloidosis, vascular purpura, hereditary hemorrhagic telangiectasia, pseudoxanthoma elasticum, vasculitis, and the Ehlers–Danlos syndrome.

A coagulopathy should be suspected when a victim of trauma develops mucosal bleeding, hematuria, petechia, bleeding from puncture wounds, or excessive bleeding into the area of injury. Coagulopathies are suspected in surgical patients when the oozing that accompanies the incision persists for more than a few minutes, when the usual methods for obtaining hemostasis are not effective, and when previously "dry" wounds fill with blood that oozes from all surfaces.

The coagulopathies encountered in surgical patients may be caused by an insufficient number of platelets or platelets with abnormal function; deficient, defective, or excessive clotting; or excessive fibrinolytic activity. If the bleeding persists, it becomes increasingly more difficult to determine the cause of the coagulopathy because platelets and coagulation factors are lost with the bleeding and may be inadequately replaced. Furthermore, the platelet, the coagulation mechanism, or the fibrinolytic mechanism rarely acts without influencing the other components responsible for hemostasis (Fig. 16-1).

PLATELETS

Platelets have a pivotal role in maintaining hemostasis and capillary integrity. Platelets adhere to exposed collagen, noncollagen microfibrils, and other substances at the site of vascular injury. Plasma proteins, calcium, fibrinogen, and von Willebrand's factor are required for platelet adhesion. The adherent platelets release adenosine triphosphate (ATP), adenosine diphosphate (ADP), serotonin, and other bioactive amines that cause additional platelets to aggregate at the site of injury and to contribute to the formation of the hemostatic platelet plug, which controls bleeding from capillaries, arterioles, and venules. The released bioactive amines cause vasoconstriction, which further contributes to the attainment of hemostasis.

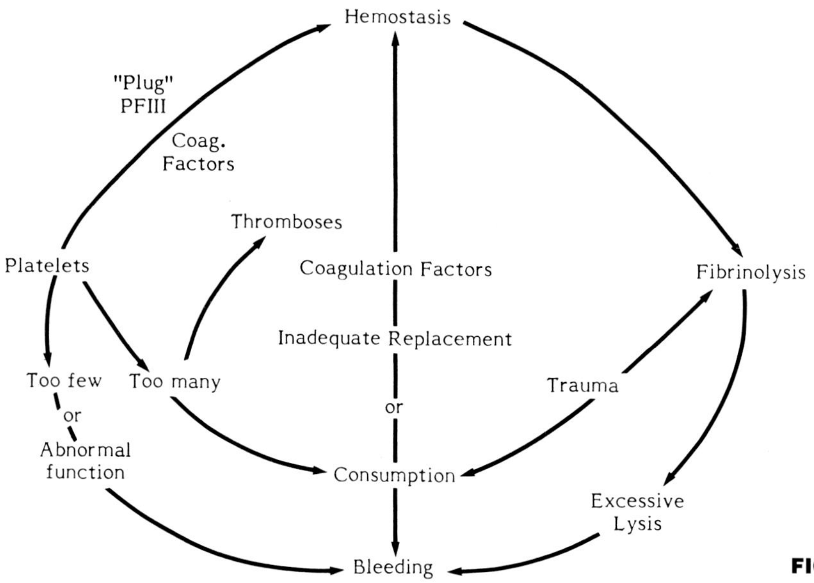

FIG. 16-1. The components of hemostasis.

The early reversible platelet aggregation becomes a permanent aggregation in the presence of additional ADP, prostaglandin endoperoxides, and thromboxane A_2. During the aggregation process, a platelet membrane phospholipoprotein (platelet factor III, PF III) becomes available and accelerates several steps of the coagulation sequence, leading to thrombin production and fibrin formation. In the late stages, the platelet plug retracts and is incorporated into and surrounded by the forming thrombus.

Bleeding may occur when too few platelets are available for hemostasis or when acquired or congenital disorders of platelet function are present. Although the number of platelets required to control bleeding varies, especially with the magnitude of bleeding, 30,000 functionally active platelets per mm^3 are generally thought sufficient for hemostasis. Too many platelets (thrombocytosis) may initiate the coagulation mechanism and lead to intravascular coagulation.

Thrombocytopenia

The most common platelet disorder that contributes to bleeding is thrombocytopenia. The clinical manifestations of thrombocytopenia, including petechia, purpura, epistaxis, and other mucosal bleeding, should alert the surgeon to the presence of thrombocytopenia preoperatively. Thrombocytopenia may be congenital or, more often, acquired. The uncommon hereditary thrombocytopenic states include the Bernard–Soulier syndrome, Wiskott–Aldrich syndrome, thrombocytopenia with absent radius, May–Hegglin anomaly, and hereditary thrombocytopenia resembling idiopathic thrombocytopenia.

Acquired thrombocytopenia may be caused by decreased or ineffective platelet production, platelet sequestration (*i.e.*, pooling of platelets in an enlarged spleen), or increased platelet destruction. Acquired thrombocytopenia may be primary or secondary to viral or other infections, drugs or toxins, consumptive coagulopathy, anaphylactoid reactions, and, not uncommonly, multiple transfusions with aged bank blood.

A decrease in the platelet number and function frequently is the cause of the uncontrollable bleeding in surgical or trauma patients who receive transfusions of massive amounts of blood. The amount of blood required before a defect in hemostasis occurs varies from patient to patient with the functional reserve of the bone marrow, but frequently a defect does not occur until several (3–6) liters of banked blood have been infused.[7, 17] Platelet counts should be monitored during the infusion of large amounts of banked blood and platelet concentrates infused when indicated.

Thrombocytopathies

Disorders of platelet function are related to alterations of adhesion, aggregation, or release, and they also may be congenital or acquired. The most common cause of a platelet adhesion defect is von Willebrand's disease, an autosomal dominant disorder. Other congenital thrombocytopathies include Glanzmann's thrombocytopenia and the reduced availability of platelet factor III. Acquired platelet dysfunction occurs with dysproteinemic states such as cryoglobulinemia, multiple myeloma, macroglobulinemia, and hypergammaglobulinemia, during which abnormal proteins coat platelets and interfere with their function. Abnormal platelet function has also been described in patients with scurvy, congestive heart failure, uremia, cirrhosis, and leukemia.

Drug ingestion is a major cause of platelet dysfunction. Many common drugs interfere with platelet adhesion or aggregation, including the following:

Aspirin
Indomethacin
Corticosteroids
Dipyridamole
Sulfinpyrazone
Theophylline
Caffeine
Papaverine
Chlorpromazine
Dextran
Antibiotics
Hydroxychloroquine
Tricyclic antidepressants
Phenothiazines
Alpha blockers
Beta blockers
Heparin
Alcohol
Antihistamines
Methysergide
Clofibrate
Cocaine
Lidocaine

Because of its widespread use, aspirin contributes to many of the acquired disorders of platelet function. Aspirin should be discontinued, if possible, 2 or more days prior to surgery to allow the patient to acquire a sufficient number of nonexposed platelets for hemostasis.

COAGULATION

Coagulation is initiated by the reaction of phospholipids with the coagulation proteins. Both the extrinsic and intrinsic coagulation pathways participate in the activation of factor X to activated factor X (Xa). Exposure of the subendothelial structures to platelets results in release of platelet factor III. The subendothelial structures also activate factor XII, which in the presence of prekallikrein and kininogens, activate factor XI (XI to XIa). XIa in the presence of calcium converts factor IX to activated factor IX (IXa). IXa, platelet phospholipids, calcium, and factor VIII convert factor X to activated factor X (Xa).

In the extrinsic pathway of coagulation, a tissue phospholipid, thromboplastin, reacts with calcium ions and factor VII (and possibly other enzymes) to convert factor X to Xa. Thus, factor VII is the unique factor involved in the extrinsic pathway of coagulation.

The final common pathway of coagulation involves the conversion of prothrombin to thrombin by phospholipids in combination with calcium, Xa, and factor V. Thrombin is the proteolytic enzyme that cleaves fibrinopeptides A and B from fibrinogen to produce fibrin monomers, which undergo spontaneous polymerization to form a gel that is "stabilized" by a fibrin stabilizing factor (factor XIII) activated by the thrombin. Thus, factor I, II, V, Xa, and XIII are utilized in the final pathway of coagulation.

All of the coagulation factors except III (thromboplastin), IV (calcium), and VIII (antihemophilic globulin) are synthesized in the liver. Hence, hepatic function determines the concentration of most of the coagulation factors. Factors II, VII, IX, and X require vitamin K for their production and may be decreased during times of diminished oral intake or times of reduced absorption of lipids. Although most coagulation factors are relatively stable in banked blood, factors V and VIII are quite labile, with only approximately 80% of factor V and 60% of factor VIII being available after 5 days of storage and 40% and 15%, respectively, after 14 days.[5, 10]

Congenital Coagulation Disorders

Acquired causes of bleeding are much more frequent in surgical and trauma patients than are congenital causes. Factor VIII and factor IX deficiencies are sex-linked recessive disorders, while the other hereditary coagulation disorders are inherited in an autosomal manner. Many patients survive very well with congenital coagulation abnormalities until the abnormalities become manifest when stressed by surgery or trauma. Deficiencies and absences of all of the coagulation factors have been reported as a cause of congenital coagulation defects.

Acquired Coagulation Disorders

Acquired coagulation disorders usually involve deficiencies of multiple coagulation factors because the factors are consumed faster than they are replaced during coagulation, because hepatic synthesis of the factors is reduced, or because components needed for the production of the factors are reduced. Most of the coagulation factors are produced in the liver, with factors II, VII, IX, and X being dependent upon an adequate level of vitamin K in the liver for their synthesis. Vitamin K is not stored to any extent in the body, and deficiencies of vitamin K occur in association with conditions that interfere with absorption of fat and the fat-soluble vitamins (e.g., common duct stones, carcinoma of the head of the pancreas, limited oral intake, and the presence of broad-spectrum antibiotics). Conditions that alter hepatic function (e.g., cirrhosis, hepatitis, hepatic toxins, etc.), can also reduce the liver's production of the coagulation factors. In hepatic insufficiency, levels of all coagulation factors may be decreased except factor VIII, but factors II, V, VII, IX, and X are the most vulnerable. If an operation is required by patients with hepatic insufficiency or if these patients sustain major trauma, they must receive fresh frozen plasma or fresh blood to ensure the presence of adequate concentrations of coagulation factors.

Transfusion-Induced Disorders

The transfusion of the large amounts of banked blood that are occasionally required during major surgery or trauma may contribute to the blood of the patient becoming similar to the banked blood. In addition to the rapid decline in number and function of platelets in banked blood, the concentrations of factors V and VIII decrease during the first few days and there is also a real, but less precipitous, decline in the other factors.[10] In addition, the fibrinolytic activity of the banked blood increases, and the degradation products of fibrinogen and fibrin, which have an anticoagulant effect, appear.

In order to prevent the adverse effects upon coagulation that follow the use of large amounts of older banked blood, many blood banks offer progressively fresher blood to patients requiring massive transfusions. The blood bank should provide blood less than a week old after each third or fourth unit of blood has been transfused. Some blood banks attempt to ensure that every third unit of blood is less than 24 hours old.[16, 17] If fresh blood is not available and platelet abnormalities are not the cause of the coagulation defect, a unit of fresh frozen plasma can be given after each third or fourth unit of older blood to replenish coagulation factors and to prevent the side-effects of excessive amounts of aged blood.

Coagulation-Induced Disorders

Coagulation usually continues until the initiating stimulus is removed and the activated components are consumed, diluted, or neutralized. If the stimulus for coagulation continues and is of sufficient intensity, the coagulation process may consume some or all of the coagulation factors and the patient's blood may become incoagulable. The stimulating factors that the surgeon is most likely to encounter include massive trauma, incompatible blood transfusions, gram-negative sepsis, large necrotic tumors, large aneurysms and vascular malformations, fat emboli, and retained products of conception. When the coagulation factors are consumed faster than they are produced, intravascular coagulation may be accompanied by bleeding from wound surfaces and into areas of trauma.

In addition to the consumption of coagulation factors, intravascular coagulation also consumes platelets and thus reduces the ability of the platelet plug to form. The intravascular coagulation also activates the fibrinolytic mechanism with the production of secondary fibrinolysis. This fibrinolysis may cause bleeding by lysing the existing thromboses in severed vessels. The products of the fibrinolytic activity, especially the fibrin and fibrinogen degradation products, have an anticoagulant effect and further enhance the bleeding.[15]

Anticoagulants

The unconscious trauma victim, the patient requiring emergency surgery, and, on rare occasions, the patient having elective surgery may bleed because the surgeon is unaware that the patient has been taking an anticoagulant. Most often, the patient or a member of the patient's family can give a history of anticoagulant use and the level of anticoagulation can be detected and corrected preoperatively if necessary.

The hypoprothrombinemic agents, especially sodium warfarin, are most often utilized for long-term anticoagulation. The level of anticoagulation can be detected by the prothrombin time and corrected by the intravenous administration of 10 mg to 25 mg of vitamin K if bleeding is not excessive or if operation can be delayed 8 to 24 hours. Fresh frozen plasma, banked blood that is less than a week old, or plasma concentrates can be utilized to correct the prothrombin time more quickly. Patients can be operated upon safely with prothrombin concentrations at 30% of normal, but it is preferable that the prothrombin concentration be at least 40% to 50% of normal prior to surgery.

More and more patients are self-administering minidose heparin as outpatients. The usual dosage of 5000 units of heparin every 8 hours to 12 hours should not produce excessive bleeding in the trauma or surgery patient. Most often, the partial thromboplastin time is normal in these patients. If it is abnormally prolonged, it can be corrected toward normal with blood, fresh frozen plasma, or small (5–10 mg) amounts of protamine sulfate given slowly intravenously.

Fibrinolytic Mechanism

The fibrinolytic system maintains the patency of blood vessels and other tubular structures by lysing thromboses and fibrin deposits within them. Fibrinolysis occurs whenever plasminogen, which is intimately bound to fibrinogen and thus is incorporated into all thromboses, is converted to plasmin by an activator. The intravascular fibrinolytic activator appears to have the major role in maintaining vascular patency and in activating intravascular plasminogen.

Plasmin is a proteolytic enzyme with a special affinity for fibrin, and it enzymatically breaks fibrin into polypeptides. Circulating inhibitors of plasmin usually inhibit the systemic effects of plasmin unless a major activation of the fibrinolytic system occurs. Plasmin is most effective in lysing fresh thromboses and has a limited effect upon thromboses more than 5 days old. Thus, during or immediately after trauma or surgery, increased fibrinolytic activity may be responsible for clinically significant bleeding. However, hyperfibrinolysis is responsible for bleeding much less frequently than the causes noted above.

Increased fibrinolytic activity occurs most often as a response to intravascular coagulation (secondary fibrinolysis). Hyperfibrinolysis also occurs in response to infusions of plasminogen activators (e.g., urokinase or streptokinase). This type of increased fibrinolytic activity is usually easily managed by stopping the infusion.

Less than 1% of the cases of nonmechanical bleeding are caused by primary hyperfibrinolysis, that is, when the fibrinolytic system is activated by stimuli other than intravascular coagulation. Primary hyperfibrinolysis has been described after sudden death, severe trauma, electric shock, and massive hemorrhage and during profound hypoxia, acidosis, or shock.

DIAGNOSTIC APPROACH TO THE BLEEDING PATIENT

Unfortunately, coagulopathies rarely become manifest in the trauma or surgical patient preoperatively but instead are encountered intraoperatively (rarely postoperatively) when the findings of the history and physical examination are less accessible. Therefore, laboratory testing becomes most important. However, if a coagulopathy is suspected before operation, and, if there is time, a careful history, physical examination, and screening battery of tests should alert the surgeon to the presence of the coagulopathy.

History and Physical Examination

The history is very important in evaluating the bleeding patient. Information should be obtained about the type of bleeding—that is, petechia, purpura, ecchymosis, or deep tissue bleeding—and whether the bleeding occurs spontaneously or is related to trauma or surgery. Spontaneous skin and mucosal bleeding is frequently associated with platelet disorders, while bleeding into deeper tissues is usually associated with coagulation-factor deficiencies. A family history of excessive bleeding should alert the surgeon to the possibility of congenital coagulation or platelet disorders. The presence of associated systemic illnesses, such as uremia, hepatic insufficiency, and so forth, should raise the possibility of bleeding. The use of drugs that affect the coagulation factors or platelet functions should be noted.

The physical examination should include a careful search for petechia, ecchymosis, telangiectasia, joint deformities, hemarthroses, splenomegaly, hepatomegaly, jaundice, abnormal elasticity of skin, or hyperextensibility of joints.

Laboratory Tests

Some believe that routine screening testing of all trauma and surgical patients is economically unsound because the tests may not cover all possible disorders and because mild disorders may not be detected. It appears, however, that a simple battery of tests will reveal most of the significant abnormalities of coagulation. The screening tests, when positive, should be followed by more definitive specific-factor testing.[1]

Although platelets are frequently evaluated by examination of the peripheral blood smear, a platelet count is more reliable. If thrombocytopenia is present, the immediate concern is to correct the thrombocytopenia to at least 30,000 platelets per mm^3 and later to determine the cause of the thrombocytopenia and correct that. If there is no thrombocytopenia, but the history suggests platelet dysfunction, the choices are qualitative platelet disorders secondary to drugs, systemic illnesses such as uremia and liver disease, and von Willebrand's disease. The Mielke template bleeding time is a useful screening test for patients with platelet dysfunction.[11] Testing for the von Willebrand factor (ristocetin-induced platelet aggregation) and factor VIII will help determine the presence of von Willebrand's disease.

The procoagulant factors are evaluated by determination of the thromboplastin time (PTT), prothrombin time (PT), and the thrombin time (TT). If clotting occurs but the clot is unstable, factor XIII should be assayed. The PTT is almost always abnormal when any of the procoagulant factors, except factor VII, are reduced to the levels that result in abnormal hemostasis. The PT is prolonged by significant reduction of factors V, VII, X, prothrombin, or fibrinogen. The TT, which measures the ability of thrombin to catalyse the transformation of fibrinogen to fibrin, is sensitive to low concentrations of fibrinogen, circulating heparin, or increases of fibrin-degradation products.

A low fibrinogen concentration may be congenital, but most often it is associated with intravascular coagulation or increased fibrinolytic activity. Several methods exist for assaying fibrinogen. To determine whether an inhibitor to one or more clotting factors exists, the patient's plasma is mixed with an equal volume of normal plasma and the PT, PTT, and TT repeated. When there are deficiencies, the normal plasma restores the PT, PTT, and TT to normal, whereas when an inhibitor is present, only partial or no normalization occurs. If clots form and then break down, the patient may be deficient in factor XIII or have increased fibrinolytic activity. If the fac-

TABLE 16-1. TESTS FOR DIFFERENTIATING BLEEDING DISORDERS

Type of Bleeding Disorder	Fibrinogen Content	Prothrombin Time	Partial Thromboplastin Time	Thrombin Time	Lysis Time	Platelet Count	Fibrin Degradation Products
Congenital coagulation deficiencies	NA	NA*	NA*	NA	N	N	N
DIC	A	A	A	NA	A	A	A
Decreased platelet number	N	N	N	N	N	A	N
Decreased platelet function	N	N	N	N	N	N	N
Hyperfibrinolysis	NA	NA	NA	NA	A	N	A
Excessive heparin	N	A†	A†	A†	N	N	N
Excessive hypoprothrombinemic agents	N	A	A	N	N	N	N
Excessive banked blood	NA	N	A	N	NA	A	A

A = abnormal; N = normal.

*A normal PT and PTT exclude hemophilia and the parahemophilias as a cause of bleeding and indicate adequate amounts of the vitamin K factors.

†The PT, PTT, and TT will return to normal, if the coagulation factors are normal, when heparin is "neutralized."

tor XIII assay is normal, a whole blood lysis time and euglobulin clot lysis time should be performed.

The screening procedures listed in Table 16-1 should detect most of the causes of surgical bleeding disorders.

Management

Bleeding that occurs early after trauma or soon after the skin incision is made during surgery usually results from deficiencies of platelet number or function, excessive anticoagulation, or a congenital deficiency of coagulation factors. Bleeding that occurs later during trauma or during an operation usually is caused by an acquired deficiency in the number of platelets or in coagulation factors, or by secondary or primary fibrinolysis. This type of bleeding may be attributed to the excessive administration of old banked blood without adequate replacement of platelets and coagulation factors, but it is frequently caused by disseminated intravascular coagulation, which consumes platelets and coagulation factors. Primary hyperfibrinolysis rarely is the cause of intraoperative bleeding.

Proper management of the bleeding patient requires identification of the cause of the bleeding. The laboratory tests noted above should be utilized in evaluating the patient with active bleeding. Specific coagulation factors should be assayed if the patients have known congenital coagulation defects or if specific testing is indicated by the screening tests.

Thrombocytopenia and defective platelet function are treated with platelet transfusions. Spontaneous bleeding rarely occurs if the platelet count is more than 30,000 per mm^3. However, after trauma or during surgery a platelet count of 50,000 per mm^3 is recommended for effective hemostasis. A single unit of platelet concentrate usually increases the platelet count by 10,000 platelets per mm^3. Platelet counts and platelet transfusions are repeated as necessary to maintain the platelet count at 50,000 per mm^3.

Platelets transfused into patients with immune-mediated thrombocytopenia do not survive longer than a few minutes and therefore should not be given unless there is life-threatening bleeding. However, if these patients are bleeding excessively, platelet transfusions are given as often as needed to control the bleeding.

Patients with multiple coagulation deficiencies (e.g., patients with cirrhosis or vitamin K deficiencies or who have received massive blood transfusions and developed the associated "wash-out" syndrome) are best managed by the administration of fresh frozen plasma or fresh whole blood. Because fresh whole blood may not be available, the patients most often receive fresh frozen plasma. Sufficient fresh frozen plasma (usually 15–20 ml/kg) is given to raise the clotting factors to 20% to 30% of normal. Fresh frozen plasma is continued at approximately one half the initial dose at 8- to 12-hour intervals until the coagulation factors stabilize and the bleeding is controlled. Dilutional thrombocytopenia is corrected with platelet transfusions. Of course, the blood bank should provide blood less than 1 week old after the first four units are infused.

The patient with a consumptive coagulopathy usually has a lower platelet count and fewer coagulation factors and more fibrinolytic activity than does a patient who has received excessive amounts of banked blood. Fresh frozen plasma and platelets will usually not correct the coagulation defect associated with a consumptive coagulopathy unless the cause for the coagulopathy has been corrected, but they will correct the defects associated with the use of excessive amounts of banked blood.

The treatment of a consumptive coagulopathy should be directed primarily at correcting or removing the underlying cause. If the cause is not corrected, the administration of fresh frozen plasma and platelets may accelerate the intravascular coagulation and compound the coagulation disorder. If the cause of the intravascular coagulation cannot be removed or reduced in a short period of time—that is, until the aneurysm or tumor is resected, abscess drained, or fetus removed—and the coagulopathy continues, attention should be directed toward reducing the intravascular coagulation with heparin. Most surgeons would prefer not to use heparin intraoperatively because the bleeding may increase. However, the administration of heparin will slow the intravascular coagulation while the cause of the intravascular coagulation is being combated. Heparin decreases the utilization of platelets and coagulation factors that are needed for functional restoration of the hemostatic mechanism. Furthermore, the platelets and coagulation factors infused will not be consumed instantly if the patient is receiving heparin. Although heparin is infrequently used intraoperatively, the usual dose for an average adult patient is 3000 units as a "loading dose" and about 400 to 600 units per hour as a constant infusion. As the hemostatic potential returns to normal and bleeding decreases, the heparin infusion can be slowed and stopped when the consumptive coagulopathy (and its cause) is controlled.

A normal platelet count or a platelet count greater than 100,000 platelets per mm^3 helps distinguish primary hyperfibrinolysis from the secondary fibrinolysis associated with an intravascular coagulation. The hyperfibrinolysis that occurs in association with intravascular coagulation usually stops when the intravascular coagulation is controlled, and it rarely requires treatment. This fibrinolysis is protective and maintains patency of the microvasculature. If the fibrinolytic activity persists after the intravascular coagulation is controlled, epsilon-aminocaproic acid (EACA) is the fibrinolytic inhibitor most often used to treat the increased fibrinolytic activity. EACA is primarily a plasminogen-activator inhibitor and therefore 30 to 60 minutes must elapse before effect can be observed.

EACA may be given intravenously to patients with primary hyperfibrinolysis and to those with continuing secondary symptomatic hyperfibrinolysis after the intravascular coagulation has been controlled. The usual initial dose for an adult is 5 g followed by 1 g an hour for 6 hours to 8 hours or until the lysis is controlled. Trauma patients or surgical patients who are at risk for deep venous thrombosis should receive EACA only during the acute lytic state. If EACA is continued after the bleeding is controlled, these patients should benefit from the administration of minidose heparin (5000 units, every 8 hours, subcutaneously) during the time of the EACA administration in order to reduce the frequency of deep venous thrombosis that is associated with prolonged EACA administration.

If large quantities of blood products are required, they should be warmed before being infused in order to help maintain the patient's temperature. A variety of blood warmers are available; however, all should be monitored to ensure that the temperature of the infusate does not exceed 40°C in order to prevent damage to the proteins or cellular materials. In addition, any particulate matter from the blood products should be removed by micropore filters. A 40-μ pore filter appears to be adequate for this purpose, but it should be changed relatively frequently (*i.e.*, after every 2 or 3 units of infusate). The filters certainly should be used in all multiple-trauma patients, all patients with chronic obstructive lung disease, and those receiving more than 4 units to 5 units of blood.

Calcium is sometimes given to patients who receive large volumes of banked blood to replace the calcium bound by the citrate and thus help the clotting. The citrate in infused blood is rapidly metabolized unless the patient has shock with reduced organ perfusion or liver failure. The calcium level rarely becomes low enough to interfere with coagulation before cardiac function is adversely affected. It is not necessary to administer calcium to improve cardiac function except during special procedures such as open-heart bypass.[8, 12]

Complications Following Splenectomy

OPERATIVE PROCEDURE

The indications for splenectomy include hematologic disorders, for example some forms of thrombocytopenia; staging for lymphomas, trauma, primary or secondary involvement with tumor, and iatrogenic injuries. In the past, all spleens with tears were removed, but now many injured spleens are salvaged.

Splenectomy may be accomplished through a left subcostal incision, an upper midline incision, or a left paramedian incision. The left subcostal incision is ideal for the removal of small spleens, but unless it is extended across the midline to the right, the subcostal incision may not allow access to the proximal portion of the splenic artery if the spleen is enlarged. I prefer a long midline incision or transverse upper abdominal incision when removing large spleens because these incisions give greater ease of access to the proximal splenic artery in case I encounter uncontrollable splenic bleeding.

The splenocolic, splenophrenic, and splenorenal ligaments, which are usually relatively avascular, may become highly vascular in patients with portal hypertension or a splenic arteriovenous fistula, and they should be divided and ligated (or clipped) with care in order to reduce operative blood loss and to reduce the possibility of postoperative bleeding. The gastrosplenic ligament containing the short gastric vessels must always be divided between clamps and the vessels securely ligated. Cautery is not utilized to control these vessels (especially in patients with hematologic disorders) because of the increased possibility of delayed bleeding. Care must be taken in placing the clamps on the gastric side of the vessels in order to avoid injury to the stomach. If the stomach is injured, the injured area should be inverted with one or two rows of permanent sutures to prevent a leak that might occur if the entire thickness of the gastric wall is damaged.

Pancreatic Injury

Because the tail of the pancreas extends toward and frequently into the hilus of the spleen, the pancreas may be injured during a splenectomy. Minimal injury to the tail of the pancreas usually requires no care, but a moderately damaged pancreas should be managed with control of bleeding, ligation of exposed ducts, and closed (sump) drainage. Extensive damage to the tail of the pancreas is usually managed by resecting the tail and closed drainage of the area. Unrecognized pancreatic injuries may be followed by pancreatitis, pancreatic cysts, or fistulas.

Drains

Drains are not recommended after an uncomplicated splenectomy because not only are they not needed, they may also serve as a portal of entry for infection. Hematomas should be prevented by obtaining adequate hemostasis rather than relying upon drains. Some surgeons recommend the use of drains, for a few days, to reduce the subphrenic accumulation of fluid that occurs in the space previously occupied by the spleen. Rather than draining the area, the fluid can be diminished by 20° to 30° elevation of the trunk of the patient. If a hematoma or effusion persists in the subphrenic space, an associated pleural effusion may develop above the diaphragm. Most often these sub- and supraphrenic effusions resolve spontaneously. If the subphrenic effusions or hematomas become infected they must be drained, usually posteriorly through the bed of the 11th or 12th rib. If a hematoma is present, it should also be evacuated. If an empyema has occurred, it should be drained.

Accessory Spleens

Fifteen to thirty percent of patients have accessory spleens. These spleens vary from a few millimeters to several centimeters in size and may become quite large in myeloproliferative disorders. The accessory spleens most often occur in the hilus, along the splenic vessels, within the attaching ligaments of the spleen and in the mesentery and omentum. If the spleen is being removed for hematologic reasons, the accessory spleens should also be removed.

Thrombocytosis

Splenectomy is frequently followed by thrombocytosis, which peaks around 7 to 10 days postoperatively and then returns toward, but rarely to, normal. The number of circulating platelets may exceed 1 million per mm^3. During thrombocytosis, the patient is at increased risk for deep venous thrombosis and small arterial occlusions. If there are no contraindications, the patient should be mobilized as soon as possible, should maintain the legs elevated while in bed or sitting, and should receive a platelet-function-inhibiting drug (*e.g.*, aspirin, 600–900 mg, twice a day, or minidose heparin, 5000 units subcutaneously every 8 hours). I frequently give 600 mg of aspirin twice a day with meals *and* 5000 units of heparin subcutaneously every 8 hours to these patients until the platelet count returns to or below 500,000 per mm^3.

Delayed Bleeding

If after splenectomy the patient becomes tachycardiac or hypotensive and has a falling hematocrit, delayed bleeding should be suspected. Most often the safest course for the patient is to evacuate the hematoma and control the source of the bleeding surgically. If the patient is bleeding from a coagulopathy, the coagulopathy should be controlled before proceeding with the operation.

POSTSPLENECTOMY SEPSIS AND SPLENIC SALVAGE

In recent years it has been established that the spleen has an important role in immunologic defenses; splenectomy increases the risk of serious, frequently fatal, sepsis—especially in children; many splenic injuries heal or can be repaired; and partial splenectomy is feasible and safe.[4, 6, 9] Singer, in a comprehensive review of postsplenectomy sepsis, found that "death from postsplenectomy sepsis is 200 times as prevalent as death due to sepsis in the population at large."[14] Even if postsplenectomy sepsis is recognized and treated aggressively, 50% to 75% of the patients with this fulminating illness die.[3]

Pneumococci have been isolated in approximately 50% of the patients with postsplenectomy sepsis; meningicocci and *Hemophilus influenzae* are the other commonly identified organisms. Streptococci, staphylococci, gram-negative, and other organisms have also been cultured. Younger patients, especially those less than 2 years of age, appear to be at greater risk for postsplenectomy sepsis than are other patients. The patient's risk for postsplenectomy sepsis is also related to why the splenectomy was needed and the subsequent management of the patient—the incidence of sepsis after splenectomy for trauma is 0.5% to 2%, while it is 10% to 25% in patients with Hodgkin's disease and thalassemia major. Patients with splenectomies who are receiving chemotherapy or radiation therapy to suppress their immune systems have a higher incidence of sepsis.

As a result of the postsplenectomy sepsis syndrome, splenectomy is no longer the treatment of choice for the injured spleen. Instead, attempts are made to salvage at least part of the injured spleen. Although the minimal amount of normal functioning spleen needed to protect a patient from postsplenectomy sepsis syndrome has not been established, immunologic protection seems likely if approximately 25% of the spleen remains perfused by either the splenic or short gastric arteries. Therefore, if possible, the portions of the injured spleens that are well vascularized should be salvaged.

The surgeon has numerous technical options during his attempts to salvage the spleen. The transverse orientation of the trabeculae and the blood supply of the spleen has helped with splenic salvage, especially with partial resection or transverse lacerations. Splenic capsular tears can be closed with fine permanent sutures. Similar sutures can be used for closing lacerations or areas after débridement or resection. Through-and-through supporting mattress sutures and even "absorbable suture ladders" have been used to stop bleeding and support the injured spleen.[2] Bleeding from areas of the spleen denuded of its capsule can frequently be controlled with pressure and with hemostatic agents (e.g., powdered gelfoam, microfibrillar collagen, cyanoacrylate adhesive, etc.). The omentum can be used to reinforce suture lines or to cover denuded areas. Splenic artery ligation will help control splenic bleeding without impairing splenic functions.

Sepsis Prophylaxis

If the spleen cannot be salvaged, all patients should be warned of the postsplenectomy sepsis syndrome and should be told to report all infectious processes to their physicians promptly for diagnosis and antibiotic management. In addition, the patient should receive a polyvalent pneumococcal vaccine (Pneumovac*), preferably preoperatively for elective splenectomies and early postoperatively otherwise. This vaccine contains polysaccharides from 14 of the common pneumococcal organisms. The duration of the protection from the pneumococcal vaccine is undetermined at present, with titers decreasing after 1 year but apparently persisting at satisfactory levels for 2 years to 8 years. It is also recommended that patients who have had a splenectomy receive prophylactic penicillin (500 mg, orally, each day or 1.2 million units of Bicillin by injection each month). Penicillin prophylaxis is especially important for all postsplenectomy patients who receive chemotherapy or radiation therapy. Because the penicillin protects the patient only against the more common organisms, all infections must be cultured and treated aggressively with appropriate antibiotics. The duration of the prophylaxis remains controversial, but certainly should be continued for the first 2 years to 5 years, when the patient is at greatest risk for infection. Postsplenectomy sepsis has occurred 20 years to 30 years after splenectomy, and, therefore, if the patients will comply, the penicillin prophylaxis should be continued indefinitely.

*Merck Sharp & Dohme, West Point, PA 19486

References

1. Bowie EJW, Owen CA Jr: The significance of abnormal preoperative hemostatic tests. Prog Hemost Thromb 5:179, 1980
2. Buntain WL, Lynn HB: Splenorrhaphy: Changing concepts for the traumatized spleen. Surgery 86:748, 1979
3. Dickerman JD: Splenectomy and sepsis: A warning. Pediatrics 63:938, 1979
4. Francke EL, Neu HC: Postsplenectomy infection. Surg Clin North Am 61:135, 1981
5. Goldstein R, Bunker JP, McGovern JJ: The effect of storage of whole blood and anticoagulants upon certain coagulation factors. Ann NY Acad Sci 115:422, 1964
6. Gopal V, Bisno A: Fulminant pneumococcal infections in 'normal' asplenic hosts. Arch Intern Med 137:1526, 1977
7. Howland WS et al: Physiologic alterations with massive blood replacement. Surg Gynecol Obstet 101:478, 1955
8. Howland WS et al: The cardiovascular effects of low levels of ionized calcium during massive transfusion. Surg Gynecol Obstet 145:581, 1977
9. King H, Shumaker HB: Splenic studies: I. Susceptibility to infection after splenectomy performed in infancy. Ann Surg 136:239, 1952
10. Limbird TJ, Silver D: Sequential changes in blood preserved with citrate-phosphate-dextrose. Surg Gynecol Obstet 138:401, 1974
11. Mielke CH Jr et al: The standardized normal Ivy bleeding time and its prolongation by aspirin. Blood 34:204, 1969

12. Perkins HA et al: Calcium ion activity during rapid exchange transfusion with citrated blood. Transfusion 11:204, 1971
13. Silver D, McGregor FH Jr: Nonmechanical causes of surgical bleeding. Curr Probl Surg (Monogr), January 1970
14. Singer DB: Postsplenectomy sepsis. Perspect Pediat Pathol 1:285, 1973
15. Triantaphyllopoulos DC, Triantaphylopoulos E: Physiological effects of fibrinogen degradation products. Thrombosis et Diathesis Haemorrhagica (Suppl)39:175, 1970
16. Wilson RF, Mammen E, Walt AJ: Eight years of experience with massive blood transfusion. J Trauma 11:275, 1971
17. Wilson WB: Emergency management of unexpected defects of hemostatic function in surgical patients. JAMA 201:123, 1967

17 Complications of Nutritional Support

Harvey J. Sugerman | H. H. Newsome, Jr.

OVERVIEW—COMPLICATIONS OF MALNUTRITION

Malnutrition is a frequent and sometimes unappreciated problem with which surgeons are faced. Either obvious protein-calorie malnutrition, resembling marasmus, or subtle protein deficiency (i.e.,) kwashiorkor), may be present in patients who must undergo major surgery. Septic, burned, or traumatized patients may lose as much as 30 g of nitrogen per day (Fig. 17-1), which is equivalent to the catabolism of 2½ pounds of wet muscle daily.[60] It is not difficult to understand how a patient with this rate of catabolism will not only lose lean muscle mass but will also lose other protein-related functions such as the enzymatic and other cellular activities important for healing of incisions and anastomoses. The leukocytes lack the energy supply to seek out, capture, and kill bacteria. Over the years great interest has been generated about the influence of undernutrition on immunologic deficiency, which might predispose surgical patients to septic complications. Hypoalbuminemia has long been considered an index of protein depletion and has been shown to be associated with an increased rate of postoperative mortality.[16, 88] Recognition and correction of malnutrition prior to elective surgery may eliminate or reduce the rates of surgical morbidity and mortality. Even in a well-nourished patient, but certainly in one already protein deficient, the trauma of surgery or septic complications of surgery may promote malnutrition. Thus, it is important for the surgeon to recognize the disastrous cycle of malnutrition → complications; complications → malnutrition.

It is critically important for surgeons to recognize the presence of and the propensity for malnutrition in their patients. The prevention or correction of these protein–calorie deficits is best managed by the assistance of a nutritional-support team that should include pharmacists, dieticians, nurses, and physicians so that the complications discussed in this chapter can be minimized or promptly recognized and expeditiously managed.

IMPAIRED WOUND HEALING

Impaired healing can probably result from malnutrition and lead to disruption of intestinal anastomoses as well as wound dehiscence and infection. Steiger

FIG. 17-1. Accelerated nitrogen excretion is noted in patients following a major burn, skeletal trauma, or sepsis. (Long CL, Schaffel N, Geiger JW: Metabolic response to injury and illness: Estimation of energy and protein needs from indirect calorimetry and nitrogen balance. JPEN 3:452, 1979)

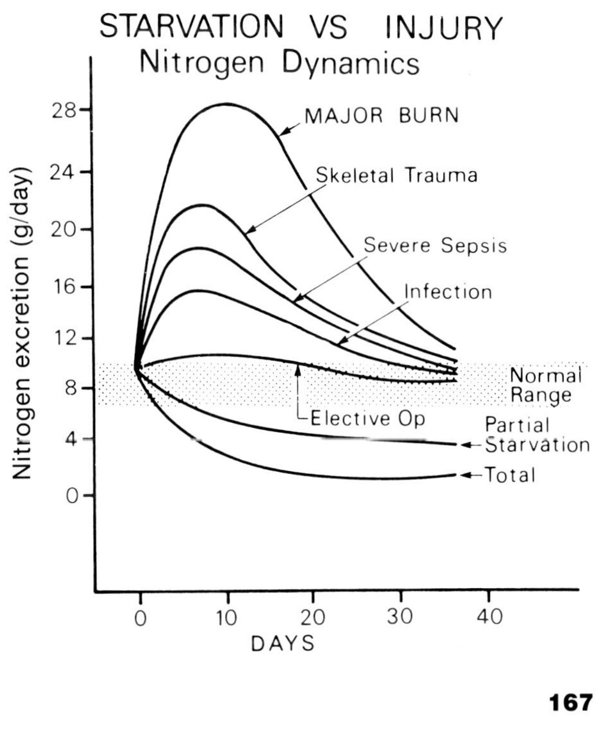

and colleagues have shown decreased tensile strength of intestinal anastomoses in malnourished rats, which could be prevented by parenteral nutritional repletion.[96] Every effort should be made, when possible, to minimize impaired wound healing by repleting, preoperatively, patients who are undernourished and by preventing postoperative starvation. Zinc, vitamin C (ascorbic acid), and vitamin A deficiencies may also lead to impaired wound healing and should be prevented.[51, 77, 86]

PULMONARY COMPLICATIONS

Malnutrition may also lead to an increased risk of respiratory difficulties such as atelectasis and pneumonia secondary to decreased strength of respiratory muscles and the inability to cough.[73] The lack of muscle strength probably decreases the patient's forced vital capacity and tidal volume and, therefore, prolongs the need for intubation and mechanical ventilation with their associated complications of pneumothorax, tracheal-innominate artery erosion, tracheal stenosis, and sepsis.[12] Impaired leukocyte function will also increase the risk of pneumonia. Although pneumonia and respiratory failure are major causes of death for persons who are starved, there is little evidence that nutritional repletion improves pulmonary function and prevents pneumonia.[58]

SEPTIC COMPLICATIONS

Several investigators have found a marked increase in septic complications in malnourished patients.[58, 75] The increase was associated in some with an impairment of delayed hypersensitivity or with neutrophil chemotaxis.[68, 69] MacLean described patients with anergy as defined by the failure of skin reactivity to four recall antigens (mumps, PPD, Varidase, and candida) and an absent primary or secondary response to dinitrochlorobenzene (DNCB).[64] "Relative anergy" was diagnosed if a patient failed to respond to one of the four antigens. The concept of relative anergy is difficult to comprehend. That a patient could respond to one recall antigen suggests that his T lymphocytes were capable of functioning. Furthermore, delayed hypersensitivity protects the body from invasion with mycobacteria and assists in the recognition and destruction of foreign cells (*i.e.*, transplant or malignant). It is not logical to ascribe the increased incidence of bacterial invasion in postoperative patients to impaired T-lymphocyte function. Perhaps impaired delayed hypersensitivity reflects a generalized immune incompetence that would include defective antibody production from B lymphocytes as well as impaired neutrophil chemotaxis in anergic surgical patients. Undernutrition alone results in depressed T-lymphocyte numbers and function.[20] Neutropenia has also been noted with copper deficiency, and impaired neutrophil chemotaxis and phagocytosis have also been found with phosphate deficiency.[22, 103] Impaired body defenses will increase the risk of pneumonia, wound infections, and intracavitary abscesses.

OTHER PROBABLE COMPLICATIONS OF MALNUTRITION

The severely debilitated, malnourished patient will be bedridden and so be increasingly vulnerable to the consequences of prolonged bed rest, such as iliofemoral venous thrombosis, pulmonary embolism, decubitus ulcers, atelectasis, and pneumonia. These patients may be obtunded or confused and unable to cooperate with nurses and physicians in their own care and rehabilitation. Intestinal mucosa, which turns over rapidly, may break down and increase the danger of stress bleeding, further impair nutrient absorption, or prolong postoperative ileus. An increased incidence of gastric erosions that could be prevented with total parenteral nutrition (TPN) was noted in nutritionally depleted monkeys.[50] Malnourished patients may also have delayed gastric emptying and prolonged intestinal transit times. Cardiac dysfunction may also be a complication of severe malnutrition.[28]

Assessment of Nutritional Status

DETECTION OF MALNUTRITION

Surgeons are now more attuned to the capability and necessity of preventing this catabolic state by the use of TPN, so that assessment of the nutritional status of each patient is important to detect undernutrition and to follow the progress of nutritional therapy. Measurement of nitrogen loss, total lymphocyte count, serum albumin, serum transferrin, and retinol binding protein permit assessment of nutritional status in surgical patients both pre- and postoperatively.[14, 110] The Harris–Benedict equation is used for calculation of basal energy expenditure (BEE).[45] The addition of a metabolic activity factor (MAF), depending on the severity of illness, enables the dietician to estimate caloric needs.[42] The response to nutritional support can be monitored with the previously mentioned blood tests as well as by measuring nitrogen balance from 24-hour urinary urea nitrogen excretion. Caloric balance should be calculated daily from estimated needs and actual calories delivered. Creatinine-height index may also be used to monitor the rate of muscle catabolism. Daily weights are helpful but can be misleading owing to excessive fluid accumulation. Anthropometric measurements are useful indices of nutritional depletion and of the response to treatment, but the low sensitivity and specificity of many of these tests limit their ability to detect small changes in nutritional status.[33, 38]

Whenever possible, the patient should be fed enterally using nasogastric, nasoduodenal, or feeding jejunostomy tubes if his gastrointestinal system is intact and he is unable or unwilling to eat. Page and colleagues suggested continuous catheter administration of an elemental diet.[83] If the gastrointestinal system is not functioning or cannot be used, TPN should be instituted.

EFFICACY OF CORRECTING MALNUTRITION

Although many studies have demonstrated the deleterious effects of undernutrition, it is difficult to find evidence that parenteral feeding eliminates the problems of malnutrition. A recent review has cited several diseases or conditions for which treatment includes parenteral nutrition, but therapeutic improvement has not been demonstrated.[40] More promise is offered by preventing perioperative complications associated with malnutrition.[47] The nonrandomized study of malnourished patients by MacLean showing restoration of immunocompetency by parenteral feeding in 17 of 43 anergic patients is an example of specific effects of parenteral feeding.[64] Mullen and colleagues showed a significant reduction of 2.5-fold for postoperative complications, 6-fold for major sepsis, and 5-fold for mortality in patients adequately nourished preoperatively over patients not receiving nutritional supplementation.[74] No randomized prospective study has yet confirmed these impressions. Intuitively, if malnutrition has been clearly shown to produce significant complications not seen in nourished individuals, then restoration of a malnourished patient's normal nutritional status should reduce the risk of significant complications.

Complications of Enteral Nutrition

GASTRIC DISTENTION, VOMITING, AND ASPIRATION PNEUMONITIS

The enteral route should be used for nutrition when possible, since this carries less risk of morbidity than does total parenteral nutrition (TPN). Nevertheless, enteral nutrition is not without problems. The greatest dangers are gastric distention, vomiting, and aspiration pneumonitis. Gastric distention alone can produce a shocklike state.[98] Aspiration pneumonitis is associated with acid burn of the alveoli with injury to the pulmonary capillary membrane and leakage of capillary fluid into the alveoli.[39] This produces either inhibition or washout of surfactant, alveolar collapse, and the perfusion of unventilated alveoli with a consequent right-to-left shunt. This results in the development of the acute respiratory distress syndrome (ARDS).

Acid aspiration pneumonitis can be diagnosed by the combination of a history of vomiting, the presence of gastric contents or acid secretions on endotracheal aspiration, the rapid onset of pulmonary dysfunction, and a diffuse, fluffy infiltrate disclosed on the chest roentgenogram.[17] ARDS can be readily differentiated from cardiogenic pulmonary edema by the absence of signs of heart failure or by the measurement of a pulmonary capillary wedge pressure (PCWP) of less than 15 torr (see Table 14-4).

The mortality of ARDS induced by aspiration of acid is high so that its diagnosis usually demands endotracheal intubation, mechanical ventilation, and the use of positive end-expiratory pressure ventilation (PEEP) to re-expand the alveoli and reduce the right-to-left shunt.[17] Pharmacologic doses of corticosteroids have been proposed to limit injury to the alveolar-capillary membrane.[99] However, their efficacy has not been proved. In addition to the immediate danger of hypoxemia and ARDS following aspiration pneumonitis, there is the problem of secondary bacterial growth in the protein fluid, which serves as a rich culture medium, with the development of lobar pneumonia.[4, 11]

Gastric distention, vomiting, and acid aspiration, therefore, must be prevented. Either bolus feeding or continuous drip infusions may be used. The head of the bed should be elevated if possible to 30°. Some cachectic patients whose fourth portion of the duodenum is constricted by the superior mesenteric artery show improved gastric emptying when they are fed in the prone position.[105] The stomach should be aspirated every 4 hours. If more than 100 ml of residual gastric contents is found, the next feeding should be withheld. The use of a long intestinal tube passed through the pylorus will also reduce the danger of gastric distention and vomiting.[24] Several commercial tubes are available for this purpose, such as the Keofed or Dobhoff catheters.

MECHANICAL COMPLICATIONS

Erosive esophagitis, pharyngeal discomfort, and otitis media are also associated with prolonged nasogastric intubation. Although they are somewhat more difficult to insert than earlier models, the newer silastic tubes are far more comfortable. It is extremely important that a nasogastric tube exit the nose inferiorly. The tube should not be brought up across the nasal ala under pressure and taped to the forehead. This can produce an unsightly necrosis of the nasal cartilage. Patients who are confused and combative may persist in removing their nasogastric tube. Placing a "circle-stitch" tied to the nasogastric tube within the oropharynx, passing out the mouth and tied again to the tube where it exits from the nose, overcomes this resistance.

Long-standing intubation of the stomach can be achieved with a cervical pharyngostomy, obviating the discomfort of a tube in the nasopharynx.[41] A feeding gastrostomy is also useful and can be performed under local anesthesia. This procedure may be associated with intraperitoneal leakage should feeding be instituted too soon after insertion of the tube. A feeding jejunostomy may also be used, either through the standard Witzel technique with a large bore, red rubber feeding tube (#18 French) or utilizing the needle-catheter jejunostomy technique.[83] Although the needle catheter is simple to insert, it limits the material that can be instilled to the expensive, high-caloric amino-acid solutions such as Vivonex. According to some reports, these solutions can be instituted in the early postoperative period. They are less expensive and associated with a lower morbidity than postoperative TPN.[82]

SECONDARY DIARRHEA

Intractable diarrhea and severe dehydration may occur when enteral feedings are advanced too rapidly in both quantity and osmolarity. This can be quite unpleasant and markedly hampers nursing care by necessitating frequent changing of linens when time could be more profitably spent in other patient-care functions. Furthermore, constant diarrhea increases the risk of skin breakdown, decubitus ulcers, and imbalances of electrolytes, water, and *p*H. The regimen used in our hospital to prevent intractable diarrhea begins with 50 ml of a commercial lactose-free enteral solution, containing 1 calorie per ml, given with 100 ml of water every 4 hours. The amount of enteral solution is advanced as tolerated over 5 days to a 400-ml feeding with 100 ml of water every 4 hours. The patient's electrolytes and blood sugar need to be carefully monitored to avoid the complications of hypernatremia, hypokalemia, hyperchloremic metabolic acidosis, hypokalemic metabolic alkalosis, and nonketotic hyperglycemic coma.

Complications of TPN

CATHETER-RELATED COMPLICATIONS

Total parenteral nutrition became possible with the development of subclavian vein catheterization by the Algerian surgeon, Aubaniac.[8] The use of a long-arm CVP catheter inserted through a peripheral vein into a main intrathoracic vein will invariably lead to thrombophlebitis and a marked increase in septic complications. The transfemoral route is also associated with an increased risk of infection as well as the danger of iliofemoral venous thrombosis and pulmonary embolism.

Although subclavian vein catheterization can and should be a safe procedure with a low risk of complications, insertion of these catheters by unskilled personnel can have disastrous consequences. The marked reduction in complications of TPN with the institution of a nutritional-support team is well established.[77] The incidence of catheter related complications, discussed below, ranges from 0.4% to 11% and is related to the experience of the insertion team.[30, 81] These complications include pneumothorax, hydrothorax, hemothorax, hemomediastinum, phrenic nerve injury, air embolism, subclavian arterial injury, internal jugular and subclavian venous thrombosis, catheter embolization, and possibly esophageal and tracheal injury.[9, 25, 30, 49, 59, 63, 67, 80, 81, 84, 89, 92, 93]

Routine auscultation and roentgenogram of the chest should be performed following subclavian venipuncture. The close proximity of the lung apex renders pneumothorax a threat. Most pneumothoraces are small and can be treated expectantly. Percutaneous aspiration will often be successful. A large pneumothorax should be treated with tube thoracostomy. A tension pneumothorax can develop rapidly in a patient receiving positive pressure ventilation, and it requires urgent chest tube insertion.

Left subclavian vein catheterization may, rarely, injure the thoracic duct and is diagnosed by the presence of a pleural effusion and chylus fluid at thoracocentesis. This should be treated by tube thoracostomy but may require ligation of the duct.

A hydrothorax results from incorrect extravascular placement of the subclavian catheter and the infusion of fluid without having checked for blood return following catheter insertion. The presence of a pleural effusion and a watery solution obtained by thoracocentesis confirm the diagnosis. Removal of the catheter is usually all that is required. Hemothorax, mediastinal hematoma, hydromediastinum, or hydropericardium may result from catheter perforation and be fatal. Hemothorax may also result from inadvertent subclavian arterial puncture or laceration. Following insertion of the needle, the barrel of the syringe should not push back spontaneously. If it does, the artery has probably been entered and the needle should be removed. The application of pressure beneath the clavicle for 5 minutes will usually prevent continued bleeding. Although arterial perforation can usually be treated simply by needle or catheter withdrawal, thoracotomy for control of bleeding may be required for life-threatening exsanguination.[59] Subclavian arterial puncture is more likely to occur in a very thin patient, in whom how rapid and how far the needle is advanced should be undertaken cautiously.

Venous air embolism can occur in a hypovolemic patient during catheter insertion or at any time following inadvertent catheter disconnection, when there is a greater risk for the aspiration of a fatal quantity of air. The development of sudden respiratory distress, wheezing, hypotension, and a "machinery wheel" murmur on cardiac auscultation confirm the diagnosis. The patient should be placed in the Trendelenburg position with the left side down to keep residual air within the right ventricle.[78] All catheter connections should be taped or of the Luer-lock type to prevent this complication.

Catheter embolism (Fig. 17-2) is a great danger when one withdraws the catheter through the needle in an attempt to reposition it.[92] The catheter tip is sheared off by the needle. This should never be allowed to happen. Rarely, the catheter may fracture and embolize. Various snares have been devised to extract embolized catheters transvenously using fluoroscopic guidance.[66]

It is not uncommon for the catheter to pass up the internal jugular vein (Fig. 17-3) or across the chest into the contralateral innominate or subclavian vein. Infusion of the TPN solution into these veins has a high incidence of venous thrombosis. The catheter must be repositioned, and fluoroscopic assistance may be necessary. Because of the risks of hydrothorax or internal jugular vein catheterization, full strength hyperalimentation solution should not be administered until one is radiographically certain of the proper placement of the catheter. Subclavian venous thrombosis can also occur (Fig. 17-4) as a complication of TPN and is diagnosed by the devel-

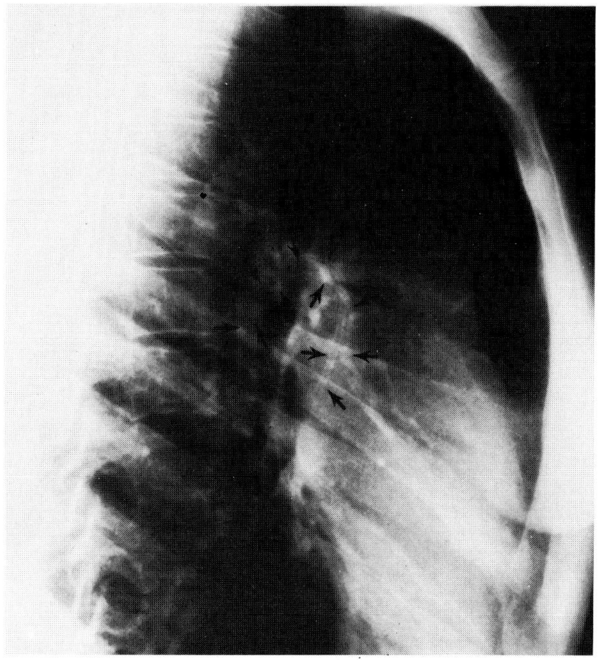

FIG. 17-2. A chest radiograph showing a severed subclavian catheter that has embolized into the pulmonary artery *(arrows)*.

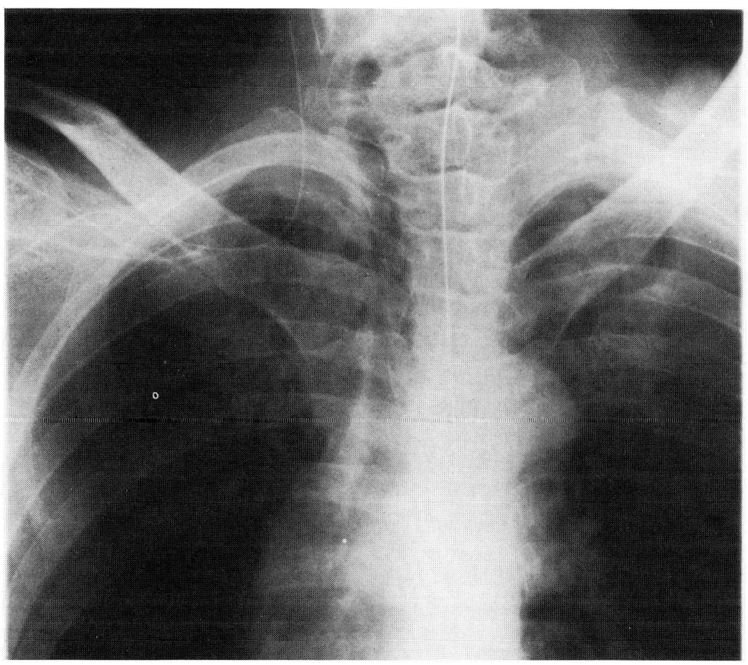

FIG. 17-3. Inadvertent passage of catheter inserted by the subclavicular route into the internal jugular vein. Infusion of hyperosmolar TPN solutions into internal jugular vein will produce venous thrombosis.

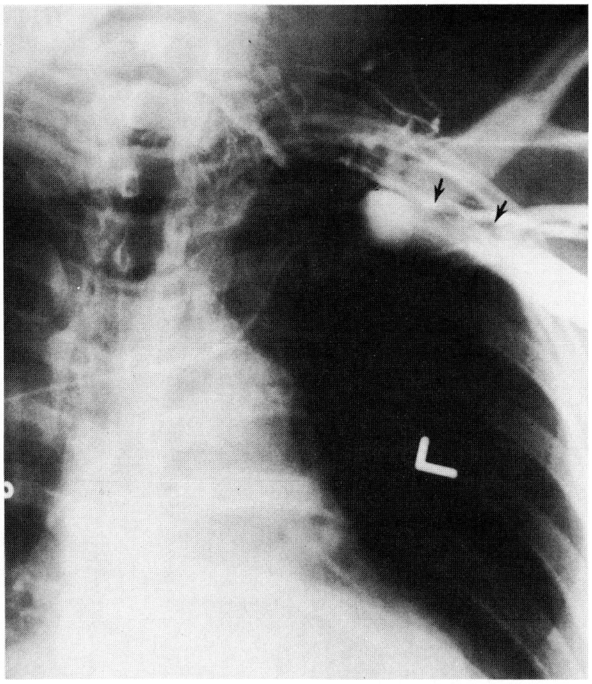

FIG. 17-4. Thrombosis of the left subclavian vein (*arrows*) demonstrated by radiopaque contrast venography in a patient following 1 month of intravenous total parenteral nutrition. This patient subsequently developed thrombosis of the right subclavian vein.

opment of edema of the ipsilateral hand, arm, or breast. The diagnosis can be confirmed with venography. The catheter should be removed and the affected arm elevated. However, we have recently had a patient with bilateral subclavian venous thrombosis in whom we continued to use the subclavian catheter without adverse sequellae. This complication may require percutaneous right atrial catheterization for TPN.[79] Clinically significant pulmonary emboli are unlikely to result from subclavian venous thrombosis.[30, 49, 81, 93]

Cardiac arrhythmias can occur with a catheter lying in the right atrium. This is easily treated by withdrawing the catheter into the superior vena cava. When using a guidewire for catheter insertion, the needle is no longer left on the catheter, and it may be necessary to cut approximately 1 inch from the standard 8-inch catheter to avoid right atrial placement.

A standard protocol for catheter insertion should be instituted to minimize the incidence of these complications. The patient should be placed in a deep Trendelenburg position so that the vein is maximally distended. A rolled sheet should be placed longitudinally between the shoulder blades so that the shoulders can externally rotate, thus opening the space between the clavicle and first rib. The skin should be thoroughly prepared with an antiseptic solution such as Betadine. The operator should wear a cap, mask, sterile gown, and sterile gloves. The area should be isolated at least with sterile towels and preferably with a sterile sheet. The skin and subcutaneous tissues are anesthetized with a local anesthetic such as 1% Xylocaine. The needle is inserted beneath the angle of the clavicle and directed slightly cephalad to the suprasternal notch. The needle should be kept parallel to the floor at all times. Traction on the syringe barrel will produce a jet of blood when the vein is entered. The bevel of the needle should be directed inferiorly. This can be assured by placing the bevel of the needle opposite to the numbers on the syringe prior to its insertion. This should minimize the chance of insertion of the catheter cephalad into the internal jugular vein. The patient's head is rotated to the opposite side. We prefer to use the Seldinger technique with a guidewire, so that the needle can be removed, thus reducing the danger of catheter embolism. One should never withdraw the catheter through the needle, since this maximizes the risk of catheter transection.[89, 92] A blood return must be present following catheter insertion. The catheter is sutured into place twice, with care taken to avoid tying the stitch too tight, which would create a stitch abscess. A gauze dressing is placed over the catheter site and the area taped nonocclusively to prevent moisture accumulation under the dressings and subsequent infection. A chest radiograph is obtained to verify the proper placement of the catheter. We have inserted such catheters through burn wound eschar. Under these circumstances, dressings are not applied to the entrance site. However, antibiotic ointments such as Sulfamylon or silver sulfadiazene are applied to the entrance site. Changing the catheter every 3 days may reduce the risk of infected catheters in these burned patients.

SEPTIC COMPLICATIONS

Infectious complications of TPN have been reported at rates of between 7% and 27%.[23, 93] Although some infections may be due to contamination of the fluids in the infusion system, most septicemias associated with TPN result from catheter wound infections. The solutions should be prepared in the central pharmacy using extreme sterile precautions including cap, mask, and a laminar flow hood.

It is not surprising that catheter-related sepsis occurs. Within 48 hours, a fibrin sleeve will envelop an intravenous catheter.[52] Skin microorganisms may migrate along the subcutaneous catheter tract to the fibrin sleeve where they can proliferate in the presence of a high glucose concentration and cause a bacteremia or fungemia.[13] Occasionally, the fibrin sleeve can be colonized during bacteremic episodes from another focus of infection.[13] Nevertheless, catheter infection is relatively uncommon. In one study more than 75% of catheters were removed unnecessarily because of the suspicion of catheter-related sepsis, although the infected focus was subsequently proven to be at another site.[93] Therefore, when fever develops in a patient receiving TPN, every effort should first be made to exclude another source. The catheter site can be readily checked by removing the catheter over a guidewire, culturing it, and inserting a new catheter.

If an unexplained fever (>101°F) should occur with TPN, the infusion should be stopped and the solution and infusion set cultured. Blood cultures should be obtained through the subclavian catheter. If the temperature returns to normal within 24 hours and remains so, TPN may be restarted while awaiting the results of blood cultures. If the temperature remains elevated and another cause not be found or should the patient develop septic shock or inflammation at the catheter site or show a positive blood or catheter culture, the catheter should be removed and cultured according to the semiquantitative method of Maki and colleagues.[65] The proximal and distal 5 cm of the catheter are aseptically cut off and rolled back and forth four times on a trypticase soy agar plate with 5% sheep blood. The number of colonies are counted at 24 to 72 hours and subsequently identified. The patient should be given a broad-spectrum antibiotic and a peripheral infusion of D_{10}/W to prevent rebound hypoglycemia. If TPN is still required, a catheter can be inserted in a new site 48 hours later.

The development of candidemia is a dangerous complication of TPN. This can, rarely, lead to disseminated fungal infections including retinal involvement with blindness. The candidemia will usually resolve upon catheter removal, but it may require therapeutic doses of amphotericin, which itself will produce fever and is extremely nephrotoxic.[91]

Extreme care should be taken to avoid septic contamination of the intravenous hyperalimentation line. These lines should not be used to infuse other intravenous solutions or to withdraw blood. The dressing over the TPN site should be changed and the skin prepared with a bactericidal solution two to three times weekly. The subclavian site is preferred since it is relatively immobile. Transcervical internal jugular venous catheterization is difficult to keep sterile. In children when this site is used, the line is tunneled subcutaneously and exited through the scalp.[27]

METABOLIC COMPLICATIONS

One of the most common and dangerous complications of TPN is the development of nonketotic, hyperglycemic coma.[57, 62] This is most likely to develop when TPN is being initiated or when a patient becomes septic while on hyperalimentation. It is extremely important for urinary glucose to be measured every 6 hours when a patient is receiving TPN. Should a patient begin to spill more than 2+ glucose in his urine, then a blood sugar level must be obtained. Marked hyperglycemia can occur extremely rapidly in the presence of infection and can precede the clinical signs of infection (Fig. 17-5).[44, 94] Nonketotic, hyperglycemic coma carries a high mortality, estimated at between 40% and 50%.[62] The mortality is thought to be related to brain shrinkage with tear-

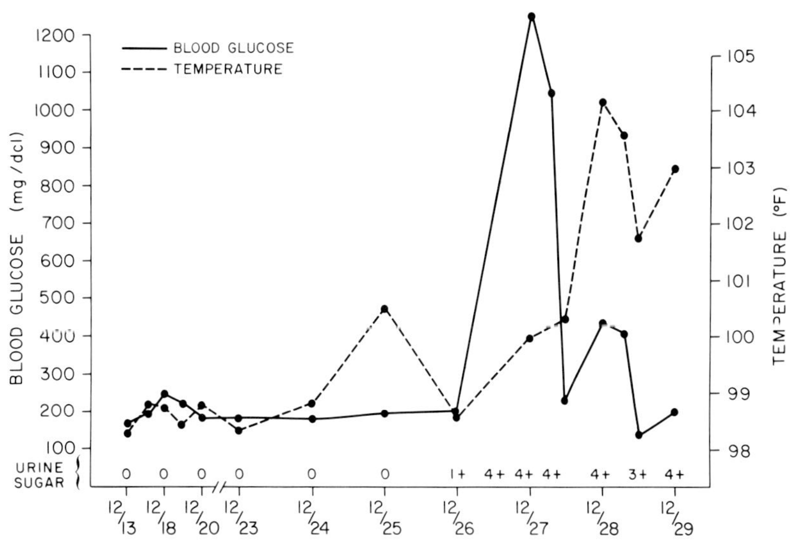

FIG. 17-5. An extremely rapid rise in blood sugar developed along with nonketotic hyperglycemic coma *preceding* the clinical signs of sepsis in a patient with subphrenic abscess. The blood sugar returned to normal over 18 hours with supplemental intravenous regular insulin. (Reproduced with permission from Sugerman HJ, Peyton JWR, Greenfield LJ: Gram-negative sepsis. In Ravitch MM et al [eds]: Current Problems in Surgery 18:405, 1981. Copyright © 1981 by Year Book Medical Publishers, Inc., Chicago)

ing of epidural and subdural veins. The patient should be treated with vigorous fluid replacement, insulin, and intravenous potassium. Should the hyperglycemia be corrected too rapidly, the serum osmolarity can fall precipitously and produce cerebral edema, uncal herniation, and death.[62] A patient's insulin dose can be titrated from a sliding scale for estimation of insulin requirements. Since the patient is receiving a continuous infusion, regular insulin is given subcutaneously or intravenously every 6 hours (rather than "qid," which is more appropriate for patients who are eating). Once the patient is getting the total estimated caloric requirement, the quantity of insulin needed can be divided equally and placed into the TPN solution. Although some of the insulin may stick to the glass or the plastic infusion bag, the administration of insulin with the TPN is smoother and proportional to the rate of glucose infusion.

A profound hypoglycemia may follow abrupt withdrawal of TPN.[26, 34, 46, 94] Continuous hyperglycemia stimulates pancreatic production of insulin. In some patients, after sudden cessation of glucose infusion, the prompt fall in blood glucose may not be matched by as prompt a drop in insulin secretion or as prompt a cessation of insulin effects. Therefore, an overshoot of insulin coupled with a sudden drop in glucose supply results in hypoglycemia. The TPN solution should be changed to 10% glucose infusion over 12 hours before the line is discontinued.

When TPN is instituted in an undernourished patient, an accelerated state of anabolism may result with a markedly increased need for potassium, the major intracellular cation. Consequently, hyperalimentation can lead to severe hypokalemia. Marked hypokalemia can cause increased cardiac irritability and ventricular fibrillation as well as produce a severe metabolic alkalosis associated with an inappropriate acidic urine that cannot be corrected without potassium supplementation.

Serum calcium may also decline during hyperalimentation and must be monitored. Supplementation by intravenous calcium is necessary to prevent neuromuscular irritability and tetany. Usually, 0.25 mEq/kg of calcium gluconate is given daily, but additional quantities may be required. A normal serum calcium level with evidence of neuromuscular irritability suggests hypomagnesemia.[95] Approximately 0.35 mEq to 0.45 mEq/kg of magnesium sulfate are infused daily, which also supplies necessary quantities of sulfate ion. Increased amounts of magnesium may be required in patients with increased gastrointestinal losses.

When hyperalimentation was first developed clinically, phosphate was not thought to be an important ion. However, a human phosphate-depletion syndrome was soon encountered that included muscle weakness, mental confusion, red cell hemolysis, and an increased affinity of the red cell for oxygen secondary to a marked reduction in 2,3-diphosphoglycerate (2,3-DPG).[53, 61, 100] In addition, impaired neutrophil chemotaxis and phagocytosis were also noted in the presence of hypophosphatemia.[22] Most commercial preparations now contain 20 mEq to 60 mEq/L of phosphate. Nevertheless, it may be necessary to supplement the amount of phosphate a patient receives. One can add 3 mM to 5 mM of potassium acid phosphate (KH_2PO_4) to each liter of TPN, if necessary.

Hyperchloremic metabolic acidosis was initially seen with the use of acidic amino-acid solutions.[48] This is now less frequent since most commercial solutions now contain acetate. Should metabolic acidosis develop, supplemental acetate can be given. Bicarbonate may cause calcium or magnesium precipitates. The amount of excess or deficit of buffer base (*i.e.*, acetate) can be calculated from the formula: mEq H_2CO_3 = (body weight in kg) × (24-plasma $H_2CO_3^-$) × 0.6.

Abnormalities of sodium balance are common in any patient receiving intravenous solutions. Nutritional repletion is usually associated with diuresis and mobilization of excess body water.[104] Should a patient have marked hyponatremia with inappropriate antidiuretic hormone secretion (SIADH), as is often seen following major surgery or multiple injuries, then free water can be restricted during TPN by using highly concentrated ($< 47\%$) dextrose solutions.

TRACE ELEMENT DEFICIENCIES

The initial hyperalimentation solutions were fibrin or casein hydrolysates that contained adequate quantities of trace minerals. The subsequent development of pure amino-acid solutions eliminated the problem of hypersensitivity reactions to the polypeptides present in hydrolysates but failed to take into account the necessity for trace mineral supplementation. Copper deficiency leads to neutropenia.[103] Chromium depletion produces insulin resistance.[55] Iodine deficiency will cause hypothyroidism. Anemia, muscular pain, weakness, and a cardiomyopathy have been described with selenium deficiency.[56]

Excessive zinc loss can be found in the presence of prolonged nasogastric suction, enteric fistulas, or prolonged diarrhea.[109] Accelerated anabolism can also increase the need for zinc. Most hospital laboratories should be able to measure zinc levels, and additional zinc, as much as 10 mg/day, may have to be provided.[109] Zinc deficiency will cause nail growth arrest and a severe skin eruption of the face and inframammary and infragluteal folds, known as acrodermatitis enteropathica, a syndrome initially described in children.[101] Zinc deficiency also leads to impaired wound healing as well as the failure of zinc-dependent enzyme systems.[77] Zinc repletion can unmask a copper deficiency which is associated with neutropenia.[13, 87]

The trace element solution should be prepared according to the AMA guidelines and administered daily if a patient has required total parenteral nutrition for more than 2 weeks.[3] Patients with intestinal fistulas or nasogastric tubes may require these solutions sooner.

FATTY-ACID DEFICIENCY

Essential fatty-acid deficiency may lead to a severe dermatitis.[37] A fat emulsion (Intralipid or Liposyn) should be provided at the rate of 500 ml twice weekly to prevent essential fatty-acid deficiency.[10] At least 3.2% of total calories should be given as fat.[10] Patients receiving large carbohydrate loads may have a greater than normal need for linoleic acid, but this has not been corroborated by others.[10, 108] Intrahepatic cholestatic jaundice associated with TPN may be related to inadequate intravenous fat.[54] Twenty percent fat emulsions that will reduce the fluid volume infused and possibly add enough calories to make peripheral parenteral nutrition more feasible are now available. The danger of excessive lipemia can be prevented by daily monitoring of the serum for turbidity.

VITAMINS

Adequate quantities of the water-soluble (B-complex and ascorbic acid) and fat-soluble vitamins (A, D, E, and K) must be provided.[43] Mild vitamin B_1 (thiamine) deficiency may produce a peripheral neuropathy and Wernicke's encephalopathy, or, when severe, high output cardiac failure; all manifestations can be prevented with 3 mg to 21 mg of the vitamin each day. Vitamin B_2 (riboflavin) deficiency will produce inflammation of the lips, cracking skin at the corners of the mouth, a seborrheic dermatitis, and ocular inflammation. Suggested requirements are 3.5 mg to 7.5 mg per day of vitamin B_2. Vitamin B_3 (pantothenic acid) is required for all acetylation reactions, and deficiency may be related to headache, nausea, vomiting, and malaise. Ten milligrams to 30 mg per day have been suggested as the normal vitamin B_3 intravenous requirement. Vitamin B_5 (niacin) deficiency leads to pellagra with weakness, anorexia, indigestion, diarrhea, dysphagia, and dermatitis. Acute toxic psychosis may also occur. Between 40 mg and 150 mg of niacin should be given daily. Vitamin B_6 (pyridoxine) deficiency produces mental changes, including irritability and depression, anemia, and skin changes. Four milligrams to 6.3 mg per day have been recommended. Biotin deficiency has recently been reported in an infant receiving TPN and was manifested by alopecia and a skin rash, which were corrected with biotin replacement.[97] The recommended dosage is 150 mg to 300 mg per day. Vitamin B_9 (folic acid) deficiency will produce a megaloblastic anemia and diarrhea, which can be prevented with 1 mg per day intravenously. Vitamin B_{12} (cyanocobalamin) deficiency will produce pernicious anemia and can be prevented with 1 mg, intramuscularly, each month.

Vitamin C (ascorbic acid) is of critical importance in wound healing, and severe deficiency will produce scurvy. Intravenous vitamin C, 100 mg to 500 mg daily, has been recommended. Vitamin A is required for epithelial regeneration and wound healing. Night blindness is one of the earliest signs of deficiency. Increased quantities are required in infections and in patients receiving corticosteroids. Suggested daily intravenous maintenance of vitamin A ranges between 2500 IU and 8000 IU. Hypervitaminosis A is associated with fatigue, malaise, anorexia, migrating arthralgias, bone pain, dry skin, alopecia, brittle nails, jaundice, and hepatomegaly. The symptoms usually resolve within 3 days after vitamin A is discontinued. Vitamin D is necessary for the mobilization of calcium and phosphate from bones. Deficiency of vitamin D leads to osteomalacia, low serum calcium and phosphate levels, and elevated alkaline phosphatase levels. Estimated daily intravenous requirements for vitamin D range between 200 IU to 420 IU. Vitamin E deficiency leads to a decreased red cell survival and anemia, skeletal muscle lesions, and increased platelet aggregation. From 2 IU to 60 IU of vitamin E intravenously per day has been suggested. Vitamin K deficiency leads to a prolongation of the prothrombin time. From 0.7 mg to 2.0 mg, intravenously, per day of vitamin K has been recommended.

RENAL FAILURE

Nutrition is extremely important but may be very difficult to maintain in patients with acute or chronic renal failure. If the patient is not on hemodialysis, the volume of intravenous fluids and protein load must be limited. Under these circumstances, 47% glucose with 1.8% amino acids should be utilized. The initial studies of TPN in acute renal failure patients by Abel and colleagues found that essential amino acids plus high-caloric (47%) glucose infusion was significantly better than a 47% glucose solution alone.[1] Recently, essential amino acids have been compared to standard amino-acid solutions, and no added benefit from the more expensive essential amino-acid solutions was found.[29, 72] Others disagree, however, and the issue is far from settled.[35] If the patient is on hemodialysis, then standard 4.25% amino-acid solutions and fluid volumes can be utilized as if the patient were not in renal failure. Urea from augmented production and the excess fluid volume can be removed with dialysis, and nitrogen balance is better maintained than when 1.8% solutions of amino acids are used.[71] In general, one should aim for no greater than a 100-g to 200-g weight loss daily in a patient with renal failure.

RESPIRATORY FAILURE

Patients with respiratory insufficiency may have difficulty eliminating the increased carbon dioxide (CO_2) produced by hypercatabolic states.[7] This is especially the case for patients with chronic obstructive pulmonary disease, who can be extremely difficult to wean from a mechanical ventilator. Under these circumstances, it may be appropriate to decrease glucose infusion and to provide a significant proportion of the caloric load in the form of an intravenous fat emulsion.[5, 15] The newer 20% fat emulsions should make this easier than it was in the past. One mole of CO_2 is produced for every mole of oxygen (O_2) utilized when carbohydrate is metabolized; whereas, only 0.8 mole of CO_2 results from the consumption of one mole of O_2 when fat is oxidized. The ratio of CO_2 production to O_2 consumption is known as the *respiratory quotient* (R/Q). With the use of fat emulsions, the R/Q can be lowered with a significant decrease in both CO_2 production and the consequent need for ventilation. Although some have noted that septic patients may preferentially utilize endogenous fat, others have found septic patients to be intolerant of supplemental intravenous fat.[5, 18] The septic patient should be followed carefully for the development of lipemic serum.

LIVER FAILURE

In severe cirrhosis, the liver's ability to metabolize the aromatic (tryptophan, phenylalanine, tyrosine) and the sulfur-containing (methionine, cysteine, and threonine) amino acids is reduced.[32] An accumulation of these aromatic and sulfur-containing amino acids may be associated with increased production of the false neurotransmitter, octopamine. The increased CNS tryptophan level leads to an increased cerebral production of serotonin. The rise in phenylalanine leads to a decreased cerebral production of catecholamines. The alterations in neurotransmitter concentrations produce a metabolic encephalopathy in cirrhosis.[32] When the branched-chain amino acids (BCAA) such as valine, leucine, and isoleucine are the primary nitrogen source, the severity of coma diminishes.[32] These BCAA solutions are available only for enteral (Hepatic-Aid) and parenteral use (Hepatamine). These solutions are quite expensive and should be used only if a patient develops hepatic coma.

TPN may be associated with acute fatty infiltration of the liver and with cholestatic jaundice, which will resolve when the TPN is discontinued.[90] The use of fat as a significant portion of the caloric load may perhaps diminish the severity of fatty infiltration of the liver.[54] The etiology of the hepatic changes is not yet known. Prolonged TPN may also lead to acalculous cholecystitis, which is thought to be a result of bile stasis.[85]

CARDIAC FAILURE

It would seem that patients with severe cardiac cachexia might benefit from nutritional repletion. However, it may be extremely difficult to provide caloric supplementation without increasing the basal metabolic rate and the need for a greater cardiac output. The increased cardiac work plus the increased fluid load may aggravate congestive heart failure. Abel and colleagues were unable to find any benefit from early postoperative TPN to cardiac patients.[2]

METABOLIC ABNORMALITIES IN SEPSIS

It may be quite difficult to achieve a positive nitrogen balance in a septic patient. In addition to the tendency toward hyperglycemia that is refractory to insulin, there may also be renal, pulmonary, and liver insufficiency. These may necessitate the use of specialized solutions and limit the availability of adequate calories and amino acids.

Wilmore and Unger and their colleagues have suggested that the hyperglycemia of sepsis is secondary to an imbalance between the catabolic hormones (glucocorticoids, catecholamines, and glucagon) and the anabolic hormone insulin.[102, 106] Cerra and colleagues have suggested that there is actual insulin resistance, since the blood sugar is proportional to the glucose load and is not responsive to increasing quantities of insulin.[18] A significant increase in lactate production occurs during sepsis. The lactate is taken up in the liver where it is converted back to glucose.[107] Similarly, there is a release of amino acids from the periphery and hepatic conversion of these compounds to glucose, owing to the markedly increased gluconeogenesis.[107] Metabolic demands upon the liver are greatly increased in the presence of sepsis, but as sepsis progresses, the production of glucose falls sharply.[31] The late deterioration in hepatic function is most likely a direct effect of bacteria or endotoxin on mitochondria.[70]

Abnormalities in protein and amino-acid metabolism are present in septic patients. Several investigators have noted a marked increase in skeletal muscle protein catabolism in sepsis as well as an increased mobilization of fat.[6–8, 21, 56] These amino acids are redistributed to tissues that take anabolic priority, namely the wound and vital organs, as well as to the liver where they undergo conversion to glucose, as mentioned above.[107] Muscle is capable of using as fuel only the BCAA. Although septic patients may have inadequate quantities of BCAA and excessive quantities of aromatic and sulfur-containing amino acids in their serum, the effectiveness of BCAA in reducing the metabolic encephalopathy or rates of morbidity or mortality has not been proven.[36] The primary defect may not be an inadequate supply of BCAA but an inadequate ability of the liver to metabolize the aromatic amino acids.[6] BCAA infusion may simply mask the symptoms of liver insufficiency without correcting the primary deficit. This would be analogous to the use of supplemental albumin to correct hypoalbuminemia in undernourished patients, which only serves to mask the presence of undernutrition rather than to correct the fundamental deficits in amino acids and calories. Prevention of muscle catabolism may require control of the septic process.[19]

In addition to abnormalities of amino-acid metabolism in sepsis, Cerra and colleagues have noted abnormalities in fatty acid and triglyceride metabolism. These patients have increased serum gamma-amino-butyric acid (GABA), oxaloacetatic acid, and beta-hydroxy-butyric acid as well as increased quantities of serum triglycerides.[18] They may be intolerant of supplemental lipid-emulsion infusions. If a septic patient is receiving a significant proportion of his caloric load in the form of fat, blood should be drawn daily, allowed to clot, and the serum examined at the bedside for gross lipemia.

References

1. Abel RM, Beck CH, Abott WM et al: Improved survival from acute renal failure after treatment with intravenous essential L-amino acids and glucose. N Engl J Med 288:695, 1973
2. Abel RM, Fischer JE, Buckley MJ et al: Malnutrition in cardiac surgical patients: Results of a prospective randomized evaluation of early postoperative total parenteral nutrition (TPN). Arch Surg 111:45, 1976
3. AMA Department of Foods and Nutrition: Guidelines for essential trace element preparations for parenteral use. JAMA 241:2051, 1979
4. Ashbaugh DG, Petty TL: Sepsis complicating the acute respiratory distress syndrome. Surg Gynecol Obstet 135:865, 1972
5. Askanzi J, Carpentier YA, Elwyn DH et al: Influence of total parenteral nutrition on fuel utilization in injury and sepsis. Ann Surg 191:40, 1980
6. Askanazi J, Carpentier YA, Michelsen CB et al: Muscle and plasma amino acids following injury. Influence of intercurrent infection. Ann Surg 192:78, 1980
7. Askanazi J, Rosenbaum SH, Hyman AI et al: Respiratory changes induced by the large glucose loads of total parenteral nutrition. JAMA 243:1444, 1980
8. Aubaniac R: L'injection intraveinneuse sous claviculaire: Avantage et technique. Presse Med 60:1456, 1952
9. Aulenbacher CE: Hydrothorax from subclavian vein catheterization. JAMA 214:372, 1970
10. Barr LH, Dunn GD, Brennan MF: Essential fatty acid deficiency during total parenteral nutrition. Ann Surg 193:304, 1981
11. Bartlett JG, Gorbach SL: The triple threat of aspiration pneumonia. Chest 68:560, 1975
12. Bassili HR, Deitel M: Effect of nutritional support on weaning patients off mechanical ventilators. JPEN 5:161, 1981
13. Bernard RW, Stahl WM, Chase RM: Subclavian vein catheterizations: A prospective study. II. Infections, complications. Ann Surg 173:191, 1971
14. Blackburn GL, Bistrian BR, Maini BS et al: Nutritional and metabolic assessment of the hospitalized patient. JPEN 1:11, 1977
15. Burke JF, Wolfe RR, Mullany CJ et al: Glucose requirements following burn injury. Ann Surg 190:274, 1979
16. Buzby GP, Mullen JL, Matthews DC et al: Prognostic nutritional index in gastrointestinal surgery. Am J Surg 139:160, 1980
17. Bynum LJ, Pierce AK: Pulmonary aspiration of gastric contents. Am Rev Respir Dis 114:1129, 1976
18. Cerra FB, Siegel JH, Border JR et al: The hepatic failure of sepsis: Cellular versus substrate. Surgery 86:409, 1979
19. Cerra FB, Siegel JH, Coleman B et al: Septic autocannibolism. A failure of exogenous nutritional support. Ann Surg 192:570, 1980
20. Chandra RK: Cell-mediated immunity in nutritional imbalance. Fed Proc 39:3088, 1980
21. Clowes GHA, Heideman M, Lindberg B et al: Effects of parenteral alimentation on amino acid metabolism in septic patients. Surgery 88:531, 1980
22. Craddock PR, Yawata Y, VanSanten L et al: Acquired phagocyte dysfunction. A complication of the hypophosphatemia of parenteral hyperalimentation. N Engl J Med 290:1403, 1974
23. Curry CR, Quie PG: Fungal septicemia in patients receiving parenteral hyperalimentation. N Engl J Med 285:1221, 1971
24. Dobbie RP, Hoffmeister JA: Continuous pump-tube enteric feeding of the malnourished patient. Surg Gynecol Obstet 143:273, 1976
25. Drachler DH, Koepke GH, Weg JG: Phrenic nerve injury from subclavian vein catheterization. Diagnosis by electromyography. JAMA 236:2880, 1976
26. Dudrick SJ, Long JM, Steiger E, Rhoads JE: Intravenous hyperalimentation. Med Clin North Am 54:577, 1970
27. Dudrick SJ, Wilmore DN, Vars HM, Rhoads JE: Can intravenous feeding as the sole means of nutrition support growth in the child and restore weight loss in an adult? Ann Surg 169:974, 1969
28. Egdahl RH: Hypertonic glucose and improved critical organ performance. Surgery 75:145, 1974
29. Feinstein EI, Blumenkratz MJ, Healy M et al: Clinical and metabolic responses to parenteral nutrition in acute renal failure: A controlled double-blind study. Medicine 60:124, 1981
30. Feliciano DV, Mattox KL, Graham JM et al: Major complications of percutaneous subclavian vein catheters. Am J Surg 138:869, 1979

31. Filkins JP: Phases of glucose dyshomeostasis in endotoxicosis. Circ Shock 5:347, 1978
32. Fischer JE, Rosen HM, Ebeid AM et al: The effect of normalization of plasma amino acids on hepatic encephalopathy in man. Surgery 80:77, 1976
33. Forse RA, Shizgal HM: The assessment of malnutrition. Surgery 88:17, 1980
34. Freeman JB, MacLean LD: Intravenous hyperalimentation: A review. Can J Surg 14:180, 1971
35. Freund H, Atamian S, Fischer JE: Comparative study of parenteral nutrition in renal failure using essential and nonessential amino acid containing solutions. Surg Gynecol Obstet 151:652, 1980
36. Freund H, Atamian S, Holroyde J, Fischer JE: Plasma amino acids as predictors of the severity and outcome of sepsis. Ann Surg 190:571, 1979
37. Freund H, Floman N, Schwartz B et al: Essential fatty acid deficiency in total parenteral nutrition. Ann Surg 190:139, 1979
38. Frisancho AR: Triceps skin fold and upper arm muscle size norms for assessment of nutritional status. Am J Clin Nutr 27:1052, 1974
39. Gareth JJ, Berry M, Hulands GH, Crawley JCW: The time course and degree of change in alveolar-capillary membrane permeability induced by aspiration of hydrochloric acid and hypotonic saline. Am Rev Respir Dis 118:1007, 1978
40. Goodgame JT Jr: A critical assessment of the indications for total parenteral nutrition. Surg Gynecol Obstet 151:433, 1980
41. Graham WP III, Royster HP: Simplified cervical esophagostomy for long-term extraoral feeding. Surg Gynecol Obstet 125:127, 1967
42. Grant JP: Handbook of Total Parenteral Nutrition, p 12. Philadelphia, WB Saunders, 1980
43. Grant JP: Handbook of Total Parenteral Nutrition, p 171. Philadelphia, WB Saunders, 1980
44. Gump FE, Long C, Killian P, Kinney JM: Studies of glucose intolerance in septic injured patients. J Trauma 14:378, 1974
45. Harris JA, Benedict FG: Biometric studies of basal metabolism in man. Carnegie Institute of Washington, Publication No. 279, 1919
46. Hays DM, Kaplan MS, Mahour GH et al: High-calorie infusion therapy following surgery in low-birth-weight infants: Metabolic problems encountered. Surgery 71:834, 1972
47. Heatley RV, Williams RHP, Lewis MH: Pre-operative intravenous feeding: A controlled trial. Postgrad Med J 55:541, 1979
48. Heird WC, Dell RB, Driscoll JM Jr et al: Metabolic acidosis resulting from intravenous alimentation mixtures containing synthetic amino acids. N Engl J Med 287:943, 1972
49. Herbst CA Jr: Indications, management and complications of percutaneous subclavian catheters. Arch Surg 113: 1421, 1978
50. Hobbs CL, Mullen JL, Buzby GP et al: The effects of nutrition on aspirin-induced mucosal ulceration in primates. Surgery 86:49, 1979
51. Hodges RE, Hood J, Canham JE et al: Clinical manifestations of ascorbic acid deficiency in man. Am J Clin Nutr 24:432, 1971
52. Hoshal VL Jr, Ause RG, Hoskins PA: Fibrin sleeve formation on indwelling subclavian central venous catheters. Arch Surg 102:353, 1971
53. Jacob HS, Amsden T: Acute hemolytic anemia with rigid red cells in hypophosphatemia. N Engl J Med 285:1446, 1971
54. Jeejeebhoy KN: Total parenteral nutrition at home for 23 months without complications and with good rehabilitation. A study of technical and metabolic features. Gastroenterology 65:811, 1976
55. Jeejeebhoy KN, Chu RC, Marliss EB et al: Chromium deficiency, glucose intolerance, and neuropathy reversed by chromium supplementation in a patient receiving long-term total parenteral nutrition. Am J Clin Nutr 30:531, 1977
56. Johnson RA, Baker SS, Fallon JT et al: An accidental case of cardiomyopathy and selenium deficiency. N Engl J Med 304:1210, 1981
57. Kaminski MV Jr: A review of hyperosmolar hyperglycemic nonketotic dehydration (HHND): Etiology, pathophysiology and prevention during intravenous hyperalimentation. J Paren Ent Nutr 2:690, 1978
58. Law DK, Dudrick SJ, Abdou NI: Immunocompetence of patients with protein-calorie malnutrition. Ann Intern Med 79:545, 1973
59. Lefrak EA, Noon GP: Management of arterial injury secondary to attempted subclavian vein catheterization. Ann Thorac Surg 14:294, 1972
60. Long CL, Schaffel N, Geiger JW et al: Metabolic response to injury and illness: Estimation of energy and protein needs from indirect calorimetry and nitrogen balance. JPEN 3:452, 1979
61. Lotz M, Zisman E, Bartter FC: Evidence for a phosphate depletion syndrome in man. N Engl J Med 278:409, 1968
62. McCurdy DK: Hyperosmolar hyperglycemic nonketotic diabetic coma. Med Clin North Am 54:683, 1970
63. McDonough JJ, Altemeier WA: Subclavian venous thrombosis secondary to indwelling catheters. Surg Gynecol Obstet 133:397, 1971
64. MacLean LD: Host resistance in surgical patients. J Trauma 19:297, 1979
65. Maki DG, Weise CE, Sarafin HW: A semiquantitative culture method for identifying intravenous-catheter-related infection. N Engl J Med 296:1305, 1977
66. Massumi RA, Ross AM: A traumatic, nonsurgical technic for removal of broken catheters from cardiac cavities. N Engl J Med 277:195, 1967
67. Mattox KL, Fisher RG: Persistent hemothorax secondary to malposition of a subclavian venous catheter. J Trauma 17:387, 1977
68. Meakins JL, Christou NV, Shizgal HM, MacLean LD: Therapeutic approaches to anergy in surgical patients. Ann Surg 190:286, 1979
69. Meakins JL, Pietsch JB, Bubenick O et al: Delayed hypersensitivity: Indicator of acquired failure of host defenses in sepsis and trauma. Ann Surg 186:241, 1977
70. Mela L, Miller LD, Diaco JF, Sugerman HJ: Effect of *E. coli* endotoxin on mitochondrial energy-linked functions. Surgery 68:541, 1970
71. Mirtallo JM, Grauer D, Ellison EC et al: Evaluation of full strength amino acid therapy in patients receiving TPN and hemodialysis (abstr). JPEN 3:522, 1979
72. Mirtallo JM, Schneider PJ, Mavko K et al: A comparison of essential and general amino acid infusions in the nutritional support of patients with compromised renal function. JPEN 6:109, 1982
73. Moore FD: Metabolic Care of the Surgical Patient, p 422. Philadelphia, WB Saunders, 1959
74. Mullen JL, Buzby GP, Matthews DC et al: Reduction of operative morbidity and mortality by combined preoper-

ative and postoperative nutritional support. Ann Surg 192:604, 1980
75. Mullen JL, Gertner MH, Buzby GB et al: Implications of malnutrition in the surgical patient. Arch Surg 114:121, 1979
76. Nehme AE: Nutritional support of the hospitalized patient. The team concept. JAMA 243:1906, 1980
77. Oberleas D, Seymour JK, Lenaghan R et al: Effect of zinc deficiency on wound healing in rats. Am J Surg 121:566, 1971
78. Oppenheimer MJ, Durant TM, Lynch P: Body position in relation to venous air embolism and the associated cardiovascular-respiratory changes. Am J Med Sci 225:362, 1953
79. Oram–Smith JC, Mullen JL, Harken AH et al: Direct right atrial catheterization for total parenteral nutrition. Surgery 83:274, 1978
80. Ordway CB: Air embolus via CVP catheter without positive pressure: Presentation of case and review. Ann Surg 179:479, 1974
81. Padberg FT, Jr., Ruggeiro J, Blackburn Gl, Bistrian BR: Central venous catheterization for parenteral nutrition. Ann Surg 193:264, 1981
82. Page CP, Carlton PK, Andrassy RJ et al: Safe, cost-effective postoperative nutrition. Defined formula diet via needle-catheter jejunostomy. Am J Surg 138:939, 1979
83. Page CP, Ryan JA, Haff RC: Continual catheter administration of an elemental diet. Surg Gynecol Obstet 142:184, 1976
84. Peters JL, Armstrong R: Air embolism occurring as a complication of central venous catheterization. Ann Surg 187:375, 1978
85. Peterson SR, Sheldon GF: Acute acalculous cholecystitis: A complication of hyperalimentation. Am J Surg 138:814, 1979
86. Pories WJ, Henzel JH, Rob CG, Strain WH: Acceleration of wound healing in man with zinc sulphate given by mouth. Lancet 1:121, 1967
87. Prasad AS, Brewer GJ, Schoomaker EB, Rabbani P: Hypocupremia induced by zinc therapy in adults. JAMA 240:2166, 1978
88. Reinhardt GF, Myslofski JW, Wilkens DB et al: Incidence and mortality of hypoalbuminemic patients in hospitalized veterans. JPEN 4:357, 1980
89. Richardson JD, Grover FL, Trinkle JK: Intravenous catheter emboli. Am J Surg 128:722, 1974
90. Rodgers BM, Hollenbeck JI, Donnelly WH, Talbert JL: Intrahepatic cholestasis with parenteral alimentation. Am J Surg 131:149, 1976
91. Rose HD: Venous catheter-associated candidemia. Am J Med Sci 275:265, 1978
92. Ross AM: Polyethylene emboli: How many more? Chest 57:308, 1970
93. Ryan JA Jr, Abel RM, Abbott WM et al: Catheter complications in total parenteral nutrition. A prospective study of 200 consecutive patients. N Engl J Med 290:757, 1974
94. Sanderson I, Deitel M: Insulin response in patients receiving concentrated infusions of glucose and casein hydrolysate for complete parenteral nutrition. Ann Surg 179:387, 1974
95. Shills ME: Experimental human magnesium depletion. Medicine 48:61, 1969
96. Steiger E, Allen TR, Daly JM et al: Beneficial effects of immediate postoperative total parenteral nutrition. Surg Forum 22:89, 1971
97. Thoene J, Baker H, Yoshino M, Sweetman L: Biotin-responsive carboxylase deficiency associated with subnormal plasma and urinary biotin. N Engl J Med 304:817, 1981
98. Thompson JC: The stomach and duodenum. In Sabiston DC Jr (ed): Davis–Christopher Textbook of Surgery, p 938. Philadelphia, WB Saunders, 1977
99. Toung TJK, Bordos P, Benson DW et al: Aspiration pneumonia: Experimental evaluation of albumin and steroid therapy. Ann Surg 183:179, 1976
100. Travis SF, Sugerman HJ, Ruberg RL et al: Alterations of red cell glycolytic intermediates and oxygen transport as a consequence of hypophosphatemia in patients receiving intravenous hyperalimentation. N Engl J Med 285:763, 1971
101. Tucker SB, Schroeder AL, Brown PW, McCall JT: Acquired zinc deficiency. Cutaneous manifestations typical of acrodermatitis enteropathica. JAMA 235:2399, 1976
102. Unger RH: Glucagon and the insulin:glucagon ratio in diabetes and other catabolic illnesses. Diabetes 20:834, 1972
103. Vilter RW, Bozian RC, Hess EV et al: Manifestations of copper deficiency in a patient with systemic sclerosis on intravenous hyperalimentation. N Engl J Med 291:188, 1974
104. Vogel CM, Kingsbury RJ, Baue AE: Intravenous hyperalimentation. A review of two and one-half years experience. Arch Surg 105:414, 1972
105. Wayne E, Miller RF, Eiseman B: Duodenal obstruction by the superior mesenteric artery in bedridden combat casualties. Ann Surg 174:339, 1971
106. Wilmore DW: Hormonal responses and their effect on metabolism. Surg Clin North Am 56:999, 1976
107. Wilmore DW, Goodwin CW, Aulick LH et al: Effect of injury and infection on visceral metabolism and circulation. Ann Surg 192:491, 1980
108. Wolfram G, Echart J, Walther B, Zöllner N: Factors influencing essential fatty acid requirement in total parenteral nutrition (TPN). JPEN 2:634, 1978
109. Wolman SL, Anderson GH, Marliss EB, Jeejeeboy KN: Zinc in total parenteral nutrition: Requirements and metabolic effects. Gastroenterology 76:458, 1979
110. Wright RA: Nutritional assessment. JAMA 244:599, 1980

18 Complications of Immunosuppression

Mitchell H. Goldman

OVERVIEW

Since the beginning of the 20th century, immunosuppression in the treatment of inflammatory disease, in allogeneic transplantation, and as a consequence of chemotherapy has created a multitude of new disease syndromes and a variety of nuances in some familiar disease processes. In addition, the recognition that some conditions are themselves immunosuppressive (e.g., aging, burns, shock, malnutrition, and cancer) has led to improved coordination of patient management to avoid the consequences of immune deficiency.

Most of the complications of immunosuppression can be related to side-effects of immunosuppressive drugs or treatments, consequences of decreasing the body's ability to respond to a foreign organism or antigen, endogenous suppression by an ongoing disease process, and suppressive effects of ancillary drugs and therapy as adjuvants to the therapy of diseases, specifically radiotherapy, anesthesia, and surgery. One of the most interesting developments of current immunologic research is the interrelationships among basic immunology, immunologic disease, and other disease states. For instance, the basic tissue typing system (HLA), located on the sixth chromosome in the human, is associated with certain diseases. The correspondence between the B-27 allele and ankylosing spondylitis and other alleles with diabetes, thyroiditis, celiac disease, and multiple sclerosis provokes interesting speculation on the role of the immune system in these diseases. On the more basic level, the interrelationships among the kallikrein; prostaglandin, clotting, and fibrinolytic systems; the maintenance of vascular integrity; the induction of the inflammatory response; circulating hormones; and the complement system with both the recognition and the effector components of the immune system have been demonstrated to be quite important in the local effects of disease processes. Although this chapter does not extensively review basic immunosuppressive mechanisms, an understanding of their action is important to an understanding of the complications.

Certain seemingly unrelated factors may have a profound effect on the immunocompetence of the surgical patient. They are, among others, cancer, malnutrition, burns and sepsis, anesthesia, surgery and trauma, and radiotherapy. Tumor-bearing patients show decreased humoral and cell-mediated responses to other nontumor antigens. Patients with lymphoma display anergy to recall antigens. This may be related, in part, to increased activation of suppressor T cells, development of blocking antibodies or antigen–antibody complexes, or decreased response to mitogens by blast cells. Uremia and diabetes result in decreased macrophage phagocytosis and neutrophil bactericidal capability, and uremia itself can cause a decrease in T-cell mitogen responsiveness. Anesthesia alone may cause temporary defects in cellular or humoral immune response. Thiopental, in vitro, inhibits the ability of sensitized leukocytes to kill tumor cells. Local anesthetics impede cell-mediated responses to antigens, as well. Halothane, in animals, suppresses the MLC response and cell-mediated lymphocytotoxicity as well as antibody-dependent cell-mediated cytotoxicity. Surgery and trauma have been demonstrated to decrease responsiveness to recall antigens and mitogens and to suppress the MLC response in a transient fashion with complete recovery of immunocompetence after at least 4 to 5 days.[9] Patients with burns may demonstrate decreased leukocyte killing, decreased numbers and reactivity of circulating B lymphocytes, and suppression of the reticuloendothelial system. Many of these changes are related to the degree and size of injury. Suppression of cell-mediated immunity has also been seen in patients on radiotherapy. Finally, both aging and malnutrition have been shown to have dramatic effects on both cell-mediated and humoral responses. In caring for the immunodepressed surgical patient, each of these factors must be taken into account, as a number of different treatment modalities and conditions may be acting synergistically toward an increased rate of morbidity and mortality. This chapter reviews a few specific immunosuppressive drugs and some of the common and uncommon complications in immunosuppression. It must be borne in mind, however, that in addition to specific regimens, other nonspecific factors may be involved as well.

Immunosuppressive Therapies

CORTICOSTEROIDS

Corticosteroids are one of the most commonly used immunosuppressive drugs. They are used in cancer chemotherapy, transplantation, and the treatment of inflammatory disorders and immunologically mediated disease, and for shock. They have both an anti-inflammatory role and a direct effect on the action and function of immunocompetent cells. Corticosteroids given in the usual clinical doses produce a transient lymphocytopenia from a redistribution of lymphocytes from the circulating pool to the extravascular pool, including the spleen, thoracic duct, lymph nodes, and bone marrow. This is especially the case with T lymphocytes. A similar effect is seen with monocytes, and, to a lesser extent, B lymphocytes. In addition, corticosteroids inhibit the accumulation of polymorphonuclear leukocytes at an inflammatory site, either by altering the cell surface properties of the neutrophil, resulting in an inability to egress from the vascular space and an adherence to the surface of the vascular endothelium, or by interfering with chemotaxis. These effects are transient but may be maintained by frequently repeated doses. At higher doses, corticosteroids stabilize lysosomal membranes, suppress cell-to-cell interaction, deplete some suppressor-cell lines, and depress the ability of responding clones to proliferate by depressing cell blastogenesis. Other functional effects of corticosteroids include depression of antibody and complement binding to macrophage and monocyte receptors and suppression of the response to macrophage-inhibition factor. Corticosteroids also have a direct effect on vessels at an inflammatory site, where they are associated with decreased capillary leakage, kinin antagonism, plasminogen activator suppression, and vasoconstriction. All of these effects have been noted in doses up to the equivalent of 60 mg per day of prednisone, doses often used in clinical practice. The immunosuppressive effects of corticosteroids result in the following general clinical effects: decreased ability to ward off infection and decreased inflammatory response to infections and intestinal perforation, which masks clinical signs and symptoms.

Some of the common nonimmunologic effects of corticosteroids are related to their metabolic effects, their suppression of the adrenal–pituitary axis, and their mineralocorticoid effects, as listed below.

Complications of Corticosteroids
- Infection
- Gastrointestinal ulceration and perforation
- Diabetes mellitus
- Pancreatitis
- Wound infection and dehiscence
- Avascular necrosis of the femoral head
- Anesthesia and stress complications
- Posterior subcapsular cataract formation
- Acne, hirsutism
- Pseudotumor cerebri
- Hypertension, edema, hypokalemia, sodium retention
- Quadriceps muscle weakness
- Increased capillary fragility and susceptibility to bruises
- Suppression of growth hormone and ACTH secretion

Protein wasting, diabetes mellitus, and suppression of growth hormone are all metabolic side-effects of corticosteroids. Sodium retention, kaliuresis, and water retention are mineralocorticoid effects seen after corticosteroid administration. Quadriceps weakness and aseptic necrosis of the hips, humerus, and thoracic vertebrae are musculoskeletal complications. In addition, patients receiving corticosteroid therapy should receive perioperative supplementation, since their ability to respond to stress by the production of native corticosteroids is generally limited. A schedule of 300 mg of hydrocortisone divided perioperatively and postoperatively and tapered over a few days is sufficient. All of the nonimmunologic complications of corticosteroids should be taken into account in the therapy of a surgical patient.

ANTITHYMOCYTE GLOBULIN (ATG)

Under the guise of specifically treating the immunoreactive clones of cells in the allograft response, the transplant field has developed a serum or an even further refined globulin in the horse, goat, or rabbit by immunizing the animal with various forms of lymphocyte preparations. Human neonatal thymocytes, cultured lymphoblasts, and T-cell membranes have been used. More recent, hybridomas have been used to produce clones of mouse myeloma cells, which make relatively large quantities of monospecific antibody to T-helper cells, T-suppressor cells, monocytes, and cytotoxic T cells. This work has vast therapeutic and diagnostic ramifications. The use of these monoclonal antibodies in cancer and transplant therapy and in diagnosis is just beginning. The common complications associated with antithymocyte globulin, or its analogues, are allergic response or anaphylaxis; local reaction in the form of pain, swelling, and tenderness from intramuscular preparations; thrombocytopenia; and infections. Anaphylaxis can generally be prevented by skin testing prior to use. However, especially with intravenous preparations, adequate preparation for immediate treatment of anaphylaxis should be available at all times. Fever occasionally occurs and can be abrogated by concomitant therapy with steroids, antipyretics, and diphenhydramine. Swelling and local tenderness can be treated by local therapy including ice-packs. Thrombocytopenia should be avoided by monitoring platelet counts and by discontinuing therapy once the platelet count drops below 50,000 to 80,000 cells per mm^3. Most antithymocyte-globulin preparations are tested for pyrogens, sterility, and antithrombocyte activity prior to human use. Although the monoclonal antibodies promise more effective immunotherapy, they represent the forefront of current research, and their efficacy, complications, and usage have not been fully elucidated.

AZATHIOPRINE

Azathioprine (Imuran), a sulfa-substituted derivative of 6-mercaptopurine, is a purine antimetabolite used in transplantation and in treatment of autoimmune and inflammatory diseases. It decreases the mitotic rate of bone marrow cells and increases the antibody production of human B lymphocytes at low concentrations, as demonstrated by the pokeweed mitogen-induced plaque-forming cell response against sheep red blood cells. It also has an effect on T-cell responses, as demonstrated by its inhibition of the mixed lymphocyte reaction and its ability to inhibit selectively the migration of labeled lymph-node cells. The subset of suppressor T cells may be sensitive to high doses of azathioprine, but helper-cell effects on B-cell responses are not affected by *in vitro* azathioprine. Many of the clinical effects of azathioprine are thought to be related to its chemical conversion *in vivo* to 6-mercaptopurine and its subsequent conversion to other biologically active nucleotides. Although azathioprine itself is minimally excreted by the kidney, a large proportion of its metabolites are excreted in the urine; the dose administrated therefore should be tailored to the creatinine clearance, so that at clearances of less than 20 ml/min, less than 1 mg/kg should be given. As in patients with normal renal function, doses should be individualized and each patient should be watched closely for evidence of toxicity.

The major side-effect of azathioprine is related to its suppression of the bone marrow and subsequent neutropenia and thrombocytopenia. Associated with this, but not always occurring pari passu, is red cell aplasia, which is usually preceded by premonitory macrocytosis, as measured by the increased mean corpuscular volume (MCV). Each of these side-effects is dose related and may be reversed by reduction of the dose or substitution of another drug. Since the individual response to azathioprine is variable, close monitoring of the peripheral leukocyte count, platelet count, and MCV should accompany azathioprine administration.

In patients with inflammatory bowel disease azathioprine and pancreatitis appear to be associated, although not as a dose dependent but rather as a hypersensitivity reaction. Changes in amylase clearance have been seen immediately after a single dose of azathioprine and have been reversed upon discontinuation. When pancreatitis is suspected to be the result of azathioprine, the drug should be stopped. Hypersensitivity to azathioprine has also been demonstrated by the development of rash, arthralgia, myalgia, nausea, vomiting, interstitial pneumonitis, and polyneuritis. In addition, hepatovenocclusive disease and intrahepatic cholestasis have been seen in conjunction with azathioprine therapy. Elevations in results of liver-function tests after treatment with azathioprine have been shown to diminish after cessation of therapy. For this reason, azathioprine should be used cautiously when other hepatotoxic drugs such as isoniazid and phenytoin (Dilantin) are used. Also, since azathioprine has a direct effect on leukocytes, simultaneous use of such antimetabolite drugs as allopurinol should be avoided. An increased risk of cancer has been alluded to, especially when azathioprine is used in conjunction with total lymphoid irradiation or cyclosporin-A.

CYCLOSPORIN-A

Cyclosporin-A is a cyclic peptide of 11 amino acids produced by the fungus *Cyclindrocarpon lucidum.*[7] It has been used both orally and parenterally in clinical and experimental cardiac, hepatic, and renal transplantation. Its effects seem to be on T cells. It works on the early stages of antigen mitogenic stimulation of immunocompetent cells so that when given at the time of stimulation, its suppression seems to be specifically directed toward the clones of cells associated with the stimulus. Nephrotoxicity, myelosuppression, lymphoma, hepatotoxicity, and an increase in viral infections have been reported, especially when cyclosporin-A is used with other immunosuppressive drugs. The correct dosage for immunosuppression and for managing the complications in cardiac and renal transplantation has not yet been defined.

CANCER CHEMOTHERAPY

In addition to the infectious complications of cancer chemotherapeutic agents, a number of agents have specific toxic side-effects, many of which affect organ function, as the list below shows.

Bone marrow
methotrexate
cytosine arabinoside
mercaptopurine
thioguanine
fluorouracil
cyclophosphamide
busulphan
chlorambucil
mustine
BCNU, CCNU
procarbazine
actinomycin D
melphalan
adriamycin
daunorubicin
mitomycin C
vinblastine

Mucosal and GI tracts
actinomycin D
adriamycin
bleomycin
methotrexate
fluorouracil
daunorubicin
cytosine arabinoside
CCNU (liver)

Cardiac system
adriamycin
daunorubicin

Pulmonary system
bleomycin

Renal system
CIS platinum
methotrexate (high dose)

Peripheral nervous system
vincristine

Urologic system
cyclophosphamide

Skin, hair
actinomycin D
adriamycin
bleomycin
cyclophosphamide

In addition, most cancer chemotherapeutic agents and radiotherapy have an immunosuppressive effect. Thus, the incidence of infectious complications in the therapy of cancer is similar to that in transplantation.

Specific Complications

PNEUMONIA

The most common serious infectious complication of immunosuppression is pneumonia. In the Medical College of Virginia series of renal and cardiac transplant recipients, it was the leading cause of mortality in the posttransplant period. Immunosuppressed patients with fever of unknown origin should always be evaluated by posterior-anterior and lateral chest films. Serial daily examinations may be necessary to make the correct and earliest possible diagnosis. Pulmonary edema must be ruled out, and other sources of fever should be sought. Again, speed is of the essence, since progression of the pneumonic process is rapid, if untreated. Although sputum and transtracheal aspiration with Gram stain, acid-fast stain, silver stains, and appropriate cultures are excellent methods of diagnosing most common infections, negative results may be misleading in the presence of opportunistic infections from *Aspergillus*, cytomegalovirus, *Pneumocystis carinii*, or *Toxoplasma gondii*.

When a localized process associated with conclusive cytologic or culture confirmation is found, appropriate antibiotic therapy should begin immediately. The choice of antibiotics and the dosage should be dictated by the results of susceptibility testing. Antibiotic therapy should be continued until the process is unequivocally resolved. Under most circumstances, immunosuppression may be continued while treating localized infection, but should the pneumonic process progress or fail to respond within 24 hours to 48 hours, immunosuppression may need to be decreased or ceased. Also, a second pathogen should be considered when there is no improvement; reculturing should be performed and more invasive procedures undertaken.

When the sputum or tracheal aspirates are not helpful in making the diagnosis or when a diffuse or progressive infiltrate is found, immediate bronchoscopy and transbronchial biopsy, transthoracic aspiration biopsy, or open-lung biopsy should be undertaken. Concomitant serum titers for cytomegalovirus (CMV), herpesvirus, Legionnaires' disease, or toxoplasmosis may be helpful, but the results are

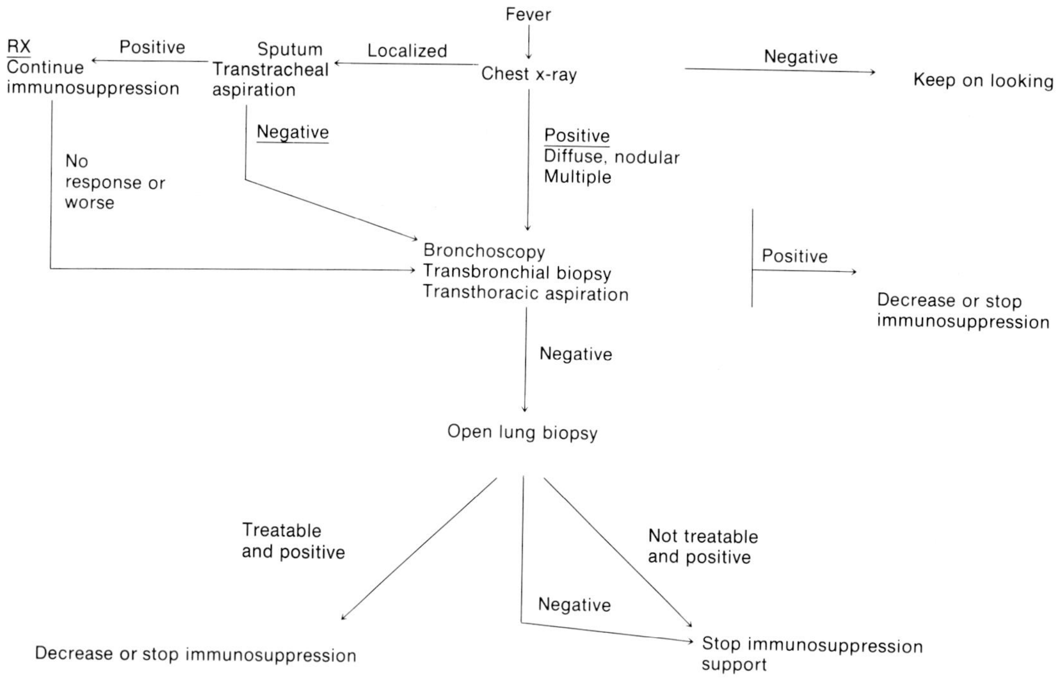

FIG. 18-1. Diagnosis and therapy of pneumonia during immunosuppression.

generally delayed. Serial arterial blood gases should be monitored. Abnormal liver-function tests, platelet count, and clotting factors may indicate disseminated infection. These tests may be helpful, but our experience indicates that time is of the essence and that early and accurate tissue diagnosis is the only way to avert a rapidly deteriorating situation. Some institutions have advocated transbronchial biopsy and brushing with the flexible fiberoptic bronchoscope or transthoracic needle biopsy, but both bear an associated 10% to 20% risk of pneumothorax and offer less consistent definitive diagnoses. Open-lung biopsy, taking generous samplings of the infected area, should be performed when the infection is rapidly progressing. The following should be undertaken: pathologic examinations for bacteria, mycobacteria, fungus, CMV or other viruses, *Pneumocystis carinii*, and toxoplasmosis; cultures for anaerobic bacteria, fungi, mycobacteria, and aerobic bacteria; touch preparations for pneumocystis, histoplasmosis, and toxoplasmosis; and silver staining for pneumocystis. The biopsy for *Legionella pneumophila* should be studied immunofluorescently and the biopsy site should be thoroughly sealed. We have found that the stapling device is the most consistent way of maintaining a good seal. A chest tube should be placed and appropriate antibiotic therapy instituted immediately.

The question of when to stop immunosuppression in the face of infection is at times difficult. In severe pneumonia, it is often necessary to avoid immunosuppressive therapy, risking the loss of an allograft or postponing cancer chemotherapy in order to abrogate the infection. Surprisingly, the allografts may not immediately be rejected and may be supported by minimum doses of prednisone (10 mg/day). Immunosuppression may be resumed after the infection is controlled. Ventilatory support should be adequate. Again, nutrition should be considered part of the total therapy for infection, and parenteral nutrition should be instituted early if prolonged ventilatory support is indicated. An algorithm used at the Medical College of Virginia for evaluating pneumonia is illustrated in Figure 18-1. It is a helpful guide through the workup procedures for a pneumonic process. Some of the microorganisms that cause pulmonary infections are listed below.

Organisms That Cause Pneumonia in Immunosuppressed Patients

Bacteria

Diplococcus pneumoniae
Escherichia coli
Klebsiella pneumoniae
Pseudomonas aeruginosa
Staphylococcus aureus
Nocardia asteroides

Mycobacterium tuberculosis
Mycoplasma pneumoniae
Legionella pneumophila
Anaerobes

Fungi
Cryptococcus neoformans
Aspergillus fumigatus
Zygomycetes (mucor)

Parasites
Pneumocystis carinii
Toxoplasma gondii
Strongyloides stercoralis

Viruses
Cytomegalovirus
Herpes simplex virus
Varicella-zoster virus
Parainfluenza and influenza virus
Adenovirus

Bacterial Agents

It is important to remember that common pathogens remain the major cause of pneumonia in the immunosuppressed patient. For instance, the pneumococcus in the immunocompromised host, and especially in the asplenic patient, frequently is the cause of pneumonia and may easily be diagnosed by a Gram stain of the sputum showing the characteristic encapsulated gram-positive diplococci. The patients are easily treated with aqueous penicillin, 600,000 to 1 million units twice daily, and occasionally as frequently as every 4 hours. Asplenic patients who are immunosuppressed should be treated prophylactically with polyvalent pneumococcal vaccine. Other bacteria, particularly the gram-negative bacteria and *Staphylococcus aureus*, may be responsible for pneumonia in the immunocompromised patient. Patients with lobar pneumonia, segmental consolidation, or cavitary lesions, and especially patients with tracheostomies or prolonged endotracheal intubation, are at risk for developing *Pseudomonas aeruginosa*, *Klebsiella pneumoniae*, and *Serratia marcescens* pneumonia. In addition, *Staphylococcus aureus* and the anaerobic organisms are important causes of necrotizing pneumonia leading to irreversible lung damage and, in many instances, death. Because the types of organisms and the antibiotic-susceptibility patterns vary among hospitals and even within individual institutions, good diagnostic material for Gram stain must be obtained so that appropriate antibiotics may be begun while awaiting culture and sensitivity results. Immunosuppression should be diminished and if possible stopped, especially if the patient shows no response to antibiotic therapy.

Still within the realm of the bacteria are the two organisms that may cause indolent, yet life threatening, pneumonia in immunosuppressed patients. Both *Nocardia asteroides* and *Mycobacterium tuberculosis* may present almost any clinical picture, ranging from diffuse bronchial pneumonia to solitary cavities. Nocardia is treated with sulfa drugs, especially sulfadiazine or sulfamethoxazole-trimethoprim in combination. Tuberculosis should be treated with isoniazid (INH) and rifampin for at least 9 months. It is noteworthy that both of these organisms may have associated unsuspected extrapulmonic disease of which the surgeon should be perpetually suspicious.

The occurrence of an epidemic pneumonia among American Legionnaires in Philadelphia, in 1978, led to the uncovering of the bacterium *Legionella pneumophila* as an etiologic agent. Retrospective studies linked the bacterium to outbreaks of pulmonary infection as far back as 1965 and to subsequent epidemics in a variety of endemic areas. *Legionella pneumophila* is a faintly staining gram-negative fastidious bacillus that must be grown in special media. At present, four antigenic groups have been recognized. Identification may be made with Gimenez stain on fresh lung, with Dieterle or Worthen–Starry silver impregnation stains, or by direct fluorescent antibody techniques. The organism seems not to be passed by person-to-person contact but to be harbored in the ground and water supply and has been associated with air conditioners, air ducts, excavation sites, showers, and water tanks.

The clinical picture in Legionnaires' disease is one of initial malaise, lethargy, weakness, fever, and a dry cough, with occasional nonpurulent sputum and mild hemoptysis. Watery diarrhea, confusion, delirium, myalgia, and relative bradycardia have been associated with the disease. Disseminated intravascular coagulopathy, thrombocytopenia, anemia, and inappropriate antidiuretic hormone have been seen in later stages. A form of the disease with minimal symptoms, known as Pontiac fever, is not usually associated with immunoincompetent patients. The radiologic picture is one of patchy alveolar infiltrates, usually in a lower lobe, progressing to lobar consolidation and even cavitation.

In patients with signs and symptoms suggestive of Legionnaires' disease, tracheal aspirates revealing a small number of leukocytes or mononuclear cells with few organisms on routine staining should lead to the suspicion of *Legionella pneumophila*. The diagnosis can be made by transtracheal aspirates, lung biopsy, and culture or by direct fluorescent antibody testing. Seroconversion in patients has been documented by indirect immunofluorescent techniques. However, there is some delay in the rise in titer of the antibody, and therefore serologic techniques may not be temporally sufficient for treatment. The treatment for Legionnaires' disease is generally erythromycin, 1 g to 2 g, every 6 hours, intravenously. Some success has been seen with tetracycline or rifampin. However, in one study the mortality for Legionnaires' disease was 24% in patients treated with erythromycin and 80% in patients not treated with erythromycin.

Fungal Infections

The fungi play the next most important role in infections in the compromised host. All of the classic mycoses occur in immunosuppressed patients, and all have a propensity for dissemination. Very often, the pneumonic process is the sentinel of systemic mycoses, especially after high-dose corticosteroids, prolonged broad-spectrum antibiotics, and in the debilitated, diabetic, or cancer patient. *Coccidioides immitis, Blastomyces dermatitidis,* and *Histoplasma capsulatum* should be suspected in the appropriate geographic areas. A good travel history is important, since endogenous reactivation may occur at the time of immunosuppression after the patient has moved from an endemic area. The opportunistic fungi causing pulmonary lesions with some regularity are the *Aspergillus* species, *Zygomycetes* (mucormycosis), and *Cryptococcus neoformans. Candida* pneumonia is rare and generally occurs when all other organ systems are failing. Both *Aspergillus* and the *Zygomycetes* infrequently invade the pulmonary vasculature, resulting in infarcts, necrosis, and rapid dissemination. Pulmonary disease due to *Cryptococcus neoformans* is much less virulent, but in the compromised host the organism may disseminate to the central nervous system. Many of the opportunistic fungi are common laboratory contaminants or saprophytes of the respiratory tree, so that a positive sputum culture is difficult to interpret. Tissue should be examined immediately for the presence of microorganisms.

The earlier antifungal therapy is started, the better the prognosis. At present, intravenous amphotericin-B is the drug of choice for fungal pulmonary infections. Therapy should be begun with a test dose of 1mg, intravenously, on the first day, and increased in increments to 20 mg to 40 mg per day until a total dose of 1.5 g to 2.0 g has been reached. Care must be taken to treat accompanying fever and chills during administration with antipyretics. In addition, serial creatinine clearances or other renal function parameters must be monitored, since amphotericin-B has a dose-related nephrotoxicity. For both cryptococcus and candida pneumonia, 5-flucytosine has been shown to be somewhat successful in treating systemic mycoses when given in conjunction with amphotericin-B. It is important that 5-flucytosine not be given by itself, since it seems to have a synergistic effect with amphotericin-B. The dose is 1.5 g to 2.0 g, parenterally or orally, every 6 hours. One should look for nephrotoxicity and bone marrow toxicity. In patients in renal failure, the dose may be tailored to blood levels but may be maintained at therapeutic levels with 25 mg to 50 mg/kg after dialysis.

Parasites

Three parasites are recognized to cause pulmonary infiltrates in the compromised host. These are *Pneumocystis carinii, Toxoplasma gondii,* and *Strongyloides stercoralis. Pneumocystis* is a protozoan from the Sporozoa class. In a patient who manifests nonproductive cough, fever, dyspnea, hypoxemia, and diffuse bilateral parenchymal abnormalities, especially in the hilar area and lower lobes, the diagnosis of *Pneumocystis* infection should be considered. Cytomegalovirus, Legionnaires', and toxoplasmosis must be ruled out. The only sure diagnosis of *Pneumocystis carinii* at present is from a biopsy demonstrating the intra-alveolar cysts on methamine-silver nitrate staining. The trophozoites can be identified by Geimsa or Wright staining. In addition, fluorescent antibody staining for *Pneumocystis carinii* antigen can be done. The treatment for pneumocystis is trimethoprim-sulfamethoxazole. Toxoplasmosis seems to have a higher incidence in patients with Hodgkins' disease and after renal and cardiac transplantation. In the transplantation population, the organism may be transmitted from the donor. Specific diagnosis is required for the parasites because therapy differs in all three. Generally, the tissue imprints are all that are needed to diagnose *Pneumocystis carinii* and *Toxoplasma gondii.* Occasionally, *Strongyloides stercoralis* can be found upon examination of a wet preparation of the sputum. *Toxoplasma gondii* requires a combination of pyrimethamine and sulfadiazine, while *Strongyloides stercoralis* can be treated with thiabendazole. Finally, the viruses may cause pneumonia as well as a myriad of other syndromes.

Viral Infections

The most common viral actors in the scenario of infections related to immunosuppression (except the hepatitis viruses) are the commensal herpesviruses, herpes simplex (HSV), varicella-zoster (VZ), and cytomegalovirus (CMV). Herpes simplex comes in two types, HSV-1 and HSV-2, the former localizing mostly in the head and neck and the latter in the genitalia. They are transmitted by personal contact. HSV-1 is associated with primary gingivostomatitis and head and neck skin vesicles, while HSV-2 is associated with genital or anal ulcerations. Reactivation of the viruses produces vesicles and ulcers. In the immunosuppressed patient, especially in patients with myeloproliferative or lymphoproliferative disorders and in transplant patients, cold sores, ophthalmic keratitis, esophageal ulcers, gastrointestinal ulcers, meningoencephalitis, paralytic bladder, and occasionally generalized infections resulting in hemorrhagic necrosis of the liver, adrenal, lungs, brain, and gastrointestinal tract have been reported. Patients with malnutrition secondary to kwashiorkor or hyperemesis gravidarium, patients with severe burns, asthmatic patients on corticosteroids, and bone marrow transplant recipients are susceptible to HSV infection and the potential of disseminated disease. Diagnosis may include serologic testing and identification of the viruses in saliva, urine, or other secretions. Treatment varies from local use of idoxuridine, 0.1%, or adenine arabinoside (vidarabine) for keratitis and local lesions to systemic treatment with adenine arabinoside, leukocyte interferon, or a cycloguanosine. Disseminated mucocutaneous HSV-1 has been successfully treated with adenine arabinoside. The use of corticosteroids for ophthalmic HSV to reduce inflammation is still controversial and should probably be avoided in the immunosuppressed patient.

Varicella-zoster virus is acquired by contact with vesicles and inhalation. The primary infection, chickenpox, is associated with a high incidence of pneumonia and fatal outcome in immunosuppressed children. The reactivation of the latent zoster infection in transplant recipients (up to 13% of patients) and in patients with lymphoma (up to 20%) and other patients with cancer is associated with a high incidence of disseminated disease. The vesicular skin lesions of zoster usually follow a sensory posterior root distribution and have a higher incidence with age. The Ramsay Hunt syndrome, facial paralysis, ear pain, and eruption in the external auditory meatus is occasionally seen. Paralysis and neuralgia may be a sequel of reactivation. Meningoencephalitis and pneumonia portend death in most immunosuppressed patients with disseminated disease. The diagnosis is made by serologic testing or by identification of herpesvirus in the vesicles. Immunosuppressed patients may be given zoster immune globulin in an effort to abort or attenuate the disease after exposure. Attenuated virus vaccine has been used to protect potentially susceptible immunosuppressed patients. Patients with disseminated disease have been successfully treated with adenine arabinoside, and cancer patients with zoster have obtained some limitation of disease with human interferon.

Cytomegalovirus (CMV) is another herpesvirus that seems to infect early in life with an increasing prevalence in poorer populations and in the aged. Presence of antibody in adults varies from 40% to 100%, depending on socioeconomic conditions. Transmission can be by the urine, saliva, breast milk, and other secretions; transfusion; and other transplanted tissues. CMV may exist in blood leukocytes banked for up to 28 days and is probably transplanted with renal allografts. The syndrome varies from mild disease with high fever, myalgia, lymphocytosis, and changes in liver enzymes, commonly associated with activation of the latent virus, to severe disease with ophthalmitis, cerebritis, fulminant hepatitis, pneumonia, leukopenia, peripheral neuritis, and myocarditis, most often ascribed to primary infection. Seroconversion; increased titers; complement fixation or immunofluorescent antibody; identification of virus shedding in the urine and saliva; or identification of the characteristic intranuclear and cytoplasmic inclusion bodies is diagnostic. Unfortunately, the treatment for severe disease in the immunosuppressed host remains supportive only, coupled with decreasing or eliminating immunosuppression. One must be aware at all times that with a diagnosis of CMV pneumonia there may be additional infectious organisms. In fact, CMV infection has been thought to be in itself immunosuppressive and to allow and even promote the development of other infections, particularly gram-negative sepsis or pneumocystis. Promising vaccines have been developed, and randomized trials are being carried out at a number of institutions in light of the fact that immunization produces seroconversion without viral shedding. Care must be taken in using attenuated viruses that there is no reactivation of latent virus and no oncogenicity.

Other viruses produce a variety of syndromes in the immunocompromised host. Papovavirus has been associated with progressive multifocal leukoencephalopathy, and both measles and herpesvirus with encephalitis. Hepatitis B and non-A, non-B hepatitis are commonly seen in transplant recipients and in chemotherapy patients who have received multiple transfusions. Parainfluenza virus has been associated with pneumonia and adenovirus with pneumonia and hepatitis in transplant recipients and in patients with severe combined immunodeficiency disease. Immunization for influenza viruses in the immunocompromised host in whom there is the potential for subsequent contact and infection seems to be safe and indicated.

WOUND INFECTIONS

The incidence of wound infection in immunosuppressed patients in noncontaminated surgical wounds varies from 5% to 15%. This high incidence is directly related to the retarded healing and suppressed collagen synthesis, epithelialization, and fibroplasia in patients on corticosteroids or in nutritionally depressed patients and to the inhibition of the immune and inflammatory response in patients on cytotoxic drugs or in patients who have received radiotherapy.[4] The local irradiation given to kidney transplant recipients also tends to decrease wound healing.

Prevention of wound infection is paramount. The surgical incision should be closed with the strictest adherence to basic principles of wound closure, including avoidance of hematoma, closure of dead space, sterile technique, and avoidance of tissue ischemia by careful technique. The incision should be copiously and frequently irrigated, including antibiotic irrigation. Septic areas should not be drained through the incision. Skin sutures in most abdominal incisions should be left in place for at least 2 weeks. We prefer using monofilament synthetic skin sutures or metal staples. Prophylactic antibiotics have been recommended, and in at least one study the complication rate was markedly diminished after routine prophylactic antibiotics.[10]

Staphylococcus aureus is the most frequent organism found in infected wounds from "clean" procedures but gram-negative organisms may also be found. In the immunosuppressed patient, complete wide drainage is important. Drainage alone may not be sufficient, and a course of appropriate antibiotic therapy is often indicated to prevent invasive or progressive infection. As with burns, débridement and diligent topical care are mandatory. We prefer wet to dry dressings with Dakin's or povidone iodine solutions with frequent changes. We also use power spraying for the débridement of dead tissue. Secondary closure is possible when adequate granulation tissue has been created.

Necrotizing fasciitis or progressive necrotizing gangrene caused by streptococci, staphylococci, or gram-negative anaerobic organisms, sometimes acting synergistically, is a fulminant and often fatal infection that may arise from operative wounds or from seemingly innocuous small wounds.[3] We have seen one case of necrotizing fasciitis arise from a venipuncture site. Violaceous, woody, edematous skin lesions with erythema, subcutaneous or fascial necrosis, and undermining of the skin are harbingers of underlying fasciitis. Cutaneous hyperesthesia indicates involvement of cutaneous nerves. Antibiotic therapy alone is usually ineffective. Wide débridement of all necrotic tissue, resection of undermined tissue, and supportive therapy of the systemic manifestations of the infection including fluid loss, anemia, and high fever are indicated. Anaerobic cultures and quantitative cultures of excised tissue pieces are vitally important because routine culture techniques may not identify microaerophilic streptococcus, clostridia, or anaerobic species. Antibiotic therapy should be aggressive. Initially, penicillin, nafcillin, gentamicin, and high doses of clindamycin may be used.

Although Meleney's gangrene classically is a superficial process, usually not involving the deep underlying fascia, in the immunosuppressed patient we have, rarely, found such a localized process, and have been sorry if we did not undertake radical excision of the infected area including well beyond the superficial erythematous margins, the undermined areas, and the deep fascia. With this disease in the immunosuppressed patient, parsimonious saving of local tissue may be fatal. The mortality rate from these infections is high, averaging 50% to 70%. Immunosuppression should be stopped when the severe necrotizing fasciitis is diagnosed.

NEUROLOGIC INFECTIONS

The headache in the nonimmunosuppressed patient may often be dismissed. However, in the immunosuppressed patient, headaches should be viewed with much suspicion. Headache associated with ocular problems, evidence of sinusitis, or localizing symptoms should be immediately evaluated with CT scan, EEG, sinus films, and lumbar puncture. Bacterial meningitis, brain abscess, cryptococcal meningitis, viral encephalitis, toxoplasmosis, fungal sinusitis, lymphoma, and pseudotumor cerebri in patients on corticosteroids should be considered in the differential diagnosis. We have seen one case of mucor meningitis originating in an infected paranasal sinus lead to the death of the patient. The characteristic findings of cells in the spinal fluid, encapsulated yeast on India ink preparation, cryptococcal antigen, and elevated protein and decreased glucose levels should lead to the diagnosis of a septic intracranial problem. Cultures should be obtained and appropriate therapy instituted immediately. Immunosuppression should be diminished if there is no observable response within 24 hours. Consideration should be given to stopping immunosuppression. Cryptococcal meningitis may require a week of treatment before there is an observable response. Viral encephalitis in the immunosuppressed patient carries a greater than 80% mortality rate. Surgical decompression may be indicated if signs of increased intracranial pressure are observed.

GASTROINTESTINAL COMPLICATIONS

Perforation

Gastrointestinal perforation, onerous as it is in the nonimmunosuppressed patient, is cataclysmic in the patient unable to mount an inflammatory response, unable to contain the perforation, and unable to control the associated sepsis. The diagnosis is often delayed, although the signs and symptoms of low-grade fever, vague abdominal discomfort or pain, nondiagnostic tenderness and tachycardia should raise the suspicion of bowel perforation. The bedrock of successful therapy is early diagnosis. Abdominal x-ray films seeking pneumoperitoneum, CT and abdominal ultrasound scans seeking a mass, contrast studies demonstrating a site of leakage, and gallium scans should be employed as quickly as possible and negative results are not conclusive. Exploratory laparotomy on the basis of a suspicion is often the tool by which the diagnosis is made.

Diverticulitis, appendicitis, perforation of cecal ulcers, and perforation of ischemic ilecolonic segments as a result of radiation, cytomegalovirus, or vascular accident are the most common bowel events. Fecal impaction has been suggested as an additional etiologic agent in some colonic perforations, especially where large doses of antacids are employed during steroid therapy. This condition can obviously be avoided. In transplant patients with diverticulitis it has been a common practice to remove all diverticula-containing colon prior to transplantation. The therapeutic surgical principle in colon perforation is exteriorization and resection of the perforated area. Proximal colostomy and drainage or primary anastomosis should be avoided because they have attendant high mortality rates. Immunosuppression should be markedly reduced or ceased. Even under the best circumstances, a 20% to 40% mortality rate has been seen.

Gastroduodenal perforation, usually secondary to peptic ulcer disease, has an 80% to 100% mortality rate if undiagnosed or treated medically. Emergency surgical intervention, consisting of closure, vagotomy, and antrectomy or pyloroplasty; resection of multiple gastric perforations; or closure and selective vagotomy, has a 25% to 50% mortality rate in the immunodepressed patient. In the transplant population, prophylactic surgery for ulcer has a 1% to 3% mortality rate. Consequently, the patient with an ulcer history should receive prophylactic surgical therapy if possible. As a second defense, medical prophylaxis with H-2 receptor blockers such as cimetidine and antacids is mandatory.

Hemorrhage

Gastrointestinal hemorrhage occurs usually as a sequel of peptic ulcer disease, gastritis, or gastrointestinal angiodysplasia, and it also occurs in colonic ulcers or diverticula. If there are hematologic abnormalities or gastric hyperacidity secondary to a disease state such as uremia or secondary to therapeutic intervention such as corticosteroid therapy or because of an infectious agent such as cytomegalovirus causing small bowel or cecal ulcers, one must be constantly alert to the possibility of gastrointestinal bleeding. In patients undergoing renal transplantation, prophylaxis is paramount.

In our institution patients with evidence of ulcer disease from their history or upper GI series usually undergo pretransplant ulcer surgery consisting of a proximal gastric vagotomy. In the patient with obstructive symptoms because of peptic ulcer disease, we prefer antrectomy and vagotomy. Although some centers have tried cimetidine alone after transplantation, no randomized trial has proven its efficacy over surgical pretransplant prophylaxis. All patients in our institution receive prophylactic antacids and cimetidine (300 mg, 3 times a day, after transplantation), especially when corticosteroid therapy is used. There may be increased rejection or at least reduced delayed hypersensitivity responses because of cimetidine therapy, but this is clinically more theoretical than proven. Patients with low platelet counts or hematologic abnormalities should receive prophylaxis for peptic ulcer disease.

The appearance of serious upper GI bleeding in the immunosuppressed patient is catastrophic, with a mortality rate of 40% to 80%. The diagnosis must be part of a differential diagnosis of any immunosuppressed patient who has suddenly become confused, hypotensive, or tachycardic. Nasogastric suction and irrigation should be begun, intravenous cimetidine started, and immediate endoscopy undertaken. Surgical intervention for gastric or duodenal ulcer or for gastritis that has been accompanied by more than five units of bleeding or that has had two temporally close, distinct episodes of bleeding should not be delayed. The situation will deteriorate and the prognosis worsen. As much correction as possible of hematologic abnormalities should occur concomitant with initial medical therapy and continue throughout surgical intervention.

Bleeding from the small bowel or colon occasionally occurs from arteriovenous abnormalities, colonic diverticula, or ulceration. The last is occasionally associated in both bowel and stomach with cytomegalovirus. The etiology of bleeding is often difficult to find, and endoscopy, barium enema, and arteriography should be rapidly employed. Delay in diagnosis and copious or frequent bleeding episodes lead to deterioration. Surgical therapy is the same as in the nonimmunosuppressed patient, relying on resection of the area of bleeding tissue.

Esophagitis, Pancreatitis, and Colitis

Esophagitis in the immunosuppressed host is usually secondary to an infectious agent. *Candida albicans* is the most common organism in the transplant recipient, but viruses, particularly herpes simplex virus, have also been implicated. Prophylaxis for *Candida albicans* with oral nystatin is indicated in the immunosuppressed host. Patients with dysphagia, heartburn, or anemia should be evaluated endoscopically by biopsy to rule out biliary reflux or peptic esophagitis and carcinoma.

Treatment is usually symptomatic with the addition of nystatin for *Candida albicans* and the reduction of immunosuppression in severe esophagitis secondary to infection. Some patients may require amphotericin-B.

Pancreatitis has been associated with steroids and with azathioprine in transplant recipients and in patients receiving immunosuppression for autoimmune disease. However, viruses, bacteria, and fungi also have been implicated as etiologic agents. In the immunocompromised host, pancreatitis carries a 50% to 60% mortality rate. The presenting signs, symptoms, diagnostic workup, and therapy are the same as for the general surgical population with a caution that the diagnosis may be more difficult if the immunosuppression masks symptoms.

Pseudomembranous antimicrobial agent-induced colitis and diarrhea have occasionally been seen in transplant recipients and in patients receiving chemotherapy for cancer. In these groups the mortality rate may be as high as 80%. Pseudomembranous colitis seems to have a higher incidence in patients with diabetes mellitus or uremia and after prolonged antibiotic therapy. The diagnosis should be suspected by diarrhea, fever, abdominal pain and distention, and systemic toxicity. However, the symptoms may be masked by the immunosuppressive regimen. Although *Staphylococcus aureus* and *Candida albicans* have been rarely implicated as etiologic agents, the most common organism found, especially in antimicrobial agent-induced colitis, is *Clostridium difficile*, which produces most of its effects by release of an enterotoxin. The physical examination, endoscopic identification of pseudomembrane plaques, and biopsy and culture of the pseudomembrane are diagnostic. In addition, *Clostridium difficile* may be identified by antibody identification of the enterotoxin in the stool. Treatment for mild *Clostridium difficile* colitis is oral vancomycin, 2 g daily for 7 to 10 days, and discontinuance of other antibiotic therapy. Antiperistaltic drugs should be avoided. The bacterial flora has been reconstituted with Lactobacillus species. If antibiotic therapy is unsuccessful and toxic megacolon ensues, the urgent surgical treatment preferred is total colectomy.

DERMATOLOGIC COMPLICATIONS

Although very rarely fatal, the dermatologic complications of immunosuppression may be lethal if unchecked, and they are occasionally harbingers of further systemic problems.[5] The direct effect on appearance from chemotherapy, such as loss of hair with cyclophosphamide or cushingoid facies with corticosteroids (which may also tend to produce acne, striae, hirsutism, and the buffalo hump appearance), may be disfiguring and have a profound psychological impact. In addition, the increased capillary fragility, decreased platelet count, and hematologic abnormalities may result in purpura, easy bleeding from injury, and poor healing of simple cutaneous lesions. Other cutaneous complications in the immunocompromised patient relate to infections and to neoplasm.

The mycoses responsible for dermatologic complications range from tinea caused by the dermatophyte *Trichophyton rubrum* or *Microsporum canis* to manifestations of more generalized opportunistic fungi, such as *Candida albicans*, producing mucocutaneous moniliasis, vulvovaginitis, or onychomycosis. *Cryptococcus neoformans* has been associated with nonhealing ulcers of the skin and with a nodular, erythematous rash from which the skin biopsy demonstrates the organism within the dermis. We have seen one case of *Allescheria boydii* mycetoma of the forefinger in a transplant patient as a result of a fishing-hook accident. Because it went untreated, the finger had to be amputated. The tineas may be treated with topical agents, particularly topical miconazole cream or ointment. Oral griseofulvin may be used for tinea capitis and onychomycosis, and nystatin mouthwash for thrush. Disseminated candidiasis must be differentiated from mucosal candida infections and treated with systemic amphotericin-B and not oral nystatin, which is not absorbed from the GI tract. Cryptococcal skin lesions always represent disseminated infection and should be treated with systemic amphotericin-B.

Bacteria may also cause cutaneous lesions such as impetigo, furuncle or abscess in injection sites, or necrotizing cellulitis. These should be treated by appropriate drainage and antibiotics. The skin lesions associated with viruses such as the herpesviruses have been discussed in another section. However, condylomata acuminata and verruca vulgaris are seen in increased numbers in immunosuppressed patients and should be treated by either local therapy or surgical excision. Diagnosis of cutaneous lesions may be made by skin biopsies; scrapings of skin and examination in 10% KOH on a slide for fungi; staining of vesicles with Gram stain, Wright stain, or PAS for identifying bacteria or intranuclear or intracytoplasmic inclusion bodies for viruses; or, finally, by culturing.

In the immunocompromised host there is approximately a 1% to 2% incidence of cutaneous malignancy, mostly squamous-cell carcinoma, basal-cell carcinoma, or malignant melanoma. Kaposi's sarcoma has also been seen in higher incidences in renal-transplant recipients. Long-term survivors of cancer chemotherapy have an additional increased incidence of second tumors, many of which are cutaneous. The basic principles of wide surgical incision should be utilized in all of these any time cutaneous cancer has been found.

MALIGNANCY

Malignancy following immunosuppression in transplantation and antineoplastic therapy and following chemotherapy for some nonmalignant disorders has been of some concern.[1, 8] An increased incidence of myeloproliferative leukemia has been noted in patients receiving radiation for localized head and neck or gynecologic cancer. In fact, one series reports a 171-fold increase in acute leukemia in patients receiving alkylating agents for ovarian cancer.[11] In another study of nontransplant, nononcology patients receiving immunosuppressive drugs for the therapy of various diseases, the incidence of non-Hodgkins' lymphoma, squamous-cell carcinoma of the skin, and sarcoma was reported to be 1.5 to 20 times that of the general population.[6] In transplanted patients receiving immunosuppression for over 6 months, there is a definite increase in lymphoma, reticulum-cell sarcoma, skin cancer, cervical cancer, and gastrointestinal cancer. While the incidence of *de novo* cancer in transplant recipients is from 2% to 13%, the probability of developing a fatal cancer seems to increase with the duration of the transplant. The risk of cancer in the immunosuppressed patient is, therefore, 200 to 300 times that of the general population, depending upon cell type. Certain immunosuppressive regimens seem to be more carcinogenic. Cyclosporin-A therapy has an increased risk of certain lymphomas.[2] Azathioprine, ATG, cyclophosphamide, and chlorambucil seem to be associated with non-Hodgkins' lymphoma, and alkylating agents and radiotherapy with acute myelogenous leukemia.

The mechanisms responsible for the increases in cancer risk are open to speculation. Evidence for loss of immune surveillance of malignant cells, loss of immunoregulation of proliferative cells, viral oncogenesis (especially the EB virus), and mutogenic effects of chemotherapy and radiotherapy is available. The mechanisms may be multifactorial and interrelated. It is noteworthy that lymphoma and reticulum-cell sarcoma seem to find some of their highest incidences in the transplant population, in whom the chemotherapy is directed toward suppressing lymphocytes, while the myeloproliferative leukemias are associated with alkylating agents and radiotherapy and with suppression of the peripheral leukocyte count. Although the mechanism of development is uncertain, cancer in immunocompromised hosts certainly acts virulently, and early detection, aggressive therapy, and, in some instances, withdrawal of immunosuppression are indicated.

References

1. Anderson JL, Bieber CP, Fowles RF, Stinson EB: Idiopathic cardiomyopathy age, and suppressor-cell dysfunction as risk determinants of lymphoma after cardiac transplantation. Lancet 2:1174, 1978
2. Crawford DH, Thomas JA, Janossy G et al: Epstein Barr virus nuclear antigen positive lymphoma after cyclosporin A treatment in patient with renal allograft. Lancet 1:1355, 1980
3. Dymock RB: Skin diseases associated with renal transplantation. Australas J Dermatol 20:61, 1979
4. Ferguson MK: The effect of antineoplastic agents on wound healing. Surg Gynecol Obstet 154:97, 1982
5. Janevicius RV, Sang–Erk H, Batt MD: Necrotizing fasciitis. Surg Gynecol Obstet 154:97, 1982
6. Kinlen LJ, Sheil AGR, Peto J, Doll R: Collaborative United Kingdom–Australasian study of cancer in patients treated with immunosuppressive drugs. Br Med J 2:1461, 1979
7. Morris PJ: Cyclosporin A. Transplantation 32:349, 1981
8. Penn I: Tumor incidence in human allograft recipients. Transplant Proc 2:1047, 1979
9. Slade MS, Simmons RL, Yunis E, Greenberg LJ: Immunodepression after major surgery in normal patients. Surgery 78:363, 1975
10. Tilney NL, Strom TB, Vineyard GC, Merrill JP: Factors contributing to the declining mortality rate in renal transplantation. N Engl J Med 299:1321, 1978
11. Zarrabi MH, Rosner F: Acute myeloblastic leukemia following treatment for non-hematopoietic cancers: Report of 19 cases and review of the literature. Am J Hematol 7:357, 1979

Suggested Reading

General

Chatterjee SN: Renal Transplantation. New York, Raven Press, 1980

Jubert AV, Lee ET, Hersh EM, McBride CM: Effects of surgery, anesthesia, and intraoperative blood loss on immunocompetence. J Surg Res 15:399, 1973

McIntosh J, Hansen P, Ziegler J, Penny R: Defective immune and phagocytic functions in uraemia and renal transplantation. Int Arch Allergy Appl Immunol 51:544, 1976

Makinodan T, Kay MMB: Age influence on the immune system. Adv Immunol 29:287, 1980

Munster AM: Immune Response in Burns and Injuries. CRC Handbook Series in Clinical Laboratory Science, Section F: Immunology. West Palm Beach, Fla, CRC Press, 1978

Slade MS, Simmons RL, Yunis E, Greenberg LJ: Immunodepression after major surgery in normal patients. Surgery 78:363, 1975

Specific Drugs

Borel JF: Cyclosporin A—Present experimental status. Transplantation Proc 13:344, 1981

DeClerck YA, Ettenger RB, Ortega JA, Pennisi AJ: Macrocytosis and pure rbc anemia caused by azathioprine. Am J Dis Child 134:377, 1980

Diethelm AG: Surgical management of complications of steroid therapy. Ann Surg 185:251, 1977

Old CW, Flannery EP, Grogan TM et al: Azathioprine-induced pure red blood cell aplasia. JAMA 240:552, 1978

Singleton JW, Law DH, Kelley ML et al: National cooperative Crohn's disease study: Adverse reactions to study drugs. Gastroenterology 77:870, 1979

Infections

Codish S, Tobias JS, Hannigan M: Combined amphotericin-B-flucytosine therapy in aspergillus pneumonia. JAMA 241:2418, 1979

Howard RJ, Simmons RL, Najarian JS: Fungal infections in renal transplant recipients. Ann Surg 188:598, 1978

Hughes WT, Kuhn S, Chaudhary S et al: Successful chemoprophylaxis for *Pneumocystis carinii* pneumonitis. New Engl J Med 297:1419, 1977

Lambert HP: Opportunistic lung infections. J R Coll Physicians Lond 13:29, 1979

Meyer RD, Finegold SM: Legionnaires' disease. Annu Rev Med 31:219, 1980

Millar JW, Horne NW: Tuberculosis in immunosuppressed patients. Lancet 1:1176, 1979

Palmer DL, Harvey RL, Wheeler JK: Diagnostic and therapeutic considerations in *Nocardia asteroides* infections. Medicine 53:391, 1974

Ryning FW, Mills J: *Pneumocystis carinii, Toxoplasma gondii, Cytomegalovirus* and the compromised host. West J Med 130:18, 1979

Timbury MC, Edmond E: Herpesviruses. J Clin Pathol 32:859, 1979

Gastrointestinal Complications

Aldrete JS, Sterling WA, Hathaway BM et al: Gastrointestinal and hepatic complications affecting patients with renal allografts. Am J Surg 129:115, 1975

George WL, Rolfe RD, Finegold SM: Treatment and prevention of antimicrobial agent-induced colitis and diarrhea. Gastroenterology 79:366, 1980

Jones RH, Rudge CJ, Bewick M et al: Cimetidine: Prophylaxis against upper gastrointestinal hemorrhage after renal transplantation. Br Med J 1:398, 1978

Lee HM, Madge GE, Mendez–Picon G, Chatterjee SN: Surgical complications in renal transplant recipients. Surg Clin North Am 58:285, 1978

Perloff LJ, Chon H, Petrella EJ et al: Acute colitis in the renal allograft recipient. Ann Surg 183:77, 1976

Schnyder PA, Brusch RC, Salvatierra O: Gastrointestinal complications of renal transplantation in children. Radiology 130:361, 1979

Welch JP, Schweizer RT, Bartus SA: Management of antacid impactions in hemodialysis and renal transplant recipients. Am J Surg 139:561, 1980

19 Complications of Antibiotic Administration

C. Glen Mayhall

OVERVIEW

Antimicrobial chemotherapy is frequently an important adjunct to the surgical therapy of infections. As in other fields of medicine, antimicrobial chemotherapy in surgery may be complicated by failure of therapy or unwanted side-effects. Application of the principles of effective chemotherapy can maximize the benefits to the patient and minimize the risks of complications.

The problems encountered in the use of antimicrobial chemotherapeutic agents can be conveniently divided into failure of therapy, hypersensitivity reactions, and direct antimicrobial toxicity on specific organ systems.

Failure of Therapy

URINARY-TRACT INFECTIONS

Bacteria that cause urinary-tract infections (UTI) usually derive from the patient's bowel flora or in the hospital from other patients or hands of health-care personnel. Most UTIs develop by the ascending route with initial infection in the bladder followed by retrograde movement of microorganisms up the ureters to the kidneys. Instrumentation or obstruction of the urinary tract potentiates the development of infection. Infections may be limited to the bladder, or pyelonephritis may occur after retrograde spread of microorganisms to the kidneys.

Failure of therapy for UTI may occur for one of several reasons. First, the causative microorganisms may be resistant to the antimicrobial agent administered to the patient. Resistance may be inherent, such as resistance of *Pseudomonas aeruginosa* to ampicillin and cephalosporins, resistance of *Klebsiella pneumoniae* to carbenicillin, or resistance of fungi to antibacterial agents.

On the other hand, microorganisms initially susceptible to a given antibiotic may acquire resistance through one of several mechanisms. Most important of these is the transfer of extrachromosomal deoxyribonucleic acid (plasmids or resistance factors) between cells. These resistance (R) factors code for the production of enzymes that either destroy or modify antibiotics, rendering them ineffective. Transfer of R factors takes place in a setting of high-antibiotic usage, particularly in the hospital.

The second cause of ineffective therapy is failure to achieve a therapeutic concentration of antibiotic in the urine. This is because the primary determinant of effective therapy for UTI is the concentration of antimicrobial agent in the urine, not in the serum.[154] Urine concentrations of antibiotics may be subtherapeutic because too low a dose has been administered or because of impairment of renal function with a decrease in renal excretion of the drug.

Diagnosis of the cause of failure of therapy for UTI rests on carefully collected culture data and on accurate assessment of renal function. If urine was not cultured prior to starting therapy, cultures should be taken to determine whether or not the causative microorganism has been eradicated. If cultures yield a urinary-tract pathogen with equal to or greater than 100,000 colonies per milliliter, infection persists, and another antimicrobial agent should be selected on the basis of antimicrobial susceptibility tests.

Even when cultures taken prior to therapy yield a microorganism that is susceptible to the antibiotic given for initial therapy, cultures should repeatedly be taken as long as the clinical response is poor. Failure of therapy may be due to superinfection with a resistant microorganism or the initial microorganism may have become resistant during therapy. When a resistant species is identified by culture, another antibiotic should be selected on the basis of susceptibility tests.

A change in therapy based on culture data assumes that the data are accurate. Contamination during collection of the specimen may occur and will frequently yield spurious results—several species may be isolated from the specimen. When more than one species is reported, the data should be discarded and another specimen sent for culture. Cultures should be collected from the catheter by aspiration with a sterile needle and syringe and not from the collection bag. Urinary-catheter tips should not be sent for culture because the results of such cultures cannot be interpreted.[70]

When adequate doses are being used to treat a UTI due to a susceptible microorganism and the infection cannot be eradicated, the patient's renal function should be assessed. Marked degrees of renal impairment have varying effects on the concentrations of various antibiotics achieved in the urine. Nitrofurantoin and chloramphenicol should not be used to treat UTI in patients with impaired renal function.[97, 142] Concentrations of aminoglycosides are considerably decreased in patients with marked renal insufficiency (creatinine clearance ≤10ml/min).[19, 110] Because of the inhibitory effect of uremic urine on the antimicrobial activity of gentamicin, many UTIs cannot be effectively treated with gentamicin in patients with a creatinine clearance of ≤10 ml per minute.

In patients whose creatinine clearance is greater than 10 ml per minute, ampicillin, cephalexin, and cefazolin all achieve therapeutic concentrations in urine.[40, 42, 94] The best antibiotics for treatment of infections in patients with severe renal insufficiency (creatinine clearance ≤10 ml/min) are ampicillin and trimethoprim-sulfamethoxazole.[18, 39] The latter drug combination provides effective therapy for UTI even in anephric patients on hemodialysis, but the package insert states that its use is contraindicated in patients with creatinine clearance of less than 15 ml per minute. Ampicillin is given in a dose of 500 mg, orally, and trimethoprim-sulfamethoxazole in a dose of one tablet (80 mg of trimethoprim and 400 mg of sulfamethoxazole), orally, both every 6 hours.[18]

Most UTIs will respond to therapy when adequate concentrations of an antimicrobial agent to which the causative organism is susceptible are attained in the urine. However, if infection persists, the patient should be evaluated for urinary-tract obstruction, calculi, or other abnormalities.

PULMONARY INFECTION

Surgical patients whose postoperative course is complicated by pneumonia will usually be infected with gram-negative bacilli or *Staphylococcus aureus* acquired from the hands of personnel, the hospital environment, or from the patients' own flora. The first step in development of infection is colonization of the oropharynx. It has been shown that the more severe the underlying illness, the more likely the patient is to develop colonization of the oropharynx with gram-negative bacilli.[82] After colonization of the oropharynx, the microorganisms are aspirated into the lower respiratory tract where they cause pneumonia. A number of factors may potentiate the development of postoperative pneumonia. These include the surgical operation, anesthesia, postoperative atelectasis, underlying pulmonary and systemic disease, lesions that cause bronchial obstruction, and instrumentation, including endotracheal tubes and tracheostomies.

Owing to the frequent presence of complicating factors in postoperative pneumonia, effective therapy may be very difficult. One problem that compromises therapy is the failure to identify the causative microorganism and obtain antimicrobial susceptibility tests. In addition to bacterial pneumonia, certain patients such as transplant patients and those treated for neoplastic diseases with steroids, cytotoxic agents, and radiation therapy may develop pulmonary infections due to opportunistic pathogens such as cytomegalovirus, *Toxoplasma gondii*, and *Pneumocystis carinii* that will not respond to antibacterial antibiotics. Further, a causative microorganism that was initially susceptible to the antibiotic chosen for therapy may become resistant or be replaced by a resistant microorganism. Finally, the antibiotic chosen for therapy may not attain concentrations in lung tissue sufficient to eradicate the causative microorganism.

The first step in determining the reason pneumonia fails to respond to therapy is to obtain bronchial secretions for microscopic examination and culture. The best specimen is obtained by transtracheal aspiration, because coughed-sputum specimens are frequently contaminated by microorganisms that colonize the oropharynx. Specimens obtained by nasopharyngeal suction or by suction through an endotracheal tube or tracheostomy may also be contaminated by microorganisms that colonize the oropharynx or the tube.

The bronchial-secretion specimens should be smeared on a slide and Gram stained, and they should be cultured for bacteria. A Gram-stained smear will be useful for choosing initial therapy and for interpretation of culture results. Polymorphonuclear leukocytes seen on Gram-stained smear indicate inflammation consistent with bacterial infection. If epithelial cells are seen on the Gram-stained smear, the specimen should be discarded, because it is contaminated with secretions from the oropharynx. When one or more microorganisms is seen on a Gram-stained smear, there are at least 100,000 microorganisms per milliliter of respiratory secretions. If the culture yields a predominant species of microorganism consistent with the morphology of microorganisms seen on Gram-stained smear, it is the likely causative agent of the infection. Therapy should be chosen on the basis of results of susceptibility tests on the isolated species. Only secretions obtained by transtracheal aspiration should be sent for anaerobic culture, since specimens collected by other means are likely to be contaminated by anaerobic bacteria from the flora of the oropharynx.

Therapy may fail even when the causative microorganism is identified and therapy is administered on the basis of antimicrobial susceptibility tests. The concentration of antibiotics in bronchial secretions may not be sufficient to eradicate the microorganism causing the infection. This is particularly the case with gram-negative infections, which require higher concentrations of antibiotics for effective therapy. Ampicillin, cephalosporins, gentamicin, tobramycin, and amikacin achieve concentrations in bronchial secretions that are only a fraction of those attained in serum.[2, 21, 22, 47, 76, 106, 171] Through much of the dosing interval, levels are below those needed to eradicate the microorganisms. Therefore, for treatment of pneumonia due to gram-negative bacilli, high doses of antibiotics should be administered parenterally, and synergistic combinations of antibiotics should be used. Gentamicin, tobramycin, and amikacin should be given in combination with carbenicillin or a cephalosporin to increase antimicrobial activity in bronchial secretions. In patients with normal renal function, ampicillin and cephalothin may be given at a total daily dose of 12 g, intravenously (IV), divided into equal doses every 4 hours. Cefazolin should be administered in a dose of 1 g, IV, every 6 hours. Gentamicin and tobramycin doses should be chosen to deliver peak serum levels of 6 μg to 8 μg/ml, and amikacin doses should be tailored to achieve peak levels of 15 μg to 30 μg/ml.[81, 147] In patients with normal renal function, carbenicillin is administered in doses of 5 g to 6 g, IV, every 4 hours.

Cefotaxime and moxalactam are third-generation cephalosporins that have recently been approved for clinical use. They are broad-spectrum antimicrobial agents and are much more active against gram-negative bacilli than first- and second-generation cephalosporins. Many gram-negative bacilli resistant to aminoglycosides are susceptible to cefotaxime and moxalactam, but many strains of *Pseudomonas aeruginosa* are resistant to these drugs. Early studies indicate that cefotaxime and moxalactam may provide effective single-drug therapy for gram-negative pneumonia.[56, 124] For patients with normal renal function, cefotaxime may be given in a dose of 1 g to 2 g, IV, every 4 to 6 hours and moxalactam may be given in a dose of 2 g to 4 g, IV, every 8 hours.

Failure of therapy for pneumonia may be due to infections caused by microorganisms that are not susceptible to antibacterial antibiotics. This is particularly likely to occur in surgical patients who are immunosuppressed. When Gram-stained smears and cultures of respiratory secretions are negative for bacteria in patients with clinical and roentgenographic evidence of pneumonitis, the patients should be evaluated for infection due to viruses, fungi, *Pneumocystis carinii*, *Toxoplasma gondii*, *Legionella pneumophila*, *Mycobacterium tuberculosis*, and *Nocardia*. In addition to preparation of a Gram-stained smear, respiratory secretions should be smeared and stained for acid-fast bacilli and with a modified acid-fast stain technique for *Nocardia*.[92] A drop of respiratory secretion should be placed on a microscope slide, under a coverslip, and examined for fungi. Respiratory secretions can be stained directly with fluorescent-antibody for *Legionella pneumophila*.[29] Respiratory secretions should be cultured for bacteria, mycobacteria, *Nocardia*, fungi, and *Legionella pneumophila*. If the results of all these studies are negative or if the patient's condition deteriorates before culture data become available, more invasive diagnostic techniques must be used. These would include transtracheal aspiration, transtracheal bronchial brushing under fluoroscopy, percutaneous aspiration under fluoroscopy, fiberoptic bronchoscopy with bronchial brushing, or transbronchial biopsy and open-lung biopsy. Fluid and tissue specimens should be examined microscopically and cultured as described above. Tissue specimens should also be submitted for histopathologic examination.

When therapy fails after a definitive microbiologic diagnosis has been reached, after therapy has been selected on the basis of susceptibility tests (when these are available), and after antibiotics have been administered in appropriate doses and combinations for maximal antimicrobial effect at the tissue level, complications of the pulmonary infection must be sought. These include bronchial obstruction, bronchopleural fistula, and empyema. Attempts at therapy will be unsuccessful until these complications are diagnosed and treated.

ABSCESSES

Most abscesses in surgical patients are caused by gram-negative bacilli including *Pseudomonas*, gram-negative bacilli mixed with anaerobes, and *Staphylococcus aureus*. These microorganisms gain entrance to tissues from traumatic or surgical disruption of the integument, rupture of organs that contain bacteria, surgical incision into organs that contain bacteria, and hematogenous seeding of tissues. An area of cellulitis may surround the abscess.

Antimicrobial therapy alone is invariably ineffective in treatment of abscesses because of the inability of antibiotics to penetrate the abscess and achieve effective levels in the purulent exudate. There is also evidence that some antibiotics are inactivated by constituents of the exudate in the abscess.[34, 160] The most important therapeutic modality for abscesses is incision and drainage. After the abscess has been incised and is draining freely, antimicrobial agents will usually eradicate microorganisms from the wall of the abscess and from the surrounding cellulitis. Antimicrobial therapy may prevent reaccumulation of the purulent exudate. Thus, antimicrobial therapy is an adjunct to incision and drainage of abscesses. As in the treatment of other infections, therapy will not be effective if the causative microorganisms are resistant to the antibiotics administered and if the antimicrobial agent does not reach sufficient concentrations at the site of infection.

In determining the cause of failure in the therapy of abscesses, the first consideration is whether or not drainage has been effective. Aside from the standard consideration of whether all loculations of exudate within the abscess have been opened, it must be determined whether all abscesses have been discovered. This is particularly important after soilage of the peritoneal cavity with bowel contents and after formation of hematogenous metastatic abscesses with microorganisms such as *Staphylococcus aureus*. When all abscesses have been identified and incised, appropriate antimicrobial therapy should be administered. Although antimicrobial chemotherapy may have been initiated prior to incision and drainage, it is very important to obtain purulent exudate for microscopic examination and culture (including cultures for anaerobic bacteria) at the time of incision and drainage. Initial therapy should be selected on the basis of a Gram-stained smear of exudate. Exudate should be collected so as to minimize the risk of contamination. Ideally, exudate should be aspirated from the abscess prior to incision. If this is not possible, great care should be exercised in avoiding contact of the sterile swab with surrounding areas, which might lead to contamination of the specimen and unreliable culture results. Therapy may not succeed if it is directed at a contaminating microorganism rather than at the causative species.

After identification and susceptibility testing of the causative microorganism, an antimicrobial agent must be selected that will achieve effective levels in tissue when given in appropriate dosage. Certain antimicrobial agents, while effective against the causative microorganism, may not achieve therapeutic levels in tissue. This is true of nitrofurantoin and indanyl carbenicillin, which are useful only for treatment of urinary-tract infections. For serious infections such as intra-abdominal abscesses due to aerobic gram-negative bacilli and anaerobes, antibiotics must be given in large parenteral doses. Such an infection could be treated with gentamicin, tobramycin, or amikacin in doses to give peak serum concentrations of 6 μg to 8 μg/ml for gentamicin and tobramycin and 15 μg to 30 μg/ml for amikacin.[147] Aminoglycoside therapy may be combined with clindamycin given in a dose of 600 mg, IV, every 6 hours. Cefoxitin, an antimicrobial agent active against both gram-negative bacilli and anaerobic bacteria, may be given as single-drug therapy in a dosage of 1 g to 2 g, IV, every 4 hours.[64, 79] Cefoxitin has been reported to attain concentrations in pus of one half to two thirds of the simultaneous serum concentrations.[114] Moxalactam has also been reported to be effective as single-agent therapy for intra-abdominal abscesses.[124] It may be administered as described above. Cefotaxime has also been approved for treatment of intra-abdominal infections. Skin and soft tissue abscesses caused by staphylococci and streptococci may be treated with dicloxacillin in a dose of 500 mg, orally, every 6 hours.

SURGICAL WOUND INFECTIONS

As with antimicrobial therapy of other infections, treatment of surgical wound infections is likely to fail if antibiotics are not administered on the basis of information obtained by appropriate cultures and susceptibility tests. Suitable material for culture cannot be obtained from some wound infections. However, whenever the causative agent cannot be identified, the therapy selected may have no effect on the pathogen. If cultures are collected improperly, they may be contaminated, and if therapy is aimed at the contaminating microorganism, the infecting microorganism may not be eradicated.

Specimens must be handled properly. If specimens containing anaerobic bacteria are left for a prolonged time in the air, the results from culture may be negative. If cultures obtained by sterile swab are allowed to dry for several hours prior to plating, some microorganisms may fail to grow on culture.

Cultures must be taken if a postoperative wound infection fails to respond to therapy. Swabbing the surface of an inflamed wound without purulent drainage may yield only contaminating bacteria or fungi that are not the etiology of the infection. When no purulent material is available for culture, therapy has to be selected empirically on the basis of the clinical setting. Thus, when evidence of a wound infection appears within 24 hours of surgery, the most likely cause is beta hemolytic group A streptococcus and the patient should be treated with penicillin. Erythromycin, clindamycin, and vancomycin could be administered to patients allergic to penicillin. When wound infection complicates laparotomy for fecal soilage of the peritoneal cavity, infection may be caused by gram-negative bacilli and anaerobic bacteria, and appropriate therapy would be gentamicin and clindamycin, or cefoxitin, moxalactam, or cefotaxime given as described above.

If the wound is draining purulent exudate, a sample should be obtained for preparation of a Gram-stained smear and culture. The culture should be taken so that microorganisms on adjacent surfaces will not contaminate the specimen. For instance, a sterile swab may be inserted into the depth of a wound so that it does not touch the wound margins. If an area of fluctuance can be palpated, the collection of exudate should be aspirated after preparation of the overlying surface with an antiseptic. A Gram-stained smear should be examined microscopically, and cultures should be sent for aerobic and anaerobic bacteria. Specimens for anaerobic cultures should be delivered in a capped syringe to the laboratory immediately or placed in a "gassed out" tube or a prereduced anaerobic-holding medium. All cultures should be transported to the laboratory promptly.

Initial antibiotic therapy should be selected on the basis of Gram-stained smear and then appropriate adjustments made after the causative microorganism has been identified and susceptibility tests performed. Antibiotics must be given in appropriate doses and by the appropriate route. Whereas aminoglycosides must be given parenterally, clindamycin can be administered orally for a mild wound infection due to *S. aureus;* however, clindamycin should be given intravenously as described above when used with gentamicin to treat an extensive surgical wound infection.

If antimicrobial therapy fails after initial clinical improvement, the wound should be recultured. The wound may have become superinfected with a resistant microorganism.

BURN-WOUND INFECTIONS

Burn-wound sepsis is a severe and often fatal complication of thermal injury. Antimicrobial therapy of burn-wound infections frequently fails, owing to the difficulty of making the diagnosis, in identifying the causative microorganism, and in achieving therapeutic antibiotic concentrations in the avascular burn eschar.

Therapy is often selected empirically or on the basis of microbial isolates from surface cultures of the eschar. The dose of antimicrobial agent given may also be empirical but it should not be surprising that the empirical approach to therapy frequently fails. The first step in attempting to improve outcome of therapy is to diagnose burn-wound infection definitively. Although quantitative burn-wound biopsy has been advocated for diagnosis, a recent study has demonstrated that this technique is not reliable in establishing the diagnosis of burn-wound sepsis.[98, 172] The only definitive approach is histopathologic examination of a biopsy that extends down to viable tissue beneath the eschar.[126] The extent of penetration of microorganisms is graded 1 to 6. Invasion of subjacent viable tissue (grade 6) is diagnostic of burn-wound infection.

Once the diagnosis has been established, the causative microorganism may be most accurately identified by culture of a biopsy. Another means of establishing the cause of burn-wound infection is by blood culture when other body sites are culture-negative for the bloodstream isolate. After identification of the cause of infection, antimicrobial therapy should be chosen on the basis of susceptibility tests.

Antimicrobial therapy of burn-wound sepsis leaves much to be desired. Many of the microorganisms that cause burn-wound infection are highly resistant to antibiotics. It is difficult to achieve high concentrations of antibiotics in burn eschar, and there are no data on the actual concentrations that can be attained in eschar by the various antibiotics used for therapy. The current approach is to administer antibiotics parenterally in doses to achieve high serum levels. It is assumed that, the higher the serum concentration, the more antibiotic will diffuse down the concentration gradient into the wound.

Burn-wound infections due to *S. aureus* may be treated with a penicillinase-resistant semisynthetic penicillin such as nafcillin, 2 g, IV, every 4 hours. *S. aureus* that is resistant to these drugs may be treated with vancomycin, 500 mg, IV, every 6 hours. Effective treatment of gram-negative burn-wound infections requires frequent tests for serum concentrations of aminoglycosides. Nomograms used to select initial doses of aminoglycosides for treatment of nonburned patients may not be applicable to therapy of infections in burn patients, because burn patients more rapidly eliminate aminoglycosides, in part because of the increased elimination by the kidneys.[81, 147, 176] Burn patients, particularly children and young adults, sustain an increase in glomerular filtration rate.[99] There is also evidence that aminoglycosides may be lost through the burn wound.[69]

Because of the decreased half-life of aminoglycosides in burn patients, doses are larger and at shorter intervals than for patients without burns. For patients with normal renal function, gentamicin may have to be given in a dosage of up to 7.2 mg/kg/day in older patients and 12.0 mg/kg/day in young adults and children.[175] To prevent gentamicin from falling to subtherapeutic levels between doses, the dosing interval may have to be shortened to 4 hours. Tobramycin will probably need to be given in similar doses.[99] In patients with normal renal function, amikacin may need be given at an initial dose of 30 mg/kg/day in four equal doses every 6 hours.[176] *It must be emphasized that, for each of these amino-*

glycosides, serum concentrations must be determined frequently and the dose modified to achieve therapeutic but nontoxic serum levels. Peak concentrations of gentamicin and tobramycin should probably be 8 μg to 10 μg/ml and peak concentrations of amikacin, 30 μg/ml. Another antibiotic to which the infecting microorgansims are susceptible should also be given. For patients with normal renal function, carbenicillin may be administered at a dose of 500 μg to 800 μg/kg/day in equally divided doses, IV, every 4 hours.[175, 176] A cephalosporin may be given at high dosage as described above for serious infections.

When therapy fails after the diagnosis has been established, after the causative microorganism has been demonstrated to be susceptible to the antibiotic selected, and after therapeutic serum concentrations have been achieved, other foci of infection should be sought and infection due to nonbacterial microorganisms considered. Septic thrombophlebitis and endocarditis also must be considered.[14, 118, 127] Nonbacterial pathogens that may cause burn-wound infection include fungi such as *Candida, Aspergillus,* and Zygomycetes.[32, 55, 101, 115, 129] Herpesvirus may also cause burn-wound infection.[54]

MENINGITIS AND VENTRICULITIS

If the infecting microorganism is resistant to the antimicrobial agent selected for therapy, treatment will be unsuccessful. Therapy will also fail if the antibiotic fails to reach therapeutic concentrations at the site of infection. This second consideration is particularly likely to explain failure of meningitis therapy, since many antibiotics do not reach therapeutic levels in cerebrospinal fluid (CSF), even when given in high intravenous doses.

In assessing the reasons for failure of therapy of meningitis and ventriculitis, the first step is to establish whether or not the causative microorganism is susceptible to the antibiotic selected for treatment. Although it is unlikely that a physician would treat meningitis without obtaining a CSF culture, it is important to perform susceptibility tests on the isolates and to choose therapy on that basis.

Another problem may arise when cultures are obtained after one or more doses of antibiotic have been given. Although the antibiotic selected may not be appropriate for the microorganism in the CSF, the presence of antibiotic in CSF may prevent recovery of the microorganism on culture. There may be no clinical response, or after an initial response, the infection may relapse. Thus, selecting effective therapy may be difficult. A lumbar puncture repeated early after initiation of antimicrobial therapy might yield CSF with a useful positive Gram-stained smear. Infections at other sites in the body may provide clues since the same microorganism could have infected the meninges hematogenously or by direct extension. The clinical setting may provide useful information. For instance, if the infection occurs after a neurosurgical operation, the most likely cause is either *S. aureus* or a gram-negative bacillus. When the cause cannot be determined or the possibilities narrowed, the patient must be treated with antimicrobial agents that cover all of the possibilities.

After identifying the infectious agent and determining its antimicrobial susceptibility, the antibiotic must be selected on the basis of susceptibility tests and whether or not therapeutic concentrations of the antibiotic can be attained in the CSF. From the outset, it must be determined whether, in addition to meningitis, there may also be infection of the ventricular system. Attaining effective concentrations of antibiotic in CSF in the subarachnoid space does not always assure therapeutic levels in CSF in the ventricles. Ventriculitis should be suspected when the patient has meningitis due to gram-negative bacilli.[1, 73, 84, 125, 143] Ventriculitis may follow seeding of the ventricles during gram-negative bacteremia or after penetrating trauma, neurosurgical operations, or placement of ventriculostomy. Although meningitis is diagnosed by culture of CSF obtained by lumbar puncture, the only way to diagnose ventriculitis definitively is by obtaining CSF directly from the ventricles for culture.

Few antimicrobial agents penetrate the blood–brain barrier in sufficient quantities to attain high CSF concentrations, even in the presence of meningeal inflammation. However, most infections due to gram-positive cocci, *Neisseria meningitidis,* and *Hemophilus influenzae* can be treated successfully with antimicrobial agents administered parenterally in high doses. Infections caused by *Streptococcus pneumoniae,* beta hemolytic group A streptococci, and meningococci respond to aqueous penicillin G, 2 million units given IV every 2 hours. These microorganisms and strains of *Hemophilus influenzae* that do not produce beta lactamase will respond to ampicillin, 2 g, IV, every 4 hours. Ampicillin-resistant *Hemophilus influenzae* meningitis is treated with chloramphenicol, 1 g, IV, every 6 hours. Meningitis due to *Staphylococcus aureus* should be treated with nafcillin at a dose of 100 mg to 200 mg/kg/day, IV, in equally divided doses every 4 hours.[86, 141] Infection due to *S. aureus* that is resistant to methicillin, nafcillin, and other semisynthetic penicillins can be treated with vancomycin, 40 mg/kg/day in four equally divided doses, IV, every 6 hours up to a maximum of 2 g per day.[38] Rifampin, 600 mg given orally every 12 hours, combined with vancomycin, may provide even more effective therapy of meningitis due to methicillin-resistant *S. aureus.*

Chloramphenicol has been used to treat meningitis due to susceptible gram-negative bacilli for many years. However, treatment failures with chloramphenicol have been frequently reported. Apparently, chloramphenicol lacks a bactericidal effect on gram-negative bacilli in CSF, which is needed for effective therapy of meningitis.[95, 132] Thus, chloramphenicol is not recommended for treatment of gram-negative bacillary meningitis.

The most effective therapy for gram-negative bacillary meningitis is provided by the aminoglycosides. However, because they cross the blood–brain barrier so poorly, they must be administered both systemically and intrathecally or intraventricularly.[26, 84] Gentamicin and tobramycin should be administered intravenously to achieve peak serum concentrations of 6 μg to 8 μg/ml.[147] Gentamicin may be given intrathecally at the lumbar level at a dose of 4 mg, every 18 hours, or 5 mg, every 24 hours.[84, 131] It has been suggested that, if cultures remain positive at 36 hours, intrathecal injections of 8 mg to 12 mg be given every 24 hours.[131]

Although good results have been reported with intrathecal gentamicin, failures have also been reported with this route of administration.[84, 104, 111] Failure of intrathecal therapy for gram-negative bacillary meningitis with ventriculitis is not surprising since the flow of CSF is unidirectional out of the ventricles to the subarachnoid space.[45] Further, whereas concentrations of gentamicin in both ventricular and the lumbar subarachnoid CSF reach therapeutic levels after intraventricular administration, concentrations in intraventricular CSF are very low when gentamicin is administered intrathecally at the lumbar level.[84, 104] Although intrathecal administration of gentamicin may be effective for gram-negative bacillary meningitis (presumably in cases without ventriculitis), when patients do not respond to intrathecal therapy, the drug should be administered intraventricularly. Gentamicin or tobramycin may be injected by way of a ventriculostomy or though an Ommaya or Rickham reservoir at a dosage of 5 mg, every 18 to 24 hours.[84]

There is less experience with intrathecal and intraventricular administration of amikacin. This drug should also be administered parenterally in doses to achieve peak concentrations of 15 μg to 30 μg/ml.[147] Amikacin has been given in doses of either 4 mg or 10 mg, every 12 hours, intrathecally.[77, 150] The drug has also been administered to pediatric patients by the intraventricular route in a variable dose of 1 mg to 8 mg per 24 hours, with the dose for each patient being selected to provide a concentration of 0.1 mg/ml in the estimated CSF volume.[168]

If the infecting microorganism is susceptible, carbenicillin may also be given intravenously in combination with parenteral and intrathecal or intraventricular aminoglycosides. The suggested dosage for neonates is 300 mg/kg per day to 800 mg/kg per day given IV in equally divided doses every 4 hours.[138] The suggested dosage for adults is 30 g to 40 g per day given IV in six equally divided doses.[130]

Cephalosporins have generally been ineffective for treatment of meningitis owing to their poor penetration into CSF. However, early studies indicate that cefotaxime and moxalactam may provide effective intravenous therapy for gram-negative meningitis [17, 56, 95, 117] This is due to the increased activity of these two drugs against gram-negative bacilli compared to first- and second-generation cephalosporins and the effective penetration of cefotaxime and moxalactam into the CSF. If additional studies confirm these results they, and other cephalosporins still being developed, may become the drugs of choice for treatment of gram-negative bacillary meningitis. The dosage of cefotaxime for treatment of gram-negative meningitis in patients with normal renal function is 2 g, IV, every 4 hours.[95] Moxalactam should be given in a dose of 2 g to 4 g, IV, every 8 hours.[95]

INFECTIONS OF THE BILIARY TRACT

Failure of therapy of infections in the biliary tract, as at other body sites, may be due to the presence of microorganisms that are resistant to the antimicrobial chemotherapeutic agent administered. Another cause for treatment failure is the absence of therapeutic concentrations of antibiotic at the site of infection. This can be due to administration of antibiotics in doses too low or by the wrong route, the inherent inability of certain antibiotics to achieve therapeutic concentrations in bile when the biliary tract is patent, and the failure of almost all antimicrobial agents to enter the biliary tract in the presence of complete obstruction of the common duct. Further, as in infections at other body sites, antimicrobial therapy will predictably fail in the face of undrained purulent exudate, such as in empyema of the gallbladder, or when there is cholangitis secondary to a stone impacted in the common duct.

When a patient with symptoms and signs of biliary-tract infection fails to respond to antimicrobial therapy, the first consideration is to rule out the possible complications of undrained purulent exudate and complete obstruction. The treatment of these complications is surgical, and antibiotics play an adjunctive role by preventing septicemia and local infectious complications in the operative wound.[88]

Although cultures of bile may be taken at operation and results of cultures used to adjust antibiotic therapy, antibiotics must be started as soon as biliary-tract infection is suspected. To maximize the likelihood that an antibiotic to which the infecting organism will be susceptible is selected for therapy, the microbiology of the diseased biliary tract must be understood. The microorganism most commonly isolated from the infected biliary tree is *Escherichia coli*. Other frequently isolated microorganisms include *Klebsiella*, enteric streptococci, and *Enterobacter*.[36, 49, 50, 60, 88, 133] Many other species have been isolated less frequently. Anaerobic bacteria may be more important than once thought. In a recent study, 41% of positive cultures from the biliary tract contained anaerobes, and *Bacteroides fragilis* was the fourth most common isolate after *E. coli*, group D streptococci, and *Klebsiella*.[49] *Clostridium perfringens* made up 5.9% of all isolates.

Although it is important to select antimicrobial agents that are excreted in therapeutic concentrations in bile, no antibiotic is excreted in the presence of complete obstruction of the biliary tract. However, even when complete obstruction or undrained purulent exudate is present, administration of antimicrobial agents is of great importance in preventing septicemia and infection of the operative wound.[60, 88]

Many antimicrobial agents currently in use attain therapeutic concentrations in gallbladder bile and common-duct bile in the absence of obstruction. These include ampicillin, cefazolin, cefamandole, clindamycin, trimethoprim-sulfamethoxazole, penicillin, tetracycline, erythromycin, rifampin, and moxalactam.[27, 28, 31, 88, 113, 121, 124, 134, 135] Gentamicin achieves therapeutic concentrations in the bile of some patients, but biliary levels may be subtherapeutic in the majority of patients.[108, 122] In spite of the relatively poor penetration of gentamicin into bile, the best combination for therapy is probably gentamicin and ampicillin. Gentamicin provides adequate therapy for gram-negative bacilli and, combined with ampicillin, for enteric streptococci. Ampicillin will be effective for *E. coli* and *Proteus mirabilis* and most anaerobic bacteria including *Clostridium perfringens*. For effective therapy, gentamicin must be given in a dose to provide peak serum levels of 6 μg to 8 μg/ml.[147] Ampicillin can be used at a dose of 1 g to 2 g, IV, every 4 hours. Alternative drugs that could be used in patients with penicillin allergy include cefazolin, cefamandole, and trimethoprim-sulfamethoxazole.

Hypersensitivity Reactions

ANAPHYLAXIS, CUTANEOUS ERUPTIONS, AND DRUG FEVER

Anaphylaxis

Anaphylaxis is the most severe reaction encountered in the treatment of patients with antibiotics. Although administration of any antibiotic may be complicated by this syndrome, anaphylactic reactions are most frequently encountered after parenteral injection of penicillin or one of its synthetic analogues.

Anaphylaxis results from rapid release of certain pharmacologically active mediators after interaction between an antigen and IgE antibody. The antigen–antibody reaction causes a release of these mediators from basophils and mast cells including histamine, slowly reacting substance of anaphylaxis, and, perhaps, serotonin and bradykinin.[89] The clinical manifestations of anaphylaxis result from action of these mediators on target organs in the body. The basic actions are bronchial constriction, increased capillary permeability, and vasodilatation.

Clinically, the reaction has its onset from 5 to 60 minutes after injection of a drug. After oral ingestion, onset of anaphylaxis may be delayed several hours or may start in minutes. Patients develop bronchial constriction manifested by a feeling of tightness in the chest or wheezing.[8] Laryngeal edema is manifested by hoarseness, stridor, or the feeling of a "lump" in the throat. Patients may sustain primary vascular collapse with hypotension. Dermal manifestations include a pruritic urticarial eruption. Many lesions may coalesce to form giant hives. Angioedema may also occur. Patients may develop nausea, vomiting, cramping abdominal pain, and diarrhea.

Since most reactions appear within minutes of parenteral injection and the clinical manifestations are dramatic, diagnosis is usually not difficult. Difficulty may arise when patients present after having received an antibiotic at another medical facility or when the offending drug is ingested at home several hours before onset of symptoms. When patients are seen with symptoms and signs compatible with anaphylaxis, a drug history should be taken while immediate therapy is prepared. Although penicillins are most frequently the cause of anaphylaxis, anaphylactic reactions have been seen with administration of most of the antibiotics. The rate of anaphylactic reactions to penicillin has been reported as 0.04% with a fatality rate of 0.0014%.[140]

The drug of choice for treatment of anaphylaxis is epinephrine, 1:1000, given at a dose of 0.3 ml intramuscularly.[89] Depending on the body site, tourniquets should be placed proximal to the injection site, and the injected site should be infiltrated with epinephrine to slow absorption of the offending drug. Epinephrine is not ordinarily given intravenously because of the risk of producing a cardiac arrhythmia. However, when anaphylaxis is very severe, epinephrine may have to be administered intravenously to achieve a clinical response. Laryngeal edema may be managed initially with epinephrine and antihistamines under close observation. Progression of the laryngeal edema is an indication for immediate tracheostomy. Endotracheal intubation may not be possible. Persistent hypotension that does not respond to epinephrine may be treated with volume expanders and vasconstrictors. Even mild symptoms of anaphylaxis such as urticaria and pruritis should be treated, because they may be forerunners of a much more serious reaction.

Prevention of anaphylaxis depends on a thorough drug history prior to administering antibiotics. When the history is in doubt, drugs to which the patient may be sensitive should be avoided. There is a lower risk of anaphylaxis when drugs can be administered orally. When drugs are given parenterally, the patient should be observed for at least 30 minutes, and emergency equipment and supplies should be readily available.

Cutaneous Eruptions

The most common manifestation of hypersensitivity to antibiotics is a dermal eruption. Although a skin eruption is most frequently associated with administration of the penicillins, allergic eruptions may be associated with most of the antibiotics currently in use. Whereas anaphylactic reactions are due to the immediate type of hypersensitivity mediated by an antigen–antibody reaction involving IgE antibodies, skin eruptions that complicate antimicrobial therapy are due to delayed hypersensitivity mediated by the cellular immune system.[163] Dermal eruptions caused by hypersensitivity to antibiotics may be morbilliform, petechial, maculopapular, or bullous. Stevens–Johnson syndrome, exfoliative dermatitis, and erythema nodosum may also occur.

Skin eruptions are most frequently associated with administration of the penicillins.[7] An allergic eruption due to penicillin may occur as early as 24 to 48 hours or as late as 5 weeks after starting therapy.[53] The eruption may also occur as late as 1 week after penicillin treatment has been discontinued. Patients who have a history of atopy have an incidence of skin reactivity to penicillin three to four times greater than that of nonatopic persons.[163] Of all the penicillins, administration of ampicillin is most frequently complicated by a cutaneous eruption. Patients who are receiving allopurinol, who have an elevated blood uric acid, who receive the drug parenterally, or who have infectious mononucleosis or chronic lymphocytic leukemia have an even greater risk of developing a cutaneous reaction to ampicillin.[53] In addition to the penicillins, other antibiotics commonly associated with dermal eruptions are the cephalosporins, vancomycin, clindamycin, trimethoprim-sulfamethoxazole, erythromycin, nitrofurantoin, gentamicin, and sulfasoxazole.[7, 38, 58, 63]

No laboratory test can diagnose drug-related skin eruptions. When a rash of any type appears during antimicrobial therapy, the possibility of a drug eruption should always be considered, particularly when the drug administered is frequently associated with skin eruptions. The drug that appears to be causing the eruption should be withdrawn. Although the skin eruption may resolve while the drug is continued, the best course of action is to discontinue administration of the drug when a dermal reaction appears. If treatment is continued, the eruption may worsen.[53] For example, when patients treated with a penicillin are continued on therapy after the appearance of an allergic eruption, they may develop laryngeal edema, hypotension, exfoliative dermatitis, or hematologic and renal manifestations of penicillin allergy.[96]

The most important approach to prevention is a careful drug history before starting antibiotic therapy and avoiding drugs to which the patient has a history of sensitivity. Use of nafcillin rather than methicillin may lessen the chance for an allergic reaction, because nafcillin therapy appears to be complicated less often by drug eruption.[85]

Another approach is to select an agent from another class of antibiotics that would be unlikely to cross react with the drug to which the patient is allergic. A class of drugs that is frequently considered for therapy of infections in patients allergic to the penicillins is the cephalosporins. Since the penicillins and cephalosporins share the beta lactam ring, cross reactivity may occur, but this probably occurs in no more than 5% to 10% of the cases.[103, 128] Cephalosporins can usually be given safely to patients allergic to penicillins, but they should be avoided in patients who have had an immediate or anaphylactic reaction to the penicillins.

Drug Fever

Drug fever may be the most difficult complication to diagnose. It may not be possible to differentiate fever due to the infection from that due to the drug administered for therapy. Further, other drugs administered simultaneously with the antimicrobial agents must also be considered possible causes of fever.

Although the pathophysiology of drug fever is not well understood, it is presumed to be a hypersensitivity reaction since it frequently occurs with other conditions known to have an allergic basis, such as drug eruption and interstitial nephritis.

Drug fever has been reported as a complication of therapy with penicillins, cephalosporins, streptomycin, kanamycin, chloramphenicol, erythromycin, sulfonamides, vancomycin, and nitrofurantoin.[38, 91, 103, 119, 128, 144–146] However, drug fever may be associated with the use of any antimicrobial agent. The fever may or may not be accompanied by eosinophilia or cutaneous eruption. Drug fever due to the penicillins may be continuous, remittent, or intermittent, and occasionally is accompanied by chills.[103] Fever usually clears in 24 to 36 hours after the penicillin is stopped. When fever is severe and sustained, the inciting drug should be discontinued immediately, because small-vessel inflammation is usually present and continued administration may lead to serious visceral or cutaneous complications.[119]

Because diagnosis of drug fever may be difficult, it should always be considered when fever is sustained or recurs in the face of apparently effective therapy. Fever that is associated with eosinophilia and a skin eruption is likely due to the antimicrobial agent administered or some other therapeutic agent such as quinidine, procainamide, the thiouracils, or anticonvulsants.[119]

Treatment of drug fever is prompt withdrawal of the suspected antibiotic. Drug fever usually can not be prevented since most patients do not give a history of previous drug fever. However, when patients have a history of any type of hypersensitivity reaction to an antibiotic, the agent should not be used.

Hypersensitivity Pneumonitis

Many drugs may cause hypersensitivity reactions in the lungs, and among these are three classes of antibiotics: the nitrofurantoins, sulfonamides, and penicillins.[137] The pathophysiology of the hypersensitivity reaction to nitrofurantoin is different from that of the reaction to the sulfonamides and penicillins. The pulmonary reaction to nitrofurantoin is characterized by an interstitial infiltrative process with thickening of the alveolar septae but no involvement of blood vessels or bronchi.[65] In contrast, sulfonamides and the penicillins cause a reaction in the lungs characterized by allergic angiitis or angiitic granulomatosis.[137]

The pneumonitis due to nitrofurantoin is characterized by fever, chills, dyspnea, and cough with onset from 2 hours to 10 days after therapy is begun. A diffuse alveolar or alveolar-interstitial infiltrate appears on chest x-ray examination. The syndrome clears within 24 to 48 hours after the drug is discontinued.[137] Eosinophilia occurs in up to 83% of patients. Patients frequently give a history of previous therapy with an adverse reaction to nitrofurantoin. The risk for developing this reaction seems to increase with age and is low in children.[80]

The pneumonitis caused by the sulfonamides and penicillins is also characterized by pulmonary infiltrates with eosinophilia.[137] Eosinophilic migrating pneumonia may occur as a complication of sulfonamide administration.[102]

The diagnosis of hypersensitivity pneumonitis should be suspected, particularly in patients who are receiving nitrofurantoin, when the patient develops fever, chills, dyspnea, and cough within a few days of starting therapy. The diagnosis is supported by the presence of eosinophilia and a history of previous treatment with nitrofurantoin. The diagnosis is highly likely if there is a previous adverse reaction to nitrofurantoin. Treatment for hypersensitivity pneumonitis is prompt withdrawal of the inciting drug. The patient should be advised not to take the drug again.

Interstitial Nephritis

Most reported cases of interstitial nephritis that complicate antibiotic therapy have been associated with the administration of methicillin. Although no controlled studies have been done, a recent publication reported that none of 29 patients treated wtih nafcillin developed interstitial nephritis while 5 of 41 patients treated with methicillin developed interstitial nephritis.[85] The only other antibiotic with which documented interstitial nephritis has been associated is penicillin G.[9]

Interstitial nephritis appears to be caused by a hypersensitivity reaction to methicillin or penicillin G.[9, 46] The dose of drug given is not related to the subsequent development of interstitial nephritis. Pathologically, interstitial nephritis is characterized by edema, mild to moderate tubular atrophy, lymphocytic infiltrates, and aggregation of plasmacytes and eosinophils to a variable degree. Glomeruli only occasionally show pathologic changes.[46]

Clinically, interstitial nephritis has its onset between 2 days and about 6 weeks after initiation of methicillin or penicillin therapy. Fever or hematuria is usually the first sign of nephritis. Other manifestations include proteinuria, leukocyturia, eosinophiluria, and eosinophilia. A generalized morbilliform cutaneous eruption or erythroderma may appear. The most serious manifestation is azotemia and renal failure, which occurs in about 50% of the adult patients. Renal failure appears to be a rare complication in patients under 16 years of age. The signs of hypersensitivity reaction are prolonged in azotemic patients compared to those who are nonazotemic. In some patients, the renal impairment is severe enough to require hemodialysis. Azotemia lasts an average of 45 days with a range of 2 to 12 months after methicillin therapy is discontinued. A few patients show signs of irreversible renal damage.[9, 46, 174] One death attributed to interstitial nephritis caused by penicillin therapy has been reported.[9]

The diagnosis of interstitial nephritis should be considered in any patient who is receiving a penicillin antibiotic, and who, after an initial response to therapy, again develops fever. It would appear from the literature that most cases of interstitial nephritis occur as a complication of methicillin therapy. The diagnosis is supported by the presence of fever, a morbilliform cutaneous eruption or erythroderma, eosinophilia, and the presence of red blood cells and white blood cells in the urine sediment. The diagnosis is essentially confirmed when eosinophils are seen on a Wright's stained smear of the urine sediment.

The most important consideration in treatment is discontinuation of the offending drug. Complete recovery of renal function occurs in 90% of the patients with this treatment alone. A high index of suspicion should always be maintained for this complication, because early recognition and withdrawal of the drug are necessary if renal function is to be preserved. The use of steroids is controversial. There are reports that suggest that steroids are effective for treatment of drug-induced interstitial nephritis, but other authors have noted no apparent benefit.[46, 68, 100, 174]

Another important consideration in management of interstitial nephritis is avoidance of other penicillin or cephalosporin antibiotics when treatment must be continued after the offending drug is withdrawn. There are reports of exacerbation of the nephritis when methicillin was replaced by ampicillin or nafcillin.[68, 120] Therapy should be reinstituted with another chemically unrelated drug such as vancomycin with the dosage appropriately adjusted for the level of renal function.[112]

The best way to prevent interstitial nephritis is to avoid use of methicillin since most of the cases reported in the literature have been due to this drug. One study indicated that methicillin is more frequently associated with adverse reactions, including interstitial nephritis, than is nafcillin.[85] A history of hypersensitivity reactions to penicillin does not seem to be important in predicting whether interstitial nephritis will occur in patients treated with methicillin.[46] Thus, a history of penicillin allergy is not associated with a higher frequency of interstitial nephritis, and the absence of a history of hypersensitivity does not preclude the development of interstitial nephritis.

Direct Organ Toxicity Caused by Antimicrobial Agents

NEUROTOXICITY OF THE PENICILLINS

Although the most common untoward effect of penicillin G is due to drug hypersensitivity, it may also have a direct toxic effect on the nervous system. The pathophysiology of neurotoxicity due to penicillin is not well understood, but it is related to the concentration of the drug in the CSF. There is some evidence that concentrations of greater than 10 μg/ml in CSF at the lumbar level may correlate with neurotoxicity.[151] Most cases of neurotoxicity have occurred at serum concentrations of at least 200 μg/ml.[33] Owing to the great capacity of the normal kidney to excrete penicillin, it is very difficult to achieve such serum concentrations in patients with normal renal function, even with massive intravenous doses. However, even moderate doses readily produce such levels in patients with marked renal impairment. Thus, most patients who develop neurotoxicity have diminished renal function. Other conditions that may predispose patients to neurotoxicity are inflammation of the meninges with greater penetration of the drug into CSF, hyponatremia, and underlying disease of the nervous system.

Clinically, the disease is manifested by the early appearance of myoclonus involving the muscles of the face and extremities and generalized hyperreflexia.[151] These signs may be followed by somnolence, coma, and tonoclonic grand mal seizures. Occasionally patients may also hallucinate.[37] Patients usually have significant renal impairment and may be overhydrated and have hyponatremia. Patients under 1 month and over 60 years of age are particularly susceptible to penicillin neurotoxicity.[162]

Treatment involves discontinuation of the penicillin. Signs of neurotoxicity usually subside within 12 to 24 hours after the dose is markedly reduced or the drug is discontinued.[151] Seizures that occur while administration of the penicillin continues will not respond even to very high doses of anticonvulsant drugs. Penicillin antibiotics other than penicillin G may also be associated with neurotoxicity, and they will also have to be discontinued when the signs appear.[37]

Prevention of penicillin neurotoxicity involves proper dosing of patients who have impaired renal function. Patients who are anephric may be treated for serious infections such as endocarditis with only 3 million units per 24 hours divided into equal doses every 8 hours; a table of doses for various levels of renal function has been published.[33] Hyponatremia should be corrected. It must be kept in mind that, even when serum creatinine is in the normal range, infants under 1 month and adults over 60 years of age have a diminished capacity to excrete penicillins.

Ampicillin dosage must be adjusted for severe renal impairment, and an appropriate dose would be 0.5 g to 1.0 g, IV, every 8 hours. Methicillin dosage must be decreased from 12 g, IV, per day for patients with normal renal function to 3 g to 6 g per day given in equally divided doses every 8 hours in patients with severe renal impairment.[4] Unlike the other penicillins, nafcillin is largely eliminated from the body by nonrenal mechanisms and requires no dosage adjustment for renal insufficiency.[44, 139] Thus, for serious infections due to *S. aureus*, all patients should be treated with 2 g, IV, every 4 hours. The usual dosage of carbenicillin for patients with normal renal function is 5 g to 6 g, IV, every 4 hours.

This dosage should be reduced by half in patients with mild renal impairment and should be reduced to 2 g, IV, every 12 hours in patients with markedly reduced renal function. Ticarcillin is also given in a reduced dosage of 2 g, IV, every 4 hours in patients with mild renal impairment and in a dose of 2 g, IV, every 12 hours when renal function is markedly reduced.[4]

CARBENICILLIN

Among the direct toxic effects of carbenicillin are overloading with sodium, hypokalemic alkalosis, inhibition of platelet agglutination, and hepatitis.

Each gram of carbenicillin disodium contains 4.7 mEq of sodium, and, thus, about 1 g of sodium is received by the patient for each 10 g of carbenicillin disodium administered. The large amount of sodium that accompanies the infusion of carbenicillin may be a problem in patients with such conditions as congestive heart failure, cirrhosis, and renal failure, and they must be observed for signs of sodium overload such as worsening congestive heart failure.

Up to 9% of patients treated with carbenicillin may develop hypokalemia.[90] Carbenicillin may induce hypokalemia by acting as a nonreabsorbable anion and by causing an increase in passive renal distal tubular potassium excretion. Hypokalemia due to carbenicillin may predispose patients to digitalis intoxication and may accentuate hypokalemia due to other causes such as steroid or diuretic therapy. Hypokalemia caused by carbenicillin may be difficult to treat and may require very large doses of potassium chloride.[35] This complication may be prevented by frequent determination of serum potassium concentrations and early administration of potassium chloride when concentrations fall below the normal range.

The inhibition of hemostasis that complicates the administration of carbenicillin has particular importance for surgical patients because it has been associated with postoperative bleeding.[30, 74] The adverse effect on hemostasis appears to be mediated by a decrease in adenosine-diphosphate-induced platelet aggregation with the defect occurring at the level of the megakaryocyte. Although it has generally been thought that abnormal hemostasis occurs only in the presence of toxic levels, particularly in patients with renal failure, a bleeding diathesis may complicate the treatment of patients who have therapeutic, nontoxic carbenicillin serum concentrations.[74]

The first indications of a hemorrhagic diathesis due to carbenicillin may be petechiae and gastrointestinal bleeding. Postoperatively, patients may develop wound oozing or severe wound hemorrhage. Treatment consists of withdrawal of the drug. Bleeding may clear within 48 hours of cessation of carbenicillin therapy. In severe cases, patients may benefit from platelet transfusions since the carbenicillin seems to act on the megakaryocytes and not on mature platelets.[74] Prevention of this complication may not be possible unless use of the drug is avoided at the time of surgery. If this antibiotic must be given prior to surgery, the dosage should be adjusted to provide serum concentrations in the therapeutic, nontoxic range. Since the same type of platelet dysfunction is induced by ticarcillin, it is unlikely that the bleeding diathesis caused by carbenicillin can be avoided by using ticarcillin.[3, 83]

The incidence of the hepatitis that complicates carbenicillin therapy is unknown, but hepatitis is probably an uncommon side-effect. The cause is also unknown, but it appears to have a direct toxic effect on the liver and not lead to a hypersensitivity reaction.[167] Clinically, hepatotoxicity is manifested by anicteric hepatitis, Patients develop nausea, vomiting, a tender liver, and sometimes hepatomegaly. There are elevations of serum glutamic-oxaloacetic transaminase, serum glutamic-pyruvic transaminase, and alkaline phosphatase, but bilirubin remains in the normal range. Liver biopsy shows minimal spotty hepatic necrosis. Treatment is withdrawal of the drug. The hepatitis appears to be reversible, at least in the early stages. It is not necessary to avoid use of other penicillins after carbenicillin hepatotoxicity because there is no evidence of cross reactivity with other penicillins. Attempts at reinstitution of carbenicillin therapy after results of liver function tests have returned to normal may lead to reappearance of the hepatitis, even when carbenicillin is given in lower doses.[167]

CEPHALOSPORINS

The only significant direct organ toxicity of cephalosporins is nephrotoxicity. Although it has been recognized for many years that cephaloridine is nephrotoxic, it has been difficult to prove that nephrotoxicity that occurs in patients treated with other cephalosporins is actually due to the cephalosporin administered.[4] Many of these patients have been concurrently treated with other nephrotoxic drugs such as aminoglycosides and frequently have been severely ill with complications such as sepsis, dehydration, hypotension, and acidosis. Thus, whether or not the use of cephalosporins other than cephaloridine is significantly associated with nephrotoxicity has been difficult to determine. With the exception of cephaloridine, cephalosporins given alone are probably rare causes of nephrotoxicity.[128, 169] There is good evidence that cephalothin potentiates the nephrotoxicity of gentamicin and tobramycin.[161] It

TABLE 19-1. DOSES OF CEPHALOSPORIN ANTIBIOTICS GIVEN INTRAVENOUSLY FOR VARYING DEGREES OF RENAL DYSFUNCTION IN ADULT PATIENTS WITH MODERATE TO SEVERE INFECTIONS

	Dosages for Varying Levels of Renal Function		
Antibiotic	*Normal*	*Mild to Moderate Failure*	*Severe Failure*
Cephalothin[20]	1–2 g every 4 hr	No change	1–2 g every 8–12 hr
Cefazolin[164]	0.5–1 g every 6 hr	0.5 g every 8 hr	100–200 mg every 8 hr
Cephapirin[4]	1–2 g every 4 hr	No change	1 g every 12 hr
Cefamandole[6]	1–2 g every 4 hr	No change	1 g every 24 hr
Cefoxitin[4]	1–2 g every 4 hr	No change	1 g every 12–24 hr
Cefotaxime[170]	1–2 g every 4-6 hr	1 g every 12 hr	0.5 g every 12 hr

is not known whether this effect occurs with other cephalosporins. Although combination therapy with an aminoglycoside and a cephalosporin may have a slightly increased risk of inducing renal damage, this should not deter the use of this combination when antimicrobial susceptibility tests indicate that the combination will provide the most effective therapy.

Cefamandole and moxalactam have been associated with bleeding abnormalities and a disulfuran-like effect.[124] The defect in coagulation is probably due to hypoprothrombinemia brought about by vitamin K deficiency. The deficiency of vitamin K is thought to be caused by reduction in the numbers of bacteria in the gastrointestinal tract that produce vitamin K. This adverse effect on bacteria in the gastrointestinal tract may be related to the high concentrations of these drugs in bile. It is not yet known how frequently this side-effect may occur and whether it poses a significant risk for intraoperative and postoperative bleeding in surgical patients. Hypoprothrombinemia can be reversed by administration of 10 mg of vitamin K. Patients with renal impairment, preexisting coagulation defects, and decreased vitamin K reserves may be at higher risk, and prophylactic vitamin K may offer some protection.

Since the primary route of excretion for cephalosporins is the kidney, all of these drugs accumulate in the serum of patients with marked renal impairment unless dosage is reduced. Dosages of cephalosporins for patients with impaired renal function are shown in Table 19-1. The dosage of moxalactam for patients with varying degrees of renal impairment may be calculated from the nomogram in the package insert or from a published nomogram.[24]

AMINOGLYCOSIDES

The newer aminoglycosides are very important drugs for treatment of infections in surgical patients. They have a broad spectrum of activity against gram-negative bacilli including *Pseudomonas*. The most important aminoglycosides are gentamicin, tobramycin, and amikacin. Owing to their limited antimicrobial spectrum, kanamycin and streptomycin are infrequently used to treat surgical infections.

All of the aminoglycosides are excreted primarily by the kidneys by glomerular filtration. Each is associated with nephrotoxicity and ototoxicity. The nephrotoxicity of the aminoglycosides is manifested pathologically by tubular necrosis.[5] Although there is no absolute proof of cause and effect, toxicity may be related to the accumulation of aminoglycoside in the kidney parenchyma, particularly in the cortex.[48, 148]

Nephrotoxicity occurs at a frequency of 2% to 10%. Clinically, it is manifested by a decrease in renal function and a rise in serum creatinine concentration. Patients have proteinuria and granular cylindruria.[5] Renal failure may be oliguric or nonoliguric. The renal impairment is reversible if the drug is withdrawn early after onset of signs of toxicity.

There are several risk factors for the nephrotoxicity due to aminoglycosides. These include diminished renal function (frequently unrecognized in elderly patients with serum creatinine levels in the normal range), previous therapy with aminoglycosides, previous renal damage, contracted intravascular volume, and concomitant treatment with the anesthetic methoxyflurane. The role of furosemide and ethacrynic acid in potentiating nephrotoxicity of aminoglycosides remains to be clarified. There is also a relationship between serum levels of aminoglycoside and toxicity. This seems to be particularly the case with trough levels because there is evidence of a significant relationship between trough levels of gentamicin greater than 2 μg/ml and of amikacin greater than 10 μg/ml and nephrotoxicity.[43, 152] It also appears that peak levels of gentamicin greater than 10 μg/ml and of amikacin greater than 38.5 μg/ml are significantly related to toxicity. Total dose administered does not seem to be related to toxicity.[152]

Nephrotoxicity due to aminoglycosides should be suspected when patients treated with these drugs develop a rise in serum creatinine levels. Other factors that should heighten the suspicion of nephrotoxicity include concomitant administration of other nephrotoxic drugs, the development of proteinuria and cylindruria, and serum aminoglycoside concentrations that exceed the upper limits of the normal range.

Treatment of nephrotoxicity is limited to withdrawal of the offending drug. When the drug is stopped early after onset of signs of toxicity, the renal damage is usually reversible. However, serum creatinine levels may continue to rise for a week to 10 days after the aminoglycoside is discontinued before starting to return toward normal. If possible, it would be appropriate to discontinue other nephrotoxic drugs as well.

Prevention of nephrotoxicity involves proper dosing with the aminoglycosides. The initial dose should be chosen using a nomogram based on the level of renal function.[81, 147] Dosage should be selected to achieve appropriate peak and trough levels, as mentioned above. After three doses, peak and trough aminoglycoside serum concentrations should be determined and the dose adjusted, when necessary, to achieve therapeutic, nontoxic levels. Serum for peak levels should be drawn 1 hour after an intramuscular dose and 30 minutes after the completion of an intravenous infusion. Serum for trough levels should be drawn just prior to the next dose.

The other major toxic effect of aminoglycosides is ototoxicity. Two percent to three percent of patients treated with gentamicin develop this complication. Both branches of the eighth cranial nerve may be involved. Damage to the vestibular system occurs more frequently with gentamicin, and cochlear damage is more common with amikacin.[5, 109] Clinical manifestations of ototoxicity include vertigo, ataxia, nystagmus, tinnitus, and high-tone hearing loss. Patients with severe vestibular toxicity may be unable to walk without assistance, and loss of hearing may progress to deafness. The toxic effect is reversible if the drug is discontinued early in the course of the toxic reaction, but it may lead to permanent deficits if the antibiotic is continued.

Risk factors for ototoxicity include renal impairment, old age, duration of therapy, total dose, high serum levels, previous aminoglycoside therapy, previous noise exposure, and use of the diuretics furosemide and ethacrynic acid.[5, 109] Early toxicity may not be apparent clinically and can be detected only by special tests including audiometry, caloric tests, and electronystagmography. The presence of ototoxicity should be suspected in any patient who develops vertigo, ataxia, tinnitus, or obvious loss of auditory acuity. Ototoxicity is treated by prompt withdrawal of the offending drug. Ototoxicity may be less likely to occur if serum aminoglycoside concentrations are maintained in the therapeutic, nontoxic range.[5, 109]

A less frequently encountered form of toxicity due to aminoglycosides is that of neuromuscular blockade.[75] This side-effect of aminoglycoside therapy may be of particular importance in surgical patients, because it seems to be potentiated by muscle-relaxing agents used during surgery. Thus, when aminoglycosides are administered postoperatively, patients may become apneic. The neuromuscular blockade can be reversed by administration of calcium.[5]

CHLORAMPHENICOL

Chloramphenicol is useful in the therapy of infections in surgical patients because of its gram-negative bacillary and anaerobic spectrum and because of its excellent tissue penetrance, particularly across the blood–brain barrier and into the parenchyma of the brain.

The most important untoward reaction that complicates the administration of chloramphenicol is hematologic toxicity. There are two types of toxicity involving the hematopoietic system. The first is reversible and dose dependent. The bone marrow of patients with this form of toxicity shows maturation arrest.[123] It is manifested by anemia, leukopenia, thrombocytopenia, and reticulocytopenia. The diagnosis of reversible bone-marrow toxicity is made by a complete blood count and platelet count. Patients who develop anemia, leukopenia, or thrombocytopenia without any other identifiable cause should be suspected of having this form of chloramphenicol toxicity. A low reticulocyte count supports the diagnosis. This toxic effect is treated by withdrawing or decreasing the dosage of the drug. The toxicity can be prevented by using a moderate dose when possible. Thus, toxicity rarely occurs at 2 g per day but occurs commonly at 4 g per day.[149] Two grams, IV, per day in equally divided doses of 500 mg given every 6 hours provides therapeutic levels for most infections. Infections of the central nervous system require at least 4 g per day, and, in this instance, reversible toxicity may be unavoidable. Since chloramphenicol is metabolized by the liver, no change in dosage is needed in patients with severe renal failure, even if they are anephric.

The second type of hematologic toxicity is that of bone-marrow aplasia, which is usually irreversible. This form of toxicity is very rare and occurs in one out of every 25,000 to 40,000 courses of therapy. The cause is unknown, but the toxic effect may be more likely to occur in patients who have damaged bone marrow prior to administration of chloramphenicol.[123] There is also evidence to suggest that the drug is more likely to cause marrow aplasia when given orally than when given parenterally. This form of toxicity is not dose related and appears between 2 weeks and 12 months after the course of therapy. The diagnosis is made by ruling out other causes of marrow aplasia. The only treatment is bone-marrow transplantation. The best prevention is to limit use of the drug to serious infections that could not be more effectively treated with other drugs. The antibiotic should probably be given only intravenously (the drug is not well absorbed from muscle) and not orally. It should not be administered to patients who have or may have preexisting marrow damage.

CLINDAMYCIN

The organ toxicity due to clindamycin is limited to the gastrointestinal tract. Clinically, toxicity is manifested as diarrhea or pseudomembranous colitis (PMC). Diarrhea has been reported to occur in from 4% to 20% of patients treated with clindamycin and PMC in from 0.001% to 10 % of patients who receive clindamycin.[156] In one study that evaluated patients treated with clindamycin for diarrhea without attempting to differentiate diarrhea alone from PMC, the incidence of diarrhea was 6.6%.[156] There were significant associations between occurrence of diarrhea and age greater than 20 years, female sex, and administration by the oral route.

The most serious side-effect of clindamycin therapy is PMC. PMC is not due to direct toxicity of clindamycin on the colonic mucosa but results from eradication of normal flora by clindamycin with overgrowth of the intestine by *Clostridium difficile*, which is not susceptible to clindamycin. *Clostridium difficile* produces a cytotoxin that causes inflammation in the colonic mucosa.[10] *Clostridium difficile* is usually present in stools from patients with PMC, and toxin in these stools can be detected by tissue-culture assay.

The clinical manifestations of PMC include diarrhea (sometimes watery), cramping abdominal pain, and fever from 100°F to 104°F. Manifestations that occur less frequently include abdominal tenderness with rebound and leukocytosis.[157, 165] It appears that the risk for PMC is greater in patients who receive the drug orally than those treated parenterally.[157, 158]

The duration of PMC is dependent on the time of onset and whether or not the syndrome is promptly diagnosed and clindamycin therapy stopped. When PMC is diagnosed early and clindamycin withdrawn, symptoms usually subside within 1 week. If PMC has its onset after clindamycin therapy has been discontinued or if clindamycin administration is continued for a prolonged period after onset of PMC, symptoms may be prolonged and continue for up to 4 weeks.[157] A few deaths have been attributed to PMC, but the long-term prognosis of this complication appears favorable.

Clindamycin-associated PMC is diagnosed by proctoscopy. At proctoscopy, the typical findings of PMC are raised yellow whitish plaques on a mucosa that is often erythematous, edematous, and sometimes friable. The diagnosis may be made by barium enema, but findings on barium enema are much less specific than those detected by proctoscopy.[165] PMC cannot be diagnosed clinically, because many patients treated with clindamycin develop diarrhea without PMC, and PMC may occur without causing gastrointestinal symptoms. It must also be kept in mind that PMC can be caused by other antibiotics including lincomycin, ampicillin, tetracycline, chloramphenicol, erythromycin, and the cephalosporins.[12, 62, 158] PMC may have to be differentiated from intra-abdominal inflammatory processes since some patients have abdominal tenderness with rebound and leukocytosis.

The most important therapeutic modality is prompt withdrawal of clindamycin (or other inciting antibiotic). Fluid replacement is important. Antimotility agents are probably contraindicated. In patients who have prolonged diarrhea after discontinuation of antimicrobial therapy, several studies indicate that vancomycin given by mouth is effective in eliminating *Clostridium difficile* from the colon with subsequent relief from diarrhea.[16, 87, 159] For adults, vancomycin is given in a dose of 500 mg orally every 6 hours. The dosage for pediatric patients has not been well defined, but 2000 mg per 1.73 m^2 per 24 hours in divided doses given orally appears effective.[16] Vancomycin is usually given for 7 to 14 days. Although effective, vancomycin therapy may be complicated by relapse, and patients should be carefully followed up after vancomycin is discontinued.[11, 66, 105] There is no effective mode of prevention for PMC other than judicious use of antimicrobial agents so that patients are not needlessly subjected to the risk of PMC.

VANCOMYCIN

Toxic effects of vancomycin include phlebitis, nephrotoxicity, and ototoxicity. Phlebitis was particularly troublesome with the early preparations of vancomycin, but the currently available drug is purer and less frequently causes phlebitis.[38, 136] Nephrotoxicity and ototoxicity occur infrequently at therapeutic serum concentrations and are uncommon in patients with normal renal function. Nephrotoxicity is usually mild and is manifested by a decrease in creatinine clearance and a rise in the serum creatinine concentration. Nephrotoxicity may also be manifested by mild hematuria, proteinuria, and cylindruria. Ototoxicity is manifested only by involvement of the auditory nerve.[67] Lost hearing may return after vancomycin is withdrawn, but in some patients there is progressive hearing loss even after the drug has been stopped.[136]

Nephrotoxicity is diagnosed by determination of the serum creatinine concentration. Ototoxicity may be diagnosed clinically by observation of hearing loss, but audiography provides early diagnosis.

The only available therapeutic modality is withdrawal of the drug, and this should be done promptly at the earliest sign of renal or auditory toxicity. Prevention of toxicity involves maintenance of therapeutic and nontoxic serum concentrations. Appearance of toxicity is highly unlikely when serum levels are kept under 30 μg/ml. Since vancomycin is eliminated almost entirely by the kidneys, dosage must be reduced in patients with renal impairment. For patients with normal renal function, the dosage is 500 mg, IV, every 6 hours. When patients are anephric, they may be treated with 1 g, IV, once each week. No modification of dosage is required for patients on hemodialysis. For degrees of renal function between normal and the anephric state, dosage may be determined by a recently published nomogram.[112] Serum creatinine concentrations should be measured frequently. Since the nephrotoxicity and ototoxicity of vancomycin and the aminoglycosides may be additive, when this combination is used, serum creatinine concentrations should be monitored and patients followed by audiography.[38]

TETRACYCLINES

Because many bacteria are so resistant, tetracyclines have few indications in surgical patients. However, when they are used, appropriate doses must be given and the patients monitored carefully. Unlike most other antimicrobial agents that inhibit protein synthesis in bacteria, tetracyclines also have a substantial inhibitory effect on protein synthesis in mammalian cells.[13] This effect may be pronounced in patients with renal failure and may lead to a catabolic state with the potential for impairment of wound healing.

Even in the presence of normal renal function, undernourished adults may develop negative nitrogen balance and weight loss when given 2 g to 3 g of tetracycline per day.[145] Thus, tetracycline administration could have a very deleterious effect on surgical patients who are malnourished to the point of requiring total parenteral nutrition.

Tetracyclines should also generally be avoided in patients with impaired renal function. Treatment with tetracyclines frequently leads to accumulation of the drugs in serum and deterioration of renal function with acidosis, hyperphosphatemia, increasing azotemia, and even death.[13, 145] The one exception is doxycycline, for which renal excretion is not an important mode of elimination. One congener of tetracycline, demeclocycline, has another adverse effect on the kidneys.[78] Persons who receive high doses may develop nephrogenic diabetes insipidus. This effect is apparently mediated by a partial blockage of endogenous antidiuretic hormone at the renal tubule. The condition is reversible and subsides within a week of stopping the medication.

Tetracyclines may also be hepatotoxic, particularly when given parenterally in a dosage of 2 g or more per day or when given orally in large doses.[145] Pathologic changes in the liver include fine vacuoles and cytoplasmic changes in hepatocytes and fatty infiltration without necrosis.[13] Hepatotoxicity is particularly likely to occur and is frequently severe in pregnant women.[145] Hepatotoxicity due to tetracyclines usually develops in pregnant patients when one of these drugs is given for urinary-tract infection. Under these circumstances, renal function may be diminished with resultant drug accumulation. Hepatotoxicity is manifested as jaundice, azotemia, acidosis, and terminal shock.[145]

Another adverse effect of tetracyclines in pregnant patients is staining of the dentition of the fetus. All of the tetracyclines are deposited in areas of the bones and teeth where calcification is taking place. The deciduous teeth may be discolored to yellow or brown.[93] Whereas tetracyclines have few indications in surgical patients, they should be altogether avoided in pregnant women.

Tetracyclines may also cause staining of teeth when given to children under 8 years of age. The occurrence of staining is dose dependent and is unlikely to be noticed unless the child receives five or more courses of one of the tetracyclines.[71] Even though it takes several courses of drug to cause visible dental staining, tetracyclines are probably best avoided in children under 8 years of age unless no other effective drug is available.

Other toxic effects of the tetracyclines include nausea, vomiting, and diarrhea.[13, 145] Nausea and vomiting can be controlled by administration of these drugs with food, but tetracyclines should not be given with milk or milk products. Antacids may also control nausea and vomiting, but only preparations that do not contain aluminum, magnesium, or calcium should be used. In some cases, the nausea and vomiting may cease while therapy with the drug is continued. Esophageal ulceration has also been reported as an adverse effect of tetracyclines and may be more likely to occur in patients with esophageal disease or when the drug is taken at bedtime.[41]

Tetracyclines should not be given to patients with esophageal obstruction caused by conditions such as stricture, enlarged left atrium, or achalasia unless no other suitable alternative therapy is available.[41] Further, the medication should not be taken during the hour prior to bedtime, particularly by patients with a history of esophageal reflux.

Pseudotumor cerebri has been reported as a complication of tetracycline therapy.[13] Most cases have been reported in infants, in whom the principal manifestation has been bulging fontanelles with normal cerebrospinal fluid. The condition clears rapidly when therapy is discontinued.[145] Pseudotumor cerebri due to tetracycline administration has been reported rarely in adults.[23]

Phototoxicity is an adverse effect of tetracycline therapy that causes a sunburnlike cutaneous eruption.[13, 145] This effect is probably due to accumulation of tetracycline in the skin. Symptoms include burning and paresthesias in areas exposed to sunlight.[59] Manifestations may be severe including edema, papules, vesicles, and onycholysis. Phototoxicity may be prevented by sunscreen preparations or ordinary window glass. Among the tetracyclines, minocycline may be least likely to cause phototoxicity.[59]

Another toxic effect of tetracycline therapy is associated with administration of outdated drug. This side-effect resembles the Fanconi syndrome and is apparently due to breakdown products of these drugs. These products probably exert their deleterious effect on the proximal tubules, which results in impaired resorption of glucose, amino acids, phosphates, potassium, and uric acid.[61] Clinical manifestations include nausea, vomiting, polydipsia, polyuria, and muscle weakness secondary to potassium depletion.[57, 61] The syndrome is treated by withdrawal of the outdated drug. Patients usually become asymptomatic within 1 month after administration of outdated medication has been discontinued. This type of toxicity can be prevented by storing tetracyclines properly to prevent deterioration and by not using tetracyclines after their expiration date.

Minocycline, one of the newer analogues of tetracycline, has been associated with a high incidence of vestibular side-effects. Several authors have noted that the incidence of this toxic effect varies between 30% and 90% of persons who receive the drug.[51, 166] The mechanism of this toxicity is unknown but would appear to be caused by an effect of the drug on the vestibular system rather than toxic action on the vestibular centers of the central nervous system.[166] Clinical manifestations include dizziness, vertigo, ataxia, weakness, nausea, vomiting, anorexia, abdominal cramps, clammy skin, hallucinations, and scotoma.[51, 166] This type of toxicity occurs in both adults and children but occurs much more frequently in women than men.[52] It has been postulated that women have a higher incidence of these side-effects because of their smaller size and higher serum concentrations when given the same dose as men,[52, 72] but although women were shown to have higher serum concentrations, the incidence of symptoms could not be related to them.[52, 72] In fact, one study has shown that lowering the dosage in women does not reduce the incidence of symptoms.[72] Symptoms usually appear within 72 hours of initiation of drug administration and subside during the 48 hours after minocycline has been stoppped.[51] The only way to avoid this type of toxicity is to avoid use of the drug.

In light of the large number of side-effects observed with tetracycline administration and the poor activity of these drugs against most microorganisms that cause surgical infections, there would appear to be few, if any, indications for use of these agents in surgical patients.

ERYTHROMYCIN

Erythromycin is an antimicrobial agent of generally low toxicity. The principal side-effects are due to its local irritative properties and to its estolate ester. The local irritative effect on the gastrointestinal tract is manifested as nausea, vomiting, and diarrhea. Nausea and vomiting are more likely to occur in children than in adults. Erythromycin also regularly causes phlebitis when infused intravenously. Virtually all patients given 1 g, IV, every 6 hours will develop phlebitis.[107] Thus, intravenous cannulas must frequently be changed to new sites.

The other major toxic effect is that of hepatotoxicity associated with administration of erythromycin estolate. Hepatotoxicity is only rarely associated with use of erythromycin base, erythromycin stearate, or erythromycin ethylsuccinate. The estolate causes cholestatic hepatitis. The mechanism by which the estolate causes hepatotoxicity is not known, but some evidence, such as the frequent occurrence of eosinophilia, suggests hypersensitivity reaction.[25] Clinically, the toxic syndrome is characterized by nausea, vomiting, severe abdominal pain, fever, jaundice, pruritis, acholic stools, dark urine, hepatomegaly, and right-upper-quadrant tenderness.[25] Results of liver-function tests, including serum bilirubin, alkaline phosphatase, and transaminases, are frequently abnormal. Hepatotoxicity usually does not occur until after the patient has been treated with the estolate for 2 weeks. It has been reported in both adults and children. Symptoms and signs clear and liver-function tests return to normal when the drug is stopped. Since there are several other oral preparations of erythromycin, the estolate should not be used.

TRIMETHOPRIM-SULFAMETHOXAZOLE

Trimethoprim-sulfamethoxazole is usually well tolerated with a very low incidence of side-effects. The most common adverse effects are nausea, vomiting, diarrhea, cramps, glossitis, stomatitis, and jaundice, but these occur in less than 3% of patients who receive the drug combination.[173]

The only toxicity clearly associated with trimethoprim alone is related to interference with folate metabolism. In normal patients who receive appropriate doses, disturbance of folate metabolism is rare. This is due to the very large difference between the affinity of the drug for bacterial and mammalian dihydrofolate reductase; the affinity for the bacterial enzyme is 50,000 times greater than that for mammalian dihydrofolate reductase.[173] Clinically, folate deficiency is manifested as a megaloblastic anemia. Although folate deficiency is a rare complication of trimethoprim-sulfamethoxazole therapy, patients who have a folate deficiency or who have depleted folate stores are more likely to experience the hematologic toxicity.[15] Patients at particular risk include those with known folate or vitamin B_{12} deficiency, pregnant women, the elderly, patients with malabsorption or malnutrition, alcoholics, patients treated with phenytoin or folic-acid antimetabolites, and patients with chronic hemolytic anemia.[173] Folinic acid given with trimethoprim-sulfamethoxazole will prevent the adverse effect on the hematopoietic system without interfering with antimicrobial activity.

The other adverse effects of the drug combination are due to sulfamethoxazole. These include erythema multiforme, the Stevens–Johnson syndrome, toxic epidermal necrolysis and exfoliative dermatitis, all of which are rare. Nephrotoxicity is due to sulfamethoxazole and may be caused by either hypersensitivity or crystalluria.[121] The latter can be prevented by a high fluid intake.

Trimethoprim can cause a rise in the level of serum creatinine by interfering with tubular secretion of creatinine, but this is not associated with renal damage. Since both trimethoprim and sulfamethoxazole are cleared from the body by renal excretion, dosage has to be decreased in patients with renal insufficiency.[121] Treatment with trimethoprim-sulfamethoxazole is contraindicated in pregnant and lactating women.[173] Children appear to tolerate the drug combination as well as do adults.[121]

NITROFURANTOIN

In addition to the acute pulmonary reaction due to hypersensitivity to nitrofurantoin discussed above, there is a chronic pulmonary reaction, which is apparently due to direct pulmonary toxicity.[80] The chronic pulmonary reaction is less common than the acute disease, and it usually occurs after long-term therapy with nitrofurantoin.[80, 137, 153, 155] Whereas the acute reaction is characterized by an alveolar or alveolar-interstitial infiltrate, the chronic reaction is manifested by interstitial fibrosis.[137, 155] The chronic syndrome has an insidious onset, usually after therapy for 6 months or longer.[137, 153, 155] Symptoms include cough and dyspnea.[91, 155] Fever and weight loss may also occur.[155] Pleural effusion and eosinophilia are absent.[137] The diagnosis is made by history of long-term therapy with nitrofurantoin in a patient with insidious onset of cough and dyspnea who has evidence of diffuse interstitial fibrosis on chest x-ray examination. Therapy includes withdrawal of nitrofurantoin and administration of corticosteroids.[137] This adverse effect of nitrofurantoin can probably be prevented to a large extent by avoiding long-term therapy. Patients on long-term therapy should be evaluated frequently with chest films, perhaps every 6 months, because symptoms may be preceded by roentgenographic changes. When symptoms of the chronic reaction to nitrofurantoin appear, the drug should be discontinued promptly, because prognosis appears to worsen with continuing administration.[155]

References

1. Adams RD, Kubik CS, Bonner FJ: The clinical and pathological aspects of influenzal meningitis. Arch Pediatr 65:354, 408, 1948
2. Alexander MR, Berglund EM, Kasik JE et al: The concentration of tobramycin in bronchial secretions. Chest 75:675, 1979
3. Andrassy K, Ritz E, Weisschedel E: Bleeding after carbenicillin administration. N Engl J Med 292:109, 1975
4. Appel GB, Neu HC: The nephrotoxicity of antimicrobial agents. N Engl J Med 296:663, 1977
5. Appel GB, Neu HC: Gentamicin in 1978. Ann Intern Med 89:528, 1978
6. Appel GB, Neu HC, Parry MF et al: Pharmacokinetics of cefamandole in the presence of renal failure and in patients undergoing hemodialysis. Antimicrob Agents Chemother 10:623, 1976
7. Arndt KA, Jick H: Rates of cutaneous reactions to drugs. A report from the Boston collaborative drug surveillance program. JAMA 235:918, 1976
8. Austen KF: Systemic anaphylaxis in the human being. N Engl J Med 291:661, 1974
9. Baldwin DS, Levine BB, McCluskey RT, Gallo GR: Renal failure and interstitial nephritis due to penicillin and methicillin. N Engl J Med 279:1245, 1968
10. Bartlett JG, Moon N, Chang TW et al: Role of *Clostridium difficile* in antibiotic-associated pseudomembranous colitis. Gastroenterology 75:778, 1978
11. Bartlett JG, Tedesco FJ, Shull S et al: Symptomatic relapse after oral vancomycin therapy of antibiotic-associated pseudomembranous colitis. Gastroenterology 78:431, 1980

12. Bartlett JG, Willey SH, Chang TW, Lowe B: Cephalosporin-associated pseudomembranous colitis due to *Clostridium difficile*. JAMA 242:2683, 1979
13. Barza M, Schiefe RT: Antimicrobial spectrum, pharmacology and therapeutic use of antibiotics. Part 1: Tetracyclines. Am J Hosp Pharm 34:49, 1977
14. Baskin TW, Rosenthal A, Pruitt BA Jr: Acute bacterial endocarditis: A silent source of sepsis in the burn patient. Ann Surg 184:618, 1976
15. Bateson MC, Hayes JPLA, Pendharkar P: Cotrimoxazole and folate metabolism. Lancet 2:339, 1976
16. Batts DH, Martin D, Holmes R et al: Treatment of antibiotic-associated *Clostridium difficile* diarrhea with oral vancomycin. J Pediatr 97:151, 1980
17. Belohradsky BH, Bruch K, Geiss D et al: Intravenous cefotaxime in children with bacterial meningitis. Lancet 1:61, 1980
18. Bennett WM, Craven R: Urinary tract infections in patients with severe renal disease. Treatment with ampicillin and trimethoprim-sulfamethoxazole. JAMA 236:946, 1976
19. Bennett WM, Hartnett MN, Craven R et al: Gentamicin concentrations in blood, urine, and renal tissue of patients with end-stage renal disease. J Lab Clin Med 90:389, 1977
20. Bennett WM, Singer I, Coggins CJ: A guide to drug therapy in renal failure. JAMA 230:1544, 1974
21. Bergogne–Berezin E: Penetration of antibiotics into the respiratory tree. J Antimicrob Chemother 8:171, 1981
22. Bergogne–Berezin E, Morel C, Bernard Y et al: Pharmacokinetic study of β-lactam antibiotics in bronchial secretions. Scand J Infect Dis (Suppl) 14:267, 1978
23. Bhowmick BK: Benign intracranial hypertension after antibiotic therapy. Br Med J 3:30, 1972
24. Bolton WK, Scheld WM, Spyker DA et al: Pharmacokinetics of moxalactam in subjects with various degrees of renal dysfunction. Antimicrob Agents Chemother 18:933, 1980
25. Braun P: Hepatotoxicity of erythromycin. J Infect Dis 119:300, 1969
26. Briedis DJ, Robson HG: Cerebrospinal fluid penetration of amikacin. Antimicrob Agents Chemother 13:1042, 1978
27. Brogard JM, Dorner M, Pinget M et al: The biliary excretion of cefazolin. J Infect Dis 131:625, 1975
28. Brogard JM Pinget M, Meyer C et al: Biliary excretion of ampicillin: Experimental and clinical study. Chemotherapy 23:213, 1977
29. Broome CV, Cherry WB, Winn WC Jr, MacPherson BR: Rapid diagnosis of Legionnaires' disease by direct immunofluorescent staining. Ann Intern Med 90:1, 1979
30. Brown CH, Natelson EA, Bradshaw MW et al: The hemostatic defect produced by carbenicillin. N Engl J Med 291:265, 1974
31. Brown RB, Martyak SN, Barza M et al: Penetration of clindamycin phosphate into the abnormal human biliary tract. Ann Intern Med 84:168, 1976
32. Bruck HM, Nash G, Foley FD, Pruitt BA Jr: Opportunistic fungal infection of the burn wound with Phycomycetes and *Aspergillus*. A clinical-pathologic review. Arch Surg 102:476, 1971
33. Bryan CS, Stone WJ: "Comparably massive": Penicillin G therapy in renal failure. Ann Intern Med 82:189, 1975
34. Bryant RE, Hammond D: Interaction of purulent material with antibiotics used to treat *Pseudomonas* infections. Antimicrob Agents Chemother 6:702, 1974
35. Cabizuca SV, Desser KB: Carbenicillin-associated hypokalemic alkalosis. JAMA 236:956, 1976
36. Chaitin H: Bacteriology of calculous cholecystitis. Int Surg 58:169, 1973
37. Conway N, Beck E, Somerville J: Penicillin encephalopathy. Postgrad Med J 44:891, 1968
38. Cook FV, Farrar WE Jr: Vancomycin revisited. Ann Intern Med 88:813, 1978
39. Craig WA, Kunin CM: Trimethoprim-sulfamethoxazole: Pharmacodynamic effects of urinary pH and impaired renal function. Studies in humans. Ann Intern Med 78:491, 1973
40. Craig WA, Welling PG, Jackson TC, Kunin CM: Pharmacology of cefazolin and other cephalosporins in patients with renal insufficiency. J Infect Dis (Suppl) 128:347, 1973
41. Crowson TD, Head LH, Ferrante WA: Esophageal ulcers associated with tetracycline therapy. JAMA 235:2747, 1976
42. Czerwinski AW, Pederson JA, Barry JP: Cefazolin plasma concentrations. J Clin Pharmacol 14:560, 1974
43. Dahlgren JG, Anderson ET, Hewitt WL: Gentamicin blood levels: A guide to nephrotoxicity. Antimicrob Agents Chemother 8:58, 1975
44. Diaz CR, Kane JG, Parker RH, Pelsor FR: Pharmacokinetics of nafcillin in patients with renal failure. Antimicrob Agents Chemother 12:98, 1977
45. DiChiro G: Cisternography: From early tribulations to a useful diagnostic procedure. Johns Hopkins Med J 133:1, 1973
46. Ditlove J, Weikmann P, Bernstein M, Massry SG: Methicillin nephritis. Medicine 56:483, 1977
47. Dull WL, Alexander MR, Kasik JE: Bronchial secretion levels of amikacin. Chemotherapy 19:526, 1981
48. Edwards CQ, Smith CR, Baughman KL et al: Concentrations of gentamicin and amikacin in human kidneys. Antimicrob Agents Chemother 9:925, 1976
49. England DM, Rosenblatt JE: Anaerobes in human biliary tracts. J Clin Microbiol 6:494, 1977
50. Engstrom J, Groth CG, Lonnqvist B: Infectious complications after surgery for biliary calculus. Acta Chir Scand 138:357, 1972
51. Fanning WL, Gump DW: Distressing side-effects of minocycline hydrochloride. Arch Intern Med 136:761, 1976
52. Fanning WL, Gump DW, Sofferman RA: Side effects of minocycline: A double-blind study. Antimicrob Agents Chemother 11:712, 1977
53. Fellner MJ: Penicillin allergy 1976: A review of reactions, detection and current management. Int J Dermatol 15:497, 1976
54. Foley FD, Greenwald KA, Nash G, Pruitt, BA Jr: Herpesvirus infection in burned patients. N Engl J Med 282:652, 1970
55. Foley FD, Shuck JM: Burn-wound infection with Phycomycetes requiring amputation of a hand. JAMA 203:596, 1968
56. Francke EL, Neu HC: Use of cefotaxime, a β-lactamase stable cephalosporin, in the therapy of serious infections, including those due to multiresistant organisms. Am J Med 71:435, 1981
57. Frimpter GW, Timpanelli AE, Eisemenger WJ et al: Reversible "Fanconi syndrome" caused by degraded tetracycline. JAMA 184:111, 1963
58. Frisch JM: Clinical experience with adverse reactions to trimethoprim-sulfamethoxazole. J Infect Dis (Suppl) 128:607, 1973
59. Frost P, Weinstein GD, Gomez EC: Phototoxic potential of minocycline and doxycycline. Arch Dermatol 105:681, 1972

60. Fukunaga FH: Gallbladder bacteriology, histology, and gallstones. Study of unselected cholecystectomy specimens in Honolulu. Arch Surg 106:169, 1973
61. Fulop M, Drapkin A: Potassium-depletion syndrome secondary to nephropathy apparently caused by "outdated tetracycline." N Engl J Med 272:986, 1965
62. Gantz NM, Zawacki JK, Dickerson J, Barlett JG: Pseudomembranous colitis associated with erythromycin. Ann Intern Med 91:866, 1979
63. Geddes AM, Bridgewater FAJ, Williams DN et al: Clinical and bacteriological studies with clindamycin. Br Med J 2:703, 1970
64. Geddes AM, Schnurr LP, Ball AP et al: Cefoxitin: A hospital study. Br Med J 1:1126, 1977
65. Geller M, Dickie HA, Kass DA et al: The histopathology of acute nitrofurantoin-associated pneumonitis. Ann Allergy 37:275, 1976
66. George WL, Volpicelli NA, Stiner DB et al: Relapse of pseudomembranous colitis after vancomycin therapy. N Engl J Med 301:414, 1979
67. Geraci JE: Vancomycin. Mayo Clin Proc 52:631, 1977
68. Gilbert DN, Gourley R, d'Agostino A et al: Interstitial nephritis due to methicillin, penicillin and ampicillin. Ann Allergy 28:378, 1970
69. Glew RH, Moellering RC Jr, Burke JF: Gentamicin dosage in children with extensive burns. J Trauma 16:819, 1976
70. Gross PA, Harkavy LM, Barden GE, Kerstein M: Positive foley catheter tip cultures—Fact or fancy? JAMA 228:72, 1974
71. Grossman ER, Walchek A, Freedman H, Flanagan C: Tetracyclines and permanent teeth: The relation between dose and tooth color. Pediatrics 47:567, 1971
72. Gump DW, Ashikaga T, Fink TJ, Radin AM: Side effects of minocycline: Different dosage regimens. Antimicrob Agents Chemother 12:642, 1977
73. Gwynn CM, George RH: Neonatal citrobacter meningitis. Arch Dis Child 48:455, 1973
74. Haburchak DR, Head DR, Everett ED: Postoperative hemorrhage associated with carbenicillin administration. Am J Surg 134:630, 1977
75. Hall DR, McGibbon DH, Evans CC, Meadows GA: Gentamicin, tubocurarine, lignocaine and neuromuscular blockade. Br J Anaesth 44:1329, 1972
76. Halprin GM, McMahon SM: Cephalexin concentrations in sputum during acute respiratory infections. Antimicrob Agents Chemother 3:703, 1973
77. Hamory B, Ignatiadis P, Sande MA: Intrathecal amikacin administration. Use in the treatment of gentamicin-resistant *Klebsiella pneumoniae* meningitis. JAMA 236:1973, 1976
78. Hayek A, Ramirez J: Demeclocycline-induced diabetes insipidus. JAMA 229:676, 1974
79. Heseltine PNR, Busch DF, Meyer RD, Finegold SM: Cefoxitin: Clinical evaluation in thirty-eight patients. Antimicrob Agents Chemother 11:437, 1977
80. Holmberg L, Boman G, Bottiger LE et al: Adverse reactions to nitrofurantoin. Analysis of 921 reports. Am J Med 69:733, 1980
81. Hull JH, Sarubbi FA Jr: Gentamicin serum concentrations: Pharmacokinetic predictions. Ann Intern Med 85:183, 1976
82. Johanson WG, Pierce AK, Sanford JP: Changing pharyngeal bacterial flora of hospitalized patients. Emergence of gram-negative bacilli. N Engl J Med 281:1137, 1969
83. Johnson GJ, White JG: Platelet dysfunction induced by parenteral administration of carbenicillin and ticarcillin (Abstr). Thromb Haemost 34:341, 1975
84. Kaiser AB, McGee ZA: Aminoglycoside therapy of gram-negative bacillary meningitis. N Engl J Med 293:1215, 1975
85. Kancir LM, Tuazon CU, Cardella TA, Sheagren JN: Adverse reactions to methicillin and nafcillin during treatment of serious *Staphylococcus aureus* infections. Arch Intern Med 128:909, 1978
86. Kane JG, Parker RH, Jordan GW, Hoeprich PD: Nafcillin concentration in cerebrospinal fluid during treatment of staphylococcal infections. Ann Intern Med 87:309, 1977
87. Keighley MRB, Burdon DW, Arabi Y et al: Randomized controlled trial of vancomycin for pseudomembranous colitis and postoperative diarrhea. Br Med J 2:1667, 1978
88. Keighley MRB, Drysdale RB, Quoraishi AH et al: Antibiotic treatment of biliary sepsis. Surg Clin North Am 55:1379, 1975
89. Kelly JF, Patterson R: Anaphylaxis. Course, mechanisms and treatment. JAMA 227:1431, 1974
90. Klastersky J, Vanderkelen B, Daneau D, Mathieu M: Carbenicillin and hypokalemia. Ann Intern Med 78:774, 1973
91. Koch–Weser J, Sidel VW, Dexter M et al: Adverse reactions to sulfisoxazole, sulfamethoxazole, and nitrofurantoin. Manifestations and specific reaction rates during 2,118 courses of therapy. Arch Intern Med 128:399, 1971
92. Koneman EW, Roberts GD: Clinical and laboratory diagnosis of mycotic disease. In Henry JB (ed): Clinical Diagnosis and Management by Laboratory Methods, 16th ed, vol 2, p 1699. Philadelphia, WB Saunders, 1979
93. Kucers A, Bennett N: The Use of Antibiotics, 2nd ed, p 398. London, William Heinemann, 1975
94. Kunin CM, Finkelberg Z: Oral cephalexin and ampicillin: Antimicrobial activity, recovery in urine, and persistence in blood of uremic patients. Ann Intern Med 72:349, 1970
95. Landesman SH, Corrado ML, Shah PM et al: Past and current roles for cephalosporin antibiotics in treatment of meningitis. Emphasis on use in gram-negative bacillary meningitis. Am J Med 71:693, 1981
96. Levine BB: Skin rashes with penicillin therapy: Current management. N Engl J Med 286:42, 1972
97. Lindberg AA, Nilsson LH, Bucht H, Kallings LO: Concentration of chloramphenicol in the urine and blood in relation to renal function. Br Med J 2:724, 1966
98. Loebl EC, Marvin JA, Heck EL et al: The method of quantitative burn-wound biopsy cultures and its routine use in the care of the burned patient. Am J Clin Pathol 61:20, 1974
99. Loirat P, Rohan J, Baillet A et al: Increased glomerular filtration rate in patients with major burns and its effect on the pharmacokinetics of tobramycin. N Engl J Med 299:915, 1978
100. Lyons H, Pinn VW, Cortell S et al: Allergic interstitial nephritis causing reversible renal failure in four patients with idiopathic nephrotic syndrome. N Engl J Med 288:124, 1973
101. MacMillan BG, Low EJ, Holder IA: Experience with *Candida* infections in the burn patient. Arch Surg 104:509, 1972
102. Mandell GL, Sande MA: Antimicrobial agents. Sufonamides, trimethoprim-sulfamethoxazole, and urinary tract antiseptics. In Gilman AG, Goodman LS, Gilman A (eds): The Pharmacological Basis of Therapeutics, 6th ed. New York, Macmillan, 1980
103. Mandell GL, Sande MA: Antimicrobial agents. Penicillins and cephalosporins. In Gilman AG, Goodman LS, Gilman A (eds): The Pharmacological Basis of Therapeutics, ed. 6. New York, Macmillan, 1980

104. Mangi RJ, Holstein LL, Andriole VT: Treatment of gram-negative bacillary meningitis with intrathecal gentamicin. Yale J Biol Med 50:31, 1977
105. Marrie TJ, Faulkner RS, Bradley BWD et al: Pseudomembranous colitis: Isolation of two species of cytotoxic clostridia and successful treatment with vancomycin. Can Med Assoc J 119:1058, 1978
106. May JR, Delves DM: Treatment of chronic bronchitis with ampicillin. Some pharmacological observations. Lancet 1:929, 1965
107. Meade RH III: Drug therapy reviews: Antimicrobial spectrum, pharmacology and therapeutic use of erythromcyin and its derivatives. Am J Hosp Pharm 36:1185, 1979
108. Mendelson J, Portnoy J, Sigman H: Pharmacology of gentamicin in the biliary tract of humans. Antimicrob Agents Chemother 4:538, 1973
109. Meyer RD: Amikacin. Ann Intern Med 95:328, 1981
110. Minuth JN, Musher DM, Thorsteinsson SB: Inhibition of the antibacterial activity of gentamicin by urine. J Infect Dis 133:14, 1976
111. Moellering RC Jr, Fischer EG: Relationship of intraventricular gentamicin levels to cure of meningitis: Report of a case of *Proteus* meningitis successfully treated with intraventricular gentamicin. J Pediatr 81:534, 1972
112. Moellering RC Jr, Krogstad DJ, Greenblatt DJ: Vancomycin therapy in patients with impaired renal function: A nomogram for dosage. Ann Intern Med 94:343, 1981
113. Mortimer PR, Mackhie DB, Haynes S: Ampicillin levels in human bile in the presence of biliary tract disease. Br Med J 3:88, 1969
114. Nair SR, Cherubin CE: Use of cefoxitin, new cephalosporin-like antibiotic, in the treatment of aerobic and anaerobic infections. Antimicrob Agents Chemother 14:866, 1978
115. Nash G, Foley FD, Pruitt BA Jr: *Candida* burn-wound invasion. A cause of systemic candidiasis. Arch Pathol Lab Med 90:75, 1970
116. Odio W, Van Laer E, Klastersky J: Concentrations of gentamicin in bronchial secretions after intramuscular and endotracheal administration. J Clin Pharmacol 15:518, 1975
117. Olson DA, Hoeprich PD, Nolan SM, Goldstein E: Successful treatment of gram-negative bacillary meningitis with moxalactam. Ann Intern Med 95:302, 1981
118. O'Neill JA, Pruitt BA Jr, Foley FD, Moncrief JA: Suppurative thrombophlebitis—A lethel complication of intravenous therapy. J Trauma 8:256, 1968
119. Parker CW: Drug allergy. N Engl J Med 292:511, 1975
120. Parry MF, Ball WD, Conte JE Jr, Cohen SN: Nafcillin nephritis. JAMA 225:178, 1973
121. Patel RB, Welling PG: Clinical pharmacokinetics of co-trimoxazole (trimethoprim-sulfamethoxazole). Clin Pharmacokinetics 5:405, 1980
122. Pitt HA, Roberts RB, Johnson WD Jr: Gentamicin levels in the human biliary tract. J Infect Dis 127:299, 1973
123. Polin HB, Plaut ME: Chloramphenicol NY State J Med 77:378, 1977
124. Polk RE: Moxalactam. Drug Intell Clin Pharm (In press)
125. Price DJE, Sleigh JD: Klebsiella meningitis—Report of nine cases. J Neurol Neurosurg Psychiatry 35:903, 1972
126. Pruitt BA Jr, Foley FD: The use of biopsies in burn patient care. Surgery 73:887, 1973
127. Pruitt BA Jr, McManus WF, Kim SH, Treat RC: Diagnosis and treatment of cannula-related intravenous sepsis in burn patients. Ann Surg 191:546, 1980
128. Quintiliani R, Nightingale CH: Cefazolin. Ann Intern med 89 (Part 1):650, 1978
129. Rabin ER, Lundbery GD, Mitchell ET: Mucormycosis in severely burned patients. Report of two cases with extensive destruction of the face and nasal cavity. N Engl J Med 264:1286, 1961
130. Rahal JJ Jr: Treatment of gram-negative bacillary meningitis in adults. Ann Intern Med 77:295, 1972
131. Rahal JJ Jr, Hyams PJ, Simberkoff MS, Rubinstein E: Combined intrathecal and intramuscular gentamicin for gram-negative meningitis. Pharmacologic study of 21 patients. N Engl J Med 290:1394, 1974
132. Rahal JJ Jr, Simberkoff MS: Bactericidal and bacteriostatic action of chloramphenicol against meningeal pathogens. Antimicrob Agents Chemother 16:13, 1979
133. Ram MD, Gharavi MA; Biliary infections and the choice of antibiotics. Am J Gastroenterol 62:134, 1974
134. Ram MD, Watanatittan S: Biliary excretion and concentration of cefazolin. Am J Gastroenterol 66:540, 1976
135. Ratzan KR, Baker HB, Lauredo I: Excretion of cefamandole, cefazolin and cephalothin into T-tube bile. Antimicrob Agents Chemother 13:985, 1978
136. Riley HD Jr: Vancomycin and novobiocin. Med Clin North Am 54:1277, 1970
137. Rosenow EC III: The spectrum of drug-induced pulmonary disease. Ann Intern Med 77:977, 1972
138. Ross S, Kraybill EN, Khan W: Treatment of *Proteus* meningitis with carbenicillin: A report of four cases. J Infect Dis (Suppl)122:62, 1970
139. Rudnick M, Morrison G, Walker B, Singer I: Renal failure, hemodialysis and nafcillin kinetics. Clin Pharmacol Ther 20:413, 1976
140. Rudolph AH, Price EV: Penicillin reactions among patients in venereal disease clinics. A national survey. JAMA 223:499, 1973
141. Ruiz DE, Warner JF: Nafcillin treatment of *Staphylococcus aureus* meningitis. Antimicrob Agents Chemother 9:554, 1976
142. Sachs J, Geer T, Noell P, Kunin CM: Effect of renal function on urinary recovery of orally administered nitrofurantoin. N Engl J Med 278:1032, 1968
143. Salmon JH: Ventriculitis complicating meningitis. Am J Dis Child 124:35, 1972
144. Sande MA, Mandell GL: Antimicrobial agents. The aminoglycosides. In Gilman AG, Goodman LS, Gilman A (eds): The Pharmacological Basis of Therapeutics, 6th ed. New York, Macmillan, 1980
145. Sande MA, Mandell GL: Antimicrobial agents. Tetracyclines and chloramphenicol. In Gilman AG, Goodman LS, Gilman A (eds): The Pharmacological Basis of Therapeutics, 6th ed. New York, Macmillan, 1980
146. Sande MA, Mandell GL: Antimicrobial agents. Miscellaneous antibacterial agents: Antifungal and antiviral agents. In Gilman AG, Goodman LS, Gilman A (eds): The Pharmacological Basis of Therapeutics, 6th ed. New York, Macmillan, 1980
147. Sarubbi FA Jr, Hull JH: Amikacin serum concentrations: Prediction of levels and dosage guidelines. Ann Intern Med 89 (Part 1):612, 1978
148. Schentag JJ, Cumbo TJ, Jusko WJ, Plaut ME: Gentamicin tissue accumulation and nephrotoxic reactions. JAMA 240:2067, 1978
149. Scott JL, Finegold SM, Belkin GA, Lawrence JS: A controlled double blind study of the hematologic toxicity of chloramphenicol. N Engl J Med 272:1137, 1965
150. Sklaver AR, Greenman RL, Hoffman TA: Amikacin therapy of gram-negative bacteremia and meningitis. Treatment in diseases due to multiple resistant bacilli. Arch Intern Med 138:713, 1978

151. Smith H, Lerner PI, Weinstein L: Neurotoxicity and "massive" intravenous therapy with penicillin. Arch Intern Med 120:47, 1967
152. Smith CR, Maxwell RR, Edwards CQ et al: Nephrotoxicity induced by gentamicin and amikacin. Johns Hopkins Med J 142:85, 1978
153. Sovijarvi ARA, Lemola M, Stenius B, Idanpaan–Heikkila J: Nitrofurantoin-induced acute, subacute and chronic pulmonary reactions. A report of 66 cases. Scand J Resp Dis 59:41, 1977
154. Stamey TA, Govan DE, Palmer JM: The localization and treatment of urinary tract infections: The role of bactericidal urine levels as opposed to serum levels. Medicine 44:1, 1965
155. Strandberg I, Wengle B, Fagrell B: Chronic interstitial pneumonitis with fibrosis during long-term treatment with nitrofurantoin. Acta Med Scand 196:483, 1974
156. Swartzberg JE, Maresca RM, Remington JS: Gastrointestinal side effects associated with clindamycin. 1000 consecutive patients. Arch Intern Med 136:876, 1976
157. Tedesco FJ: Clindamycin and colitis: A review. J Infect Dis (Suppl) 135:95, 1977
158. Tedesco FJ, Barton RW, Alpers DH: Clindamycin-associated colitis. A prospective study. Ann Intern Med 81:429, 1974
159. Tedesco F, Markham R, Gurwith M et al: Oral vancomycin for antibiotic-associated pseudomembranous colitis. Lancet 2:226, 1978
160. Vaudaux P, Waldvogel FA: Gentamicin inactivation in purulent exudates: Role of cell lysis. J Infect Dis 142:586, 1980
161. Wade JC, Smith CR, Petty BG et al: Cephalothin plus an aminoglycoside is more nephrotoxic than methicillin plus an aminoglycoside. Lancet 2:604, 1978
162. Weinstein L, Lerner PI, Chew WH: Clinical and bacteriologic studies of the effect of "massive" doses of penicillin G on infections caused by gram-negative bacilli. N Engl J Med 271:525, 1964
163. Weinstein L, Weinstein AJ: The pathophysiology and pathoanatomy of reactions to antimicrobial agents. Adv Intern Med 19:109, 1974
164. Welling PG, Craig WA, Amido GL, Kunin CM: Pharmacokinetics of cefazolin in normal and uremic subjects. Clin Pharmacol Ther 15:344, 1974
165. Wells RF: Clindamycin-associated colitis. Ann Intern Med 81:547, 1974
166. Williams DN, Laughlin LW, Lee Y: Minocycline: Possible vestibular side-effects. Lancet 2:744, 1974
167. Wilson FM, Belamaric J, Lauter CB, Lerner AM: Anicteric carbenicillin hepatitis. Eight episodes in four patients. JAMA 232:818, 1975
168. Wirt TC, McGee ZA, Oldfield EH, Meacham WF: Intraventricular administration of amikacin for complicated gram-negative meningitis and ventriculitis. J Neurosurg 50:95, 1979
169. Wise R: Use of antibiotics. Cephalosporins. Br Med J 2:40, 1978
170. Wise R, Wright N, Wills PJ: Pharmacology of cefotaxime and its desacetyl metabolite in renal and hepatic disease. Antimicrob Agents Chemother 19:526, 1981
171. Wong GA, Pierce TH, Goldstein E, Hoeprich PD: Penetration of antimicrobial agents into bronchial secretions. Am J Med 59:219, 1975
172. Woolfrey BF, Fox JM, Quall CO: An evaluation of burn wound quantitative microbiology. I. Quantitative eschar cultures. Am J Clin Pathol 75:532, 1981
173. Wormser GP, Keusch GT: Trimethoprim-sulfamethoxazole in the United States. Ann Intern Med 91:420, 1979
174. Zacherle B: Medical staff conference: Methicillin-induced interstitial nephritis. West J Med 123:380, 1975
175. Zaske DE, Sawchuk RJ, Gerding DN, Strate RG: Increased dosage requirements of gentamicin in burn patients. J Trauma 16:824, 1976
176. Zaske DE, Sawchuk RJ, Strate RG: The necessity of increased doses of amikacin in burn patients. Surgery 84:603, 1978

20 Complications of Anesthesia

S. K. Kallar | R. L. Keenan | A. Aghdami

OVERVIEW

Surgical anesthesia—by its very nature—is hazardous, since it obtunds normally protective reflexes and disrupts physiologic control systems. Nevertheless, anesthetic morbidity and mortality rates have been kept acceptably low over the past half century largely through increasing knowledge of cardiovascular and respiratory physiology, improvements in intraoperative physiologic monitoring, and the increasing availability of well-trained anesthesia personnel. Moreover, the benefits of surgery have now been extended to severely ill patients who were considered inoperable previously. Renal transplantation and myocardial revascularization, for instance, would be unthinkable without modern anesthesiology.

Still, anesthetic deaths and complications do occur. Deaths due to anesthesia alone are believed to occur once in every 5,000 to 10,000 operations performed under anesthesia.[21] If this number is combined with an overall operative mortality rate of approximately 2%, then of the 200 patients expected to die after 10,000 operations, two will die solely as a result of anesthetic complications.[11] Though the number is small, anesthetic deaths are often disturbing because many—some would say most—are the result of simple mistakes or oversight and thus, in theory, might have been prevented.[29]

The complications and problems described below include the most common (such as sore throat after tracheal intubation) and the most dramatic or catastrophic (such as malignant hyperthermia). For the sake of brevity and practicality, complications that are both minor and rare have been omitted.

Complications of the Respiratory System

MINOR UPPER AIRWAY PROBLEMS

SORE THROAT is common after an operation is performed with general anesthesia and is not necessarily related to laryngoscopy and intubation. Trauma to the mucous membrane of the pharynx and trachea, the tongue, and the tonsillar pillars may be caused by the use of an oropharyngeal airway, the insertion of a nasogastric tube, packing, and, of course, laryngoscopy and intubation. Contributing factors are drying of the mucous membranes due to the administration of antisialogogue drugs, breathing dry anesthetic gases, and general dehydration.

The actual incidence of postoperative sore throat is unclear. Hartsell and Stephen reported an incidence of only 6% in patients questioned postoperatively, while in another study the incidence was in excess of 50%.[15, 30] Fortunately, sore throat is not long lasting; it usually disappears within 24 hours. Specific therapy is not necessary.

HOARSENESS may result from prolonged abduction of the cords; it is then of short duration. However, if hoarseness persists, one must watch for the formation of a *laryngeal granuloma*. This is one of the rare complications of endotracheal intubation and is caused by prolonged pressure of the tube on the posterior portion of the vocal process of the arytenoid cartilage, causing ulceration with subsequent infection and formation of granulation tissue. If indirect laryngoscopy confirms the presence of an ulcer, complete voice rest is necessary to permit healing. If a granuloma has already developed, laryngoscopic excision is indicated.[25] In recent years the use of sterile, disposable tubes has virtually eliminated the incidence of granuloma.

COMPLICATIONS RELATED TO INTUBATION

Intubation complications include trauma to lips and teeth. If a tooth is dislodged or fragmented, the fragments must be recovered, since the most serious consequence would be aspiration into a bronchus. If a tooth or fragment is missing, chest roentgenogram is mandatory.

The rare complication of *subglottic sloughing and stenosis* may be caused by a cuff inflated too tightly and for too long. This complication, however, is seen only after prolonged intubation.

Laceration of the pharyngeal mucosa may result in extensive *surgical emphysema* and later *mediastinal infection,* which can be catastrophic. It demands immediate surgical exploration, repair, and drainage.

Mucosal drying and *loss of body heat* result when dry inspired gases bypass the nasal mucosa. The use of a low-flow anesthetic circuit or a heated humidifier provides moisture and helps to maintain body temperature.[13]

Hypoxia during laryngoscopy and intubation will occur after 30 seconds of apnea if the lungs are filled with air. For this reason inhalation of pure oxygen for at least 2 minutes prior to intubation should be carried out. When this is done, apneic periods for more than 2 minutes can be allowed without the danger of hypoxemia.[63]

Misplacement of the endotracheal tube is serious and entirely preventable. Correct placement of the tube within the trachea must be ascertained immediately following intubation and whenever position is changed. To make sure that both lungs are ventilated both lung fields should be ascultated immediately after inflation of the cuff. Too deep an insertion of the tube will result in the loss of breath sounds in one (usually the left) chest. The tube should be withdrawn until both lungs are equally ventilated. If the endotracheal tube is mistakenly placed into the esophagus and positive pressure ventilation is begun, the air movement in and out of the stomach can easily be misinterpreted as lung ventilation. The stethoscope should be placed over the stomach to detect sounds of air movement. If there is any question at all, the glottis must be reexposed to confirm correct placement of the tube. Alternatively, it is often prudent to extubate the patient, ventilate by mask, and reintubate under direct vision. An inappropriately placed or nonfunctioning endotracheal tube is lethal.

Laryngospasm

Laryngospasm may be encountered during any type of operation with any agent but is seen most frequently in infants and children. Secretions, light anesthesia, and painful stimuli are predisposing factors. It is also seen immediately following tracheal extubation and is the result of reflex adduction of the vocal cords. Laryngospasm is recognized by the impairment of inspiration or the inability to provide positive pressure inspiration; expiration is typically unimpaired. Fortunately it is usually short-lived, and some air exchange will commonly occur within 30 seconds if oxygen is applied with gentle, continuous positive pressure; ordinarily, this will be adequate to maintain oxygenation. If the laryngospasm persists, it will be necessary to administer a rapid-acting muscle relaxant like succinylcholine to paralyze the vocal-cord musculature and allow the patient to be ventilated passively. Treatment of laryngospasm by inexperienced personnel is extremely hazardous.

Airway Obstruction

Anesthetic causes of airway obstruction can be divided into normal and abnormal groups. Nonpathologic (normal) airway obstruction occurs when the airway collapses as a result of unconsciousness, and it is common. The tongue may fall back and, by occluding the hypopharynx, will interfere with respiratory exchange. To prevent this, the postoperative or nonsurgical patient should be placed in the semiprone or "tonsil" position with an oral or nasal airway in place until all reflexes and muscle tone return. Excessive secretions may also obstruct the airway in the course of anesthesia, especially during the period that the patient is emerging from anesthesia. Suctioning and turning the patient on his side while lowering the head to drain the secretions toward the mouth are useful routines.

Pathologic (abnormal) airway obstruction may be due to congenital abnormalities such as choanal atresia, Pierre–Robin syndrome, and laryngeal stenosis; tumors, inflammation, and foreign bodies; to enlarged tonsils and adenoids. The anesthesiologist must anticipate these problems and secure a patent airway before unconsciousness is produced. "Awake" intubation under topical pharyngeal and tracheal analgesia is usually employed. "Blind" intubation, direct laryngoscopy, and intubation over a flexible fiberoptic bronchoscope are all recognized methods. Tracheostomy is indicated if all other methods fail, and a tracheostomy set should be available for use whenever trouble is suspected.

Bronchospasm

Bronchospasm implies the reflex constriction of bronchiolar smooth muscle typically seen in an asthmatic attack. Bronchospasm under anesthesia occurs most frequently in known asthmatic patients, but occasionally it is seen in patients with no history of asthma. Anesthetically related bronchospasm is typically the result of stimulation of the respiratory tract with either irritant vapor or the placement of an artificial airway or tube before adequate analgesia is established. In known asthmatics, bronchospasm is best avoided by a careful, smooth induction and the production either of deep anesthesia or topical analgesia prior to instrumentation of the airway. Occasionally bronchospasm occurs spontaneously, despite the best preventive efforts of the anesthetist.

In diagnosing bronchospasm, it is critically important to rule out other causes of increased airway resistance that might cause "wheezing." A partially kinked endotracheal tube will cause the breathing bag to feel "stiff" and will be associated with high-pitched breath sounds. It can usually be differentiated from bronchospasm on the basis of the expiratory wheezing associated with bronchospasm and the inspiratory and expiratory squeaks that come from a kinked tube. A tube mistakenly placed in the esophagus rather than in the trachea may also fool the unwary anesthetist; the bag will be "stiff," and high-pitched sounds will be heard in the chest. But the sounds will be coarse, and loudest over the stomach. A kinked or misplaced tube must be withdrawn and replaced immediately, while with bronchospasm the tube is best left in place.

Once bronchospasm is diagnosed, treatment must be prompt and aggressive, and it does not differ materially from the management of status asthmaticus in the emergency room or intensive-care unit. Endotracheal intubation (usually already performed) and positive pressure ventilation with oxygen should be undertaken while specific bronchodilator therapy is begun. The positive pressure delivered by an anesthetic machine and ventilator normally does not exceed 40 torr. In most cases this will maintain ventilation during an episode of bronchospasm, but if it does not (as documented by a rising $PaCO_2$) then an intensive-care ventilator may be brought into the operating room to maintain ventilation while anesthesia is continued with intravenous drugs.

Of the anesthetic agents, halothane appears to be a specific bronchodilator and has been used successfully to prevent or abort bronchospasm during anesthesia and surgery. It has also been used to treat status asthmaticus for prolonged periods. Halothane therefore is specifically indicated for anesthesia in an asthmatic patient. All depressant drugs appear to be helpful in relieving bronchospasm, even if they are not specific bronchodilators. Muscle relaxants, perhaps because they prevent coughing, have also been found useful in treating status asthmaticus and can be valuable in bringing an episode of bronchospasm under control in the operating room.

Specific bronchodilator therapy during anesthesia is similar to that used in a medical setting. Aerosolized beta agonists delivered into the airway are often effective. Parenteral epinephrine and terbutaline administration may also be attempted (although epinephrine may be risky in the presence of halothane because of myocardial irritability). When all else fails, glucosteroid therapy is indicated. In almost all instances, bronchospasm can be relieved without the need to abort the proposed operation. Monitoring of the adequacy of ventilation and gas exchange is best achieved with serial arterial blood-gas analysis, and the early insertion of an indwelling radial artery cannula should be considered. The anesthetist may detect improvement of airway resistance from the feel of the breathing bag (or the surgeon may detect it, by observing the relieved look on the anesthetist's face), or, by a reduction in the peak airway pressure required to deliver a tidal breath during mechanical ventilation with a volume-limited device. Once airway resistance has returned to normal or near-normal, the operation may proceed if it has been interrupted. Therapy with aminophylline or steroids, once begun, should be continued in adequate dosage well into the postoperative period, since emergence from anesthesia and extubation are as much a stimulus to bronchospasm as are induction and intubation.[66]

POSTOPERATIVE RESPIRATORY DEPRESSION

If a patient's ventilation is depressed at the end of surgery, for whatever reason, mechanical ventilatory assistance is necessary until the patient regains full exchange. If the respiratory depression is due to the *effects of narcotics*, antagonists like naloxone, 0.2 mg, IV, can be used and repeated hourly if necessary (the pediatric dose is 5–10 μg kg of body weight). But it is far safer (and more comfortable for the patient) to continue mechanical ventilation.

Depression from the *persistent effect of nondepolarizing muscle relaxants* (such as curare or pancuronium) can, in theory, be reversed by giving an anticholinesterase such as neostigmine in combination with atropine. Succinylcholine, a depolarizing muscle relaxant, normally results in paralysis for about 10 minutes. But one may see a prolonged response from overdose, from preoperative long-term anti-cholinesterase therapy (as used for glaucoma), or, most common, from the presence of atypical plasma-cholinesterase enzyme activity.[45] The last is a congenital, inherited trait. Persistent neuromuscular blockade can readily be diagnosed with a nerve stimulator and, in the case of atypical enzyme activity, with appropriate laboratory tests. But the safe procedure in all cases of postoperative respiratory depression is to continue mechanical ventilation and administer sedation for as long as is required. Given adequate ventilatory support, muscular paralysis will ultimately dissipate spontaneously.

Other factors contributing to prolonged paralysis in the immediate postoperative period are inadvertent *hypothermia* following long surgical procedures, the use of large doses of *antibiotics* (especially if used intraperitoneally), and *hypoperfusion states* (hypovolemia and cardiac depression).[54]

PULMONARY ASPIRATION

Normal protective reflex mechanisms that prevent foreign material from entering the tracheobronchial tree are obtunded by anesthesia. The danger of pulmonary aspiration of stomach contents is particularly common in patients who are elderly, obese, or pregnant; during induction and recovery from anesthesia; in the later recovery period after gastrointestinal surgery; and in patients with hiatal hernias, full stomachs, or high intestinal obstructions. Aspiration may be the result of passive, silent, and often unrecognized regurgitation or the active reflex process of vomiting.

The clinical picture of pulmonary aspiration depends on the nature of the material aspirated. Solid particulate matter will occlude various parts of the tracheobronchial tree, producing physical signs of collapse localized to the area distal to the blockade. Hypoxic cardiac arrest may occur quickly following tracheal or bronchial obstruction if solid or semisolid aspiration is voluminous. Aggressive suctioning should be attempted, but it is often in vain. Massive solid aspiration is therefore almost hopeless once it occurs. It is best avoided by strict adherence to an "NPO" rule when possible, and awake or rapid-sequence intubation where delay is not possible.

"Mendelson's syndrome," or chemical aspiration pneumonitis, is caused by aspiration of liquid stomach contents. Its severity is related to the chemical composition of the liquid and the volume aspirated. Although the full-blown picture of aspiration pneumonitis is generally thought to be seen only if the pH of the aspirate is 2.5 or less and the volume is on the order of more than 0.4 ml per kg of body weight, severe lung injury may also occur after aspiration of stomach contents with a much higher pH value.[50] Antacid pretreatment of patients at risk appears to help but cannot be relied upon to eradicate the problem.[64] The mortality rate for this complication is extremely high even with first-class treatment. Symptoms include dyspnea, cyanosis, and tachycardia, usually occurring within 15 to 30 minutes of aspiration. Auscultation reveals generalized rales and expiratory rhonchi; sometimes asthmalike wheezing is noticed. Usually the patient manifests symptoms of pulmonary edema, hypotension, and elevated pulmonary artery pressure. Blood gas studies show hypoxia, mild hypercapnia, and metabolic acidosis. The hypoxia is not relieved by oxygen supplementation alone. A chest x-ray examination will reveal interstitial pulmonary edema, while the heart is not enlarged.

Although aspiration of infected material may result in a superimposed component of infection and contribute to a higher rate of mortality, more commonly sterile aspiration pneumonitis is followed in 3 to 5 days by secondary infection in devitalized lung tissue. The rapid spread and dilution of the gastric aspirate (in less than a minute) is such that any attempt at dilution and removal by endotracheal instillation of saline or sodium bicarbonate will not be effective and may indeed be harmful.

Treatment for aspiration includes mechanical ventilation for at least 24 hours, using continuous positive end expiratory pressure (PEEP) as required to maintain an acceptable arterial oxygen tension. Since early aspiration pneumonitis is purely chemical in nature and is noninfective, antibiotic therapy is not helpful. The prophylactic use of antibiotics has not been proven to prevent the subsequent development of infection. Although steroids have been suggested, there is no hard evidence to show that the process is altered by the use of large doses of steroids immediately after aspiration has occurred. Steroid use may result in an increased incidence of endotoxic shock and late pulmonary granulomata.[47, 65, 68]

POSTOPERATIVE ATELECTASIS AND PNEUMONIA

Despite a better understanding of pulmonary pathophysiology, improved preparation of the patient for surgery, and better intraoperative and postoperative care, the incidence of postoperative atelectasis and pneumonia remains high. The occurrence varies widely; some studies show 2% to 3%, others as high as 75%. Obviously, many factors play a role: the type and length of surgery, the site of operation, the patient's own physical condition, preexisting disease, the anesthesia used, and the quality of postoperative care. Despite many improvements and attention to detail, there remains an overall incidence of 5% to 10% in most large series, not much different from what it was 50 years ago. However, it has become clear that the site of surgery and the preoperative pulmonary status of the patient are the two main contributors to postoperative atelectasis and pneumonia.

In the postoperative period the normal mechanisms that ensure patency of alveoli and small airways and promote clearance of secretions are interrupted. Shallow breathing and cough suppression because of pain lead to retention of secretions and the collapse of small airways with subsequent decreased lung volumes and compliance. These in turn lead to a reduction in vital capacity, increased ventilation/perfusion inequality, and hypoxemia. Airway closure and microatelectasis also result, a process that will eventually lead to gross atelectasis and pneumonia. These changes in pulmonary function are especially severe after thoracic and upper abdominal surgery, less so following lower abdominal surgery, and least after superficial operations.[43]

Anesthesia probably does contribute to postoperative respiratory complications by reducing lung volume and by its drying properties and influence on surfactant. However, the choice of technique is of little importance. As early as 1946, Dripps and Deming showed that with aggressive "stir-up" recovery-room care there is no higher incidence of postoperative pulmonary complications after general inhalation anesthesia than after spinal anesthesia.[17]

The most important contributing factors lie with the patient. Pulmonary dysfunction existing at the time of surgery will increase the risk of postoperative complications. Even minimal respiratory infections increase that risk, and it is important to delay surgery, if possible, until any respiratory tract infection, even the common cold, has subsided. A careful preoperative evaluation and the inclusion of pulmonary function tests will identify patients at risk for developing complications postoperatively. Using simple pulmonary function tests, Stein and Cassara found a 3% complication rate in patients with normal tests versus a 70% rate in those with one or more abnormal tests.[57] Expiratory flowrate measurements seem to be the best predictors of whether patients will be able to cough adequately to clear secretions postoperatively.

Cigarette smokers have a higher incidence of pulmonary complications following surgery. Chalon and co-workers found that even in the absence of demonstrable pulmonary disease, the smoker's risk is much higher.[11] Smoking alters the cytologic picture of the respiratory epithelium, and poor ciliary activity together with more viscous mucus makes the smoker more than the nonsmoker dependent on an effective cough mechanism to clear secretions, a mechanism known to be impaired following anesthesia and surgery. In Chalon's study of 111 patients, the incidence of postoperative pulmonary complications ranged from 7.9% in nonsmokers, to 23% in moderate smokers, and to 43% in very heavy smokers.

Obesity also increases the risk of postoperative pulmonary complications, since chest wall compliance is decreased and the work of breathing increased. However, airway closure also contributes to the marked hypoxemia of obese subjects under anesthesia.[31]

A somewhat higher incidence of postoperative respiratory complications can also be seen in the elderly, and the sex of the patient makes no difference.

The emphasis of therapy lies on prevention and early treatment.[57] The objectives are to identify preoperatively patients who are at increased risk, to improve impaired pulmonary function, to control secretions, and to prevent hypoxemia and atelectasis by aggressive treatment. Preoperative and postoperative chest physical therapy of patients with abnormal pulmonary function can reduce the incidence and severity of respiratory complications. Small-airway obstruction may be relieved by treating any reversible element with bronchodilators, helping the patient to clear secretions as much as possible and treating culture-proven purulent secretions with antibiotics, postural drainage, and chest physical therapy. Cessation of smoking at least for several days prior to surgery is perhaps the single most effective means of decreasing the risk of postoperative pulmonary complications. Breathing exercises, chest physical therapy, and incentive spirometry should all improve lung expansion in principle and are used widely. However, their efficacy remains to be proven scientifically. Intermittent positive pressure breathing (IPPB) therapy with aerosol and bronchodilators is now considered ineffective except in the few patients who have proven reactive airway disease, such as bronchial asthma or chronic bronchitis with a bronchospastic component.

Postoperative management consists of aggressive nursing care, emphasizing frequent deep breaths and coughing; frequent change in position; and clearing of secretions by suctioning. The use of analgesics may allow deep breathing and coughing, which will overcome the reduced lung volumes due to pain and reluctance to breathe deeply. However, narcotic analgesics themselves cause respiratory depression, so their administration must be judicious. Intercostal nerve block and epidural analgesia can be very effective in restoring pulmonary function without central depression. Voluntary deep breathing is a simple method to reduce the incidence of postoperative pulmonary complications. Multiple, slow, and deep breaths held at peak inspiration for several seconds and repeated several times are most useful.

If retention of secretions proves to be particularly stubborn, tracheobronchial suctioning should be attempted. When all else fails, reintubation of the trachea may be required to facilitate frequent suctioning. This is usually best accomplished in an intensive-care environment. In patients with chronic lung disease with impaired mucus clearance, emphasis should be on hyperventilation. In addition to the maneuvers already mentioned, postural drainage with chest percussion or vibration will be helpful in moving secretions to large airways where they are more easily cleared. Early ambulation, if feasible, is important.

Cardiovascular System Complications

MYOCARDIAL INFARCTION AND REINFARCTION

Myocardial infarction is perhaps the most feared cardiovascular complication of the perioperative period. This risk is increased in patients with a history of previous myocardial infarction. Classic studies at the Mayo Clinic by Tarhan and Steen and their colleagues revealed that 6.1% of patients who had had myocardial infarction had a reinfarction during the first postoperative week.[55, 59] More important, the incidence varied according to how recent the previous infarct was. Patients who were operated on within 3 months of previous infarction had a 27% reinfarction rate: those between 3 to 6 months, 11%. After 6 months, the incidence was stabilized at 4% to 5%. The overall mortality rate of patients with recurrent myocardial infarction was 69%.

Risk factors associated with reinfarction include preoperative hypertension requiring medical treatment; an intraoperative hypotensive episode; site of surgery (great vessels, noncardiac intrathoracic and upper abdominal); duration of anesthesia (2% for under 1 hour versus almost 17% for more than 6 hours); and duration of surgery. The most common time of occurrence of perioperative myocardial infarction is the third postoperative day, possibly owing to the stress of atelectasis and hypoxemia.[59]

The diagnosis is made by clinical signs (hypotension and arrhythmias), ECG, and enzyme studies. Chest pain at this time may be absent or obscured because of narcotics and sedatives. Serial ECG tracings performed daily for up to a week after the operation should be considered in patients with hypertension, known coronary disease, or a history of previous infarction.

Management

Obviously elective surgery should be postponed to at least 6 months beyond infarction. In emergencies, delay may be impossible but the sharply increased risk must be recognized. Tachycardia, hypoxemia, hypotension, and especially hypertension should be avoided. In addition to the routine monitoring, these patients should have precordial (V4 or 5) ECG monitoring for changes in S-T segment and T waves. Direct arterial pressure monitoring should be performed during major surgery, and pulmonary artery catheterization for monitoring of wedge pressure and cardiac output should be considered if there is any possibility of left ventricular dysfunction.[34]

DYSRHYTHMIAS

Dysrhythmias are common in the operating room, with a reported incidence as high as 30%.[2, 36] They are so common, in fact, that most need not be viewed as complications. Only about 1% of patients under anesthesia have life-threatening dysrhythmias, according to one study.[62] Preexistent heart disease and treatment with digitalis both predispose surgical patients to serious dysrhythmias. Dysrhythmias most commonly occur during endotracheal intubation and with manipulation of the heart during intrathoracic procedures. The most common dysrhythmias seen during anesthesia are supraventricular slow rhythm such as nodal rhythms (usually benign) and premature ventricular contractions (not so benign). For purposes of discussion as well as of management, anesthesia-related dysrhythmias are best classified as tachyarrhythmias and bradyarrhythmias.

Tachyarrhythmias

Perioperative causes of sympathetic stimulation and catecholamine release abound: hypoxemia, hypercarbia, light anesthesia with stimulation, fluid deficits or excesses, anxiety, and postoperative pain. All cause sinus tachycardia, which is best managed by control of the underlying cause. Ventricular irritability with frequent premature beats, bigeminy, or ventricular tachycardia may be induced by sympathetic stimulation as well, but are more ominous. If the ventricular beats are not too frequent and are unifocal, specific therapy with antiarrhythmia drugs may be safely delayed while the underlying cause is treated. For instance, a unifocal bigeminy is frequently seen during endotracheal intubation, but with the reestablishment of ventilation after intubation and the deepening of anesthesia, the bigeminy usually reverts spontaneously to sinus rhythm in 2 or 3 minutes.

However, multifocal ventricular beats or ventricular tachycardia should be regarded as precursors of ventricular fibrillation and should be treated promptly with an intravenous bolus of lidocaine (normally 1.5 mg/kg) while the underlying cause is determined and if possible corrected. Ventricular tachycardia also may be effectively treated with electric countershock. It is always wise to call for the defibrillator when ventricular tachycardia occurs, not only because countershock can treat it but also because ventricular fibrillation may occur. Persistent or recurrent ventricular irritability may require the use of continuous-drip lidocaine.

Anesthetic agents that "sensitize" the myocardium to the arrhythmogenic effect of epinephrine—either endogenous or injected—include cyclopropane (now rarely used) and halothane. In the presence of these agents, dosages of epinephrine used surgically to curtail bleeding should be sharply reduced. Fortunately the newer halogenated agents enflurane and isoflurane do not share this property with halothane.

Patients with ischemic heart disease are prone to ventricular irritability. Under anesthesia, therefore, factors that are known to increase irritability should be especially avoided; hypoxemia, hypercarbia, hypertension, and hypokalemia.[35] Hypokalemia can result in enhanced automaticity and reentry and thereby contribute to ventricular irritability. Where time permits, it should be corrected prior to surgery, especially in patients already at risk for the development of ventricular tachyarrhythmias.

Paroxysmal atrial tachycardia occurs rarely under anesthesia, but it can be disturbing, especially if hemodynamics are altered. It is best treated conservatively first, for example, gentle pressure over the eye or carotid bifurcation. If these fail, small doses of intravenous propranolol (0.5–2 mg) are usually effective in lowering the pulse rate. Paroxysmal atrial tachycardia may occur in otherwise healthy patients. In contrast, the appearance of atrial fibrillation or flutter during anesthesia may well be a sign of heart failure, particularly in patients with valvular heart disease. Their treatment may require digitalis to control heart rate.

Bradyarrhythmias

Bradyarrhythmias occurring in the perioperative period may be divided into functional, toxic/hypoxic, and organic. Functional bradyarrhythmias are the result of vagal stimulation, which in turn may be caused by reflex activity. Classic examples well-known to surgeons and anesthesiologists include upper-abdominal traction and manipulation of the carotid sinus. The hallmark of reflex vagal bradycardia is the suddenness of its onset and the promptness of its reversion to normal when the reflex is blocked, either with local anesthesia to its sensory limb or with atropine, which blocks the motor limb. The suddenness and intensity of bradycardia associated with vagal stimulation tends to terrorize the anesthetist, but because it is readily reversed, it is usually benign. Drugs that have vaguslike properties include the muscle-relaxant antagonists neostigmine and pyridostigmine. They may cause profound bradycardia unless an anticholinergic drug is administered concomitantly. The relaxant succinylcholine may also produce a transient but profound bradycardia, especially in children. Pretreatment with atropine reduces the incidence and intensity.

Toxic/hypoxic bradyarrhythmias are due either to the overdose of a drug that depresses the heart (which includes all potent inhalation anesthetics) or to severe hypoxemia. The former is seen typically in infants with severe congenital heart disease who cannot tolerate the usual induction concentrations of halothane or other inhalant, but it may also be seen when dosage is miscalculated or the vaporizer tips over and spills liquid agent into the breathing system. The latter, hypoxic bradycardia, is typically seen when a hypoxic gas mixture is administered inadvertently or when a breathing system disconnection is not discovered. The feature of a toxic or hypoxic bradycardia that differentiates it from vagal reflex bradycardia is its relatively slow onset. It does not begin abruptly (although it may be discovered suddenly); rather, it develops gradually over a period of 1 or 2 minutes. Obviously, treatment is directed at the underlying cause and must be prompt if it is to be effective, since the bradycardia tends to progress to arrest. Atropine may be useful in restoring the heartbeat to normal, but only if the underlying cause is corrected.

Organic bradyarrhythmias consist of various types of heart block and are the responsibility of the cardiologist. It should be noted, however, that patients who are known to have complete heart block or any of its immediate precursors, such as "sick sinus syndrome," trifascicular block with a history of Stokes–Adams attacks, and perhaps Mobitz type II blocks, should have a pacemaker implanted under local anesthesia prior to major surgery.[67] Should heart block occur during anesthesia, it may be treated with isoproterenol.[35]

HYPERTENSION

The most common cause of hypertension in the perioperative period is preexisting hypertension. As many as one third of patients presenting for surgery have severe arterial hypertension (180/110 torr or more).[22] There is a high incidence of ischemic heart disease in these patients, and with long-standing untreated hypertension there may be cerebral and renal disease too. Preexisting hypertension can be exaggerated during the perioperative period and, if not properly recognized or treated, may lead to myocardial infarction, intracerebral hemorrhage, or cardiac failure. It is now well recognized by anesthesiologists that severe hypertension, like tachycardia, can be a major stress to an ischemic myocardium and is especially to be avoided in patients with coronary artery disease.

Anesthetic management of hypertension begins with thorough preoperative assessment including a medical history, physical examination, a full 12-lead ECG chest x-ray examination, and serum electrolytes. Cerebral, renal, and cardiac disease should be suspected and ruled out. Contrary to the old belief, it is now established that antihypertensive drug therapy should be maintained up to and including the day of surgery. This is particularly the case with propranolol. Special mention should also be made of clonidine. Sudden rebound hypertension has been reported after preoperative withdrawal of clonidine; therefore, it should be replaced by hydralazine preoperatively unless clonidine can be restarted within 4 hours postoperatively.[10] It is generally accepted that elective surgery should be postponed in patients with severe, untreated hypertension until the blood pressure has been brought under reasonable medical control, especially if there are major organ complications.[24]

Operative management should include the careful avoidance of hypertensive episodes, especially during the stressful periods of endotracheal intubation and initial incision. Numerous anesthetic methods have been used successfully, but all avoid anesthesia that is too light for the anticipated times of sympathetic stimulation. Should the arterial pressure rise to unacceptable levels despite adequate anesthesia, the use of vasodilators such as nitroglycerine or sodium nitroprusside given as an intravenous drip is indicated. Intravenous propranolol in small doses (0.5–2 mg) has also been recommended both for prophylaxis and for therapy in patients with good myocardial function.[22]

Hypertension continues to be a problem in the postoperative period. Factors contributing to postoperative hypertension include pain, hypoxemia, emergence excitement, hypercarbia, hypothermia, and reaction to an endotracheal tube. Most postoperative hypertension occurs in patients with preexistent hypertensive disease, and it tends to be self-limiting if the contributing factors are removed. Pain relief with intravenous narcotics, rewarming, attention to ventilatory function, and timely tracheal extubation will "cure" most postoperative hypertension within 2 hours of the end of surgery.[23] When, rarely, hypertension persists, hemodynamic abnormalities such as fluid overload should be considered. Vasodilator therapy with small doses of chlorpromazine (2.5–10 mg, IV) can be very effective. Sodium nitroprusside, hydralazine, or diazoxide should be employed only as a last resort, when severe hypertension persists despite the above measures.[46]

HYPOTENSION

Hypotension, often defined as a fall in arterial blood pressure 30% below the patient's normal range, is perhaps the most common problem that confronts the anesthesiologist. The cause of hypotension is more important to the anesthesiologist than is the degree, since certain forms of hypotension can be beneficial. The question that underlies any unintentional hypotension in the operating room is, "Is perfusion adequate?" The answer to the question, in practice, lies with identification of the cause. Anesthetic or drug-induced arteriolar dilatation will result in hypotension, while at the same time cardiac output remains normal or actually increases. Hypotension of this type will not be harmful, provided cerebral perfusion pressure is maintained (normally a mean arterial pressure of 50 torr is sufficient to maintain cerebral perfusion).

However, when hypotension is the result of a fall in cardiac output, perfusion may well be impaired. Myocardial depression, hypovolemia, or venous pooling, alone or more frequently in combination are the typical causes of low cardiac output seen intraoperatively.

With invasive monitoring, cardiac output can be measured directly and identification of the direct cause of hypotension (arteriolar dilatation *versus* low cardiac output) is easy. Furthermore, if cardiac output is low, left atrial or pulmonary capillary wedge pressure will readily define whether myocardial depression (high wedge pressure) or hypovolemia or venous pooling (low wedge pressure) is the culprit. But the vast majority of hypotensive episodes occur when the insertion of a pulmonary artery catheter is not indicated. The surgical team, and particularly the anesthetist, must then rely on their knowledge of the patient, their understanding of the pharmacology of the drugs employed, and their clinical judgment.

Some basic principles useful in determining the probable cause and most likely cure of hypotension include the following: (1) Potent inhalation anesthetics tend to be vasodilators as well as myocardial depressants; fortunately their effects are readily reversible. Myocardial depression is normally a problem only in patients with severely impaired myocardial reserve. (2) Intravenous drugs used in anesthesia, notably the narcotics and benzodiazepines, are not normally myocardial depressants. Thiopental is only a slight depressant. However, all are powerful vasodilators. (3) In addition to anesthetic drugs, other aspects of routine anesthesia that contribute to venous pooling include positive pressure ventilation and hypocarbia. (4) In the presence of hypovolemia or even mild dehydration, vasodilators will cause not only arteriolar dilatation but also venous (capacitance) dilatation, which results in a fall in cardiac output due to venous pooling. Hypotension so induced can readily be reversed with the rapid infusion of a moderate volume (250–500 ml) of intravenous fluids or a very small dose of alpha-adrenergic drug. (5) Although large doses of alpha-adrenergic drugs such as phenylephrine produce arteriolar vasoconstriction, small doses produce significant venous vasoconstriction. Thus hypotension during anesthesia that responds dramatically to a small dose (0.1–0.5 mg IV) of phenylephrine is likely to be due to hypovolemia or venous pooling. Hypotension *not* so responding can be considered much more serious; it may be caused by severe myocardial depression. (6) When severe myocardial depression or pump failure is suspected, beta adrenergic drugs such as dopamine or dobutamine are indicated. Larger doses of phenylephrine or the use of a more powerful alpha stimulant may be harmful. (7) Not every fall in blood pressure indicates hypotension. Because of his apprehension, the patient's blood pressure on admission and immediately preceding induction may not be his normal value. Hypotension should not be considered serious until the blood pressure is below the patient's normal resting or sleeping blood pressure, which should be known to the anesthetist. Thus, a precipitous fall on induction of anesthesia may simply be a fall *to normal* and alone does not justify aggressive therapy.[16, 53, 60]

Neurologic Complications

HYPOXIC BRAIN INJURY

Whatever the cause of brain hypoxia, the end result is neuronal damage, differing only in extent, which is directly related to the degree and duration of suboxygenation. Essentially no cerebral oxygen storage is possible, and stores of high-energy phosphates in the form of ATP, ADP, and phosphocreatine are sufficient to maintain tissue availability for only a few minutes. Since the brain is extremely sensitive to loss of its oxygen supply, it is important to qualify the severity of an hypoxic event.

A reduction of oxygen delivery may be caused by either a reduction in oxygen content of arterial blood or by a reduction in blood flow. In the latter case, flow might decrease either to the entire brain (global) or to a portion of the brain (focal or regional). In the event of a reduction in arterial oxygen content, the initial response is a global increase in cerebral blood flow. This is triggered at a PaO_2 of about 50 torr and is probably mediated by a developing cerebral lactic acidosis. Hypoxic brain damage will first be manifested in the most metabolically active areas, the cortical and subcortical grey matter. Clinically, a reduction in oxygen delivery due to reduction of cerebral blood flow is the most common cause of brain hypoxia. The critical level of cerebral blood flow is approximately 18 ml to 20 ml per 100 g per minute (normal is about 50 ml/100 g/min). At flows below the critical level, EEG changes are demonstrable and neuronal death may eventually result. Consciousness is lost when cerebral venous PO_2 (normally above 30 torr) falls below 20 torr. Irreversible damage usually occurs after 4 to 5 minutes of total ischemia or anoxia in the brain, but under proper circumstances, the brain's tolerance to total ischemia can apparently be extended.

Hypoxia due to anesthesia may occur in the operative or postoperative period. Operatively it may be the result of hypoperfusion incident to hypotension, the inadvertent delivery of hypoxic mixtures of oxygen, and anesthetic equipment disconnection or failure. Postoperatively, causes include hypoventilation secondary to the depressant effect of anesthetic drugs or muscle relaxants, hypoperfusion due to persistent cardiovascular depression, sudden position change, and overdose of sedatives or narcotics for postoperative pain. The elderly and patients with electrolyte imbalance are more vulnerable to these complications.

The pathophysiologic changes in the brain seen after hypoxia include tissue acidosis, loss of pressure autoregulation, brain swelling, hypoperfusion, hypermetabolism, and neurotransmitter changes progressing to multifocal neuronal death.

Treatment

Prevention is without question the most effective means of dealing with brain hypoxia, and many of the details of clinical anesthesiology are directed to this end. When preventive measures fail, prompt recognition of hypoxia and correction of the underlying cause are the next best treatment. To this end, an anesthetist alert to color changes of the skin and changes in vital signs is most valuable. Particularly noteworthy in hypoxia due to a falling blood oxygen content (as from a ventilator disconnect or a loss of oxygen supply to the breathing system) is bradycardia, which gradually develops and continues to worsen over a 1- to 2-minute period. *Prompt* review of the oxygen-delivery system, from the patient's lungs back to the supply source, and immediate correction of the fault is indicated. Administration of atropine simply wastes valuable time.

With regard to prevention, continuous monitoring of a vital sign, usually the ECG signal, is widely practiced. An audible "beep" that can be heard by all members of the surgical team improves the odds that a decelerating heart rate will be recognized.

When patients remain unconscious after an acute hypoxic episode, active treatment may result in partial or complete recovery, although the outlook is guarded. Methods of brain protection that are currently under investigation include ones intended to diminish brain swelling or edema such as hyperventilation, hyperosmolar drying agents, and steroids. Control of blood pressure at near-normal levels is important since autoregulation of cerebral blood flow may be impaired. Hypothermia or barbiturate coma may be useful in protecting the brain even after an insult, although these modalities remain controversial.[48]

AWARENESS DURING OPERATION

Pain with awareness during operation and its later recall are obviously the result of inadequate anesthesia. This may be caused by unintentional anesthetic errors, such as leaks within the breathing system, unnoticed changes in gas flows, or malfunctioning vaporizers. It may also be the result of inadequate dosage or inappropriate selection of intravenous drugs. Occasionally anesthesia may be decreased or discontinued in an effort to treat severe hypotension, air embolism, and so forth. Awareness is seen mostly with the "balanced" or relaxant technique, but there have been reports with inhalation agents, too. It is often difficult to assess the depth of anesthesia in a patient who is paralyzed. Tolerance to CNS depressants develops in patients who are heavy drinkers and in narcotic or tranquilizer users.

Memory also improves as the importance to the patient of a triggering event (e.g., an anesthetic crisis or surgical complication) increases. Chances of recall are increased at the beginning of the operation (between induction of anesthesia and onset of operation) and at the end when levels of anesthesia are light. Unfortunately, the noise level in the operating room increases with loud conversation at the end of operation too, and the semiconscious patient may believe that this noise can be heard during the intraoperative period.[18, 20]

Operating-room personnel should always be mindful that even the unconscious patient may hear offhand remarks. Therefore, conversation should be quiet and disciplined.

Diazepam and scopolamine have been used as premedicants for their amnesic action. Lorazepam seems even more promising; 4 mg administered orally usually produces amnesia persisting for 8 to 10 hours.[44] During the operation it should be kept in mind that nitrous oxide is a *powerful* amnesic. If it is to be discontinued for any reason during "balanced" anesthesia, substitution with an intravenous agent with known amnesic properties (diazepam, ketamine) is indicated. Narcotics are notoriously poor amnesics.

In some patients recall presents little problem, while in others it may lead to a traumatic neurotic syndrome with symptoms of anxiety, irritability, and preoccupation with death.[3] Although these patients are reluctant to discuss it or even believe that what they remember really happened, it is important that the cause of such symptoms be explored with them. A direct and honest explanation gives a dramatic cure.

POSTANESTHETIC EXCITEMENT/DELIRIUM

Postoperative excitement, characterized by restlessness, disorientation, or irrational talking, represents a stage between surgical anesthesia and complete orientation. The most common stimulus for this behavior is pain, but a distended urinary bladder may also be a cause. It is most common in children and healthy young adults. Other contributory factors include barbiturate premedication, the type of operation (breast biopsy is typical), the preoperative psychological state, and chronic alcoholism. Hypoxia, hypercarbia, or cerebral ischemia may also be a factor and should be ruled out before analgesics are administered.

Delirium (wild thrashing, with shouting and screaming) is seen after administration of anticholinergic drugs, especially scopolamine, if they are not supplemented with narcotic premedication. Emergence from inhalation anesthesia and intravenous diazepam may also result in postoperative delirium in children.

Treatment

Postanesthetic excitement should be treated with small intravenous doses of narcotics to relieve pain, where indicated. Delirium due to anticholinergics or benzodiazepines (diazepam) can be successfully reversed by intravenous physostigmine (1–3 mg).[19, 32]

NEUROLOGIC SEQUELAE OF SPINAL AND EPIDURAL ANESTHESIA

Headache

"Spinal headache" is mostly seen after spinal anesthesia and sometimes after epidural analgesia. The opening in the dura made by lumbar puncture causes the escape of cerebrospinal fluid (CSF), thus decreasing intracranial pressure. This loss of CSF permits traction on intracranial pain-sensitive structures. Headache is typically postural (*i.e.*, worse on sitting or standing up); is occipital in location; and is relieved by lying flat in bed. It may be accompanied by difficulty in hearing and vision.

The incidence of headache is directly related to the size of the needle. Greene has shown that with a 22-gauge spinal needle the incidence of headache is 26% and with a 26-gauge needle it drops to 0.4%.[26]

Conservative treatment of spinal headache consists of rest to discourage more CSF leak, hydration with intravenous or oral fluids to encourage CSF formation, a tight abdominal binder to increase extradural venous pressure, and systemic analgesics to relieve pain.

Active measures of treatment include the administration of extradural saline, 40 ml to 60 ml every 6 hours for the first 24 hours if an epidural catheter is in place. An epidural blood patch has been shown to have a success rate of 94% to 100%.[1] Blood-patch therapy consists of the administration of 10 ml of the patient's own blood into the epidural space directly over the site of the previous lumbar puncture. Although it appears safe in trained hands, blood-patch therapy should be used only when headache is unusually persistent or severe.

Neurologic Deficit

The incidence of neurologic complications after spinal and epidural anesthesia is less than one in 10,000.[61] Neurologic lesions can be grouped according to the mechanisms that cause nerve dysfunction: trauma, toxic agents and infection, ischemia, exacerbation of previous pathology, and unknown.

TRAUMA is one of the most common causes of neurologic complications following spinal or epidural anesthesia. The lesions may be neural (spinal cord and nerve roots) or vascular (arteries and veins), or they may include vertebrae and ligaments. Trauma to the cord and roots often produces neurologic deficit, which recovers poorly. Trauma to the vessels may result in compression-hematoma formation, which requires evacuation. Bone and ligamentous lesions usually are followed by backache, which lasts only a few days. If a patient complains of persistent backache after a difficult puncture, an x-ray examination can be used to rule out damage to the intervertebral disc or signs of infection.

TOXIC AGENTS AND INFECTION. Chemical damage from contaminants such as soaps and detergents and infections used to be very common, when "cold" sterilization (soaking of ampules in alcohol or formalin) was in practice, but with proper selection of drugs and better sterilization of equipment, they are now virtually nonexistent.

ISCHEMIA. Of all the postanesthetic spinal-cord syndromes, those caused by vascular pathology are now the most common. There is scarcity of arterial anastomosis in the spinal cord, which renders it vulnerable to vascular insufficiency. Spinal and epidural anesthesia can cause hypotension, and, in an already compromised patient, spinal-cord ischemia and damage may result. Nevertheless, this is rare.

EXACERBATION OF PREVIOUS PATHOLOGY. Patients suffering from degenerative neurologic diseases, intervertebral disc disease, or epidural tumors may suffer neurologic deterioration after spinal or epidural anesthesia. Whether or not the acceleration of symptoms is due to the anesthetic is never clear. Although there is little evidence to establish cause and effect, most anesthesiologists consider it legally prudent to avoid the issue by avoiding spinal anesthesia in patients with preexistent neurologic disease.[7, 41]

COMPLICATIONS OF NERVE BLOCKS

The complications from nerve blocks range in degree from minor, such as bleeding with or without hematomas, to catastrophic, such as pneumothorax, apnea, and cardiac arrest. They result from misplaced needles or injection of excessive doses of the drug. These complications are reversible. Therefore, monitoring the patient is essential not only during the block but for at least 30 minutes after its completion. Also, drugs and equipment to prevent or correct cardiopulmonary collapse, as well as adequate personnel to assist in their use, must be immediately available.

Some of the commonly used blocks are intercostal nerve block and brachial plexus block. *Intercostal nerve block* is a remarkably safe and effective procedure in expert hands. The most important hazard of this block is pneumothorax, the incidence of which ranges from 0.092% to 19%, depending on the skill of the operator.

Brachial plexus block is frequently performed. The brachial plexus is closely related to the subclavian artery and vein, to the cupula of the pleura, and to small vessels and nerves, so that various techniques have been advocated to avoid these structures and thereby minimize the complications. Of these, the axillary block is very easy to perform and has few complications. Hematoma from inadvertent puncture of the artery is common but does not seem to produce sequelae. When the supraclavicular approach is chosen, one may encounter complications such as Horner's syndrome, phrenic nerve block, arterial puncture, and pneumothorax. To prevent these complications it is advisable to use a 25-gauge needle, stay in close proximity to the bone, instruct the patient not to move or cough, and aspirate before injecting the drug. The interscalene route has recently been advocated for brachial plexus block. Reported complicatons include hematoma formation, recurrent laryngeal nerve and unilateral phrenic nerve blocks, and Horner's syndrome.

Neuropathy is a rare complication. Clinically, complete recovery of nerve function usually occurs after local anesthetic block, but signs of neuropathy have been reported. It is not clear whether they were due to the needle or to the anesthetic agent. Symptoms usually appear 1 week or more after the block, are maximal in about 3 weeks, and diminished after 2 to 3 months.[58]

SYSTEMIC REACTIONS DUE TO LOCAL ANESTHETIC DRUGS

Systemic reactions are the result of high blood levels of local anesthetic drugs due to inadvertent intravascular injection, overdosage, or rapid systemic absorption. Intravascular injection is probably the most common cause of toxicity from local anesthetics. Symptoms and signs appear very rapidly—within 30 seconds—and often before the injection has been completed. Aspiration of blood prior to injection is recommended but may not always be positive, since small veins collapse when suction is applied. It is better to give a test dose of 2 ml to 3 ml of local anesthetic, wait, and then inject the rest of the drug.

Overdosage may also result in toxicity. The total amount of drug should be noted in advance and should not exceed that recommended. It should be reduced in the sick and elderly. Signs and symptoms of toxicity due to overdose appear in 5 to 20 minutes after completion of injection.

Systemic absorption from the mucosa of the nose, pharynx, and respiratory tract is rapid, similar to that following intravenous administration. For transcutaneous local anesthetic, absorption depends on tissue blood supply. Plasma levels are highest after intercostal nerve block and lowest after infiltration of subcutaneous tissues of the abdomen.

Clinical features of toxicity include effects on the central nervous and cardiovascular systems. Usually CNS signs appear first. Early evidence of toxicity includes garrulousness and personality changes, followed by numbness of the tongue and circumoral tissues, which is diagnostic. Others include tinnitus, visual disturbances, and muscular twitching. These may rapidly progress to clouded consciousness, convulsions, and coma with respiratory arrest.

Cardiovascular depression may be directly produced by a high blood level of local anesthetic but more commonly is secondary to respiratory depression and arrest.

Treatment of systemic toxicity should be directed toward prevention of hypoxia, control of convulsions, and cardiovascular support. Mild, early signs of toxicity require the administration of oxygen and the reassurance of the patient. Respiration should be carefully observed, and positive pressure ventilation with oxygen initiated promptly when required. Convulsions are typically short-lived and usually cease spontaneously. However, intravenous diazepam, small doses of barbiturates, and succinylcholine can be useful if convulsions are prolonged. Cardiovascular depression should be anticipated during a reaction; blood pressure and pulse should be monitored. Intravenous therapy with fluids and vasopressors should be available and employed if cardiovascular depression persists after hypoxia has been corrected.

These measures, which if promptly applied will prevent serious consequences in even the most severe toxic reaction, imply that a local anesthetic injection should be administered only when resuscitative drugs and equipment are immediately available. This equipment includes a source of 100% oxygen, a means of delivering positive pressure ventilation, intravenous infusion equipment, a blood-pressure cuff and an electrocardiograph, and drugs, including epinephrine and barbiturates or diazepam.

A special form of systemic reaction to local anesthetics involves epinephrine, which is commonly added to local anesthetics. Its absorption can result in sweating, apprehension, tachycardia, and palpitation. It should not be confused with local anesthetic toxicity or "allergy." Epinephrine overdose is usually self-limiting but may occasionally cause hypertension or ventricular irritability severe enough to require treatment.[52]

Toxic and Metabolic Problems

TOXICITY OF POTENT INHALATION ANESTHETICS

Halothane

Halothane has been implicated as the causative agent in postoperative hepatitis. Halothane hepatitis is rare, with an incidence of fatal hepatic necrosis of 1 per 35,000.[11]

ETIOLOGY. About 20% of inhaled halothane is normally biotransformed to nontoxic products by an oxidative pathway. It is now known that the hepatotoxicity of halothane is the result of metabolic degradation of the parent molecule to a toxic product, a mechanism similar to that seen with chloroform and acetaminophen.[40] A free radical is formed by a reductive pathway that bonds covalently to, and destroys, liver cell membranes. With halothane, the toxic pathway is not normally present, but animal studies have shown that prior enzyme induction and liver hypoxia during anesthesia are routinely followed by the syndrome.[8] Halothane causes centrilobular necrosis, and the liver pathology in cases of jaundice following halothane anesthesia is indistinguishable from that of viral hepatitis.

CLINICAL FEATURES. Typically, there are unexplained low-grade fever, nausea, myalgia, and leukocytosis within 3 to 10 days of operation.[37] Jaundice may not appear for several days. Approximately 10% of patients develop a skin rash, arthralgia, and eosinophilia. Liver chemistries show very high transaminase and bilirubin levels. Prolongation of prothrombin time or evidence of encephalopathy indicates severe liver necrosis and a poor prognosis. Mild cases are accompanied by low-grade fever and elevation of transaminases but without jaundice. It is important to recognize these milder cases, because fulminant hepatitis can be precipitated with subsequent administration of halothane.

DIAGNOSIS. There are no laboratory tests or histologic features specific for halothane hepatitis. Pathologic findings are indistinguishable from those of viral hepatitis. Therefore, diagnosis is based on clinical features and the exclusion of other causes. Differential diagnosis includes viral hepatitis, hepatitis from other drugs, shock, or exacerbation of preexisting liver disease. A careful drug history and examination of the medical record for evidence of preexisting liver disease are vital. Schemel reported that healthy patients scheduled for surgery have an incidence of unsuspected liver disease of 1:750, and visible jaundice of 1:2540.[49]

There is no specific treatment for halothane hepatitis, other than supportive therapy. Mortality rates are high. It has been suggested that halothane should be avoided in patients with unexplained fever or jaundice after a previous halothane anesthetic. It is generally believed that an interval of 4 to 6 weeks decreases the risk from repeated halothane exposure.[9]

Methoxyflurane

Methoxyflurane can cause renal damage because its biotransformation produces inorganic fluoride ion, which damages renal tubules.[39] Toxicity is directly related to the plasma level of fluoride ion: when it exceeds 150 to 200 μ/L, clinical evidence of renal dysfunction occurs. Toxicity typically produces renal insufficiency with polyuria that is resistant to vasopressin. Obesity, enzyme-inducing drugs like phenobarbital, and preexisting renal disease are other contributing factors. For these reasons, the use of methoxyflurane has all but disappeared from practice.

Enflurane

Enflurane is also metabolized to inorganic fluoride, but much less so than is methoxyflurane. Enzyme induction with phenobarbital does not usually lead to nephrotoxic levels in animals given enflurane. Worsening of preexisting renal disease has been reported following enflurane anesthesia, so its use in patients with abnormal renal function should be limited.[38]

Isoflurane

Isoflurane is a new inhalation agent with a potency between that of halothane and enflurane. Since isoflurane undergoes almost no biotransformation, (less than 0.3%) it may prove nontoxic.[33] No significant organ toxicity has been reported to date, and animal models that routinely produce organ toxicity with halothane or methoxyflurane fail to do so with isoflurane.[8]

THYROTOXICOSIS AND THYROID STORM

Thyroid storm is an extreme accentuation of both the signs and symptoms of thyrotoxicosis.[56, 69] If untreated, mortality rates from this rare but serious complication exceed 70%. It has an abrupt onset that is usually triggered by the stress of injection, trauma, or surgery in a patient with previously unrecognized and untreated hyperthyroidism.

Thyroid storm when related to surgery develops intraoperatively or within 6 to 18 hours postoperatively. It is characterized by hyperpyrexia, tachycardia, arrhythmias, profuse sweating, and severe hypotension. Treatment is both supportive and specific. Supportive therapy includes the use of high inspired oxygen concentrations, aggressive cooling, adequate fluid replacement and caloric intake, and close observation in an intensive care unit.

Specific therapy consists of the following:

1. Propranolol in doses of 2 mg to 5 mg should be carefully titrated intravenously every 30 to 120 minutes. It is important to recognize that most of the symptomatology of hyperthyroidism (hypermetabolism, tachycardia, tremor, sweating) is mediated by the sympathetic nervous system and is blocked by propranolol.
2. Large doses of propylthiouracil to prevent further thyroid hormone synthesis (200 mg every 4–6 hr).
3. Sodium iodide, 1 g to 2 g, should be given by slow intravenous infusion every 12 hours.
4. Large intravenous doses of hydrocortisone should be given (300 mg a day).
5. Rarely, hypertension that can be treated with nitroprusside occurs.

Additionally, if surgery has begun, it should be interrupted as soon as possible. Elective surgery should be postponed in all hyperthyroid patients until they have been rendered euthyroid by medical therapy. Propranolol should be given to hyperthyroid patients who require emergency surgery. The dose varies with each patient, ranging from 10 mg to 40 mg every 6 hours, and it must be adjusted individually. Intravenous propranolol, 2 mg to 5 mg every 10 to 30 minutes, can be administered in the intra- and postoperative period.

MALIGNANT HYPERTHERMIA

Malignant hyperthermia (MH) is a genetically determined syndrome characterized by high fever, tachycardia, arrhythmias, rigidity (not always), cyanosis, skin mottling, and profuse sweating.[5, 12, 27, 28] It has been reported in patients whose ages range from 3 months to 72 years. The incidence is 1:15,000 in children and 1:50,000 in adults with a mortality rate of 60% when associated with anesthesia.

The accepted etiology of MH is a defect in calcium transfer that leads to an elevated intracellular calcium level. There is evidence for a myogenic etiology. MH-susceptible patients manifest a high incidence of clinical muscle abnormalities such as ptosis, squint, generalized muscle bulk, joint hypermobility (especially knee), and clubfoot. Measurements of blood creatine phosphokinase (CPK) levels are 70% reliable and provide a basic screening tool, but definite diagnosis requires muscle biopsy. Two types of syndrome have been observed, rigid and nonrigid, but treatment for both is the same.

DIAGNOSIS. The appearance of the sudden generalized hypermetabolic state of MH is unique. The most common presentation is development of muscle rigidity following administration of succinylcholine or a potent inhalation agent. MH also may present as bizarre ventricular arrhythmias. Unexplained tachycardia, fever, tachypnea, sweating, or cyanosis should suggest MH. One should then look for signs of increased metabolism, acidosis, or hyperkalemia. If arterial blood gas studies show metabolic acidosis with a negative base excess of greater than -5 mEq/L and an arterial blood PCO_2 greater than 60 torr despite adequate ventilation, the diagnosis of MH can be established. Therefore the combination of hyperthermia, muscle stiffness, and acidosis calls for immediate treatment.

TREATMENT. A plan of treatment is outlined below:

1. Stop anesthesia. Change rubber tubing and anesthesia machine.
2. Administer dantrolene sodium, which inhibits its calcium release into the muscle cell from the sarcoplasmic reticulum. The dose is 1 mg to 10 mg/kg, IV, with an average dose of 3 mg/kg, depending upon the patient's response. In animals dantrolene is effective in preventing as well as aborting MH syndrome.
4. Administer sodium bicarbonate, 100 mEq initially and up to 600 mEq over a period of time, guided by arterial *p*H and PCO_2. It is highly effective in reversing the severe hyperkalemia. Use of THAM has been associated with a high mortality rate and should be avoided.
5. Actively cool the patient with iced saline, intravenously, through peritoneal and thoracic cavities if possible, and by stomach and bladder lavage. Extracorporeal circulation and heat exchangers have been utilized but normally take too long.
6. Maintain urine output at more than 2 ml/kg/hour. High urine output prevents myoglobin from forming casts in the kidney, which can lead to renal failure. Give mannitol, 12.5 g, IV, or furosemide, 50 mg, IV, up to four doses each.
7. Administer 20% dextrose and 10 units of regular insulin to provide an exogenous energy source and lower hyperkalemia.
8. Use procainamide to stop arrhythmias, 15 mg/kg diluted in 500 ml of isotonic saline, administered over a period of 10 minutes with ECG monitoring. Do not use procaine HCL because in this dose it causes severe cardiovascular instability.
9. Monitor ECG, temperature, arterial blood gases, serum electrolytes, urinary output, and central venous pressure.

Despite appropriate initial therapy, there may be late complications including acute renal failure, consumption coagulopathy, inadvertent hypothermia, and neurologic sequelae.

In providing anesthesia for MH-susceptible patients, their anxiety and stress should be allayed in the preoperative period. Atropine should be given intravenously in small doses if needed. Dantrolene, 4 mg/kg, may be given orally in three or four divided doses in the 24-hour period before anesthesia. Use of potent inhalation agents (halothane, enflurane, isoflurane), succinylcholine, amide local anesthetics, and phenothiazines must be avoided. Ester-type local anesthetics, barbiturates, neuroleptanesthetics, opiates, and pancuronium have been used without incident and are recommended for anesthesia.

Accurate diagnosis of MH susceptibility preoperatively requires a skeletal muscle biopsy. Contractility in the presence of several drugs including caffeine and halothane is tested, and therefore the test must be performed on fresh muscle. Unfortunately the test is available in only a few centers at present. It is important, however, to attempt a positive diagnosis whenever a patient appears susceptible to MH. Exposing a susceptible patient to triggering agents may be fatal; yet withholding such important drugs as muscle relaxants and volatile anesthetics is a severe limitation that is hardly justifiable without adequate evidence of MH susceptibility.

Other less specific signs often seen in patients with MH susceptibility include a family history of MH, an elevated serum CPK in the patient or in relatives, and muscle abnormalities (squint, ptosis, kyphosis, joint hypermobility). Although any one of these may not be associated with MH, the occurrence of several in one patient should alert the clinician to its possibility. At the very least, a careful family history should be a routine part of the preanesthetic evaluation of all patients.

HYPOTHERMIA

The most common cause of hypothermia in surgical patients is air-conditioned operating rooms in which measures have not been taken to maintain the body temperature, especially in lengthy intra-abdominal surgery or in extensive dissection.[42] Hypothermia is also seen in children and debilitated elderly patients. Hypothermic patients seem too depressed for the amount of anesthetic used and may exhibit bradycardia, hypotension, and a low minute volume ventilation. Because of vasoconstriction, they may have masked hypovolemia, which becomes apparent upon rewarming.

Intense vasoconstriction results in impaired tissue perfusion and metabolic acidosis. Shivering in a hypothermic patient with coronary artery disease can lead to myocardial infarction because these patients cannot meet the increased demand of oxygen by the myocardium. Therefore, oxygen and respiratory support must be given until normothermia is achieved and to prevent shivering with sedation and muscle relaxants when indicated. Arterial blood gases should be checked periodically, and ventilation assisted when necessary.

Although moderate hypothermia can be readily treated with supportive measures, deeper hypothermia is extremely hazardous, since ventricular fibrillation frequently occurs when the temperature falls below 29°C and is difficult to reverse without rewarming.

PREVENTION. Temperature should be monitored whenever hypothermia is suspected or expected. Prevention in adults includes the use of circulating water warming blankets on the operating-room table and the infusion of all intravenous fluids and blood through warming coils.[4] Equally important is heated humidification of breathing gases, since the vaporization of the patient's own body water to humidify dry inhaled gases results in significant loss of body heat.[15] These methods, plus the warming of the operating room to 30°C and the use of warming lamps, are widely practiced in children. Once hypothermia has occurred, treatment consists of supportive measures, especially continued ventilatory assistance, as body temperature is slowly returned to normal with warming blankets.

Minor Problems of the Unconscious Patient

SKIN COMPLICATIONS

Anesthesia does obtund normal protective reflexes, and injuries to skin can occur. Pressure-related sores in already poorly perfused areas or over bony promontories may occasionally be seen. More common are burns sustained from defective or improperly grounded diathermy machines. Prompt attention and treatment will lead to success and lessen the chances of later litigation.

Muscular pains, involving mostly the neck, shoulder, and calf muscles, are a minor complication, most probably due to the fasciculations following the administration of depolarizing muscle relaxants such as succinylcholine. Pretreatment with a small dose of a nondepolarizing relaxant drug is said to prevent this complication.[66]

NERVE PALSIES

Peripheral nerve palsies are usually the result of pressure or stretching of a nerve in the course of anesthesia and surgery. Other causes of peripheral nerve injury, such as direct damage to a nerve by a needle or irritant solution, should also be kept in mind. Generalized debility, hypothermia, and hypotension may aggravate the problem. Certain preexisting diseases can predispose patients to these complications; diabetes and alcoholic neuritis come to mind, besides preexisting neurologic disorders.

Brachial plexus palsy may result from improper shoulder support during Trendelenburg position, excessive abduction of the arm causing stretching of the plexus, and bringing the arm to a position behind the coronal plane.

Ulnar nerve palsy is especially easily sustained because the ulnar nerve is unprotected in its path over the medial epicondyle of the humerus and may inadvertently be compressed between the bone and the edge of the operating-room table by the surgeon or his assistants.

Radial nerve injury is less frequent but can occur in the lateral position when the arm sustains pressure over the inner surface of the upper arm. Facial nerve palsy is also rare but may occur from compression of the jaw owing to faulty placement of headstraps to secure a facemask.

Common peroneal nerve damage is encountered frequently following incorrect placement of the legs in stirrups during lithotomy position. The nerve is compressed between the poles and the head of the fibula when the legs are placed inside the stirrups. A faulty lithotomy position or inadequate padding may also cause damage to the saphenous nerve.

An extravenous injection of irritant solution around the cubital veins can easily reach the median nerve and cause damage. For this reason, other venipuncture sites are preferred, although the extravasation of an irritant solution such as thiopental at the wrist may also cause injury to the radial nerve.

Peripheral nerve injuries can be prevented by paying meticulous attention to positioning of the patient and by having all members of the operating-room team focus on possible problems. When a nerve palsy is found, a thorough neurologic examination should be done to determine the correct diagnosis and to assess the severity of the injury. Active exercises and splinting to prevent deformities are indicated. Analgesics may be needed for pain. The extent of the injury will be dependent upon the amount of pressure and the length of time it was exerted on the nerve. Prognosis is good when there is no preexisting neurologic disease. Recovery is slow (up to 6 months for full recovery) but usually complete. Large muscles recover power faster than do small ones. Immediate attention, close follow-up, and support for the anxious patient and family will help to minimize legal consequences.[6]

OPHTHALMIC COMPLICATIONS

In the absence of the protective lid reflex, the eye can easily sustain injury during anesthesia. To prevent trauma to the open eye by drapes, dust, solutions, instruments, and fingers, it is important to keep the eyelids closed. Using some eye ointment will eliminate drying, which in itself can cause damage. In special situations, such as exophthalmos, prone positions, and head and neck surgery, the eyelids should be taped or sewn shut. These measures will largely prevent such complications as conjunctivitis, corneal abrasions, and ulcers. However, when abrasions have occurred, rest and an eyepatch will usually promote healing within 12 hours.

Patients with preexisting ophthalmic conditions may sustain an exacerbation of their disease, especially if periods of hypotension and hypoxia are superimposed. Thus one may see, though rarely, blindness due to acute glaucoma or thrombosis of the central retinal artery. The pressure of the facemask may aggravate ischemia and cause pain in the region of the supraorbital nerve.[66]

The use of atropine in acute narrow-angle glaucoma is not necessarily contraindicated. Small doses (e.g., 0.5 mg) given intramuscularly normally will not dilate the pupil, especially when narcotics or myotic eyedrops are used at the same time.[51]

References

1. Bart AJ, Wheeler AS: Comparison of epidural saline placement and epidural blood placement in the treatment of post-lumbar-puncture headache. Anesthesiology 48:221-223, 1978
2. Bertrand CA, Steiner NV, Jameson AG et al: Disturbances of cardiac rhythm during anesthesia and surgery. JAMA 216:1615-1617, 1971
3. Blacher RS: On awakening paralyzed during surgery: A syndrome of traumatic neurosis. JAMA 234:67-68, 1975
4. Boyan CP, Howland WS: Cardiac arrest and temperature of bank blood. JAMA 183:58-60, 1963
5. Britt BA (ed): Malignant hyperthermia. Int Anesthesiol Clin 17(4):1–168, 1979
6. Britt BA, Gordon RA: Peripheral nerve injuries associated with anesthesia. Can Anaesth Soc J 11:514-536, 1964
7. Bromage PR: Epidural Analgesia, pp 654-715. Philadelphia, WB Saunders, 1978
8. Brown BR Jr: Pharmacogenetics and the halothane hepatitis mystery. Anesthesiology 55:93-94, 1981
9. Bruce DL: What is a "safe" interval between halothane exposure? JAMA 221:1140-1143, 1972
10. Bruce DL, Croley TF, Lee JS: Preoperative clonidine withdrawal syndrome. Anesthesiology 51:90-92, 1979
11. Bunker JP, Forrest WH, Mosteller F, Vandam LD (eds): National halothane study. A study of the possible association between halothane anesthesia and postoperative hepatic necrosis, Washington, DC, US Government Printing Office, 1969
12. Cain PA, Ellis FB: Anesthesia for patients susceptible to malignant hyperpyrexia. Br J Anaesth 49:941-944, 1977
13. Chalon J, Patel C, Ali M et al: Humidity and the anesthetized patient. Anesthesiology 50:195-198, 1979
14. Chalon J, Tayyab MA, Ramanathan S: Cytology of respiratory epithelium as a predictor of respiratory complications after operation. Chest 67:32-35, 1975
15. Cronin M, Redfern PA, Utting JE: Psychometry and postoperative complaints in surgical patients. Br J Anaesth 45:879-886, 1973
16. Cullen DJ: Recovery room care of the surgical patient. Int Anesthesiol Clin 18(3):39-52, 1980
17. Dripps RD, Deming MV: Postoperative atelectasis and pneumonia: Diagnosis, etiology and management based upon 1,240 cases of upper abdominal surgery. Ann Surg 124:94-110, 1946
18. Dubovsky SL, Trustman R: Absence of recall after general anesthesia: Implications for theory and practice. Anesth Analg (Cleve) 55:696-701, 1976
19. Eckenhoff JE, Kneale DH, Dripps RD: The incidence and

etiology of postanesthetic excitement. A clinical survey. Anesthesiology 22:667-673, 1961
20. Eisele V, Weinreich A, Bartle S: Preoperative awareness and recall. Anesth Analg (Cleve) 55:513-518, 1976
21. Epstein RM: Morbidity and mortality from anesthesia: A continuing problem. Anesthesiology 49:388-389, 1978
22. Foex P, Prys–Roberts C: Anesthesia and the hypertensive patient. Br J Anaesth 46:575-588, 1974
23. Gal TJ, Cooperman LH: Hypertension in the immediate postoperative period. Br J Anaesth 47:70-74, 1975
24. Goldman L, Caldera DL: Risks of general anesthesia and elective operation in the hypertensive patient. Anesthesiology 50:285-292, 1979
25. Gray TC, Nunn JF, Utting JE: General Anaesthesia, vol. II, pp 1082-1083. London, Butterworths, 1980
26. Greene BA: A 26 gauge lumbar puncture needle: Its value in the prophylaxis of headache following spinal analgesia for vaginal delivery. Anesthesiology 11:464-469, 1950
27. Gronert GA: Malignant hyperthermia. Anesthesiology 53:395-423, 1980
28. Gronert GA: Puzzles in malignant hyperthermia. Anesthesiology 54:1, 1981
29. Hamilton WK: Unexpected deaths during anesthesia: Wherein lies the cause? Anesthesiology 50:381-383, 1979
30. Hartsell CJ, Stephen CR: Incidence of sore throat following endotracheal intubation. Can Anaesth Soc J 11:307-312, 1964
31. Hedenstierna G, Santesson J, Norlander O: Airway closure and distribution of inspired gas in the extremely obese, breathing spontaneously and during anesthesia with intermittent positive pressure ventilation. Acta Anaesth Scand 20:334-342, 1976
32. Hill GE, Stanley TH, Sentker CR: Physostigmine reversal of postoperative somnolence. Can Anaesth Soc J 24:707-711, 1977
33. Holaday DA, Fiserova–Bergerova V, Latto IP et al: Resistance of isoflurane to biotransformation in man. Anesthesiology 43:325-332, 1975
34. Kaplan JA: Hemodynamic monitoring. In Kaplan JA (ed): Cardiac Anesthesia, pp 71-153. New York, Grune & Stratton, 1979
35. Katz RL, Bigger JT: Cardiac arrhythmias during anesthesia and operation. Anesthesiology 33:193-213, 1970
36. Kuner J, Enescu V, Utsu F et al: Cardiac arrhythmias during anesthesia. Dis Chest 52:580-587, 1967
37. Lamont JT, Isselbacher KT: Postoperative jaundice. JAMA 288:305-307, 1973
38. Loehning RW, Mazze RI: Possible nephrotoxicity from enflurane in a patient with severe renal disease. Anesthesiology 40:203-205, 1974
39. Mazze RI, Trudell JR, Cousins MJ: Methoxyflurane metabolism and renal dysfunction: Clinical correlation in man. Anesthesiology 35:247-252, 1971
40. McLain GE, Sipes IG, Brown BR: An animal model of halothane hepatotoxicity: Role of enzyme induction and hypoxia. Anesthesiology 51:321-326, 1979
41. Moore DC: Regional Block. Springfield, Ill, Charles C Thomas, 1965
42. Morris RH, Wilkey BR: The effects of ambient temperature on patient temperature during surgery not involving body cavities. Anesthesiology 32:102-107, 1970
43. Otto CW: Respiratory morbidity and mortality. Int Anesthesiol Clin 18(3):85-106, 1980
44. Pandit SK, Heisterkamp DV, Cohen PJ: Further studies of the anti-recall effect of lorazepam: A dose-time-effect relationship. Anesthesiology 45:495-500, 1976
45. Pantuck EJ: Ecothiopate iodide eye drops and prolonged response to suxamethonium. A case report. Br J Anaesth 38:406-407, 1966
46. Prys–Roberts C, Meloche R: Management of anesthesia in patients with hypertension or ischemic heart disease. Int Anesthesiol Clin 18(4): 181-217, 1980
47. Roberts RB (ed): Pulmonary aspiration. Int Anesthesiol Clin 15(4):595–597, 1977
48. Safar P: Pathophysiology and resuscitation after global brain ischemia. Int Anesthesiol Clin 17(2,3):239-284, 1979
49. Schemel WH: Unexpected hepatic dysfunction found by multiple laboratory screening. Anesth Analg (Cleve) 55:810-812, 1976
50. Schwartz DJ, Wynne JW, Gibbs CP et al: Pulmonary consequences of aspiration of gastric contents at pH values greater than 2.5. Am Rev Respir Dis 121:119-126, 1980
51. Schwartz H, Deroetth A, Jr, Popper EM: Preanesthetic use of atropine and scopolamine in patients with glaucoma. JAMA 165:144-146, 1957
52. Scott DB, Cousins MJ: Clinical pharmacology of local anesthetic agents. In Cousins MJ, Bridenbaugh PO (eds): Neural Blockade in Clinical Anesthesia and Management of Pain, pp 104-115. Philadelphia, JB Lippincott, 1980
53. Smith NT, Corbascio AN: The use and misuse of pressor agents. Anesthesiology 33:58-95, 1970
54. Sokoll MD, Gergis SD: Antibiotics and neuromuscular function. Anesthesiology 55:148-159, 1981
55. Steen, PA, Tinker, JH, Tarhan S: Myocardial reinfarction after anesthesia and surgery. JAMA 239:2566-2570, 1978
56. Stehling LC: Anesthetic management of the patient with hyperthyroidism. Anesthesiology 41:585-595, 1974
57. Stein M, Cassara EL: Preoperative pulmonary evaluation and therapy for surgery patients. JAMA 211:787-790, 1970
58. Swerdlow M: Complications of local anesthetic neural blockage. In Cousins MJ, Bridenbaugh PO (eds): Neural Blockage in Clinical Anesthesia and Management of Pain, pp 526-542. Philadelphia, JB Lippincott, 1980
59. Tarhan S, Moffit EA, Taylor WF et al: Myocardial infarction after general anesthesia. Anesth Analg (Cleve) 56:455-461, 1977
60. Theye RA, Perry LB, Brzica SM: Influence of anesthetic agent on response to hemorrhagic hypotension. Anesthesiology 40:32-40, 1974
61. Usubiaga JE: Neurological complications following epidural anesthesia. Int Anesthesiol Clin 13(3):3, 1975
62. Vanik PE, Davis HS: Cardiac arrhythmias during halothane anesthesia. Anesth Analg (Cleve) 47:299-308, 1968
63. Weitzner SW, King BD, Ikezono E: The rate of arterial oxygen desaturation during apnea in humans. Anesthesiology 20:624-627, 1959
64. Whittington RM, Robinson JS, Thompson JM: Fatal aspiration (Mendelson's) syndrome despite antacids and cricoid pressure. Lancet 2:228-230, 1979
65. Wolfe JE, Bone RC, Ruth WE: Effects of corticosteroids in the treatment of patients with gastric aspiration. Am J Med 63:719-722, 1977
66. Wylie WD, Churchill–Davidson HC: A Practice of Anesthesia, p 872. Philadelphia, WB Saunders, 1978
67. Wynands JE: Anesthesia for patients with heart block and artificial cardiac pacemakers. Anesth Analg (Cleve) 55:626-632, 1976
68. Wynne JW, Modell JH: Respiratory aspiration of stomach contents. Ann Intern Med 87:466-474, 1977
69. Zonezein J, Santangelo RP, Mackin JF et al: Propranolol therapy in thyrotoxicosis. A review of 84 patients undergoing surgery. Am J Med 66:411-416, 1979

Part Three

Complications of Thoracic Surgery and Trauma

21 Complications of Intubation, Tracheal Surgery, and Trauma

Ronald C. Elkins

OVERVIEW

The acute complications associated with orotracheal or nasotracheal intubation include injury to the nasopharynx, oropharynx, larynx, and trachea with associated hemorrhage and misplacement or occlusion of the endotracheal tube. A complete discussion of the acute complications is detailed in Chapter 20. This chapter deals primarily with the late complications of endotracheal intubation that involve injury to the larynx or trachea.

The response of the larynx or trachea to the presence of an endotracheal tube may include the development of significant edema, ulceration, granulation tissue, membrane formation, adhesions, and fibrous strictures. The incidence and etiology of these complications have been reviewed by Harrison and Tonkin.[8] There appears to be no "safe period" for endotracheal intubation, since granulomas have occurred after a 15-minute period of intubation. However, prolonged intubation and traumatic intubation are among the factors associated with an increased risk of complications.

Orotracheal and Nasotracheal Intubation

The complications of intubation are present at the time of extubation, when the patient's symptoms may vary from a sore throat or hoarseness to acute upper-airway obstruction requiring emergency reintubation or tracheostomy. In the patient with a sore throat or hoarseness, resolution usually occurs without specific treatment. Those with severe symptoms of persistent hoarseness, aphonia, or stridor, in which the pathologic lesion is one of superficial laryngeal ulceration, supraglottic edema, or a mild case of subglottic edema, can usually be managed conservatively. Treatment with humidification of inspired air, antibiotics, and corticosteroids should be instituted immediately. Avoidance of further traumatic injury from the injudicious use of nasotracheal suction and avoidance of overhydration will usually allow improvement over a 24-hour period. If respiratory status does not improve over this time period or if airway injury requires early reintubation or tracheostomy, investigation of the airway injury by direct laryngoscopy and bronchoscopy should be undertaken. Usually this is best accomplished in the operating room and can be done at the time of tracheostomy.

Patients in whom direct laryngoscopy shows uncomplicated subglottic or supraglottic edema or laryngotracheal membrane can usually be managed conservatively with early resolution and successful decannulation of their tracheostomy. An occasional patient will require release of vocal-cord adhesions or removal of the membrane by bronchoscopy.

Patients with persistent laryngeal obstruction, particularly those in whom there is granulation tissue in the subglottic areas or in the interarytenoid space, may heal with fibrous-stricture formation. The result is subglottic stenosis or fixation of the cords in close apposition because of immobility of the arytenoids. Repeated laryngeal dilatation, operative mobilization of the arytenoids, or direct operative treatment of the laryngeal stenosis may be required. When the cartilagenous framework of the larynx is intact, the stenosis can be relieved by a combination of stenting and mucosal grafting. When destruction and collapse of the cartilages of the upper airway are part of the pathology, stenting has not been as successful. In these situations, division of the cartilage at the point of stenosis and interposition of new cartilage or bone have been helpful to restore an adequate lumen.[25]

The use of carbon dioxide laser for repair of subglottic and upper tracheal stenosis has been advocated by several authors; however, its success to date would suggest that it should be viewed as an experimental surgical procedure.[11,12] Further long-term results will be needed to clarify its indications and usefulness.

Tracheostomy

The complications of tracheal surgery have received considerable attention over the past 20 years because of the widespread use of mechanical ventilators and increased frequency of tracheostomy. Complications have been associated with technical aspects of the operation as well as the late complications from use of the cuffed tracheostomy tube. The complications of tracheostomy have been nicely summarized by Kennan in a symposium on reconstruction of the larynx and trachea.[10] Grillo and Cooper have provided the basic understanding for the mechanism of injury and the pathology of tracheal injury secondary to mechanical ventilation and prolonged intubation with a cuffed tracheostomy tube.[2,3] The fatal complications of tracheostomy have been reviewed by Stemmer and colleagues, who found that the most common complication was hemorrhage.[21] In 10 deaths due to hemorrhage, 9 were secondary to injury to venous or arterial vessels at the time of the tracheostomy. Intraoperative complications can be minimized through attention to certain operative details:

1. Tracheostomies should be performed in the operating room over an endotracheal tube or ventilating bronchoscope with an anesthesiologist in attendance. The operating surgeon or assistant should be a senior surgeon well acquainted with the operative procedure. Local or general anesthesia may be used depending on the clinical problem.
2. Adequate illumination should be obtained. For many patients, this will require the use of a fiberoptic headlight.
3. The patient should be carefully positioned so that the trachea can be readily exposed. Overextension of the head and neck should be avoided.
4. The skin incision may be transverse or vertical. It should be of adequate length to allow exposure of the trachea without undue traction.
5. Sharp dissection should be used for exposure of the trachea with careful attention to hemostasis. Adequate hemostasis should be obtained prior to opening the trachea. Prior endotracheal intubation facilitates this part of the operative procedure.
6. The trachea should be gently retracted with a tracheal hook prior to opening. Vigorous traction on the trachea can produce vagal stimulation with resultant bradycardia and cardiovascular collapse.
7. The incision into the trachea must be tailored to the patient. For infants and young children, I prefer a short vertical incision through one or occasionally two tracheal rings. For adults, a short inferiorly based U-shaped flap works well. The trachea is incised between the second and third tracheal ring and then vertically across the third tracheal cartilage.
8. The diameter of the tube must be individualized. The tube should pass readily into the trachea and should provide little to no resistance to ventilation. A tube that is small for the patient and requires forced expiration increases the risk of development of significant subcutaneous emphysema.
9. A chest x-ray film should be obtained at the completion of the procedure.

OPERATIVE COMPLICATIONS

Careful attention to these details should prevent the common operative complications, which include hemorrhage; bradycardia, hypotension, or cardiac arrest associated with vagal stimulation; false passage into or around the trachea with subsequent injury to the adjacent structures; injury to the recurrent laryngeal nerves; injury to the posterior tracheal wall; injury to the pleura with resultant pneumothorax; and injury to a major vein with air embolism as well as hemorrhage.

As mentioned, intraoperative complications are best avoided, but when they do occur each must be managed as indicated. Adequate exposure and lighting are essential for successful management. Hemorrhage should be dealt with directly, and if it is venous in origin, ligation or suture ligation will suffice. Laceration of the innominate or carotid arteries may be managed by local compression and direct suture repair of the lacerated vessels. If the inferior thyroid artery is the source of the injury, ligation of the vessel will control the bleeding; however, the possibility of an associated recurrent laryngeal nerve injury must be assessed by local inspection or by direct laryngoscopy attentive for vocal cord function at a later date. Techniques for surgical management of the patient with unilateral or bilateral vocal cord palsy have been developed.[15]

Injury to the esophagus as as a result of posterior laceration of the trachea should be managed by direct suture repair. I prefer the use of fine, monofilament, nonabsorbable suture tied on the inside of the trachea. Following healing of the laceration, the patient should be examined bronchoscopically; if the sutures are visible, they can be readily removed.

The neck should be drained with a paraesophageal drain. The patient should not take anything orally and the stomach should be kept empty with a nasogastric tube on low intermittent suction until healing has occurred.

Inadvertent laceration of the pleura is most likely to be detected on the postoperative chest x-ray film. The identification of a pneumothorax requires the placement of a chest tube. Even small pneumothoraces should be treated by tube thoracotomy since many patients will be managed by mechanical ventilators or assisted ventilation.

Air embolism results from a sucking wound in a large vein. Local compression and placement of the patient in a *Trendelenburg position* will allow repair of the venous injury without continued risk of further air embolism. Most episodes of minor air embolism will resolve without specific treatment; however, occasionally massive air embolism is associated with cardiovascular collapse. Immediate closed-chest cardiopulmonary resuscitation should be instituted; if the patient does not respond, open-chest resuscitation with evacuation of air from the pulmonary circulation and heart will often allow successful resuscitation of the patient.

EARLY POSTOPERATIVE COMPLICATIONS

In the immediate postoperative period, the most common complication is recurrent hemorrhage. Persistent bleeding should be managed by returning the patient to the operating room. Under adequate exposure and lighting, hemostasis can be obtained.

The second most common and frequently difficult problem to manage is the development of interstitial air. This may present as subcutaneous emphysema, pneumothorax, pneumomediastinum, pneumopericardium, or pneumoperitoneum.

Subcutaneous emphysema usually occurs in patients not on a ventilator in whom there is a discrepancy between the tracheostomy tube and the opening made in the trachea with an associated tight skin closure around the tracheostomy tube. Usually removal of skin sutures and, if necessary, replacement of the tracheostomy tube with a larger one will allow resolution of the subcutaneous emphysema. Occasionally it will be necessary to insert a cuffed endotracheal tube, control the patient's ventilation with a mechanical ventilator, and adequately sedate the patient so that the tracheostomy tract will heal and subcutaneous emphysema will not develop.

Interstitial air in other sites usually occurs in patients on mechanical ventilators and is secondary to a ruptured subpleural bleb. If the rupture is into the pleural space, the patient will develop a pneumothorax. Frequently this is under tension and should be suspected in any patient on a ventilator who develops sudden cardiovascular deterioration. Tube thoracostomy is the treatment for *all* patients who develop a pneumothorax while on a ventilator.

Pneumomediastinum, pneumopericardium, and pneumoperitoneum are usually the result of intrapulmonary rupture of a bleb or alveoli with dissection of the air in the subpleural planes along the bronchi to the mediastinum, the pericardium, or the peritoneum. Usually these result when patients are "fighting their respirators." Patient anxiety, inadequate ventilation, or attempts by the patient to clear endobronchial secretions results in markedly elevated airway pressures with subsequent parenchymal rupture. Attention to better management of the patient's ventilation, adequate sedation, and good nursing will frequently avoid these complications. The development of these complications in patients being treated with positive end expiratory pressure (PEEP) ventilation can frequently be very difficult to manage. In general, reduction in the level of PEEP with placement of chest tubes as indicated will allow resolution.

LATE POSTOPERATIVE COMPLICATIONS

Infection

Significant infections are rare following tracheostomy, although most of the wounds become colonized with *Staphylococcus aureus* or *Pseudomonas aeruginosa*. Except in the compromised host, they rarely require antibiotic treatment. However, in the intensive-care unit a colonized tracheostomy may be the source for significant nosocomial infections. Occasional patients will develop a severe tracheitis or an invasive infection at the stoma. Organism-specific antibiotics, local wound care, and careful attention to tracheal toilet will allow resolution.

Obstruction

Obstruction of the tracheostomy tube is usually the result of retained, thickened, or inspissated secretions. Frequently secretions act as a ball valve over the end of the tube, producing severe respiratory embarrassment. The tube should be changed whenever this is suspected. If this is the first tube change or if previous tube changes were difficult, the tube may be changed over a small rubber catheter, which will act as a guide for the new tube into the trachea and avoid misplacement into the mediastinum.

Granulation tissue at the tip of the catheter may be the cause of the tracheostomy tube obstruction. If suspected, a rigid bronchoscope will allow definition of the extent of the lesion and appropriate therapy. Localized granulation tissue may be removed through the bronchoscope; however, extensive lesions and destruction of tracheal cartilage will usually require surgical resection and repair at a later date. Most areas of tracheal necrosis are secondary to balloon damage, but occasional damage is produced by the tip of the tracheostomy tube owing to the anatomy of the patient and the geometry of the tube, causing local pressure by the tube tip. A different or longer tracheostomy tube or a tube with a different curvature may be required to allow healing at the site of erosion.

Hemorrhage

Late hemorrhage secondary to an acquired tracheainnominate artery fistula should be considered in any patient with intratracheal bleeding following tracheostomy. Such bleeding usually occurs in patients whose tracheostomy has been in place for more than 1 week. However, it may occur during the first or second postoperative day if injury to the innominate artery was not recognized during surgery. The most helpful diagnostic aid is endoscopy. It should be performed in the operating suite, first through the tracheostomy tube and then through the tracheostomy stoma with the tube removed. Occasionally arteriography will demonstrate the presence of a false aneurysm or evidence of intimal injury in the patient in whom a diagnosis cannot be made at the time of endoscopy.

The etiology of injury to the innominate artery and the operative management of this complication have been discussed by several authors.[1, 14, 17, 20, 24] The sudden onset of exsanguinating or asphyxiating hemorrhage is a dire emergency. Management is as follows: Generally the hemorrhage can be controlled by insertion of the gloved finger adjacent to the tracheostomy and compressing the ruptured vessel against the back wall of the sternum. Ventilation can be maintained through the tracheostomy tube with the balloon kept inflated to minimize aspiration. Occasionally it is necessary to remove the tracheostomy tube to compress the vessel adequately; however, this should not be done until an orotracheal tube has been positioned through the vocal cords so that it can be rapidly positioned below the tracheostomy stoma upon removal of the tracheostomy tube. This latter maneuver is usually best accomplished in the operating room while preparing the patient for definitive repair of the arterial injury. A median sternotomy gives good exposure of the arterial injury, allowing one to gain proximal and distal control of the vessel and then occlude, débride, and oversew the two ends.

Authors are divided on the necessity of reconstructing the innominate artery in this desperate setting. The operative field is septic, and primary reconstruction carries significant risk of anastomotic breakdown and recurrent hemorrhage. In a number of patients ligation of the innominate artery has not been associated with permanent sequelae, and this should generally be the procedure of choice. In closure of the wound, thymic tissue or a viable muscle flap should be placed between the tracheostomy stoma and the arterial suture lines. Management of the tracheostomy stoma will depend on the etiology of the tracheo-innominate artery fistula. This has been reviewed by Grillo.[4]

Tracheoesophageal Fistula

Tracheoesophageal fistula is usually suggested when a nurse notes gastric contents in the tracheal aspirate. Occasionally it is suspected when gastric distention occurs and auscultation over the stomach reveals air movement occurring synchronously with the ventilator. Increased tracheal secretions or the necessity to increase the balloon volume to provide an adequate seal for ventilation may be the presenting sign. Confirmation can be obtained by having the patient swallow dilute methylene blue and noting its prompt appearance in the trachea.

The fistula should be localized by endoscopy. Frequently both esophagoscopy and bronchoscopy are required; however, bronchoscopy will usually identify the site. Often there is other evidence of balloon injury in the trachea. Contrast studies should not be performed owing to the risk of aspiration.

If the patient's condition will permit, the fistula should be closed surgically. Most fistulas secondary to a tracheostomy tube can be closed through a cervical incision. The edges of the fistula should be primarily closed in the esophagus and the trachea. A muscle flap should then be placed between the two closures to lessen the likelihood of recurrence. If continued ventilator support is required by the patient, an attempt should be made to position the balloon on the tracheostomy tube at a different site in the trachea. The patient should not take anything orally, and a gastrostomy should be performed to avoid any need for a nasogastric tube. In the few patients who cannot tolerate a major surgical procedure, delayed repair can be carried out by performing esophageal diversion in the neck with an end esophagostomy and a gastrostomy for gastric decompression.

This complication is often lethal in patients who continue to require ventilatory support and is best prevented. Use of a low-pressure, large-volume cuff on the tracheostomy tube and insistence on early removal of the nasogastric tube with gastrostomy placement if prolonged gastric decompression is required should be part of the management of any patient requiring prolonged ventilatory support.

Postextubation Complications

GRANULOMAS

Granulomas most frequently form at the site of the tracheal stoma, but they also occur occasionally at the cuff or tip site where localized injury may have occurred. Granulomas may be removed successfully endoscopically with a low rate of recurrence. Although this problem is more difficult in children, cryosurgical removal has been reported by Rodgers and Talbert with good results.[18]

STENOSIS

Tracheal stenosis occurs at two sites, the stoma and the cuff. Local damage due to the tube, the cuff pressure, or occasionally sepsis plays a role in the development of local cartilage destruction with healing by stricture formation. The stricture usually presents in 2 to 5 weeks following extubation but may occur years later. The first symptom is usually dyspnea on exertion followed by wheezing and stridor. The presumptive diagnosis of stenosis should be made in any patient with upper-airway obstruction and a recent history of tracheal intubation. Radiographic study of the trachea, especially tomography, will confirm the level and length of the stenosis. If tracheomalacia is suspected, this can be confirmed by fluoroscopy. Bronchoscopy should be avoided until definitive management of the stricture is undertaken. Surgical management for tracheal stricture has been outlined, and proper surgical excision of the lesion has a high likelihood of success. Some lesions may be managed by the conservative approach of reinstituting the tracheostomy, dilatation of the stricture, and internal stenting. This approach should be used in any patient who is not a good candidate for operative management.

PERSISTENT STOMA

Persistent stoma is rarely seen except in patients who have required intubation for long periods. An epithelialized tract from skin to tracheal mucosa is present, and this prevents complete healing. Surgical closure should be entertained if the stoma persists for more than 2 to 3 months. Closure by excision of the skin edges, careful closure of the trachea, reapproximation of the strap muscles, and closure of the platysma and skin will nearly always cure this complication.

Tracheal Resection

The frequency of tracheal resection has increased as the incidence of severe tracheal stenosis unresponsive to other therapy has increased. Patients whose severe blunt trauma involves laryngotracheal or bronchial injury are now surviving to reach the hospital, where definitive surgical repair is accomplished at the time of injury. In these patients, the most common late complication is tracheal stenosis, and, in general, surgical resection is required for treatment. Although the most common etiology of tracheal stenosis is prolonged intubation, a better understanding of the pathophysiology and improved design of the endotracheal tubes have decreased the frequency of tracheal stenosis. The surgical management of patients with tracheal stenosis or tracheal tumors has evolved through excellent, detailed descriptions of these procedures.[5, 6, 18, 19] Attention to these details will lower the incidence of major complications, but one must be alert to the possibilities of dehiscence, granulation-tissue formation, recurrent stenosis, recurrent laryngeal-nerve injury, or superior laryngeal-nerve injury.

DEHISCENCE

Dehiscence usually occurs as the result of too much tension on the anastomosis or improper mobilization of the trachea, which sacrifices the vascular supply of the distal trachea. Early postoperative episodes of dehiscence are usually the result of significant tension due to an inadequately planned operation or the inadequate identification of the extent of disease. Several techniques for increased mobilization of the larynx and trachea have been described, and these include laryngeal release by a supralaryngeal approach; release by division of the omohyoid and thyrohoid muscles; and mobilization of the carina and right main-stem bronchus either through a right anterior thoracotomy or a median sternotomy. A right thoracotomy will also allow division of the inferior pulmonary ligament for additional mobility of the trachea. The early dehiscence, especially if it involves more than one third of tha anastomosis, should be treated by immediate reoperation with attention to technical maneuvers that will relieve tension. The development of subcutaneous mediastinal emphysema is an indication for immediate bronchoscopy to assess the need for reoperation. Small areas of disruption may be treated by drainage and allowing the area to heal by secondary intention.

Later suture-line disruption is usually due to devascularization of a tracheal cartilage. The cartilage will hold sutures long enough so that adjacent soft tissues have healed and an air leak does not occur, and airway obstruction from a recurrent stricture is the presenting problem. Management of the recurrent stricture is discussed under Restenosis.

The need for continued ventilatory support in a patient who has undergone a tracheal resection markedly increases the likelihood of dehiscence. Several authors have suggested that patients with tracheal stenosis who require ventilator support have their tracheal resection delayed until they can be weaned from the ventilator. If a tracheal resection must be performed on a patient who requires the support of a ventilator, the patient should be intubated with a low-pressure, high-volume cuff tube and efforts made to place the cuff above or below the suture line.

In a tracheal resection for malignancy following irradiation, anastomotic dehiscence is often fatal. In this setting, dehiscence is usually associated with necrosis and separation of the tracheal ends so that reanastomosis is not possible. A mediastinal tracheostomy should be performed by resection of the upper sternum, the two clavicular heads, and the upper two costal cartilages, and then developing skin flaps that can be brought to the tracheal stoma without tension. This often will allow healing to occur.

GRANULATION TISSUE

Granulation tissue usually occurs at the site of imperfect healing. It is frequently asymptomatic and only is detected at bronchoscopy. In this setting, granulation tissue has no long-term significance and healing with epithelialization will occur. At other times the granulation tissue can produce coughing spasms, wheezing, and minor hemoptysis. The diagnosis can be confirmed by bronchoscopy. This complication is treated by endobronchial resection. Sutures that are frequently at the base of the granulation tissue should be removed. Treatment of granulation tissue by the use of cryosurgery or carbon dioxide laser has been advocated by several authors.[9, 18] The absence of hemorrhage and the ability to be very exact in the area of resection make this technique appealing, especially in a child or a patient who has undergone a resection for a subglottic stricture and has a laryngotracheal or a cricotracheal anastomosis.

RESTENOSIS

Restenosis usually follows a delayed dehiscence of a previous resection, but occasionally it is the result of very localized scar formation. Resection and anastomosis are required for cure in most patients. However, in patients with subglottic stenosis there have been several reports of successful management with use of the carbon dioxide laser.[9, 11] In patients in whom there is recurrent stenosis following an extensive primary resection, the adequacy of the remaining trachea is of paramount importance. Occasionally extensive reconstructive procedures will be required, even including the use of a tracheal prosthesis.[13, 15] When resection and primary anastomosis are being planned, a delay of 3 to 4 months is usually advisable. A tracheostomy should be performed for safety since frequently the degree of airway obstruction is rapidly progressive and can be fatal.

RECURRENT LARYNGEAL NERVE INJURY

It is best to avoid surgical injury of the recurrent laryngeal nerve. In dealing with a benign stricture, the recurrent laryngeal nerve is best avoided by not attempting to identify the nerve in the area of significant scarring immediately adjacent to the stricture. In this area, dissection is kept close to the trachea, especially that portion to be removed. Knowledge of the course and anatomical location of this nerve will prevent injury to it. If the lesion is malignant and resection of the tumor requires resection of one nerve, avoidance of injury to the remaining nerve will prevent the respiratory embarrassment that occurs from bilateral nerve injury and avoid aphasia.

Recent advances in surgical management of patients with unilateral and bilateral laryngeal nerve damage provide hope for many of these patients.[9]

SUPERIOR LARYNGEAL NERVE INJURY

Injury to the superior laryngeal nerve produces difficulty in swallowing with recurrent aspiration as the patient's complaint. Injury to these nerves usually occurs in patients undergoing tracheal resection in whom a laryngeal-release procedure is necessary. A technique of division of the greater cornu of the laryngeal cartilage has been described by Ross to avoid this complication.[19] In most patients with a laryngeal release, swallowing dysfunction is frequently present for up to 6 weeks. Preoperative preparation of the patient and reassurance and patience will allow for resolution of the problem. Permanent injury to the superior laryngeal nerves is a major complication, and management must be tailored to each patient. In some patients, laryngectomy with permanent tracheostomy may be the only recourse for control of the patient's aspiration.

Trauma

Several authors have discussed the importance of early recognition and prompt early surgical management of tracheal injury as the hallmarks of successful treatment.[7, 16, 22] Injuries to the intrathoracic trachea and bronchi are more common than injuries to the cervical trachea.

INTRATHORACIC TRACHEAL INJURY

Disruption of the intrathoracic trachea or bronchus presents in two distinct ways, depending on whether the disruption communicates with the pleural space or is contained by the peritracheal or peribronchial tissues. The patient with a disruption that communicates with the pleural space presents with a pneumothorax and frequently has associated pneumomediastinum and subcutaneous emphysema that begins in the neck and may rapidly expand to involve the face and anterior chest wall. The pneumothorax is usually complete and is rarely under tension since the pleural communication generally is large and does not obstruct the egress of air during exhalation. Closed-tube thoracostomy usually does not produce complete expansion of the lung, and a major air leak is noted. If after insertion of a chest tube, the extent of subcutaneous emphysema is increasing and there is to be a delay before definitive treatment of the injury, a tracheostomy should be performed. This will decrease the resistance to exhalation in the upper airway and tend to decrease further development of subcutaneous emphysema.

Surgical management of the intrathoracic tracheal disruption or laceration consists of surgical repair or, in patients in whom the injury is so severe that repair cannot be accomplished, pulmonary resection. The complications of primary repair include granulation-tissue formation, stricture with atelectasis of the involved lung, and dehiscence. Granulation tissue can be managed as previously discussed. Its presentation is similar irrespective of its site or location.

Stricture formation should be suspected in any patient who develops persistent atelectasis in the postoperative period. The diagnosis can usually be confirmed by bronchoscopy, but bronchography is the most valuable diagnostic test. It will delineate the extent of the lesion and often provides information about the likelihood of reexpansion of the atelectatic segment. In almost all patients, the stricture should be resected or managed by a bronchoplastic procedure. Reexpansion and improvement in pulmonary function will occur in most patients. However, some will have developed bronchiectasis in the atelectatic segment, and these patients should be treated by pulmonary resection. Patients in whom the bronchial stenosis cannot be surgically corrected should undergo pulmonary resection, since persistent stenosis is frequently associated with recurrent infection in the distal pulmonary tissue.

Dehiscence of the tracheal or bronchial suture line results in a recurrent pneumothorax and a bronchopleural fistula. If closed-tube thoracostomy is successful in expanding the lung and the air leak is not massive, healing of the dehiscence or fistula may occur without further operative intervention. Frequently this healing is associated with some degree of bronchial stenosis, and close long-term observation of the patient is indicated. In patients with a persistent bronchopleural fistula, surgical management should follow the principles for management of this thoracic surgical problem. In patients with a massive air leak, pulmonary resection with reinforcement of the bronchial or tracheal closure by a pleural, pericardial, or muscle flap is frequently required.

Patients in whom the tracheal or bronchial disruption is contained by the peribronchial or peritracheal tissue have their airway maintained by these tissues, and although a small pneumomediastinum is usually present, it is frequently undetected. Healing of the site of disruption is usually associated with some stenosis and, depending on its site, the patient may present with an asymptomatic atelectatic lobe or lung or the patient may develop recurrent distal infection. In the case of atelectasis of one lung, significant respiratory embarrassment may occur. This complication frequently does not present until months or years after the original injury. The possibility of bronchial or tracheal stenosis should be considered in any patient with a history of significant chest trauma. Bronchography is the ideal diagnostic test, and management is dependent upon the site of stenosis and the status of the distal pulmonary tissue. In almost all patients, resection of the area of stenosis with primary anastomosis is the procedure of choice.

CERVICAL TRACHEAL INJURY

Cervical tracheal injury from blunt trauma is more common in women and usually results from impact of the neck on the padded dashboard. Complete transection of the trachea with laryngotracheal discontinuity is the usual injury. The patient presents in acute respiratory distress and frequently has severe subcutaneous emphysema of the neck and face. Orotracheal intubation utilizing a flexible bronchoscope as a guide to bridge the gap between larynx and trachea will relieve the respiratory distress and allow surgical repair of the lesion. Primary anastomosis is the preferred treatment, and the complication rate is quite low. The complications are similar to those described in the section on tracheal resection. Management of patients with penetrating trauma of the cervical trachea is dependent upon the extent of injury to the trachea and the degree of injury to adjacent structures. The management of these injuries has been summarized by Urschel and Symbas.[22, 23] Many of these injuries require tracheostomy or tracheal resection for repair, and the complications of the injury are similar to those previously described. Owing to the frequency of associated vascular or esophageal injury in these patients, late complications involving these organs are more frequently seen in patients with penetrating trauma than in patients having a primary operation on their trachea. Management of these complications has been described.

Tracheostomy in the Pediatric Patient

Although most of the preceding discussion relates to the adult patient, the material can be applied to the pediatric age group with few exceptions. Nowhere is there a greater need for meticulous surgical and nursing care than in these young patients, particularly those less than 1 year of age. In this population the need for tracheal intubation and for tracheostomy has increased, particularly with the growth of neonatal intensive-care units and as the ability to sustain these tiny infants increases.

A feared complication in patients under 1 year of age who require tracheostomy has been the inability to decannulate the infant. In patients in whom the original tracheostomy was properly performed and in whom a silastic tracheostomy tube was utilized, the following approach to decannulation has proved uniformly successful. The patient whose respiratory status allows decannulation is bronchoscoped under general anesthesia to ensure the absence of endotracheal pathology. The following day, in the intensive-care unit and under close observation, the tracheostomy tube is removed, leaving the stoma open. Tracheal suction is avoided, since the patient who is ready for decannulation can handle his own secretions. Progressive reduction in the size of the tracheostomy tube or occlusion of the lumen of the tracheostomy tube, forcing the infant to ventilate around the tube, is avoided. Over the next 24-hour period the stoma will usually close, and successful decannulation will be accomplished. If respiratory distress should develop, orotracheal intubation is accomplished. The tracheostomy stoma is then reopened in the operating room and the tracheostomy reestablished. After an additional period of respiratory support, decannulation can again be attempted.

References

1. Brantigan CO: Delayed major vessel hemorrhage following tracheostomy. J Trauma 13(3):235-237, 1975
2. Cooper JD, Grillo HC: The evolution of tracheal injury due to ventilatory assistance through cuffed tubes: A pathologic study. Ann Surg 169(3):334-348, 1969
3. Cooper JD, Grillo HC: Experimental production and prevention of injury due to cuffed tracheal tubes. Surg Gynecol Obstet 129(6):1235-1241, 1969
4. Grillo HC: Surgery of the trachea. Curr Probl Surg 7:3-59, 1970
5. Grillo HC: Reconstruction of the trachea. Experience in 100 consecutive cases. Thorax 28(6):667-679, 1973
6. Grillo HC: Tracheal tumors: Surgical management. Ann Thorac Surg 26(2):112-125, 1978
7. Grover FL, Ellestad C, Arom KV et al: Diagnosis and management of major tracheobronchial injuries. Ann Thorac Surg 28(4):384-391, 1978
8. Harrison GA, Tonkin JP: Prolonged (therapeutic) endotracheal intubation. Br J Anaesth 40(4):241-249, 1968
9. Hybels RL: Selected new techniques of laryngeal surgery. Surg Clin North Am 60(3):637-647, 1980
10. Kennan PD: Complications associated with tracheostomy: Prevention and treatment. Otolaryngol Clin North Am 12(4):807-816, 1979
11. Lyons GD, Owens R, Lousteau RJ, Trail ML: Carbon dioxide laser treatment of laryngeal stenosis. Arch Otolaryngol 106(5):255-256, 1980
12. McGee KC, Nagel JW, Toohill RJ: CO_2 laser repair of subglottic and upper tracheal stenosis. Otolaryngol Head Neck Surg 89(1):92-95, 1981
13. Neville WE, Bolanowski PJP, Soltanzadeh H: Prosthetic reconstruction of the trachea and carina. J Thorac Cardiovasc Surg 72(4):525-538, 1976
14. Nunn DB, Sanchez–Salagon AA, McCullogh JM et al: Trachea-innominate artery fistula following tracheostomy. Successful repairs using an innominate vein graft. Ann Thorac Surg 20(6):698-702, 1975
15. Pearson FG, Henderson RD, Gross AE et al: The reconstruction of circumferential tracheal defects with a porous prosthesis. An experimental and clinical study using heavy Marlex mesh. J Thorac Cardiovasc Surg 55(5):605-625, 1968
16. Potter CR, Sessions DG, Ogura JH: Blunt laryngotracheal trauma. ORL J Otorhinolaryngol Relat Spec 86(6ptl):909-923, 1978
17. Revilla AG Jr, Donahoo JS, Cameron JL: Tracheal-innominate artery fistula after tracheal reconstruction. A case of successful repair. J Thorac Cardiovasc Surg 67(4):629-633, 1974
18. Rodgers BM, Talbert JL: Clinical application of endotracheal cryotherapy. J Pediatr Surg 13(6):662-668, 1978
19. Ross JA: Techniques in the surgical repair of tracheal stenosis. Otolaryngol Clin North Am 12(4):893-899, 1979
20. Silen W, Spieker D: Fatal hemorrhage from the innominate artery after tracheostomy. Ann Surg 162(6):1005-1012, 1965
21. Stemmer EA, Oliver C, Carey JP, Connolly JE: Fatal complications of tracheostomy. Am J Surg 131(3):288-290, 1976
22. Symbas PN, Hatcher CR Jr, Boehm GAW: Acute penetrating tracheal trauma. Ann Thorac Surg 22(5):473-476, 1976
23. Urschel HC Jr, Razzuk MA: Management of acute traumatic injuries of the tracheobronchial tree. Surg Gynecol Obstet 136(1):113-117, 1973
24. Utley JR, Singer MM, Roe BB et al: Definitive management of innominate artery hemorrhage complicating tracheostomy. JAMA 220(4):577-579, 1972
25. Ward PH, Canalis R, Fee W et al: Composite hyoid sternohyoid muscle grafts in humans. Its use in reconstruction of subglottic stenosis and the anterior tracheal wall. Arch Otolaryngol 103(9):531-534, 1977

22 Acute Respiratory Failure Following Surgery and Trauma

Joseph M. Civetta | Jeffrey S. Augenstein

OVERVIEW

So often in medicine a "new" concept represents a continued evolution of observations and ideas formulated, tested, and improved. This often involves synthesizing varied ideas and methodologies until the most workable and clinically effective constellation of theory and practice are attained. Acute respiratory failure (ARF) represents a classic example of the process. Today, treatment probably has outstripped our understanding of the actual pathophysiologic changes and of why present treatment methods are effective.

It may be helpful to review this process of evolution as applied to acute respiratory failure following surgery and trauma in order to appraise not only the effectiveness of our current therapy but also to examine each step as a basis for future development. In the following discussion, our bias is unmistakably a factor in the development and selection of a coordinated approach to ARF.

ARF seems to have been discovered in the past few decades. It has been given a wide variety of names, initially being called congestive atelectasis and often the catch-all phrase, "the adult respiratory distress syndrome."[26, 32] *For the purpose of this discussion, ARF describes the pathophysiologic processes that begin with the characteristic blood gas abnormalities, arterial hypoxemia, and associated hypocarbia. This disease process has diverse etiologies, including aspiration, pancreatitis, thoracic trauma, sepsis, near drowning, and fat embolism. It is often discussed in relation to other less clear-cut etiologic agents such as shock, disseminated intravascular coagulation, and multiple transfusions.*

From the list of antecedents, it is clear that the patient who has undergone extensive elective surgery or has suffered multiple traumatic injuries may be at high risk for developing ARF. A patient under the influence of alcohol who is involved in a vehicular accident may well aspirate, suffer direct thoracic trauma, require many blood transfusions, and develop shock. After extensive elective surgery, patients may develop severe septic complications or pancreatitis as well as have been recipients of multiple transfusions. In fact, one of the more common appellations for respiratory failure following trauma is "shock lung." The presence of shock alone has been found in equal frequency in patients who do and who do not develop ARF.[24] *Although direct thoracic trauma can result in the subsequent development of ARF, the etiologic agents in cases of severe sepsis are still to be clearly established. Increased cappillary permeability has often been postulated in septic complications, but alternative explanations linking sepsis and respiratory failure have been offered. These include an increase in the osmotic forces in the interstitium following bacterial degradation of mucopolysaccharides as well as an increased capillary surface area for filtration caused by the vasodilatory effects of severe sepsis. Despite these unknowns, ARF in the surgical and post-traumatic patient requires therapy now; further investigations are necessary but treatment cannot await elucidation of the fundamental mechanisms.*

As ventilatory support has evolved, therapy has been directed more appropriately at an earlier stage and the decision to employ mechanical ventilatory support has been replaced by a desire to encourage spontaneous ventilation. One of the most important developments in this process has been the introduction of intermittent mandatory ventilation (IMV). As a mode of ventilatory support, it eliminated for the first time the distinction between continuous mechanical ventilation and total spontaneous ventilation. Support could then be defined by the patient's demonstrated need *for increased alveolar ventilation, not a physician's* decision *to provide ventilation for a patient. This difference in perspective took a number of years to evolve; during this period there has been a gratifying, although possibly merely concomitant, decrease in the morbidity and mortality rates from ARF.*

HISTORICAL DEVELOPMENT

In the 1950s and 1960s, mechanical ventilators were used quite appropriately to ventilate patients who had insufficient alveolar ventilation and who thus presented with elevated arterial CO_2 tension. The reasons varied: in patients with poliomyelitis, muscle weakness was the cause; in patients with advanced chronic obstructive pulmonary disease (COPD), abnormalities of ventilation and perfusion resulted in CO_2 retention; in the group of patients who are now recognized to have ARF, mechanical ventilation was usually instituted late in the course of the disease.[2, 4, 17] At this point, pulmonary compliance was markedly decreased, chest radiographs usually showed advanced infiltrative disease, and pathologic specimens showed the "liver lung" picture (Fig. 22-1). The term *adult respiratory distress syndrome* evolved because, despite the diverse etiologies, the end-stage pulmonary pathologic picture appeared the same. Marked pulmonary congestion, interstitial fibrosis, cellular infiltrates, and, in some situations, hyaline membranes were noted in the alveolar spaces similar to the disorder seen in neonates. It is no wonder that inadequate ventilation resulted; the decrease in compliance made effective alveolar ventilation impossible by the patient alone, and marked increases in dead space/tidal volume ratios (VD/VT) reduced the effectiveness of any spontaneous breath to perhaps only 30% of the tidal volume. With these physiologic and pathologic determinants, it was entirely appropriate to supply mechanical ventilation for these patients. Unfortunately mechanical ventilation *per se* had little effect upon the primary disorder, but this was not realized until some years later.

DEFINITIONS

In order to understand cardiorespiratory pathophysiology, it is necessary to define a number of terms that are in common usage. The most common basic abbreviations are defined in Table 22-1. These can be combined in various ways and expanded to relate to oxygenation (Table 22-2) and to describe various parameters of ventilatory function (Table 22-3). As the concepts of ventilatory support have been expanded, so too have the modalities available for initiating such support. The commonly used types of ventilatory support are defined in Table 22-4. The simultaneous occurrence of cardiovascular and respiratory disease is most prominent in the traumatic and severely ill surgical patient. It is therefore necessary to understand the cardiovascular data base and the calculations necessary for interpretation of

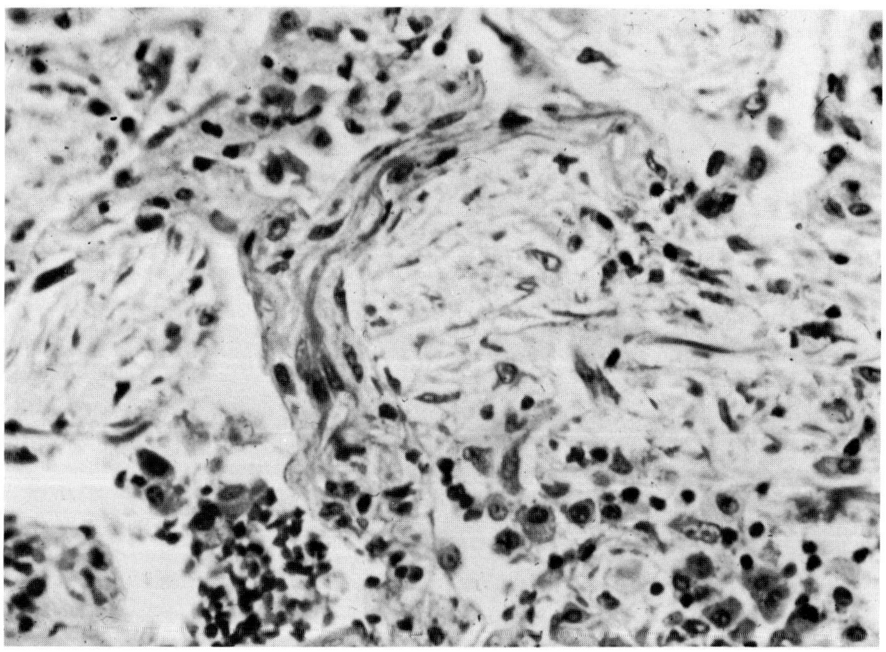

FIG. 22-1. Microscopic examination of the lung reveals essentially no normal features. The epithelium is cuboid; the interstitial space is widened and filled with fluid and collagen. The capillaries are engorged, and the alveoli are filled with debris and hyaline membranes. Extensive white cell infiltration is also present.

TABLE 22-1. ABBREVIATIONS

Abbreviation	Meaning
F_I	Fraction of inspired gas content
C	Content
P	Partial pressure
A	Alveolus
a	Arterial
v	Venous
V	Ventilation
Q	Blood flow

TABLE 22-2. SYMBOLS RELATED TO OXYGENATION

Symbol	Meaning
F_IO_2	Fraction of inspired oxygen content; e.g., room air: F_IO_2 = 0.21; 100% oxygen: F_IO_2 = 1.0
PaO_2	Partial pressure of oxygen in arterial blood; e.g., breathing room air, normal PaO_2 = 80–100 torr
CaO_2	Arterial oxygen content. Used to calculate oxygen consumption and arterial–venous content difference, e.g., Fick principle: cardiac output = O_2 consumption/A − VO_2 content difference
CvO_2	Mixed venous oxygen content; obtained from pulmonary artery blood
V/Q	Ventilation/perfusion; abnormalities arise from unequal distribution of gas and blood to same alveoli
Qt	Cardiac output
Qs	Shunted blood; a method of quantitating pulmonary dysfunction in terms of oxygenation
Qsp/Qt	Physiologic right to left intrapulmonary shunt; total shunt is comprised of Anatomic shunt (normal): veins entering left atrium or pulmonary veins Anatomic shunt (abnormal): direct pulmonary artery flow to pulmonary veins that have been seen in humans and experimental animals Perfusion or blood flow to nonventilated alveoli so that pulmonary capillary blood is not exposed to alveolar oxygen Perfusion to underventilated alveoli so that insufficient oxygen is present to fully oxygenate capillary blood; often called "shunt-like effect" since contributes to arterial hypoxemia

cardiac function. These terms are defined in Table 22-5. The formulas from which these variables may be calculated are displayed in Table 22-6. These symbols and definitions represent a sizable body of knowledge, and these tables may be of value if unfamiliar terminology is encountered in the ensuing discussion.

TABLE 22-3. TERMS RELATED TO VENTILATION

Term	Definition
Vital capacity (VC)	Total amount that can be exhaled from maximal inspiration to maximal expiration; normally 10–15 ml/kg necessary for spontaneous ventilation (normal values, however, are 70–100 ml/kg)
Tidal volume (VT)	Amount exhaled from end of a normal inspiratory effort to normal expiratory state
Dead space ventilation (VD)	Amount of inspired gas that does not reach perfused alveoli; this is sum of anatomic dead space—and physiologic dead space—ventilation of nonperfused alveoli; normal VD/VT = 0.3; ventilation usually requires assistance when ratio exceeds 0.6
$PaCO_2$	Partial pressure of CO_2 in arterial blood; normally approximately 40 torr
Residual volume	Amount of air in lungs at end of forced expiration
Functional residual capacity (FRC)	Volume of air in lungs at end of normal expiration
Spontaneous ventilation	Breathing unassisted
Assisted ventilation	Patient initiates respiratory effort, ventilator supplies predetermined tidal volume
Controlled ventilation (CMV)	Ventilator automatically supplies tidal volume at predetermined rate
End-expiratory pressure (EEP) (Positive EEP = PEEP)	Used to increase airway pressure by maintaining pressure higher than 0 at end of expiration; can be applied during spontaneous ventilation or assisted respiration
Compliance	Measurement of distensibility of lung; measured in terms of volume of gas introduced by a known change in airway pressure (ml/cm)

Pathophysiology

CURRENT HYPOTHESES

Although all of the specific details of etiology and response to therapy are not certain, a workable hypothesis has been formulated (Fig. 22-2). ARF is as-

TABLE 22-4. MODES OF VENTILATORY ASSISTANCE

Mode	Definition
Pressure limited ventilator	Gas flows until present pressure reached; changes in compliance thus cause marked changes in tidal volume
Volume limited ventilator	Preset volume is delivered; pressure changes adjusted by varying flow patterns; advantage is minute ventilation can be maintained relatively constantly
Time cycled ventilator	Time of inspiration preset; inspiratory flow rate may also be varied; tidal volume is product of inspiration time in seconds and inspiratory flow rate (TV = Ti (secs) × IFR (ml/sec) = ml); this type of ventilator very useful in patients with severe respiratory failure
"Weaning"	Transition from assisted respiration to spontaneous breathing; guidelines for oxygenation and mechanics should be followed
IMV	Intermittent mandatory ventilation; patient breathes spontaneously between predetermined mechanical breaths from ventilator
PEEP	Positive end-expiratory pressure, used during spontaneous or mechanical ventilation; pressure can be zero or subambient during inspiratory phase
CPAP	Continuous positive airway pressure; applies to spontaneous breathing—airway pressure remains positive during entire ventilatory cycle
SPEEP	Spontaneous PEEP: positive end-expiration pressure during spontaneous ventilation
HFPPV	High-frequency positive pressure ventilation: a technique using small tidal volume at rates of 60–3000 breaths per minute
ILV	Independent lung ventilation: separate tidal volume and PEEP to each lung field

TABLE 22-5. CARDIOVASCULAR PARAMETERS

Data Base	Calculations
Cardiac output	Stroke volume/index
Systolic blood pressure	
Diastolic blood pressure	
Mean arterial pressure	
Systolic pulmonary artery pressure	
Diastolic pulmonary artery pressure	Cardiac index
Mean pulmonary artery pressure	Right ventricular stroke work/index
Heart rate	
Pulmonary artery occlusion pressure	Left ventricular stroke work/index
Central venous pressure	
Body surface area	Systemic vascular resistance
	Pulmonary vascular resistance
	Myocardial oxygen consumption correlate
	Arterial–venous oxygen content
	Oxygen delivery
	Oxygen consumption
	Oxygen utilization

TABLE 22-6. FORMULAS FOR CARDIOVASCULAR PARAMETERS

Parameter	Formula
MAP	DP + 1/3 (SP − DP) (normal = 80–90 torr)
SV	CO/HR (normal = 50–60 ml)
CI	CO/BSA (normal = 3.5–4 ICU population)
SI	SV/BSA (normal = 35–40 ICU population)
RVSW	SV × (MPA − CVP) × 0.0136 (normal = 10–15 g–M)
LVSW	SV × (MAP − PAO) × .0136 (normal = 60–80 g–M)
SVR	$\frac{(MAP - CVP) \times 80}{CO}$ (normal = 1200 dynes cm^{-5})
PVR	$\frac{(MPA - PAO) \times 80}{CO}$ (normal = 200 dynes cm^{-5})
MVO_2C	$\frac{SP \times HR}{100}$ (higher values = greater consumption)
O_2Del	Ca × CO × 10 (normal = 1000 ml/min)
Ca − Cv	Ca − Cv (normal = 3.5–4.5 ml/100 ml)
O_2 Cons	(Ca − Cv) × CO × 10 (normal = 250 ml/min)
% Util	$\frac{Ca - Cv}{Ca}$ (normal = 0.3)
O_2 Cont	dissolved oxygen + oxygen bound to hemoglobin
O_2 Cont	(gas tension × .0031) + (Hb × 1.39 × Sat)
Ca	(PaO_2 × .0031) + (Hb × 1.39 × Art Sat)
Cv	(PvO_2 × .0031) + (Hb × 1.39 × Ven Sat)

(Data from Hurst JW, Logue RB [eds]: The Heart, 2nd ed. New York, McGraw-Hill, 1970)

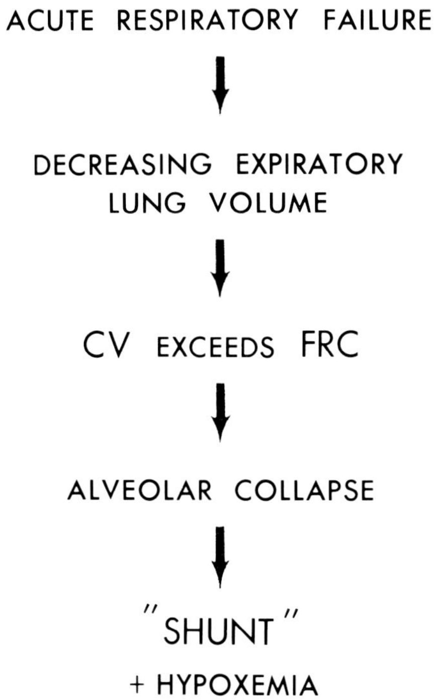

FIG. 22-2. A simplified schema outlining the process that results in ARF. The disease is characterized by decreasing functional residual capacity (*FRC*) until closing volume (*CV*) exceeds FRC. At this point the alveoli collapse, an event that is measured as an increased intrapulmonary shunt, which results in arterial hypoxemia.

sociated with decreased functional residual capacity (FRC): FRC is comprised of residual volume and expiratory reserve volume. It is primarily the latter that is diminished in acute respiratory insufficiency. When FRC is diminished sufficiently that closing volume occurs during tidal respiration, alveolar collapse will occur, thus creating intrapulmonary shunt, which in turn results in arterial hypoxemia. It is now appreciated that the application of positive end-expiratory pressure (PEEP) reverses this process. It has been shown to increase FRC particularly by increasing expiratory reserve volume.[18] The plane of tidal respiration is elevated so that closing volume is not reached (Fig. 22-3). This increase in FRC represents air now remaining in the lung at the end of exhalation (in the previously collapsed alveoli, we suppose); thus ventilation is restored to the areas of perfusion, intrapulmonary shunt is diminished, and arterial hypoxemia is corrected. Although this hypothesis is convenient and has, in fact, been demonstrated with modest levels of PEEP (5–15 cm), it must be stated at the outset that this hypothesis probably will not explain the extremely critical lev-

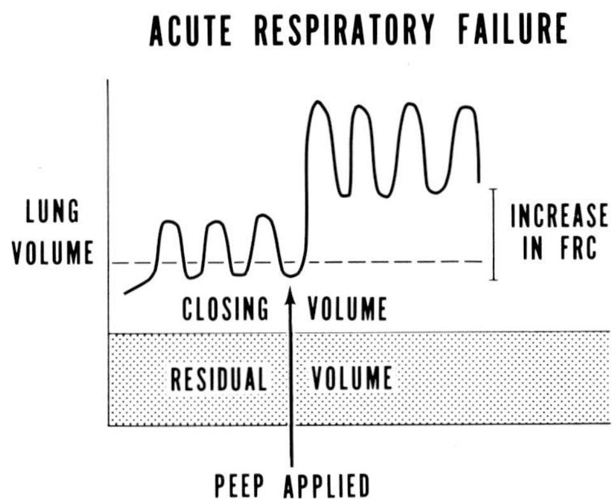

FIG. 22-3. A diagrammatic representation of the effect of applying PEEP in cases of ARF. By promoting alveolar recruitment and improvement in functional residual capacity, PEEP elevates tidal respiration so that closing volume no longer occurs during normal respiration.

els of effective PEEP that are encountered clinically and the sudden response at very high levels. Thus it is common to see dramatic changes in arterial oxygen tension with the addition of 2 cm or 3 cm of water of PEEP in a particular patient after 20 cm had been totally ineffective. Yet the fundamental applicability of this hypothesis has withstood the test of time and permitted the evolution of our treatment perspective for ARF.

Mechanical Ventilation

Acute respiratory failure, though described by Jenkins as congestive atelectasis after the Korean War, became more specifically recognized and treated during the 1960s.[26] In fact, its treatment parallels the growth and development of intensive care. It is important to realize that most patients were admitted to ICUs late in the course of their disease. Although arterial hypoxemia was extreme in most instances, because of the associated hypercarbia, tachypnea, obvious respiratory distress, infiltrative disease on chest x-ray films, and extremely poor compliance, mechanical ventilation was selected as the primary and only therapy.

After Gregory reported the gratifying response of the infant respiratory distress syndrome to continuous positive airway pressure (CPAP), Ashbaugh and colleagues reported the application of PEEP to mechanical ventilation with subsequent improvement in oxygenation.[1, 23] In the late 1960s and 1970s others confirmed these results and demonstrated the association among improvement in FRC, decreased shunt, and improved arterial oxygenation.[33] However, the failure of mechanincal ventilation was not truly appreciated nor was PEEP applied in an early

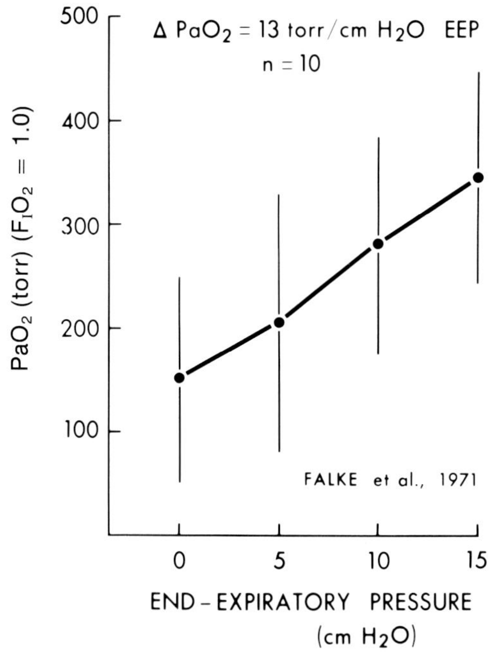

FIG. 22-4. The relationship between end-expiratory pressure (*EEP*) and arterial oxygen tension. Zero EEP represents controlled mechanical ventilation. Note that oxygenation is far below expected levels for patients breathing 100% oxygen. This represents a failure of mechanical ventilation to correct the underlying abnormality. Improvement in this group of 10 patients occurred after the application of EEP. (Data from Falke K, Pontoppidan H, Kumar A et al: Ventilation with end-expiratory pressure in acute lung disease. J Clin Invest 51:2315, 1972)

phase to improve oxygenation. Rather it was added as a last resort—after conventional therapy, usually continuous mechanical ventilation—had failed to improve oxygenation. Mortality rates during the era of mechanical ventilation were 60% to 80%. The reason for the failure of mechanical ventilation is obvious, since arterial oxygenation was still markedly impaired. The zero point in most graphs illustrating the effect of PEEP confirms the failure of mechanical ventilation to improve oxygen tension (Fig. 22-4). This is not surprising, since mechanical ventilation can affect alveolar collapse only during the inspiratory phase. Thus during expiration the factors leading to the decreased FRC recur, the alveoli collapse again, and the shunt is not affected. However, in the late stage of the disease process, CO_2 retention is present, and there is need for mechanical ventilation.

Other studies confirm that PEEP added to mechanical ventilation often decreased cardiac output, most probably due to the increased intrathoracic pressure produced.[33, 39] Recently "stretch" receptors in the lung have been postulated to decrease cardiac output through an unidentified blood-borne factor. The myocardial depression did not occur if PEEP or mechanical ventilation alone were tested but only when PEEP was imposed in addition to mechanical ventilation. The results unfortunately have been interpreted as an effect of PEEP alone. The mistake in emphasis stems from attributing the decreased cardiac output solely to PEEP rather than to an additive effect to the already high intrathoracic pressures created during mechanical insufflation of stiff lungs. An alternative approach suggests that PEEP can only be considered the culprit in such a situation if the effect of mechanical ventilation is ignored. Of course, when patients were treated late in the course of the disease and mechanical ventilation was necessary, this distinction was not even considered because both modalities of therapy appeared mandatory—in fact, the order of application and degree utilized were concepts that had not evolved.

The Development of "Optimal" PEEP

In the early 1970s three changes occurred that, when put together, would provide a more satisfactory plan of therapy in terms of both efficacy and ease in practice. First, IMV, introduced as a weaning technique, became employed as a new mode of ventilation.[14] The ease in weaning due to the small decrements in machine-supplied ventilation was reassessed in the reverse: mechanical ventilation need *only* provide the necessary increment of ventilation in a patient who still maintained some spontaneous ventilatory activity. The sum of mechanical and spontaneous ventilation are adjusted to provide total alveolar ventilation. If a patient retains the ability to provide 70% of this need, one need *not* begin therapy at the 100% mechanical level and *wean* but, rather, provide only the 30% lacking, eliminating most pressure-related effects and encouraging the salutory effects of spontaneous ventilation upon V/Q relationships and cardiac output.[31, 42] As experience was gained, it became clear that if treatment of these patients was instituted earlier, far less mechanical ventilation was necessary.

Second, it was during this era that oxygen toxicity became recognized, and, therefore, the primary therapeutic effect of PEEP was considered to be related to its ability to improve oxygenation to avoid potentially toxic levels of oxygen. Quite often PEEP was withheld until arterial PO_2 fell to 50 torr at an F_IO_2 of 1.0. The impetus to utilize PEEP to treat the disease process itself was not fully appreciated until 1973 when Downs and colleagues introduced the concept of incremental PEEP.[15] Thus the combination of IMV and PEEP shifted attention from the hope that mechanical ventilation alone would provide satisfactory therapy for ARF to the perspective that PEEP reversed the pathophysiologic changes

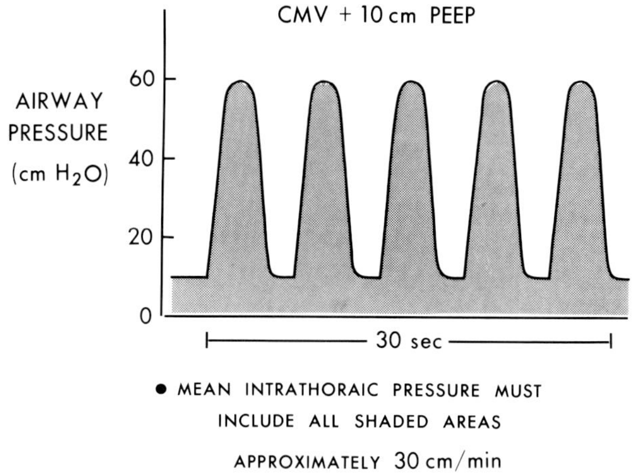

FIG. 22-5. The effect of CMV and PEEP in a patient with ARF and reduced compliance. Inspiratory pressures are higher than normal. The most significant finding, however, is that 10 cm of PEEP does not emphasize the marked increase in mean minute intrathoracic pressure (30 cm/min) generated by the combination of CMV and PEEP.

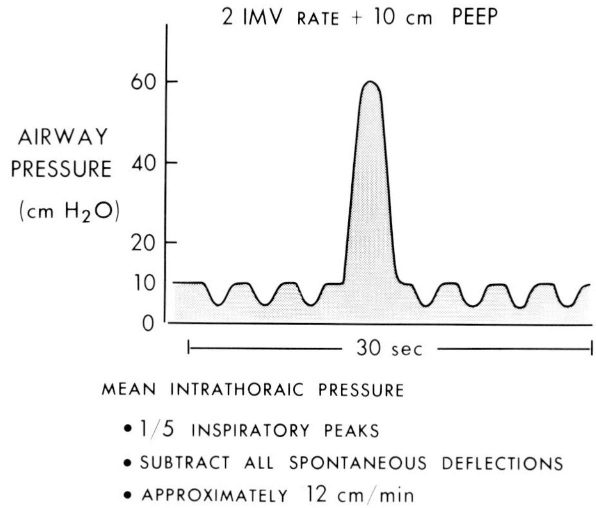

FIG. 22-6. The combination of IMV and PEEP results in a marked diminution of mean minute intrathoracic pressure. Both the decreased number of inspiratory peaks and the salutory effect of the spontaneous breaths on intrathoracic pressure contribute to lowering mean minute intrathoracic pressure.

and that mechanical ventilation should be provided only to help normalize CO_2 elimination. In a quasi-quantitative way, PEEP could be applied at higher levels, since overall mean thoracic pressure would be diminished owing to the decreased mechanical ventilation empirically delivered when controlled mechanical ventilation (CMV) was employed (Figs. 22-5 and 22-6).

The last development that permitted the evolution of this therapeutic regimen was the advent of the Swan–Ganz thermodilution catheter and cardiac output computer.[21, 40] Most patients with severe ARF had numerous reasons to develop ventricular compromise or at least ventricular disparity such that right atrial pressure measurements were of relatively little value in determining left ventricular filling pressures.[10] The simplicity and reliability of the thermodilution cardiac output measurements enabled clinicians to monitor the cardiovascular system with a specificity hitherto unknown in clinical care. Measurement of systolic, diastolic, and mean pulmonary artery pressure; systolic, diastolic, and mean arterial pressure; central venous pressure; pulmonary artery occlusion pressure; heart rate, cardiac output, and hemoglobin concentration; and inspired oxygen tension, arterial oxygen tension, arterial carbon dioxide tension, and mixed venous oxygen tension gave fundamental information necessary to calculate both cardiac and respiratory variables important to determine the relationships of cardiac output, PEEP, and intrapulmonary shunt. A further technological step was the advent of inexpensive, programmable calculators so that the calculations, though simple mathematically but cumbersome in practice, could be handled rapidly at very little cost or effort.[6] Thus myocardial function could be delineated as preload, as evidenced by pulmonary artery occlusion and right atrial pressure; contractility, as inferred from the relationships among left ventricular stroke work, cardiac output, stroke volume and heart rate; and afterload, from direct calculations of systemic and pulmonary vascular resistance. The effects of the particular type of ventilatory support could be quantitated and interventions directed to improve cardiac function—whether compromised primarily or adversely affected by the ventilatory support employed. At this point, the synthesis of these three techniques could be applied to ARF. This approach was termed "optimal PEEP" (Fig. 22-7), and it involves three separate facets of applied physiology.[8]

PEEP is introduced or titrated until satisfactory oxygenation occurs. As experience with the technique evolved, the "hyperoxic–hypoxic" indications for PEEP were abandoned. Experimental and clinical data suggested that inspired oxygen tensions of greater than 0.5 (50% oxygen concentration) could lead to increased pulmonary damage. From inspection of the oxyhemoglobin dissociation curve, arterial oxygen tensions in excess of 60 torr produced nearly complete saturation of the hemoglobin and thus facilitated oxygen transport. We identify this as a hyperoxic–hypoxic goal of therapy. The emphasis

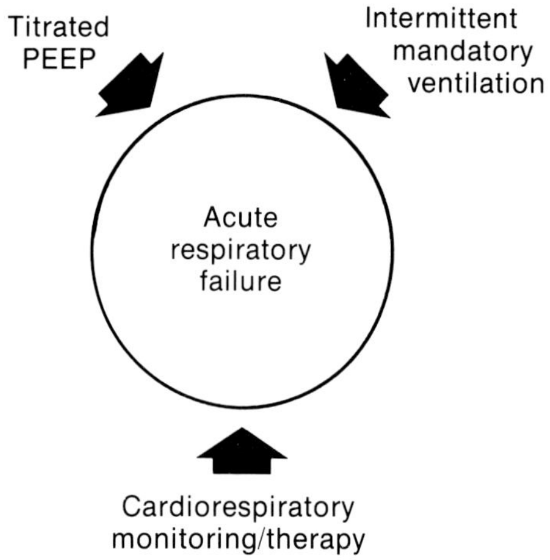

FIG. 22-7. Schematic representation of the application of PEEP, IMV, and cardiorespiratory monitoring to form a coordinated approach to the treatment of ARF.

on utilizing nontoxic (less than 50% oxygen) supplementation in ventilatory support techniques while yet providing at least adequate arterial oxygenation ($PaO_2 > 60$–70 torr) actually left the patient with a significant and severe impairment of gas exchange. With normal cardiac output, this would imply an intrapulmonary shunt in excess of 35% to 40%. Optimal PEEP, on the other hand, attempts to reduce intrapulmonary shunt to a value of 15% to 20%. Although this end point appears somewhat arbitrary, it does represent a level of pulmonary function compatible with unassisted and unsupplemented ventilatory support. In other words, if functional blood gas abnormalities can be reversed early to a level compatible with totally adequate spontaneous ventilatory activity, then therapy need not be delayed until advanced disease necessitates major interventions. The patient's improvement is then gauged by the elimination of the ventilatory support rather than by further improvement in blood gas exchange. In practice, most patients now undergoing treatment have relatively normal blood gases, although they may require application of IMV and PEEP therapy. Previously, patients with the same disease entities were maintained at critically compromised blood gas values as a direct result of the clinically selected end points.

IMV is utilized as the primary mode of mechanical ventilatory support in most patients. The desirability of maintaining even minor spontaneous respiratory excursions is difficult to quantify, but this technique avoids the necessity for paralysis and heavy sedation and obviates the relearning of breathing during the weaning process. However, the most significant advantage to IMV is only discernible in a negative way: if continuous mechanical ventilation is not supplied, then the patient must perform some spontaneous breathing. If therapy is instituted early and progression of the disease has not occurred, the increment provided by the patient can be much more significant than previously appreciated. Patients with severe arterial hypoxemia can generate 90% or more of the mechanical work necessary to eliminate CO_2 without laboring. The advantages to this approach are numerous. Controlled mechanical ventilation usually results in at least a modest degree of respiratory alkalosis. Even if paralyzing agents are used, dead space employed, and slow ventilator rates selected, most patients will be observed to have $PaCO_2$ levels of 30 to 34 torr. The resultant alkalemia increases oxygen consumption and hemoglobin's affinity for oxygen, resulting in a greater oxygen demand and lessened availability—the opposite of what should be desirable in critically ill patients.[11, 27] Mechanically supplied positive pressure breaths increase VD/VT.[19] If one chooses to override the patient's own ability to breathe, the result may be to worsen ventilation perfusion relationships in patients whose primary disease process is characterized by abnormal V/Q ratios.[42] Each mechanical breath raises intrathoracic pressure above the baseline and impedes venous return. Each spontaneous breath results in a negative intrathoracic pressure with respect to the patient's therapeutic baseline and in some measure aids venous return and lowers mean intrathoracic pressure. The increased number of breaths seen with controlled mechanical ventilation also increases the risk of pneumothorax, since it is the high peak inflation pressure that ruptures the lung. If the patient can tolerate only a certain level of mean intrathoracic pressure, it seems reasonable to utilize this as PEEP, which affects the pathophysiologic process rather than to "use up" the patient's tolerance as ineffective mechanical breaths. Finally, cardiovascular function will be less affected.[29]

Since the definition of optimal PEEP requires an understanding of cardiorespiratory physiology and response to therapy, cardiorespiratory monitoring was the third necessary development to be applied in practice. Many of our potent therapeutic interventions have both positive and negative effects. The present therapeutic milieu is usually defined as a negotiated balance between these effects. Although mechanical ventilation and PEEP both have adverse effects on cardiovascular function, they are neither uniform nor predictable. In practice, the introduction of the thermistor-tipped pulmonary artery catheter provides much of the necessary information.[6] Although the theoretical effect of cardiac output on arterial oxygenation has been known for many years, it was not until the application of IMV and PEEP became widespread that the absolute necessity for discrimination became so clear-cut.[28]

The Fick principle is one of the fundamental concepts of cardiovascular physiology that has achieved its proper level of understanding since precise cardiovascular monitoring became available at the bedside. Arterial oxygen tension is not uniquely determined by the degree of ventilatory insufficiency. In fact, *venous oxygen content* also has a major role in determining arterial oxygen tension. The Fick principle is

$$\text{Cardiac output} = \frac{\text{Oxygen consumption}}{\text{Arteriovenous } O_2 \text{ content difference}}$$

Although oxygen consumption may vary with increased or decreased perfusion, pH, or septic states, in the 10 or 15 minutes in which equilibration occurs after ventilatory support is changed, it is probably reasonable to assume that oxygen consumption remains fairly constant. In such an instance, then, there will be an inverse relationship between cardiac output and arteriovenous oxygen content difference. Since oxygen content of the arterial blood is determined primarily by arterial oxygen tension and can be maintained in a range sufficient to provide near total hemoglobin saturation, changes in cardiac output will be reflected by changes in arteriovenous oxygen content induced almost entirely by increased extraction. Therefore a decreased venous oxygen content, when "shunted" through perfused and unventilated alveoli, will "dilute" the oxygen tension of blood from pulmonary capillaries that still are ventilated (*i.e.*, fully saturated). The lower the venous oxygen content, the more the arterial PO_2 will be lowered. Thus, in the presence of a modest or increased intrapulmonary shunt, changes in cardiac output will have a major effect on the actual arterial oxygen tension. If therapy such as PEEP (or mechanical ventilation) should decrease cardiac output, a lower PaO_2 will result—even though intrapulmonary shunt may be favorably decreased. Documentation of the cardiovascular response to therapy therefore is crucially important. If physiologic reserves are sufficient to maintain cardiac output, no further therapy is necessary: the application of sufficient PEEP to reduce shunt is often possible without any cardiovascular manipulations. However, if cardiac output does fall, the physiologic profile of the cardiovascular system should suggest therapeutic interventions.

CARDIOVASCULAR INTERVENTIONS

It is crucial to remember that most surgical and trauma patients who develop ARF may also have compromised cardiovascular function because of their primary disease process. ARF is commonly seen in patients who have undergone lengthy reconstructive vascular procedures, the prolonged stress of multisystem trauma, or have developed severe sepsis. Disparity between right and left ventricular filling pressures and altered systemic and pulmonary vascular resistances make this population subject to significant disorders of cardiovascular function.

Major advances have occurred in augmentation of cardiac function through all three factors: preload, contractility, and afterload.

Preload

The importance of balanced electrolyte solutions in correcting intravascular and extracellular fluid deficits has been emphasized, while the maintenance of serum oncotic pressure and attempts to retrieve interstitial pulmonary edema have not found experimental or clinical validation.[5, 41, 43] Although an extensive discussion of pulmonary interstitial fluid is beyond the scope of this discussion, certain principles have found clinical utility. Pulmonary edema occurs when net filtration from the pulmonary capillaries exceeds the lung's capacity to remove the filtered fluid.[7] Much attention has been focused on the importance of oncotic pressures as a determinant of net filtration.[12] It appears that this factor has been overemphasized, since interstitial oncotic pressure in the lung apparently approaches 70% to 80% of the serum oncotic pressure.[3, 43] Therefore, oncotic factors exert a relatively minor influence upon fluid flux. Furthermore, it has been difficult to change oncotic pressure gradients. If serum oncotic pressure is increased, so is lung lymph oncotic pressure.[13] If oncotic pressure in the serum decreases there is a concomitant fall in lymph oncotic pressure.[43] Finally, if there are changes in capillary permeability, no oncotic gradient can be established.[3] Thus it is nearly impossible to affect oncotic gradients for a protracted time. Various manipulations have been attempted, such as the use of potent intravenous diuretics and administration of concentrated albumin solutions. These seem to be ill advised, since most often pulmonary interstitial edema is not affected by such maneuvers and there can be significant deleterious effects. In both the post-traumatic and septic surgical patient, effective intravascular volume is usually decreased. Administration of potent diuretics can exacerbate this problem and can result in further impairment in cardiovascular function. This might actually result in further deterioration in oxygenation as outlined in the previous section. The administration of concentrated albumin solutions may have a transient effect upon serum oncotic pressure, but interstitial oncotic pressure will soon establish equilibrium. The net effect only increases the dollar cost to the patient without therapeutic benefit. Therefore, if fluid therapy is deemed necessary to restore effective left ventricular filling pressure, red cells or balanced electrolyte solutions seem appropriate. Red cells are administered if the hematocrit is low and serve to increase oxygen transport. If the hematocrit is acceptable, balanced electrolyte solutions alone should be utilized.

Contractility

Methods of enhancing contractility have undergone considerable revision in the past few years. In the compromised patient, the balance between oxygen delivery and oxygen demand caused by the use of inotropic agents has been more effectively measured.[22] Agents that markedly increase oxygen consumption in the compromised heart may actually be more deleterious than helpful. Thus the use of isoproterenol in elderly patients has generally fallen out of favor because it induced major increments in the heart's need for oxygen. Digoxin has been shown to increase cardiac performance and decrease oxygen consumption in the failing heart and therefore often seems indicated.[25] Agents such as dopamine or dobutamine may influence contractility more than heart rate and therefore may produce the necessary increment in cardiac work without inducing an overwhelming oxygen burden. Studies relating serum ionized calcium to cardiac performance have some fascinating connotations for the critically ill patient.[16] Although the mechanisms are not yet entirely clear, "hypo-ionized calcemia" is a common finding in critical illness. Animal experimentation has revealed that in both sepsis and trauma interstitial ionized calcium levels may be markedly decreased. Since interstitial calcium is one of the prime determinants of myocardial contractility, depression of cardiovascular function may result. Although the influence of multiple transfusions upon ionized calcium seems to be related to the rapid infusion of banked blood (a rate of 1 unit in 5 minutes), it is not uncommon in the postresuscitative period to find that cardiac contractility is depressed. The clinical response to the infusion of 1 g to 2 g of calcium chloride may well be related to the hypoionized calcemia seen in experimental shock and sepsis. Since ARF has been long associated with these disease states, restoration of ionized calcium levels is a simple way to improve cardiovascular performance so that ventilatory manipulations can be performed safely.

Afterload

The importance of increased impedance to outflow, commonly termed afterload, has been recently advanced with studies of specific drugs that decrease arteriolar resistance or venous capacitance.[35, 38] Various combinations of the two types of drugs have also been investigated. Decrease in afterload does more than merely decrease the pressure–work generated by the left ventricle. If the mean arterial pressure is high, pre-ejection period is lengthened. During the pre-ejection period, myocardial muscle fibers contract without producing any external work. This is extremely costly in oxygen consumption. After the aortic valve opens, the ejection period commences and the stroke volume is ejected. This period will be shortened if mean arterial pressure is high because the aortic valve will open at a later time in the cardiac cycle and close more rapidly (Fig. 22-8). When mean aortic pressure is lowered (Fig. 22-9), the duration of the pre-ejection period is shortened, thus decreasing the time that the myocardial muscle contracts without performing any external work. Oxygen consumption is thereby decreased. In addition, left ventricular ejection time will be prolonged since the aortic valve will open earlier and close later because mean aortic pressure is diminished. The heart benefits from ejecting earlier and longer while requiring less oxygen because less wall tension is necessary. Should left ventricular filling pressure diminish as a result of the increase in contractility or from combined arteriolar and venular vasodilatation using an agent such as nitroprusside, the decrease in filling pressure will result in a decrease in ventricular end-diastolic radius. Through the law of

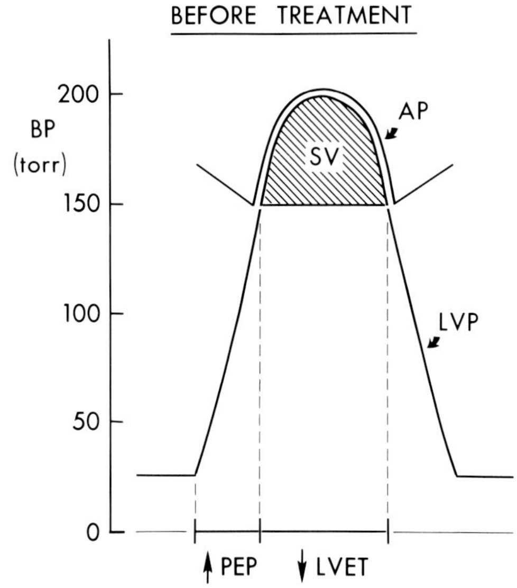

FIG. 22-8. Schematic representation of aortic pressure (*AP*) and left ventricular pressure (*LVP*) before treatment. In this instance, aortic pressure is markedly elevated, thus prolonging the pre-ejection period (*PEP*) and simultaneously decreasing the stroke volume (*SV*) ejected because the left ventricular ejection time (*LVET*) is necessarily shortened.

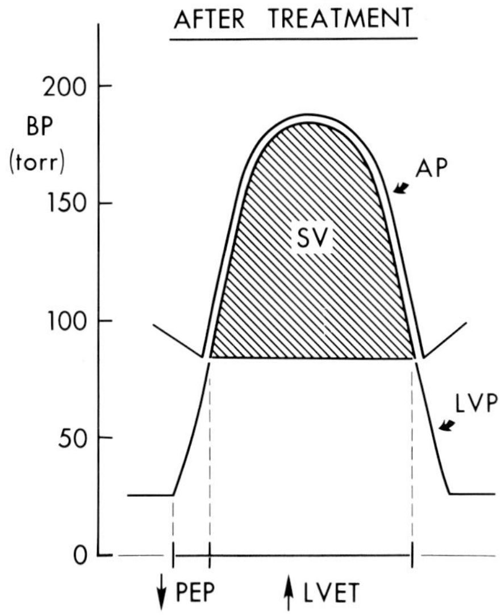

FIG. 22-9. After mean arterial pressure has been reduced, the left ventricle requires a shorter pre-ejection period (*PEP*) to exceed aortic pressure (*AP*) and open the aortic valve. The aortic valve stays open longer, and thus there is a marked increase in stroke volume (*SV*) ejected. *LVET*, left ventricular ejection time; *LVP*, left ventricular pressure.

LaPlace, this will permit the heart to generate the same pressure with less muscle shortening—and less oxygen consumption. The law of LaPlace relates the tension necessary to produce a given pressure to the radius, which is an inverse relationship,

$$P = T \times (1/R_1 + 1/R_2)$$

Therefore, the longer the radius (an overdistended ventricle), the greater the muscle tension.

It is fortunate that programmable calculators can provide the necessary cardiovascular variables, now that new drugs and new approaches to therapy allow sustaining or augmenting cardiovascular function during necessary ventilatory manipulations.

THERAPEUTIC USE

Perhaps optimal PEEP should be defined as the time when technology and physiology could be applied in practice. Previous data suggesting that more than 15 cm of PEEP should not be applied to a patient receiving CMV had to be reevaluated. IMV permitted the patient to provide spontaneous ventilation for 80% of the time, ventilation perfusion abnormalities were diminished, intrathoracic pressure was lessened, and cardiac function was enhanced. With monitoring and augmentation of cardiovascular function, levels of end-expiratory pressure in excess of those previously accepted could also be utilized. Thus in 1975 Kirby and colleagues reported on a series of patients in whom higher levels of end-expiratory pressure were used.[29] It is interesting to note that, first, these patients were encountered late in the course of their disease and required extremely careful monitoring of both cardiovascular and respiratory parameters to achieve improvement in arterial oxygenation, and that, second, this approach was associated with a higher survival rate than had been anticipated. Once the technique was established, its true utility became evident: application of such goal-directed therapy could be instituted earlier in the course of the disease. In a later series of 315 patients approximately 80% of the patients treated immediately upon arrival in the intensive-care unit did not require such major interventions.[20] If the mechanical ventilatory rate was decreased according to the ability of the patient to ventilate spontaneously and PEEP was instituted to reduce intrapulmonary shunt to the preselected 15% shunt criterion, it was only the occasional patient who required more aggressive intervention. IMV, PEEP, and cardiorespiratory monitoring now constitute a practical approach to acute ventilatory insufficiency.

Diagnosis and Treatment

The most important concept in successful treatment of ARF as a complication following surgery and trauma is that early therapy is easier and more effective than therapy instituted late in the course of the disease. As a corollary, it is obvious that one must establish the diagnosis, and this requires preformed expectations and adequate observation of all patients who are at high risk of developing ARF.

For the patient with traumatic injuries, there are three major factors associated with the development of severe ARF: the presence of direct thoracic trauma, the number of associated injuries, and late septic complications.

Penetrating thoracic trauma is often associated with hemopneumothorax. It is not as often stated that any thoracic trauma may be associated with the late development of pneumothorax. In our experience approximately one third of the patients with blunt trauma develop pneumothorax after admission to the hospital. This is in contrast to a rate of less than 5% in patients with ARF secondary to other factors. ARF associated with blunt thoracic trauma is usually more severe than that encountered in patients who have suffered only penetrating injuries.

While "flail chest" is often considered to be a distinct entity due to the paradoxical movement of the flail segment, the underlying pulmonary contusion is probably the most important component. Controlled mechanical ventilation for periods in excess of 2 weeks has usually been utilized in the treatment of these patients because internal stabilization of the chest could be achieved without the necessity for cumbersome external fixation devices. However, even in flail chest the characteristic blood gas abnormalities of arterial hypoxemia and hypocarbia are usually present early in the patient's hospital course. In such instances the addition of mechanical ventilation *per se* would seemingly have little impact on a disease process characterized by intrapulmonary shunting and increased alveolar ventilation demonstrated by the decreased $PaCO_2$. We consider that the arterial hypoxemia serves as a stimulus to increase ventilation. When minute ventilation is markedly increased, both in terms of tidal volume and respiratory rate, the flail segment becomes obvious. However, if positive end-expiratory pressure is used as a primary form of therapy, arterial hypoxemia can be corrected, the need for increased minute ventilation diminishes, and the flail segment is no longer as obvious. Thus, the same treatment principles apply to flail chest with rib fractures or in pulmonary parenchymal contusion alone. In fact, arterial hypoxemia may often be seen in the trauma patient without discernible x-ray abnormalities early in the patient's hospital course. We believe that therapy for hypoxemia should be instituted at this time where hypoxemia is defined as an arterial PO_2 less than 55 torr while the patient is breathing room air.

The incidence of ARF rises in proportion to the number of associated injuries. Long bone fractures, in particular, may be associated with ARF owing to fat embolism without any other injuries. Closed head injury has been associated with respiratory failure secondary to neurogenic pulmonary edema. However, significant neurogenic pulmonary edema rarely is evident unless massive head injury has occurred. Since therapy involves manipulation of airway pressure, one must be aware of the relationship between increasing intrathoracic pressure and impaired venous return and the potential for increasing intracranial pressure. Concomitant severe head injury and respiratory failure therefore require monitoring not only of the cardiac and respiratory system but also of intracranial pressure. Although many drugs are capable of reducing intracranial pressure, venting of cerebral spinal fluid is another method of rapidly reducing intracranial pressure. In addition, the subarachnoid bolt may not reflect the magnitude of intracranial pressure, and for both of these reasons an intraventricular catheter should be considered.

When more than three other injuries are sustained, the incidence of ARF is approximately 33%. Initial observation should detect the early onset of ARF due to direct thoracic trauma or that associated with other injuries. However, careful observation is necessary during the entire phase of critical illness since sepsis due to a pulmonary, abdominal, or a wound source can occur later.

The patient with possible or documented aspiration, a reaction to a transfusion, compromised myocardial function, or subjected to a long operation is also at high risk for developing ARF. With these factors in mind, careful observation should include the obvious clinical parameters of respiratory function such as respiratory rate, particularly in association with small tidal volumes; anxiety; and restlessness. The most sensitive indicator of all is sequential monitoring of arterial blood gases.

It is difficult to define absolute values for the diagnosis of ARF; however, if arterial oxygen tension falls below 55 torr while the patient is breathing room air, significant impairment of oxygenation has occurred. If hypocarbia without a markedly increased respiratory rate is present, PEEP alone may be effective therapy. If the first blood gas reveals severe arterial hypoxemia or if clinical observation shows respiratory rates in excess of 40 to 50 per minute, then the "early-warning system" has not been employed. Since the majority of the patients at high risk have undergone an operation under general anesthesia administered through an endotracheal tube, the safest course is to maintain intubation during the early postoperative period. If sequential blood gas analyses do not document initial hypoxemia or progressive diminution in oxygen tension, the endotracheal tube can be removed. The time of observation will vary with the number of antecedent factors and the severity of the insult. After only a prolonged elective operation, perhaps 2 to 3 hours would suffice. If multiple injuries are present, particularly if direct thoracic trauma has been sustained, it is probably safer to delay extubation for 24 hours. During this period we commonly use an IMV rate of 2 breaths per minute and maintain 5 cm of water of PEEP. Further weaning is easily accomplished if ARF does not supervene. However, when progressive blood gas abnormalities occur or the patient's clinical condition deteriorates, it is then possible to escalate therapy without the necessity for emergency reintubation.

CLINICAL GUIDELINES FOR PEEP

The principles are simple: first, increase PEEP in increments of 2 to 3 cm of water until the shunt is reduced to approximately 15%. When there is neither cardiovascular compromise nor severe degrees of ventilatory insufficiency the guideline should be when arterial PaO_2/F_IO_2 approximates 300 torr. Cardiorespiratory monitoring should be considered necessary if more than 15 cm of water of PEEP is needed. Patients whose PaO_2 is restored to 90 to 110 torr while breathing 30% oxygen would therefore fit the criterion for adequate oxygenation.

Second, the IMV rate is determined by the patient's need: "normocapnea" actually is the normal for an individual patient. Patients with chronic obstructive pulmonary disease (COPD) must be treated carefully, because one must make every effort to maintain a normal but elevated $PaCO_2$. Weaning from textbook normal levels ($PaCO_2$ = 40 torr) is very difficult in COPD patients, since 40 torr actually represents weaning from controlled ventilation with a relative respiratory alkalosis. In fact, *p*H criteria have been found a satisfactory alternative from which to infer the patient's normal $PaCO_2$.[20] As long as the *p*H exceeds 7.35, one has probably maintained the normal $PaCO_2$ for this patient, unless a concomitant cause for metabolic alkalosis can be discerned by careful review of the patient's record. Thus, the usual determinant of the adequacy of the supplied mandatory breaths rests on three criteria: $PaCO_2$ that is normal for the patient, *p*H greater than 7.35, and spontaneous respiratory rate of 30 or less. It is perfectly clear that some patients can maintain a normal $PaCO_2$ by breathing 40 to 50 times per minute. However, this in no way should be considered adequate ventilatory support. Although certain patients with CNS injury will ventilate at excessive rates no matter what IMV rate is supplied, the average patient breathing spontaneously with a low IMV rate will have none of the stigmata of ventilatory insufficiency. No matter what the blood gas criteria, should any patient appear to be laboring, anxious, or combative, one must assume that there is an inadequate level of ventilatory support. A simple therapeutic trial of an increased IMV rate should resolve the complicated cases in which CNS factors or other metabolic phenomena may confuse the picture.

The third determinant of therapy is the adequacy of cardiovascular response. As a general rule, cardiovascular monitoring is instituted whenever compromise is considered likely. In patients who have cardiovascular instability, IMV seems to provide protection from the detrimental effects of PEEP on cardiovascular function until at least 15 cm of water is applied. Actual or relative hypovolemia may precipitate an adverse reaction to lower levels of PEEP so that adequate fluid replacement in multisystem insults must always be encouraged. At this arbitrary point, 15 cm of water of PEEP, invasive cardiovascular monitoring is instituted to be sure that no compromise in cardiovascular function occurs while respiratory manipulations are continued. A demonstrated decrease in cardiovascular function requires further investigation to determine therapy of the cardiovascular depression rather than retreating from effective ventilatory support.

ARF in its earliest stages reflects functional disruption of the normal ventilation and perfusion relationships. PEEP improves FRC and provides alveolar recruitment that should improve the V/Q abnormalities, since ventilation is restored to the areas of maintained perfusion. The fact that positive pressure ventilation produces a 60% increase in VD/VT in normal patients must not be overlooked. Areas of overventilation are created as well as true shunt (*i.e.*, perfusion of nonventilated alveoli). But the most significant change is the appearance of areas with marked excess of perfusion where some ventilation is still maintained. It would appear that PEEP not only affects alveolar recruitment but provides ventilation to areas with extremely low V/Q ratios. IMV in this circumstance can be considered a supplemental form of therapy. No longer is control of ventilation desirable; ventilation must be supplied only when the ventilatory status of the lungs is so compromised that overall CO_2 elimination is impaired. This is extremely rare in the early stages of all forms of ARF.

We avoid imposing an *a priori* decision to override the patient's ability to ventilate spontaneously. The actual "wasted" breaths inherent in selecting CMV should serve to bring the point home. Should a patient receive 2 breaths per minute from an IMV system in contrast to continuous ventilation at the rate of 12, there would be a net saving of 10 breaths per minute, 600 per hour, or 14,400 breaths per day. If the mechanical breaths serve no useful function in CO_2 elimination, if they are truly ineffective in correcting hypoxemia, and if they increase intrathoracic pressure and worsen ventilation–perfusion abnormalities, it is hard to understand why CMV should be advocated as the primary therapy for ARF. The decreased likelihood of pulmonary barotrauma is also important, since eliminating over 14,000 inflations per day of any balloon certainly decreases the risk of rupture. Weaning is already nearly completed if mechanical ventilation is not utilized to a significant degree, but this should not be interpreted to indicate the superiority of one weaning technique over another. Rather, IMV reinforces the principle that clinical support should supply what the patient requires.

Fluid therapy should not be focused on theories related to possible but *not demonstrated* effects of colloids; rather, it should be directed more appropriately to correct the deficits encountered in the disease states that created ARF. For instance, translocation of functional extracellular volume has been documented in both shock and septic cases. Maintenance and augmentation of cardiovascular function in these states is crucial. Left ventricular filling pressure should be adjusted to the range expected to enhance cardiovascular function. It appears that pulmonary artery occlusion pressure or left ventricular filling pressure can be increased to a range of 13 to 17 torr in patients with documented cardiovascular dysfunction.[10] If oxygen delivery and cardiovascular performance appear sufficient, as evidenced by normal PvO_2 (35 torr) and the absence of metabolic acidosis, arbitrary manipulation of wedge pressure to achieve a preselected range (*i.e.*, 13–17 torr) should not even be considered. Augmentation of cardiac function is necessary only if the ventilatory support actually decreases cardiac output. Red cells or balanced electrolyte solution should be administered in a dose sufficient to maintain a reasonable cardiac output for the patient. In most circumstances this is higher than that observed in the resting patient and reflects the stress state associated with ARF. Inotropic agents and manipulations of afterload follow similar therapeutic directions.

NEWER MODALITIES OF THERAPY

Prolonged Inspiration

Once the flexible concept of ventilatory support using IMV and PEEP was introduced, other changes in the pattern of ventilatory support were considered. The demonstrations that CO_2 elimination can be enhanced by providing mechanical ventilation when necessary and that PEEP can be instituted if gas exchange is impaired suggested other possibilities. Can the inspiratory/expiratory (I/E) pattern be further modified? Prolongation of the inspiratory phase of the mandatory breaths has received considerable attention.[34] This might be redefined as "pulsed PEEP." In other words, if inspiratory time is prolonged to 4 to 5 seconds, during the last 2 or 3 seconds there is a high mean intrathoracic pressure but only intermittently during a minute of ventilatory time. For instance, if 27 cm of water of PEEP is applied with an inspiratory time of 5 seconds, mean intrathoracic pressure for the last 2 or 3 seconds might exceed 50 cm to 60 cm of water. Patients continue spontaneous breathing during this time, and since the PEEP effect occurs only two or three times a minute, the overall effect upon cardiovascular function is minimized. However, there may be alveoli that require such sustained pressures for reinflation. Furthermore, ventilation–perfusion abnormalities in other sections of the lung may also be corrected. Patients for whom this technique has been utilized include infants with the idiopathic respiratory distress syndrome and adults who have severely compromised ventilatory function with markedly decreased compliance. Since the pressure generated during delivery of a tidal volume is related to compliance, standard mechanical ventilation may produce extremely high peak airway pressures because of the rapid inspiratory flow rates. Prolongation of the inspiratory time may promote more even distribution so that alveolar areas of slow filling receive a portion of the tidal volume. With this technique, it has been possible to lower peak inspiratory pressures by one third, and PEEP by one half and yet maintain oxygenation, CO_2 elimination, and cardiovascular function. These patients are usually seen late in the course of this disease and have marked infiltrative changes on x-ray examination. They usually require inspiratory pressures greater than 100 cm of water prior to alteration of I/E patterns.

Positioning of the Patient

Other techniques have been tried to improve perfusion as well as ventilation. The Roto bed, designed for orthopaedic and neurosurgical patients with spinal cord injuries, has been utilized in conjunction with IMV and PEEP to alter pulmonary perfusion.[36] In this application, a patient with one-sided pulmonary pathology, albeit rare, can be preferentially positioned so that the diseased lung is elevated and the good lung is dependent. In this fashion, both ventilation and perfusion will be delivered to the "good" lung, resulting in two effects: first, with less perfusion of nonventilated areas in the diseased lung, intrapulmonary shunt must decrease, and, second, there should be decreased pulmonary microvascular pressure and egress of fluid. One-sided pulmonary pathologic processes include both infectious and traumatic insults. Direct pulmonary contusion resulting from a shotgun blast is one obvious example (Fig. 22-10). Utilization of this technique resulted in rapid resolution of a pulmonary contusion in only 8 hours (Fig. 22-11).

Independent Lung Ventilation

If this technique is not effective, simultaneous independent lung ventilation (SILV) can be used. This technique finds application in patients with recurrent atelectasis unresponsive to bronchoscopy or conventional IMV and PEEP therapy, patients with large bronchopleural-cutaneous fistulas, and patients with unilateral pulmonary consolidation. To employ this technique, a Carlen's tube is inserted so that each lung may be ventilated independently. High-volume, low-pressure cuffs and implant-tested tubes are presently available so that the risks of the older Carlen's tubes are eliminated. In order to employ the technique, two ventilators with synchronous timing devices or a single ventilator employing two separate ventilatory circuits can be employed. Both tidal volume and PEEP can be varied so that one may select an appropriate level of ventilation and PEEP for each lung independently. In cases of atelectasis, larger tidal volumes and higher levels of

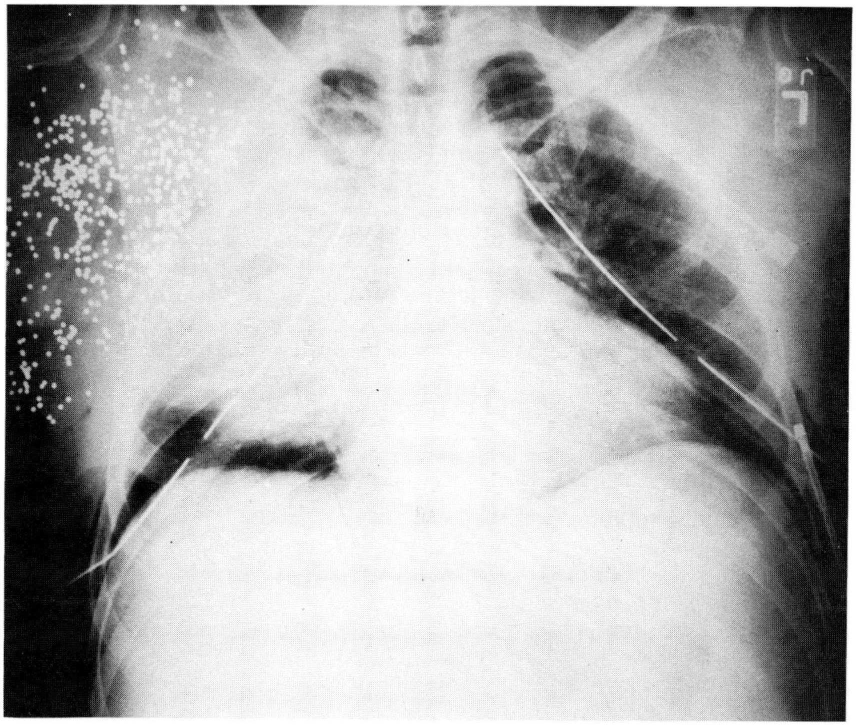

FIG. 22-10. A chest radiograph obtained 1 hour after the patient sustained a shotgun blast injury to the right axilla. Note the severe pulmonary contusion in the right lung. Intrapulmonary shunt at this time was 61% of the cardiac output.

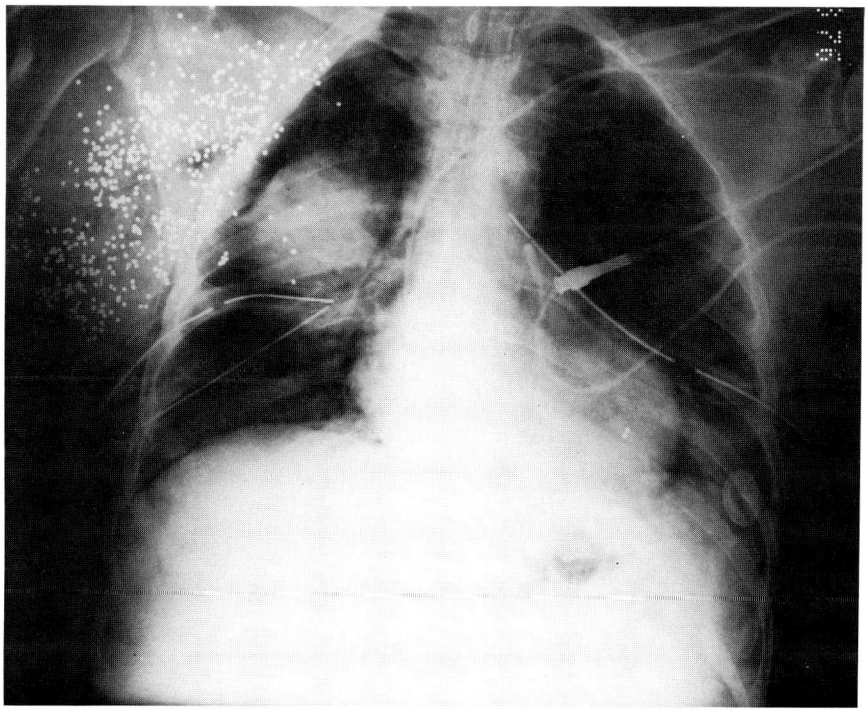

FIG. 22-11. A second radiograph of the patient dicussed in Figure 22-10 obtained 8 hours after IMV, PEEP, and a Roto bed were utilized in the treatment of the pulmonary contusion. Marked resolution of the contusion occurred, and intrapulmonary shunt was calculated to be 17%.

PEEP are usually employed to aid in the reexpansion of the atelectatic segments. In a solitary consolidated lesion, however, smaller tidal volumes are used in the affected lung because the markedly diminished compliance would cause excessive airway pressures. Ventilation in this instance is directed toward the uninvolved lung. In a patient with a severe bronchopleural-cutaneous fistula, the tidal volume delivered by a conventional volume ventilator exits through the bronchopleural-cutaneous fistula and alveolar ventilation is inadequate. SILV is not the only applicable form of therapy and should be reserved for patients who do not respond to other techniques (discussed below). In patients requiring SILV, the principle can be stated: direct the largest tidal volume to the uninvolved lung.

Inspiratory Chest Tube PEEP or Occlusion

Bronchopleural-cutaneous fistula may occur after penetrating or blunt thoracic injury as well as during therapy for ARF. Generally, manipulation of the IMV rate and PEEP suffices to provide adequate oxygenation and CO_2 elimination. Other techniques that can be employed include maintaining PEEP despite the leak from the chest tubes employing a Venturi PEEP device. If gas leaks from the lung during the expiratory time, additional gas will be entrained into the ventilator circuit to maintain airway pressure. PEEP may also be applied directly to the chest tubes to prevent a gas leak during exhalation. If the gas leak occurs during inspiration, valves can be placed between the chest tube and the suction device. The chest suction will then be eliminated during the inspiratory phase of the ventilator cycle and reopened automatically during exhalation. This technique has been termed *intermittent inspiratory chest tube occlusion* and is applicable when bilateral bronchopleural fistulas are present. SILV can be employed in patients with unilateral involvement.

High-Frequency Positive Pressure Ventilation

Finally the technique of high-frequency positive pressure ventilation (HFPPV) has been developed and can be used in massive bronchopleural-cutaneous fistulas as well as other forms of ARF. HFPPV is one of the most radical departures from conventional mechanical therapy. This technique has been used to provide ventilation to patients undergoing bronchoscopy and others in Europe for the past 10 years. It should still be considered largely experimental for the treatment of ARF, and no standardization of equipment has been achieved. However, the common features include utilization of ventilatory rates far in excess of normal (*i.e.*, 90–900 per minute); delivered tidal volumes *less* than the patient's *anatomic* dead space volume; extremely small airway pressure changes between the expiratory and inspiratory phase, usually less than 4 cm; maintenance of normal $PaCO_2$ despite the fact that the supplied mechanical tidal volume is less than the patient's anatomic dead space; and maintenance of adequate arterial oxygen tension.

There are many theories presently under scrutiny to explain how this technique works, since it seems to violate physiologic principles; however, there is no satisfactory explanation except the clinical results! Since airway pressure changes are minimal, very little gas is lost through the bronchopleural-cutaneous fistula. Other attractive possibilities for this technique include patients with severely compromised compliance in whom major changes in airway pressures affect cardiovascular performance. If gas exchange can be maintained without necessitating markedly increased intrathoracic pressures, cardiovascular performance may be preserved.

Continuous Positive Airway Pressure

If, indeed, PEEP exerts significant therapeutic benefits in ARF and mechanical ventilation is relegated to a supportive role, further investigation into provision of total spontaneous ventilation with manipulation of expiratory airway pressures is also in order. If airway pressure and flows are adjusted, it is possible to create a pattern of spontaneous breathing in which airway pressure is always positive. This has been termed continuous positive airway pressure (CPAP). "Prophylactic" CPAP using a noninvasive technique of a close fitting mask can eliminate the need for endotracheal intubation in early ARF.[30, 37] Since the patient's mechanics of ventilation are not impaired during this phase, there is no need for a mechanical ventilator. This is most attractive because it preserves the patient's natural defenses, which are violated by endotracheal intubation. Since it requires inexpensive and simple devices, it can be used to assist in the management of a large number of patients who are at high risk for developing ARF. It has found its greatest application in the early postoperative period when oxygenation may be impaired because of decreased FRC, resulting from abdominal surgery or from the lingering effects of anesthetic agents. CPAP can also be used in patients who have suffered direct thoracic trauma, long bone fractures, near drowning, and aspiration judged to be of minor degree if used soon after the incident.

References

1. Ashbaugh DG, Petty TL, Bigelow DB et al: Continuous positive pressure breathing CPPB in adult respiratory distress syndrome. J Thorac Cardiovasc Surg 57:31, 1969

2. Bjork VO, Engstrom CG: The treatment of ventilatory insufficiency after pulmonary resection with tracheostomy and prolonged artificial ventilation. J Thorac Cardiovasc Surg 30:356, 1955
3. Brigham KL, Woolverton WC, Blake LH et al: Increased sheep lung vascular permeability caused by pseudomonas bacteremia. J Clin Invest 54:792, 1974
4. Burke JF, Pontoppidan H, Welch CE: High output respiratory failure, an important cause of death ascribed to peritonitis or ileus. Ann Surg 158:581, 1963
5. Carrico CJ, Canizaro PC, Shires GT: Fluid resuscitation following injury: Rationale for the use of balanced salt solutions. Crit Care Med 4:46, 1976
6. Civetta JM: A rapid, simple and inexpensive technique (abstr). Intensive Care Med (Berlin) 3:208, 1977
7. Civetta JM: A new look at the Starling equation. Crit Care Med 7:84-91, 1979
8. Civetta JM, Flor RJ, Smith LO: Aggressive treatment of acute respiratory insufficiency. South Med J 69:749, 1976
9. Civetta JM, Gabel JC: Flow-directed pulmonary artery catheterization in surgical patients: Indications and modifications of technic. Ann Surg 176:753, 1972
10. Civetta JM, Gabel JC, Laver MB: Disparate ventricular function in surgical patients. Surg Forum 22:136, 1971
11. Comroe JH: Physiology of Respiration. Chicago, Year Book Medical Publishers, 1965
12. Da Luz PL, Shubin H, Weil MH et al: Pulmonary edema related to changes in colloid osmotic and pulmonary artery wedge pressure in patients after acute myocardial infarction. Circulation 51:350, 1975
13. Demling RH: Fluid distribution during overload edema (abstr). Crit Care Med 6:123, 1978
14. Downs JB, Klein EF, Desautels DA et al: Intermittent mandatory ventilation: A new approach to weaning patients from mechanical ventilation. Chest 64:331, 1973
15. Downs JB, Klein EF, Modell JH: The effect of incremental PEEP on PaO_2 in patients with respiratory failure. Anesth Analg (Cleve) 52:210, 1973
16. Drop LJ: Interdependence Between Plasma Ionized Calcium and Hemodynamic Performance. Boston, Massachusetts General Hospital Printing Office, 1974
17. Engstrom C: Treatment of severe cases of respiratory paralysis by the Engstrom university respiratory. Br Med J 3:666, 1954
18. Falke K, Pontoppidan H, Kumar A et al: Ventilation with end expiratory pressure in acute lung disease. J Clin Invest 51:2315, 1972
19. Froese AD, Bryan AC: Effects of anesthesia and paralysis on diaphragmatic mechanisms in man. Anesthesiology 41:242, 1974
20. Gallagher TJ, Civetta JM, Kirby RR: Terminology update: Optimal PEEP. Crit Care Med 6:323, 1978
21. Ganz W, Donoso R, Marcus HS et al: A new technique for measurement of cardiac output by thermodilution in man. Am J Cardiol 27:392, 1971
22. Glass DD: Cardiovascular drugs in intensive care units. In Civetta JM (ed): Intensive Care Drug Therapeutics. New York, Appleton-Century-Crofts, 1980
23. Gregory GA, Kitterman JA, Phibbs RH et al: Treatment of the idiopathic respiratory-distress syndrome with continuous positive airway pressure. N Engl J Med 284:1333, 1971
24. Horovitz JH, Carrico CJ, Shires GT: Pulmonary response to major injury. Arch Surg 108:349, 1974
25. Hurst JW, Logue RB (eds): The Heart, 2nd ed. New York, McGraw-Hill, 1970
26. Jenkins MT, Jones RF, Wilson B et al: Congestive atelectasis—A complication of the intravenous infusion of fluids. Ann Surg 132:327, 1950
27. Karetzky M, Cain S: Effect of carbon dioxide on oxygen uptake during hyperventilation in normal man. J Appl Physiol 28:8, 1970
28. Kelman GR, Nunn JF, Prys–Roberts C et al: The influence of cardiac output on arterial oxygenation—A theoretical study. Br J Anaesth 39:450, 1967
29. Kirby RR, Downs JB, Civetta JM et al: High-level positive end-expiratory pressure (PEEP) in acute respiratory insufficiency. Chest 67:156, 1975
30. Kirby RR, Smith R, Gooding JM et al: PEEP therapy by face mask. ASA Abstracts of Scientific Papers, p 195, 1977
31. Manny J, Patten MT, Liebman PR et al: The association lung distention, PEEP and biventricular failure. Ann Surg 187:151, 1978
32. Petty TL: IMV versus IMC (editorial). Chest 67:630, 1975
33. Powers SR Jr, Mannal R, Neclerio M et al: Physiologic consequences of positive end-expiratory pressure (PEEP) ventilation. Ann Surg 178:265, 1973
34. Reynolds EO: Pressure waveform and ventilator settings for mechanical ventilation in severe hyaline membrane disease. Int Anesthesiol Clin 12:259, 1976
35. Ross J Jr, Braunwald E: The study of left ventricular function in man by increasing resistance to ventricular ejection with angiotensin. Circulation 29:739, 1964
36. Schimmel L, Civetta JM: A new mechanical method to influence pulmonary perfusion in critically ill patients. Crit Care Med 5:277, 1977
37. Schmidt GB, O'Neill WW, Kotb K et al: Continuous positive airway pressure in the prophylaxis of the adult respiratory distress syndrome. Surg Gynecol Obstet 143:613, 1976
38. Schultz C, Holloway E, Derby G et al: Effect of nitroprusside and chlorpromazine on left ventricular function during the early postoperative period. Circulation (Suppl) 48:859, 1973
39. Sugerman HJ, Rogers RM, Miller LD: Positive end-expiratory pressure (PEEP): Indications and physiologic considerations. Chest 62:865, 1972
40. Swan HJC, Ganz W, Forrester J et al: Catheterization of the heart in man with use of a flow-directed balloon-tipped catheter. N Engl J Med 283:477, 1970
41. Virgilio RW, Rice CL, Smith DE et al: Crystalloid vs. colloid resuscitation: Is one better? Surgery 85:129, 1979
42. West J: Ventilation/Blood Flow and Gas Exchange, 2nd ed. Oxford, Blackwell Scientific Publications, 1970
43. Zarins CK, Rice CL, Smith DE et al: Role of lymphatics in preventing hypooncotic pulmonary edema. Surg Forum 27:257, 1976

23 Complications of Esophageal Surgery and Trauma

Mark B. Orringer

OVERVIEW

ANATOMY AND PHYSIOLOGY

Knowledgeable surgeons have at times referred to the esophagus as the "pancreas of the chest," an allusion to the similarly devastating physiologic effects of surgical complications involving these two organs. Certain unique features of esophageal anatomy and physiology readily account for many of the problems associated with esophageal surgery and trauma. A familiarity with these characteristics permits the well-informed esophageal surgeon to "think defensively," avoiding complications before they occur.

There are three naturally occurring sites of narrowing of the esophagus: the upper esophageal introitus, or cricopharyngeal sphincter; the level of the aortic arch and left main-stem bronchus; and the lower esophagus as it joins the stomach. Knowledge of this normal anatomy is essential in performing esophagoscopy. Another unique feature of the esophagus is its submucosa, the fat content of which permits unusual mobility of the overlying squamous mucosa. This must be borne in mind during performance of every esophageal anastomosis lest a carelessly placed suture fail to transfix the mucosal edge, which has retracted 1 cm to 1.5 cm away from the cut esophageal margin (Fig. 23-1). Failure to recognize this is responsible for a large percentage of postoperative anastomotic leaks. There is no substitute for meticulous technique and attention to detail in esophageal surgery.

The extensive submucosal lymphatic drainage of the esophagus, communicating freely with paratracheal, posterior mediastinal, cervical, perigastric, and periaortic lymph nodes, has direct implications for resectional procedures. Not only is cure of esophageal malignancies seldom achieved, but also careful pathologic evaluation of esophagi resected for carcinoma has documented repeatedly the presence of tumor cells in submucosal lymphatics 4 cm to 6 cm beyond gross neoplasm. Thus, whenever possible, unless the surgeon is prepared to perform an anastomosis through tumor, a 6 cm- to 10-cm margin beyond an intrathoracic esophageal carcinoma should be obtained. An intrathoracic anastomosis should be avoided whenever possible both to prevent the possibility of recurrent obstruction from the tumor at the suture line and to minimize the mortality and morbidity rates of an anastomotic disruption.

The esophageal wall is also unique in that it lacks a serosal layer. Although there are available for suturing two layers of esophageal muscle, an inner circular and an outer longitudinal, this muscle is frequently quite soft and tenuous. As a result, hiatal hernia repairs that rely upon the ability of esophageal sutures to "hold" are often jeopardized. The lack of the usual serosal layer present for most gastrointestinal anastomoses emphasizes the imperative that when performing an anastomosis *each* suture transfix *every* available layer of the esophageal wall.

The major blood supply of the intrathoracic esophagus is from four to six aortic esophageal arteries, supplemented by collaterals with the inferior thyroid, intercostal and bronchial, inferior phrenic, and left gastric arteries. While the segmental "poor" blood supply of the esophagus has often been incriminated as the cause of anastomotic disruptions, clinical experience has demonstrated repeatedly that virtually all of the thoracic esophageal aortic branches can be divided, and yet the esophagus will remain viable. It is apparent, therefore, that, in most instances, poor *technique,* rather than poor blood supply, is the explanation for complications of esophageal anastomotic disruption. The extensive venous circulation of the esophagus, emptying into

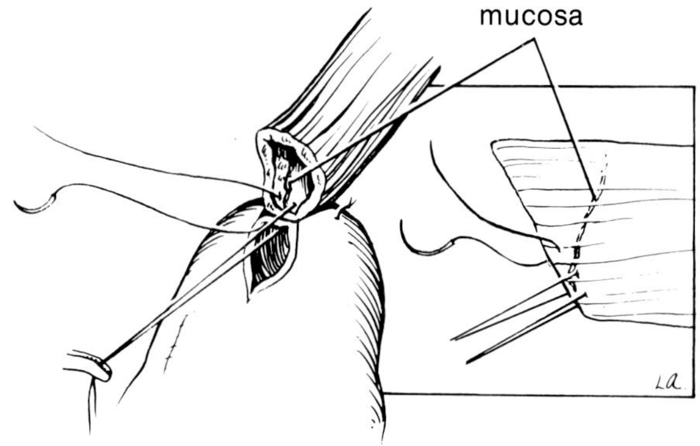

FIG. 23-1. Misplacement of the esophagogastric anastomotic suture. The relatively great mobility of the esophageal mucosa over the fatty submucosa permits the cut mucosal edge to retract proximally. Unless you take care to identify the mucosa with each suture placed in order to be certain that it is being transfixed, you will not achieve mucosal apposition, and an anastomotic disruption will follow.

the azygos, hemiazygos, intercostal, or gastric veins, provides communication between the portal and systemic venous systems and is the basis for esophageal varices in portal hypertension.

The esophagus receives both sympathetic and parasympathetic innervation. The sympathetic nerves are mediastinal branches of the thoracic sympathetic trunk and recurrent sympathetic branches from the celiac axis. Their functional importance has not been established. The parasympathetic nerve supply is from the vagus nerves, with the recurrent laryngeal nerve supplying the upper portion of the esophagus and the remainder of the vagi supplying the rest of the esophagus. Thus, injury to the recurrent laryngeal nerves (e.g., during pulmonary surgery, laryngectomy, thoracic aortic operations, or thyroid operations) may result in upper esophageal (cricopharyngeal) muscle dysfunction and subsequent incapacitating cervical dysphagia and aspiration.[7, 15] Similarly, injury to the vagal nerve trunks adjacent to the distal esophagus may produce lower esophageal motor dysfunction resembling achalasia or esophageal spasm (see below, Dysphagia of Hiatal Hernia Repair).

GASTROESOPHAGEAL REFLUX

Incompetence of the distal esophageal sphincter mechanism with the development of gastroesophageal reflux and secondary reflux esophagitis has direct bearing on the results of antireflux operations (Fig. 23-2). The incidence of recurrent reflux in patients undergoing the standard Belsey Mark IV transthoracic hiatal hernia repair in the presence of esophagitis or a stricture, for example, is between 25% to 75%.[5, 27] The intramural inflammation jeopardizes the reliability of sutures placed into the distal esophagus, and the esophageal shortening that so often accompanies reflux esophagitis prevents the *tension-free* reduction of the prerequisite distal 3 cm to 5 cm of esophagus below the diaphragm (Fig. 23-3). These same considerations must also apply to the Nissen fundoplication and Hill median arcuate ligament repairs as well, since these operations also strive to reduce the esophagogastric junction into the abdomen and require sutures into either esophageal or periesophageal tissues. These considerations have led to use of the esophageal lengthening Collis-gastroplasty in combination with a fundoplication for control of gastroesophageal reflux and its complications (Fig. 23-4).[14, 28–31, 34, 35] The new distal esophagus, the gastroplasty tube, provides healthy, resilient tissue—the gastric wall—around which to perform the fundoplication, and it also eliminates tension on the repair by providing additional "esophageal length" (Fig. 23-5). Reflux esophagitis with peptic stricture may also greatly complicate the antireflux procedure if the stricture is perforated during attempted dilatation.

Gastroesophageal reflux plays a major role in the morbidity of an intrathoracic esophagogastric anastomotic leak, since refluxed bile and gastric contents drain into the mediastinum and thorax and contribute to ongoing sepsis and mediastinal inflammation. This is but another justification for the cervical esophagogastric anastomosis, whenever feasible. For although gastroesophageal reflux is the rule with an *intrathoracic* anastomosis—since half the stomach is above and half below the diaphragm (*i.e.*, there is a hiatal hernia)—when the entire stomach has been mobilized into the chest for a *cervical* anastomosis, clinically significant reflux is seldom encountered. Further, a cervical esophagogastric anastomotic leak may be converted to a controlled cervical salivary fistula by simply opening the neck wound, without the need for thoracotomy and attempted repair or drainage.

Finally, the potential morbidity from gastro-

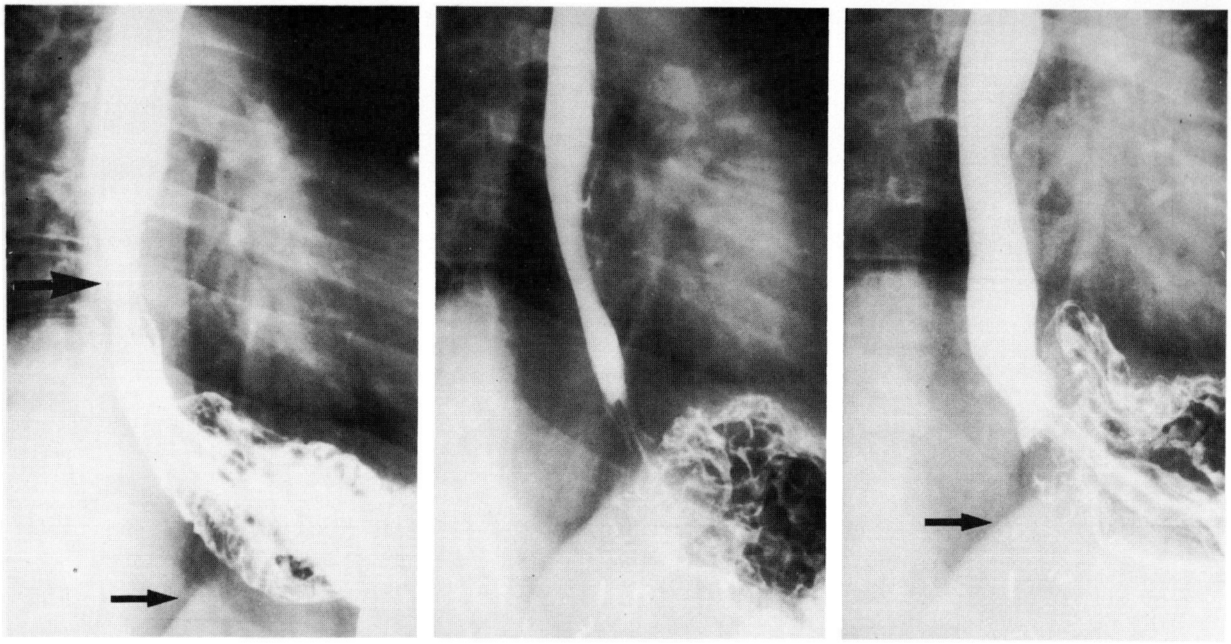

FIG. 23-2. Recurrent hiatal hernia following a Hill posterior gastropexy for reflux esophagitis with stricture. (*Left*) A large sliding hiatal hernia above the diaphragm (*small arrow*). This patient was obese and had distal esophagitis, a stricture (*large arrow*), and relative esophageal shortening. (*Center*) Immediately after a Hill repair, there was little evidence of an intra-abdominal distal esophageal segment. (*Right*) One year later, the repair, which had been performed under tension, had pulled loose, and stomach can again be seen above the diaphragm (*arrow*).

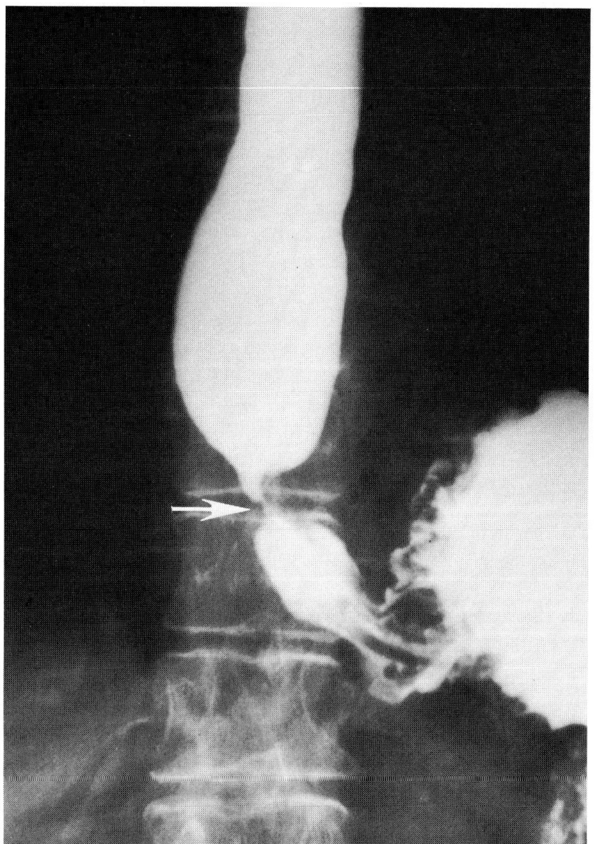

FIG. 23-3. A sliding hiatal hernia with a peptic stricture at the esophagogastric junction (*arrow*). Standard antireflux operations (Hill, Belsey, or Nissen) require reduction below the diaphragm not only of the esophagogastric junction but also of the distal 3 cm to 5 cm of esophagus. The relative esophageal shortening associated with the distal esophagitis in this patient prevented a tension-free standard repair.

esophageal reflux following esophageal resection and esophagogastric anastomosis in the immediate postoperative period merits careful gastric decompression, initially with a nasogastric tube, as well as 30° to 45° head-up posturing, to prevent aspiration of gastric contents into the tracheobronchial tree. Respiratory therapists must be cautioned not to tip the patient for postural therapy within 1 to 2 hours of meals to avoid unexpected massive regurgitation and aspiration.

Refinements in objective methods of evaluating esophageal function with manometric techniques and the intraesophageal *p*H electrode have increased awareness of the role of abnormal esophageal motility in numerous conditions affecting the esophagus. In esophageal scleroderma, for example, not only is distal esophageal sphincter tone lost so that gastroesophageal reflux is common, but also normal, progressive esophageal peristalsis is replaced by absent or weak, simultaneous, nonprogressive contractions after swallowing.[25] This results in prolonged contact between gastric acid and the esophageal mucosa, so that acclerated severe reflux esophagitis, often with a stricture, occurs. The pulmonary complications in these patients may therefore be related not only to scleroderma of the lungs, but also to aspiration of esophageal and gastric contents. Despite their systemic disease, however, *carefully selected* scleroderma patients may benefit greatly from antireflux operations, particularly the combined Collis-gastroplasty-fundoplication procedures.[16, 26]

In the patient with achalasia and an advanced megaesophagus, aspiration of retained esophageal secretions on induction of general anesthesia may be life threatening. Awareness of this possibility leads to prevention by adequate preoperative preparation of the patient (see under Esophagomyotomy for Achalasia or Esophageal Spasm).

ESOPHAGEAL PERFORATION

Esophageal perforation has numerous etiologies that may be summarized as follows:

- I. Instrumental
  - A. Endoscopy
    1. Direct injury
    2. During removal of a foreign body
  - B. Dilatation
  - C. Intubation (esophageal, endotracheal)
- II. Noninstrumental
  - A. Barogenic trauma
    1. Postemetic
    2. Blunt chest or abdominal trauma
    3. Other (labor, convulsions, defecation, etc.)
  - B. Penetrating neck, chest, or abdominal trauma
  - C. Postsurgical
    1. Anastomotic disruption
    2. Devascularization following pulmonary resection, vagotomy, or repair of a hiatal hernia
  - D. Corrosive injuries (acid or alkali ingestion)
  - E. Erosion by adjacent infection with resulting fistula with the tracheobronchial tree, pericardium, pleural cavity, or aorta

In all of these etiologies, the pathophysiology and consequences of the resulting mediastinitis are linked by a common denominator that emphasizes the urgency of prompt recognition and treatment of disruption of esophageal continuity, regardless of the cause. The diagnosis and treatment of esophageal perforation is discussed under Esophagoscopy but also is considered throughout the remainder of this chapter.

Procedural Complications

ESOPHAGOSCOPY

Certain basic principles of esophageal surgery bear emphasis. *No esophagoscope should ever be passed without a prior barium swallow,* and the surgeon should have the results of that study with him in the operating room during esophagoscopy. Advances in flexible fiberoptic esophagogastroscopy have simplified endoscopic procedures and increased the number of outpatient studies. Along with this increase in the number of esophagoscopies has come a rather cavalier attitude toward this procedure. Esophagoscopy, particularly with dilatation, is one of the most dangerous operations in thoracic surgery. Nothing can condone perforating a cervical esophageal diverticulum, for example, because the presence of a lesion had not been detected by barium swallow examination.

The leading and most serious complication of esophagoscopy, with or without dilatation of a stricture, is perforation, occurring in 1% to 2% of patients, even in the hands of the most experienced endoscopist. In most cases, common errors are responsible for the perforation:

1. *Inadequate pre- and intraoperative sedation and anesthesia.* It is foolhardy to persist with attempts at esophagoscopy in an anxious, combative, noncooperative patient. It is *not* a sign of defeat to request general anesthesia, which is preferred when performing the initial endoscopic evaluation of an obstructing esophageal lesion. Esophageal dilatation is a painful procedure that requires the complete concentration of the surgeon on the operative field, *not* on a struggling patient.

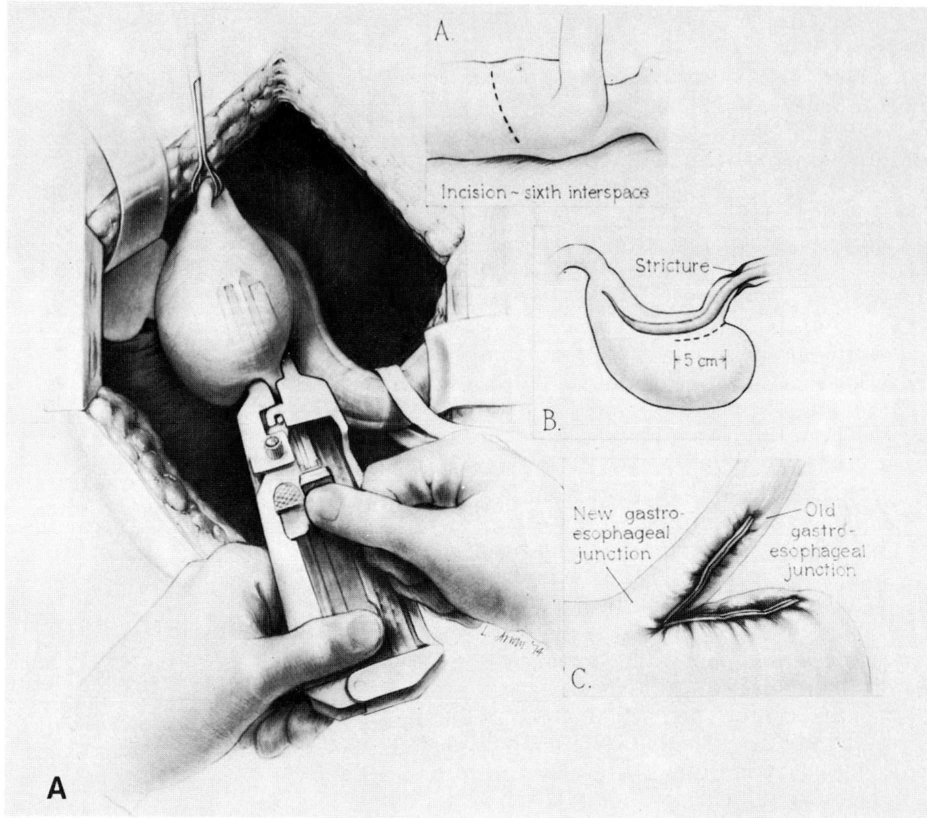
A.
Incision ~ sixth interspace
Stricture
5 cm
B.
New gastro-
esophageal
junction
Old
gastro-
esophageal
junction
C.
A

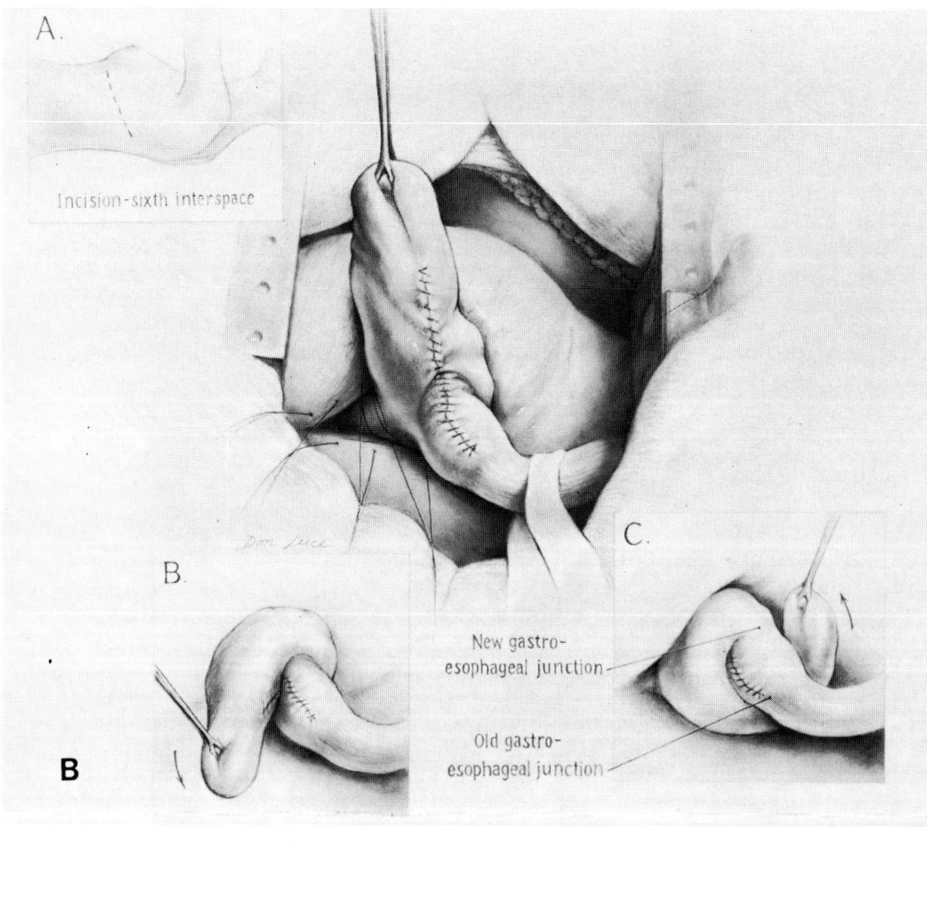
A.
Incision-sixth interspace
B.
C.
New gastro-
esophageal junction
Old gastro-
esophageal junction
B

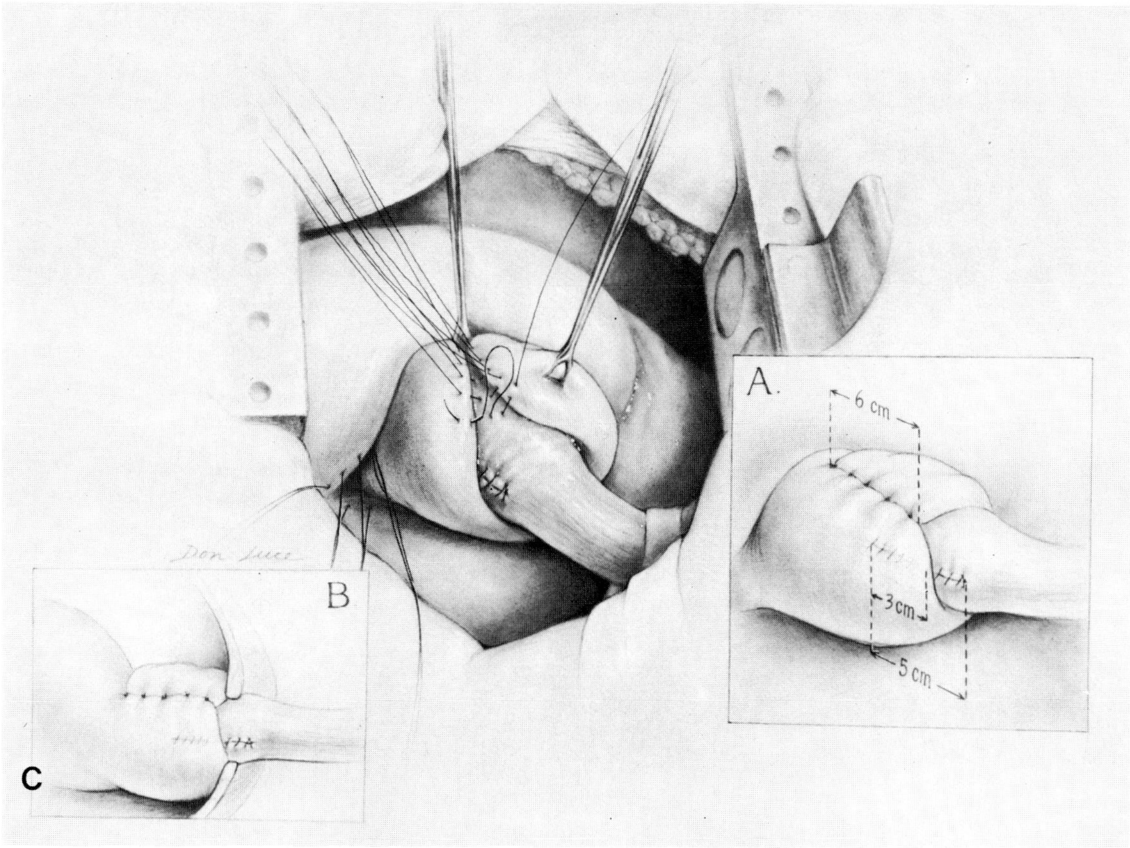

FIG. 23-4. (*A*) The Collis gastroplasty using the GIA surgical stapler. (*Inset A*) The esophagus and fundus of the stomach are mobilized through a lateral thoracotomy in the 6th left intercostal space. (*Inset B*) A 56 or 58 French Hurst–Maloney dilator is passed through the esophageal stricture and displaced against the lesser curvature of the stomach as the stapler is applied. The knife assembly is advanced (*main figure*), and the stapler is removed. (*Inset C*) The result is a 5-cm-long gastric tube extension of the esophagus. An additional 2 cm to 3 cm can be gained by a second, partial application of the stapler. (*B*) The elongated, narrowed gastric fundus available for fundoplication after completion of the Collis procedure. (*Inset A*) Placement of the incision through the 6th left intercostal space. (*Insets B and C*) The gastric fundus is wrapped around the gastroplasty tube and adjacent stomach. Note that the posterior crural sutures are left untied for the moment. (*C*) Placement of the seromuscular sutures from the gastric fundus to the gastroplasty tube to the gastric fundus for the proximal 3 to 4 sutures, and from the gastric fundus to the anterior stomach wall and then to the gastric fundus for the distal 3 to 4 sutures. After these sutures are tied, the fundoplication includes the distal 3 cm to 4 cm of gastroplasty tube and the proximal 3 cm to 4 cm of stomach. (*Inset A*) The fundoplication, reduced in the abdomen, rests below the diaphragm without tension on the distal esophagus after the posterior crural sutures are tied (*Inset B*). (*A*, Orringer MB, Sloan H: An improved technique for the combined Collis–Belsey approach to dilatable esophageal stricture. J Thorac Cardiovasc Surg 68:298, 1974; *B* and *C*, Orringer MB, Sloan H: Combined Collis–Nissen reconstruction of the esophagogastric junction. Ann Thorac Surg 25:16, 1978)

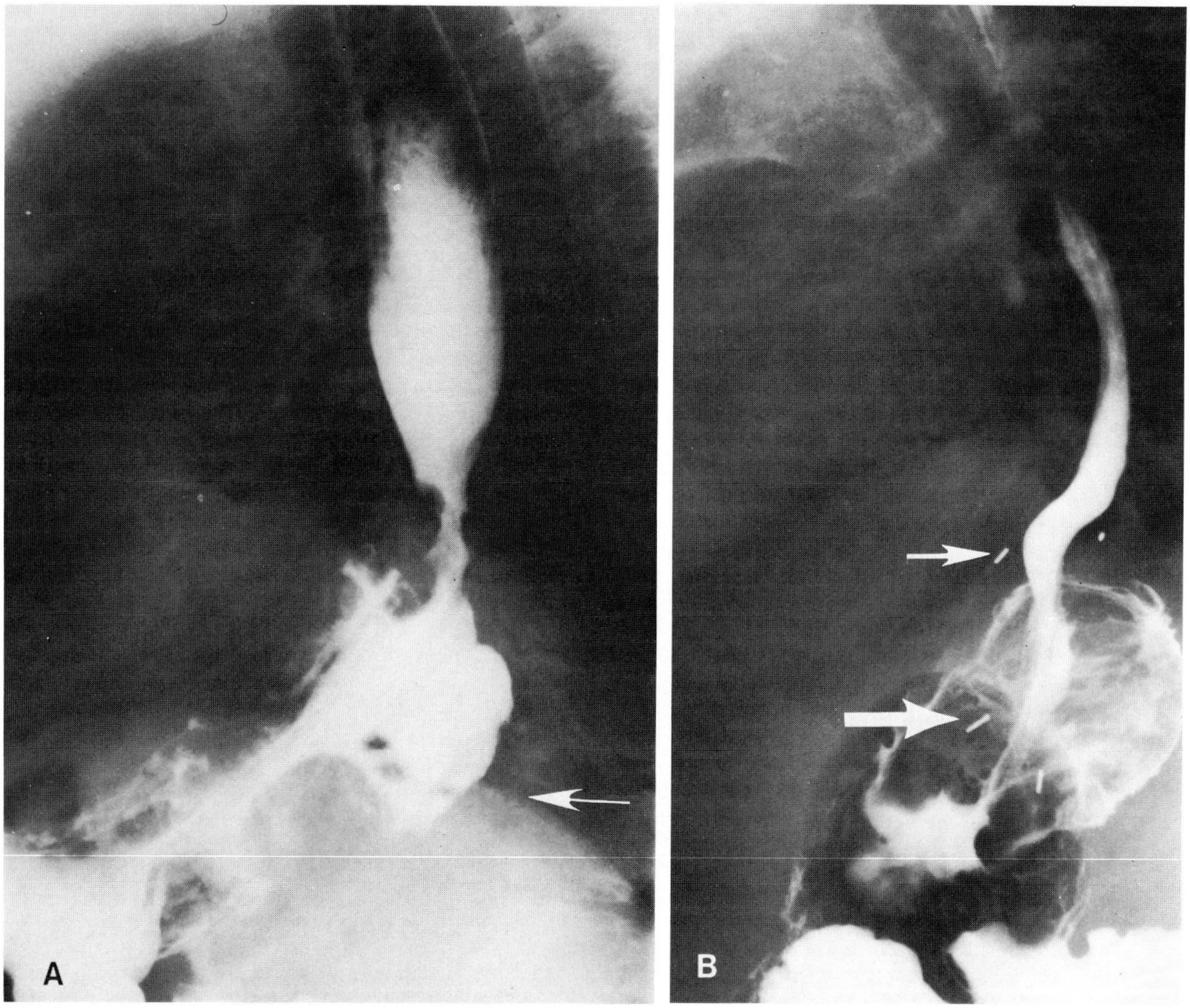

FIG. 23-5. (*A*) This lateral view from a preoperative esophagogram shows a large, sliding hiatal hernia with half of the stomach above the left hemidiaphragm (*arrow*), a proximal stricture, and esophageal dilatation from the obstruction. (*B*) Postoperative appearance of the reconstructed distal esophagus following intraoperative dilatation of the stricture and a Collis–Nissen repair. The horizontal gastric folds in the fundoplication around the distal 5 cm to 7 cm of the functional esophagus can be seen. Also visible are the silver clips (*small arrow*) marking the diaphragmatic hiatus and those at the new esophagogastric junction (*large arrow*). There is no evidence of esophageal stenosis, and the dilation proximal to the obstruction has resolved.

2. *Lack of appreciation of the extent or nature of the existing esophageal pathology as a result of failure to obtain a preoperative barium swallow examination.* As a corollary, when removing an obstructing foreign body from the esophagus of a patient with no known esophageal history, the foreign body should *always* be extracted, *never* pushed into the stomach, lest a tear of the esophagus proximal to a benign stricture or carcinoma occur.
3. *Improper introduction of the esophagoscope through the upper esophageal cricopharyngeal sphincter.* Because of the natural "pull" of the upper sphincter muscle against the cricoid cartilage (making this the narrowest point of the gastrointestinal tract), unless upward displacement of the larynx by the ad-

vancing esophagoscope is maintained, a posterior perforation by the instrument can occur (Fig. 23-6). The esophageal lumen must be kept in view at all times. Use of a flexible gum-tipped bougie as a guide through the upper sphincter is often helpful.

4. *Failure to visualize the esophageal lumen at all times during the endoscopy.* The esophagoscope should *never* be advanced unless there is a clear view of the lumen. Preoperative atropine to reduce oral secretions and the availability of adequate suction are essential.
5. *Lack of knowledge of normal anatomy.* The upper esophageal sphincter and distal esophagus, two of the naturally occurring sites of esophageal narrowing, are also the most common sites of endoscopic perforation. The distal esophagus courses anteriorly and to the left as it joins with the stomach, and it is necessary to direct the esophagoscope accordingly to avoid a perforation.
6. *Improper techniques of dilatation.* Dilatation of a stricture should be performed with the patient under general anesthesia for both the patient's and the physician's benefit. Further, the *rigid* esophagoscope, *not* the flexible instrument, should be used for the initial evaluation. The rigid esophagoscope is carefully advanced through the stricture, and, by using flexible gum-tipped bougies, gently passed through the stricture under direct vision, the pliability and extent of the stenosis is assessed (Fig. 23-7). If the stricture is very mild, dilatation with the rigid esophagoscope advanced through the stenosis may be possible. With a dense, high-grade stenosis, however, progressive dilators should be passed through the esophagoscope. The 26-French is the largest dilator that will pass through most rigid esophagoscopes. After this, if the stricture is relatively soft and pliable, the esophagoscope is removed and dilatation continued with progressively larger, flexible, rubber mercury-filled, *tapered* Hurst–Maloney dilators passed "blindly" through the stricture per oram.

With a *dense* stricture, it is possible that "curling" of the dilator within the esophagus proximal to the stenosis may result in a perforation (Fig. 23-8). To avoid this, a special-order 45-cm rigid esophagoscope (Pilling Company), which will accept up to a 50-French bougie, is carefully introduced through the upper esophageal sphincter and advanced to the stricture, which then can be dilated *under direct vision* (Fig. 23-9). If the patient has a stricture secondary to reflux esophagitis and a subsequent antireflux operation is planned, dilatation at this point beyond a 40-French bougie is unnecessary, because virtually every stricture that can be dilated to this size per oram can be more safely dilated later *intraoperatively* to the 56- to 58-French range, with the surgeon's hand supporting the mobilized esophagus from without. We have found Hurst–Maloney tapered esophageal dilators to be the most reliable and safest instruments for dilating esophageal strictures, and we seldom resort to the Eder–Puestow wire, blunt Hurst dilators, or retrograde Tucker dilators.

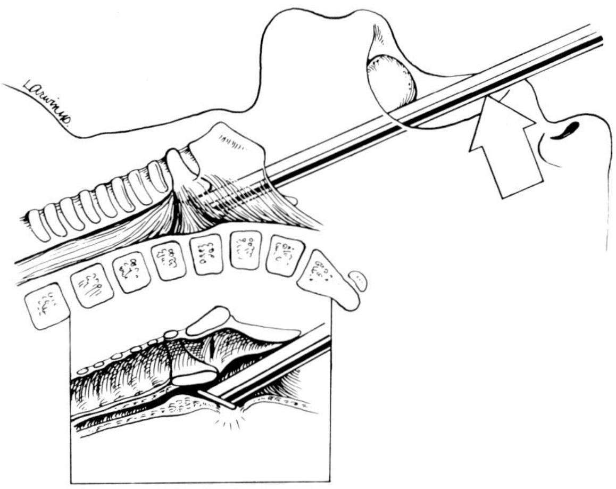

FIG. 23-6. The mechanism of endoscopic cervical esophageal perforation. In performing rigid esophagoscopy, it is essential that a gentle, steady, lifting force be exerted in order to displace forward the larynx and cricoid cartilage. Failure to overcome the natural pull of the upper esophageal sphincter against the cricoid cartilage results in a typical posterior perforation (*inset*).

Diagnosis of Esophageal Perforation

Pain or fever after esophageal instrumentation or operation represents an esophageal perforation until proven otherwise and is an indication for an immediate esophagogram. Following any esophageal procedure, an aggressive "defensive" attitude toward diagnosing a perforation must be adopted, for the morbidity and mortality rates associated with perforation are directly related to the time between diagnosis of the injury and its repair or drainage. The surgical house officer may approach such a patient in a routine fashion and work up the standard "five Ws of postoperative fever":

1. Wind (pulmonary atelectasis)
2. Water (urinary tract infection)

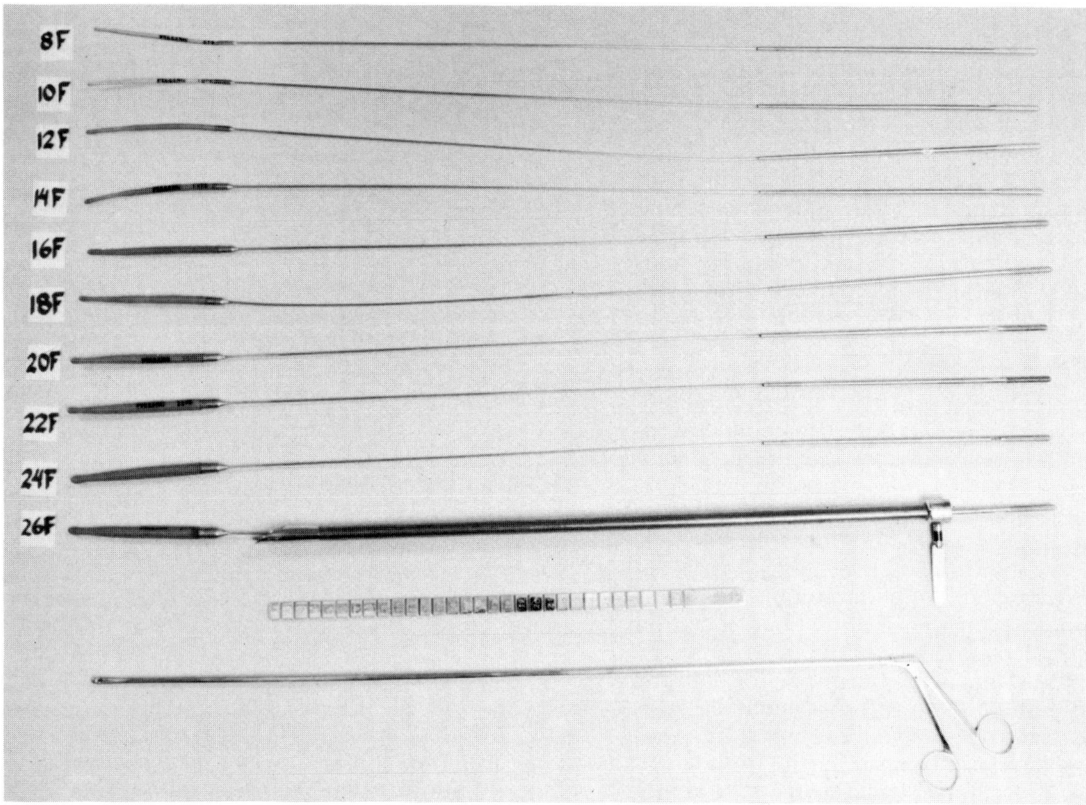

FIG. 23-7. The instruments required for evaluating peptic esophageal stricture. Precisely measured localization of the stricture (in centimeters from the incisor teeth) and adequate biopsies and brushings from the stricture must be obtained. The gum-tipped Jackson dilators, gently manipulated through the stenosis, permit evaluation of the extent and pliability of the obstruction. The 26-French dilator is the largest one that will pass through the standard 45-cm rigid esophagoscope.

3. Walk (phlebitis)
4. Wound (wound infection)
5. "Wonder drugs" (allergic reactions to antibiotics, etc.)

But *CAUTION* in a patient who has had esophageal surgery! Fever must never be attributed to any of the five Ws until perforation has been excluded with an esophagogram. Traditionally, a water-soluble contrast agent (for example, Gastrografin) is used to evaluate the esophagus for the presence of a perforation because barium extravasating into the mediastinum through the site of the injury might induce a severe reactive mediastinitis. Yearly, we see patients in whom perforations were "missed" with Gastrografin and only detected later when a barium swallow was performed (Fig. 23-10). Thus, when a contrast study with Gastrografin fails to show a suspected perforation, confirmation should be obtained with swallowed barium. The risk of barium leaking into the chest is far less than failing to recognize the perforation.

If a perforation is suspected, a chest roentgenogram may help confirm the diagnosis by demonstrating air in the soft tissue of the neck or mediastinum, or a hydro- or pneumothorax. A normal chest roentgenogram, however, does not exclude an esophageal perforation. As indicated above, contrast studies of the esophagus are mandatory if perforation is suspected, not only to establish a diagnosis, but also to demonstrate the exact site of the injury so that appropriate therapy can be instituted.

Unless the esophageal perforation is contained by preexisting periesophageal fibrosis, dissection of saliva and gastric contents into the fascial planes of the neck and mediastinum will occur. The inevitable presence of oral bacteria in these fluids, except in edentulous patients, initiates infection. Respiratory movements and negative intrathoracic pressure "suck" the esophageal and gastric contents into the

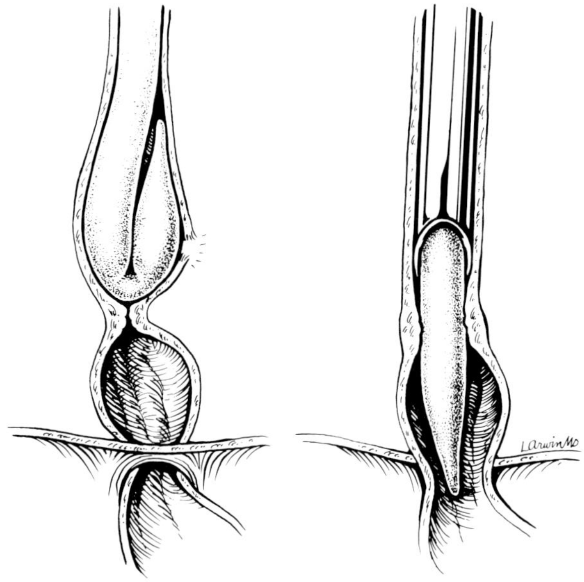

FIG. 23-8. Esophageal perforation during an attempt at blind passage of a dilator through a tight stricture. (*Left*) The dilator has curled proximal to the stenosis, and as the bougie is advanced, disruption of the esophagus may occur. (*Right*) Using a special-order, large esophagoscope that will accommodate up to a 50-French dilator (see Fig. 23-9), you can visualize the stricture directly for dilatation.

FIG. 23-9. Tapered Hurst–Maloney esophageal dilators and a 45-cm Pilling esophagoscope, which accommodates up to a 50-French bougie, thus permitting progressive dilatation of severe peptic strictures under direct vision.

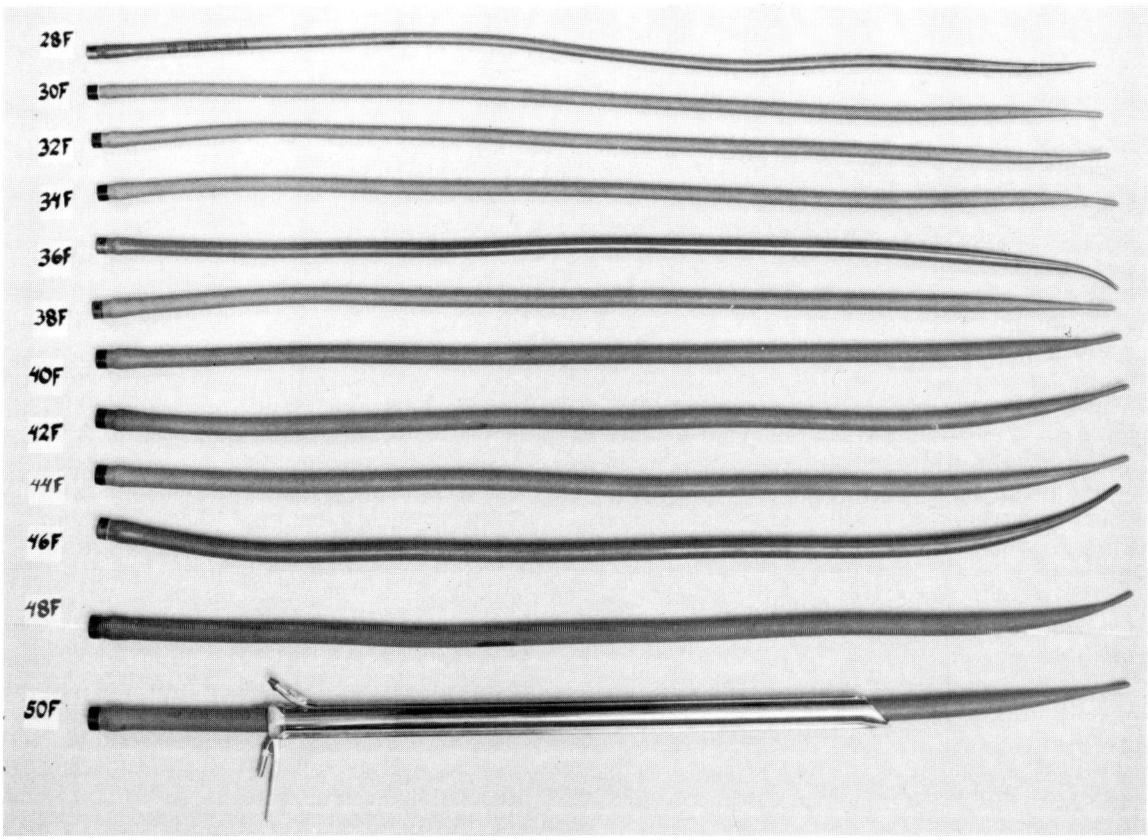

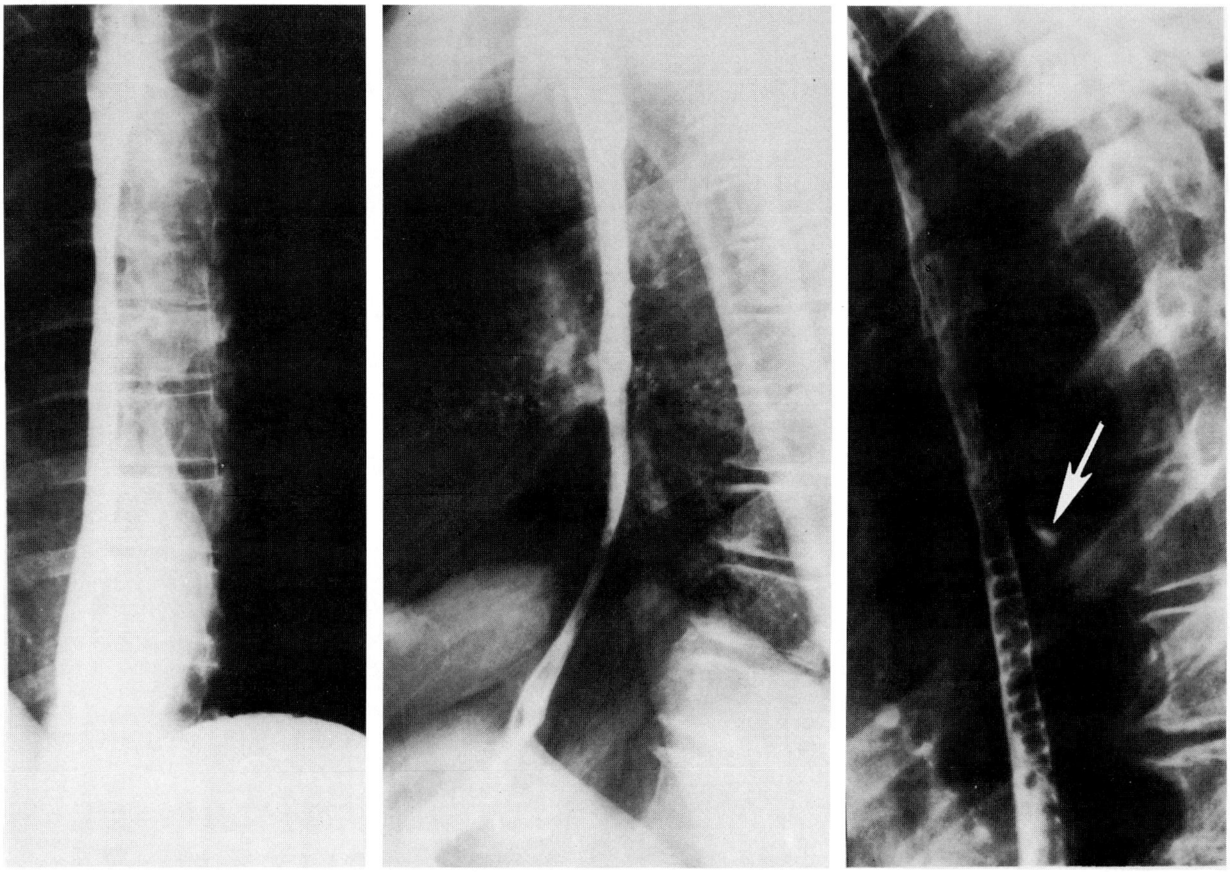

FIG. 23-10. Meglumine diatrizoate (Gastrografin) fails to demonstrate an esophageal perforation in these PA (*left*) and lateral (*center*) Gastrografin esophagograms of a patient with an acute caustic burn who was dilated wrongly and prematurely within 10 days of ingesting Drāno. Despite the development of fever and chest pain, no perforation was seen in this study. (*Right*) A barium esophagogram demonstrated a perforation (*arrow*) in the middle third of the thoracic esophagus.

mediastinum. Salivary digestive enzymes, as well as gastric acid, bile, and food enter the chest and contribute further to the fulminant inflammatory response. This mediastinal "burn" is associated with massive fluid accumulation, which may displace the trachea, heart, or lungs. The response of the tracheobronchial tree to surrounding mediastinitis is not unlike that seen with blunt chest trauma and pulmonary contusion (*i.e.*, there is a reflex bronchorrhea that results in copious pulmonary secretions and noisy, wet respirations contrally, with relatively clear breath sounds peripherally). With loss of circulating extracellular fluid volume into the mediastinum, neck, or adjacent pericardial, pleural, or peritoneal spaces, hypovolemia and respiratory distress are superimposed upon existing sepsis. The entire process is, of course, aggravated by any preexisting esophageal disease producing obstruction distal to tho porforation.

CLINICAL PRESENTATION. The hallmarks of esophageal perforation are cervical or thoracic pain, pain or difficulty swallowing, respiratory distress, and fever. Cervical thoracic esophageal perforations will generally cause cervical or high retrosternal pain, while those of the mid or distal esophagus produce anterior thoracic, posterior, interscapular, or epigastric pain. Upper thoracic esophageal perforations may result in signs of a right pleural effusion, while a left pleural effusion is often seen with a distal perforation.

Treatment of Esophageal Perforations

With the diagnosis confirmed, the patient should not take anything orally and should be instructed not to swallow his saliva. A disposable oral dental suction at the bedside is helpful for evacuating oral secretions. Vigorous intravenous volume replacement may be required if there is associated mediastinitis and fluid sequestration associated with an intrathoracic esophageal perforation. Broad-spectrum intravenous antibiotic coverage is instituted using a combination of a cephalosporin (cefazolin or cefamandole, 1 g, every 4 hr) and an aminoglycoside (gentamicin or tobramycin, 1–1.5 mg/kg every 8 hr). Attention to oral hygiene is important in the patient with an esophageal perforation because swallowed bacteria from carious teeth increase the morbidity of the injury. This explains why some elderly, edentulous patients will at times tolerate a chronic esophageal fistula extremely well.

The treatment of choice in the patient with an esophageal perforation is controversial. Although nonoperative management occasionally suffices in patients with preexisting periesophageal and mediastinal fibrosis that "contains" the injury, such conservative therapy, in the opinion of most surgeons, is more radical than surgical intervention. If an acute esophageal tear in an otherwise normal esophagus is recognized and repaired within 6 to 8 hours of the injury, the morbidity may be the same as from elective esophagotomy and primary esophageal closure. If, on the other hand, operation is delayed beyond 6 to 8 hours of the injury, the local inflammatory response associated with a perforation may be so great that primary healing of the repaired esophagus is unlikely.[9, 24] If delay has occurred, the intrathoracic esophageal suture line should be reinforced with either a pedicled intercostal muscle flap, adjacent pleura or pericardium, or diaphram.[3, 6, 10, 18, 36, 39] The mediastinal pleura should be opened widely to permit adequate drainage, and the chest tube should be left in place in case a suture-line disruption with subsequent esophagopleural cutaneous fistula occurs.[41]

Perforations of the cervical and upper thoracic esophagus are explored or drained through an oblique cervical incision paralleling the anterior border of the left sternocleidomastoid muscle.[33] This muscle and the carotid sheath are retracted laterally and the trachea and thyroid gland, medially. If closure of the perforation is possible, nonreactive, monofilament polypropylene (Prolene) is used. If the injury cannot be visualized for repair, the prevertebral space behind the esophagus is bluntly developed with the finger, and two 1-inch Penrose rubber drains are inserted into the superior mediastinum and brought out the neck incision. Despite the relatively dependent position of an upper thoracic esophageal perforation in relation to the cervical skin incision, adequate drainage and spontaneous closure with this method are usual. Perforations in the mid thoracic esophagus are approached through a right thoracotomy, and those of the distal third, through a left thoracotomy.

Regardless of the site of perforation, associated esophageal pathology *must* be considered and treated. Thus, it may be necessary to perform an esophagectomy and either primary or delayed esophageal reconstruction when confronted with such a perforation proximal to a carcinoma or caustic stricture.[17] Alternatively, if a benign stricture can be dilated intraoperatively so that the distal obstruction is relieved, closure of a proximal perforation may be feasible. Even if a leak again ensues, so long as dilatation of the stricture is continued, healing should follow. Similarly, a perforated esophageal pulsion diverticulum may be resected within several hours of the injury, but the underlying neuromotor esophageal dysfunction responsible for formation of the pouch must be relieved by performing an esophagomyotomy, lest the suture line be disrupted (see Esophageal Diverticulectomy).

Minor Complications

Minor complications of rigid esophagoscopy include fractured or dislodged teeth and lip lacerations. These can be avoided by carefully padding the lip and teeth with a moistened gauze square before introducing the esophagoscope and by being certain that the upper lip is not compressed between the esophagoscope and incisor teeth during the instrumentation.

HIATAL HERNIORRHAPHY

The complications of hiatal herniorrhaphy include the following:

- Perforation (following esophagoscopy, disruption of a stricture, or at the site of an esophageal suture)
- Dysphagia secondary to too tight a fundoplication
- Vagal nerve injury (resulting in either postoperative dysphagia from distal esophageal neuromotor dysfunction or delayed gastric emptying)
- Disruption of the posterior crural sutures with migration of the fundoplication into the chest
- Chylothorax

Esophageal perforation in association with hiatal hernia repair may occur as a result of endoscopy performed at the time of the antireflux operation, disruption of the distal esophagus during attempts at intraoperative dilatation of a stricture, and leak from placing too deeply the esophageal sutures required in either the standard Belsey Mark IV or Nissen fundoplications. We believe that patients with peptic strictures undergoing antireflux operations should be approached transthoracically to enable optimal esophageal mobilization and the most reliable hiatal hernia repair.

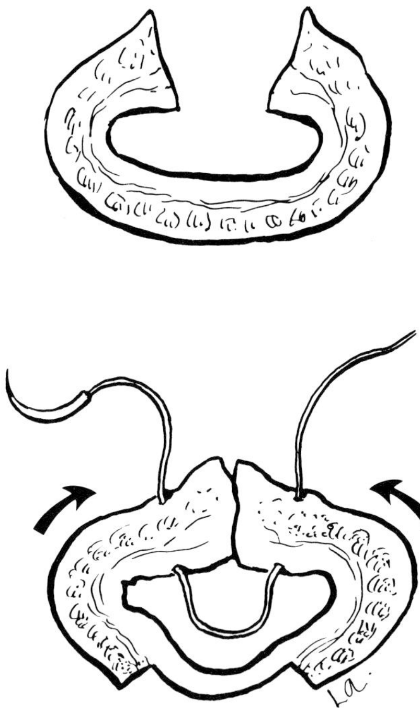

FIG. 23-11. Use of limited esophagomyotomy opposite an esophageal perforation in order to facilitate closure. (*Top*) The edges of an esophageal perforation associated with mural edema and friability may be difficult to approximate. (*Bottom*) A limited esophagomyotomy performed 180° on the opposite esophageal wall may increase lateral mobility sufficiently to permit a tension-free closure.

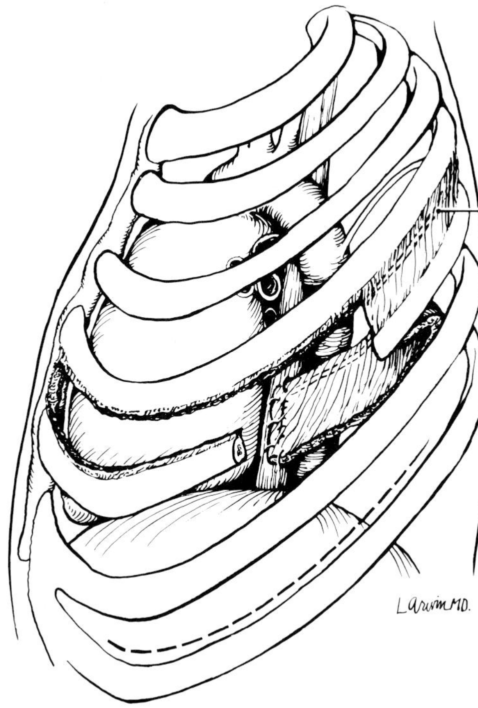

FIG. 23-12. Pedicled intercostal muscle-flap reinforcement of the esophageal suture line. An intercostal muscle from one or two interspaces above the thoracic incision is carefully dissected from the adjacent ribs, leaving intact its neurovascular bundle posteriorly. The flap is gently curved into the chest so that when the lung is re-expanded, the muscle will not be pulled off the esophagus. The end of the muscle pedicle is "tacked" over the esophageal suture line as an "onlay patch" with interrupted absorbable sutures. The esophagus should not be encircled with the pedicle, lest periosteal regeneration result in anular constriction and obstruction. (For purposes of illustration, a portion of rib overlying the muscle pedicle has been removed.)

Acute injuries recognized at the time of the operation should, of course, be repaired. Closure of the disrupted distal stricture may be extremely difficult because of the friability and relative immobility of the fibrotic tissue. Nevertheless, closure should be attempted. We have found that a limited esophagomyotomy performed 180° on the side of the esophagus opposite the injury may permit enough advancement of adjacent esophageal wall for an adequate repair of the perforation (Fig. 23-11). If the tear is limited to the esophagogastric junction and there is no significant esophageal shortening, the suture line should be buttressed with either a Belsey or Nissen fundoplication. A traditional two-layered esophageal closure may be impossible in the inflamed, thickened esophageal wall. We prefer a single layer of interrupted monofilament 3-0 Prolene for the repair because this reduces local ischemia. The repair should be reinforced with an onlay, pedicled, intercostal muscle graft or adjacent pleura or pericardium (Figs. 23-12, 23-13). An esophageal lengthening Collis-gastroplasty will provide healthy "distal esophagus" around which the fundoplication can be performed (see Fig. 23-4). Should the esophageal closure be disrupted postoperatively, with adequate drainage of the chest and repeated dilatations of the distal stricture, a controlled esophagopleural cutaneous fistula will occur. So long as there is no significant distal obstruction and reflux has been controlled, spontaneous closure will occur. Once a fistula is established, oral intake need not be withheld, since many patients will be able to maintain far superior caloric intake if they are permitted to eat with the understanding that a portion of what they swallow may come out the chest drain.

We oppose use of the Thal fundic patch esophagoplasty, since this procedure relies on the healing of the extensively opened, inflamed distal esophagus to which the stomach is sutured and expected to heal.[46, 47] Further, if a fundoplication is added in an attempt to control reflux (Thal–Woodward procedure), this requires leaving an intrathoracic portion of gastric fundus—in effect, a manmade paraesophageal hiatus hernia.[48, 50] The recognized mechanical complications from this condition condemn this procedure. Similarly, we oppose use of an intrathoracic fundoplication (without a Thal procedure) for control of reflux as this is also fraught with potential complications.[37, 40]

If during the first week after hiatal hernia repair, fever, chest pain, or respiratory distress leads to a diagnosis of distal esophageal perforation, treatment is dictated by the patient's condition, but generally involves reoperation. If possible, the site of perforation is identified (occasionally this necessitates insufflating air intraoperatively down an intraesophageal nasogastric tube). A leak from a fundoplication esophageal suture may occasionally be closed and reinforced with adjacent tissue. With a transthoracic repair, an intercostal muscle flap or pericardium is used (see Figs. 23-12, 23-13). If this is not feasible, the area is irrigated and drained well to permit establishment of a controlled fistula. A jejunostomy feeding tube provides the safest means of nourishment until normal swallowing is possible. At times, a "silent" walled off "leak" in the area of the fundoplication is noted on the routine barium swallow taken 1 week after operation. No treatment of this abnormality may be required.

Dysphagia after an antireflux operation may be secondary either to distal esophageal motor dysfunction from manipulation of the vagus nerves (see below) or to a relative obstruction of the distal esophagus produced by constructing too tight a fundoplication.[42] This latter complication is avoided by performing the fundoplication around a large (46 French or greater) intraesophageal dilator. Since the earliest reports of dysphagia following truncal vagotomy, it has been apparent that manipulation of the vagus nerves at the level of the distal esophagus may result in transient disruption of normal innervation to this segment.[4, 11, 12, 23] This may occur during an antireflux operation and is more likely to occur with transthoracic, as opposed to transabdominal, repairs, which more often require identification and displacement of the main vagal trunks. The resulting clinical picture may resemble either achalasia or spasm and manifest itself as dysphagia immediately following an antireflux operation. The distal esophagus may appear radiographically to be narrowed to varying degrees. Reassurance and maintenance of a mechanical soft diet for several days is generally adequate therapy. Occasionally passage of an esophageal dilator may be required for this generally self-limited process.

Vagal-nerve injury during hiatal hernia repair may result in delayed gastric emptying and pylorospasm with secondary gastric dilatation, a disastrous complication following an operation designed to establish a competent distal esophageal sphincter mechanism. Such gastric dilatation may disrupt the esophageal sutures of the fundoplication and thus disrupt the repair (Fig. 23-14). A 7- to 10-day trial of gastric decompression with a nasogastric tube is warranted, but persistent gastric distention from pylorospasm is a definite factor in subsequent unsatisfactory results from antireflux operations. At times, an anticholinergic (e.g., atropine, 0.4 mg, either PO or IM every 4–6 hr) may relieve the pylorospasm. However, the patient's best interest is not to permit this problem to persist, and an early gastric drainage procedure (pyloromyotomy or pyloroplasty) should be considered.

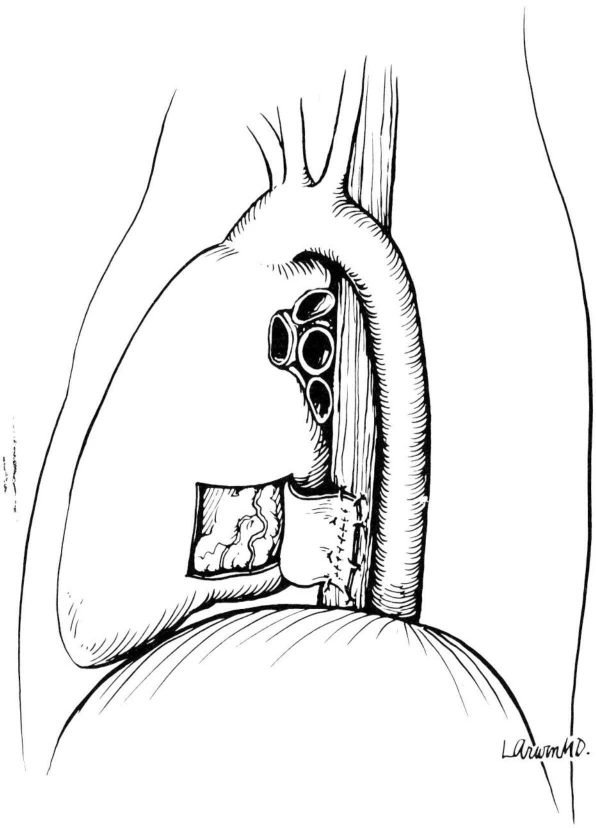

FIG. 23-13. Reinforcement of an esophageal suture line with adjacent pericardium.

Approximately 1 week after a hiatal hernia repair, prior to discharge from the hospital, a routine barium swallow should be obtained to demonstrate the postoperative appearance of the reconstructed esophagogastric junction. Unfortunately, on rare occasions, in an absolutely asymptomatic patient, the fundoplication or gastric fundus will be found to have slipped into the chest as a result of disruption of the posterior crural sutures (Fig. 23-15). *Reoper-*

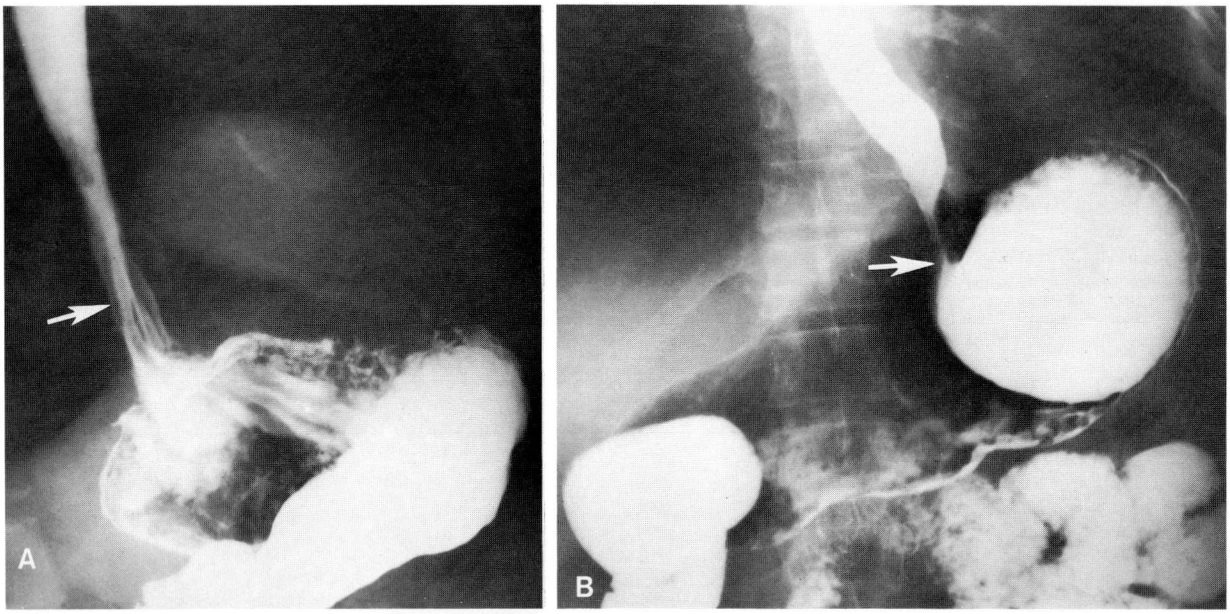

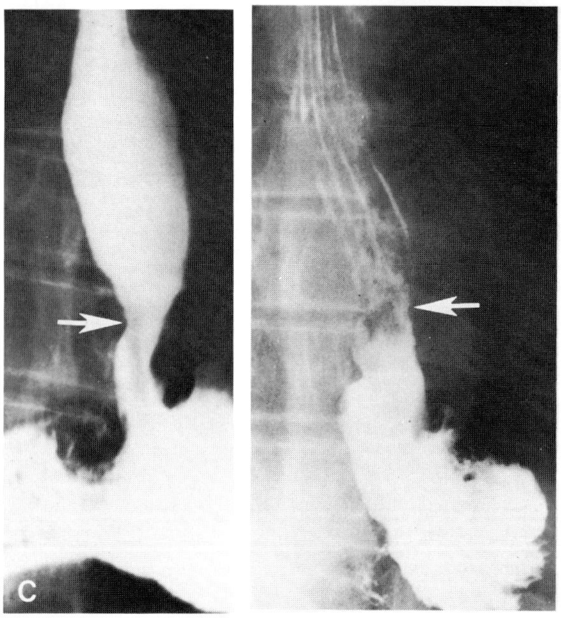

FIG. 23-14. Disruption of hiatal hernia repair owing to postoperative gastric dilatation. (*Arrows* indicate the esophagogastric junction.) (*A*) A preoperative esophagogram shows a small, recurrent sliding hiatal hernia. (*B*) A postoperative esophagogram taken 1 week after a Belsey mark IV repair shows not only good reduction of the esophagogastric junction below the diaphragm, but also gastric dilatation due to poor emptying. (*C, left* and *right*) A recurrent hiatal hernia 1 year after the initial operation, with the esophagogastric junction above the diaphragm. Vagal nerve injury at the time of repair of the recurrent hiatal hernia produced delayed gastric emptying, which should have been treated with a pyloromyotomy or pyloroplasty.

ation is indicated to prevent the mechanical complications of this iatrogenic paraesophageal hiatal hernia, and it is best not to delay this decision. It is far easier to reoperate and reduce the fundoplication into the abdomen *before* postoperative adhesions form between the herniated gastric fundus and adjacent tissues. The conservative wait-and-see approach has no place here.

Chylothorax is a rare but recognized complication of hiatal hernia repair, occurring as a result of injury to the thoracic duct, which courses along the right side of the aorta, anterior to the spine, as it traverses the aortic hiatus. Injury may occur during placement of crural sutures. This complication should be suspected whenever there is excessive prolonged drainage from the chest tube following a transthoracic repair. Until the patient is eating a fairly substantial diet containing fat, the chest drainage may remain serosanguineous. If a chylothorax is suspected, oral administration of 4 oz to 6 oz of cream will produce a definite change in the character of the chest tube drainage to the typical opalescence of chyle. Fat stains of the fluid with Sudan Red will demonstrate the diagnostic globules of fat. Treatment consists of continued chest-tube suction and maintenance of caloric intake with an elemental, low-residue diet (for example, Vivonex). Concern about the development of an empyema related to the need for prolonged chest-tube drainage is unfounded, as chyle is bacteriostatic. The rare chylothorax following a hiatal hernia repair resolves spontaneously in virtually every case.

ESOPHAGEAL RESECTION AND VISCERAL ESOPHAGEAL SUBSTITUTION

Complications
- Anastomotic disruption
- Postoperative respiratory insufficiency
- Delayed emptying of the intrathoracic stomach
- Herniation of abdominal viscera through enlarged diaphragmatic hiatus
- Chylothorax
- Massive aspiration
- Pancreatitis
- Delayed splenic rupture

The two leading causes of death following standard esophagectomy and visceral esophageal substitution with either stomach or intestine are sepsis from mediastinitis resulting from disruption of an intrathoracic anastomosis and respiratory insufficiency following a combined thoracoabdominal operation in a nutritionally depleted patient. As indicated above, the safest esophageal anastomosis is a *cervical* anastomosis, where a leak means little more than a transient salivary fistula and is treated by simply opening the neck wound to establish adequate drainage. In our experience with more than 100 patients requiring esophageal resection, the technique of blunt transhiatal esophagectomy without thoracotomy has also decreased postoperative mortality rates by reducing the operative physiologic insult to the patient.[32] This approach exemplifies the concept of "thinking defensively" in esophageal surgery—avoiding the complication before it occurs. Similarly, insertion of a feeding jejunostomy is performed routinely after every esophagectomy and esophageal reconstruction in the event that an anastomotic disruption occurs and an alternative means of nourishment is needed. If it is not used postoperatively, the tube is removed after several weeks. On the other hand, if a leak does occur, a jejunostomy is infinitely safer and more effective in providing calories than is intravenous hyperalimentation, which we virtually never use.

If disruption of an intrathoracic esophagogastric anastomosis occurs during the critical first 10 days after the operation, the event is heralded by the characteristic signs and symptoms of mediastinitis: fever, chest pain, tachycardia, tachypnea, respiratory distress, peripheral cyanosis, vasoconstriction, hypotension, and shock. A chest roentgenogram showing the development of a hydro- or pneumothorax postoperatively leaves no doubt about the diagnosis.

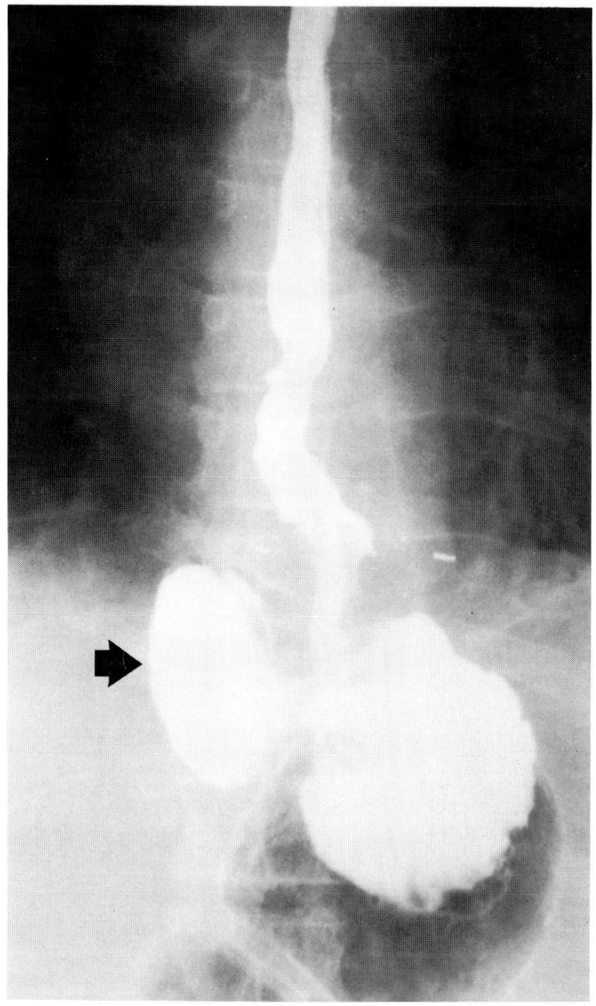

FIG. 23-15. An esophagogram taken 1 week after a combined Collis gastroplasty–Nissen fundoplication. A portion of the fundoplication (*arrow*) has slipped into the chest through the diaphragmatic hiatus because of disruption of the posterior crural sutures. Although this patient was asymptomatic, reoperation and reduction of the herniated fundus below the diaphragm were carried out to prevent the potential complications of this "paraesophageal" hernia.

Treatment consists in immediate reexploration, irrigation of the chest and mediastinum, and chest-tube drainage. If a localized, limited anastomotic leak with viable adjacent tissue is found, suture closure may be possible, but the likelihood of primary healing is small. The closure should therefore be reinforced with an intercostal muscle flap, pleura, or pericardium. Nasogastric tube decompression of the stomach, a feeding jejunostomy, and antibiotic coverage complete the therapy. The chest tube is not removed until the barium swallow after 10 days confirms healing. Alternatively, if the inevitable leak again becomes evident, chest-tube drainage is continued to allow development of a controlled esophagopleural-cutaneous fistula. Aspirated gastric contents may be returned to the gastrointestinal tract by way of the jejunostomy tube to minimize electrolyte and fluid imbalance. If, on initial exploration for anastomotic disruption, extensive gastric or esophageal necrosis with a major anastomotic dehiscence is found, the only hope of salvage is to resect the nonviable stomach and return it to the abdomen, resect nonviable esophagus, perform an *end*-cervical esophagostomy, and insert a feeding jejunostomy. This, of course, is the worst possible course that can occur after esophagectomy, for it leaves the patient unable to eat normally. In debilitated patients, a later attempt at esophageal reconstruction is unlikely to be successful. The maximum length of remaining esophagus should be preserved in constructing the esophagostomy, since this may aid in future reconstructive efforts using a colonic interposition.

FIG. 23-16. A barium study of a patient with regurgitation and dilatation of the intrathoracic stomach following esophagectomy for distal-third carcinoma. This complication was the result of two technical errors: failure to enlarge the diphragmatic hiatus sufficiently, and failure to perform a gastric drainage procedure. *Large arrow,* relative obstruction at the diaphragmatic hiatus; *small arrow,* obstruction at the pylorus.

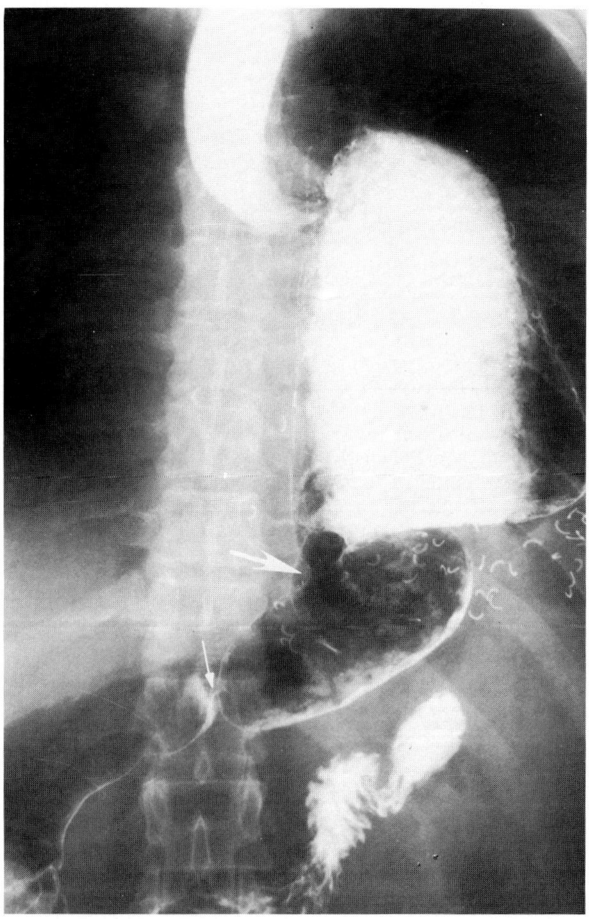

Similar considerations apply to esophageal reconstruction using colon or jejunum. Anastomotic disruption may be localized and respond well to drainage and attempted closure. Alternatively, major disruption may result from either ischemia or venous infarction of the intestinal graft, which must be removed with performance of an esophagostomy and insertion of a feeding tube. Later reconstruction can be attempted when septic complications have been successfully treated.

It is *wrong* to "take down" a disrupted anastomosis, oversew "healthy" remaining distal intrathoracic esophagus, leave this closure in the chest, and perform a side cervical esophagostomy. The distal esophageal closure performed in an infected field will inevitably disrupt, resulting in continued sepsis. After the surgical attack on the intrathoracic esophageal anastomotic leak, postoperative support with mechanical ventilatory assistance, intravenous volume replacement, broad-spectrum antibiotic coverage, and vigorous nutritional support from the feeding jejunostomy will be required.

As indicated above, respiratory insufficiency following esophageal resection and reconstruction is minimized if the physiologic insult to a debilitated patient is reduced by avoiding a thoracotomy and resecting the esophagus bluntly.[32] Equally important, however, is a careful preoperative assessment of the patient's pulmonary reserve and vigorous pulmonary physiotherapy, if necessary, for 1 to 2 weeks prior to the operation. Cigarette smoking should be eliminated for at least 2 weeks before the operation. The preoperative investment of time to improve and optimize the patient's pulmonary status is amply rewarded by reduced postoperative morbidity from respiratory complications.

When the stomach is used as an esophageal substitute, the danger of delayed gastric emptying with secondary regurgitation and massive aspiration must be recognized. Although many patients will have no difficulty with gastric outlet obstruction following the vagotomy that accompanies thoracic esophagectomy, the disastrous consequences of this complication are, in my opinion, a mandate to perform a gastric drainage procedure in every patient undergoing such an operation (Fig. 23-16). We prefer a

Ramstedt-type extramucosal pyloromyotomy because a Heinecke–Mikulicz pyloroplasty results in a gastric suture line at right angles to the axis of the stomach, which is being pulled upward into the chest for anastomosis with the remaining esophagus. Following the pyloromyotomy, silver clip markers are placed at the level of the pylorus to aid in subsequent radiographic studies, and the site of the pyloromyotomy is covered with adjacent omentum or fat, secured in place with several sutures. In more than 150 such pyloromyotomies performed during esophageal bypass or replacement with stomach, we have experienced no leaks or septic complications from this method of gastric drainage. Intrathoracic gastric outlet obstruction may also result from failure to enlarge the diaphragmatic hiatus before mobilizing the stomach into the chest (see Fig. 23-16). We do not routinely incise the diaphragmatic crura, however, and we prefer simply to dilate the hiatus manually until it freely admits the entire hand of the surgeon (size-7 glove) into the chest.

Following esophagectomy and esophageal substitution with either stomach or intestine, the abdominal viscera may herniate through the enlarged diaphragmatic hiatus (Fig. 23-17). This complication may occur acutely, during the first several days after operation, or years after the esophagectomy. Most often, the hernia is an asymptomatic finding on a postoperative chest roentgenogram, where it presents as extraneous collections of air above the diaphragm in the region of the hiatus, or on routine contrast studies taken to assess the function and position of the esophageal substitute. Occasionally, as with chronic traumatic diaphragmatic hernias, patients may present with vague left upper abdominal or lower thoracic cramping pain, nausea, and vomiting. Because of the risks of incarceration and strangulation of the herniated organs, reduction of the hernia is indicated whenever the diagnosis is established. As is the case when repairing acute traumatic diaphragmatic hernias, the transabdominal approach is used for hernias occurring during the first week or so after esophagectomy. Chronic hernias, on the other hand, are approached transthoracically because of the almost inevitable adhesions between the herniated intestines and the lungs, pericardium, and pleura. Again, avoidance of this complication is central to prevention. Once the esophageal substitute has been brought through the diaphragmatic hiatus and is positioned in the chest, several interrupted sutures between the edge of the diaphragmatic hiatus and adjacent stomach or colon interposition should be placed to discourage migration of other intra-abdominal viscera through the hiatus into the chest.

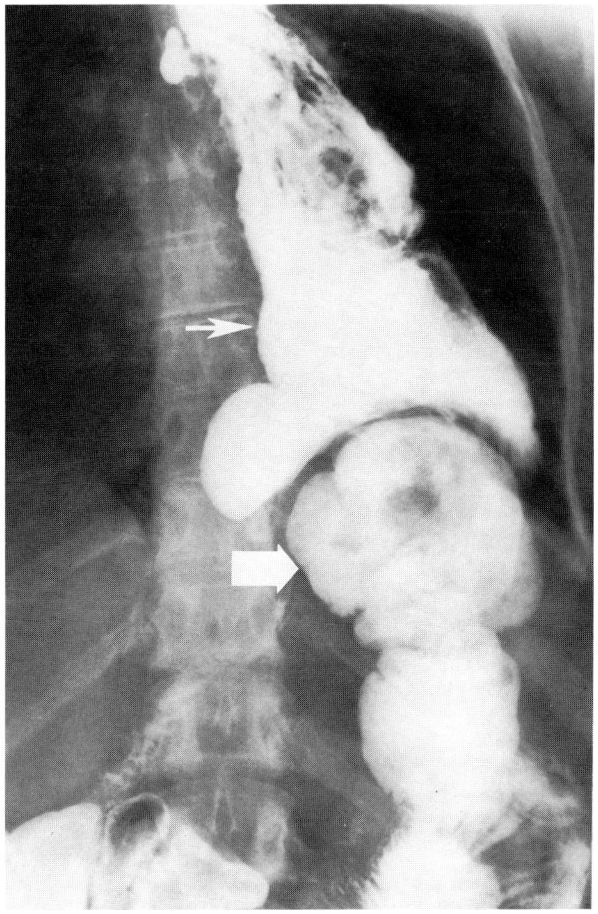

FIG. 23-17. Herniation of the splenic flexure of the colon (*large arrow*) through the diaphragmatic hiatus following esophageal replacement with stomach for a caustic stricture. No sutures had been placed between the intrathoracic stomach (*small arrow*) and the edge of the diaphragmatic hiatus to prevent this complication.

Chylothorax may complicate esophagectomy if injury to the thoracic duct occurs in the upper thorax as it crosses from the right to the left of the midline, hugging the vertebral bodies and the left posterolateral wall of the esophagus. If the injury is recognized intraoperatively, the duct should be ligated. If chylothorax becomes manifest several days after the operation, it should be treated as described previously. Unlike the relatively healthy patient who sustains a chylothorax postoperatively, the debilitated patient with esophageal carcinoma, particularly in the presence of obstructed intrathoracic lymphatics, may not respond to conservative therapy. If the chest drainage does not subside significantly with a regimen of chest tube suction and a low-residue diet (or intravenous hyperalimentation) after 7 to 10 days, reoperation and direct ligation of the torn thoracic duct are indicated. The patient should receive 4 oz to 6

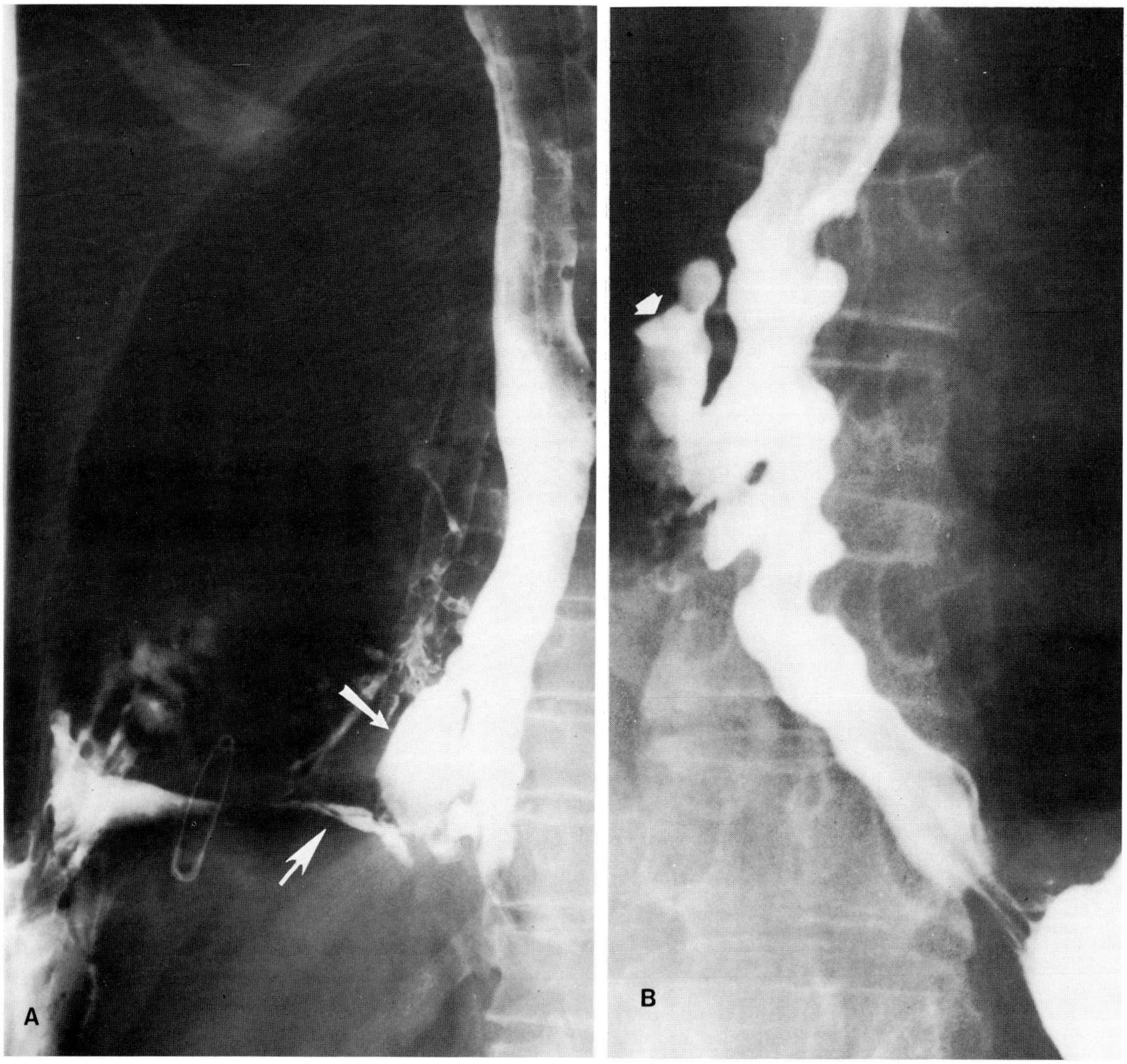

FIG. 23-18. (*A*) This esophagogram shows an esophagopleural cutaneous fistula (*large arrow*) and a recurrent esophageal diverticulum (*small arrow*) in a patient who had undergone prior resection of the diverticulum *without* an esophagomyotomy. (*B*) The patient's underlying esophageal neuromotor problem is evident in this view from the same esophagogram, showing a typical corkscrew esophagus. The relative obstruction secondary to intermittent spasm distal to the esophageal suture line had not been relieved when the diverticulum was resected, hence disruption of the suture line with fistula formation and recurrence of the diverticulum (*arrow*) followed.

oz of cream by way of the jejunostomy tube 1 hour before exploration of the chest. There will then be no difficulty identifying extravasation of milky chyle from the torn lymphatic channel.

As with any operation, postoperative pancreatitis may occur following esophagectomy and esophageal reconstruction. The likelihood of this complication is increased by the pancreatic manipulation during performance of the Kocher maneuver or by direct trauma to the pancreas during division of the short gastric and left gastroepiploic vessels while mobilizing the stomach. Serum amylase and calcium levels should be followed serially for the first several days after the operation, particularly with the development of unexplained fever, respiratory distress, hypotension, or increased intravenous fluid requirements so that the diagnosis of postoperative pancreatitis is not overlooked and institution of appropriate standard therapy delayed.

Delayed rupture of the spleen during the first week after esophageal resection and reconstruction is heralded by the sudden onset of an acute abdomen and hypovolemic shock. This occurs when an inadvertent splenic capsular tear sustained while mobilizing the stomach is contained intraoperatively, only to disrupt later. Treatment is immediate abdominal exploration and splenectomy.

ESOPHAGEAL DIVERTICULECTOMY

Whether operating upon oropharyngeal (Zenker's) or intrathoracic esophageal diverticula, suture-line disruption is a major complication if the underlying neuromotor abnormality responsible for formation of the pulsion diverticulum is not dealt with at the time of diverticulectomy (Fig. 23-18). That is, a concomitant *esophagomyotomy* is an integral part of the operation (Figs. 23-19, 23-20).

Should a leak occur after cervical esophageal diverticulectomy and esophagomyotomy, the neck wound must be reopened and irrigated and a 1-inch Penrose drain placed anteriorly to the prevertebral fascia. Nutrition may be maintained with feedings through a nasogastric tube or intravenously. Antibiotics that cover intraoral flora are administered. So long as an esophagomyotomy has been performed, spontaneous closure of the cervical salivary fistula within 7 to 10 days is the rule. With an intrathoracic esophageal leak following diverticulectomy, immediate reexploration of the chest with identification of the site of perforation, closure if possible, and reinforcement with muscle or pleura as described above are indicated (Figs. 23-12, 23-13).

ESOPHAGOMYOTOMY FOR ACHALASIA OR ESOPHAGEAL SPASM

Aspiration of esophageal contents retained in a megaesophagus of achalasia is a potentially lethal perioperative complication that may occur at the time of induction of general anesthesia before the skin incision is ever made. The esophagus in such a patient must be emptied prior to induction to prevent this complication. Rather than requiring the patient to contend with an intraesophageal nasogastric tube (and its pulmonary complications) for 2 to 3 days before the operation, we prefer to restrict the diet to clear liquids for 2 days and then, immediately before the operation, to pass a nasogastric tube, with the patient sitting upright in the operating room, and aspirate the esophagus. A skilled anesthesiologist can then either perform endotracheal intubation under topical anesthesia with the patient awake and upright, or a rapid sequence "crash" induction may be used, maintaining constant pressure on the cricoid cartilage to prevent regurgitation into the pharynx until the endotracheal tube balloon is inflated. Rigid esophagoscopy with direct suctioning should then be performed to allow completion of esophageal emptying, though few retained secretions will be encountered after evacuation with the nasogastric tube.

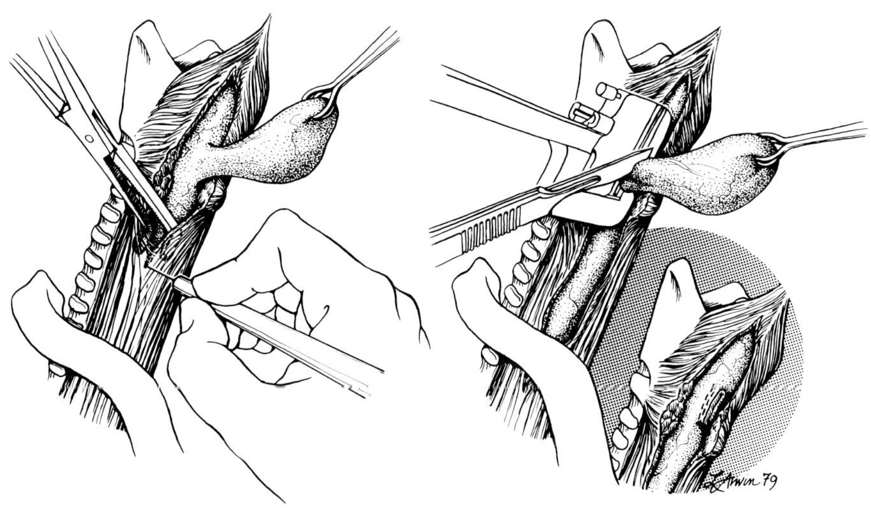

A B

FIG. 23-19. Cervical esophagomyotomy and concomitant resection of Zenker's diverticulum. (*A*) After mobilization of the diverticulum, the esophagomyotomy is performed in either direction from the base of the pouch to the level of the superior cornu of the thyroid cartilage above and to 1 cm to 2 cm behind the clavicle below. (*B*) After the esophagomyotomy is completed, the base of the diverticulum is crossed with a TA-30 stapler and amputatod. (Orringor MB: Extended cervical esophagomyotomy for cricopharyngeal dysfunction. J Thorac Cardiovasc Surg 80:669, 1980.)

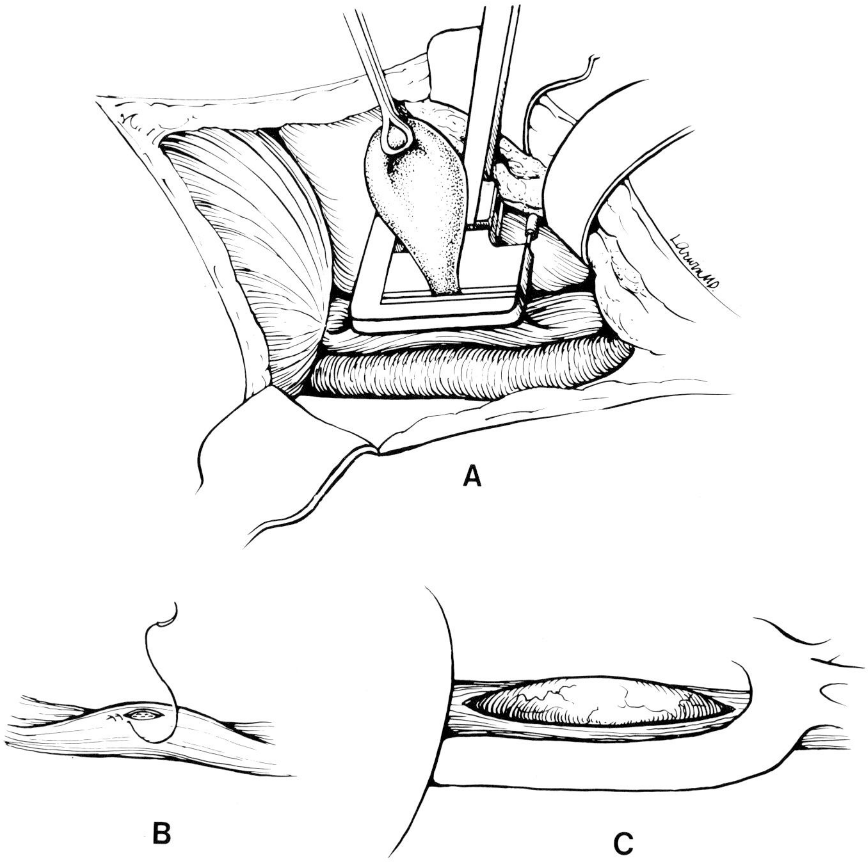

FIG. 23-20. Resection of thoracic esophageal diverticulum and concomitant esophagomyotomy. (*A*) The diverticulum is mobilized to its base and amputated with the TA-30 surgical stapler. (*B*) The staple suture line is oversewn. (*C*) A long esophagomyotomy from the esophagogastric junction to the aortic arch is performed 180° on the opposite wall of the esophagus.

After completion of the esophagomyotomy for achalasia or spasm, integrity of the esophageal mucosa should always be documented by having the anesthesiologist insufflate air into the esophagus through an intraesophageal nasogastric tube. The esophagus is submerged under saline, and the escape of air is watched for while the mucosa is distended (Fig. 23-21). If a small mucosal tear is identified, it is sutured closed with a fine 5-0 or 6-0 Prolene stitch; this is generally adequate treatment. A perforation occurring during the first week of operation is approached in the same fashion as described above for leaks following diverticulectomy. At reexploration, because of the esophageal dilatation in achalasia, closure of the perforated mucosa in one layer reinforced by a second muscle layer closure is usually possible if an esophagomyotomy 180° from the injury is performed (see Fig. 23-11).

Persistent dysphagia and regurgitation in the immediate postoperative period after esophagomyotomy suggest that an incomplete esophagomyotomy has been performed and that the distal obstruction has not been relieved. Reoperation may be the only means of dealing with this problem, if it is severe.

Esophageal Trauma

With both penetrating and blunt thoracic and abdominal trauma, the magnitude of associated injuries may overshadow an esophageal wound and lead the examining physician to fail even to consider it (Fig. 23-22).[43] Particularly with penetrating wounds of the cervicothoracic area or posterior chest, however, if the patient's general condition permits, a Gastrografin swallow using 60 ml to 120 ml of contrast while taking a posterolateral and lateral chest roentgenogram may be diagnostic of an esophageal tear. Alternatively, esophagoscopy at the time of thoracic or abdominal surgical exploration should be performed so that an esophageal injury will not be overlooked.

With "clean" esophageal lacerations due to knife or similar wounds, direct suture repair of the tear will most often result in primary healing. In the case of bullet wounds, small holes (e.g., from a .22 caliber bullet) should be débrided and closed primarily. A decompressing gastrostomy and feeding jejunostomy may be performed in the event that a leak occurs, but this is not routine if the esophageal

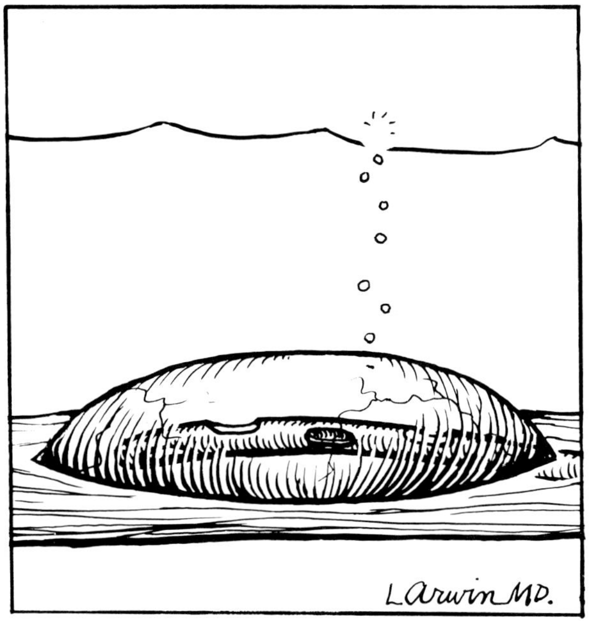

FIG. 23-21. Testing for inadvertent esophageal perforation following esophagomyotomy. The esophageal mucosa is distended by insufflating air down an intraesophageal nasogastric tube. Air bubbles escaping from the esophagus submerged under saline indicate a perforation.

closure is satisfactory. More extensive wounds, with surrounding tissue necrosis, present a much greater threat to survival, and rather than risking a repair in the hope that partially devitalized tissue will heal, the safer course may be an esophagectomy, end cervical esophagostomy, and gastrostomy until the patient has recovered from the original injury. Esophageal reconstruction can be performed at a later date.

Esophageal rupture due to blunt chest trauma is rare, but it mimics spontaneous esophageal rupture both in pathogenesis and presentation. The tears are generally vertical and linear and involve the distal third.[21] During rapid deceleration motor vehicle accidents in which the driver is thrown forward against the steering wheel, intraesophageal pressures may be markedly elevated while the upper and lower esophageal sphincters are in their normally closed positions. Esophageal rupture with dissection of air, gastric contents, and saliva into the mediastinal planes results in mediastinitis. The patients present with dyspnea, cyanosis, upper abdominal and thoracic pain, hypotension, and cervical or anterior thoracic subcutaneous emphysema. The chest roentgenographic findings include hydro- or pneumothorax and subcutaneous or mediastinal emphysema. The esophagogram provides the definitive diagnosis and location of the injury. Early thoracotomy and repair of the injury, if possible, are performed as described above—"defunctionalizing" the esophagus by means of an intraesophageal sump nasogastric tube inserted through a lateral pharyngostomy and a gastrostomy to prevent gastroesophageal reflux (Fig. 23-23). A feeding jejunostomy is also performed. With extensive tissue necrosis, esophagectomy may be required.

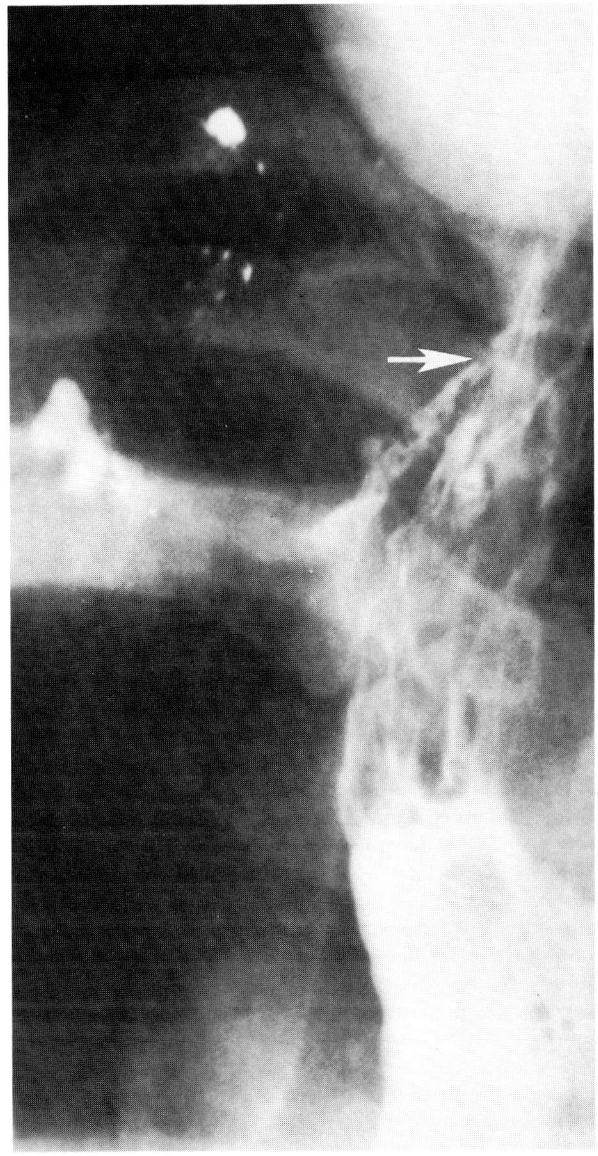

FIG. 23-22. Cervicothoracic esophageal fistula (*arrow*) following a gunshot wound to the neck. At initial exploration a tracheostomy was performed and vascular injuries repaired. The esophageal wound was unrecognized until septic complications led to this meglumine diatrizoate (Gastrografin) swallow 6 days later. Bullet fragments can be seen in the right side of the neck above the clavicle.

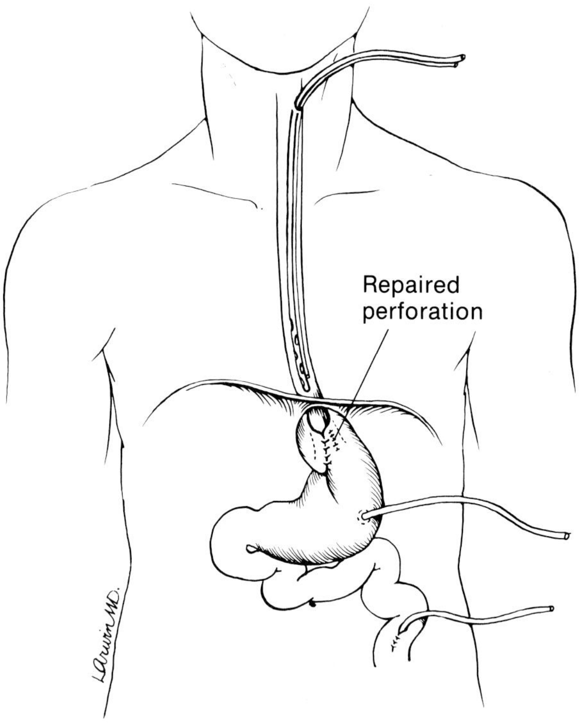

FIG. 23-23. Repair of a distal esophageal tear and reinforcement of the suture line with fundoplication. A decompressing gastrostomy and feeding jejunostomy are performed. A sump-type nasogastric tube positioned in the esophagus above the injury effectively diverts swallowed oral secretions and is far more efficient than a standard nasogastric tube.

Postemetic ("spontaneous") perforations are most often associated with underlying esophageal pathology (spasm or reflux esophagitis), and surgeons who attempt to deal with these injuries must bear this in mind. The rupture usually occurs just above the diaphragm.[1, 45] Although prompt recognition of the tear with direct transthoracic suture is usually successful, a repair of such a tear beyond 6 to 8 hours in the presence of surrounding tissue inflammation is unlikely to result in primary healing.[13, 22, 38] If a leak again ensues and the patient has associated gastroesophageal reflux, the morbidity from the resulting gastroesophagopleural cutaneous fistula may be enormous and ultimately fatal. Unfortunately, many of these perforations are diagnosed late, an inebriated patient or concern about a cardiac or abdominal cause for the presenting symptoms being responsible for delay in recognition.

Our approach to postemetic perforations is transthoracic. Perforations localized to within several centimeters of the esophagogastric junction are repaired, if possible, and the suture line is buttressed with a fundoplication (either Belsey or Nissen), which is then reduced below the diaphragm (see Fig. 23-23). The mediastinal pleura is opened widely and the chest drained with a large-bore (36 French) catheter after copious irrigations. Repairs that cannot be completely covered by a fundoplication are buttressed with either an intercostal muscle flap (see Fig. 23-12) or pleura or pericardium (see Fig. 23-13). If there is serious concern about the likelihood of primary healing of the suture line, a feeding jejunostomy and placement of an intraesophageal sump nasogastric tube through a lateral pharyngostomy are performed.

Large, necrotic, inflamed spontaneous ruptures have little chance of healing per primum. The numerous operations devised for management of these injuries attest to the generally unsatisfactory outcome of any single approach. I have already expressed my opposition to the Thal fundic patch or Thal–Woodward procedures, because these operations involve construction of a paraesophageal hernia, which may lead to serious later complications.[47, 48, 50] Various T tubes positioned in the esophagus through the perforation in order to establish a controlled esophagopleural cutaneous fistula relegate the patient to a protracted hospital course and frequent septic complications.[1] Exclusion of the perforated thoracic esophagus by means of a cervical esophagostomy and ligation of the distal esophagus was proposed by Johnson and colleagues.[19] Alternatively, exclusion with removable silastic tapes placed around the esophagogastric junction and the cervical esophagus, proximal lateral cervical esophagostomy, and feeding gastrostomy have been used to treat some esophageal perforations.[49] These approaches obviously involve reoperation either to remove the tapes or to reanastomose the esophagus, but they may salvage the patient's esophagus. Esophagectomy with end cervical esophagostomy and gastrostomy, rather than the more conservative procedures, again may represent the safest, most expeditious means of treating extensive esophageal injuries. This is the only way of guaranteeing absolute control of continued mediastinal sepsis. Improved techniques of esophageal replacement enable later excellent restoration of swallowing ability when the patient's general condition permits. The choice of the operative approach to the patient with a spontaneous perforation is clearly influenced by the surgeon's experience in dealing with this problem as well as by the condition of the patient.

Esophageal perforation resulting from inadvertent trauma during operations on adjacent structures (for example, devascularization during pulmonary resection or a vagotomy) must be approached as described above.[2, 8, 44] Once the diagnosis is established, unless the fistula is well drained by existing chest tubes and the patient is not toxic, reoperation, attempted closure, drainage, and irrigation are indicated. Primary healing of the esophageal wound is unlikely to be successful, since the injury is not acute. With an established esophagopleural-cutaneous fistula, so long as there is no intrinsic esophageal disease, healing will usually eventually occur.

The highly corrosive drain and oven cleaners now available commercially result in far more severe esophageal injuries than those that in the past followed ingestion of household lye solutions. These newer agents cause almost instantaneous tissue necrosis, frequently involving the full thickness of the esophageal or gastric wall. Failure to recognize the implications of such injuries in the initial evaluation and treatment may be disastrous. Our approach to caustic esophageal injuries has been reviewed.[20] Suffice it to say that if esophagoscopy reveals the presence of a third-degree burn or if the patient develops signs of peritoneal or pleural inflammation, it must be assumed that there is full-thickness gastric or esophageal destruction, and exploration is indicated. Nonviable stomach and esophagus should be resected to prevent the later development of major intrathoracic or abdominal infections. We have utilized the technique of blunt transhiatal esophagectomy in patients with severe caustic injuries, irrigating the mediastinum through the cervical incision and reconstructing the esophagus at a later time. We believe that treatment of these esophageal burns with steroids is absolutely contraindicated because these drugs simply mask the septic complications that may develop. Further, unlike the dilute sodium hydroxide (household lye) burns, bougienage earlier than 4 to 6 weeks after the injury should not be performed, since the transmural inflammation that exists greatly increases the risk of perforation (see Fig. 23-6).

References

1. Abbott OA, Mansour KA, Logan WD Jr et al: A traumatic so-called "spontaneous" rupture of the esophagus: A review of 47 personal cases with comments on a new method of surgical therapy. J Thorac Cardiovasc Surg 59:67, 1970
2. Benjamin I, Olsen AM, Ellis FH Jr: Esophagopleural fistula: A rare postpneumonectomy complication. Ann Thorac Surg 7:139, 1969
3. Bryant LR, Eiseman B: Experimental evaluation of intercostal pedicle grafts in esophageal repair. J Thorac Cardiovasc Surg 50:626, 1965
4. Dagradi AE, Stempien SJ, Seifer HW, Weinberg JA: Terminal esophageal (vestibular) spasm after vagotomy. Arch Surg 85:955, 1962
5. Donnelly RJ, Deverall PB, Watson DA: Hiatus hernia with and without esophageal strictures; Experience with the Belsey Mark IV repair. Ann Thorac Surg 16:301, 1973
6. Dooling JA, Zick HR: Closure of an esophagopleural fistula using onlay intercostal pedicle graft. Ann Thorac Surg 3:553, 1967
7. Duranceau A, Jamieson G, Hurwitz AL et al: Alteration in esophageal motility after laryngectomy. Am J Surg 131:30, 1976
8. Engelman RM, Spencer FC, Berg P: Postpneumonectomy esophageal fistula. J Thorac Cardiovasc Surg 59:871, 1970
9. Foster JH, Jolly PC, Sawyers JL et al: Esophageal perforation: Diagnosis and treatment. Ann Surg 161:701, 1965
10. Grillo HC, Wilkins EW Jr: Esophageal repair following late diagnosis of intrathoracic perforation. Ann Thorac Surg 20:387, 1975
11. Grimson KS, Baylin GJ, Taylor HM et al: Transthoracic vagotomy. JAMA 134:925, 1947
12. Guillory JR Jr, Clagett OT: Postvagotomy dysphagia. Surg Clin North Am 47:833, 1967
13. Hardy JD, Tompkins WC Jr, Ching EC, Chavez CM: Esophageal perforations and fistulas: Review of 36 cases with operative closure of four chronic fistulas. Ann Surg 177:778, 1973
14. Henderson RD: Reflux control following gastroplasty. Ann Thorac Surg 24:206, 1977
15. Henderson RD, Boszko A, van Nostrand SWP: Pharyngoesophageal dysphagia and recurrent laryngeal nerve palsy. J Thorac Cardiovasc Surg 68:507, 1974
16. Henderson RD, Pearson FC: Surgical management of esophageal scleroderma. J Thorac Cardiovasc Surg 66:686, 1973
17. Hendren WH, Henderson BM: Immediate esophagectomy for instrumental perforation of the thoracic esophagus. Ann Surg 168:997, 1968
18. Jara FM: Diaphragmatic pedicle flap for treatment of Boerhaave's syndrome. J Thorac Cardiovasc Surg 78:931, 1979
19. Johnson J, Schwegman CW, Kirby CK: Esophageal exclusion for persistent fistula following spontaneous rupture of the esophagus. J Thorac Cardiovasc Surg 32:827, 1956
20. Kirsh MM, Peterson A, Brown JW et al: Treatment of caustic injuries of the esophagus: A ten year experience. Ann Surg 188:675, 1978
21. Kirsh MM, Sloan H: Tracheobronchial disruption and injuries of the esophagus. In Kirsh MM, Sloan H (eds): Blunt Chest Trauma, pp 107–129. Boston, Little, Brown & Co, 1977
22. Loop FD, Groves LK: Esophageal perforations. Ann Thorac Surg 10:571, 1970
23. Moses WR: Critique on vagotomy. N Engl J Med 237:603, 1947
24. Nealon TF Jr, Templeton JY III, Cuddy VD et al: Instrumental perforation of esophagus. J Thorac Cardiovasc Surg 41:75, 1961
25. Orringer MB, Dabich L, Zarafonetis CJD, Sloan H: Gastroesophageal reflux in esophageal scleroderma: Diagnosis and implications. Ann Thorac Surg 22:120, 1976
26. Orringer MB, Orringer JS, Dabich L, Zarafonetis CJ: Combined Collis–gastroplasty–fundoplication operations for scleroderma reflux esophagitis. Surgery 90:624, 1981
27. Orringer MB, Skinner DB, Belsey RHR: Long-term results of the Mark IV operation for hiatal hernia and analyses of recurrences and their treatment. J Thorac Cardiovasc Surg 63:25, 1972
28. Orringer MB, Sloan HE: An improved technique for the combined Collis–Belsey approach to dilatable esophageal strictures. J Thorac Cardiovasc Surg 68:298, 1974
29. Orringer MB, Sloan HE: Collis–Belsey reconstruction of the esophagogastric junction. J Thorac Cardiovasc Surg 71:295, 1976

30. Orringer MB, Sloan H: Complications and failings of the combined Collis–Belsey operation. J Thorac Cardiovasc Surg 74:726, 1977
31. Orringer MB, Sloan H: Combined Collis–Nissen reconstruction of the esophagogastric junction. Ann Thorac Surg 25:16, 1978
32. Orringer MB, Sloan H: Esophagectomy without thoracotomy. J Thorac Cardiovasc Surg 76:643, 1978
33. Payne WS, Larson RH: Acute mediastinitis. Surg Clin North Am 49:999, 1969
34. Pearson FG, Henderson RD: Long-term follow-up of peptic strictures managed by dilatation, modified Collis gastroplasty, and Belsey hiatus hernia repair. Surgery 80:391, 1976
35. Pearson FG, Langer B, Henderson RD: Gastroplasty and Belsey hiatus hernia repair. J Thorac Cardiovasc Surg 61:50, 1971
36. Petrovsky BV: The use of diaphragm grafts for plastic operations in thoracic surgery. J Thorac Cardiovasc Surg 41:348, 1961
37. Polk HC Jr: Fundoplication for reflux esophagitis: Misadventures with the choice of operation. Ann Surg 183:645, 1976
38. Quintana RO, Bartley TD, Wheat M: Esophageal perforation analysis of 10 cases. Ann Thorac Surg 10:45, 1970
39. Rao KVS, Mir M, Cogbill CL: Management of perforations of the thoracic esophagus: A new technique utilizing a pedicle flap of diaphragm. Am J Surg 127:609, 1974
40. Richardson JD, Polk HC Jr: Intrathoracic fundoplication for shortened esophagus: A treacherous solution to a challenging problem. Presented at the Society for Surgery of the Alimentary Tract. New York, May 19-20, 1981
41. Rosoff L, White EJ: Perforation of the esophagus. Am J Surg 128:207, 1974
42. Skinner DB: Complications of surgery for gastroesophageal reflux. World J Surg 1:485, 1977
43. Symbas PN, Tyras DH, Hatcher CR et al: Penetrating wounds of the esophagus. Ann Thorac Surg 13:552, 1972
44. Takaro T, Walkup HE, Okano T: Esophagopleural fistula as a complication of thoracic surgery. J Thorac Cardiovasc Surg 40:179, 1960
45. Tesler MA, Eisenberg MM: Spontaneous esophageal rupture: A collective review. Surg Gynecol Obstet 117:1, 1963
46. Thal AP: A unified approach to surgical problems of the esophagogastric junction. Ann Surg 168:542, 1968
47. Thal AP, Hatafuicu T: Improved operation for esophageal rupture. JAMA 188:826, 1964
48. Thomas HF, Clarke JM, Rayl JE, Woodward ER: Results of the combined fundic patch-fundoplication operation in the treatment of reflux esophagitis with stricture. Surg Gynecol Obstet 135:240, 1972
49. Urschel HC Jr, Razzuk MA, Wood RE et al: Improved management of esophageal perforation: Exclusion and diversion in continuity. Ann Surg 179:587, 1974
50. Woodward ER: Sliding esophageal hiatal hernia and reflux peptic esophagitis. Mayo Clin Proc 50:523, 1975

24
Complications of Pulmonary and Chest Wall Resection

James W. Brooks

OVERVIEW

Patients undergoing elective pulmonary or chest wall resections require initial evaluation of their pulmonary status, and measures should be taken preoperatively to improve any deficiencies. The most frequent complications following pulmonary or chest wall resection involve the respiratory system, namely, atelectasis and pneumonia. These must be prevented to minimize postoperative problems.[53]

Complete pulmonary function studies, including ventilatory and blood gas determinations before and after exercise and ventilation–perfusion scans, when coupled with an adequate respiratory history, can provide insight into the patient's ability to lose functioning pulmonary tissue. If an adequate assessment is established preoperatively as to the limit of functioning lung tissue the patient can sacrifice without developing postoperative respiratory insufficiency, then the respiratory insufficiency induced by surgical resection can be minimized.[19]

Many patients with lung disease have pulmonary infection or chronic obstructive pulmonary disease. Proper management of the infection preoperatively will minimize atelectasis and pneumonia.[31]

Active pulmonary physiotherapy, including chest wall, diaphragm, and arm and shoulder exercises, needs to be taught preoperatively as well as stressed twice daily postoperatively. The use of endotracheal suction to clear the airway periodically throughout each postoperative day can avoid many of the most difficult postoperative problems.

Patients undergoing pulmonary surgery must have good fluid balance, and their crystalloid infusions postoperatively need to be carefully monitored in order to avoid an overload. On the other hand, dehydration tends to thicken pulmonary secretions and make their removal by cough more difficult. Therefore, a carefully monitored fluid balance pre- and postoperatively is essential.[51]

A more complete and thorough discussion of these problems is provided in Chapter 12.

Respiratory Problems

AIR LEAK

Air leakage from the site of pulmonary resection is very common initially, but usually it does not produce difficulty or hazard to the patient.[53] Following all pulmonary resections, two chest tubes should be placed within the pleural space, one going from the diaphragm level to the apex anteriorly, and the second from the diaphragm level to the apex posteriorly (Fig. 24-1). These will drain air and allow the lung to remain completely expanded. Serum, blood, or pus is adequately eliminated from the pleural space by this same drainage technique. Underwater drainage is always supplemented by suction to provide a more efficient and continuous evacuation of air or fluid from the pleural space.

Most pulmonary fissures are not complete, and, therefore, lobectomy or segmental resection is almost always accompanied by an initial air leakage that will generally stop within the first 3 to 4 days postoperatively. We make it a policy to repleuralize all raw surfaces of remaining lung tissue to minimize air leakage. Repleuralization is not carried out where lung distortion might prevent adequate inflation and space filling.[10]

A major bronchiolar, segmental, or larger bronchial air leak should not occur until later in the postoperative course. The methods of dealing with this problem are detailed in a later section of this chapter.

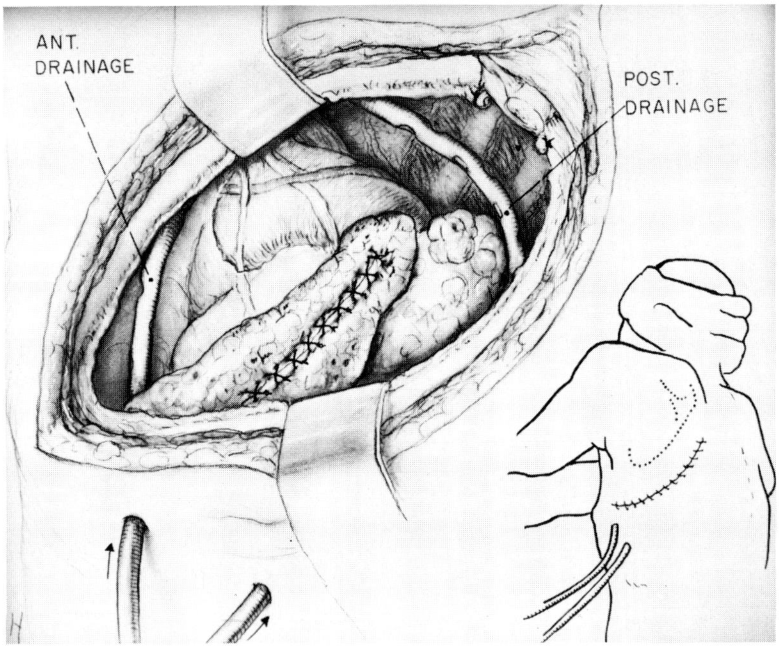

FIG. 24-1. Proper placement of chest tube in all thoracotomies ensures complete, continuous air and fluid drainage from the pleural space and optimal expansion of the pulmonary tissue. At least 15 cm of continuous suction is attached to the underwater drainage system. Note that the tubes are positioned in such a way that patient does not occlude in the supine position.

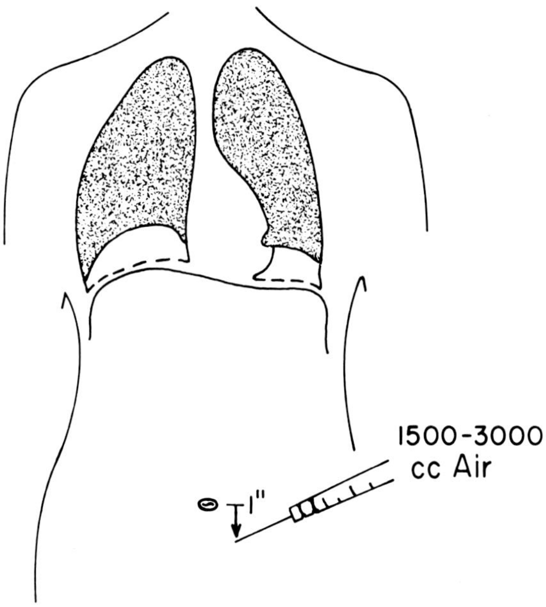

FIG. 24-2. Therapeutic pneumoperitoneum.

If air leaks beyond 7 days postoperatively, it is usually advisable to remove the chest tubes, allow the lung to collapse somewhat, and reinsert a tube through a new site. At times, the chest tube may be responsible for the continued air leak, and the insertion of a tube through a new site may eliminate the problem.

Elimination of suction is acceptable at this stage postoperatively only if the lung does not collapse to a position lower than that attained with good suction. Increasing the suction to pressures that approach 50 cm of water may be helpful in stubborn small air leaks. Should the air space remaining be small and the air leak persist, treatment by open drainage is acceptable. If the air leak still persists, a space-closing procedure, such as thoracoplasty, will become necessary in order to obliterate the space and treat or prevent an empyema.

If an early air leak is prominent, the use of therapeutic pneumoperitoneum may be advantageous (Fig. 24-2). Under these circumstances, 1500 cc of air is placed in the peritoneal cavity; the following day another 1500 cc is added to maintain between 3000 cc and 4000 cc of air within the peritoneal cavity. This will elevate both diaphragms, reducing the space in the operative hemithorax and facilitating sealing of the air leak (Fig. 24-3). Seldom does this amount of air within the peritoneal cavity interfere with the patient's overall function, and therefore its use can be liberal for a prominent initial air leak that is not coming from the main bronchial stump.[90] Ideally therapeutic pneumoperitoneum should be administered within the first 12 to 24 hours postoperatively. Extension beyond that time reduces the effect of the pneumoperitoneum because of the formation of adhesions that will not allow the lung to move upward.[24]

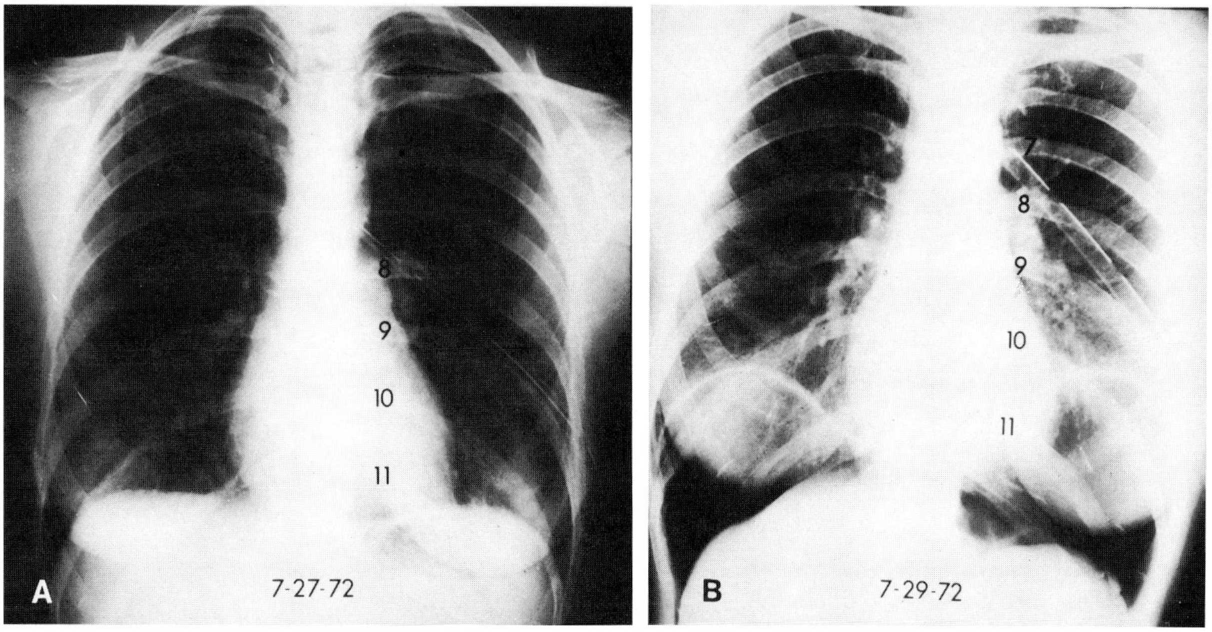

FIG. 24-3. Tube drainage for spontaneous left pneumothorax (*A*) before pneumothorax and (*B*) after pneumothorax. Note the decrease in the size of each hemithorax and the crowding of the lung parenchyma.

The most serious complication from therapeutic pneumoperitoneum is air embolism. Careful positioning of the needle in the left lower quadrant of the abdomen and frequent checks of this position during the administration of the air will avoid this complication. If air embolism is suspected, the patient should be placed in deep Trendenlenburg position while oxygen is administered.

Mechanical ventilatory support (MVP) is often used in the immediate postoperative management of patients following pulmonary resection.[17] Our preference is a volume-cycled respirator, which tends to cope with air leaks and abnormal pulmonary compliance well in the postoperative patient. Positive end-expiratory pressure (PEEP) may prolong air leaks, decrease cardiac output, increase the incidence of pneumothorax, and lead to infection (the same as MVP without PEEP) by bypassing protective mechanisms.[5, 82]

Pneumothorax may also result in a pneumoperitoneum.[48] Air from ruptured alveoli will dissect toward the hilus along the pulmonary vessels and bronchi. Once in the mediastinum, this air leak will dissect toward the neck and inferiorly toward the diaphragm. Once in the retroperitoneal space, it may rupture into the free peritoneal cavity and present on x-ray examination as free air under the diaphragm. Congenital openings in the diaphragm will also allow air to pass directly into the peritoneal cavity. Continued air leak under pressure into the lung substance may also allow mediastinal air to accumulate to such a degree that rupture into the pleural space results in a pneumothorax, either ipsilateral or contralateral.

TORSION OF LOBE OR SEGMENT

Following removal of pulmonary tissue, one of the remaining lobes or segments may twist on its bronchial pedicle, causing total bronchial obstruction of the lobe or segment; there is also obstruction of the venous outflow, while arterial (bronchial or pulmonary artery) inflow is seldom hampered (Fig. 24-4). Massive enlargement of that segment or lobe will result. This type of torsion must be recognized quickly and dealt with, because of the threat of gangrene.[75]

Prevention of torsion of lung tissue can usually be attained by suturing contiguous lung tissue at the end of the operative procedure. The most common area subject to torsion is the right middle lobe after either upper or lower lobectomy. At the time of segmental resection, the remaining segments are also candidates for this type of complication. Suturing them to the surrounding lung tissue will prevent such a complication.

Pulmonary torsion is usually recognized on

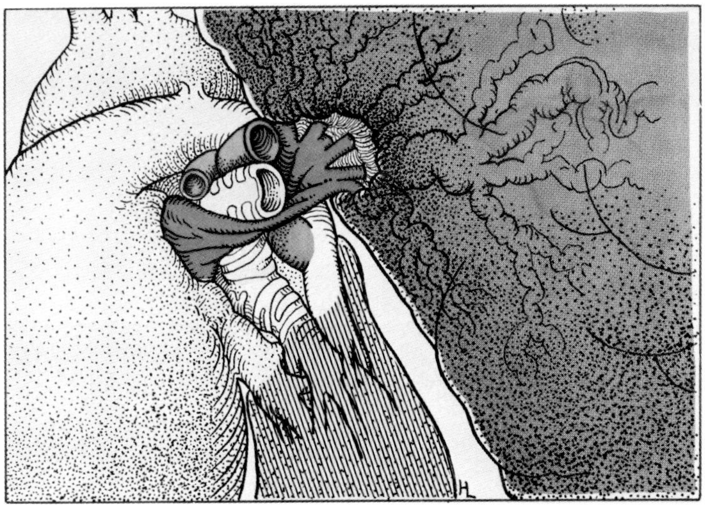

FIG. 24-4. Traumatic torsion of the left upper lobe of the lung. Note the greater obstructive effect on the veins, with less obstruction of the bronchus and artery. The result is outflow obstruction with "wet gangrene" and bloody drainage into the bronchus.

chest x-ray examination by an area of homogeneous density in the operative hemithorax. This density will continue to expand on subsequent films. Not infrequently the patient will have hemoptysis, dyspnea, and elevated temperature, pulse, and respiratory rate. One radiologic clue to the possibility of torsion is the outline of the blood supply to the affected lung area on a posterolateral chest x-ray film. The blood vessels are traveling toward the apex rather than toward the base, as would be normal.

Bronchoscopy will usually show twisting and closure of the affected bronchus.

Management is immediate thoracotomy with release of the torsion, and in many cases lobectomy will be required because of the destruction of lung tissue.

GANGRENE OF REMAINING LUNG

Gangrene of the lung results when the venous drainage of the remaining lung has been totally interrupted or when pulmonary arterial thrombosis is coupled with bronchial artery insufficiency.[64] This usually produces signs of sepsis, with a rapid rise in temperature, chills, and quite frequently hemoptysis and foul-smelling purulent sputum. The chest x-ray will demonstrate an area of homogenous density, and foul-smelling, purulent material will drain from the chest tube or be obtained from thoracentesis as fluid accumulates in the involved hemithorax.

The management is immediate repeat thoracotomy with resection of the involved portion of lung followed by liberal pleural space drainage. Prevention of this complication requires meticulous attention to the anatomical features of each case and gentle, precise dissection.

MEDIASTINAL SHIFT

Following all pulmonary resections the mediastinum shifts to compensate for volume loss in the involved hemithorax. This shift should not encroach upon functioning lung tissue but rather should be a part of the compensatory mechanism to obliterate the space following partial or complete lung removal. The other mechanisms at work during this postoperative readjustment phase are further expansion of the remaining lung on the ipsilateral side, elevation of the ipsilateral diaphragm, and narrowing of the interspaces between ipsilateral ribs (Fig. 24-5).

Excessive postoperative mediastinal shift is frequently an indication of ipsilateral lobar atelectasis or contralateral pulmonary overexpansion, fluid accumulation, or even pneumothorax on the side opposite that of the surgery. Careful physical examination to elucidate these findings in coordination with the chest x-ray film will help to establish the priorities.

Most common, loss of volume in the remaining ipsilateral lung tissue is the cause of excessive shift of the mediastinum, and this should be prevented. The complication of collapse of remaining lung tissue can best be avoided by prompt attention to postoperative physiotherapy and endotracheal suction. This having failed, or if the amount of collapse is severe, the secretions are thick, and the lung does not reexpand, it is wise to consider therapeutic bronchoscopy followed by nasotracheal tube insertion and volume respirator support with PEEP.

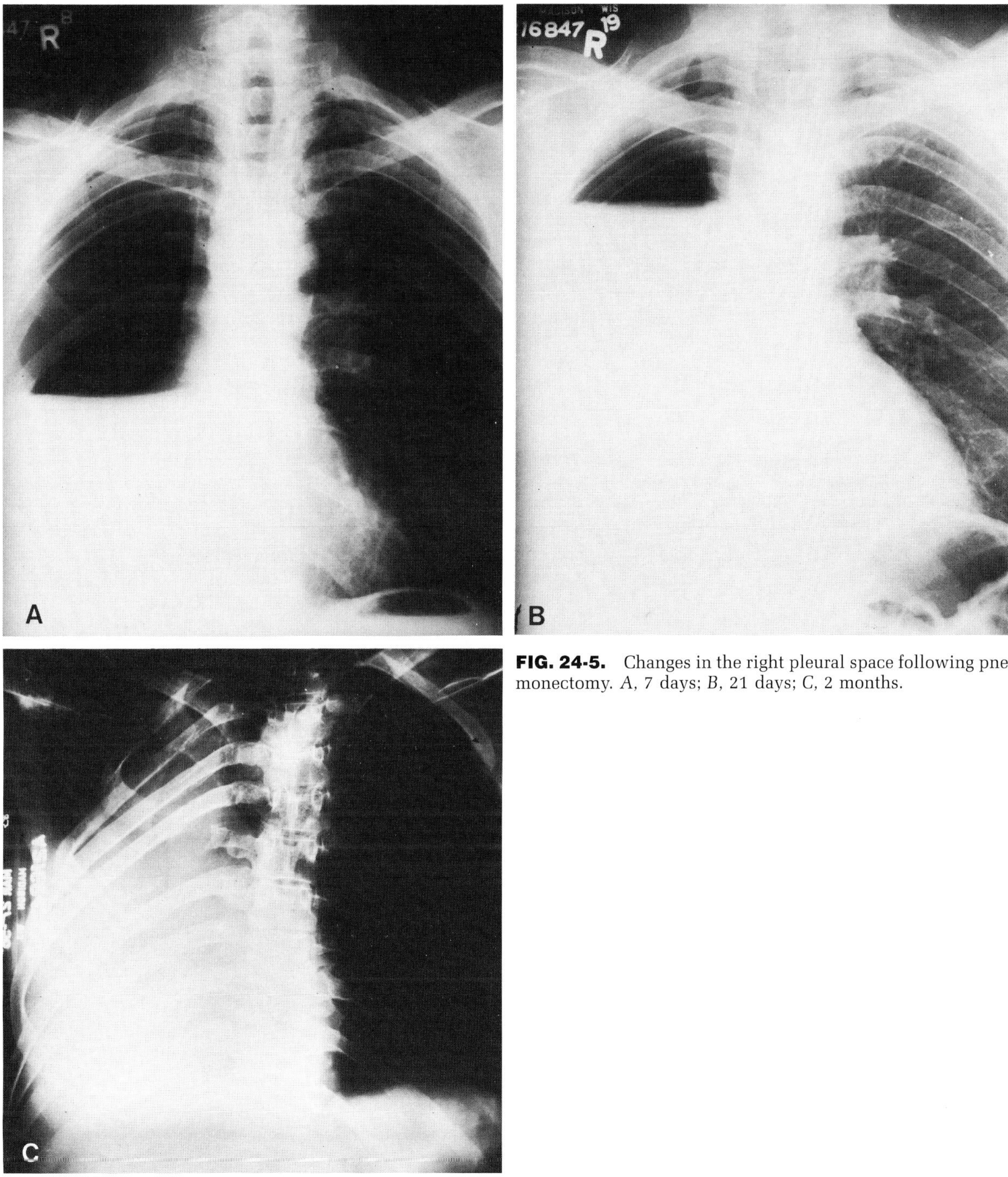

FIG. 24-5. Changes in the right pleural space following pneumonectomy. *A*, 7 days; *B*, 21 days; *C*, 2 months.

MECHANICAL AIRWAY OBSTRUCTION

Mechanical airway obstruction following pulmonary resection is most commonly due to retained blood, blood clot, or thick secretions that were allowed to accumulate during or following an operative procedure. The use of a double-lumen endotracheal (Carlen's) tube during thoracotomy tends to prevent this postoperative complication (Fig. 24-6).[27] With the double-lumen airway, secretions from the operative side will not be allowed to drift into the opposite lung. One can thus maintain a cleaner ipsilateral and contralateral bronchial tree during resection.

Mechanical airway obstruction may occur postoperatively if upper airway secretions are allowed to be aspirated into the bronchial tree during the reactive phase.

Frequent postoperative bedside auscultation of the lungs will reveal the early signs of airway secretions, consisting of wheezing, ronchi, stridor or decreased to absent breath sounds. Tachypnea and dyspnea will increase, and chest x-ray film will reveal air trapping, various stages of atelectasis, or pneumonia. Prompt attention to these findings by the liberal use of endotracheal suction (Fig. 24-7) and bronchoscopy is the most prudent approach to this problem, and can avoid long-term postoperative management problems (Fig. 24-8).

Any evidence of gastric dilatation on physical examination postoperatively or a large gastric air bubble on x-ray film requires immediate gastric intubation and emptying to avoid regurgitation and aspiration of gastric contents. Chemical bronchitis or pneumonitis is a grave postoperative complication most effectively avoided rather than treated. Treatment should include immediate bronchoscopy (to remove solid material), steroids (to reduce bronchial mucosal edema), nasotracheal intubation with mechanical ventilation support, and PEEP (to ventilate the patient effectively and avoid alveolar collapse).

Patients undergoing left upper lobe lobectomy

FIG. 24-6. Proper placement of Carlen's tube. Such a tube allows the total collapse of the ipsilateral lung during thoracotomy, thus allowing maximal exposure of all structures with minimal trauma to the lung. The contralateral lung is protected from endobronchial secretions that may otherwise drain into its bronchus. (Brooks JW: Complications following pulmonary lobectomy. In Cordell AR, Ellison RG [eds]: Complications of Intrathoracic Surgery. Boston, Little, Brown & Co, 1979)

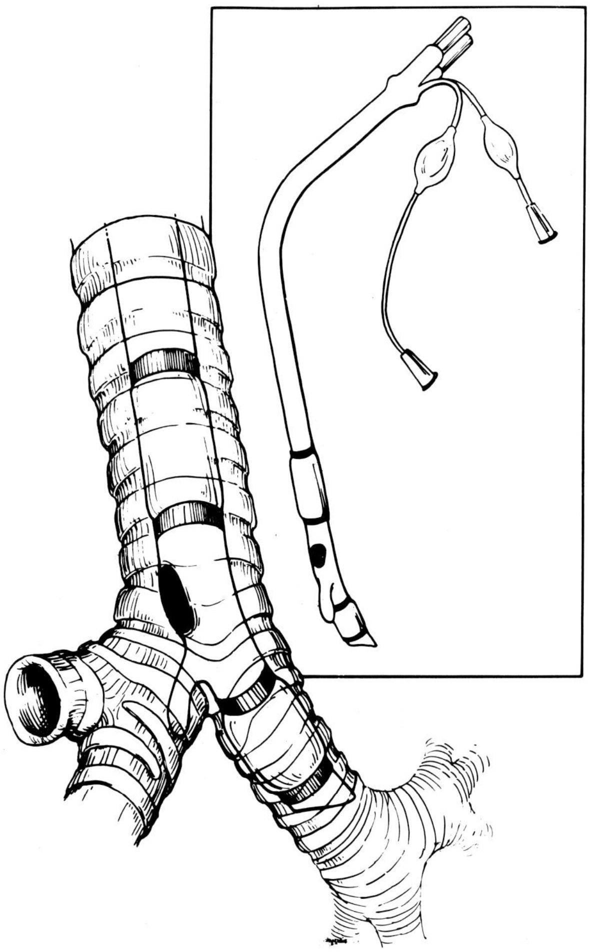

FIG. 24-7. Endotracheal suction is used liberally to ensure a clean tracheal and bronchial airway. Soft rubber (not plastic) catheters with an end opening are essential for maximal efficiency. (Brooks JW: Complications following pulmonary lobectomy. In Cordell AR, Ellison RG [eds]: Complications of Intrathoracic Surgery. Boston, Little, Brown & Co, 1979)

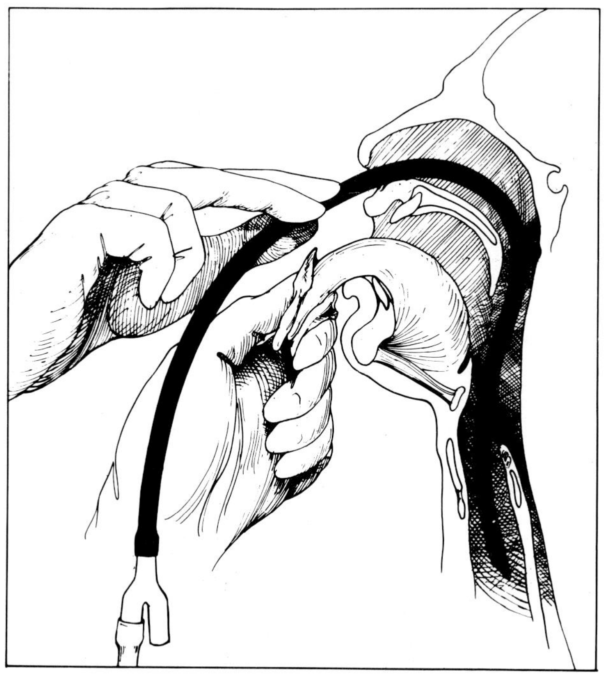

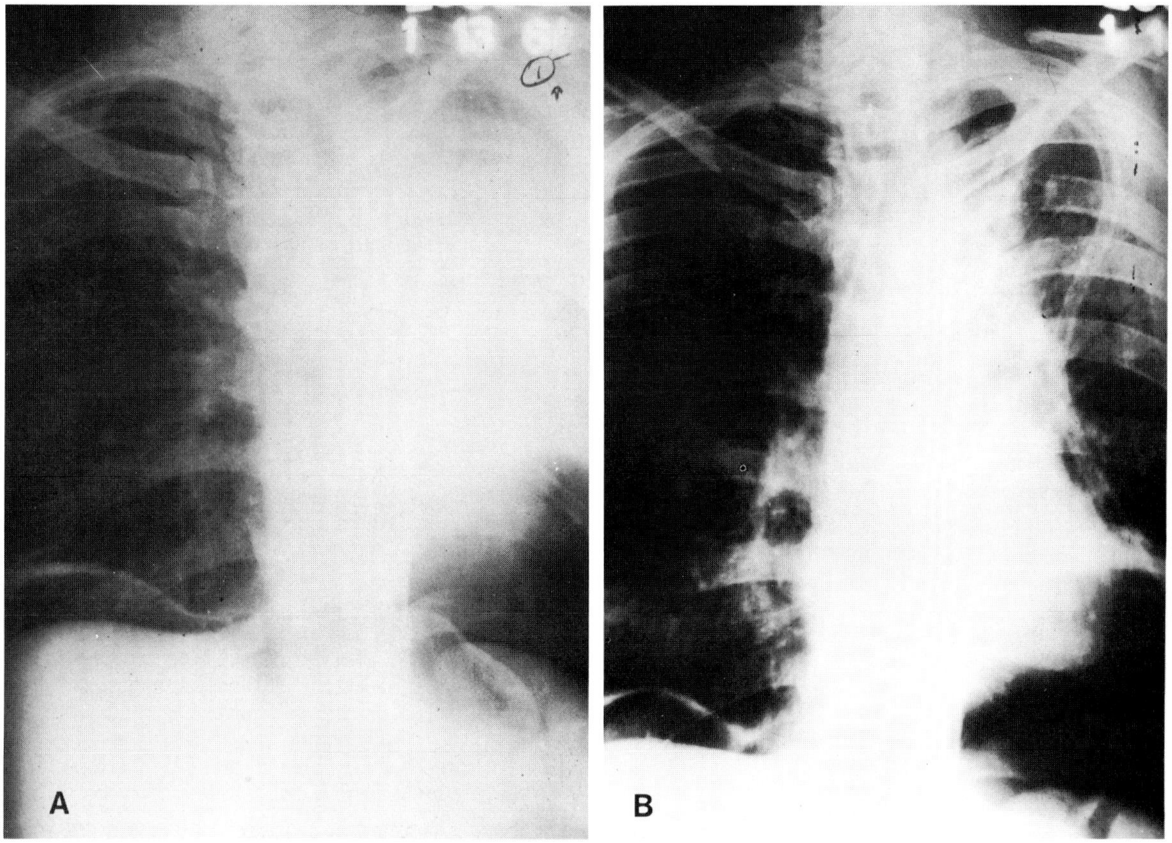

FIG. 24-8. (*A*) Total atelectasis of the left lower lobe of the lung after a left upper lobectomy. (*B*) Complete re-expansion after good endotracheal suction. Note the use of therapeutic pneumoperitoneum.

need more constant postoperative suctioning and physiotherapy than others because as the left lower lobe of the lung rises in the left hemithorax, the long left bronchus tends to kink as it passes under the aortic arch, thus adding one more mechanical obstacle to free and easy ventilation.

Bronchial Stump Problems

BRONCHOPLEURAL FISTULA

A major bronchopleural fistula occurs within 1 to 7 days postoperatively because of an inadequate initial bronchial closure. Great care must be exercised during operative dissection to preserve the delicate bronchial blood supply to the remaining bronchial stump. Whether one uses staples or suture technique for bronchial closure, careful attention to detail at the time of placement is essential.[14, 36] The bronchial stump should be long enough to accept these sutures without tension and with an adequate bite (5–8 mm) back from the edge so that sufficient tissue has been grasped for healing. Simple end-over sutures avoid strangulation of the vascular supply. The bronchial stump closure is tested by filling the hemithorax with saline and having the anesthesiologist maintain a pressure within the bronchial system of 35 cm to 40 cm of water. If no air leakage occurs, the bronchial stump should be considered properly closed.[80]

Reinforcement of the closure is advisable by suturing pleura, azygos vein, pericardium, or mediastinal fatty tissue over the stump after it has been properly closed (Fig. 24-9).[22]

The most common causes of bronchial stump disruption are the following:

- Improper initial closure
- Inadequate blood supply, due to stripping the bronchus too vigorously at the time of resection and necrosis at the suture line
- Infection of the bronchial stump
- Malignant tumor in the bronchial stump

Late bronchial fistulas usually occur because of the last three causes.

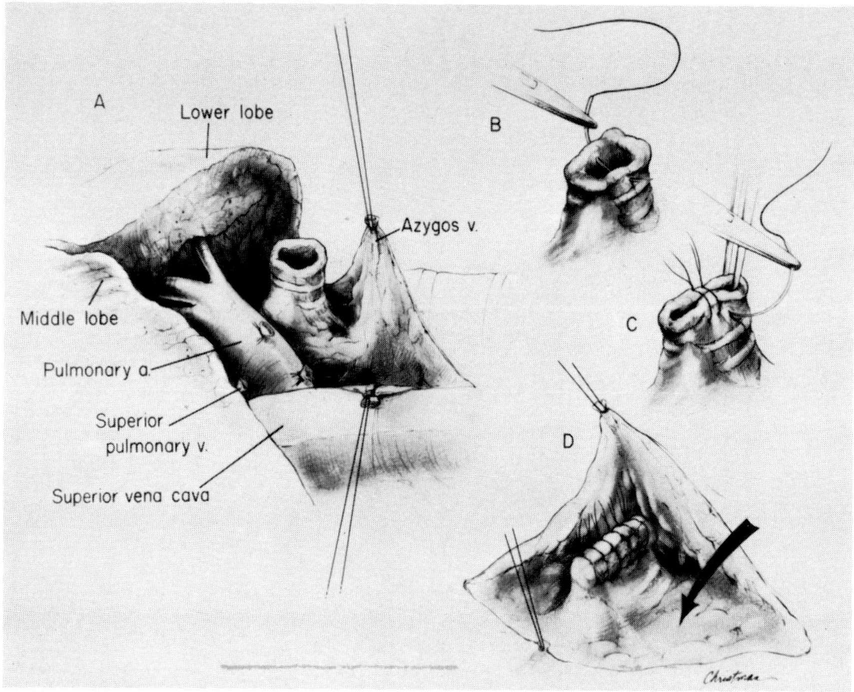

FIG. 24-9. Azygos vein–pleural reinforcement of a right-upper-lobe bronchial stump closure using the interrupted-suture technique. The azygous vein–pleural flap is raised (*A*) and, after suture closure of the bronchial stump (*B,C*), brought over the stump for suture fixation (*D*). (Brooks JW: Complications following pulmonary lobectomy. In Cordell AR, Ellison RG [eds]: Complications of Intrathoracic Surgery. Boston, Little, Brown & Co, 1979)

The early fistula can be recognized by an abrupt, sudden increase in air leak from the chest tube, accompanied by the sudden appearance of hemoptysis and coupled with an x-ray film revealing a new air–fluid configuration in the involved hemithorax (Fig. 24-10). Confirmation is gained by bronchoscopy and the placement of radiopaque material through the bronchoscope at the level of bronchial closure to demonstrate by x-ray film the anatomical site of the leak. A confirmed leak suggests immediate thoracotomy with reclosure as the treatment of choice.[7]

In late bronchial breakdown, one may find that the patient's general condition is not suitable for immediate open thoracotomy. Therefore, drainage with intercostal tube suction will be the immediate course of action. Weeks later repeat thoracotomy and the application of a viable muscle flap over the stump will provide the best method for correction.[39, 42, 59, 66]

EXCESSIVE BRONCHIAL STUMP LENGTH

When the bronchial stump is amputated, the length should be no greater than 1 cm. At the time of closure, that portion of bronchial lumen that is exposed to the remaining bronchial tree should be no greater than several millimeters. If the bronchial stump is excessively long, secretions will accumulate, ulceration may occur, and ultimate breakdown of the bronchial stump can result. Chronic infection within a long stump can be a constant postoperative problem and should be avoided. Ulceration with hemorrhage may occur.

If an excessively long bronchial stump is recognized as a problem several months after initial surgery because of serious purulent bronchitis or hemoptysis, consideration must be given to reamputation of the stump.

Pleural Space Problems

EXCESSIVE POSTOPERATIVE BLOOD LOSS

Following thoracotomy, loss of blood into the pleural space should be considered excessive if over 500 ml of blood drains within the first 24 hours. Blood loss after thoracotomy is generally from the systemic circulation. Rarely do pulmonary sources of blood loss affect initial blood drainage. Common sources of systemic blood loss are vessels in the chest wall, such as the intercostal artery; vessels within the mediastinum along its posterior aspect; vessels within the inferior pulmonary ligament; bronchial arteries and their branches; vessels in the superior mediastinum; periocardiophrenic vessels; and vessels in the azygos system.

Rarely, there will be postoperative bleeding from a major pulmonary artery or vein. These vessels should be managed at the time of surgery by the application of a vascular clamp and oversewing with a double row of arterial suture. They may also be

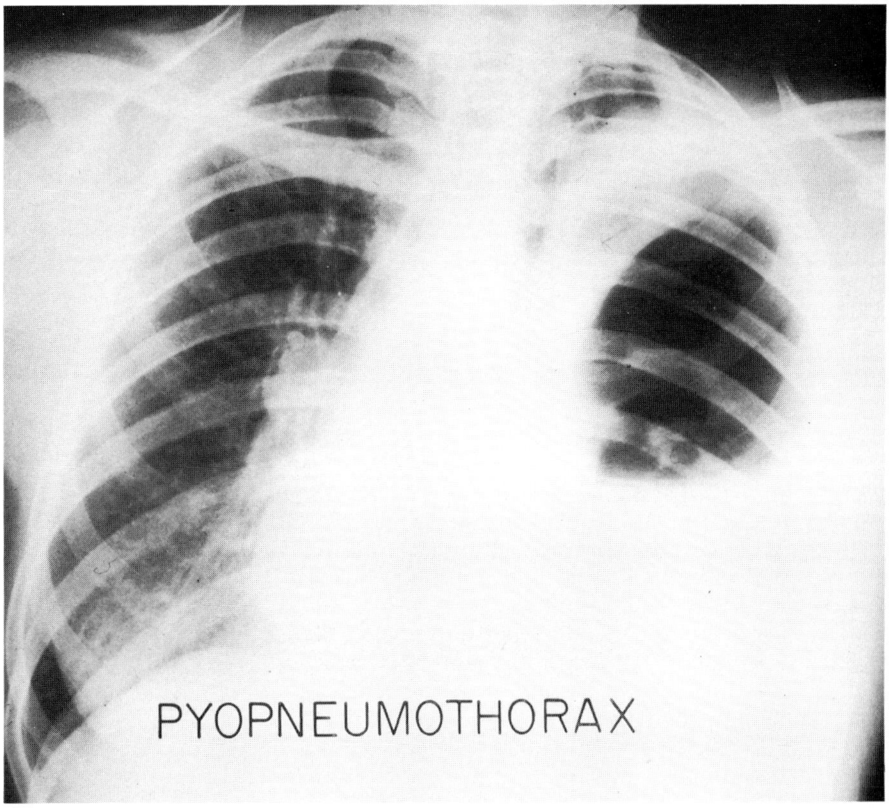

FIG. 24-10. A small bronchial leak in this patient produced a sudden cough, hemoptysis, and collapse of the left upper lobe leading to left pyopneumothorax.

managed by a proximal tie, followed by a ligature of permanent suture material. With these techniques vessel breakdown is rare but can occur owing to an unrecognized tear.

If excessive bleeding follows surgery, one can monitor it adequately through double-chest-tube drainage and careful inspection of postoperative x-ray films. When excessive blood is lost through the tubes, there is almost invariably clot and accumulation of blood within the hemithorax, causing compression of remaining lung tissue and heralding the necessity for immediate thoracotomy to stop the bleeding, remove the clot, and reexpand the remaining lung tissue.

After the first 24 hours following thoracotomy, blood loss is very unusual, but its occurrence usually signifies infection that has eroded a vessel at a point of suture placement or a pressure point from rib or chest tube complicated by infection. This type of late post-thoracotomy bleeding must be approached by emergency thoracotomy.

FAILURE OF REMAINING LUNG TO FILL SPACE

Failure of the remaining lung tissue to fill the ipsilateral hemithorax after pulmonary resection is usually due to the presence of fibrosis within the remaining lung tissue. It is rare to have a failure to fill the ipsilateral pleural space if the remaining lung tissue is healthy. The shifting mediastinum, expansion of the remaining lung tissue, elevation of the diaphragm, and narrowing of the rib interspaces usually suffice. The most common examples of failure to fill the space were seen in the days of pulmonary surgery for tuberculosis, where the scar in the remaining lobes made it impossible for residual lung tissue to fill the space adequately. Problems result if any of the mechanisms used by nature to fill the remaining pleural space fail. A fixed mediastinum from preexisting disease or a fixed diaphragm or chest wall because of thickened pleura will contribute to postresection air space.[8, 78] Such air spaces can be anticipated at the original surgery and steps taken then to compensate for these factors. Methods include creating a pleural tent, performing a Bjork osteoplastic thoracoplasty, reattaching the diaphragm at a high level, or allowing the space to develop and treating it only if it becomes infected.[9, 16, 21, 23–25, 69]

An empty pleural space may contribute to a continued air leak and empyema. Therefore, any measures taken at the time of surgery to prevent its formation are to the patient's advantage. A postoperative therapeutic pneumoperitoneum can play an important role in the management of such spaces. If the space does become a problem postoperatively, the most frequent surgical procedure to fill the space is thoracoplasty.

Should an air space exist at the apex of the hemithorax without a persistent air leak into it from the remaining lung, it will usually fill with fluid and later undergo organization and retraction without complication. Therefore, air spaces not below the fourth rib posteriorly usually require no surgical intervention.[53]

EMPYEMA

Postoperative infection within the pleural space occurs rarely unless there is a continuing air leak, failure of the remaining lung to fill the space, or overwhelming operative contamination. Proper preoperative preparation of the patient should reduce or eliminate pulmonary infection. Selection of the proper surgical approach will minimize operative contamination; and drainage will obliterate the pleural space. If empyema does develop postoperatively, the source of the infection must be located, that is, pulmonary leak, communication with the gastrointestinal tract, bronchopleural fistula, or chest wall infection. Immediate drainage of an empyema space is essential.[1, 32, 33, 40, 42, 44, 61, 71–73, 81, 91] Pre- and postoperative antibiotics are important in pulmonary resection cases, but they are supportive and do not replace appropriate surgical judgment.[37]

If the remaining lung tissue and chest wall will not allow for complete obliteration of the space after insertion of the chest tube, and in all cases of postpneumonectomy empyema, open pleural drainage 2 to 3 weeks after the initial drainage will be needed. Dependent rib removal is necessary for open drainage, and irrigations using saline, Dakin's solution, or Betadine will allow for total cleansing of the pleural space to lessen the systemic infection.

In the nonpneumonectomy patient with or without a bronchopleural fistula, thoracoplasty ultimately will be required to close the space, stop purulent drainage, and permit tube removal.

In the postpneumonectomy patient, the Clagett procedure may avoid thoracoplasty in the patient without a bronchopleural fistula.

CHYLOTHORAX

Chylothorax occurs as a complication of thoracotomy for lung disease more often on the left when dissection is carried between the aorta and esophagus.[13, 76] Chyle escapes into the pleural cavity from a disrupted major lymphatic branch or the thoracic duct itself. Bacterial infections of chylous effusions are infrequent since chyle is sterile and bacteriostatic.

The signs and symptoms are those of pleural effusion, usually leading to dyspnea if no postoperative tube is still in place. Low-grade fever may be noted, and the severity of symptoms depends on the volume and rate of fluid accumulation.

The chylothorax can be drained with the usual postoperative chest tubes, and if it continues in an excessive manner, intravenous hyperalimentation will become necessary. A persistent chylous fistula may be fatal because the loss of fat and fat-soluble vitamins is poorly tolerated. As a final resort, to stop chyle leakage, it is necessary to approach the fistula directly for suture closure or closure of the thoracic duct through a right thoracotomy. Usually it is ligated where it emerges from the abdomen into the mediastinum between the aorta and azygos vein against the vertebral column.

ESOPHAGOPLEURAL FISTULA

Esophagopleural fistula is most commonly associated with pneumonectomy for tuberculosis or suppurative lung disease and rarely, if ever, occurs after thoracotomy for lobectomy.[11, 45, 83] Ninety percent occur following right pneumonectomy and result from interference with the blood supply of that portion of the esophagus near the tracheal carina. Suppurative mediastinal node disease secondary to lung infection and surgical trauma may produce this esophageal vascular problem with necrosis and fistula. An unrecognized traction diverticulum of the esophagus also may be accidentally opened. Such a fistula generally is ushered in by the development of sepsis and the accumulation of foul-smelling pus (empyema) within the right pleural space.

The diagnosis is established if food particles or gastric contents are found in the empyema drainage. Proof is obtained from the results of a barium swallow, since a bronchopleural fistula may still be included in the differential diagnosis. In the case of a late fistula in patients with a primary diagnosis of malignancy or where a malignant complication must be ruled out, both bronchoscopy and esophagoscopy will be needed.

After adequate pleural drainage to control sepsis, temporary defunctionalizing of the esophagus is necessary to minimize soilage both by saliva and regurgitated gastric contents. Improvement in nutrition is accomplished by intravenous or alimentary-tract routes.

Closure of the esophageal opening is first attempted by direct suture and reinforcement. Should this fail, replacement of the esophagus by stomach or colon will become necessary. Ultimate closure of the empyema space may be accomplished by either thoracoplasty or the method of Clagett.[32]

Cardiac Problems

ARRHYTHMIAS

The incidence of cardiac arrhythmias following thoracic surgery may be as high as 30% in the age group above 60 years. Arrhythmias occurring after thoracotomy are usually atrial flutter, atrial fibrillation, or paroxysmal atrial tachycardia.[47, 63] They can be suspected at the time of postoperative examination, both by pulse and by auscultation and confirmed by the electrocardiogram, using routine and rhythm strips. These arrhythmias respond most promptly to digitalization, and only rarely is it necessary to consider the use of electrical defibrillation or quinidine.

The cause of such arrhythmias is unknown but may be secondary to one or a combination of factors such as increased pulmonary vascular resistance, mediastinal shift, myocardial (atrial) irritation due to major vein ligations and resulting inflammatory reaction, increased vagal tone, hypoxemia, preexisting cardiovascular disease, age above 50, and extent of surgery (there is a greater incidence following pneumonectomy). Digitalization prior to or at the time of surgical decision for pneumonectomy seems to lessen the severity of the arrhythmia and make it easier to control.[12, 26, 56, 77, 86]

PULMONARY HYPERTENSION

Pulmonary hypertension may be adequately determined by cardiac catheterization preoperatively and should be suspected in patients in whom a right heart strain is demonstrated on the preoperative electrocardiogram and in far advanced, long-standing chronic obstructive pulmonary disease (COPD).

Pulmonary hypertension should be suspected in patients who have a long history of COPD, and preoperative cardiac catheterization is of value, particularly when one is considering pneumonectomy. With special inflatable balloon catheters, one can obtain the pressures in the pulmonary circuit before and then after occlusion of the artery that will be resected.[79, 88] If the initial mean pressure within the pulmonary circuit is 35 cm of water, mean pressure, or higher, pulmonary hypertension is present. If the pressure in the remaining pulmonary artery rises 5 cm or more after balloon occlusion, pneumonectomy is not advisable.[70]

If these pressures were not obtained, by preoperative catheterization prior to pneumonectomy, direct measurements should be made at the operating table.[29] Rarely, if ever, will pulmonary hypertension preclude lobectomy or segmental resection. It is only at the time of pneumonectomy that one must be very careful not to resect in the face of significant pulmonary hypertension.

Once pulmonary hypertension has been found following resection, no management is better than fluid restriction and supportive measures, since digitalis has little or no supportive effect in these circumstances.

PULMONARY EMBOLISM

A thrombus that develops in a long pulmonary artery stump may dislodge and embolize to the contralateral lung, increase in size and propagate into the remaining pulmonary artery, or even cause right ventricular outflow obstruction.[3, 30] It is not surprising that this is described more often following a right pneumonectomy than left, since a long stump on the right is more likely. Suspicion of such a complication should prompt cardiac catheterization and selective angiogram of the right ventricular outflow tract and pulmonary arterial tree. Treatment is reamputation of the pulmonary artery stump and removal of the thrombus. Extracorporeal pump bypass should be available. Prevention of this complication requires meticulous original dissection with vascular control near the bifurcation of the main pulmonary artery and suture closure of the proximal pulmonary artery, thus achieving the shortest possible pulmonary artery stump with the smoothest intimal surface.

Pulmonary embolism from peripheral sites in the systemic venous circulation may occur following thoracic surgical procedures. The diagnosis of such events and the treatment by suction embolectomy, open-heart surgery, and vena-caval filters is discussed in detail in Chapter 30.

SYSTEMIC EMBOLISM

Systemic arterial embolism from thrombi in pulmonary vein stumps following resections are not documented, but they seem possible if such stumps are unduly long. However, tumor emboli dislodged at the time of tumor manipulation in surgery are documented.[57] They can be recognized by peripheral pulse examination, central nervous system evaluation after reaction from anesthesia, or signs and symptoms of visceral abnormalities by abdominal examination. Treatment is anticoagulation (heparin) followed immediately by appropriate embolectomy. Prevention requires a very cautious approach to the pulmonary venous drainage, initial venous ligation, and maintenance of the shortest possible pulmonary vein stump by taking some left atrial wall if indicated.

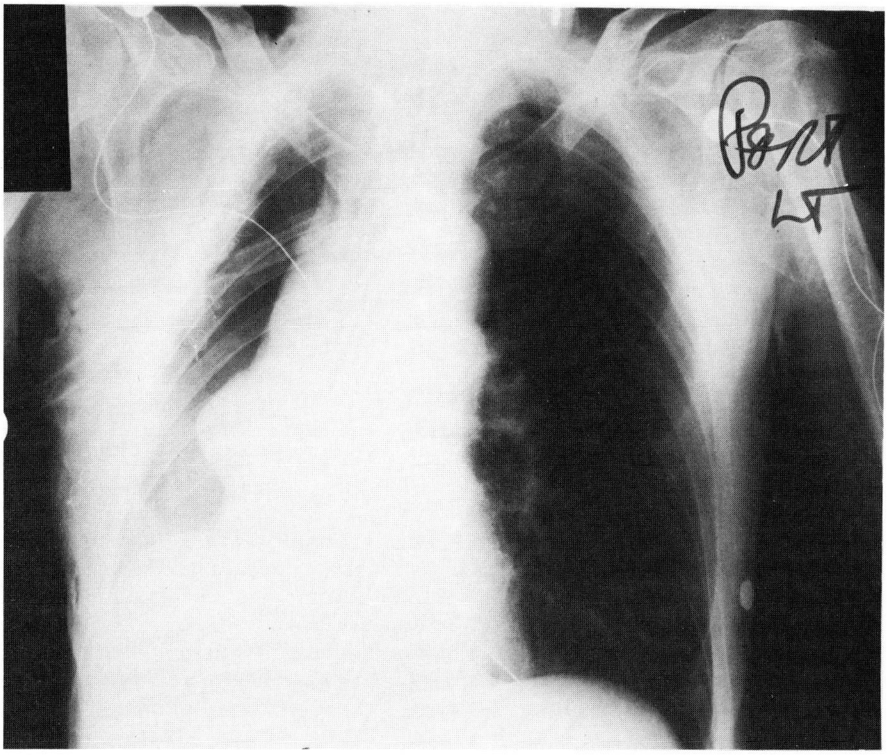

FIG. 24-11. Partial cardiac herniation after right pneumonectomy with removal of a portion of the pericardium.

CARDIAC HERNIATION

When pulmonary resection on the left or right is accompanied by removal of a portion of the pericardium, herniation of the heart may occur (Fig. 24-11).[38, 41, 46, 53, 67] In such herniation, twisting of the vena cava may interfere with atrial filling, or emptying of the ventricles may be impaired.

Herniation usually occurs in the immediate postoperative period. The onset is sudden and dramatic. With right-sided herniation, tachycardia, hypotension, cyanosis of the upper half of the body, and elevation of venous pressure are seen (twisted superior vena cava with poor emptying into atria). Left-sided herniations show only hypotension and tachycardia. X-ray films show the heart displaced abnormally into the operative hemithorax. The peculiar clinical picture and abnormal x-ray appearance of the cardiac silhouette provide adequate indication for immediate thoracotomy. However, thoracoscopy will provide an absolute diagnosis.

Prevention includes closure of any pericardial defect created by surgery using direct-suture techniques or replacement of the removed pericardium by prosthetic material. The differential diagnoses are massive intrathoracic hemorrhage, atelectasis of the remaining lung due to a bronchial plug, tension pneumothorax, acute cardiac tamponade, and acute myocardial infarct.

MYOCARDIAL FAILURE

Myocardial failure can occur postoperatively in a patient with chronic heart disease or secondary to a major myocardial infarction. If a major myocardial infarction is responsible, the patient will be managed as with any other myocardial infarct during the postoperative pulmonary recovery. If failure alone has occurred without infarction, it is treated with digitalis, diuretics, and fluid restriction. The underlying cause must be sought and corrected.[51]

MYOCARDIAL INFARCT

Myocardial infarct following pulmonary surgery is not seen any more frequently than after any operative procedure.[35, 43, 60, 74] It is managed as any myocardial infarct would be, without surgery, by careful monitoring and medication as required. The indications for coronary angiogram and saphenous vein coronary bypass are the same as for the patient who has not had surgery.

Patients who have suffered a myocardial infarct prior to elective major thoracic surgery should usually have this surgery delayed until at least 1 year following the infarct. In proven pulmonary malignancy, at least 3 months should elapse following a myocardial infarct before major pulmonary resection is undertaken. However, each case must have the benefit of individualized consideration.

Infection Problems

Tuberculosis, actinomycetic infections (actinomycosis and nocardiosis) and fungal infections (histoplasmosis, coccidioidomycosis, North American blastomycosis, cryptococcosis, and aspergillosis) usually respond to appropriate current antimicrobial therapy. Thus surgical therapy is usually not necessary in routine management. However, surgical removal may sometimes be necessary to prevent complications or to allow complete removal of a focus not totally responsive to the nonsurgical management. In addition, it is sometimes impossible to differentiate such lesions from primary pulmonary malignancies.

All patients with proven tuberculosis need adequate management initially with appropriate antituberculous drugs, often as many as three given simultaneously, before consideration for surgery. The aim of all therapy is to convert a positive sputum to negative; if this can be accomplished, surgery is less likely to be necessary.

Lobectomy and pneumonectomy have fewer complications than do segmental resections and thus are preferred. Complications postoperatively are the same as for any pulmonary surgical procedure, but their incidence is somewhat increased over those for malignancy due to the prominent vascular inflammatory reaction. In tuberculosis complications of bronchial stump breakdown, empyema, and spread of pulmonic disease are greatly enhanced in the face of persistent positive sputum at the time of surgical intervention.

Actinomycosis produces an indolent, inflammatory reaction characterized by abscess, sinus tracts, and dense scarring that destroys tissue planes and will involve chest wall, pleura, and mediastinum. "Sulfur granules" found in the pus are pathognomonic of actinomycosis. In all known cases, penicillin in doses of 20 million units per day should be administered several days preoperatively, intraoperatively, and for an extended period postoperatively.

Nocardiosis behaves much as actinomycosis does in that the chest wall is involved, causing subcutaneous abscesses and draining sinuses. Sulfonamides are the drugs of choice prior to drainage of abscesses or empyema, or thoracotomy to rule out malignancy.

Most fungal disease is subjected to surgical intervention because of persistent disease foci (mainly cavitary) after adequate therapy with amphotericin B. When such drug therapy is indicated, it should also be maintained postoperatively to minimize complications. Again, lobectomy and pneumonectomy will yield fewer postoperative complications than will segmental or wedge resections.

Aspergillosis deserves special consideration because even though it may be allergic or invasive, its most prominent form in clinical problems is saprophytic. In this circumstance it forms a "fungus ball" within preexisting cavitary lesions. Such fungus-ball lesions have a relatively high incidence of hemoptysis, which may be massive, causing death. Thus, the usual indication for surgery is significant blood loss at the time of hemoptysis. Broad-spectrum antibiotics are given to reduce secondary invaders, but no drug is effective against the aspergillus. Complication rates tend to be higher than with other forms of pulmonary disease owing to the patients' general poor state of health and the lack of adequate time to prepare patients prior to surgery.

ACQUIRED POSTOPERATIVE INFECTION

Infection acquired following thoracic surgery is usually the result of intraoperative contamination or a persistent bronchopleural fistula. Under these circumstances, management of the bronchopleural fistula and obliteration of the pleural space are mandatory.

Infection of thoracotomy incisions is rare.[65, 85] It may signify contamination at the time of surgery, hematoma formation within the wound, or fat necrosis in the subcutaneous tissue. Once the infection is discovered, the wound must be opened widely, properly débrided, and carefully packed and sprayed daily for débridement in order to allow healthy granulation tissue to form. Small wounds may granulate to closure; larger ones need to develop clean, healthy granulations and then undergo secondary closure in the operating room.

Any wound infection must be managed in a fashion that will preserve the pleural integrity and function of the lung beneath it.

Chest Wall Problems

PARADOX

Paradoxical chest wall motion occurs in all instances of resection of bony elements of the thorax. The influence on the patient's overall respiratory function is directly proportional to the amount of chest wall support sacrificed at the time of resection and the patient's preoperative pulmonary-function status. Thus, the patient with good lungs and no evidence of emphysema or COPD will fare much better with a large chest wall resection than will the patient who has poor pulmonary function. The state of the mediastinum is also an important consideration. Patients with a fixed mediastinum due to previous pleural pathology on either the ipsilateral or contralateral mediastinal pleura will have less adverse effect from paradox than will the patient with a virgin mediastinum.

When chest wall resection is anticipated as a part of surgery, that portion of wall resected should be replaced and stabilized using plastic mesh, fascia lata, musculocutaneous chest wall flap, or a combination.[16, 50, 54] A stabilizing metal strut will add further support. This increases the competencé of the chest wall and minimizes the paradox, thus making more efficient that portion of lung remaining.

Most patients with this type of resection, regardless of the operative measures that are taken to minimize the paradox, will be managed in the initial postoperative period using an indwelling nasotracheal or orotracheal tube and ventilatory volume respirator support, with or without the use of PEEP. Postoperative stabilization of the affected chest wall will usually allow removal of ventilator support within 24 to 48 hours, but such support may be maintained for a much longer period if necessary.

MEDIASTINAL AND SUBCUTANEOUS EMPHYSEMA

Mediastinal and subcutaneous emphysema occur after pulmonary surgery in a large number of patients (Fig. 24-12). Air leakage into the pleural space may gain access to the mediastinum because of pleural interruption at the time of surgery and then dissect along the mediastinal structures into the supraclavicular and suprasternal areas of the neck. Chest wall subcutaneous emphysema can also occur postoperatively, as the air within the pleural space finds its way between the ribs and into the muscle layer of the chest. Obviously, an adequate number of well-placed chest tubes will minimize this occurrence.

After pneumonectomy, the pleural space is initially filled with air. As fluid (blood and serum) replaces the air, the air is pushed out of the pleural space into the subcutaneous and mediastinal structures.

Mediastinal and subcutaneous emphysema postoperatively are not harmful to the patient unless they signify persistent air leak from a raw pulmonary surface, a bronchial breakdown, or leakage from the esophagus, which could have been injured during the operative procedure. Adequate steps need to be taken to ensure that intrapleural drainage is proper and that no major extrapulmonic structure is responsible for the air accumulation.

HEMATOMA

Hematomas that occur in a chest wall closure should be evacuated once discovered. This evacuation can be accomplished by needle aspiration or by opening of the wound, evacuation, and secondary closure in the operating room. Obviously very small hematomas will usually absorb without drainage.

Frequently hematomas in the wound are initially recognized at the time of a wound breakdown

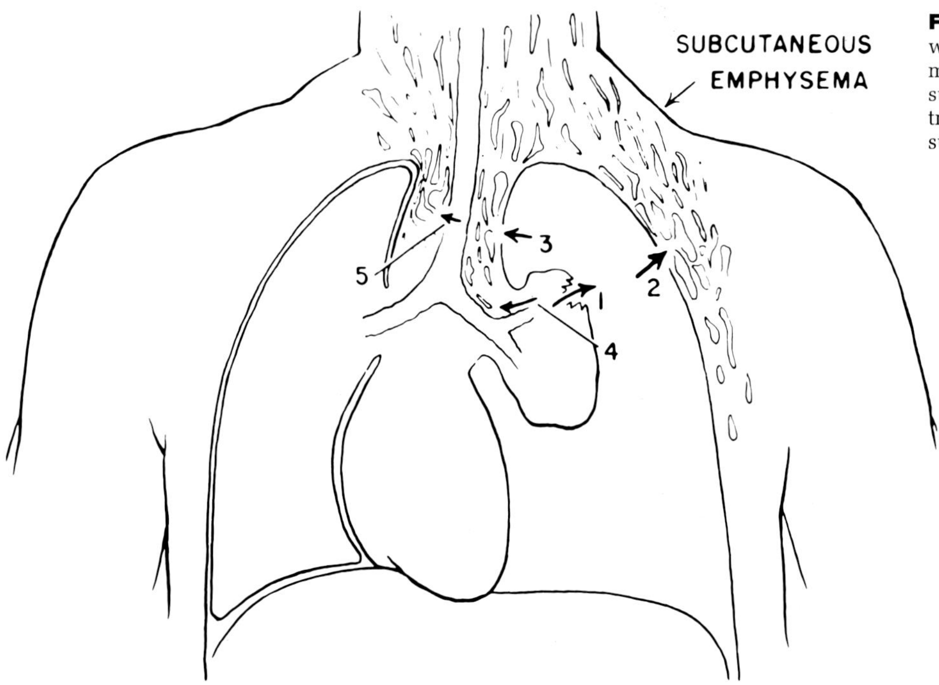

FIG. 24-12. The routes by which air can gain access to the mediastinum (3,4,5) and the subcutaneous tissue (1,2) after trauma or surgery and cause subcutaneous emphysema.

because of infection, Under these circumstances the wound must be treated as an infected wound with open drainage, mechanical cleansing daily, and secondary closure after the wound infection has come under control and granulations are healthy. Maintenance of pleural space integrity throughout this management is essential in order to prevent lung collapse and intrapleural infection secondary to the wound problem.

WOUND HEALING WITH DEHISCENCE

Faulty wound healing with dehiscence of the wound muscle and subcutaneous layers is most frequently secondary to infection, seroma, hematoma, improperly sutured layers, or generally poor health.[20, 58] This seldom occurs because of the rich vascular supply of the muscles of a thoracotomy incision. However, when it does occur, that portion of wound that has dehisced must be laid open, the area cleansed, and the wound prepared over a period of days or weeks for secondary closure. A healthy granulating wound is always sought before a secondary closure is attempted.

Poor wound healing in the greatly debilitated patient is more of a problem than it is in patients not showing weight loss and general deterioration.[58] In debilitated patients one must address the problem of pleural space integrity more frequently, because an open sucking wound may occur. Immediate steps to close the wound and expand the lung with adequate drainage of the pleural space must be taken at the time such a dehiscence is discovered. Preoperative as well as postoperative steps to enhance nutritional status are essential in avoiding and treating faulty wound healing.

INFECTION OF SOFT TISSUE, BONE, AND CARTILAGE

Infection in the soft tissues of the chest wall has been discussed previously and may be complicated by the involvement of bone or cartilage. If there is exposed cartilage in the area of infection, total resection of that involved cartilage is necessary before the wound will heal, since the poor blood supply to cartilage causes it to act as a sequestrum. Once cartilage is detected in the open, infected wound, steps must be taken for its resection prior to undertaking secondary closure to allow complete wound healing.[55, 62, 89]

In the case of exposed bone, unless it is truly sequestered, cleaning of that area with débridement of the exposed bone back to the point of good periosteal covering is usually all that is necessary.

Again, adequate drainage and cleansing of the wound to stimulate good healthy granulation tissue is imperative prior to a secondary closure effort.

PAIN

Pain following thoracotomy is generally more unpleasant and persistent than that following other types of surgery. This pain is secondary to the transection of major muscles: to ribs being removed, cut, or broken; and to the spreading of ribs by the metal retractor. The mechanical rib spreader pulls, tears, disrupts, and possibly fractures areas of ligamentous attachment to the vertebral body posteriorly as well as to the sternal cartilage attachments anteriorly.

To lessen postoperative discomfort, long-acting local anesthetics may be injected into the intercostal nerves prior to closure. The great disadvantage of this method is that it must be repeated every 10 to 12 hours postoperatively and eight to ten ribs must be blocked for genuine benefit to the patient.

Vigorous postoperative cough, deep breathing, and exercise activities by the patient, under the direction of a properly instructed physiotherapist, are the best methods to overcome pain and discomfort postoperatively. With this approach and with the judicial use of mild narcotics, most patients will overcome their discomfort and do quite well. The possibility of intercostal neuroma must always be considered, but it is certainly rare. Properly instructed patients following exercise regimes for 6 months after surgery seldom have the pain complaint that patients without this vigorous physiotherapy might experience.

DIMINISHED SENSATION

Diminished sensation along the pathway of the dermatome of the fifth or sixth intercostal nerve is a very frequent postoperative complaint. This arises from trauma to the nerve at the time the rib is spread by the rib spreader. Frequently the intercostal bundle, including intercostal artery, vein, and nerve, are divided between clamps in order to avoid this trauma, and the skin dermatome of those nerves will be numb. Patients should be warned of this and advised that it will last forever.

KELOID

Keloid formation in scars can occur in the thoracic area, and its management is discussed more completely in Chapter 1, Complications of Wound Healing.

TUMOR IMPLANTS

Patients undergoing thoracotomy for malignant tumor may develop nodules within their chest incision secondary to seeding of malignant cells in the wound at the time of thoracotomy This unfortunate occurrence may manifest itself in patients undergoing nonresectable thoracotomy or in patients having resection of a lesion with no evidence of spread at the time of thoracotomy.

One possible prophylaxis for this type of complication is the vigorous washing of the pleural space with 3 L to 4 L of warm saline at the completion of every operation for malignant resection. Nitrogen mustard wash has been used, but with little evidence of benefit.

The malignant nodules within a thoracotomy incision may appear within several months of the initial resection or years later. It is unusual for these nodules to appear in a wound without evidence of other areas of recurrent malignant disease. Once these nodules appear, specific diagnosis must be sought by direct open biopsy.

Management is either by irradiation or chemotherapy. Should a single nodule appear, its total resection is warranted in hopes that it will not spread.

Nerve Injuries

INTERCOSTAL NERVES

Intercostal pain following thoracotomy has been discussed previously. Alleviation of this discomfort can be effected temporarily by the application of local anesthetics and, on occasion, the injection of steroids. However, intercostal nerve interruption or dissection surgically for a neuroma is rarely, if ever, indicated.

PHRENIC NERVE

The phrenic nerve should be preserved carefully at every thoracotomy, regardless of the purpose of the thoracotomy. Should the phrenic nerve be directly involved with malignant disease, it should be resected if the tumor itself can be totally resected. Under all other circumstances, the phrenic nerve must be protected from injury to preserve diaphragmatic function.

A flail diaphragm on the ipsilateral side of surgical resection, whether the resection is for lobectomy or pneumonectomy, is a deterrent to rapid uncomplicated postoperative recovery. This flail diaphragm acts as a flail chest wall and interferes with proper ventilatory action, respiratory function, and effective cough. In the case of pneumonectomy, the diaphragm soon becomes fixed by scar in an elevated position, whether the nerve has been interrupted or not. If the pneumonectomy patient has COPD or emphysema in his only remaining lung, a flail diaphragm can pose a severe management problem during the first 2 to 3 weeks postoperatively.

VAGUS NERVE

The vagus nerve is easily identifiable during all thoracotomies, and it should be protected. Branches leaving the vagus nerve and entering the hilus of the lung are individually clamped and ligated while protecting the main vagal trunk. Unilateral interruption of the vagus nerve in the chest may result in pyloric obstruction and require postoperative gastroenterostomy or pyloroplasty. This is a rare but possible occurrence that must be watched for carefully if such an interruption is necessary at the time of thoracotomy.

It is most important not to interrupt the vagus nerve proximal to the recurrent laryngeal nerve, for total paralysis of the ipsilateral vocal cord will result. This not only interferes with the patient's phonation, but causes problems from aspiration of secretions from the pharynx and interferes with good postoperative cough.

Intentional sacrifice of a vagus nerve is justified in nonresectable lung malignancy resulting in hypertrophic pulmonary osteoarthropathy. Such action will relieve the joint signs and symptoms and thus aid in palliation of the patient's disease.

RECURRENT LARYNGEAL NERVE

The left recurrent laryngeal nerve is more likely to be interrupted at the time of thoracotomy than is the right. The left recurrent laryngeal nerve leaves the vagus in the region of the aortic arch and passes beneath the arch at the level of the ligamentum arteriosum, traveling back up the mediastinum to the left vocal cord in the neck. Careful dissection in the area is indicated to define the left recurrent laryngeal nerve and to protect it at the time of resection. If there are malignant nodes involved in the area of the left main bronchus as it passes beneath the aortic arch, one may voluntarily sacrifice the recurrent laryngeal nerve in order to perform a proper node dissection in this area. This is the only acceptable alternative when resecting malignant nodes and is the only acceptable intentional sacrifice of the recurrent laryngeal nerve. Once this nerve has been interrupted, careful postoperative management of the patient is necessary because of the patient's inability to cough well and clear secretions. Aspiration from the pharyngeal area is more common and troublesome under these circumstances.

No repair of the recurrent laryngeal nerve is feasible routinely to regain function of the left vocal cord when interruption occurs in the thoracic cavity.

On the right side, the right recurrent laryngeal nerve leaves the vagus near the innominate artery and passes beneath either the innominate or the subclavian artery to travel back into the neck and right vocal cord area. This nerve is seldom at risk during dissection because of its location, but on occasion it may become involved when the dissection of the peritracheal nodes is carried out in the presence of inflammation, scar, or malignant nodes in that area. The same precautions postoperatively are necessary when one knows that the nerve has been interrupted.

Hoarseness following thoracotomy is not unusual because of the nasotracheal or orotracheal tubes that are in place during surgery; therefore, if one doubts the etiology of the hoarseness, careful mirror inspection (indirect laryngoscopy) of the cords is necessary to differentiate paralysis from edema.

Diagnostic Thoracic Procedures

BRONCHOSCOPY

Serious complications following rigid bronchoscopy are rare. The most common postoperative complication following bronchoscopy is hoarseness and sore throat brought about by irritation from the procedure. Generally these complaints subside within 12 to 24 hours and do not require any specific therapy other than mild analgesia of a nonnarcotic nature. There are times when the use of steroids after bronchoscopy may be beneficial in reducing vocal cord edema, for example, when the procedure has been exceptionally long or traumatic. Vocal-cord granulations may occur from cord injury by forceful, traumatic insertion of the bronchoscope. Injury to the upper incisor teeth or to bridgework is likely in any patient in whom careful attention is not directed at this area of contact, but it is more frequent in patients with small mouths, receding lower jaws, or a pronounced anterior placement of the larynx. The best way to prevent such accidents is to keep the bronchoscope always on the endoscopist's thumb while the middle finger is kept in the roof of the patient's mouth. Other aids in difficult cases are the use of a laryngoscope to aid insertion or passing the scope through the side of the mouth rather than along the midline. Abnormalities of the cervical or thoracic spines may make passage of a rigid scope impossible.

Bronchoscopic manipulations in patients with tracheal lumen narrowing responsible for dyspnea and tracheal stridor can be more safely carried out under well-performed local anesthesia, saving general anesthesia for later when the airway is completely assessed.

Bronchoscopy can initiate considerable irritation of the bronchial tree, particularly if brushings are performed, and therefore postoperative cough in excess of the preoperative cough may be noticed. However, in patients who are undergoing diagnostic workup for malignant disease, this deep cough may be most beneficial in obtaining cells for analysis.

Elevation of temperature following bronchoscopy is not unusual, because pulmonary infection may be precipitated by the procedure itself. This may lead to a transient bacteremia, causing temperature elevation. In patients with lung abscess, such transient bacteremia may actually induce septicemia. Widespread abscess formation may follow, including the greatly feared brain abscess. In patients who have infection as the primary problem, antibiotics for several days before and particularly intravenous antibiotics during the bronchoscopy may prevent bacteremia and subsequent complications. Elevated temperatures in some may be related to improper sterilization of the bronchoscopic equipment.

Hemoptysis following bronchoscopy is common and due to the mechanical irritation from the tube or suction tip at the time of bronchial washings, irritation from brushings of lesions, and biopsy of raw surfaces.

Significant bleeding may follow biopsy of tumors such as a bronchial adenoma or vascular malignant lesions. Careful monitoring of such patients at the time of bronchoscopy will avoid serious complications. If bleeding is a major problem at the time of biopsy, one must maintain the airway for proper ventilation. If one is not very careful in tamponading the area of brisk bleeding, asphyxiation can occur from blood clotting in the major bronchi. Vasoconstrictor pledgets may prove helpful. Before removing the bronchoscope following such bleeding, it must be judged controlled and a careful search made bilaterally for retained blood clots, which must be removed.

Immediate thoracotomy is necessary if the bleeding cannot be controlled. Should thoracotomy be necessary, the rapid insertion of a double-lumen endotracheal tube (Carlen's tube) to maintain the blood on the ipsilateral side of biopsy is essential to survival. One clear lung (the contralateral one) is usually adequate to sustain life during surgery. Brisk bleeding will occur at the time of bronchial biopsy, if the biopsy is too deep and actually encompasses a portion of the pulmonary artery or bronchial artery.

With the present enthusiasm for bronchoscopy brushing and blind peripheral biopsy taken endoscopically in the diagnosis of pulmonary disease, a pneumothorax or hemothorax may develop owing to perforation of the visceral pleura.[2, 15, 34] Under such circumstances, the pneumothorax or hemothorax must be treated in the usual manner with insertion of a chest tube, evacuation of material from the pleural space, and complete reexpansion of the lung.

Mediastinal emphysema following bronchoscopy may occur when biopsies are full thickness through the bronchus, allowing air to escape into the peribronchial tissues and then into the mediastinum and even into the neck. Generally this does not cause serious problems.

Complications associated with flexible fiberoptic bronchoscopy are much the same as those with the rigid scope except that epistaxis may occur owing to the nasal passage of the tube.

If the ventilating rigid bronchoscope is always utilized or general anesthesia is employed with the flexible scope passed through a special adapter to allow continuous control of ventilation, hypoxemia is not apt to occur. In both methods of bronchoscopy, anesthesia complications must be taken into account, whether local or general anesthesia is employed.

MEDIASTINOSCOPY

At the time of mediastinoscopy, careful attention to the details of the anatomy is essential to avoid complications.[4, 28, 46, 49, 68, 84] The superficial neck veins must be carefully observed and retracted or tied. After the strap muscles have been dissected laterally and the region of the pretracheal fascia is approached, careful attention to the inferior thyroid veins is essential. These veins may cause serious difficulties if not properly managed with clamp and tie, and even suture ligatures may be used. There are occasional patients in whom the isthmus of the thyroid gland is in the way and must be carefully retracted or even transected to gain access to the proper pretracheal plane.

The arteries of concern in mediastinoscopy are the innominate or its branches, the subclavian, and the carotid. Any of these may be tortuous, and require careful dissection.

Once the operator's finger has been placed in the pretracheal fascia, the dissection should proceed in a careful, orderly manner posterior to the innominate artery and into the deep structures of the mediastinum. Careful palpation will alert the surgeon to other vascular structures in the area and their relationship to any masses felt within the mediastinum.

When the mediastinoscope is inserted into the mediastinum, careful monitoring of the carotid pulses in the head (superficial temporal artery) is essential. Absence of pulse in this area for periods longer than 1 minute should be avoided and the surgeon so advised by the monitoring anesthesiologist. The surgeon must also be certain that his metal mediastinoscope is not causing pressure or distortion on the artery that might result in disruption. This is most important when arteriosclerotic plaques are palpated in the innominate artery.

If pathology in the mediastinal area is present, the surgeon usually can palpate it with his finger. Once the mediastinoscope has been inserted, the area of abnormality is sought and biopsies obtained. Careful attention to the structures in the mediastinum through the narrow, limited focus of the mediastinoscope is essential. The innominate artery, the superior vena cava, and the pulmonary artery are of utmost importance in the relationship of biopsies taken. One can easily enter the pleural space by traumatizing the parietal pleura. It is of paramount importance to avoid pneumothorax, injury to the phrenic nerve, injury to the recurrent nerve, and vascular injury of any structure in the area.[87] Needle aspiration prior to biopsy is advisable for structures that are not clearly demarcated lymph nodes. It is also advisable not to exert excessive traction on nodes, which may be adherent to the pulmonary artery and produce a tear in its fragile wall.

Many complications of mediastinoscopy can be minimized if one avoids dissecting along the left main bronchus under the arch of the aorta. Probably this route should never be explored. If one needs more detail of the left hilus, a Chamberlain procedure (anterior mediastinotomy) is the best choice.[52]

If minor bleeding occurs, it may be managed by tamponade, electrocoagulation, or even silver-clip application through the mediastinoscope. If vascular structures such as the innominate artery, aorta, pulmonary artery, or superior vena cava are injured, immediate thoracotomy is the procedure of choice. This may best be managed by median sternotomy.

SCALENE-NODE BIOPSY

Scalene-node biopsy is still an important part of staging in malignant disease of the lung and in diagnosis of benign conditions that occur within the mediastinum, such as sarcoidosis.[6, 18] When scalene-node biopsies are taken, the structures of greatest importance are the internal jugular vein, the subclavian vein, the subclavian artery, the transverse cervical artery and vein, and the phrenic nerve (Fig. 24-13). On the left side, special attention must be directed to the region of the thoracic duct. All structures defined in the area must be carefully dissected free and protected. The nodes are removed and cultures and microscopic study performed.

If there is injury to a major vascular structure, careful attention to its closure is necessary. Rarely will incision extension for control of vessel bleeding be required. In dealing with lacerations of the internal jugular vein, great care must be exercised to prevent air embolism; therefore, finger pressure of the opening with careful control by vascular clamps is preferable to suctioning and allowing air embolism to occur.

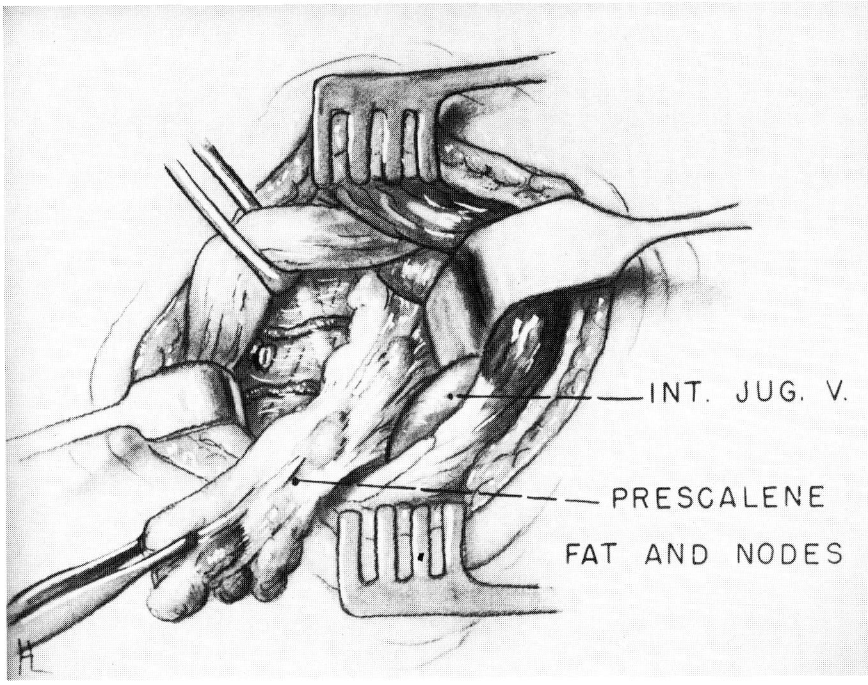

FIG. 24-13. The essential anatomy of the right scalene node biopsy site. The labeled structures are those that must be identified and preserved.

The phrenic nerve must be protected because its paralysis following thoracic surgical procedures is devastating to the management of the patient. Should a phrenic nerve be transected, the nerve should be carefully sutured immediately, even though the efficacy of this is questionable.

Major thoracic duct leaks during the operative procedure must be controlled by suture ligature before the procedure is terminated. If no such leaks occur, or if their control seems complete at the time of surgery and then massive thoracic duct leak occurs postoperatively, the management must be by immediate reoperation and suture ligature. Pressure dressings are ineffective and cannot be expected to help, since the opening in the thoracic duct will lie beneath the level of the clavicle and pressure cannot be applied adequately.

All scalene-node biopsies should be drained for 24 hours in order to prevent hematoma and seroma formation. It also provides a clue whether or not chyle is draining. Delayed hematomas and seromas should be drained if excessive. Infection in scalene-node incisions is rare, but it should be treated the same as infection elsewhere, with proper, adequate, dependent drainage.

THORACOCENTESIS

The complications of thoracocentesis are those of injury to structures in the pathway of the needle. The greatest single complication following thoracocentesis is pneumothorax, which can occur when the needle perforates the visceral pleura at the time of insertion or when the lung reexpands and comes against the needle during the phase of withdrawal of fluid or air from the pleural space. If the pneumothorax allows 1 cm collapse of the lung from apex to base, a chest tube should be inserted for proper, continuous removal of air and total reexpansion of the lung.

Hemothorax can occur after thoracocentesis by injury to the pulmonary vessels, the internal mammary artery or vein, the intercostal artery or vein, or a major muscular branch in the pathway of the needle as it passes through the chest wall. If the bleeding is excessive, such as more than 500 ml of blood drainage, one needs to consider open incision for control.

Injury to the intercostal nerve is rare, but it can occur with anesthesia in the dermatome area of that nerve.

Constant drainage of intrapleural fluid through the needle hole from thoracocentesis can occur in patients with large effusions under pressure, but generally, this does not occur over an extended period of time. A pressure dressing usually is effective in stopping any drainage. If the drainage is excessive and persistent, a suture placed at the skin level will bring it under control.

At the time of thoracocentesis, so-called pleural shock may occur. The patient generally feels faint and weak and manifests a drop of blood pressure and a severe pallor to the face and mucous membranes. The patient should be placed in the supine position with the feet elevated and the thoracocentesis promptly terminated. Pleural shock may be avoided or minimized if the patient is adequately medicated preoperatively with a narcotic and atropine sulfate.

COPE-NEEDLE BIOPSY

The complications of Cope-needle biopsy are essentially the same as those from thoracocentesis. The complications with Cope-needle biopsy may be more pronounced since a large needle is used for the procurement of tissue. Care must be exercised to keep the tip of the needle pointing down, away from the intercostal artery. The greatest complication of Cope-needle biopsy of the pleura is failure to obtain pleura and rather to obtain only chest wall muscle.

CHEST-TUBE INSERTION

When it is necessary to insert a large chest tube for the evacuation of air or any type of fluid from the pleural space, complications from this tube insertion may arise. Each chest-tube insertion must be preceded by a successful thoracocentesis (air, blood, pus, fluid). The trocar technique for chest-tube insertion is superior to that requiring the use of surgical clamps to ram the tube through the chest wall, thus creating more trauma and dead space in the muscles of the chest wall. The clamp technique leads to excessive dead space, hematoma, and a fertile field for bacterial growth.

Injury to major vessels in the path of the tube may lead to bleeding severe enough to require open closure of the bleeding point. Frequently bleeding from small vessels at the skin edge or subcutaneous tissue is encountered, and this is easily controlled by a stitch to hold the tube in place. Bleeding from vessels within the muscle is unusual, but should a large hematoma form, it may require open suture of the injured vessel.

Bleeding from the intercostal artery must be controlled by open thoracotomy and suture. The same would be required for major injury to the internal mammary artery.

Posteriorly placed chest tubes are to be avoided to guard against injury to the thoracic aorta on the left (4th–10th interspaces) and to the azygos system on the right. Also, posteriorly placed tubes are most uncomfortable to the patient and drain poorly.

Perforation of the diaphragm and injury to the liver, colon, spleen, or stomach must be avoided. Such injury will require laparotomy. Anteriorly on the left side or laterally below the sixth interspace (if cardiac displacement laterally may have occurred) knowledge of position of the heart is essential to avoid its injury by chest-tube placement.

The chest tube may lacerate the lung, causing some bleeding and air leak, but this is rarely significant. However, occasionally when chest tubes are improperly placed they may enter the lung itself and cause severe hemorrhage from a major pulmonary vessel or a severe air leak from a major bronchus. Under these circumstances, immediate thoracotomy is necessary. There are instances in which a chest tube is inserted into pulmonary tissue and causes a persistent air leak that is not discovered until many days later. Removal of the tube will usually allow healing to occur, or if it does not, thoracotomy may be necessary for closure.

If there is hematoma or seroma formation in the chest wall at the site of tube insertion, infection may occur, allowing sepsis to dissect along subcutaneous and muscle tissues in the region of the tube-insertion site. These circumstances require tube removal and open drainage of the chest-wall infection. A tube placed through a new site will then care for the intrathoracic problem.

Some chest-tube insertions result in considerable air leakage into the chest wall because the most proximal tube hole lies within the chest wall itself. If this happens, the tube should be removed and replaced by a new tube. The pushing in or pulling out of chest tubes after their initial insertion is courting infection. Therefore, tube rearrangement is best done by the insertion of a new tube.

One of the dilemmas in chest-tube insertion is the radiographic evidence of a very poor position or a very abnormal curvature. This should not annoy the operator, because if the tube is effective in removal of fluid or air, its position and appearance on x-ray film are of minimal concern. One exception to this occurs if there is evidence of tube pressure on major vascular or bronchial structures. In the face of infection and pressure, such a malpositioning could cause erosion and major complications. Under these circumstances, tube repositioning is vital.

After the tube has performed its function of removing air or fluid from pleural space adequately, it should be removed. The tube-insertion site through the skin can be well managed with a figure-of-eight suture placed at the initial insertion and then pulled up and tied when the tube is removed. Alternatively, an oily dressing may be applied with pressure to prevent air from being sucked through the wound.

Almost all tube-insertion sites will have an element of infection after the tube is removed, but this rarely causes any problem. If abscess formation does occur after the removal of the chest tube, adequate drainage is the management of choice.

CHEST WALL INJURY

Rib Fracture

The most common chest wall injury is rib fracture, which varies from a painful but innocuous injury to a sufficient disruption to cause hemopneumothorax. More severe multiple fractures may produce flail chest and extensive internal injuries. The principal symptom from an isolated rib fracture is pain on inspiration, which can be managed adequately either by strapping the chest wall with adhesive tape or by intercostal nerve block and analgesics. Complications are most commonly related to associated organ injury, although there is particular concern for the elderly in whom rib fracture can lead to a cycle of complications including atelectasis, pneumonia, and sepsis. For this reason, it is preferable in the elderly to utilize intercostal nerve block rather than immobilization techniques in order to preserve adequate ventilation and a productive cough. Further discussion of the management of the complications of hemothorax and pneumothorax can be found in Chapter 24.

Flail Chest

Flail chest can usually be diagnosed from inspection of the chest wall when paradoxical motion is seen during inspiration, reflecting the lack of rib stability in that region of injury. The presence of multiple fractures isolates that segment of chest wall, and its paradoxical motion can produce severe reduction in ventilatory efficiency. Obviously the magnitude of the disorder is determined by the size of the flail segment and the extent of underlying pulmonary contusion. Although flail chest is due most commonly to the presence of at least two fractures of the same rib, bilateral costochondral separation and sternal fracture can also produce a flail segment.

The diagnosis of flail chest is often delayed or missed because of attention to resuscitation, muscle spasm producing some degree of fixation of the isolated segment, or the presence of extensive soft tissue hematoma obscuring the underlying motion. The force transmitted to the underlying lung often produces initial radiographic evidence of hemorrhage, which is followed within 24 to 48 hours by more extensive pulmonary interstitial edema and the characteristic blood gas deterioration of respiratory distress, as discussed earlier.

The management of flail chest evolved from the initial efforts at external fixation of the chest wall by means of orthopaedic devices, to a period when mandatory tracheostomy and prolonged positive pressure ventilation were employed, and finally to selective application of ventilation therapy based on important clinical determinants of outcome. The major factors that warrant a more aggressive approach to the management of a flail chest include advanced age of the patient, presence of associated injuries, and initial blood gas abnormalities. Older patients have more difficulty adjusting to the work requirements of inefficient ventilation with a flail chest and are obviously more likely to develop the secondary problems of atelectasis and pneumonitis. The presence of more than one associated injury also compounds the difficulty of adjustment to ventilatory work requirements, and, in this situation, nasotracheal intubation is advisable with mechanical ventilation to stabilize the chest wall, minimize the extent of interstitial edema, and facilitate tracheal toilet. Under some circumstances, especially with fractures of the sternum, fixation of the chest wall by pins or other orthopaedic appliances can be very useful to avoid problems with nonunion and to reduce the amount of time for endotracheal intubation and positive pressure ventilation.

A common and potentially very serious complication is the development of pneumothorax during positive pressure ventilation, especially when end expiratory pressure has been added. The risk is increased when the lung is exposed to multiple jagged rib fracture sites. For this reason, bilateral chest tubes may be advisable prophylactically if the number and position of the rib fractures suggest this possibility. As well demonstrated by Trinkle and his associates, many of these patients can be managed effectively without mechanical ventilation, resulting in lessened morbidity rates and shortened periods of hospitalization.[83a] This approach requires experienced and frequent observation of the patient in an intensive-care unit with limited fluid administration, diuretics, broad-spectrum antibiotics, and measures to control pain. Intensive pulmonary physiotherapy is required with humidification of inspired air, incentive spirometry, and tracheal suctioning. Using humidified nasal or mask oxygen, it should be possible to maintain the PaO_2 at levels of 80 to 100 torr. If the PaO_2 falls to less than this level with supplemental oxygen or to levels below 60 torr on room air or if the $PaCO_2$ rises above 45 torr, then endotracheal intubation and mechanical ventilation should be undertaken. Ventilatory treatment for flail chest should be controlled rather than assisted and, if necessary, paralyzing agents should be used. Once intubation has been performed, it is usually advisable to maintain it for a minimum of 4 to 5 days without any efforts at further weaning. If there is injury to more than one organ system or body cavity, then it is inadvisable to risk nonventilatory management. These patients should have early tracheal intubation and ventilatory control while resuscitation and evaluation of other injuries are performed.

References

1. Adler RH, Plaut, ME: Postpneumonectomy empyema. Surgery 71:210, 1972
2. Andersen HA, Miller WE, Bernatz PE: Lung biopsy: Transbronchoscopic, percutaneous, open. Surg Clin North Am 53:785, 1973
3. Arciniegas E, Coates EO: Massive pulmonary arterial thrombosis after pneumonectomy. J Thorac Cardiovasc Surg 61:487, 1971
4. Ashbaugh DG: Mediastinoscopy. Arch Surg 100:568, 1970
5. Ashbaugh DG, Petty TL: Positive end-expiratory pressure. J Thorac Cardiovasc Surg 65:165, 1973
6. Baker NH, Hill L, Ewy, HG et al: Pulmonary lymphatic drainage. J Thorac Cardiovasc Surg 54:695, 1967
7. Barker WL, Faber LP, Ostermiller WE, Langston HT: Management of persistent bronchopleural fistula. J Thorac Cardiovasc Surg 62:393, 1971
8. Barker WL, Langston HT, Naffah P: Postresection thoracic spaces. Ann Thorac Surg 2:299, 1966
9. Bell JW: Management of the postresection space in tuberculosis. I. Following segmental and wedge resection. J Thorac Cardiovasc Surg 29:649, 1955
10. Bell JW: Reconstitution of the lung. J Thorac Cardiovasc Surg 32:198, 1956
11. Benjamin I, Olsen A, Ellis FH Jr: Esophagopleural fistula: A rare postpneumonectomy complication. Ann Thorac Surg 7:139, 1969
12. Bergh NP, Dottori O, Malmberg R: Prophylactic digitalis in thoracic surgery. Scand J Respir Dis 48:197, 1967
13. Bessone LN, Ferguson TB, Burford TH: Chylothorax. Ann Thorac Surg 12:527, 1971
14. Betts RH, Takaro T: Use of a lung stapler in pulmonary resection. Ann Thorac Surg 1:197, 1965
15. Bibbo M, Fennessy JJ, Lu C et al: Bronchial brushing technique for the cytologic diagnosis of peripheral lung lesions. A review of 693 cases. Acta Cytol (Baltimore) 17:245, 1973
16. Björk VO: Thoracoplasty. A new osteoplastic technique. J Thorac Cardiovasc Surg 28:194, 1954
17. Björk VO, Engström CG: The treatment of ventilatory insufficiency after pulmonary resection with tracheostomy and prolonged artificial ventilation. J Thorac Cardiovasc Surg 30:356, 1955
18. Blair CR, Hughes JH: Scalene node biopsy: A reevaluation. J Thorac Cardiovasc Surg 52:595, 1966
19. Block AJ, Olsen GN: Preoperative pulmonary function testing. JAMA 235:257, 1976
20. Boyd AD, Gonzales LL, Altemeier WA: Disruption of chest wall closure following thoracotomy. J Thorac Cardiovasc Surg 52:47, 1966
21. Brewer LA III: Pleural partition procedure: A technic for management of large intrapleural dead space following lobectomy. Bull Soc Int Chir 17:305, 1958
22. Brewer LA, Bai AF: Surgery of the trachea and bronchi: Experience with the pericardial fat graft reinforcement. Am J Surg 89:331, 1955
23. Brewer LA, Gazzaniga A: Phrenoplasty: A new operation for the management of pleural dead space following pulmonary resection. Ann Thorac Surg 6:119, 1968
24. Buechner HA, Ziskind MM, Strug LH: Pneumoperitoneum as a space-occupying procedure in conjunction with pulmonary resection. J Thorac Cardiovasc Surg 33:229, 1957
25. Burdette WJ: Transplantation of the diaphragm for obliteration of dead space following pulmonary resection. J Thorac Cardiovasc Surg 33:803, 1957
26. Burman SO: The prophylactic use of digitalis before thoracotomy. Ann Thorac Surg 14:359, 1972
27. Carlens E: A new flexible double-lumen catheter for bronchospirometry. J Thorac Cardiovasc Surg 18:742, 1949
28. Carlens E: Mediastinoscopy: A method for inspection and tissue biopsy in the superior mediastinum. Dis Chest 36:343, 1959
29. Carlens E, Hanson HE, Nordenström B: Temporary unilateral occlusion of the pulmonary artery. A new method of determining separate lung function and of radiologic examination. J Thorac Cardiovasc Surg 22:527, 1951
30. Chaung TH, Dooling JA, Connally JM, Shifts LM: Pulmonary embolization from vascular stump thrombosis following pneumonectomy. Ann Thorac Surg 2:290, 1966
31. Churchill ED: The surgical treatment of carcinoma of the lung. J Thorac Cardiovasc Surg 2:254, 1933
32. Clagett OT, Geraci JE: A procedure for the management of postpneumonectomy empyema. J Thorac Cardiovasc Surg 45:141, 1963
33. Conkhn WS: Post-pneumonectomy empyema. J Thorac Cardiovasc Surg 55:634, 1968
34. Credle WF Jr, Smiddy JF, Elliott RC: Complications of fiberoptic bronchoscopy. Am Rev Respir Dis 109:67, 1974
35. Dack S: Symposium on cardiovascular–pulmonary problems before and after surgery. II. Postoperative problems. Postoperative myocardial infarction. Am J Cardiol 12:423, 1963
36. Dart CH, Scott SM, Takaro T: Six-year clinical experience using automatic stapling devices for lung resections. Ann Thorac Surg 9:535, 1970
37. Davia JE, Sienisen AW, Anderson RW: Uremia, deafness and paralysis due to irrigating antibiotic solution. Arch Intern Med 125:135, 1970
38. Deiraniva AK: Cardiac herniation following intrapericardial pneumonectomy. Thorax 29:545, 1974
39. Demos NJ, Timmes JJ: Myoplasty for closure of tracheobronchial fistula. Ann Thorac Surg 15:88, 1973
40. Dieter R, Pifarre R, Neville WE et al: Empyema treated with neomycin irrigation and closed chest drainage. J Thorac Cardiovasc Surg 59:496, 1970
41. Dippel WF, Ehrenhaft JL: Herniation of the heart after pneumonectomy. J Thorac Cardiovasc Surg 65:207, 1973
42. Dorman JP, Campbell D, Grover FL, Trinkle JK: Open thoracostomy drainage of postpneumonectomy empyema with bronchopleural fistula. J Thorac Cardiovasc Surg 66:979, 1973
43. Driscoll AC, Hobika JH, Etsten BE et al: Clinically unrecognized myocardial infarction following surgery. N Engl J Med 264:633, 1961
44. Eloesser L: An operation for tuberculosis empyema. Surg Gynecol Obstet 60:1096, 1935
45. Engelman RM, Spencer FC, Berg P: Postpneumonectomy esophageal fistula: Successful one-stage repair. J Thorac Cardiovasc Surg 59:871, 1970
46. Gates GF, Setle RS, Cope JA: Acute cardiac herniation with incarceration following pneumonectomy. Radiology 94:561, 1970
47. Ghosh P, Pakrashi BC: Cardiac dysrhythmias after thoracotomy. Br Heart J, 34:374, 1972
48. Glauser FL, Bartlett RA: Pneumoperitoneum in association with pneumothorax. Chest 66:536, 1974
49. Goldberg EM, Glicksman AS, Khan FR et al: Mediastinoscopy for assessing mediastinal spread in clinical staging of carcinoma of the lung. Cancer 25:347, 1970
50. Graham J, Usher FC, Perry JL et al: Marlex mesh as a prosthesis in the repair of thoracic wall defects. Ann Surg 151:469, 1960

51. Hutchin P, Terzi RG, Hollandsworth LA et al: Pulmonary congestion following infusion of large fluid loads in thoracic surgical patients. Ann Thorac Surg 8:339, 1969
52. Jolly PC, Hill LD III, Lawless PA et al: Parasternal mediastinotomy and mediastinoscopy. Adjuncts in the diagnosis of chest disease. J Thorac Cardiovasc Surg 66:549, 1973
53. Kirsh MH, Rotman H, Behrendt DM: Complications of pulmonary resection. Ann Thorac Surg 20:215, 1975
54. LeRoux BT, Stemmler P: Maintenance of chest wall stability. A further report. Thorax 26:424, 1971
55. Lewis FJ: Chondritis as a postoperative complication. Lancet 87:247, 1967
56. Lown B, Black H, Moore FD: Digitalis, electrolytes and the surgical patient. Am J Cardiol 6:309:1960
57. MacMahon H, Forrest JV, Weisz D, Sagel SS: Massive tumor embolism occurring during pneumonectomy. Ann Thorac Surg 17:395, 1974
58. MacLean LD, Meakins JL, Taguchi K et al: Host resistance in sepsis and trauma. Ann Surg 182:207, 1975
59. Malove G, Foster ED, Wilson JA, Munro RD: Bronchopleural fistula. Present-day study of an old problem. Ann Thorac Surg 11:1, 1971
60. Mauney FM Jr, Ebert PA, Sabiston DC Jr: Postoperative myocardial infarction: A study of predisposing factors, diagnosis and mortality in a high risk group of surgical patients. Ann Surg 172:497, 1970
61. Michelson E: Partial scapulectomy with subscapular muscle-flap operation for post-pneumonectomy empyema. Surg Gynecol Obstet 111:234, 1960
62. Moschcowitz AV: The treatment of diseases of the costal cartilages. Ann Surg 68:168, 1918
63. Mowry F, Reynolds EF: Cardiac rhythm disturbances complicating resectional surgery of the lung. Ann Intern Med 61:688, 1964
64. Nullin MJ, Zumbro GL, Fishback ME, Nelson TG: Pulmonary lobar gangrene complicating lobectomy. Ann Surg 175:62, 1972
65. Nelson JC, Nelson RM: The incidence of hospital wound infection in thoracotomies. J Thorac Cardiovasc Surg 54:586, 1967
66. Pacheco CR, Gongora E, Rivero O et al: Conservative treatment of bronchopleural fistula after pulmonary resection. J Thorac Surg 34:196, 1957
67. Patel DR, Shrivastav R, Sabety AM: Cardiac torsion following intrapericardial pneumonectomy. J Thorac Cardiovasc Surg 65:626, 1973
68. Pearson FG: Mediastinoscopy. Surg Annu 2:95, 1970
69. Rainer WG, Newby JP: Prevention of residual space problems after pulmonary resection. Am J Surg 114:744, 1967
70. Rams JJ, Harrison RW, Fry WA et al: Operative pulmonary artery pressure measurements as a guide to postoperative management and prognosis following pneumonectomy. Dis Chest 41:85, 1962
71. Robinson CLN: Pyogenic postpneumonectomy empyema. Can Med Assoc J 95:1294, 1966
72. Samson PC: Empyema thoracis. Essentials of present-day management. Ann Thorac Surg 11:210, 1971
73. Samson PC: Discussion of Zumbro GL Jr, Treasure R, Geiger JP, Green DC: Empyema after pneumonectomy. Ann Thorac Surg 15:620, 1973
74. Saunders GA, Carey RJ, Hewitt GC et al: Myocardial infarction in the elderly surgical patient. Geriatrics 26:122, 1971
75. Schuler JG: Intraoperative lobar torsion producing pulmonary infarction. J Thorac Cardiovasc Surg 65:951, 1973
76. Selle JG, Snyder WH III, Schreiber JT: Chylothorax: Indications for surgery. Ann Surg 177:245, 1973
77. Shields TW, Yjiki GT: Digitalization for prevention of arrhythmias following pulmonary surgery. Surg Gynecol Obstet 126:743, 1968
78. Silver AW, Espinas EE, Byron FX: Fate of the postresection space. Ann Thorac Surg 2:311, 1966
79. Sloan H, Morris JD, Figley M et al: Temporary unilateral occlusion of the pulmonary artery in the preoperative evaluation of thoracic patients. J Thorac Surg 30:591, 1955
80. Smith DE, Karish AF, Chapman JP et al: Healing of the bronchial stump after pulmonary resection. J Thorac Cardiovasc Surg 46:548, 1963
81. Stafford EG, Clagett OT: Postpneumonectomy empyema: Neomycin instillation and definitive closure. J Thorac Cardiovasc Surg 63:771, 1972
82. Stein M, Ching N, Robert EB, Nelson T: Pneumothorax complicating continuous ventilatory support. J Thorac Cardiovasc Surg 67:17, 1974
83. Symes JM, Page AJF, Flavell G: Esophagopleural fistula: A late complication after pneumonectomy. J Thorac Cardiovasc Surg 63:783, 1972
83a. Trinkle JK, Richardson JD, Franz JL et al: Management of flail chest without mechanical ventilation. Ann Thorac Surg 19:355,1975
84. Utley JR, Montgomery S, Sanderson RG: Atrial fibrillation induced by coagulating suction tip during mediastinoscopy. N Engl J Med 284:106, 1971
85. Walter CW, Kundsin RB: The airborne component of wound contamination and infection. Arch Surg 107:588, 1973
86. Wheat MW, Burford TH: Digitalis in surgery: Extension of classical indications. J Thorac Cardiovasc Surg 41:162, 1961
87. Widstrom A: Palsy of the recurrent nerve following mediastinoscopy. Chest 67:365, 1975
88. Wiederanders RE, White SM, Saichek HB: The effect of pulmonary resection on pulmonary artery pressures. Ann Surg 160:889, 1964
89. Williams CD, Cunningham JN, Falk EA et al: Chronic infection of the costal cartilages after thoracic surgical procedures. J Thorac Cardiovasc Surg 66:592, 1973
90. Wright GW, Place R, Princi F: The physiological effects of pneumoperitoneum upon the respiratory apparatus. Am Rev 60:706, 1949
91. Zumbro GL, Treasure R, Geiger JP, Green DC: Empyema after pneumonectomy. Ann Thorac Surg 15:615, 1973

25
Complications of Pediatric Thoracic Surgery

Arnold M. Salzberg | Kevin Ducey

OVERVIEW

Many complications of pediatric noncardiac thoracic surgery are similar to the ones reviewed in the adult chapter (Chap. 24). This section emphasizes those that are more specific to the pediatric patient.

Avoiding complications begins preoperatively with careful attention to associated anomalies of the cardiac, nervous, gastrointestinal, and genitourinary systems. The likelihood of various abnormalities should be appreciated and their presence established by specific diagnostic maneuvers. Not infrequently, the preoperative approach and risks of morbidity and mortality will be altered by the presence of additional, serious embryologic defects. Prior to surgery, newborns receive vitamin K and antibiotics. In infants and children, antibiotics are restricted to documented, suspected, or predictable sepsis; high-risk operation; or disease.

Intraoperative complications are either anesthetic or surgical. Specialized, experienced anesthesiologists are total partners and a first-priority, since proper airway and hemodynamic management, temperature monitoring, and protection from hypother-

FIG. 25-1. Right lung agenesis.

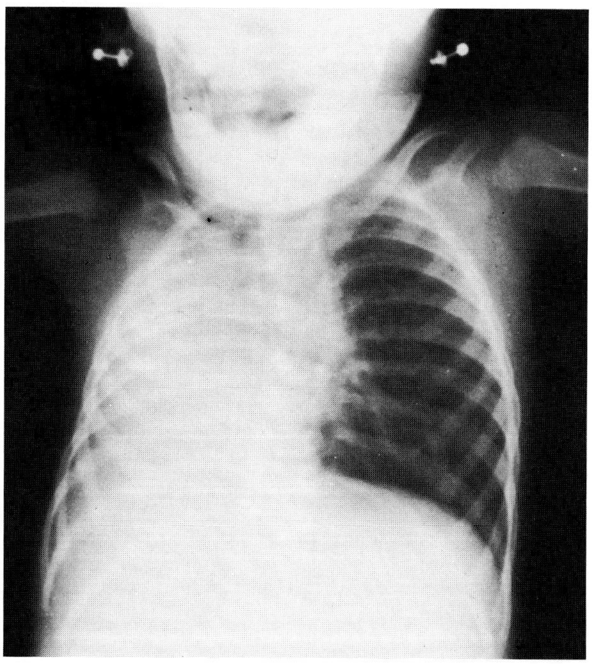

FIG. 25-2. Confirmation of right lung agenesis by pulmonary arteriography.

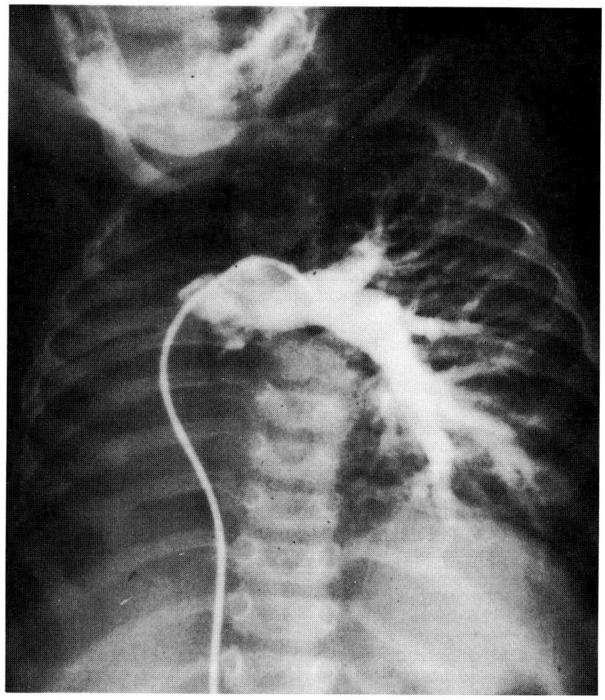

mia are essential, especially in neonates. Then, the orderly management of the operation with meticulous technique becomes a major factor in the success of the operative and postoperative course.

Congenital Lung Malformations

Congenital malformations of the lungs include an interesting array of clinical problems. The exact anatomy of each depends on the embryologic stage of respiratory foregut development during which the defect occurs.[14, 28, 38, 82] Early in extrauterine life, these lesions are space occupying with mediastinal shift, ipsilateral and contralateral lung compression, and respiratory distress. Later, infection is the clinical problem. Complications in this area are both diagnostic and operative.[53]

PULMONARY AGENESIS

Pulmonary agenesis presents as mild respiratory distress, critically aggravated by airway infection. A foreign body may be fatal. The chest radiograph is often interpreted as complete unilateral lung atelectasis with mediastinal and tracheal shift (Fig. 25-1). The issue can be resolved, if agenesis is considered, by bronchography, bronchoscopy, or pulmonary arteriography (Fig. 25-2). Arteriography is most desirable, since additional cardiac anomalies will be uncovered about 50% of the time.[96]

PULMONARY CYSTIC DISEASE

Pulmonary cystic disease may be bronchogenic, alveolar, or the more complex anomaly, cystic adenomatoid malformation.[100] Bronchogenic cysts occur as

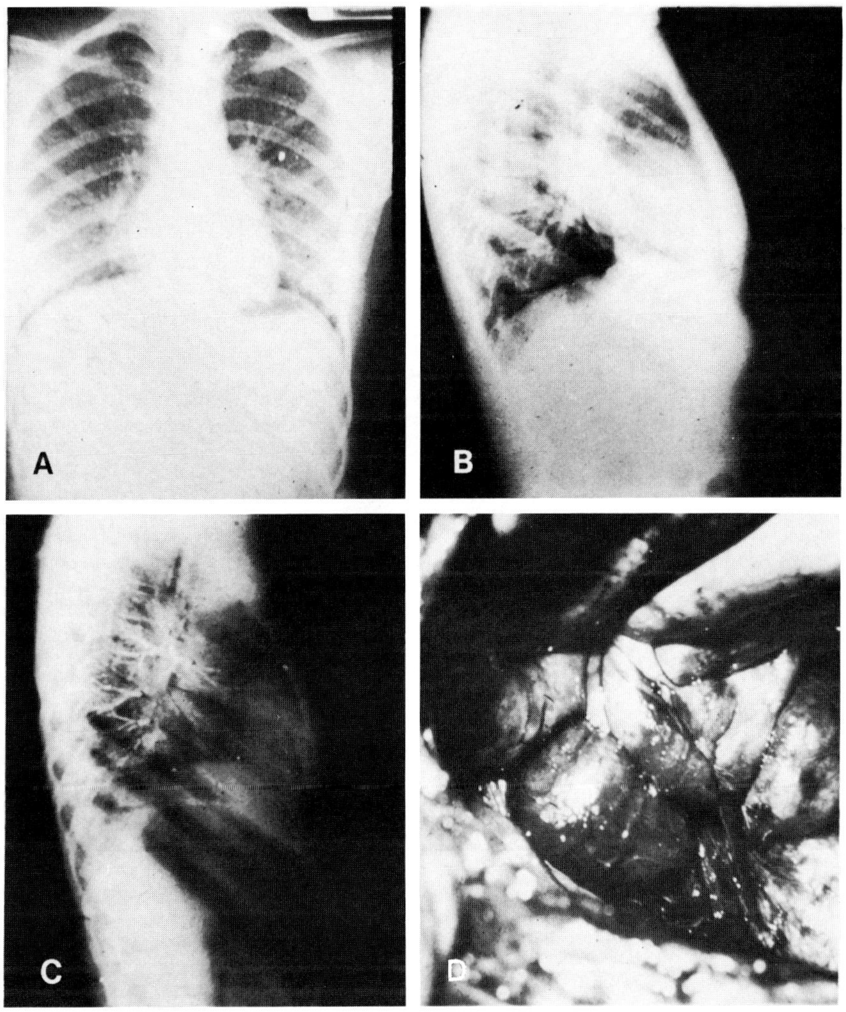

FIG. 25-3. A right mediastinal mass in a 10-year-old girl with a positive tuberculin skin test who did not respond to antituberculous therapy. The posteroanterior (*A*) and lateral (*B*) chest films show a mass posterior to the border of the heart, beneath the right hilum. The lateral bronchogram (*C*) failed to fill the middle lobe bronchus. (*D*) A bilobate bronchogenic cyst was found in the region of the inferior pulmonary vein and ligament. (Salzberg AM, Erlich FE: Congenital malformations of the lower respiratory tract. In Kendig EL, Jr., Chernick V [eds]: Disorders of the Respiratory Tract in Children, 3rd ed. Philadelphia, WB Saunders, 1977)

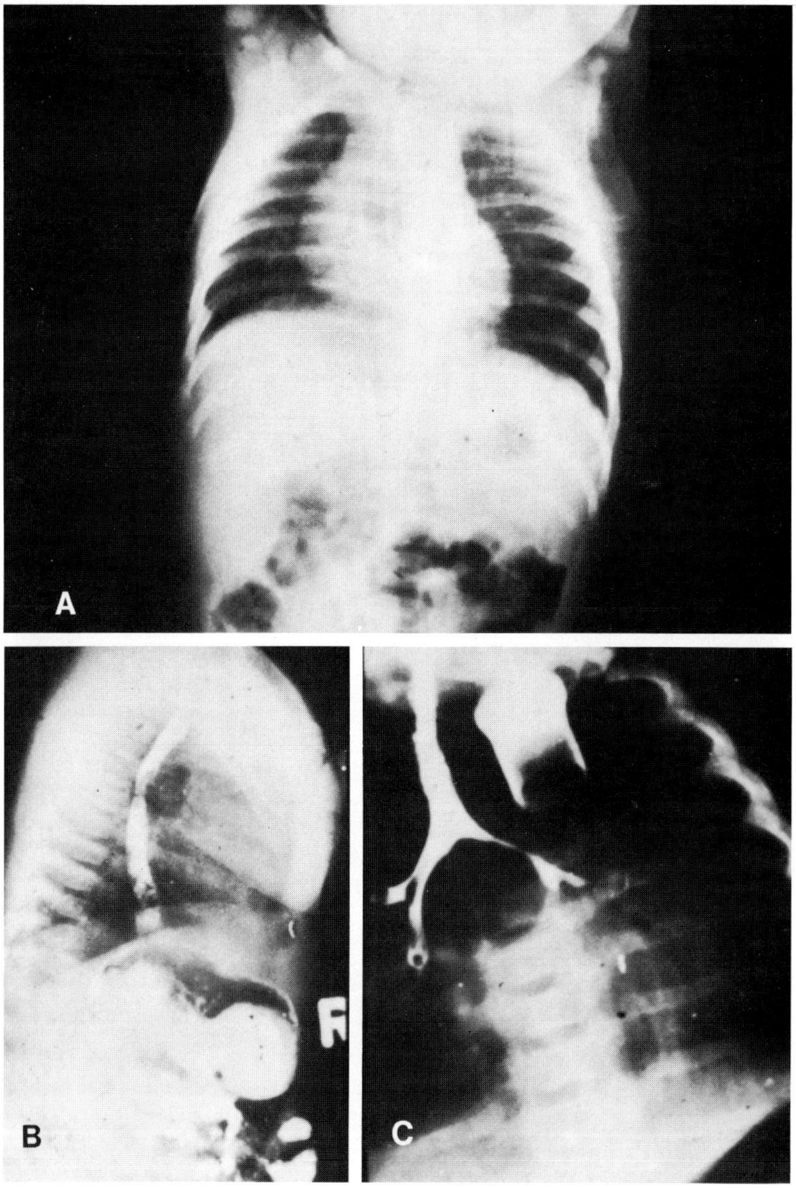

FIG. 25-4. A 2-month-old infant with intermittent severe respiratory distress. (*A*) The posteroanterior film shows radiolucency in the mid-mediastinum. The esophagogram (*B*) shows narrowing of the esophagus, and the tracheobronchogram (*C*) demonstrates widening of the bifurcation and narrowing of the left main-stem bronchus by an air-filled bronchogenic cyst. The cyst was resected from the left mainstem bronchus. (Salzberg AM, Erlich FE: Congenital malformations of the lower respiratory tract. In Kendig EL, Jr, Chernick V [eds]: Disorders of the Respiratory Tract in Children, 3rd ed. Philadelphia, WB Saunders, 1977)

mediastinal or paramediastinal masses. Accurate localization by tomograms, esophagograms, bronchoscopy, and bronchogram makes resection easier (Fig. 25-3). In this regard, it should be noted that bronchography is an adventure in infants, especially below 6 months of age. The contrast material should be oily Dionosil concentrated by removing one half of the supernatant, and its volume limited to 1 ml delivered unilaterally. Alveolarization should be minimal and with postoperative suction and parenchymal absorption, clearing will occur within 24 hours. Cyst removal usually does not pose any peculiar problems, and parenchymal resection is highly unlikely.

An uncomfortable and morbid location for a bronchogenic cyst is subcarinal.[72] Here, bronchial compression results in marked respiratory distress and should provoke urgent diagnostic and therapeutic steps. Intraoperative airway management for the subcarinal cyst must include preparation for one-

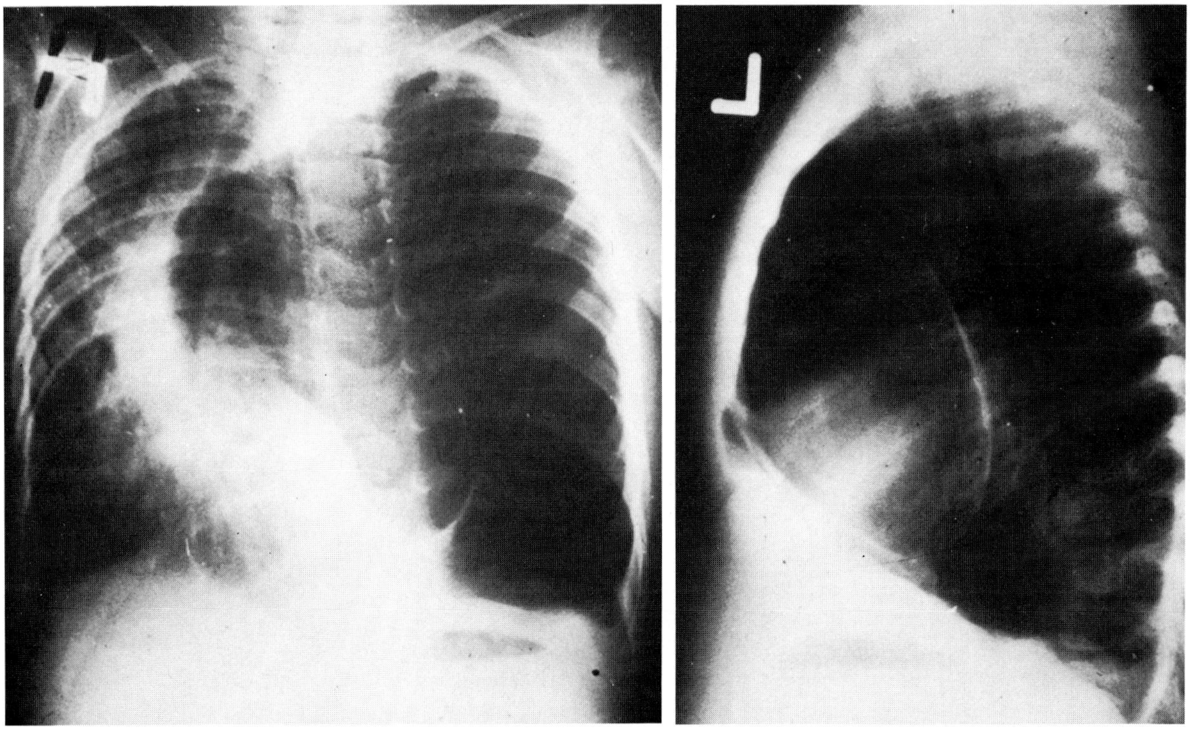

FIG. 25-5. A 1-year-old infant with minimal respiratory distress and gross hyperlucency of the left hemithorax. The mediastinum and left lung are herniated to the right, and there is compression of the right lung. (Sides are marked incorrectly.) *Left*, posteroanterior view; *right*, lateral view. (Salzberg AM, Erlich FE; Congenital malformations of the lower respiratory tract. In Kendig EL, Jr., Chernick V [eds]: Disorders of the Respiratory Tract in Children, 3rd ed. Philadelphia, WB Saunders, 1977)

lung anesthesia for resection and reconstruction, not unlike anesthesia for tracheal resection. The operative goal is complete resection of the cyst with maximum preservation of functional lung tissue (Fig. 25-4).

Alveolar or parenchymal pulmonary cysts will produce symptoms by pressure or sepsis (Fig. 25-5). Mediastinal and pulmonary decompression is best performed by thoracotomy with careful anesthetic precautions during induction, as described for obstructive emphysema (Fig. 25-6). The contaminated pulmonary cyst is in essence a lung abscess for which all appropriate medical therapy should have been tried and exhausted. Transbronchial surgical drainage with a catheter accurately placed under fluroscopy into the abscess through a Storz bronchoscope has been described by Groff.[34] Failure here logically leads to resection after accurate mapping of the diseased parenchyma by bronchography. Every step must be taken to avoid contralateral intraoperative bronchogenic spread of contaminated secretions (see Pulmonary Abscess). Again, preservation of functional lung tissue is mandatory.

CONGENITAL CYSTIC ADENOMATOID MALFORMATION

Congenital cystic adenomatoid malformation (CCAM) is a related but more complex anomaly, generally affecting a single lower lobe that is massively enlarged with displacement, compression, and distortion of adjacent structures (Fig 25-7).[39] Grossly, the lobe looks and feels like liver, and if respiratory distress is produced in the newborn, urgent thoracotomy is required. However, CCAM must be differentiated from congenital diaphragmatic hernia since the operative approach is dissimilar although the radiographic appearance of these conditions may be similar. Generally, the positions of gastrointestinal gas will differentiate the two. However, in a recent case, the subdiaphragmatic location of the stomach

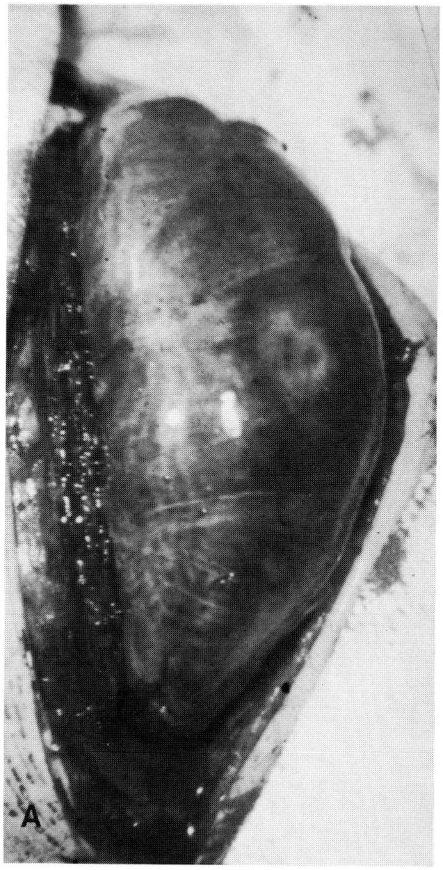

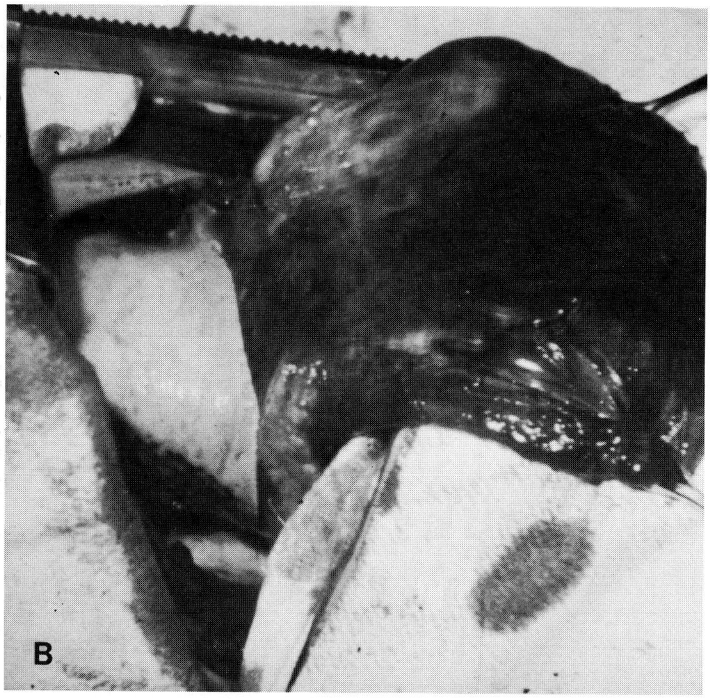

FIG. 25-6. (*A*) Extrusion of a tense left upper lobe pulmonary cyst through an intercostal incision with relief of respiratory distress, accentuated during induction of anesthesia. (*B*) The resulting deflated multilocular cyst with lower-lobe reexpansion. (Salzberg AM, Erlich FE: Congenital malformations of the lower respiratory tract. In Kendig EL, Jr., Chernick V [eds]: Disorders of the Respiratory Tract in Children, 3rd ed. Philadelphia, WB Saunders, 1977)

FIG. 25-7. A 2-day-old infant with critical respiratory distress and a mediastinum shifted to the right. In the left mid- and lower thorax there are multiple cystlike areas intermingled with consolidation. There is a normal gastric air bubble. An unnecessary upper GI series confirmed the preoperative diagnosis of CCAM. (Salzberg AM, Erlich FE: Congenital malformations of the lower respiratory tract. In Kendig EL, Jr., Chernick V [eds]: Disorders of the Respiratory Tract in Children, 3rd ed. Philadelphia, WB Saunders, 1977)

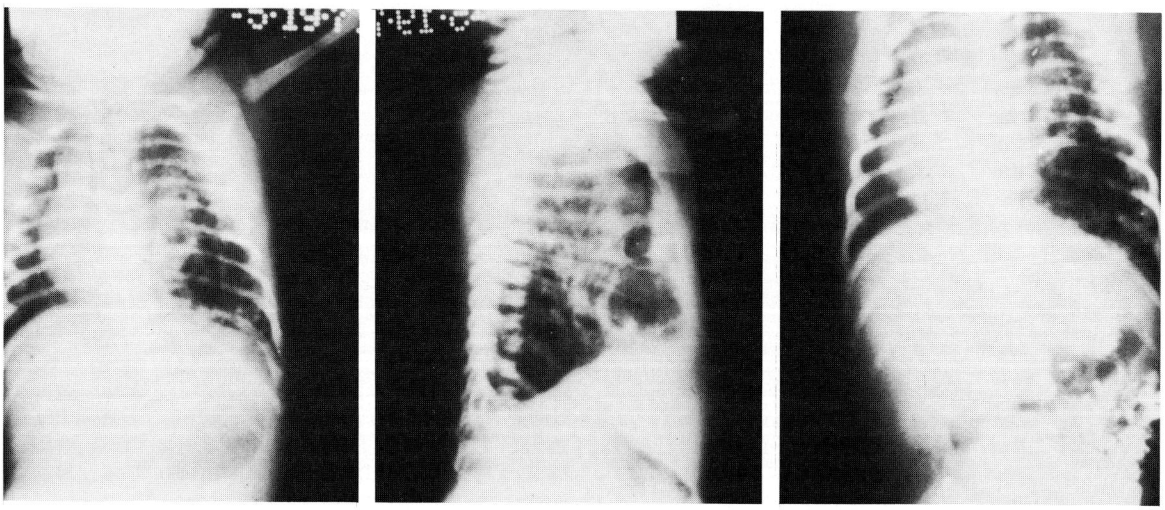

and bowel led to the referral diagnosis of CCAM in a neonate with respiratory distress in whom contrast studies were not feasible (Fig. 25-8). Exploratory thoracotomy revealed a small posterolateral diaphragmatic hernia with several loops of jejunum in the chest. The typical Bochdalek hernia is more expeditiously repaired by laparotomy, but if the distinction between the two is in doubt, thoracotomy is the route, since both can be handled from above the diaphragm.

The treatment of CCAM is lobectomy. Massive enlargement of the affected lobe makes exposure and dissection difficult. In one case, CCAM of a right lower lobe was adherent to and displacing the right middle lobe bronchus. Inadequate exposure resulted in a laceration of the middle lobe bronchus and loss of this lobe (Fig. 25-9). Despite an otherwise satisfactory surgical result, this is an avoidable complication. The distinction between CCAM and intralobar pulmonary sequestration may be unclear during the operation, since both may possess a systemic arterial supply to the involved lobe. Cavalier division of the inferior pulmonary ligament in the presence of such an artery can result in significant hemorrhage.

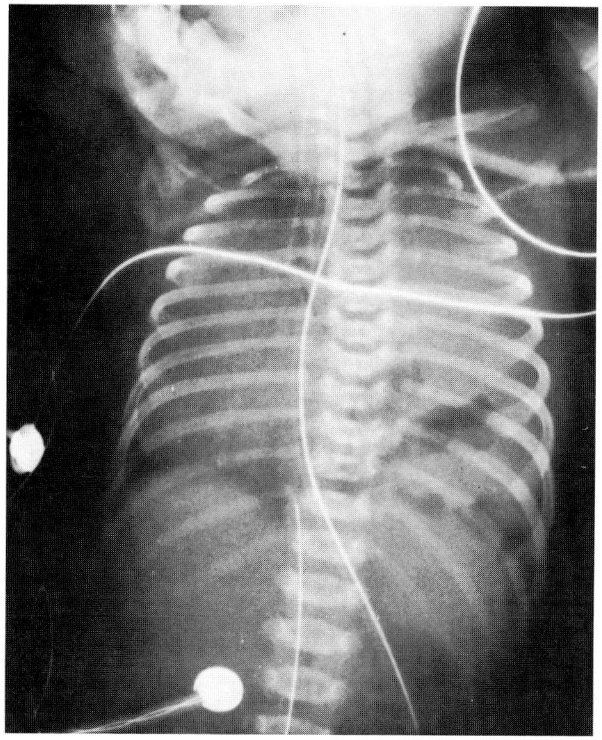

FIG. 25-8. A newborn in severe respiratory distress with a preoperative diagnosis of CCAM, not a Bochdalek hernia.

CONGENITAL LOBAR EMPHYSEMA

Congenital lobal emphysema is a more frequent reason for respiratory distress in the newborn.[60, 64, 92] Overexpansion of the involved lobe results in me-

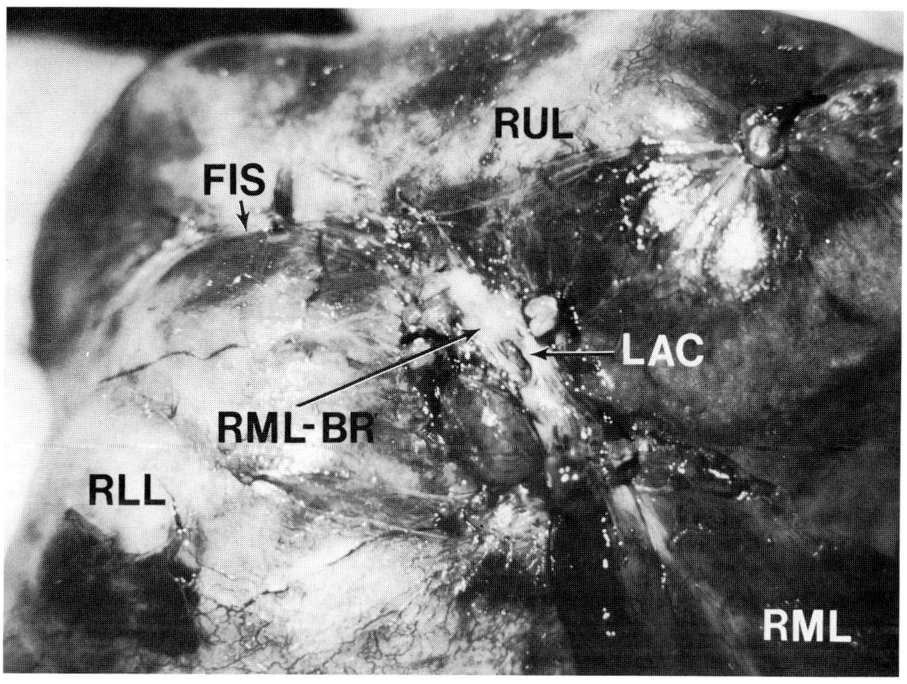

FIG. 25-9. A close-up view of a case of CCAM shows the right upper lobe (*RUL*), the middle lobe (*RML*), and the right lower lobes (*RLL*). Both fissures (*FIS*) were fused secondary to a severe inflammatory reaction. Difficult exposure led to a laceration (*LAC*) of the middle lobe bronchus (*RML-BR*).

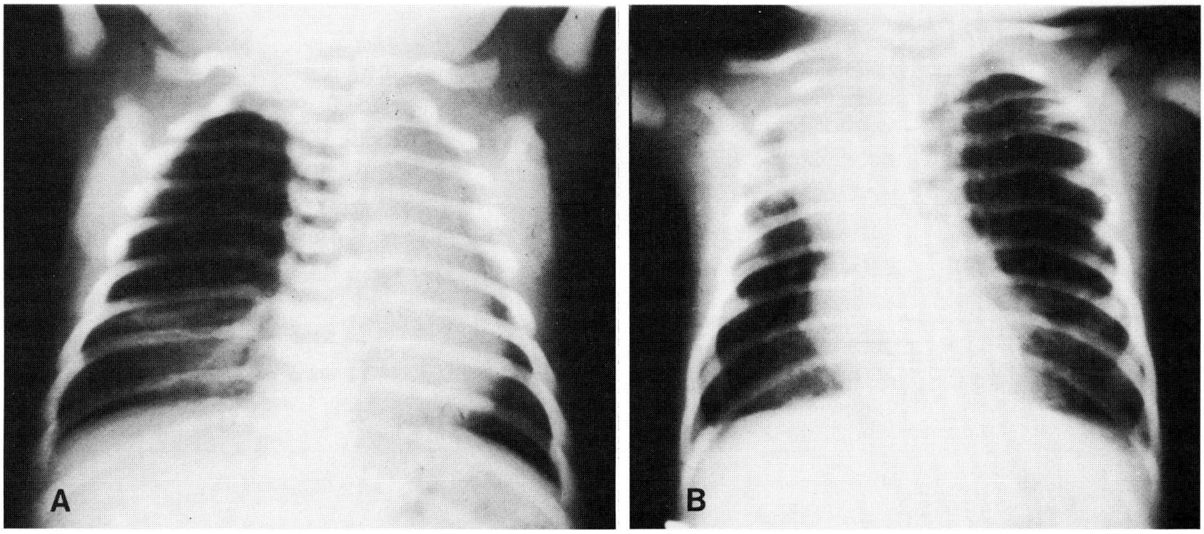

FIG. 25-10. Two newborns with respiratory distress due to congenital lobar emphysema. (*A*) Right upper lobe obstructive emphysema, a mediastinal shift to the left, and compression in the contralateral lung and right lower lobe are evident. (*B*) In the second infant there is left upper lobe emphysema without similar mirror-image findings.

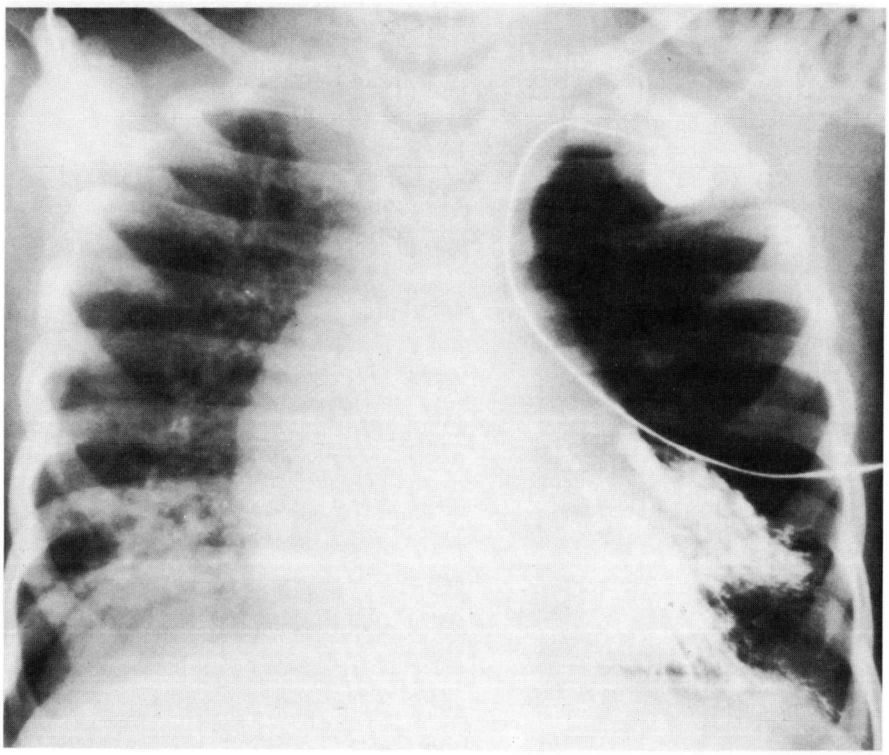

FIG. 25-11. An 8-month-old infant with congenital lobar emphysema. This infant had respiratory distress, bilateral wheezing, and air trapping in the left upper lobe. There is compression of the left lower lobe, a mediastinal shift to the right, and some compression of the right lung. The bronchogram further illustrates the unilateral compression.

diastinal shift and compression of remaining lung tissue (Fig. 25-10). Most cases have no discernible intraluminal bronchial obstruction, although Murray and colleagues feel that preoperative bronchoscopy may be curative occasionally by removing a mucous plug producing the problem.[69] The hyperlucent parenchyma is almost always a unilateral upper or middle lobe. This must be differentiated from asthma, pneumothorax, simple lung cyst, unilateral hyperlucent lung syndrome, and extrinsic bronchial compression.[16, 24, 101] Bronchoscopy and bronchograms are helpful in this task.

The diagnosis of congenital lobar obstructive emphysema should be made with some hesitation when the child is over 6 months of age because asthma with excessive lobar bronchospasm can mimic it. The radiographic findings of mediastinal shift and ipsilateral and contralateral pulmonary compression secondary to upper lobe overexpansion are similar in both. A bronchogram confirms these findings, while bronchoscopy is not helpful (Fig. 25-11). Nevertheless, with increasing respiratory distress, thoracotomy becomes mandatory to relieve the compression. With asthma, the operative finding is a large overexpanded, but not emphysematous lobe. There is postoperative relief, but symptoms recur from migratory lobar distention.

Observation and whether or not there is improvement determine the need for thoracotomy in congenital obstructive lobar emphysema. Induction of anesthesia is the crucial event and should forestall further overexpansion of the involved lobe and sudden respiratory deterioration. Similarly, thoracotomy is performed rapidly and herniation of the emphysematous lobe quickly relieves the worrisome situation. Treatment is lobectomy and is usually straightforward, although some have advocated segmental resection.[59] There is prompt respiratory relief, and the long-term prognosis is excellent.

PULMONARY SEQUESTRATION

In pulmonary sequestration the affected lung tissue has no normal bronchial communication, but it does have a systemic arterial supply. (Fig. 25-12).[78, 79] Extralobar sequestration is totally separate from the lung and is usually encased in pleura between the diaphragm and the lower lobe. It is asymptomatic and discovered fortuitously on a chest roentgenogram performed for other reasons. Removal is for diagnosis. Intralobar sequestration is contained within the lung substance, with venous drainage occasionally into the cava. Both evolve as distinct second lower respiratory buds from the foregut.

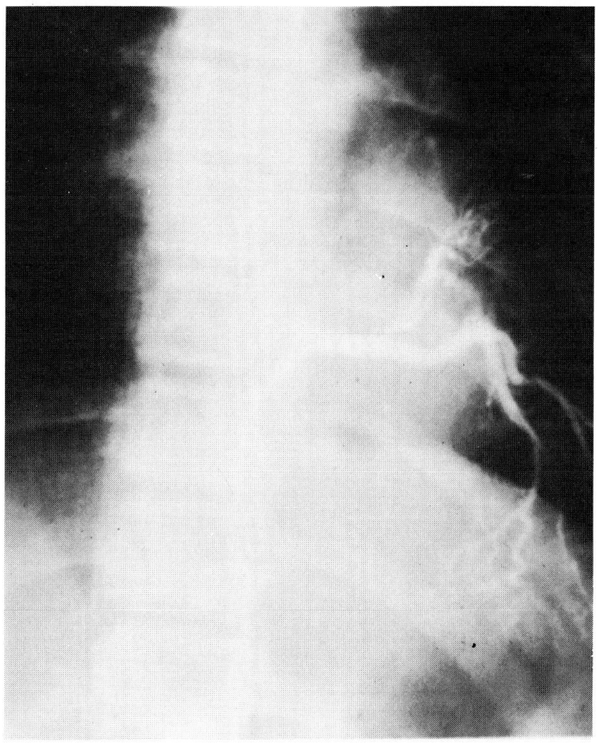

FIG. 25-12. A preoperative aortogram demonstrates the large systemic arterial supply to the left lower lobe in a case of intrapulmonary sequestration.

Intralobar sequestration is more frequent and nocuous, presenting during the first 5 years of life with repetitive suppuration in one lobe, preferentially the left lower and with or without abscess formation. There are characteristic bronchographic findings consisting of elevation and concavity of the lower lobe bronchus over the sequestered parenchymal mass (Fig. 25-13). Simultaneously, bronchoscopy will rule out the presence of a foreign body. Occasionally, sequestration will displace the adjacent lung and mediastinum with respiratory distress.

Systemic arteries from the thoracic and abdominal aorta are very likely and will be found within the inferior pulmonary ligament or as direct branches from the adjacent aorta. Preoperative aortography will demonstrate the size and number of abnormal vascular channels and confirm the diagnosis. However, this procedure is not mandatory and not utilized universally.

Hemorrhage from the systemic arterial supply is the major operative risk. Careful inspection and dissection of the inferior pulmonary ligament and ad-

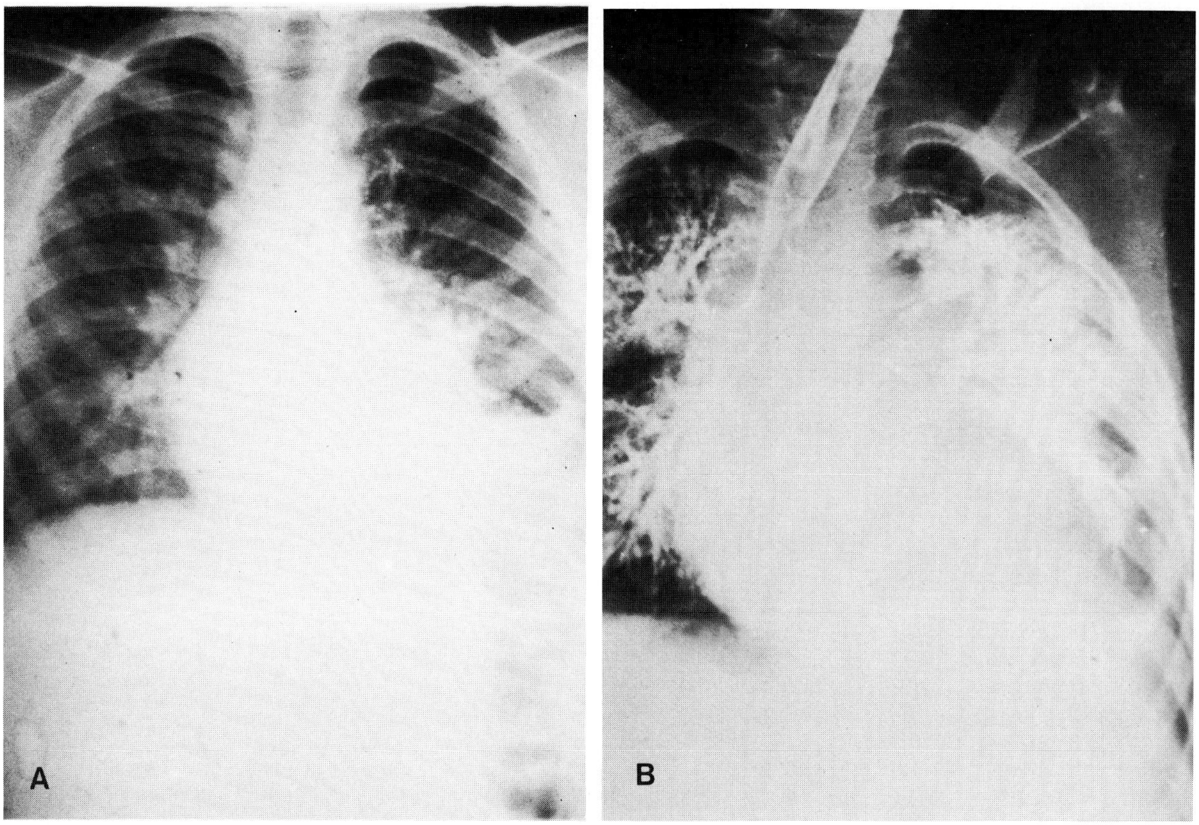

FIG. 25-13. (*A*) This 5-year-old child had repeated pulmonary infection for 2 years. The posteroanterior film shows intrapulmonary sequestration and abscess in the left lower lobe. (*B*) A bronchogram of the same child shows typical elevation of the left main-stem bronchus and lower lobe bronchi. (Salzberg AM, Erlich FE: Congenital malformations of the lower respiratory tract. In Kendig EL, Jr., Chernick V [eds]: Disorders of the Respiratory Tract in Children, 3rd ed. Philadelphia, WB Saunders, 1977)

jacent aorta will clarify the anatomy, and this step must be done with diligence and care. Arteries arising from the abdominal aorta and supplying the sequestration from this direction can retract into the abdomen if inadvertently severed without ligation. After these vascular maneuvers, the intralobar sequestration is managed with standard lobectomy. No attempt should be made to remove the sequestration from within the lower lobe (Fig. 25-14).

It is likely that sequestration arises from the primitive foregut as a second lower distinct respiratory diverticulum below the main, normal pulmonary anlage. This communication with the esophagus may persist and lead the operator to a dissection in juxtaposition to the esophagus. The placement of a nasogastric tube helps in the proper orientation and differentiation between esophageal and pulmonary tissue. Successful separation is then accomplished with the esophagus clearly in view (Fig. 25-15).

Chest Infections

The majority of serious pediatric chest infections are treated medically. However, several suppurative conditions may have significant surgical complications both in diagnosis and management.

MEDIASTINITIS

Mediastinitis is a potentially fulminant and life-threatening infection. Insidious spread through cervical and mediastinal fascial planes leads to extensive contamination prior to diagnosis. Most com-

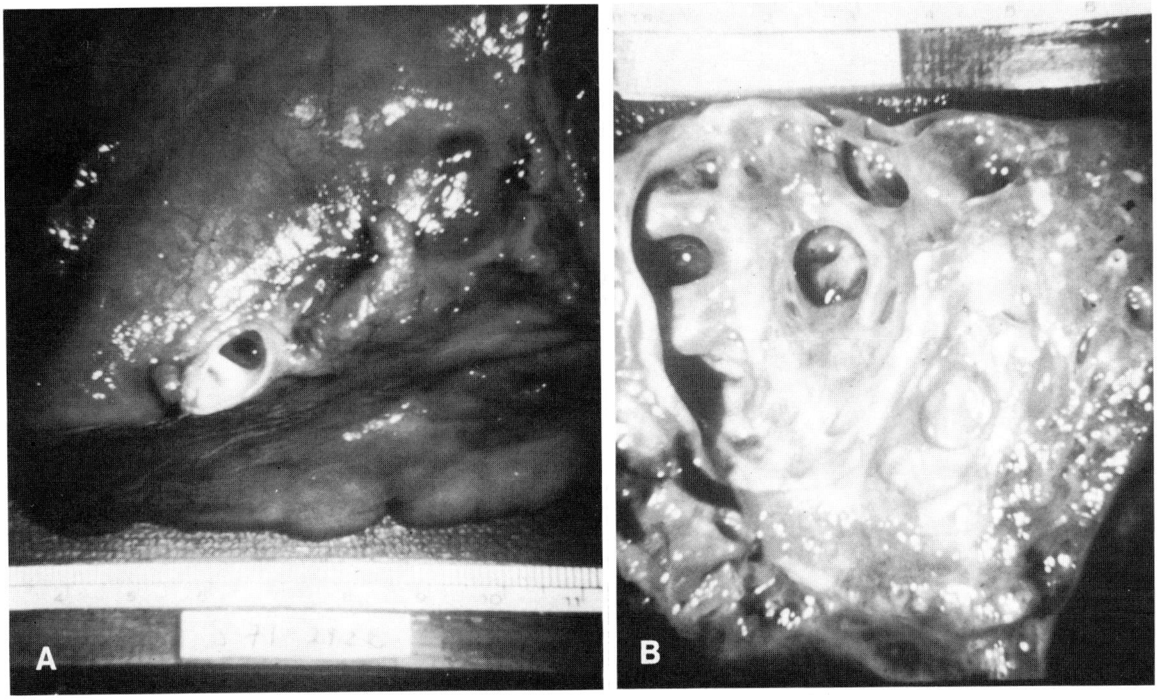

FIG. 25-14. (*A*) Intrapulmonary sequestration of the left lower lobe with an aberrant systemic artery in the lower left corner. (*B*) A cut specimen shows multiple cysts and compressed surrounding lung parenchyma.

monly, disruption of the pharynx or esophagus is produced by foreign bodies, instrumentation, or anastomotic leak. Modern aggressive neonatal intensive care requires frequent manipulation of the pharynx and esophagus with laryngoscopes and endotracheal and nasogastric tubes.

Perforations generally occur in low-birth-weight premature infants. Typically, a nasogastric tube perforates the hypopharynx and courses along the esophagus until it reperforates the medial parietal pleura into a pleural space (Fig. 25-16). Tubes terminating in the pericardium and retroperitoneum have been reported. The diagnosis is suspected if intubation is difficult or if excessive blood-tinged oropharyngeal secretions are noted. An abnormal location of the nasogastric tube on x-ray examination is the usual first indication. Pneumomediastinum or pneumothorax is common. The diagnosis is confirmed by esophagogram but occasionally is delayed, and sepsis may be the first sign. The mortality rate can vary between 17% to 70%.[20, 71, 99]

Prevention by the education of physicians and nurses to the potential hazards of traumatic, careless intubations is the first step in avoiding this complication. Early diagnosis is the next priority. In the neonate, questionably located airway, esophageal,

FIG. 25-15. A Penrose drain beneath the esophagus, which had a thick fibrous connection to the clamped residual sequestrated pulmonary tissue.

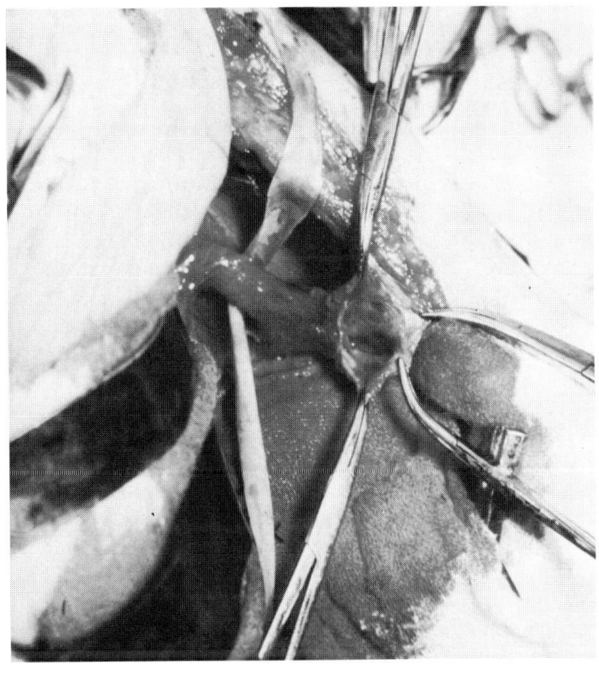

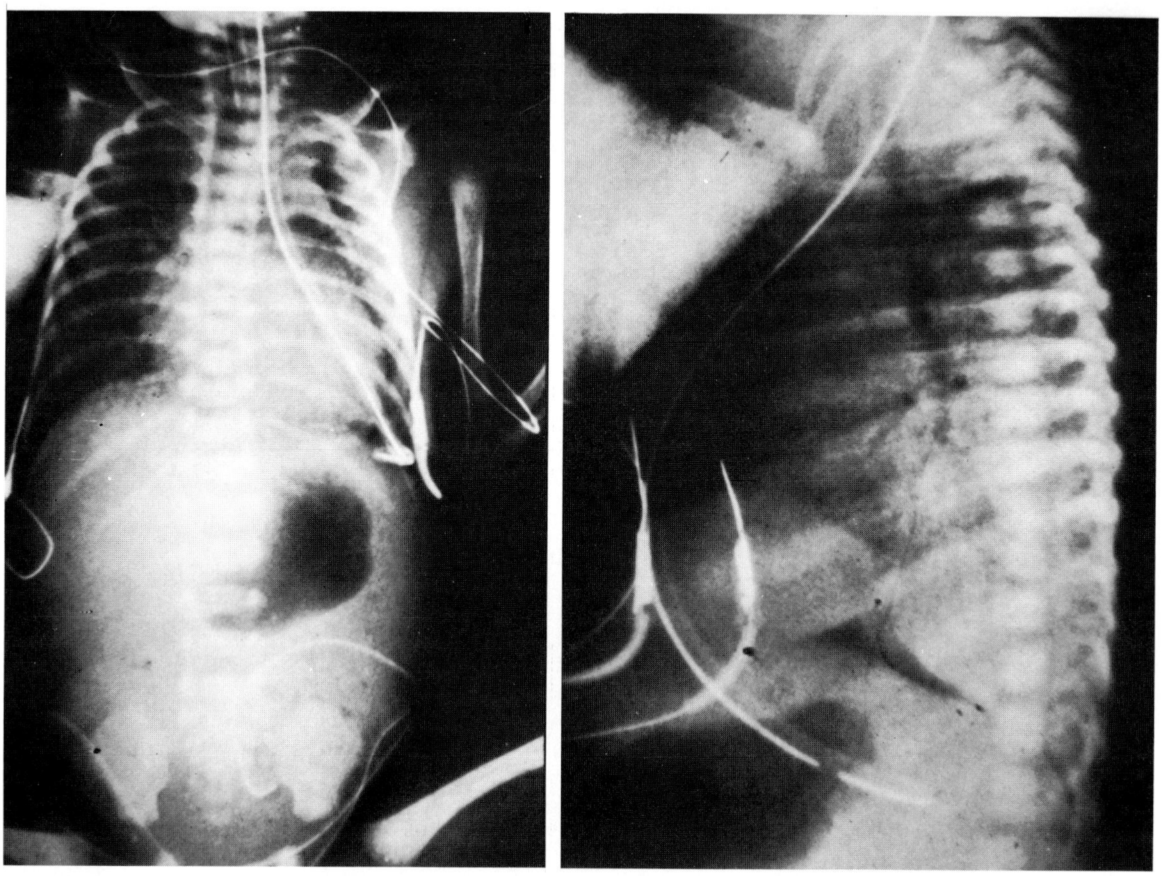

FIG. 25-16. High esophageal perforation in a newborn by a nasogastric tube. The extraesophageal and anterior thoracic location of the tube is obvious in both the posteroanterior (*left*) and lateral (*right*) views. The infant survived with nonsurgical therapy.

and gastric tubes should be confirmed radiographically. When the diagnosis of pharyngoesophageal perforation is made quickly, antibiotics, gastric decompression, and hyperalimentation are utilized and may suffice. Surgical intervention is required for uncontrolled local or systemic sepsis. Drainage of the medistinum through a cervical incision is generally adequate. Rarely, thoracotomy is required for low esophageal perforations with malignant mediastinitis.

Diagnostic errors can lead to unnecessary or misplaced thoracic incisions. First, esophageal perforation may be mistaken for esophageal atresia.[11] The esophagogram should discriminate between these two. Second the esophagogram may be misinterpreted to indicate an intrathoracic esophageal perforation when, in fact, a cervical injury is present. In Figure 25-17 contrast material was incorrectly interpreted as normal esophagus with low intrapleural perforation. This led to a thoracotomy for a supposedly intrathoracic perforation, when actually a typical cervical injury was present with contrast material in a paraesophageal mediastinal false tract.

PULMONARY ABSCESS

Pulmonary abscess is primarily a medical disease with surgical implications. It may occur in many clinical settings, including bacterial and fungal pneumonias, cystic fibrosis, bronchiectasis, immune deficiencies, foreign-body aspiration, lung cysts, sequestration, and chronic granulomatous disease of childhood. Chalasia, achalasia, hiatal hernia, and dysphagia secondary to brain damage may play a significant etiologic role.

The initial and often only treatment is specific antibiotics with postural drainage and chest physiotherapy. Inadequate drainage may be improved by bronchoscopy alone or transbronchial insertion of a catheter through a Storz bronchoscope into the abscess cavity under fluoroscopic control.[34] Bronchoscopy with removal of an obstructing foreign body may be curative for the distal abscess.

Surgical resection is required for extralobar sequestration, life-threatening hemorrhage, and abscesses recalcitrant to medical therapy. The peculiar pediatric surgical threat is endobronchial spill with contralateral contamination. The possibility of this complication, which has occurred twice in our experience, is exaggerated by the lateral decubitus operative position and the regrettable lack of a pediatric Carlen's tube. Obviously, the incidence of spill may be lessened by anterior or posterior (Overholt) thoracotomy. Unfortunately, the posterolateral approach, by habit, remains the basic incision. Under these circumstances, selective bronchial blocking by a Fogarty or Swan–Ganz catheter may assume greater importance.[102] This can be accomplished bronchoscopically under anesthesia and fluoroscopy prior to thoracotomy. In addition, intraoperative manipulation of the abscess should be minimized prior to bronchial division. Finally, for large abscesses that prevent exposure, intraoperative needle aspiration, as suggested by Clatworthy, seems reasonable.[21]

EMPYEMA

Today empyema is uncommon because bacterial pneumonias are promptly eradicated with appropriate antibiotics. When it is present, treatment consists of urgent drainage of the pleural abscess by dependent-tube thoracostomy after needle localization, followed by readjustment of antibiotics, depending on culture and sensitivity. Satisfactory drainage may be prevented by multiple loculations not accessible to a tube in the primary space. These septic pockets can be localized by cross-sectional imaging with computed tomography or sonography. Drainage is then accomplished with one or more additional tubes under sonographic control. Rarely is thoracotomy or decortication required.[68]

FIG. 25-17. A cervical esophageal perforation with contrast material in a paraesophageal mediastinal false tract. *Left*, posteroanterior view; *right*, lateral view.

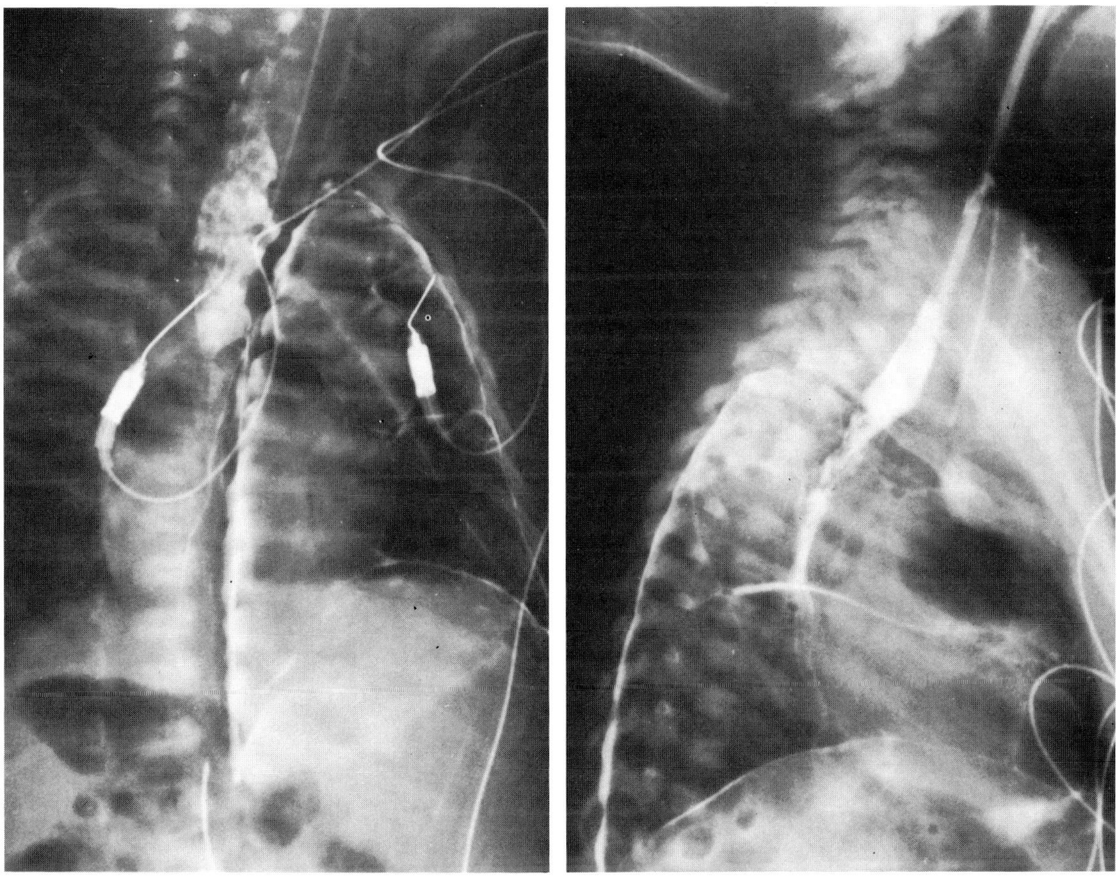

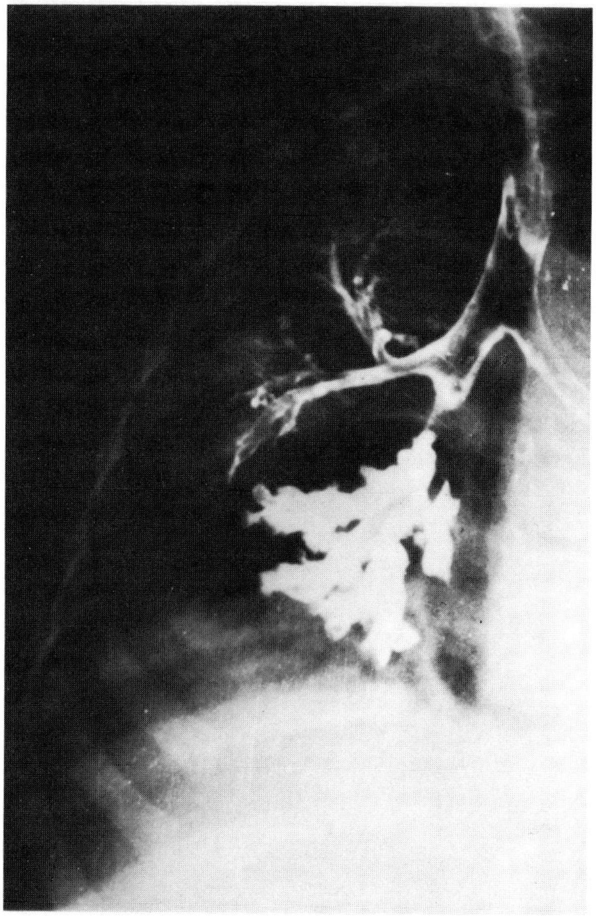

FIG. 25-18. Lower lobe bronchiectasis in a markedly symptomatic 7-year-old requiring resection.

BRONCHIECTASIS

Bronchiectasis is also uncommon because chronic childhood pulmonary disease has been prevented. Treatment is primarily postural drainage and antibiotics, but surgery may be required for persistent hemoptysis, atelectasis, and recurrent, localized suppuration with irreversible distortion of bronchopulmonary architecture that is not responsive to current medical therapy.

Resectional surgery is predicated on accurate localization of recalcitrant lobar and segmental bronchial disease. Bronchography under general anesthesia then becomes indispensable and should include the entire tracheobronchial tree in two stages in patients under 4 years of age. In children over 4 years, bilateral bronchograms without alveolarization can be performed with warm oily Dionosil with half the supernatent discarded (Fig. 25-18). The pediatric anesthesiologist must then aspirate the contrast through the endotracheal tube at the conclusion of the procedure. The case for pulmonary resection is strengthened if destruction of function and anatomy coexist. This at times can be documented with ventilation–perfusion radioisotope scans.

Finally, preoperative chest physiotherapy, postural drainage, and antibiotics can diminish the postoperative pulmonary complication rate.

CYSTIC FIBROSIS

Cystic fibrosis is hereditary and transmitted by a mendelian recessive gene.[91] The pulmonary component is its major cause of morbidity. Inability to clear thick inspissated bronchial secretions produces obstruction, infection, and eventually a spectrum of pulmonary and pleural pathology including pneumonitis, bronchiectasis, abscess, fibrosis, atelectasis, emphysema, hemorrhage, and pneumothorax. Aggressive medical management has resulted in significant prolongation of life with a corresponding increase in the complications that require surgical consultation.

The persistent, tenacious purulent bronchial secretions are often the basis for exacerbations that are expressed symptomatically by fever, sepsis, and dyspnea and pathologically by radiographic progression of the pulmonary disease (Fig. 25-19). Surgical drainage and lavage through contemporary bronchoscopic equipment complements antibiotic therapy, postural drainage, and physiotherapy, clearing the tracheobronchial tree of secretions and temporarily interrupting the deterioration of pulmonary function. Symptomatic improvement is noted in over 90% of patients after this procedure. However, objective changes in arterial blood gases and radiographs are usually not concomitant.[25, 31, 80]

The maneuver is performed through a Storz bronchoscope under general anesthesia after hyperventilation. The hazard is cardiac arrhythmia from hypoxia and hypercarbia secondary to compromised pulmonary function, instillation of lavage fluid, and the presence of an airway (bronchoscope) that is often down one main bronchus and does not always provide a closed anesthetic system. Preoperatively, cardiac monitors are applied, venous and arterial lines established, and lidocaine kept nearby. The lavage is performed with large volumes of 10% acetylcysteine followed by saline irrigation. At the conclusion, residual fluid is removed from the bronchial tree, and this is continued through an endotracheal tube postoperatively because of difficulty in spontaneous clearing of retained lavage fluid. The endotracheal tube is left in place until all excess tracheobronchial secretions are removed and the tube can no longer be tolerated. All patients are managed in the pediatric intensive-care unit for 24 hours.

Pneumothorax complicates cystic fibrosis, especially in the older child, adolescent, and young adult. The initial episode is treated with tube thoracostomy. Recurrences with either unilateral or contralateral pneumothoraces are high and may approach 50%. Instillation of sclerosing agents or thoracotomy with pleural abrasion has been done for repetitive pneumothoraces that occur in spite of adequate tube drainage.[62, 94]

Hemoptysis is potentially life threatening, since it occurs with far advanced bilateral disease. The sources are enlarged, tortuous bronchial arteries. When hemorrhage is massive or persistent or interferes with pulmonary function, invasive management should be considered. Bronchoscopy and angiography are jointly employed to localize the site of bleeding, and if facilities and personnel are available, bronchial artery embolization should be attempted, as suggested by Fellows and Schuster.[32, 97] In the series of Fellows and colleagues, over 90% of bleeding episodes were controlled. Recurrences were frequent (40%) but minor in degree. Ischemia of the spinal cord or inadvertent embolization to other vessels is a hazard but did not occur in their 13 patients. Without embolization, thoracotomy is a possibility, but the mortality will be excessive in the presence of a predictably fatal illness.

Respiratory Foreign Bodies

Complications can occur in the diagnosis and management of aspirated respiratory foreign bodies.[58]

No matter how classic the symptoms and physical findings, chest roentgenograms in various positions are indispensable for the diagnosis and should include posterior–anterior, lateral, and bilateral decubitus films.[13, 17] The presence of a radiopaque object poses no problem. The majority of foreign bodies, however, are not opaque, and more often diagnostic criteria depend upon obstructive emphysema rather than upon atelectasis (Fig. 25-20). Although emphysema may be a gross finding in many

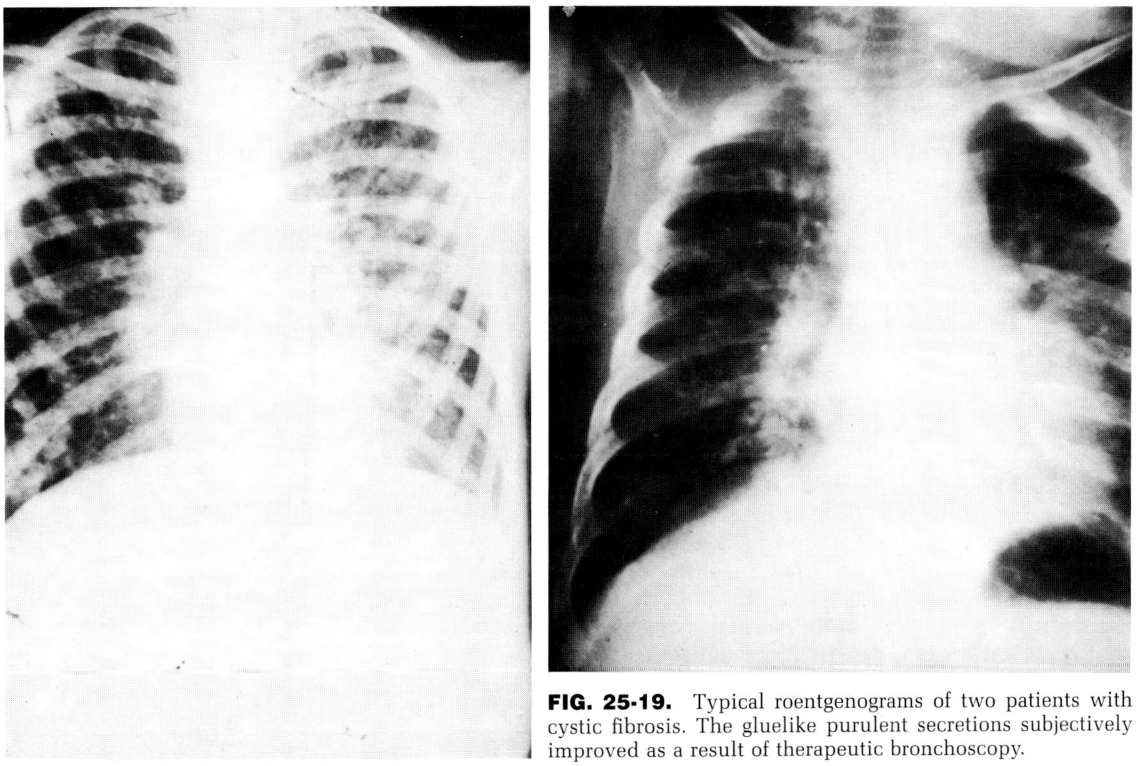

FIG. 25-19. Typical roentgenograms of two patients with cystic fibrosis. The gluelike purulent secretions subjectively improved as a result of therapeutic bronchoscopy.

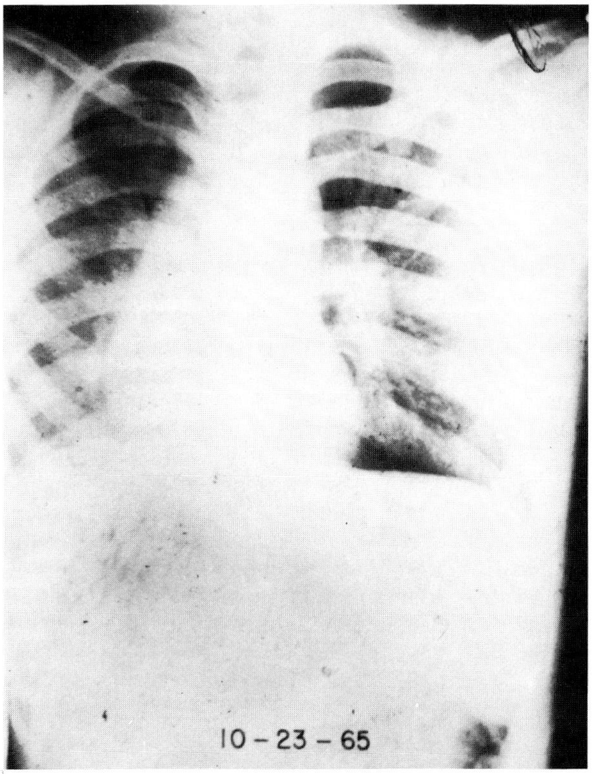

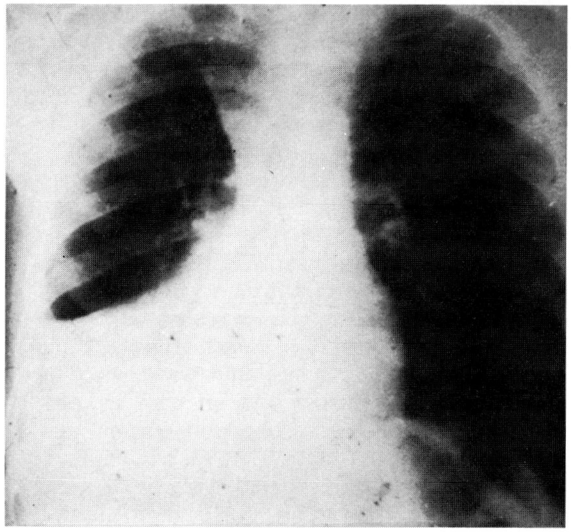

FIG. 25-20. (*Left*) There is a peanut in the left main-stem bronchus, with obstructive emphysema. (*Right*) A peanut is completely obstructing the intermediate bronchus, and there is distal atelectasis.

children, the overexpansion at times is subtle, and confirmation of this air trapping by fluoroscopy in a dyspneic, uncooperative infant is difficult. Therefore, the lateral decubitus films assume great importance. In normal decubitus chest x-ray films, the down, dependent lung will be smaller than it is in the posterior–anterior film because of immobility and fixation. With a partially obstructing, air-trapping, nonopaque foreign body, the space occupied by the dependent lung remains the same as it is in the posterior–anterior film. This is a dependable, sensitive finding in questionable cases and will avoid some diagnostic complications (Fig. 25-21).

Chronic respiratory foreign bodies may present as fever, hemoptysis, and superimposed pneumonia or abscess.[4, 26, 47, 50, 54, 63] Even more disconcerting is the normal chest x-ray film, including the decubitus films. The dictum to follow is to consider foreign body and bronchoscopy in patients with unexplained, chronic, nonspecific pulmonary disease, undiagnosed hemoptysis and in patients with normal roentgenograms but with a suspicious history, physical examination, and symptomatology.

Respiratory distress from aspiration is not confined to foreign bodies in the tracheobronchial tree. Acute and chronic dyspnea may accompany foreign bodies of the upper esophagus impinging on the trachea. If the trachea is deformed on the x-ray film, and dysphagia concurrent, esophagoscopy should be done[15, 59]

Endoscopic management of chronic foreign bodies can be complicated by granulation tissue, stenosis, bleeding, infection, and purulent secretions. The extraction should always be through contemporary endoscopic equipment that provides a closed, safe route for general anesthesia and ventilation, a separate instrument channel in the bronchoscope sheath for instruments and suction, and continuous telescopic magnification unobstructed by aspirating catheters or foreign-body forceps (Fig. 25-22).[12, 33, 51] Even under these improved circumstances, extraction can be difficult and tedious, especially with foreign bodies such as peanuts that tend to crumble with metal forceps. In order to avoid this annoying complication, these aspirated objects are best removed by a Fogarty catheter inserted through the instrument channel. The balloon is inflated distally to the foreign body and drawn against the object, which is then impinged into a metal pouch created by the withdrawal of the telescope for 1 cm from the tip of the sheath (Fig. 25-23).[48, 57]

Last, difficulty has been encountered on two

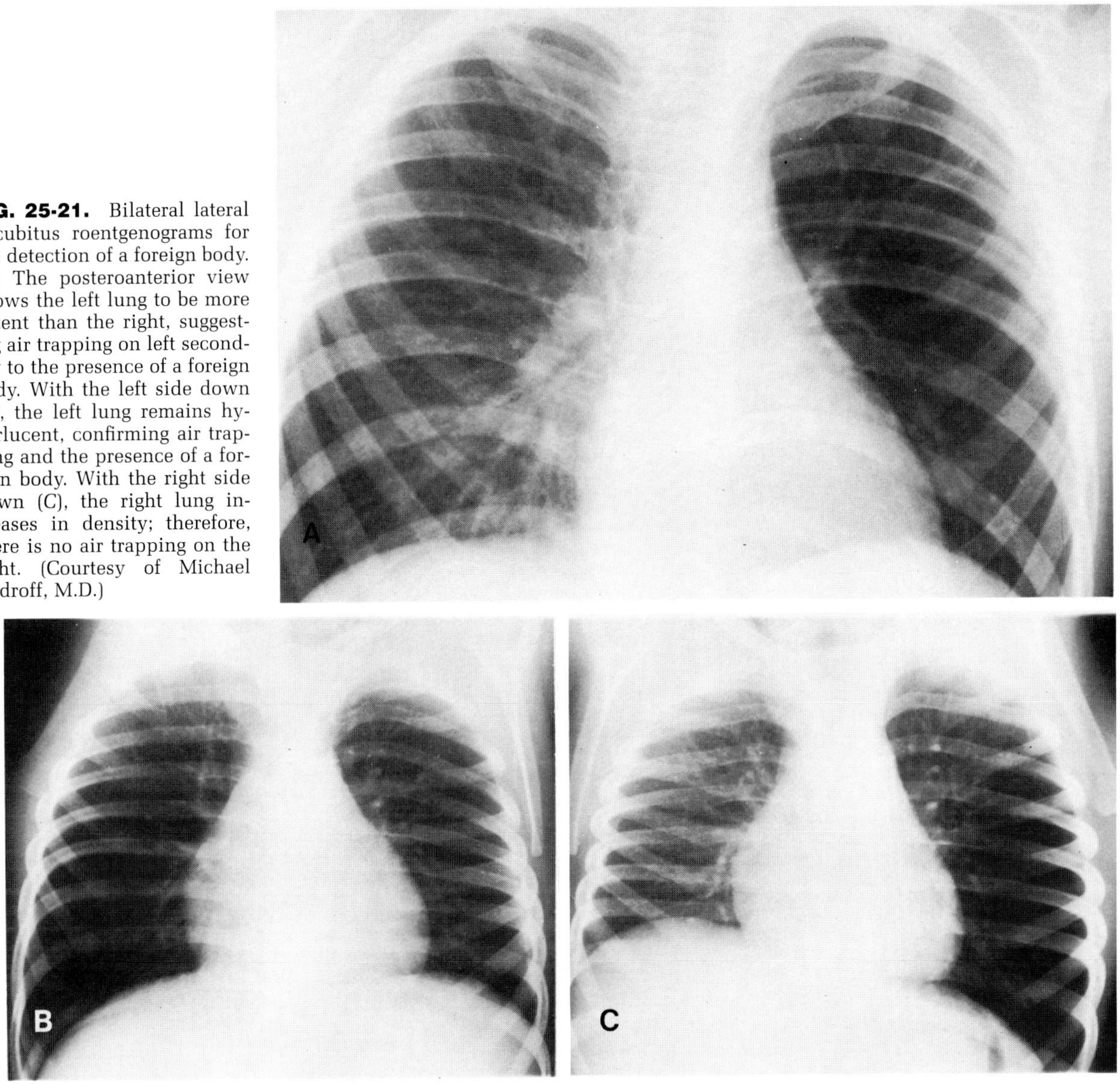

FIG. 25-21. Bilateral lateral decubitus roentgenograms for the detection of a foreign body. (*A*) The posteroanterior view shows the left lung to be more lucent than the right, suggesting air trapping on left secondary to the presence of a foreign body. With the left side down (*B*), the left lung remains hyperlucent, confirming air trapping and the presence of a foreign body. With the right side down (*C*), the right lung increases in density; therefore, there is no air trapping on the right. (Courtesy of Michael Kodroff, M.D.)

occasions with sharp-pointed metal foreign bodies, such as a straight pin, which can pass into tertiary bronchi and pulmonary parenchyma. Endoscopic visualization in children, under these circumstances, is impossible and should be performed under biplane fluoroscopy. The tip of the bronchoscope is placed in the lobar position and the foreign-body forceps inserted under fluoroscopic control into the segmental or tertiary bronchus that contains the foreign body. This may be the only method available for removal in this location, short of thoracotomy (Fig. 25-24).[18, 43]

Esophageal Atresia

Esophageal atresia with and without tracheoesophageal fistula is an important category of congenital lesions producing respiratory distress in the newborn (Fig. 25-25). Intensifying the risks of mortality and morbidity are prematurity, pneumonia, and other serious congenital malformations that exist in about one third of these babies. Since mortality now is at a very respectable level, considerable energy must be devoted to the prevention and management of complications.[36, 45, 84, 104]

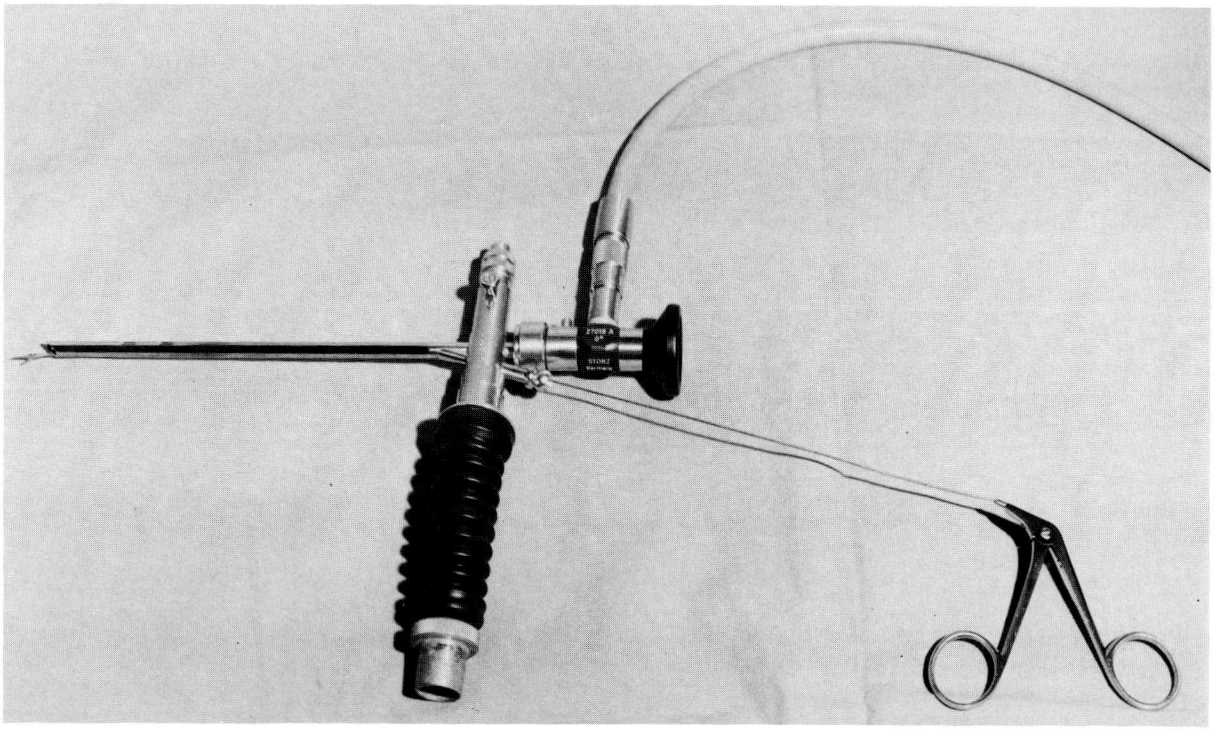

FIG. 25-22. A Storz–Hopkins pediatric bronchoscope with anesthetic connector and a foreign-body forceps inserted through a separate instrument channel to avoid obstructing the magnified vision.

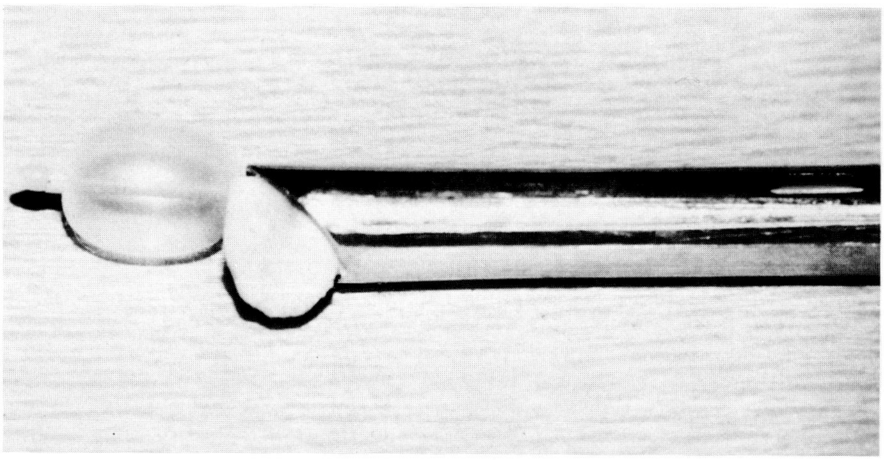

FIG. 25-23. A simulation of how the inflated Fogarty balloon can be used to trap a peanut fragment in a shallow pouch in the distal sheath by withdrawing the telescope.

DIAGNOSIS

The diagnosis of esophageal atresia can invariably be confirmed radiologically by a radiopaque catheter coiled in the proximal pouch. The use of contrast material should be avoided since it can be aspirated (Fig. 25-26). The rare laryngotracheal cleft, although presenting symptomatically like esophageal atresia, will be ruled out by the catheter and, if necessary, endoscopy.

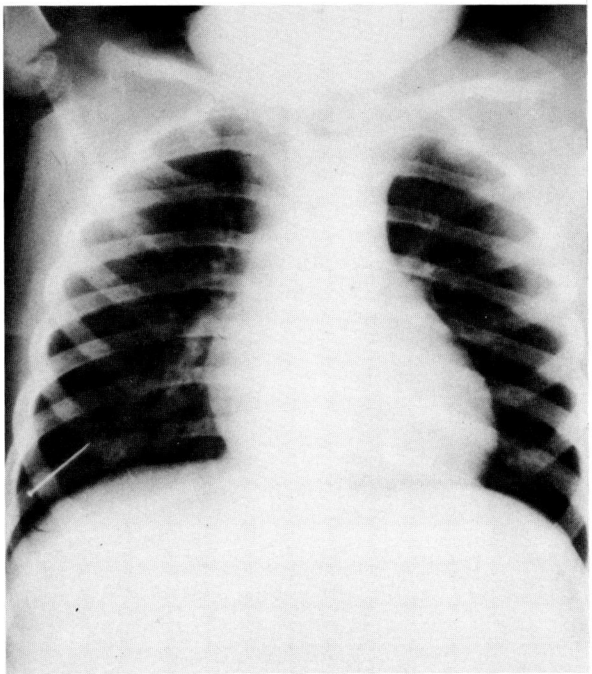

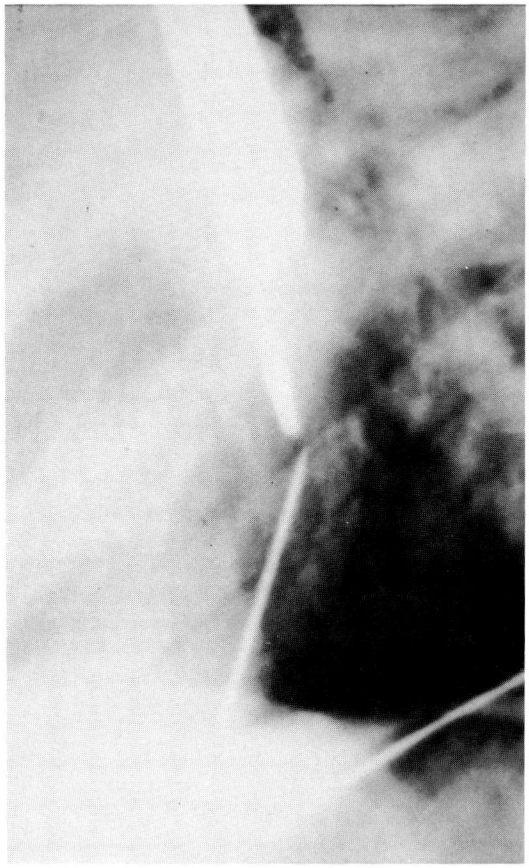

FIG. 25-24. (*Left*) A straight-pin in the distal bronchial tree. (*Right*) A foreign body forceps, visualized under anesthesia and fluoroscopy, approaching the foreign body in the tertiary bronchus.

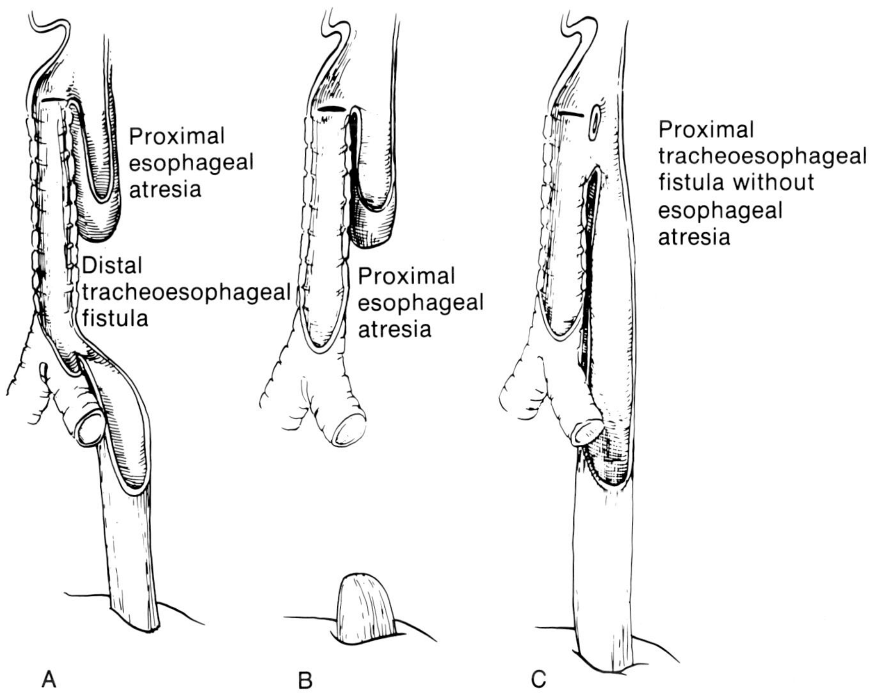

FIG. 25-25. The three most common forms of esophageal atresia and TEF. *A* constitutes 85% of the total, while *B* and *C* together make up another 10%. The rarer types are not depicted.

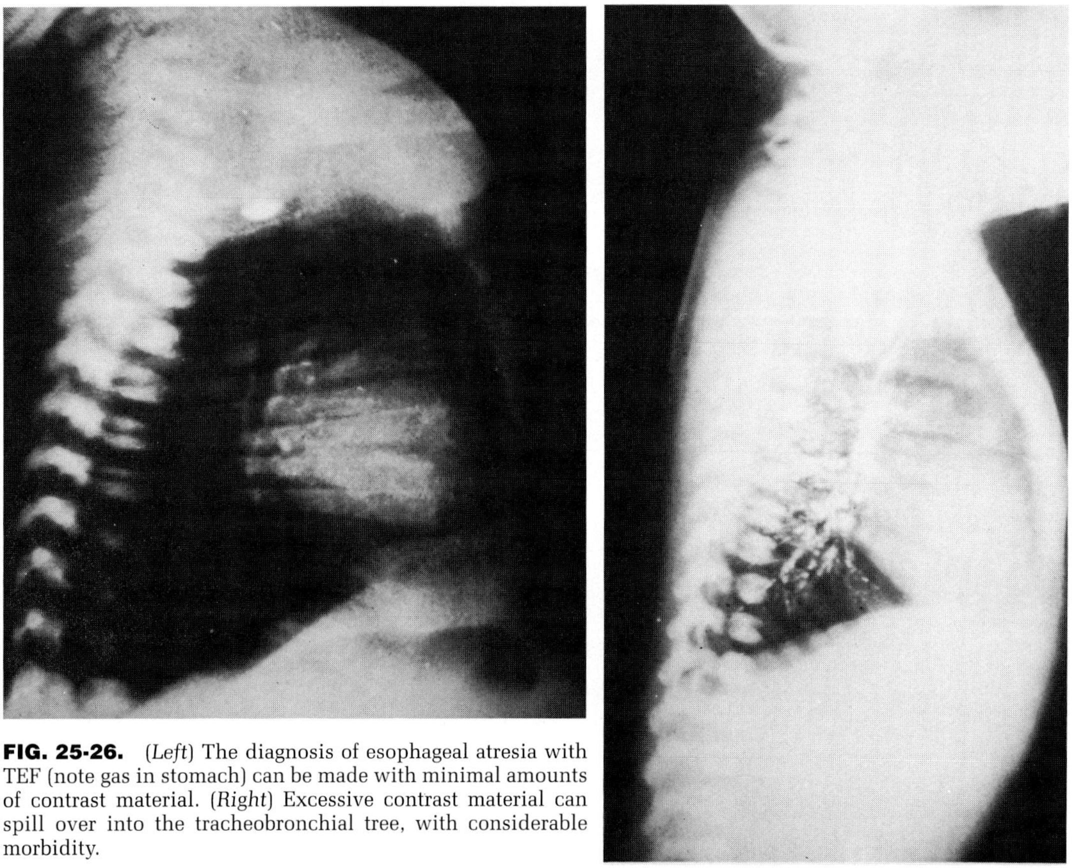

FIG. 25-26. (*Left*) The diagnosis of esophageal atresia with TEF (note gas in stomach) can be made with minimal amounts of contrast material. (*Right*) Excessive contrast material can spill over into the tracheobronchial tree, with considerable morbidity.

The thoracoabdominal x-ray films that confirm the diagnosis can provide much additional information. The length of the proximal pouch is measured against the thoracic vertebral bodies. A pouch at or below the level of the second thoracic vertebra can usually be anastomosed, and if one descends to the third or fourth vertebra, a common muscular wall may be found between the proximal and distal esophageal segments. A pouch at T1 or higher, in contrast, may post a difficult anastomotic problem and such should be explained to the parents.

It is vital to assess the presence of aspiration pneumonia, most likely in the right upper lobe, since the operative approach and timing may in part be determined by this complication. The location of the aortic arch should be identified, and if this cannot be done with certainty, additional views with higher kilovoltage and echocardiograms must be obtained.[7, 41] The abdominal x-ray film has, on one occasion, supplied the answer by the presence of the abdominal aorta to the right of the vertebral column, and some have advocated the insertion of an umbilical catheter to make the decision. The eventual thoracic incision must be made on the side opposite the arch. If not, the operator is trapped into conducting the delicate esophageal dissection and anastomosis underneath an arch that at best can be only poorly mobilized anteriorly. The other alternative is closure and contralateral thoracotomy.

The abdominal portion of the roentgenogram must be carefully scrutinized, especially for duodenal obstruction. The management of the obstruction must then be incorporated into the total operative plan. Imperforate anus is especially frequent and should have been detected during the initial physical examination.

OPERATIVE TREATMENT

Preoperatively, normothermia must be maintained, cardiac and renal function evaluated, and the lungs protected. The baby should be positioned in an isolette with the head up to lessen gastric reflux. A nasoesophageal pouch sump catheter can be inserted after the radiologc examination, positioning its tip at the bottom of the pouch and connecting it to intermittent suction.[93] In addition, pharyngeal suction should be carried out every 10 minutes. Antibiotics are essential at this time. If aspiration pneumonia occurs, these maneuvers are continued along with gastrostomy under local anesthesia to allow the pulmonary lesion to resolve.

The details of the thoracic approach remain controversial. The transpleural technique is quick and affords excellent exposure. Pulmonary retraction and overexpansion uncontrolled by a restricting pleural membrane can lead to extensive parenchymal trauma. An anastomotic leak with intrapleural tamponade and sepsis is often lethal. Accordingly, the extrapleural approach is probably favored by most, even though it adds a few minutes to the operative time. Pleural nicks are often made anteriorly during the extrapleural dissection. Repair of these is difficult, and additional tearing by sutures can lead to larger defects. Exposure is adequate if the dissection is carried far enough anteriorly and inferiorly. Iatrogenic pulmonary trauma is less, and suture-line disruption is much better handled in the extrapleural space.[46]

At operation the distal esophagus in the region of the tracheoesophageal fistula (TEF) is found about where the medial stump of the ligated azygos vein and right vagus nerve intersect (Fig. 25-27).[3, 70, 81] The exact site of the TEF, at the carina or high on the right main-stem bronchus, must be seen precisely without major dissection of the distal esophagus and interruption of its radial blood supply. This is accomplished by protection of the aortic side of the distal esophagus from whence the intercostals arise. Excessive ligation of these could lead to necrosis of the future suture line. Therefore, when the fistula is divided, the distal esophagus should not have been excessively stripped inferiorly.

After fistula division, two fine silk sutures should be placed at the margins of the distal esophagus and used in the eventual anastomosis. If done later, more instrumental manipulation is required for exposure and placement of these angle anastomotic sutures. The flimsy, poorly nourished distal esophagus is vulnerable to such trauma, and anastomotic complications can conceivably be lessened by minimizing contact between this tissue and forceps.

Two lateral fine silk sutures can also be placed on the esophagus attached to the trachea, prior to fistula division. Enough esophagus must remain on the trachea to provide substantial tissue for closure without encroaching on the airway lumen. Insufficient esophagus here will lead either to inadequate approximation with risk of tracheal leak or recurrent fistula or to more reasonable bites with narrowing of the trachea or bronchus. Surrounding areolar tissue

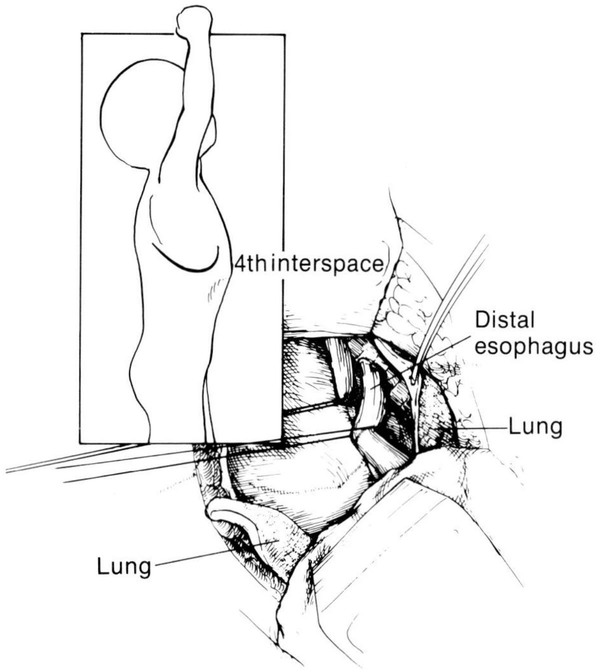

FIG. 25-27. Transpleural view of the operative field in correction of a TEF. The distal esophagus has been excessively mobilized inferiorly, jeopardizing its blood supply. (*Inset*) The one-layer completed anastomosis.

is used to cover the closure, which should be tested for leak by positive pressure ventilation. Excessive esophagus remaining on the trachea compromises the length of the distal esophagus and, if it is not obliterated by sutures, will remain an airway diverticulum for secretions, pulmonary soiling, sepsis, and cough.

The proximal esophagus is quickly located with the help of a catheter inserted from above and its end transfixed by suture. Approximation of the two segments depends on thorough mobilization by sharp dissection of the atretic esophagus. Inferior tension on the transfixation suture allows the plane of tissue between trachea and esophagus to be recognized and divided. A proximal fistula, although rare, should be anticipated during this part of the operation, which is carried circumferentially into the neck. A preliminary judgment about ease of anastomosis is now possible, on the basis of the initial radiograph that verified the anomaly and the operative location of the distal fistula and proximal segment. In about 20%, the two segments touch. The remainder will be separated by varying distances. Now, with moderate downward and minimal upward traction on sutures, the segments are approximated. Further length of the distal esophagus can be

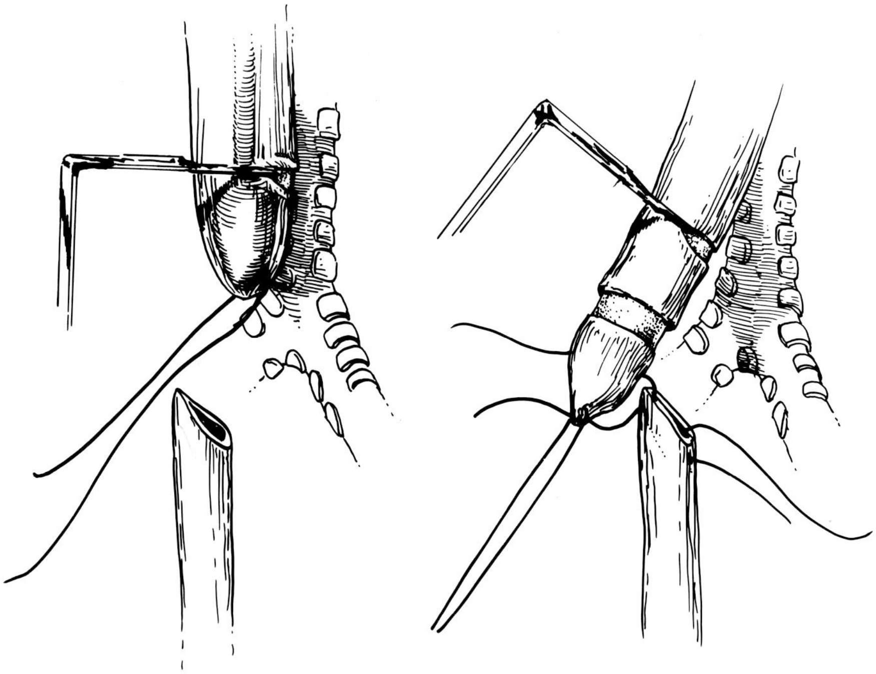

FIG. 25-28. The two 5-0 silk sutures at the margins of the distal esophagus that will be used as lateral sutures in the anastomosis in correction of TEF. The end of the proximal esophagus is transfixed. The circular esophagomyotomy has been performed over a distended Fogarty balloon and may be repeated for additional length, which in this illustration appears unnecessary.

obtained by careful division of one intercostal artery below the cut end and a lower dissection on the antiaortic wall. These maneuvers are all performed under magnification. If approximation without tension is still doubtful, circular myotomy, 2 cm proximal to the atretic tip, should be done over a distended Fogarty catheter with a right-angle knife handle (Fig. 25-28).[30, 61] The straight handle, because of the overhanging thoracic cage, may produce an oblique rather than right-angle cut of the muscle. If tension is still a factor, this maneuver can be repeated above the original myotomy for further length. The tip of the proximal esophagus must now be opened. If tension is exerted on the traction suture and the tip amputated, the critical and strong submucosal layer will retract upward and pose a minor problem in retrieval during the anastomosis. In addition, the upper opening may be made too large in proportion to the lower lumen. Therefore, with modest downward traction, the muscle alone is circumcised and discarded just above the traction suture and the submucosa and mucosa then entered without excision so that the edge of submucosa extends just a bit beyond muscle in this opening, which should correspond in circumference to its lower mate.

The distal esophagus is catheterized to avoid the embarrassment of overlooking a stenosis farther down, and the two esophageal ends are approximated under magnification in one layer with interrupted sutures of 5-0 silk.

POSTOPERATIVE COMPLICATIONS

Postoperatively, emphasis on avoiding pulmonary complications continues. The environment is an isolette with oxygen and humidity. The endotracheal tube should not be removed prematurely and at times remains for 24 hours or longer. Following this, oropharyngeal suction is performed several times an hour with a catheter carefully marked 6 cm from its tip so that accidental penetration of the esophageal anastomosis is avoided. A small, fairly stiff catheter is inserted daily for 2 days into the trachea under laryngoscopic control and more frequently if clinical assessment and daily chest roentgenograms show significant atelectasis.

Infants with persistent total lung consolidation on either side not relieved by tracheal catheter suction should undergo prompt bronchoscopy for aspiration and selective hyperventilation with the Storz equipment. Visualization of the tracheal suture line may reveal critical airway narrowing at this site, and this must be retrieved by operation. Prompt reentry is also indicated in the very rare instance of the immediate postoperative tracheal leak.

The most frequent catastrophic complication, occurring from the fourth to the eighth postoperative day, is disruption of the esophageal anastomosis with massive pleural tension and soiling (Fig. 25-29). The characteristic features are usually sudden, gross respiratory distress, hypotension, and significant sepsis. The chest tube may mirror the patho-

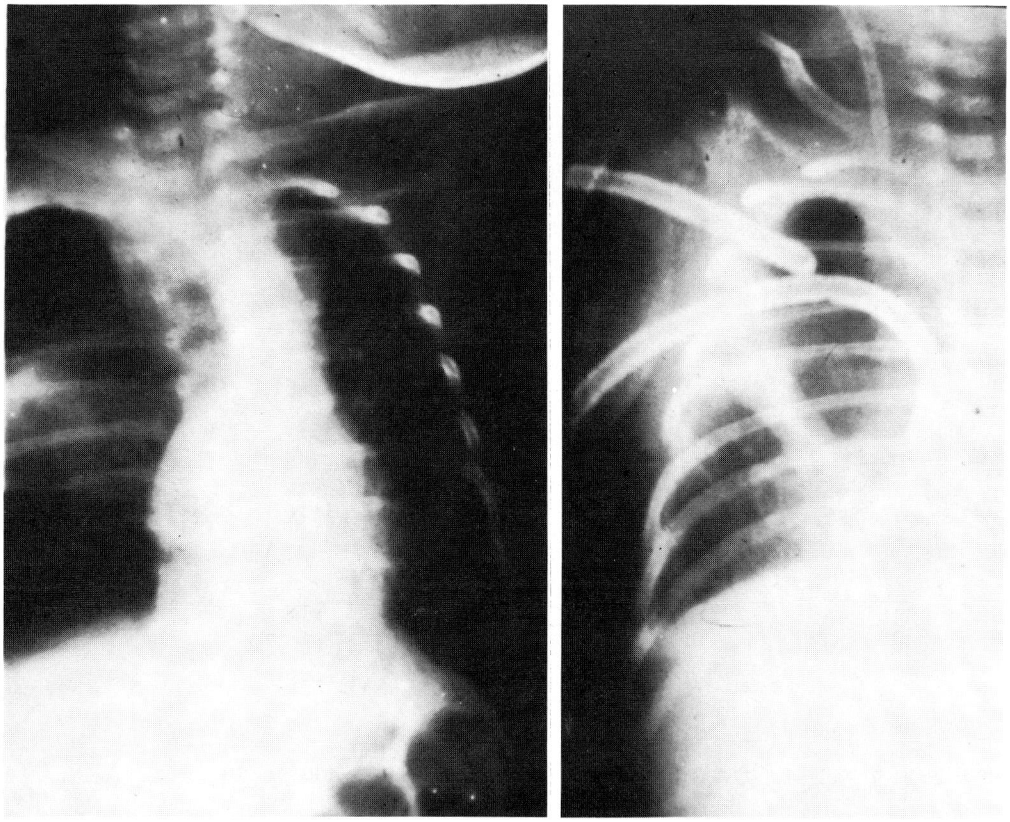

FIG. 25-29. (*Left*) Anastomotic disruption on the sixth postoperative day after transpleural esophagoesophagostomy, with mediastinal shift and tension pneumothorax. (*Right*) Two chest tubes have been inserted, as well as a central venous pressure line in the right side of the neck.

logic event with drainage of saliva and air. The quick insertion of additional chest tubes often is required for pleural and mediastinal decompression, and provision must be made for total antibiotic coverage, nutrition, and control of the mediastinal contamination. The last requires continuous sump suction of the proximal pouch and a gastrostomy tube, since gastric reflux can occur with every Valsalva maneuver. Central hyperalimentation completes the necessary therapeutic maneuvers. Unfortunately, the mortality still remains high, although it is lower with the extrapleural approach. Morbidity with survival consists of anastomotic stricture, which usually responds to one or more dilatations, always done over an endless circle string. The recalcitrant stricture must be resected with another esophagoesophagostomy.

Smaller anastomotic leaks are seen without systemic symptoms during the contrast swallow 8 to 10 days after the operation (Fig. 25-30). This appears as a pseudodiverticulum at the anastomosis, usually located posteriorly, and it empties promptly on follow-up films. Feedings by mouth should be delayed for 7 to 10 days, hyperalimentation maintained, and a repeat esophagogram obtained, which will usually show absence of leak but narrowing of the anastomosis. Postoperative feedings are started slowly and increased as tolerated. Dilatations over a string are done for dysphagia and not because of narrowing seen radiologically. These strictures almost always respond to dilatations. Strictures, of course, can develop without leak and are handled in the same fashion, dilating only for symptoms and not prophylactically.

Recurrent tracheoesophageal fistula fortunately is rare, but it is more likely to occur following an anastomotic leak. Although symptoms are reasonably obvious, the diagnosis is usually delayed and respiratory morbidity results from the continuous pulmonary soiling. The diagnosis should be entertained when there is persistent or quickly recurrent pneumonia associated with coughing, choking, or cyanosis after eating. Gastrostomy feedings are handled with less difficulty, and the gastrostomy tube

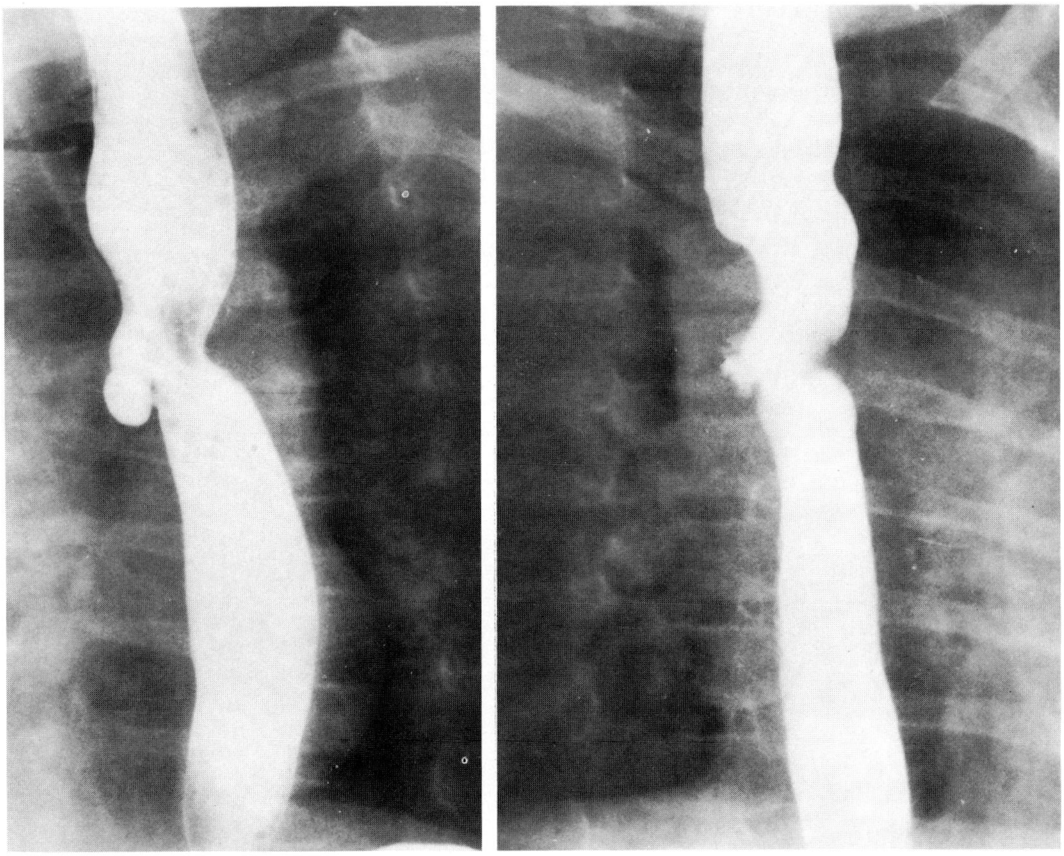

FIG. 25-30. (*Left*) A small, contained anastomotic leak, with gradual obliteration of the fistulous tract (*right*).

under water produces almost continuous bubbling. Visualization of the fistula by endoscopy or radiographically permits diagnosis (Fig. 25-31).[19] Overflow aspiration with stricture or abnormal peristalsis in the distal esophagus must be ruled out as well as chalasia, achalasia, hiatal hernia, and bacterial pulmonary disease.

Transpleural repair should be done with a confirmed preoperative diagnosis. The lumen of the trachea or right main-stem bronchus must not be compromised, and formal reanastomosis is a possibility, although the majority of such cases in the literature have simply required division of the fistula and closure of defects in both airway and esophagus.

ASSOCIATED ANOMALIES

Two concomitant anomalies that must receive simultaneous surgical repair with esophageal atresia are duodenal obstruction and imperforate anus. Both occur more than coincidentally and should always be sought in the preoperative workup. Imperforate anus will be noted during the initial physical examination, and the duodenal obstruction is seen on the early thoracoabdominal x-ray films because of the characteristic double-bubble sign or absent distal gas (Fig. 25-32).

The imperforate anus can be managed by colostomy after performance of the gastrostomy. Thoracotomy should be delayed for 24 to 48 hours with special nursing attention to proximal esophageal pouch sump drainage. The duodenal obstruction can be bypassed with the usual duodenoduodenostomy or jejunostomy followed by gastrostomy with, again, a delay of a day or two prior to thoracotomy. If the esophageal atresia is without fistula, the imperforate anus can be diagnosed but not the duodenal obstruction since air contrast is not available. Under these circumstances, both the unused stomach and colon are more difficult to localize, and the stomach especially is fragile and tears with manipulation during gastrostomy. Two bites of the eventual outer purse-string suture placed near the greater curvature provide the initial traction to bring the stomach into the operative field. Following gastrostomy, air-con-

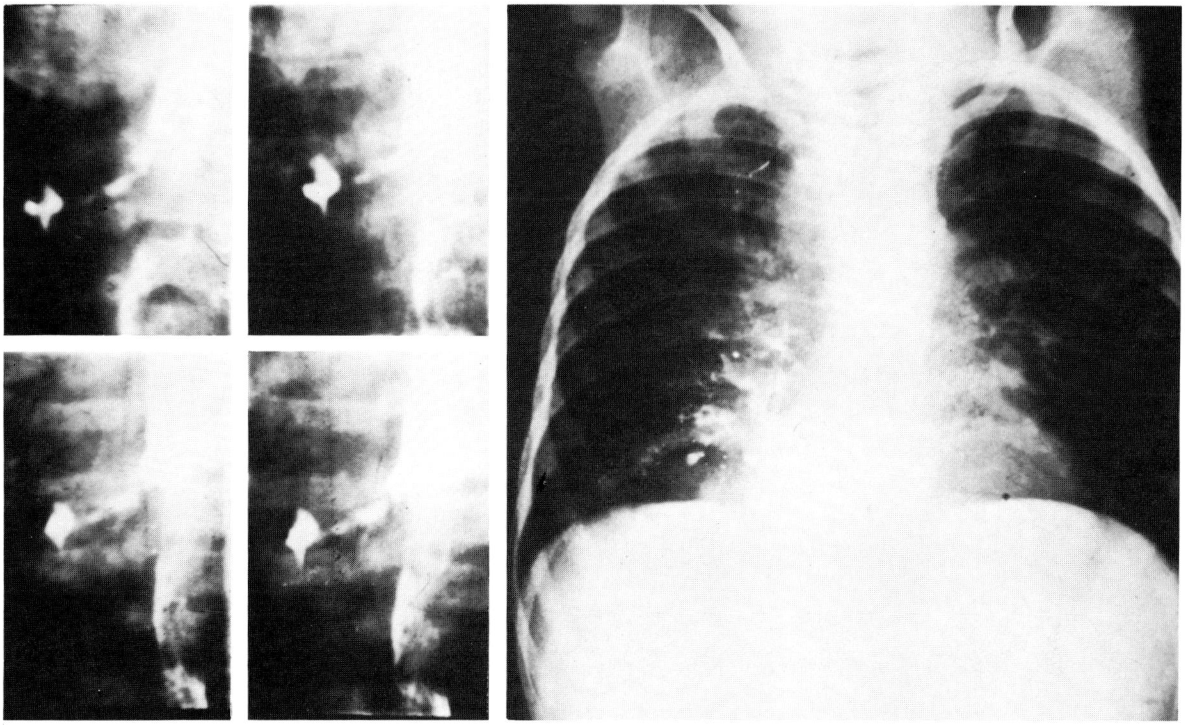

FIG. 25-31. Recurrent TEF as demonstrated on an esophagogram.

trast radiographs should document gastrointestinal patency prior to the initiation of feedings.

LATE COMPLICATIONS

Longer-term postoperative problems are largely restricted to upper airway and digestive tracts. Tracheal or bronchial diverticula, granuloma, stricture, and tracheomalacia with or without anterior compression from aortic arch or innominate artery are the offending lesions in this most strategic area, and treatment is basically conservative.[27] A tracheal diverticulum can probably be managed with postural drainage and occasionally antibiotic coverage. A granuloma here could be removed through the Storz scope with the biopsy forceps but stricture in the lower trachea should await enlargement with time without local manipulation, if at all possible. Tracheomalacia at times can be decompressed by suturing aortic arch to posterior sternum.[98]

Postoperative dysphagia and vomiting are not uncommon. Stricture, of course, must be ruled out and dilatations usually suffice (Fig. 25-33). Rarely, resection is required. Obstruction at the anastomosis by impacted food or a foreign body can be seen without stricture, but more often it follows anastomotic narrowing. Poorly chewed hot dogs, hamburger, other meats, and bread often are incriminated and should be avoided by continuing strained foods

FIG. 25-32. Proximal atresia and distal fistula with right upper lobe pneumonia and duodenal obstruction.

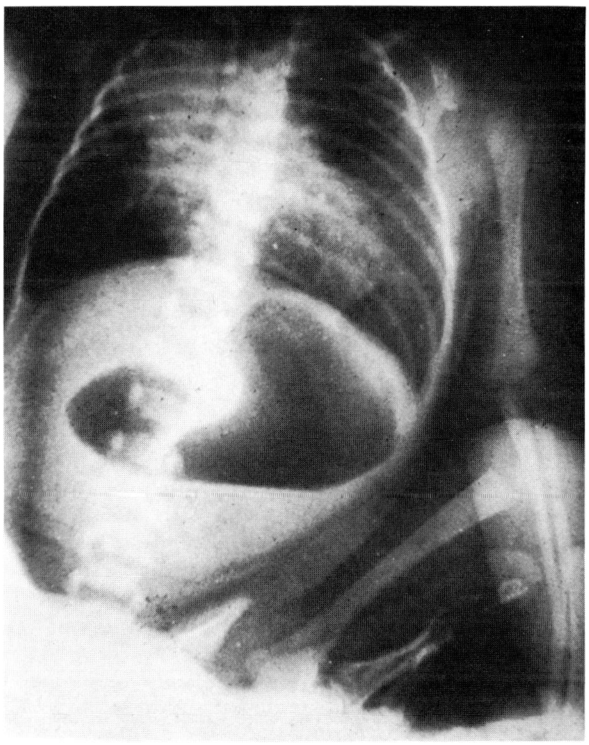

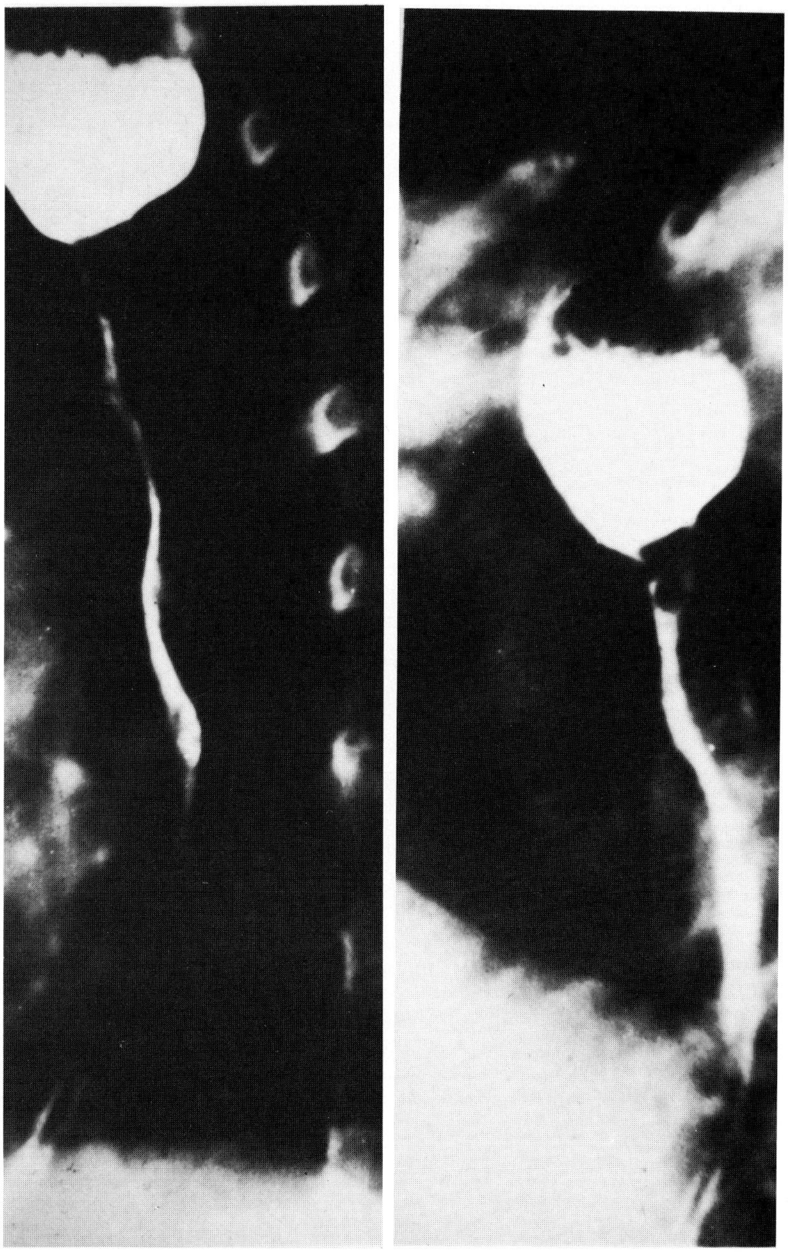

FIG. 25-33. Postoperative stricture requiring multiple dilatations for relief of dysphagia.

past the usual age for intake of solids. Sudden inability to swallow even saliva in a previously asymptomatic patient with postoperative TEF is characteristic of obstruction, and x-ray confirmation is followed by endoscopic removal, which can be tedious. The Fogarty catheter should not be overlooked as an efficient ally. Repeated episodes may require dilatation.

Abnormal peristalsis in the distal esophagus is observed routinely by esophagogram and can be associated with a high degree of regurgitation or vomiting.[45, 52] The treatment is cardiac chair positioning and oral or gastrostomy feedings with a high expectation that it will resolve with time. In this regard, the gastrostomy tube becomes most useful and should not be removed until feedings by mouth are well tolerated.

Reflux esophagitis with or without hiatal hernia with vomiting and regurgitation is not unusual. Failure of medical therapy will lead to unwholesome sequelae such as aspiration pneumonia, poor weight gain, esophagitis, stricture, and bleeding. Accordingly, persistence of these complications requires fundoplication.[74, 76]

Finally, gastric outlet obstruction must be considered with vomiting. Most frequent, unremitting pylorospasm secondary to vagal nerve injury is the etiologic factor. Again, conservative therapy including anticholinergics and nasojejunal tube feedings should be exhausted prior to considering pyloroplasty. Pyloric stenosis should not be overlooked as a coincidental possibility.

Pectus Excavatum

Indications for the surgical treatment of pectus excavatum in children and adolescents include evidence of cardiopulmonary disease, a cosmetic deformity that is psychologically oppressive, and deep and relentlessly progressive concavities.

The operation popularized by Ravitch (1949) and subsequently modified in stages by Haller, Stonesifer, and Sanford is preferred by many because it fulfills the technical principles of cartilage resection, dividing sternal attachments and overcorrection and splinting without external or internal appliances.[86–88]

Complications are basically restricted to the operative procedure and postoperative course, both acute and long-term. It is unfortunate that an operation often performed for cosmetic reasons must be initiated by vertical or transverse incisions that at times are not aesthetic. This must be explained to the parents and the older patient. Injection of steroids locally prior to skin closure or even scar revision has not been predictably preventive or therapeutic. Steroids in the skin incision and subcuticular closure are most favored.

OPERATIVE TREATMENT

After exposure of sternum and cartilages by elevation of soft tissue flaps including the rectus, the magnitude of the deformity must be assessed and the extent of cartilage resection planned. As Ravitch emphasizes, compromising the lateral, upper, or lower extent of cartilage removal relates directly to the results.[89] Accordingly, if the operator has the slightest doubt, the cartilage should be resected. Subperichondrial resection usually extends from sternum to costochondral junction and will frequently involve the third through the seventh cartilages bilaterally. Some have suggested removal of cartilage with perichondrium, but this can lead only to greater blood loss, more frequent pleural penetration, prolonged paradox, gross subcutaneous cardiac impulse, and less acceptable cosmetic results.[90] Therefore, subperichondrial resection is essential and can be accomplished with a Sayre or Freer type elevator after an initial perichondrial incision with scalpel rather than the cutting current. The cutting current often and easily penetrates cartilage as well during this maneuver and makes perichondrial elevation difficult.

A minor technical point is the fate of the posterior-pointing xiphoid, which is surgically separated from the manubrium during the course of the operation. Sparing it at times can leave an unsightly postoperative upper abdominal bulge and, in one instance in our experience required a separate procedure for its removal. Xiphoid resection should perhaps be a routine part of the initial procedure.

After elevation of the sternum from its mediastinal attachments, the intercostal bundles are divided at the sternum. Counting from above, the lowest normal cartilage that has not been resected, usually the second or third, is divided obliquely from medial to lateral. The posterior sternal osteotomy is performed in the next higher interspace and overcorrected with a wedge of bone from an adjacent rib. The medial tip of the obliquely divided cartilage can now be made to override the tip of its lateral mate and they are sutured in this position, further immobilizing the repaired pectus. On two occasions in our series, however, the anteriorly placed medial cartilage segment has created an annoying postoperative prominence, especially at its chondrosternal junction. Recently, this has been shaved and thinned prior to fixation. Closure is then accomplished by suturing pectoralis to pectoralis with an intervening bite in the sternum (Fig. 25-34).

Wound drainage is controversial. However, since the pleura can be nicked without recognition and fluid does accumulate in the mediastinal space, there is no harm in tube drainage connected to mild negative pressure for 24 to 48 hours following the operation.[106] Omission of this has necessitated an occasional postoperative needle aspiration for either fluid or pneumothorax if a pleural defect has been overlooked.

COMPLICATIONS

Pectus, recurring 5 or more years after correction, is perhaps the most serious postoperative complication.[105] Reoperation requires sternal fixation and consists of a Kirschner wire passed horizontally behind the sternum in a shallow posterior osteotomy groove, with ends resting and sutured onto the ribs of the anterior chest wall.[75] It is removed electively in 1 year if it is asymptomatic and stationary. Complications of metallic internal fixation, requiring more urgent operative removal, consist of dislodge-

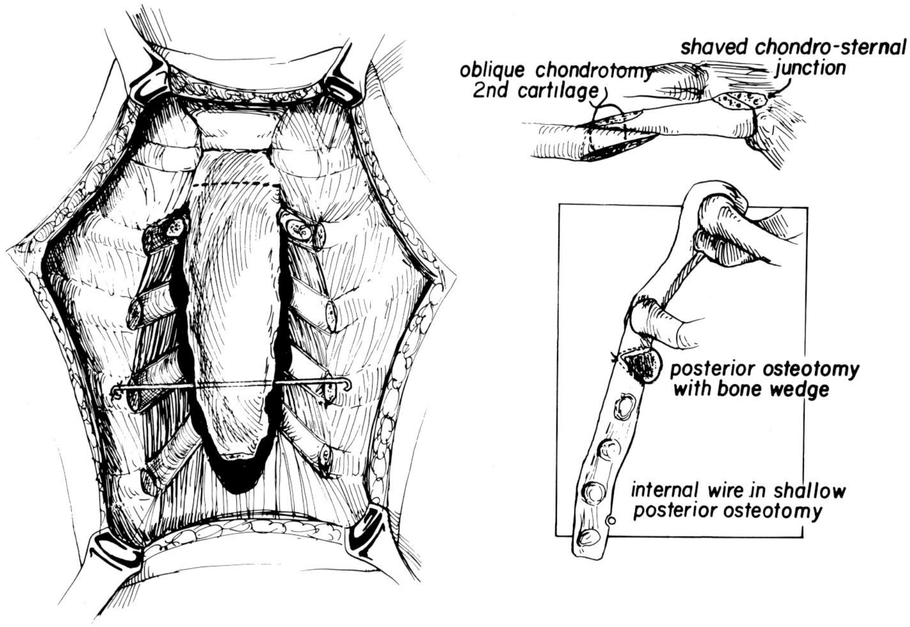

FIG. 25-34. Correction of pectus excavatum. (*Left*) The *dotted transverse line* is the posterior wedge osteotomy above the highest divided cartilage. Cartilages 3, 4, and 5 have been resected bilaterally, and the intercostal bundles have been separated from the sternum. The Kirschner wire lies in a shallow posterior osteotomy sutured to the ribs and supporting the lower sternum. (*Upper right*) The bilateral oblique overriding chondrotomy of the second cartilage is sutured, and the knob of chondrosternal junction is shaved.

ment, migration, percutaneous presentation, and pain. Nevertheless, in spite of these minor hazards, such fixation in these circumstances is almost mandatory.

As with any major thoracic wall procedure involving bone and cartilage, respiratory complications, especially left lower lobe atelectasis, occur because of diminished ventilation secondary to pain as well as to chronic preoperative pulmonary compression. Judicious use of narcotics, incentive spirometry, early ambulation, moist air, and tracheal suction all have their place. Frequent chest x-ray films help determine the degree of aggressiveness required. Antibiotics for 72 hours have become customary.

Postoperatively, a light anterior chest brace is worn for 8 weeks and contact sports avoided for 8 additional weeks. Passive and then active physiotherapy begins at 2 months and is continued for another 2 months.

With this operative and postoperative regimen, recurrence rates after 10 years that require surgery should be well below 10%, with serious wound complications such as chondritis exceedingly low and pleuropulmonary problems even lower. The appearance of the skin incision remains a nuisance.

Bochdalek Hernia

Posterolateral diaphragmatic hernia is an urgent thoracoabdominal emergency that even today, in spite of "state of the art" therapy, carries a particularly excessive rate of mortality (Fig. 25-35).[1, 10] Predictable complications can be divided into diagnostic, preoperative, operative, and postoperative areas.[42]

DIAGNOSIS

Roentgenograms taken in conventional views without contrast will show signet-ring lucencies in the chest suggestive of air-filled bowel loops, a loss of bowel gas in the abdomen, and a markedly displaced mediastinum with apparent dextrocardia (Fig. 25-36). It may be impossible and unnecessary to isolate a Bochdalek hernia from eventration and phrenic nerve paralysis since therapy is similar and surgical if symptoms are overwhelming. Congenital pulmonary cysts and pneumatoceles are usually listed in the differential diagnosis, but both are exceedingly rare at this time. CCAM can be an annoying differential problem and is an indication for an upper GI series to establish the presence of a normal intra-abdominal configuration if this is not apparent on plain film. In one newborn with this problem, contrast studies were not feasible. A left thoracotomy was utilized to avoid the embarrassment of an abdominal approach for thoracic pathology.[95]

Associated lesions occur with some regularity and must be uncovered preoperatively or anticipated. These would include hypoplastic lung, midgut malrotation, congenital heart disease, and extralobar sequestration. The preliminary radiographs should, of course, include abdominal views. Restriction of the gas pattern to stomach and duodenum with even perhaps a double-bubble sign would be pathognomonic of duodenal obstruction. Rapid cardiac evaluation, including ECG and ultrasound, would provide some insight into the cardiac operative and postoperative prognosis. Hypoplastic lung and sequestration are encountered and recognized during the operation.

PREOPERATIVE CARE

Prompt and urgent preoperative resuscitation and preparation for generalized metabolic problems such as hypothermia and acidosis must be mainly directed toward the peculiar, specific pulmonary abnormality. Ventilation and oxygenation are difficult in the presence of hypoplastic lungs with abnormal pulmonary arterioles. Oxygen desaturation, acidosis, and pulmonary hypertension are uniformly present. A right-to-left shunt through ductal, cardiac, and pulmonary pathways increases venoarterial admixture. The hypoxia and acidosis are worsened, and the cycle deepens (Fig. 25-37).[8, 29, 41] Unfortunately, in many neonates operative correction of the diaphragmatic defect does not alter this malignant chain of events.

Preoperative preparation in the isolette under controlled temperature begins with constant nasogastric suction through a pediatric sump catheter, which may relieve or prevent further intrathoracic gastrointestinal distention. Ventilatory support must be done through an orotracheal tube to avoid a face mask and further dilatation of the intrathoracic gastrointestinal tract at the expense of lung space. How-

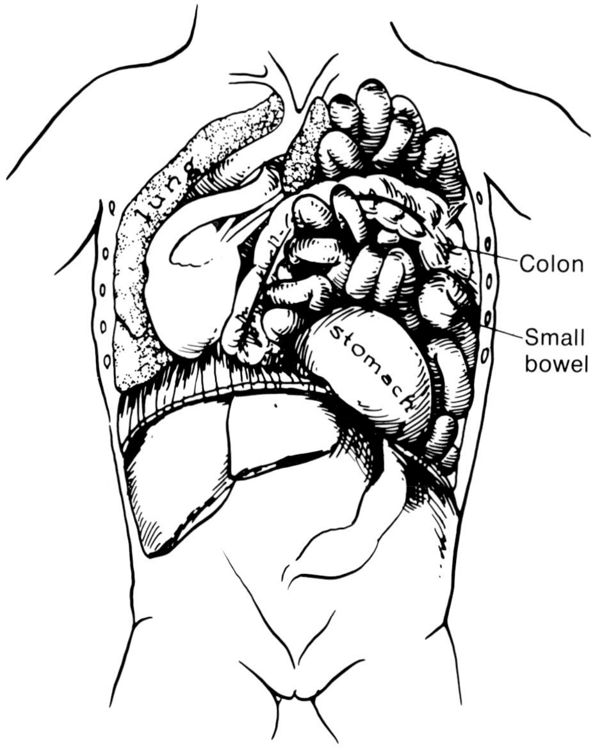

FIG. 25-35. A left-sided Bochdalek hernia with the stomach, bowel, and spleen in the chest. The right lung is critically compressed, and the left lung is a residual nubbin. The pulmonary hypoplasia and its cardiovascular repercussions contribute largely to an excessive early mortality.

FIG. 25-36. (*Left*) A typical preoperative roentgenogram of a left-sided Bochdalek hernia with a loss of abdominal bowel gas, the mediastinum shifted to the right, compression of the right lung, and the stomach and loops of bowel situated in the left side of the chest. (*Center*) A postoperative roentgenogram shows the mediastinum in the midline and good expansion of both lungs. A tube is present in the left side of the chest. (*Right*) A postoperative roentgenogram of a patient with a right Bochdalek hernia in whom there was failure of the ipsilateral lung to reexpand, contralateral pneumothorax, and lung compression. A tube is present in the right side of the chest.

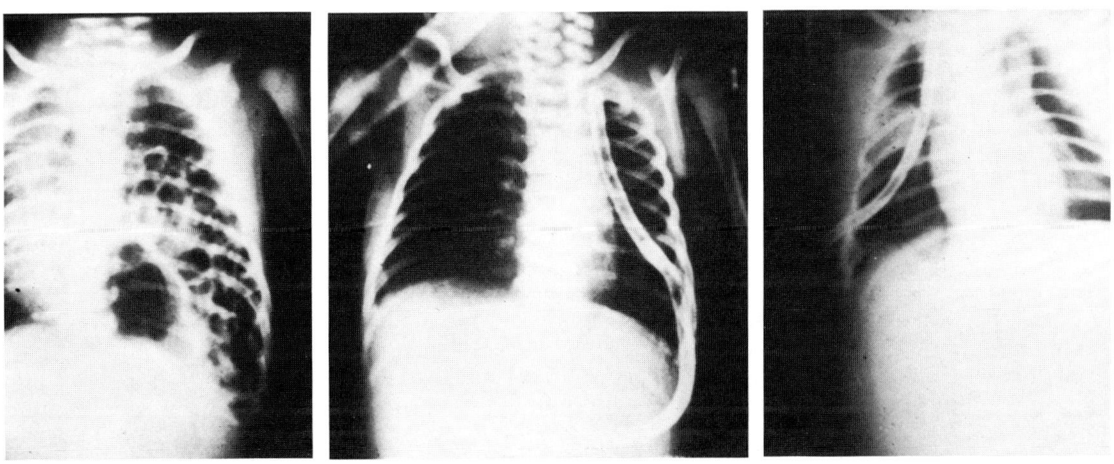

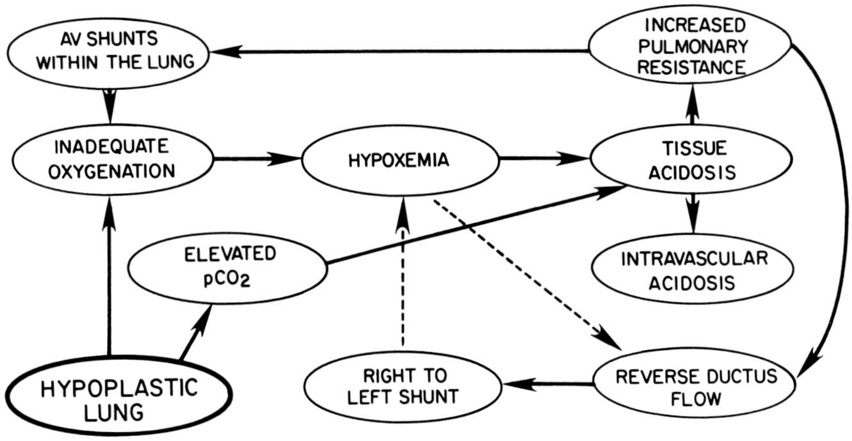

FIG. 25-37. Pathophysiology of diaphragmatic hernia in the neonate.

ever, overenthusiastic manual inspiratory pressures may produce unilateral or bilateral pneumothorax.

Serial blood gas and pH monitoring are vital at this time, during operation, and well into the postoperative period; vigorous management of the acidosis is always necessary. Umbilical and right radial-artery catheters are necessary for the evaluation of right-to-left shunting. These determinations become vital in orderly postoperative therapy.

OPERATIVE TREATMENT

An abdominal subcostal or vertical incision under most circumstances may minimize complications now and later.[37] Exposure of the defect, the abdominal and thoracic bowel, and the ipsilateral lung is highly adequate. As Potts has pointed out, it is much easier to reduce the intrathoracic viscera by pulling down from below than pushing from above.[77] Anomalies of rotation are easily determined and corrected. If space is a problem, the abdominal parietes can be stretched, a ventral hernia created, and gastrostomy performed.[22, 44, 83] The thoracic approach might be restricted to Bochdalek hernias presenting months later when intrathoracic adhesions require division.

Once the peritoneal cavity has been entered, air is inserted or allowed to enter the involved pleural cavity, usually the left. Intra-abdominal contents are gently withdrawn from the chest with special care devoted to the spleen. Once the left chest is cleared, the defect becomes obvious. Further exposure requires gentle retraction of the liver. Nothing is worse at this stage than a subcapsular hematoma of the liver or spleen. It can truly demolish the operation.

Intrathoracic exposure from below will demonstrate the pulmonary remnant and its expansion capabilities with inspiratory pressures not exceeding 30 ml of saline. Unfortunately, prognosis cannot be based on this observation. At this time, the hernial sac, present about 10% of the time, should be conscientiously sought because failure to remove it will provide an incarcerating membrane, which may be the decisive factor in preventing vital lung reexpansion. While this exposure is maintained, a lateral chest tube is inserted anteriorly with its tip near the mediastinum and connected to appropriate drainage.

The majority of congenital posterolateral diaphragmatic defects can be closed primarily with one or preferably two layers of 3-0 silk. A rim of muscle is usually present anteriorly, and this can be sutured to the posterior segment (Fig. 25-38). With insufficient tissue in back, sutures between the anterior muscle and around the posterior ribs should be attempted. If the tension is too great, rib fractures anteriorly will provide additional mobility, which may bridge the gap with less tension. If this fails, a Marlex or Silastic prosthesis should be applied with special attention devoted to the sutures medially. The esophagus is located with its nasogastric tube and, of course, avoided. The left adrenal gland should be identified so that these sutures, too, can be placed laterally. Finally, thoracic-duct injury can occur at this stage of the operation, and even with loop magnification, iatrogenic trauma may occur. A Stamm gastrostomy will provide postoperative gastrointestinal decompression and avoid respiratory distress from this source.

Prior to replacement of the viscera into the peritoneal cavity, the abdominal wall is stretched manually and a layered closure assayed. If tension is obvious, skin closure alone is usually adequate. If not, a Marlex silo is constructed. Insertion of a contralateral chest tube will circumvent the untoward sequelae of a postoperative pneumothorax secondary to high inspiratory pressures through the ventilator.

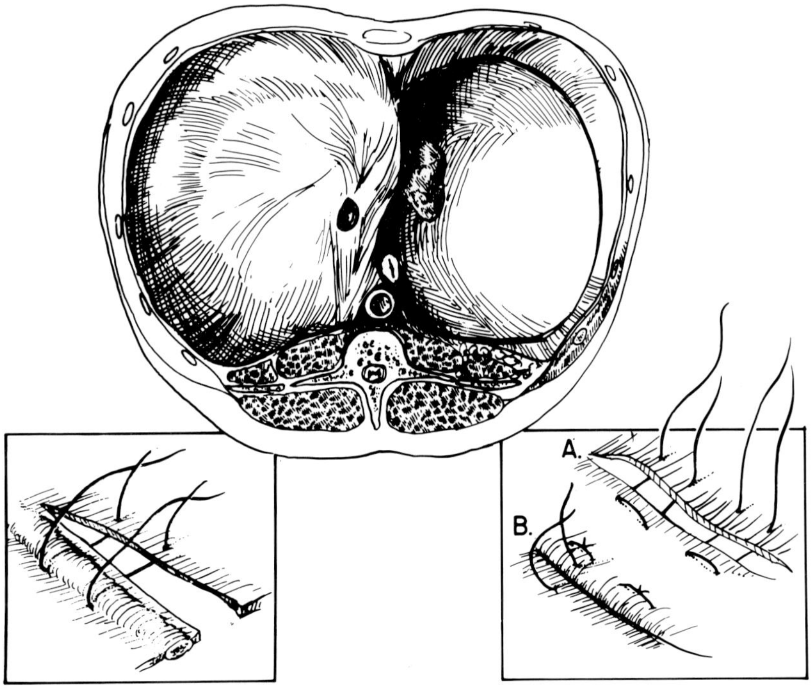

FIG. 25-38. (*Top*) A diaphragmatic defect with a severely hypoplastic left lung, seen from below. (*Right inset, A*) Horizontal mattress sutures imbricate the posterior muscle rim beneath the anterior diaphragmatic segment. (*Right inset, B*) Simple sutures of 3-0 silk tack the free margin of the anterior rim to the posterior diaphragm. (*Left inset*) Approximation of the anterior diaphragm around the posterior ribs.

COMPLICATIONS

In the majority of newborns diagnosed within 8 hours of birth and quickly repaired, persistent fetal circulation associated with relentlessly progressive acidosis, hypoxemia, and cardiovascular instability is followed by irreversible pulmonary failure and death. Early identification of these infants with severe but still reversible pulmonary failure would permit orderly conventional resuscitative measures, including pulmonary arteriolar dilators such as Priscoline.[9, 66, 73] If pulmonary failure persists in spite of maximal medical therapy, as manifested by (A-a) DO_2 of greater than 620 torr for 10 to 12 hours, the mortality rate will be 100%.[85] Under these circumstances, extracorporeal membrane oxygenation using the internal jugular vein and common carotid artery for access to the right atrium and aortic arch seems justified (Fig. 25-39). Ductus ligation can be added if a large right-to-left shunt persists.[23] This type of mechanical extracorporeal ventilatory support in patients with Bochdalek hernia may purchase the critical time necessary for resolution of the underlying parenchymal disease including the pulmonary hypertension. Its application in several dozen patients after exhaustion of standard therapy has been accomplished safely and successfully with acceptable levels of morbidity.[6, 40, 56]

Unfortunately, as with all hernias, there are recurrences (Fig. 25-40). Abdominal reentry would require an extensive and dangerous dissection of liver and spleen from the defect. Accordingly, the second operation should be transthoracic, through the sixth or seventh interspace. Visualization is ideal, dissection minimal, and repair usually uncomplicated.

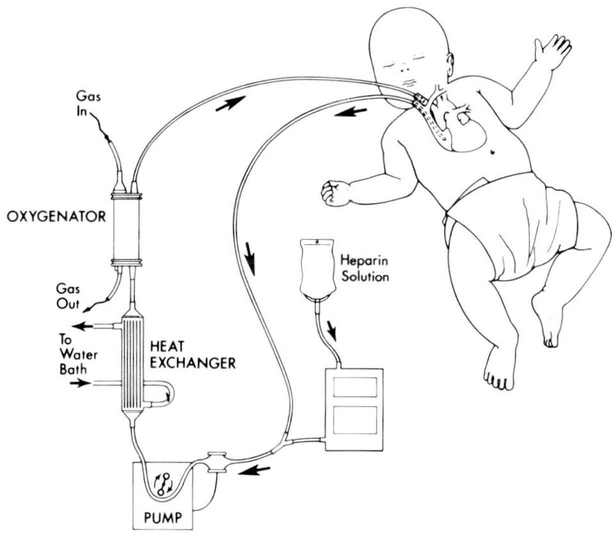

FIG. 25-39. An extracorporeal membrane-oxygenation circuit.

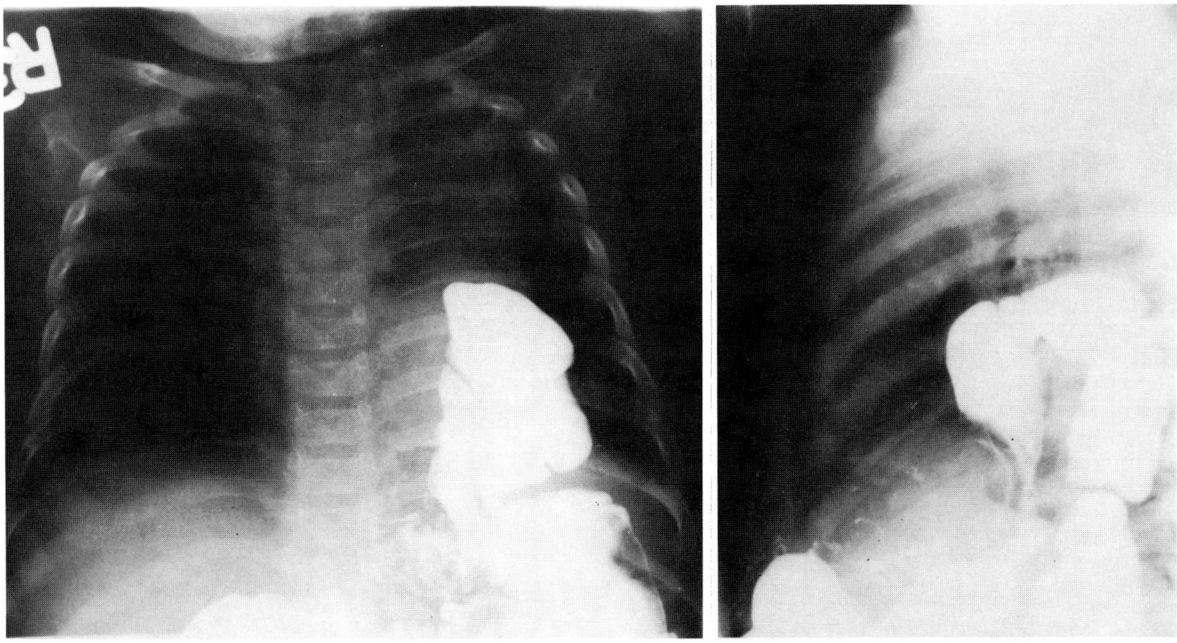

FIG. 25-40. A recurrent left Bochdalek hernia 6 months after initial repair. *Left,* posteroanterior view; *right,* lateral view.

FIG. 25-41. Insertion of a chest tube in a newborn in respiratory distress. (*Left*) A posteroanterior chest radiograph shows a posterior tube and demonstrates a lateral pneumothorax, in addition to the anterior and subpulmonic collections. (*Right*) With an additional anterior tube, there is no subpulmonic collection and minimal anterior pneumothorax. The catheter hole outside the pleura was corrected.

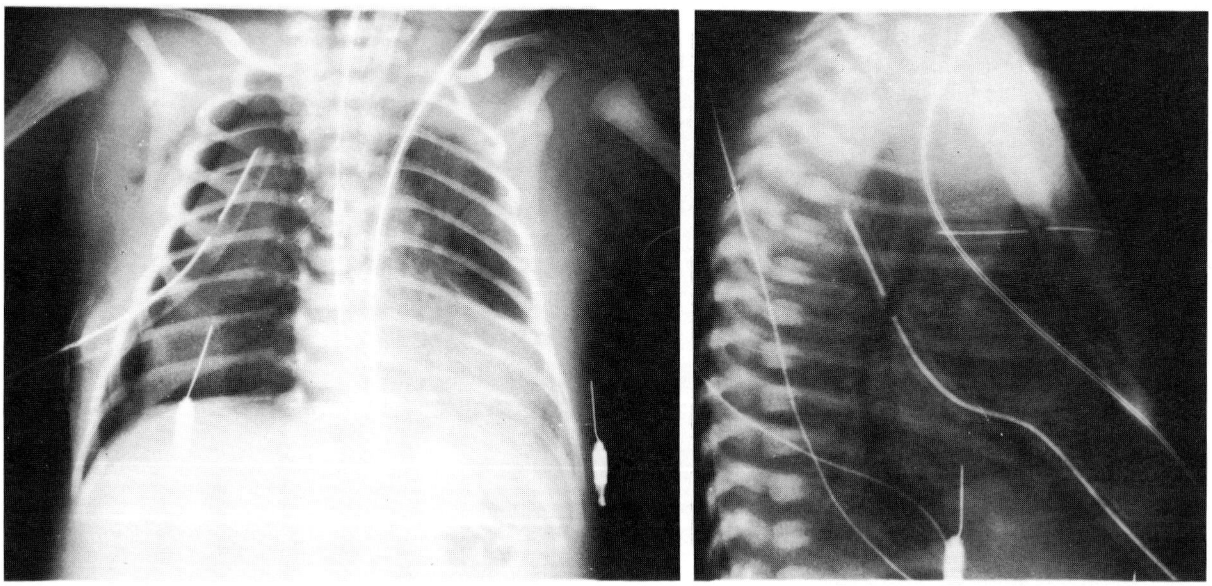

The ipsilateral lung is still hypoplastic and has a high propensity for atelectasis, perhaps secondary to inefficient management of secretions. Resort to bronchoscopy should be quick and repetitive if necessary. Several days of postoperative positive end expiratory pressure through a nasotracheal tube may be prophylactic.

Newborn Respiratory Distress

Management of the respiratory distress syndrome almost uniformly includes an endotracheal tube and ventilators set at high inspiratory pressures. Under these circumstances tension pneumothorax is predictable.[55] The insertion of an intercostal tube in children with this disease is a frequently employed thoracic surgical procedure with avoidable complications.[2]

The initial diagnosis usually offers no problems with a lateral pneumothorax on the posterior–anterior film requiring decompression. A No. 10 to No. 12 plastic tube for newborns should be inserted through the fourth or fifth interspace in the mid or anterior axillary line with the involved hemithorax slightly elevated on towels from hips to shoulders. The interspace in the line of the nipples is appropriate. The skin incision under local anesthesia just above the rib below is deepened with the tip of a curved mosquito hemostat opening and closing parallel and touching the rib below. This will avoid the intercostal vessels just above. Once the pleura is penetrated, a second similar hemostat grabs the tip of the intercostal tube and, with the tip of the hemostat pointing upward toward the anterior chest wall, the tube is pushed through the stab wound after withdrawal of the first hemostat. The trocar should never be used for insertion of chest tubes in children because of the possibility of lung trauma, and it is equally essential that the tube be placed anteriorly since pneumothoraces here with the patient always on his back are invariably anterior and medial as well as lateral.[5, 35, 65, 67] A lateral thoracostomy tube that is unguided during insertion will most likely terminate posteriorly, and, trapped by the expanding lung, it will fail to evacuate the anterior pneumothorax, which continues to prevent lung expansion (Fig. 25-41).[49, 103] Both posterior–anterior and lateral chest roentgenograms after the insertion should demonstrate no extrapulmonary air. Equally effective in achieving this result is the anterior–superior tube thoracostomy advocated by Allen and colleagues.[27]

Other more generalized precautions for children are to avoid inadvertent low-tube insertion into high-riding liver, spleen, and diaphragm and catheter holes outside the chest.

References

1. Adelman S, Benson CD: Bochdalek hernias in infants: Factors determining mortality. J Pediatr Surg 11:569, 1976
2. Allen RW et al: Effectiveness of chest tube evacuation of pneumothoraces in neonates. J Pediatr 99:629, 1981
3. Ashcraft KW, Holder TM: Esophageal atresia and tracheoesophageal malformations. In Holder TM, Ashcraft KW (eds): Pediatric Surgery, p 266. Philadelphia, WB Saunders, 1980
4. Aytac A et al: Inhalation of foreign bodies in children. Report of 500 cases. J Thorac Cardiovasc Surg 74:145, 1977
5. Banagale RC et al: Lung perforation: A complication of chest tube insertion in neonatal pneumothorax. J Pediatr 94:973, 1979
6. Bartlett RH et al: Extracorporeal membrane oxygenation (ECMO) support in neonatal respiratory failure. J Thorac Cardiovasc Surg 74:826, 1977
7. Beardon WE et al: Plain film detection of right aortic arch in infants with esophageal atresia and tracheo-esophageal fistula. J Pediatr Surg 14:436, 1979
8. Bloss RS et al: Congenital diaphragmatic hernia: Pathophysiology and pharmacologic support. Surg 89:418, 1981
9. Bloss RS et al: Tolazoline therapy for persistent pulmonary hypertension after congenital diaphragmatic hernia repair. J Pediatr 97:984, 1980
10. Boix–Ochoa J et al: Acid-base balance and blood gases in prognosis and therapy of congenital diaphragmatic hernia. J Pediatr Surg 9:49, 1974
11. Boles ET, Amoury R: Discussion of Nagaraj HS: Iatrogenic perforation of the esophagus in premature infants. Surg 86:583, 1979
12. Brooks JW, Salzberg AM: Foreign bodies in the air passages. In Kendig EL, Chernick V (eds): Disorders of the Respiratory Tract in Children, p 513. Philadelphia, WB Saunders, 1977
13. Brown BSJ et al: Foreign bodies in the tracheo bronchial tree in childhood. J Can Assoc Radiol 14:158, 1963
14. Buntain WL et al: Lobar emphysema, cystic adenomatoid malformation, pulmonary sequestration, and bronchogenic cyst in infancy and childhood: A clinical group. J Pediatr Surg 9:85, 1974
15. Camarata SJ, Salyer JM: Management of foreign bodies in air passages and esophagus under general anesthesia. Am Surg 31:725, 1965
16. Canty TG: Congenital lobar emphysema resulting from bronchial sling around a normal right main pulmonary artery. J Thorac Cardiovasc Surg 74:126, 1977
17. Capitanio MA, Kirkpatrick JA: The lateral decubitus film: An aid in determining air-trapping in children. Radiology 103:460, 1972
18. Carter R: Bronchotomy: The safe solution for an infarcted foreign body. Ann Surg 10:93, 1970
19. Chrispen AD et al: Aspiration pneumonia and dysphagia after technically successful repair of esophageal atresia. Thorax 21:104, 1966
20. Clarke TA et al: Esophageal perforations—premature infants and comments on the diagnosis. Am J Dis Child 134:367, 1980
21. Clatworthy HW Jr: Intrathoracic tumors and cysts. In Ariel M, Pack GT (eds): Cancer and Allied Disease of Infancy and Childhood, p 143. Boston, Little, Brown & Co, 1960

22. Collins DL: Diaphragmatic hernia. In Holder TM, Ashcraft KW (eds): Pediatric Surgery, p 232. Philadelphia, WB Saunders, 1980
23. Collins DL et al: A new approach to congenital posterolateral diaphragmatic hernia. J Pediatr Surg 12:149, 1977
24. Cummings GR et al: Unilateral hyperlucent lung syndrome in children. J Pediatr 78:250, 1971
25. Dahm LS et al: Comparison of three techniques of lung lavage in patients with cystic fibrosis. Chest 72:793, 1977
26. Daniilides J et al: Foreign body in the airways. A review of 90 cases. Arch Otolaryngol 103:570, 1977
27. Davies MR, Cywes S: The Fiaccid trachea and tracheoesophageal anomalies. J Pediatr Surg 13:363, 1978
28. Demos MJ et al: Congenital lung malformations, a unified concept and a case report. J Thorac Cardiovasc Surg 70:260, 1975
29. Dibbins AW, Weiner ES: Mortality from neonatal diaphragmatic hernia. J Pediatr Surg 9:653, 1974
30. Erakles AJ et al: Circular esophagomyotomy of upper pouch in primary repair of long segment esophageal atresia. J Pediatr Surg 11:709, 1976
31. Ewing CW: Role of the fiberoptic bronchoscope in lung lavage in patients with cystic fibrosis. Chest 73:750, 1978
32. Fellows KE et al: Bronchial artery embolization in cystic fibrosis, technique and long-term results. J Pediatr 95:959, 1979
33. Gans SO, Austin E: Foreign bodies. In Holder TM, Ashcraft KW (eds): Pediatric Surgery, p 116. Philadelphia, WB Saunders, 1980
34. Groff DB et al: Treatment of lung abscess by transbronchial catheter drainage. Radiology 107:61, 1973
35. Grosfeld JL, Ballantine TVN: Surgical respiratory distress in infancy and childhood. Curr Probl Pediatr 6:5, 1976
36. Grosfeld JL, Ballantine TVN: Esophageal atresia and tracheoesophageal fistula. Effect of delayed thoracotomy on survival. Surgery 84:394, 1978
37. Gross E: An Atlas of Children's Surgery. Philadelphia, WB Saunders, 1970
38. Haller JA et al: Surgical management of lung bud anomalies. Ann Thorac Surg 28:33, 1979
39. Halloran GL et al: Congenital cystic adenomatoid malformation of the lung. Arch Surg 104:715, 1972
40. Hardesty RL et al: Extracorporeal membrane oxygenation. J Thorac Cardiovasc Surg 81:556, 1981
41. Harrison MR et al: The significance of right aortic arch repair of esophageal atresia. J Pediatr Surg 12:861, 1977
42. Harrison MR, deLorimier AA: Congenital diaphragmatic hernia. Surg Clin North Am 61:1023, 1981
43. Hight DW et al: The treatment of retained peripheral foreign bodies in the pediatric airway. J Pediatr Surg 16:694, 1981
44. Holder TM, Ashcraft KW: Congenital diaphragmatic hernia. In Ravitch MM et al (eds): Pediatric Surgery, 3rd ed, p 438. Chicago, Year Book Medical Publishers, 1979
45. Holder TM, Ashcraft KW: Developments in the care of patients with esophageal stenosis and tracheo-esophageal fistula. Surg Clin North Am 61:1050, 1981
46. Holder TM et al: Esophageal atresia and tracheoesophageal fistula: A survey of its members by the Surgical Section of the American Academy of Pediatrics. Pediatrics 34:542, 1964
47. Holinger LD, Callins WO: Endobronchial foreign body removal. Arch Otolaryngol 103:564, 1977
48. Hunsicker RC, Gartner WS: Fogarty catheter technique for removal of endobronchial foreign body. Arch Otolaryngol 103:103, 1977
49. Ivey RM et al: Subvisceral pleural air in neonates with respiratory distress. Pediatr Res 14:600, 1980
50. Jackson C: Grasses as foreign bodies in the bronchus and lung. Laryngoscope 62:897, 1952
51. Johnson DG: Endoscopy. In Ravitch MM et al (eds): Pediatric Surgery, 3rd ed, Vol 1, p 513. Chicago, Year Book Medical Publishers, 1979
52. Jolly SG et al: Patterns of gastroesophageal reflux in children following repair of esophageal atresia and distal trachaeoesophageal fistula. J Pediatr Surg 15:857, 1980
53. Kendig EL et al: Disorders of the Respiratory Tract in Children. Philadelphia, WB Saunders, 1977
54. Kim KG et al: Foreign body in the airway: A review of 202 cases. Laryngoscope 83:347, 1973
55. Kirkpatrick BV et al: Complications of ventilation therapy in respiratory distress syndrome. Am J Dis Child 138:496, 1974
56. Krummel T et al: Clinical use of an extracorporeal membrane oxygenator in neonatal pulmonary failure. J Pediatr Surg (in press)
57. Law D, Kosloske AM: Management of tracheobronchial foreign bodies in children: A re-evaluation of postural drainage and bronchoscopy. Pediatrics 58:362, 1976
58. LeJeune FE: Foreign bodies in the tracheobronchial tree and esophagus. Surg Clin North Am 46:1501, 1966
59. Lilly JR et al: Segmental lung resection in the first year of life. Ann Thorac Surg 22:16, 1976
60. Lincoln JCR et al: Congenital lobar emphysema. Ann Surg 173:55, 1971
61. Livaditis A et al: Esophageal end-to-end anastomosis. Reduction of anastomotic tension by circular myotomy. Scand J Thorac Cardiovasc Surg 1:206, 1972
62. Luck SR et al: Management of pneumothorax in children with chronic pulmonary disease. J Thorac Cardiovasc Surg 74:834, 1977
63. Major NS et al: Lower airway foreign body aspiration in children. Clin Pediatr 16:13, 1977
64. Mitchelson E: Clinical spectrum of infantile lobar emphysema. Ann Thorac Surg 24:182, 1977
65. Moessinger AC et al: High incidence of lung perforation by chest tube in neonatal pneumothorax. J Pediatr 92:635, 1978
66. Moodie DS et al: Use of tolazoline in newborn infants with diaphragmatic hernia and severe cardiopulmonary disease. J Thorac Cardiovasc Surg 75:725, 1978
67. Moskourtz PS, Griscon NT: The medial pneumothorax. Radiology 120:143, 1976
68. Murphy D et al: Pneumococcal emphysema. Am J Dis Child 134:659, 1980
69. Murray GF et al: Obstructive lobar emphysema of the newborn infant: Documentation of the "mucus plug syndrome" with successful treatment by bronchoscopy. J Thorac Cardiovasc Surg 53:886, 1967
70. Myers NA, Aberdeen E: Congenital esophageal atresia and tracheo-esophageal fistula. In Ravitch MM et al (eds): Pediatric Surgery, 3rd ed, vol 1, p 446. Chicago, Year Book Medical Publishers, 1979
71. Nagaraj HS et al: Iatrogenic perforation of the esophagus in premature infants. Surgery 86:583, 1979
72. Opsahl T et al: Bronchogenic mediastinal cysts in infants. Pediatrics 30:376, 1962
73. Ormazabal M et al: Alteration of alveolar-arterial O_2 gradient (A-a DO_2) in response to tolazoline as a prediction of outcome in neonates with persistent pulmonary hypertension. Pediatr Res 14:607, 1980

74. Parker AF et al: Incidence and significance of gastroesophageal reflux following repair of esophageal atresia and tracheoesophageal fistula and the need for anti-reflux procedures. J Pediatr Surg 14:5, 1978
75. Peters RM, Johnson G: Stabilization of pectus deformity with wire stint. J Thorac Cardiovasc Surg 47:814, 1964
76. Pieretti R et al: Resistant esophageal stenosis associated with reflux after repair of esophageal atresia: A therapeutic approach. J Pediatr Surg 9:355, 1974
77. Potts WJ: The Surgeon and the Child. Philadelphia, WB Saunders, 1959
78. Pryce DM: Lower accessory pulmonary artery with intralobar sequestration of lung: A report of seven cases. J Pathol 58:457, 1946
79. Pryce DM et al: Intralobar sequestration of lung associated with an abnormal pulmonary artery. Br J Surg 35:18, 1947
80. Quick CA et al: Bronchoscopy and lavage in management of pulmonary complications of cystic fibrosis. Chest 73:755, 1978
81. Raffensperger JG: Esophageal atresia and tracheoesophageal fistula. In Raffensperger JG (ed): Swenson's Pediatric Surgery, 4th ed, p 650. New York, Appleton-Century-Crofts, 1980
82. Raffensperger JG et al: Swenson's Pediatric Surgery, p 695. New York, Appleton-Century-Crofts, 1980
83. Ramenofsky ML, Luck SR: Diaphragmatic anomalies. In Raffensperger JG (ed): Swenson's Pediatric Surgery, 4th ed, p 679. New York, Appleton-Century-Crofts, 1980
84. Randolph JD et al: Selective surgical management used upon clinical status in infants with esophageal atresia. J Thorac Cardiovasc Surg 76:335, 1977
85. Raphaely RC, Downes JJ: Congenital diaphragmatic hernia: Prediction of survival. J Pediatr Surg 8:815, 1973
86. Ravitch MM: Congenital Deformities of the Chest Wall and Their Operative Correction, p 78. Philadelphia, WB Saunders, 1977
87. Ravitch MM: Congenital Deformities of the Chest Wall and Their Operative Correction, p 172. Philadelphia, WB Saunders, 1977
88. Ravitch MM: Congenital Deformities of the Chest Wall and Their Operative Correction, p 174. Philadelphia, WB Saunders, 1977
89. Ravitch MM: Congenital Deformities of the Chest Wall and Their Operative Correction, p 175. Philadelphia, WB Saunders, 1977
90. Ravitch MM: Technical problems in the operative correction of pectus excavatum Ann Surg 162:29, 1965
91. Ravitch MM et al: Pediatric Surgery. Chicago, Year Book Medical Publishers, 1979
92. Raynor AC et al: Lobar emphysema of infancy. Ann Thorac Surg 4:374, 1967
93. Replogle PL: Esophageal atresia: Plastic sump catheter for drainage of the proximal pouch. Surgery 54:296, 1963
94. Rich RH et al: Open thoracotomy and pleural abrasion in the treatment of spontaneous pneumothorax in cystic fibrosis. J Pediatr Surg 13:237, 1978
95. Salzberg AM, Ehrlich FE: Congenital malformations of the lower respiratory tract. In Kendig EL Jr, Chernick V (eds): Disorders of the Respiratory Tract in Children, p 213. Philadelphia, WB Saunders, 1977
96. Salzberg AM, Ehrlich FE: Congenital malformations of the lower respiratory tract. In Kendig EL, Chernick V (eds): Disorders of the Respiratory Tract in Children, 3rd ed, p 241. Philadelphia, WB Saunders 1977
97. Schuster SR et al: Management of major hemoptysis in patients with cystic fibrosis. J Pediatr Surg 12:889, 1977
98. Schwartz MZ, Filler RM: Tracheal compression as a cause of apnea following repair of tracheoesophageal fistula: Treatment by aortopexy. J Pediatr Surg 15:842, 1980
99. Stein RT et al: Neonatal anterior esophageal perforation. Pediatrics 60:744, 1977
100. Stocker JT et al: Cystic and congenital lung disease in the newborn. In Rosenberg HS, Boloade RP (eds): Perspectives in Pediatric Pathology, vol 4, p 93. Chicago, Year Book Medical Publishers, 1978
101. Swyer PR et al: A case of unilateral pulmonary emphysema. Thorax 8:133, 1953
102. Vale R: Selective bronchial blocking in a small child. Br J Anaesth 41:453, 1968
103. Volberg FM et al: Radiologic features of inferior pulmonary ligament air collections in neonates with respiratory distress. Pediatr Radiol 130:357, 1979
104. Waterston DJ et al: Esophageal atresia: Tracheoesophageal fistula: A study of survival in 218 infants. Lancet 1:819, 1962
105. Welch KJ: Chest wall deformities. In Holder TM, Ashcraft KW (eds): Pediatric Surgery, p 171. Philadelphia, WB Saunders, 1980
106. Welch KJ: Satisfactory surgical correction of pectus excavatum deformity in childhood. J Thorac Cardiovasc Surg 36:697, 1958

Part Four

Complications of Cardiovascular Surgery and Trauma

26 Complications of Cardiopulmonary Resuscitation

Lazar J. Greenfield

OVERVIEW

Cardiopulmonary resuscitation (CPR) is currently practiced widely by nonmedical as well as medical personnel as a result of the efforts of many national organizations and secondary-school programs. The principles of resuscitation can be traced to the biblical era with attempts to resuscitate newborn infants. The evolution of both open- and closed-chest methods progressed rapidly as knowledge of the pathophysiology of respiratory and circulatory arrest improved. Since cardiopulmonary arrest can occur in any patient whose level of activity may range from vigorous exertion to deep, general anesthesia, the response of a rescuer must be virtually automatic in order to minimize the period of hypoxemia and resultant complications. Whether or not the sequence of events is initiated by ventilatory or cardiac dysfunction, the cause of death is always asyphyxiation when circulation fails. This concept is important because the restoration of circulation without adequate oxygenation is doomed to failure.

The surgeon is most likely to be confronted with the need for CPR in a patient in the operating room or intensive-care unit. Estimates of the actual incidence vary widely, but as more complex procedures are performed on an older population, the frequency would appear to be increasing. The initial response depends upon whether the arrest was witnessed or not. For the unwitnessed arrest, the decision algorithm outlined in Figure 26-1 should be followed. It emphasizes the need for adequate ventilation prior to initiating closed-chest cardiac compression. Since the hospital environment should provide for monitoring and support personnel competent to initiate CPR, the surgeon will usually become involved after resuscitation has been initiated. Under this assumption, the surgeon will then be expected to manage the resuscitation and deal with its complictions.

Antecedent Factors

With the exception of the sudden effects of pulmonary thromboembolism or massive myocardial infarction, most episodes of cardiorespiratory arrest occur in a setting of serious organ dysfunction. Prompt recognition and management of these underlying factors can provide the best protection against cardiorespiratory arrest. Their management is also often the key to successful resuscitation should the recognition be delayed.

RESPIRATORY FACTORS

VENTILATORY INSUFFICIENCY may be due to excessive doses of paralytic drugs or the synergistic effects of some antibiotics with muscular relaxation agents used during anesthesia. It is essential to monitor carefully the effects of the administration of neuromuscular-blockade-reversing agents, since their duration of effect may not be sufficient to prevent delayed muscular paralysis. Other less common disorders that increase the vulnerability to respiratory failure include myasthenia gravis, poliomyelitis, and the muscular dystrophies. Monitoring of $PaCO_2$ levels is essential.

CENTRAL DEPRESSION may be due to head injury, stroke, hypercapnia, or anesthesia, as mentioned above. The stastistical likelihood of cardiac arrest during anesthesia is approximately 1 in 1500. In addition, overdosage of narcotics, barbiturates, or tranquilizer drugs, particularly in the elderly or in patients with chronic obstructive lung disease, may occur. In patients with chronic obstructive lung disease, the well-known loss of sensitivity to carbon dioxide levels may lead to respiratory depression when the chronic hypoxemia is corrected by oxygen administration.

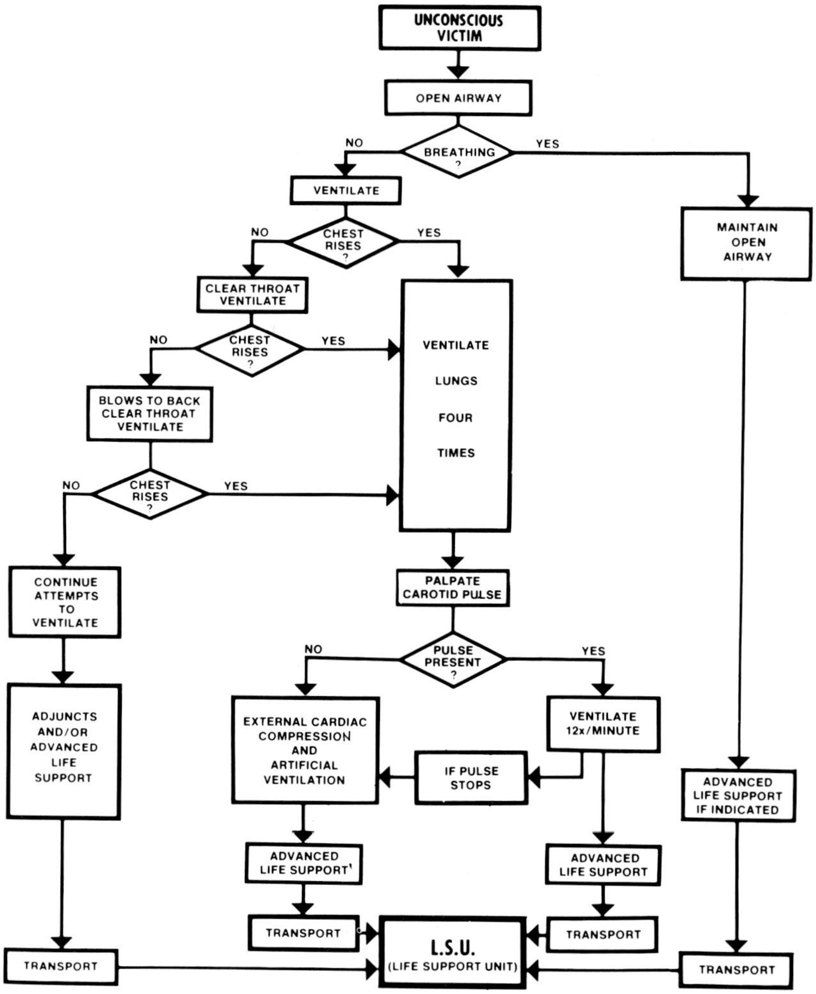

FIG. 26-1. The management sequence for an unwitnessed cardiac arrest is shown as a life-support decision tree. (Reproduced from the Supplement to the Journal of the American Medical Association, August 1, 1980. Copyright © 1980, the American Medical Association. Reproduced with permission from the American Heart Association.)

AIRWAY OBSTRUCTION may be due to mucus, laryngeal spasm, or aspiration of blood, vomitus, or a foreign body. It is important to recognize that gastric distension often precedes major aspiration and that any regimen of tube feeding should include measures to confirm that gastric emptying has occurred prior to additional feeding. Also, airway obstruction and inadequate ventilation that might otherwise have been averted can result from esophageal intubation from emergency tracheal procedures or other mechanical problems.

HYPOXEMIA is the result of the aforementioned ventilatory problems and also may be the result of more localized pulmonary pathology. The susceptibility to cardiorespiratory arrest is increased, usually in proportion to the degree of blood gas derangement, from extensive atelectasis, chest trauma, and other disorders.

Extensive atelectasis is a factor, especially when it occurs in the immediate postoperative period. The use of high F_IO_2 tends to wash out the less soluble pulmonary nitrogen and allow the readily absorbable oxygen to promote atelectasis.

Chest trauma sufficient to produce hemothorax, pneumothorax, flail chest, or contused lung is a factor. The splinting from multiple rib fractures and resistance to painful coughing also promote atelectasis. The latter often can be improved by intercostal nerve block rather than by heavy sedation.

Other disorders such as pneumonia, inhalation burn, congestive heart failure, and asphyxiation from carbon monoxide, smoke inhalation, or excess anesthetic gas mixtures are significant. Pulmonary vascular perfusion problems can result from thrombus, air or fat embolism, or the particulate microembolism that occurs after multiple transfusions and with septicemia. Genuine arteriovenous shunting can occur in the presence of congenital heart disease, but the most common demonstrable derangement from all of these factors is an imbalance between ventilation and perfusion.

CARDIAC FACTORS

REDUCED CARDIAC OUTPUT secondary to arrhythmia, shock, myopathy, cardiac tamponade, myocarditis, or direct trauma is important. The reduction in diastolic pressure leads to inadequate coronary perfusion with most of the vulnerability in the subendocardial region.

CORONARY OCCLUSION may result from thrombus, air, contrast medium injection, coronary artery ligation, or dissection of the arterial wall. The effect may include a serious rhythm disturbance as well as reduced output.

ELECTROMECHANICAL STIMULATION by catheter manipulation, electrode, pericardiocentesis, inotropic drugs, electrocution, or operative manipulation should be minimized. The presence of a monitoring catheter in the right ventricle reduces the resistance to random current since it is an effective conductor. Pacemaker malfunction also may result in ventricular arrhythmias and fibrillation.

METABOLIC DISTURBANCES such as the hyperkalemia associated with renal failure, rapid infusion of stored blood, or of intravenous fluid containing potassium can lead to arrest. Similarly, acidosis increases myocardial vulnerability and is associated with starvation, high intestinal fistula, diabetes mellitus, hypothermia, or hypocapnea. Extremes of core temperature also increase vulnerability and can be seen after environmental exposure, extracorporeal circulation, and long operative procedures, especially when more than one body cavity is entered.

Pathophysiology

The end result of the progression of the adverse factors described in the previous section is cessation of cardiac function in one of the following ways:

Ventricular fibrillation most commonly follows acute myocardial infarction. Often it may be preceded by the development of multifocal premature ventricular contractions. It is strong justification for continuous electrocardiographic monitoring of patients with ventricular irritability.

Mechanical asystole results from arrest in diastole. It is seen in the operating room from anesthetic overdose, as a result of hyperkalemia, and after a vasovagal event as can follow tracheal suctioning in tetraplegic patients since their compensatory sympathetic activity has been lost.

Ineffective ventricular contraction is seen in association with rhythm disturbances or hypoxemia. In this situation the electrocardiogram may be misleading with maintenance of a QRS complex in the absence of cardiac output. The complexes are usually widened and "agonal' in appearance.

Following cessation of the circulation, the pupils begin to dilate in 30 to 45 seconds, and the respiratory drive is lost after approximately 60 seconds as the medulla is depressed. An adult at normothermia can usually tolerate only 4 minutes of this ischemia before irreversible central nervous system damage occurs. Tolerance is increased with hypothermia and at younger ages, allowing the occasional remarkable recovery of children apparently drowning in cold water for more than 30 minutes. The tolerance to respiratory arrest is more difficult to predict, since circulation continues for several minutes with variable levels of oxygen availability and extraction.

Drowning

Although large numbers of healthy people die each year as a result of drowning, asphyxia is suspected to be the cause in only about 10% of cases. The effects on the victim depend on the quantity and quality of the fluid aspirated.[5] In fresh water, large volumes can enter the circulation, producing massive hemolysis and hemodilution.[9] The combination of hypoxia and hypervolemia results in ventricular fibrillation. Sea water, however, draws fluid into the lung by osmosis, resulting in hypovolemia and hypotension. Ventilation with air can prevent pulmonary edema and death from near-drowning but does not prevent the ventricular fibrillation associated with fresh water drowning.[6]

Accordingly, management of near-drowning should begin with mouth-to-mouth ventilation as soon as the victim is in shallow water, and basic life support is continued on land. Resuscitation is not possible in deep water. No attempt should be made to evacuate water from the lungs, but ventilation with high F_IO_2 should be started as soon as possible. A pulmonary arterial catheter is useful to monitor wedge pressures and intrapulmonary shunt. Aseptic tracheobronchial toilet and antibiotics should be used to control bacterial superinfection. Transfusion of red blood cells may be needed after aspiration of fresh water if hemolysis has occurred. Frequent measurement of arterial blood gases allows selective control of appropriate levels of pulmonary end-expiratory pressure (PEEP) and F_IO_2 as outlined in Chapter 22.

Diagnosis

Respiratory arrest can be recognized readily by the absence of any thoracic movement or audible breath sounds. The diagnosis of cardiac arrest depends on the absence of a palpable pulse at the carotid or femoral level unless the surgeon is operating in the abdomen, where the abdominal aorta is readily available to palpation. More distal pulses such as the radial are not reliable for the diagnosis, although obviously a functioning radial artery catheter that indicates no pulse wave should be investigated. Further support for the diagnosis can be found in the loss of perfusion. As indicated previously, the electrocardiogram can be misleading with persistent agonal activity, but the appearance of ventricular tachycardia or fibrillation is sufficient to initiate resuscitation. In the absence of monitors, resuscitation should also be started rather than awaiting electrocardiographic confirmation. Delay is catastrophic to the central nervous system, and there is little risk in initiating basic life support, as described below.

Management

The standards for cardiopulmonary resuscitation (CPR) and emergency cardiac care (ECC) have been established by the American Heart Association.[7] The objective is to maintain circulation and oxygenation until advanced life support is available or vital function is restored. The mnemonic A-B-C has been used to establish the priority for airway, breathing, and circulation, as was outlined in Figure 26-1.

In the absence of suspected cervical trauma, the airway is opened by tilting the victim's head backward as far as possible, using one hand on the forehead and the other behind the neck (Fig. 26-2). This lifts the tongue from the back of the throat to open the airway. If the airway is not cleared by this maneuver, the jaw can be displaced further forward by traction or pushing on the angles of the mandible. In the absence of breathing efforts, mouth-to-mouth or mouth-to-nose ventilation must be started. The F_IO_2 of expired air of 0.16 is more than adequate for respiratory exchange. In the hospital environment, an oral airway, self-inflating bag, and facemask

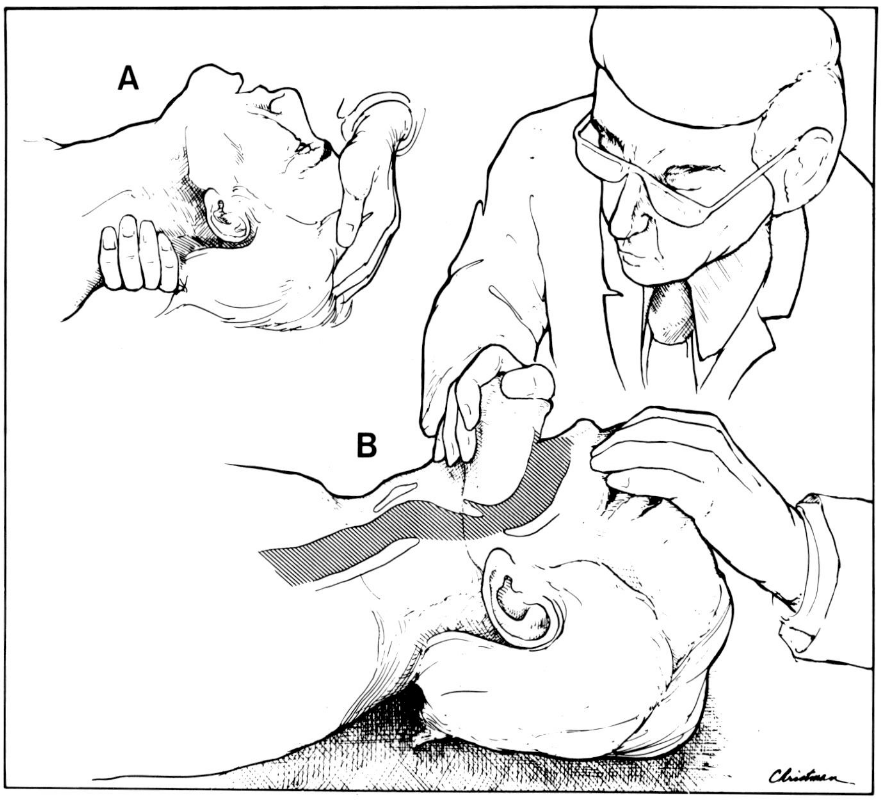

FIG. 26-2. (*A*) In the absence of suspected cervical injury, the initial step in resuscitation is to open the airway by tilting the head back and, if necessary, by elevating the jaw to displace the tongue forward. (*B*) Mouth-to-mouth resuscitation can be facilitated by closing the nose by compression. If the mouth cannot be opened, ventilation through the nose is possible if the lips are held closed. (Greenfield LJ: Cardiac arrest. In Sabiston D [ed] Davis–Christopher Textbook of Surgery, p 2209. Philadelphia, WB Saunders, 1981)

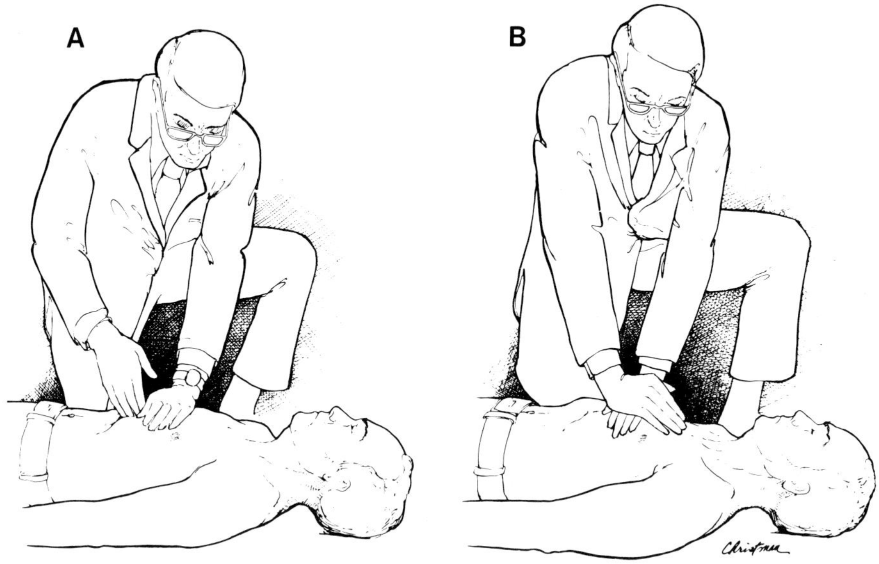

FIG. 26-3. (*A*) The correct hand position for cardiac compression is determined by palpating the xyphoid with one hand and placing the other above that level on the sternum. (*B*) External cardiac compression requires depression of the sternum approximately 2 inches with the heels of the hands and the weight of the rescuer. (Greenfield LJ: Cardiac arrest. In Sabiston D [ed] Davis–Christopher Textbook of Surgery, p 2210. Philadelphia, WB Saunders, 1981)

should be available and can improve ventilation until an endotracheal tube can be inserted.

Ventilation by bag or breathing should be provided every 5 seconds and the victim allowed to exhale passively, which verifies the effectiveness of ventilation. Over-inflation of infants and children can be avoided by smaller breaths and more rapid cycles, closer to every 3 seconds. Also, the infant's head does not need to be tilted backward as much. If thoracic expansion and passive exhalation do not occur, the airway must be checked for possible foreign material. This can be cleared manually or by suction apparatus if it is available.

The sequence of management for an unwitnessed arrest is to ventilate for four or five breaths while the carotid pulse is palpated. If no pulse is present, external cardiac compression is started (Fig. 26-3). Effective ventricular compression requires sternal displacement of about 2 inches, which can be accomplished best using the heels of both hands over the lower half of the sternum. The arms should be kept straight and the compression maintained for about 60% of each cycle. If there is only one rescuer, he should perform two quick lung inflations after every 15 chest compressions, since compressions alone do not provide adequate air exchange. The rate of chest compression also must be increased to 80 per minute in order to average 60 per minute when the ventilation time is interposed. When there are two rescuers, ventilation should be performed after every fifth beat without interrupting cardiac compression. If the rescuers are on opposite sides of the victim, they can trade places easily to avoid fatigue. For infants, only two fingers are used for chest compression at rates of 80 to 100 beats per minute, and for children only one hand is applied at the level of midsternum because of the higher position of the heart in the chest.

In the event of a witnessed cardiac arrest, which is more likely in the intensive-care unit, effective cardiac and ventilatory support will be readily available. Although a "precordial thump" has been recommended in the past, it is just as likely to cause ventricular fibrillation as it is to restore cardiac action, and it is not indicated in the presence of anoxia, as with an unwitnessed arrest, or in children. Cardiac compression in a hospital bed is less effective than on a firm surface, and therefore a board should be placed behind the patient as soon as possible. Other measures for advanced life support also should be utilized, such as supplemental oxygen by mask or tube if a tube is in the trachea. An oropharyngeal airway can be inserted if personnel experienced in the insertion of an endotracheal tube are not immediately available. It is often wiser to use this approach rather than risk misplacement or pharyngeal injury with hurried attempts by the inexperienced to insert a tube. As more assistance becomes available, intravenous lines can be inserted, electrocardiographic monitoring established for dysrhythmia management, and a defibrillator obtained. Definitive drug therapy for inotropic support and correction of acidosis can be started.

Manual or automatic chest compression devices are available but are relatively awkward to use and limited to use in adults. Effective cardiac compression provides sufficient circulation for drug action in all tissues, and therefore intravenous injection usually is adequate for drug administration. Direct intracardiac injection not only introduces the pos-

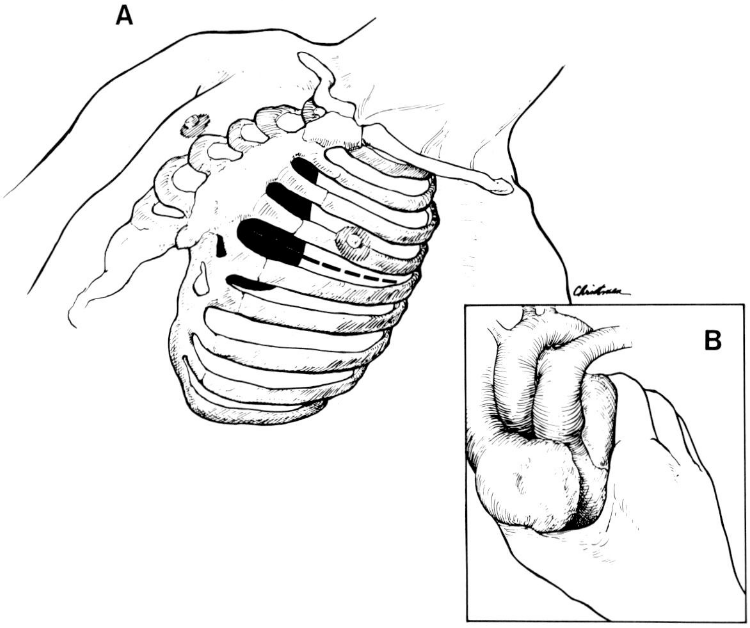

FIG. 26-4. (*A*) The incision for open cardiac compression should be made anteriorly in the left fifth intercostal space. (*B*) After the pericardium is opened, direct cardiac compression may be performed with either hand, but the surgeon should be careful to avoid excessive pressure on the right ventricle, which can be perforated. (Greenfield LJ: Cardiac arrest. In Sabiston D [ed] Davis–Christopher Textbook of Surgery, p 2211. Philadelphia, WB Saunders, 1981)

sibility of cardiac tamponade, coronary artery injury, or pneumothorax, but it obligates cessation of cardiac compression. In the absence of reliable intravenous access, epinephrine can be administered by intratracheal instillation. If an intracardiac injection is felt to be necessary, the needle should be inserted under negative pressure to ensure placement in the ventricular cavity. A complete description of the drugs useful in cardiac resuscitation can be found in Chapter 28.

Once the resuscitative effort is considered optimal, an effort should be made to differentiate between cardiac standstill and ventricular fibrillation. The availability of miniaturized oscilloscopes that are battery powered and packaged with a defibrillator unit has made the task more rapid and efficient. Generally, capacitance–discharge (DC) defibrillation is used today with the electrode-pasted paddles applied to the right upper sternal border and at the apex of the heart. For an adult, the unit should be set to deliver the maximum of 400 watt-seconds. In children 60 to 100 watt-seconds should be used. After defibrillation, basic life support should be resumed immediately for sufficient oxygenation to permit another 5-second pause to determine the cardiac rhythm. Repetitive defibrillations can produce superficial burns, but the effect can be minimized by insuring adequate contact surface with electrode paste. Failure to defibrillate may be due to inadequate electrical current, acidosis, or hypoxemia, which are amenable to treatment. Less favorable causes such as massive infarction or pulmonary thromboembolism reduce the chances for survival.

Complications

The most serious complication of standard closed-chest resuscitation is, of course, failure to restore effective cardiac action. In some patients, such as those with chest or spinal deformities, closed-chest compression is predictably ineffective and even dangerous. In these patients, including those with the barrel-chest deformity of severe emphysema, open-chest cardiac compression is required. Open compression is also advisable after penetrating wounds of the heart or blunt chest injury when cardiac tamponade, tension pneumothorax, or other intrathoracic injuries are suspected.

When closed-chest compression fails to provide effective circulation, the chest should be opened through the left fifth intercostal space and the pericardium opened to allow direct manual cardiac compression (Fig. 26-4). An increased cardiac output can be obtained because only the ventricles are compressed and not the atria, as in closed-chest massage. Even under optimal circumstances, closed-chest compression provides only 30% of normal cardiac output, and for this reason it should be maintained without interruption of more than 10 to 20 seconds at a time, even for tracheal intubation.

During open thoracotomy, it is advisable to insert a rib spreader to relieve the pressure on the surgeon's hand and also to allow the insertion of the opposite hand to compress the ascending aorta during diastole. This provides more coronary perfusion, and the improved access allows assessment of cardiac tone and the direct application of electrodes for defibrillation. When the cardiac arrest occurs in the operating room during laparotomy, the heart may be palpated and compressed through the diaphragm against the sternum. It is relatively easy to open the diaphragm for more direct access to the ventricles, beginning at the anterior aspect of the diaphragm, which preserves sterility during an abdominal procedure.

The unsterile thoracotomy is subject to infection, and if the resuscitation is successful, the patient should be transported to the operating room for closure of the wound under sterile conditions. This allows precise control of bleeding points and copious wound irrigation. Chest-wall infections are usually superficial and well tolerated.

The other serious complication of direct ventricular massage is perforation of the right ventricle, usually by the thumb of the surgeon. The vulnerability of the right ventricle is related to the fact that it is thinner than the left ventricle and often distended from fluid resuscitation. Being aware of this vulnerability obligates the surgeon to use care with preference for two hands for compression. It is also advisable to keep the digits flat rather than curled. A perforation can be repaired by sutures buttressed with Teflon felt, but the ventricle is highly friable under these circumstances, and this complication usually portends an unsuccessful outcome. Rarely, the pericardial space may be obliterated by adhesions, making its opening hazardous; in this case no attempt should be made to incise the pericardium.

The complications of closed-chest massage are most frequently related to chest-wall damage and include rib fractures and costochondral separation, risking aortic and cardiac injury, pneumothorax, or hemothorax. Compression of the xiphoid, if it angles downward, can produce laceration of the liver. Less common, rupture of the stomach or fracture of the spleen can occur, and fat embolism has been described.[2] These adverse effects can be minimized by steady rhythmical compression of the chest wall using the heels of the hands rather than the fingers. The frequency of intrathoracic complications, however, requires that a chest film be obtained as soon as possible after resuscitation. Particular attention should be paid to the position of the endotracheal tube, since it is easy to have it inserted so deeply that it enters the right bronchus and fails to ventilate the left side.

Another serious complication is failure to resuscitate in time to prevent brain damage or to resuscitate a patient who has an irreversible terminal illness. The latter problem can be minimized by leaving instructions with the nursing staff not to resuscitate the patient and documenting by written note in the patient's chart that this decision has been discussed with the family. It is more difficult to decide when to terminate resuscitative efforts, and the physician must assess the cerebral and cardiovascular status of the patient in relationship to the time that has elapsed since the arrest. Generally, nonreactive pupils and lack of respiratory effort persisting in excess of 30 minutes reflect cerebral death, and absence of cardiac electrical activity after 10 minutes of resuscitation offers a poor prognosis. When the arrest is known to have occurred for longer than 10 minutes before effective resuscitation, the outlook for resuscitation is bleak.

Results

In a general hospital setting, resuscitation will be successful initially in about 35% of patients.[1] The incidence of additional episodes of arrest is very high, however, so that only about 10% to 20% of patients survive to leave the hospital. Their subsequent course is encouraging, however, since in one series 74% were alive at the end of 1 year, and 51% were alive at the end of 3 years.[4]

The mechanism of arrest is a major determinant of survival. Ventricular standstill is particularly ominous, and the likelihood of resuscitation after asystole is remote.[1] It is more encouraging to find ventricular fibrillation, probably because it occurs earlier with residual muscular viability. Approximately 30% of patients in ventricular fibrillation can be resuscitated and survive.[8] In contrast to other major complications, younger age has an adverse effect on survival, which was only 17% after 1 month in a group of patients 40 to 49 years of age.[10] Since cardiac arrest may be the presenting sign of coronary artery disease, coronary angiography must be considered in the younger survivers. The results of aggresive management, including early intra-aortic balloon placement and coronary artery bypass grafting, have improved outlook for these patients.[3] Further improvement in the results of resuscitation will occur when more of the population learns basic CPR. It is well established that bystander CPR and trained paramedics significantly improve the likelihood of survival.

References

1. Castagna J, Wed MH, Shubin H: Factors determining survival in patients with cardiac arrest. Chest 65:527, 1974
2. Clark DT: Complication following closed chest massage. JAMA 181:337, 1962
3. Kaiser GA, Ghahramani A, Bolooki H et al: Role of coronary artery surgery in patients surviving unexpected cardiac arrest. Surgery 78:749, 1975
4. Kouwenhoven WB, Jude JR, Knickerbocker GG: Closed chest cardiac massage. JAMA 173:1064, 1960

5. Madell JH, Graves SA, Ketover A: Clinical course of 91 consecutive near drowning victims. Chest 70:231, 1976
6. Redding JS, Voigt GC, Safar P: Drowning treated with intermittent positive pressure breathing. J Appl Physiol 15:849, 1960
7. Standards for Cardiopulmonary Resuscitation (CPR) and Emergency Cardiac Care (ECC). JAMA 227:837, 1974
8. Stiles QR, Tucker BL, Meyer BW et al: Cardiopulmonary arrest, evaluation of an active resuscitation program. Am J Surg 122:282, 1971
9. Swann HG, Spafford NR: Body salt and water changes during fresh and sea water drowning. Tex Rep Biol Med 9:356, 1951
10. Wildsmith JA, Dennyson WG, Myers KW: Results of resuscitation following cardiac arrest. Br J Anaesth 44:716, 1972

27 Complications of Vascular Surgery and Trauma

Paul R. Liebman | Robert W. Barnes

OVERVIEW

Sergeant P. B. Messenger, Co. A, 111th Pennsylvania, aged 33 years, was wounded at Lookout Mountain, November 24, 1863. Sergeant B. Woodward, 22nd Illinois, described the case. . . .

> The injury consisted of a compound comminuted fracture of the right lower jaw, the ball passing in at the angle of the mouth. . . . and making its exit close by the cervical column. By December 2nd the wound was discharging freely [and there was a] . . . great amount of swelling. At noon the patient fed himself with soup; but at 1:30 P.M. I was called to him and found four quarts of blood collected in a large tin basin. Arterial blood was also pouring in torrents from his mouth. On introducing the finger it was found that the internal carotid had sloughed, ... I pressed lint soaked with solution of persulphate of iron firmly back against the bleeding artery, and, holding it there with my finger directed Assistant Surgeon H. Pierce, 150th New York, to cut down and take up the common trunk, which he did. . . . Before the artery was taken up the patient had a severe convulsion from the loss of blood, rendering the operation very difficult [but after the ligation] . . . the blood ceased to pour from the artery . . .; pulse at the wrist [was] imperceptible; breathing gasping. . . . [He] was allowed to lie on the table for four hours, . . . wrapped in hot blankets . . . [and was] made to swallow pure extract of beef. . . . The following morning his pulse was 160 and very feeble . . . [but by] 8:00 P.M. his pulse was 130 and fuller . . . he was given one drachm of wine and two drachms of extract of beef every two hours. . . . [The] next night he slept well; pulse 120 and growing fuller; no hemorrhage; wound . . . suppurating well . . . [on] December 5th . . . [he was] doing well; . . . appetite good; craves oysters . . . [but by December 7th he showed] evidences of cerebral symptoms . . . such as hebetude and listlessness, breathing very feeble, slight divergence of the right eye. Coma came on at 8:00 P.M. [December 8th] and complete paralysis of the left side. Death occurred at 1:00 A.M. on December 9th, 1863. The autopsy showed . . . the brain to be covered with lymph [pus]. Dissecting out the carotid . . . a firm clot [was found] . . . extending . . . above the ligature. The internal carotid was completely filled with . . . clot as far as the entrance into the skull. . . .
>
> —Medical and Surgical History of the War of Rebellion, 1883[49]

Thromboembolism, sepsis, and ischemia so plagued early attempts at even the most elementary vascular surgery that its development was delayed many years longer than that of other fields of surgery. Despite dramatic advances in technique, materials, antibiotics, anticoagulation, and perioperative care, these complications, as well as others, still persist in operations upon blood vessels.

Although complications may be related and peculiar to a particular operation or anatomical area, several complications are common to all arterial reconstructive procedures.

General Complications of Arterial Surgery

EARLY THROMBOSIS

Every operation that involves arterial reconstruction requires the use of some index of patency in the postoperative period. This may involve distal pulse palpation and the examination of the color and temperature of the involved extremity. However, the recording of a segmental (usually ankle) Doppler arterial pressure provides an objective, quantitative, physiologic value. This measurement can be followed sequentially to identify early thrombosis. A deterioration of the segmental pressure in the postoperative period may identify impending graft failure. As soon as early graft thrombosis is detected,

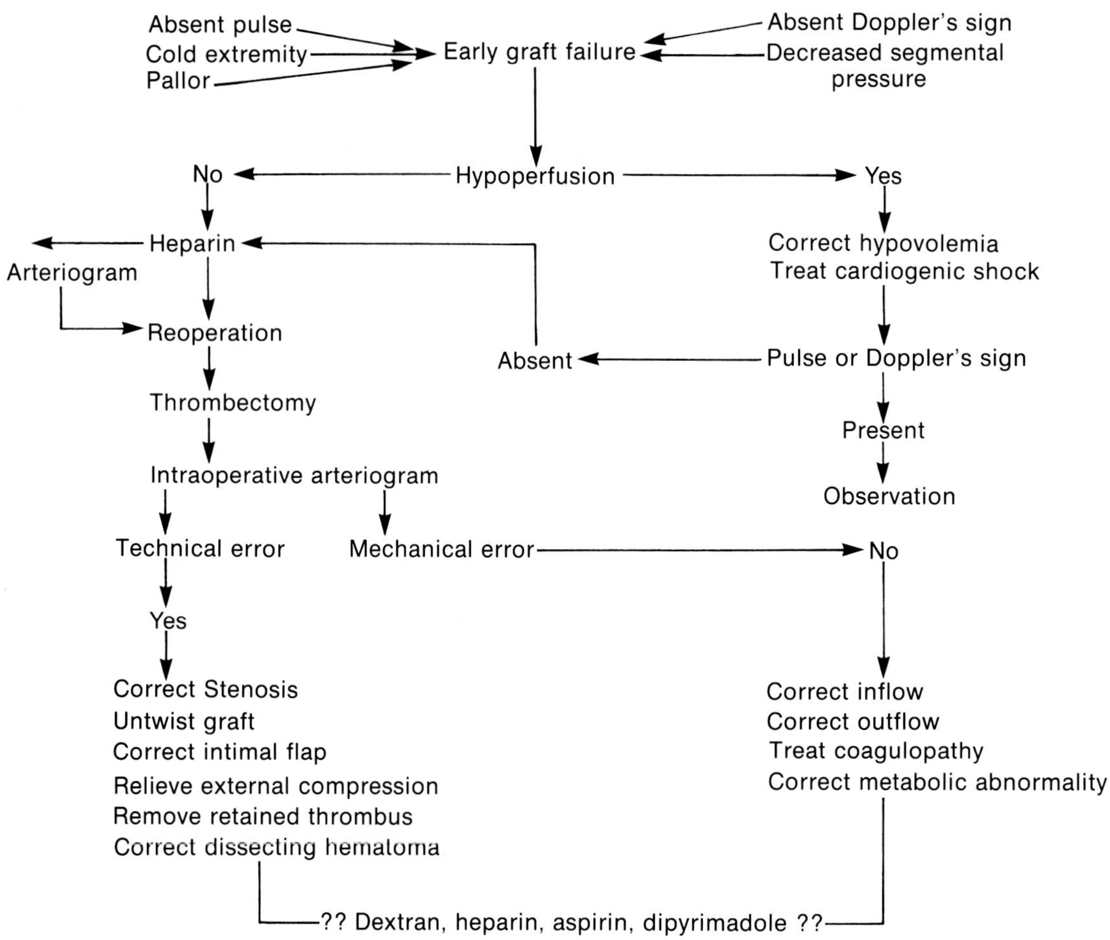

FIG. 27-1. An approach to early graft failure.

the patient should be heparinized systemically in an attempt to prevent clot propagation and returned to the operating room. Occasionally an arteriogram is indicated prior to reoperation, but usually the graft or endarterectomized vessel needs to be cleared of clot before the problem can be localized.

After thrombectomy with a Fogarty catheter, an intraoperative arteriogram will usually reveal a mechanical cause of the early graft failure. Causes of early postoperative failure are listed below.

Mechanical
Stenotic anastomosis
Twisted graft
Thrombus
Perigraft hematoma
Intimal flap
Dissecting hematoma
External compression (suture, tunnel, etc.)

Hemodynamic
Inadequate inflow
Inadequate outflow
Hypoperfusion (cardiogenic, hypovolemia)

Hematologic and Metabolic
Hypercoagulable state
Prolonged ischemia → thromboplastin, ↓ *p*H
Massive blood transfusions

An approach to early graft thrombosis is outlined in Figure 27-1. Most early graft failures are secondary to technical errors and could, therefore, be prevented.[84] Proper illumination with a head lamp or other auxiliary sources is important for precise vascular anastomosis. Magnification using 2.5 × loupes should be routine for vascular reconstruction, especially of those below the inguinal ligament. Careful attention should be paid to placing the graft where it will not be compressed by muscle, kinked at a joint, or twisted. Technical errors may be detected by a variety of methods: electromagnetic flow measurements, pulse volume recordings, segmental plethysmography, Doppler ultrasound assessment, and intraoperative angiography. Intraoperative angiography has the advantage of requiring no special equipment or preparation and of being particularly sensitive to the technical errors found responsible for most early graft failures (Fig. 27-2).[42]

By properly selecting the operative procedure, early graft failure due to inadequate inflow or outflow can be avoided. A common clinical problem is determining the significance of aortoiliac disease in the patient with symptomatic femoropopliteal occlusion. The hemodynamic significance of aortoiliac stenosis may be evaluated using noninvasive diagnostic techniques or by intra-arterial measurement of aortoiliac pressure gradients at rest and during hyperemia (reactive or pharmacologically induced). Intra-arterial pressure may be measured at the time of arteriography or the operation. Finally, multiple views (including oblique views) of the aortoiliac and femoral arterial segments are useful to evaluate the need for correction of inflow arterial disease prior to more distal bypass. Thus, methods to determine the significance of aortoiliac disease include the following:

Multiple view arteriograms
Segmental Doppler pressure
Pulse volume recording
Doppler signal analogue trace
Doppler signal spectral analysis
Direct catheter pull-back pressures

The need for an outflow procedure following aortofemoral reconstruction can be predicted by noting the increase in ankle pressure postoperatively or through examining the preoperative pulse volume plethysmographic thigh–ankle ratio.[9, 55] It is important to correct profunda femoris stenosis at the time of the inflow procedure.

With developing experience and the availability of percutaneous transluminal angioplasty, the correction of isolated iliac stenosis prior to femoropopliteal bypass or femoral stenosis prior to aortoiliac reconstruction will allow correction of compromised inflow or outflow without the need for extensive combined or sequential procedures.[2, 86]

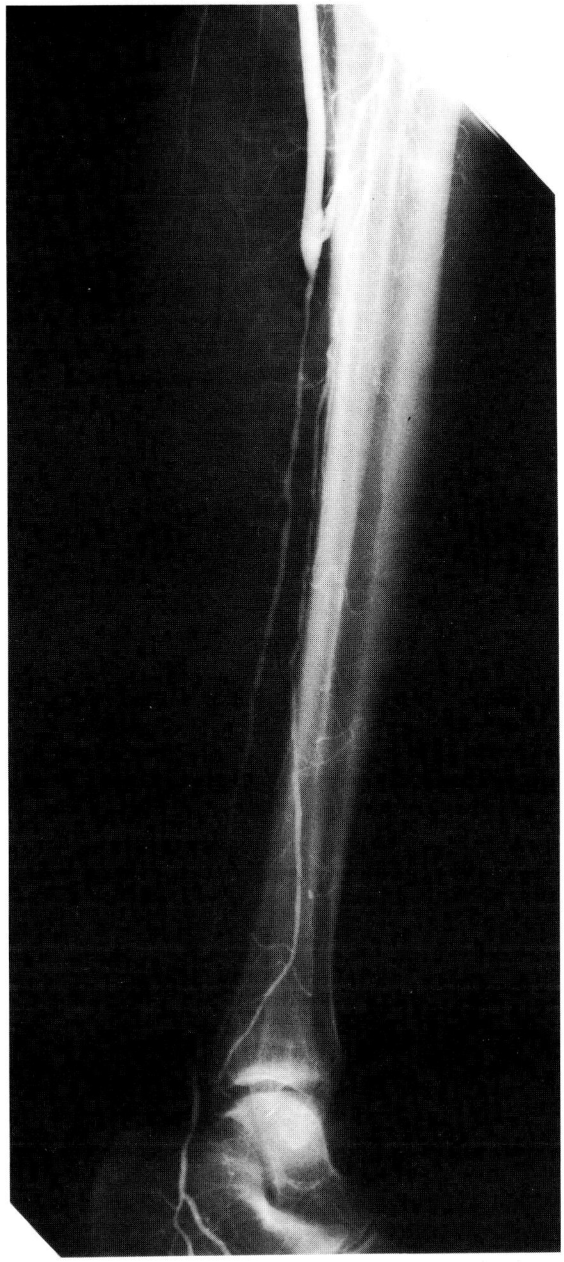

FIG. 27-2. An intraoperative arteriogram taken following a femoroposterior tibial bypass reveals technically satisfactory anastomosis.

GRAFT SEPSIS

A devastating complication of arterial reconstruction that threatens both life and limb is infection in a prosthetic graft. Fortunately this complication occurs rarely (less than 2% of grafts limited to the abdomen, less than 5% of grafts that involve the groin), because when it occurs, the rate of limb loss and mortality are quite high despite aggressive therapy.[43]

The predominance of skin organisms isolated from infected prosthetic grafts suggests that many of these infections result from either a break in technique or a superficial skin infection at or remote from the operative site.

Organisms Isolated from Prosthetic Graft Infections (%)
Staphylococcus Aureus, 50
Escherichia coli, 13
Streptococcus, 9
Klebsiella, 5
Proteus, 5
S. albus, 4
Others, 14

A prosthetic graft as a foreign body will become infected from a bacterial inoculum that might be resisted in the presence of an autologous vein or endarterectomized vessel. Accumulation of blood and lymph around the graft, particularly if the lymph contains organisms drained from an infected distal site, predisposes the patient to graft sepsis.

Prophylaxis is the most important way to deal with the problem of graft sepsis. Large exposed areas of skin should be covered with plastic adherent drapes to prevent contamination of the graft on exposed skin. No groin with dermatitis or in which a recent arteriogram has created a groin hematoma should be subjected to an operation. Distal infection should be drained and controlled as much as possible prior to reconstruction. Appropriate antibiotics should be continued through the postoperative period. Both prophylactic topical and systemic antibiotics will serve to reduce the incidence of graft infection.[61] Prophylactic antibiotics must be begun before the operation and should be appropriate for the common organisms, especially *Staphylococcus aureus* and coliform bacteria. Meticulous attention to technique, particularly for hemostasis, and the control of lymph channels in the groin and around the infrarenal aorta are important. Wound irrigation with saline or antibiotic solutions serves to reduce bacterial contamination.

Prosthetic grafts may be seeded by bacteremia in the postoperative period. Experimental evidence suggests that this susceptibility may decrease with time, perhaps when a pseudointimal lining is complete.[53] These facts should be considered when dealing with ischemic ulcers, intravenous catheters, bladder drainage catheters, and complications that might produce bacteremia.

Prosthetic graft infections can be divided by their presentation into three often overlapping categories: early graft sepsis, late graft sepsis, and graft contamination secondary to wound breakdown.

Early graft sepsis is often noted in the groin associated with wound abscess. When the abscess is drained, the underlying graft is found bathed in pus. Less frequently early graft sepsis is noted in the groin by acute hemorrhage, usually occurring between the fifth to tenth postoperative day without gross evidence of pus. Attempts to repair this "anastomotic leak" will be disastrous, and the situation must be recognized for what it is, a prosthetic graft infection. Early graft sepsis rarely occurs in an abdominal graft, but it should be considered in the postoperative patient who shows systemic signs of sepsis and intra-abdominal inflammation, particularly persistent postoperative ileus. Hemorrhage rather than thrombosis is usually an accompaniment of early graft sepsis.

Early graft sepsis is much more easily recognized than is the late presentation. Late graft infection is usually caused by organisms of low virulence and may be manifest by a thrombosed graft or anastomotic pseudoaneurysm. Associated findings that may suggest late graft sepsis are fever, leukocytosis, and an elevated erythrocyte sedimentation rate. Unfortunately, these are nonspecific observations that are usually present with infection anywhere and help very little in identifying graft sepsis. Positive blood cultures further support the suspicion of graft sepsis, but they also may result from other septic foci. Distal septic embolization appears as petechiae that contain organisms that can be demonstrated on Gram stain, but it is rarely present. This finding in a patient with a graft is pathognomonic of an infected prosthesis.

The principles involved in treating graft sepsis are the same for both early and late presentation and are listed below:

- High-dose antibiotics
- Removal of infected graft
- Heparinization to prevent distal thrombosis
- Closure of proximal and distal arteries with monofilament suture material
- Provision of soft tissue coverage over sutured arteries (muscle, omentum, etc.)
- Provision of adequate drainage of abscess
- Extra-anatomical bypass by clean operative fields if limb viability in question

Infection in a graft that has not thrombosed may remain localized, but an occluded graft is quickly and completely involved in the septic process. The first priority is to remove all infected graft. Thus an occluded graft should be completely removed. If it is patent, the infected limb of a bifurcation graft may be removed, preserving the unaffected limb. At the time of reoperation the unaffected limb must show signs of good tissue incorporation and no evidence of fluid collection around the graft. The next step is to provide perfusion distally. With adequate collateral circulation, the extremity may survive without need for additional reconstruction. However, usually a new bypass will be required by means of an extra-anatomical route remote from the septic sites. The preferred routes of extra-anatomical bypass appropriate to a given infected site are listed in Table 27-1.

Graft contamination secondary to wound breakdown may sometimes be handled differently. Rather than viewing these grafts as infected, they may be thought of as being contaminated as a result of wound breakdown secondary to seroma, hematoma, lymphocele, or technical error of wound closure. The contamination may occur either in the early or late postoperative period. In the late presentation, this complication most commonly occurs in the long limb of an axillobifemoral graft when the graft erodes through the skin. The most common site of such erosion is at a counter incision. This complication is best treated by establishing coverage before the graft is exposed. Once the graft is exposed, the patient should be promptly brought to the operating room for aggressive débridement and primary closure. Graft coverage with muscle is important. The sartorius muscle may be detached from its origin to cover an exposed prosthesis in the groin. The experience and ingenuity of plastic surgeons can be helpful to plan myocutaneous coverage elsewhere. Catheters for antibiotic irrigation and drainage are useful adjuncts in such procedures. Appropriate systemic antibiotics are also indicated. Personal experience and two small series demonstrate that contaminated grafts can be salvaged using these techniques.[33, 66]

ANASTOMOTIC ANEURYSMS

An anastomotic aneurysm is the result of anastomotic disruption with a pulsating hematoma contained by surrounding fibrous connective tissue. These are by definition false or pseudoaneurysms because they contain no elements of the arterial wall. Anastomotic aneurysms occur in 3% of femoral anastomoses, about 1% of iliac and popliteal anastomoses, and less than 1% of aortic and carotid anastomoses.[78] The natural history of anastomotic aneurysms is unclear. Some will remain small, nonprogressive, and uncomplicated and probably do not need operative intervention. Others will progressively enlarge and may produce various complications. Anastomotic aneurysms have been implicated in graft thrombosis and peripheral embolization. Ureteral obstruction has been noted secondary to an aortoiliac anastomotic aneurysm.[16] Both consumptive coagulopathy and pathologic fibrinolysis have been attributed to anastomotic aneurysms.[3, 64] Rarely, these aneurysms will rupture, producing massive hemorrhage (Fig. 27-3).

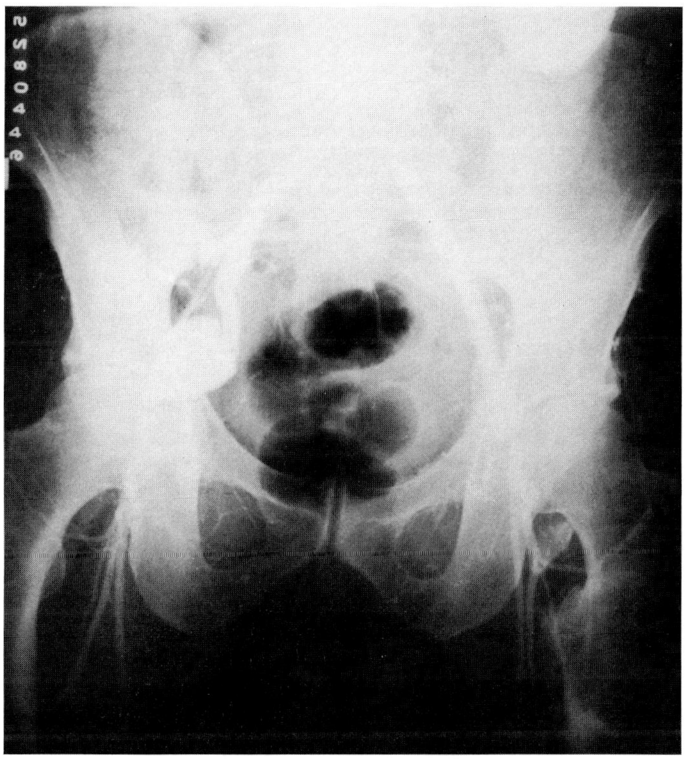

FIG. 27-3. A large anastomotic aneurysm in the right side of the groin following an aortobifemoral graft.

Historically, false aneurysms were thought to be due to the use of silk in vascular anastomosis. A prosthetic graft will not heal with a native artery so that a suture must be permanent to maintain anastomotic integrity. Silk, a biologic substance, is "permanent" for most surgery, but not for vascular anastomoses. Even with the development of newer permanent synthetic suture materials false aneurysms have still been found. Therefore most of these aneurysms are the result of technical errors. Inadequate depth of suture placement in the arterial wall and excess tension on the anastomosis have been cited as etiologic factors. End-to-side anastomosis, failure of graft material, and systemic hypertension have all been implicated in the development of false aneurysms. Graft infection may weaken the adjacent artery with resultant anastomotic disruption. Indeed, any false aneurysm may be infected, and specimens from all must be cultured at the time of repair. If frank pus or suspicious fluid is found to surround the graft or if the graft is poorly incorporated into surrounding tissue, an immediate Gram stain of the fluid should be obtained. If the fluid contains organisms, the graft should be resected and an extra-anatomical bypass performed. Finally, arteriosclerotic degeneration of the arterial wall itself may so weaken the anastomosis that a false aneurysm develops.

Small false aneurysms may be observed, especially in the groin where inspection is easy. Large lesions should be treated surgically. Principles of operative repair include initial proximal control, early culture and Gram stain of suspicious fluid, endoaneurysmal approach to preclude much dissection in the heavily scarred surrounding tissue, resection of aneurysmal tissue back to normal artery, replacement of the distal graft, and anastomosis with sutures incorporating large bites of healthy arterial wall.

POSTOPERATIVE HEMORRHAGE

Hemorrhage in the early postoperative period has several etiologies, most commonly a technical error. A tie may have come off a vein graft side branch; an anastomosis may be leaking; or an incised vessel in the subcutaneous tissue or retroperitoneum may have been overlooked. If it is apparent that the hemorrhage is secondary to a technical error, immediate reoperation is indicated. If, however, the problem is a generalized ooze or if reoperation fails to reveal an error that can be corrected, a coagulopathy may be present. The presence of residual heparin activity must be considered. Acute and chronic consumptive coagulopathy as well as depressed fibrinogen levels have been associated with abdominal aortic aneurysms.[45, 47, 69] The approach to the patient with an abnormal bleeding mechanism is discussed in Chapter 16.

Complications of Aortoiliac Surgery: Aneurysm, Occlusive Disease, and Trauma

The complications that accompany surgery and trauma of the abdominal aorta are the most varied, spectacular, and serious of peripheral vascular surgery. These complications may be divided into complications of aortic disease itself, complications of aortic surgery, and complications of aortic trauma.

Complications of Disease
Ischemia: claudication, rest pain, tissue loss, emboli
Abdominal aortic aneurysm, rupture
Abdominal aortic aneurysm, aortoenteric fistula, primary
Abdominal aortic aneurysm, aortocaval fistula

Early Complications of Surgery
Hemorrhage
Myocardial infarction
Respiratory failure
Renal failure
Paraplegia
Intestinal ischemia
Chylous ascites
Peripheral ischemia

Late Complications of Surgery
Aortoenteric fistula
Infected prosthetic graft
Anastomotic aneurysm
Graft thrombosis
Sexual dysfunction

COMPLICATIONS OF AORTIC DISEASE

The complications of aortic occlusive disease are the everyday presentations of chronic ischemia, claudication, rest pain, and ischemic ulceration. The signs of aneurysmal disease are sometimes more varied and urgent.

Unusual Presentation and Complications of Abdominal Aortic Aneurysm
Ureteral obstruction
Peripheral ischemia
Peripheral emboli
Aortocaval fistula
Aortoenteric fistula
Duodenal obstruction
Femoral neuropathy
Inferior vena cava obstruction

Fortunately, most abdominal aortic aneurysms are

discovered before these devastating complications occur. The natural history of abdominal aortic aneurysms and the rate of rupture have been studied, and the clear superiority of surgery over observation has been established.[77]

An abdominal aortic aneurysm may rupure into the free peritoneal cavity and rapidly exsanguinate. More common, the leak initially occurs into the retroperitoneum, which may tamponade the hemorrhage. Abdominal, flank, or back pain; hypotension; and the presence of a tender, pulsatile abdominal mass establish the diagnosis. An expanding abdominal aortic aneurysm may cause ureteral obstruction as periaortic inflammation and fibrosis encase the ureter.[20] Treatment involves aneurysm resection and ureterolysis. Infrequently an abdominal aortic aneurysm will present with symptoms of occlusive disease. Thrombosis of the aneurysm should be considered in the patient with acute aortic occlusion who presents with evidence of an abdominal mass that is nonpulsatile.[56] Emboli that cause major vessel occlusion as well as microemboli responsible for the "blue toe syndrome" may be the initial signs of an abdominal aortic aneurysm.[44, 67]

Aortoenteric fistulas, usually duodenal, are more commonly associated with prosthetic aortic grafts. However, primary aortoduodenal fistulas do occur in association with gastrointestinal bleeding and a pulsatile abdominal mass. There may be premonitory minor upper or lower gastrointestinal bleeding before an exsanguinating hemorrhage develops. Unfortunately, an aortogram is rarely useful in making the diagnosis. Endoscopy and gallium-67 citrate or CT scanning may be more helpful, but a high index of suspicion is necessary.[60] Although primary repair of aortoduodenal fistula has been suggested, the more conventional approach involves closure of the duodenum, oversewing the abdominal aorta, and extra-anatomical bypass with an axillobifemoral graft through an uncontaminated operative field.[21, 41]

Rarely, an abdominal aortic aneurysm will rupture into the inferior vena cava or the iliac or renal vein, producing a spontaneous massive arteriovenous fistula. Such fistulas are associated with the rapid appearance of congestive heart failure, including dyspnea, edema, ascites, pleural effusion, and hepatomegaly. Abdominal pain, harsh abdominal bruit, venous engorgement, and peripheral arterial insufficiency may also occur, but these signs are frequently absent.[19] Hematuria may be a consistent finding.[12] The diagnosis is confirmed by aortogram. The surgical approach involves closure of the fistula from within the aneurysm followed by interposition of an aortic prosthesis.[5]

Expanding or retroperitoneal rupture of an abdominal aortic aneurysm may rarely present as evidence of duodenal obstruction, femoral neuropathy, or inferior vena cava obstruction.[1, 28, 71]

TABLE 27-1. PREFERRED EXTRA-ANATOMICAL BYPASSES FOR GRAFT SEPSIS

Infected Site	Preferred Bypass Route
Aorta, groin uninvolved	Axillobifemoral
Aorta and groin	Axillosuperficial femoral or popliteal tunneled lateral to anterior superior iliac spine
Groin, aorta uninvolved	Aortosuperficial femoral by obturator foramen

Operative Complications of Aortic Surgery

Upon opening the abdomen for a contemplated aortic operation, a thorough examination of the viscera must be undertaken. If there is any evidence of unsuspected active diverticulitis, cholecystitis, appendicitis, or any other septic process, the placement of a prosthetic graft must be delayed. The concomitant performance of aortic prosthetic surgery with colectomy for cancer, cholecystectomy for inactive gallbladder disease, and incidental appendectomy is controversial. Proponents believe that such surgery may be done with minimal risk of contaminating the graft. If such concomitant surgery is contemplated, it should be done following the aortic surgery after the retroperitoneum is closed. Recent evidence suggests that major surgery in the presence of an abdominal aortic aneurysm may predispose the patient to rupture through elevation of serum collagenase activity. Such data suggest that aneurysm repair should be done prior to or concomitant with other indicated intra-abdominal procedures.[14, 75]

The duodenum should be mobilized to the right by incising the peritoneum on the duodenal wall in an attempt to preserve the maximal lappet of peritoneum to be imbricated behind the duodenum and over the aorta, thus excluding contact of duodenum from the prosthesis and reducing the possibility of development of late aortoduodenal fistula.

Minimal surgery need be done to control the aorta. By avoiding circumferential dissection around the aorta or iliac arteries, injury to the vena cava, lumbar veins, iliac veins, or an aberrant left renal vein that courses behind the aorta will also be avoided. Care should be taken when dissecting the retroperitoneum to control small vessels and lymphatics. The aorta should be disturbed as little as possible during this dissection to avoid dislodgment of atheromatous laminated thrombus. Clamps on the iliac vessels should be placed before the aorta is clamped to avoid dislodgment of such emboli to the lower extremities.

A preoperative arteriogram is of course a necessity in aortoiliac occlusive disease, but it is also important when dealing with abdominal aortic aneurysmal disease. Such arteriograms will define arterial abnormalities as well as the presence of significant renal artery or mesenteric artery stenosis. If the arteriogram reveals a dominant inferior mesenteric artery or if at aneurysmal surgery this vessel appears quite large or does not back bleed when transected, consideration should be given to implanting this vessel into the graft.

The colon, especially the sigmoid, should be carefully inspected for adequate perfusion at the conclusion of the procedure. Routine systemic heparinization should be employed during aortic cross clamping to avoid thrombotic complications of the lower extremities.

Venous anomalies complicate abdominal aortic surgery. Although not common, each presents a problem in intraoperative management and in protection from injury. These anomalies include transposition of the inferior vena cava, duplication of the inferior vena cava, circumaortic venous collar, and retroaortic left renal vein. Transposition of the inferior vena cava is easily recognized at the operating table and presents a problem in exposure of the aorta immediately below the renal arteries. To gain exposure, the cava or the right renal vein bearing the right adrenal and spermatic vein may be divided. Duplication of the inferior vena cava may pose no problem in exposure. If needed, the left-sided cava (often rudimentary) may be sacrificed. Division of the left renal vein may afford exposure of the aneurysmal neck so that renal blood will drain freely into the left-sided cava. A circumaortic venous collar poses a special danger of injury. The normal preaortic left renal vein will be observed, and the retroaortic component to the collar, often located more caudad, might not be noticed until it is torn by dissection or aortic clamping. A retroaortic left renal vein is subject to the same type of injury. Avoiding circumferential aortic dissection should preclude injury to this anomalous left renal vein. Occluding the aorta with a vertical clamp also helps to avoid this complication.[11]

Horseshoe kidney represents another developmental abnormality that requires special preoperative and intraoperative care. Preoperative aortography followed by intravenous pyelography will confirm the diagnosis as well as delineate the arterial supply. During the operation, division of the isthmus *versus* placement of the graft behind this renal bridge must be decided. The reimplantation of renal arteries involved in the aneurysm or occlusive disease is required to preserve renal function.[72]

Care should be taken when dissecting around the aortic bifurcation to avoid disruption of the preaortic autonomic plexus. (Detailed discussion of sexual dysfunction after aortic surgery follows.)

Tunnels for the graft limb to the iliac or femoral vessels should be made using blunt dissection. Placement of the grafts behind the ureters is important. A ureter caught between the graft and the native iliac artery will be compressed.

Hypotension as a result of declamping of the aorta has been greatly reduced through the routine use of a pulmonary artery or a central venous catheter to monitor heart filling pressures and, thus, allow precise fluid preloading.[13, 85]

At the conclusion of the procedure, reperitonealization should be performed to leave the third and fourth portions of the duodenum within the peritoneal cavity. Reperitonealization should also help to isolate the graft from any future intraperitoneal septic complications such as appendicitis or diverticulitis.

Early Complications of Aortic Surgery

HEMORRHAGE. Early postoperative hemorrhage is a common complication of aortic surgery. The sources of this hemorrhage are the anastomosis, particularly the posterior aortic suture line; overlooked retroperitoneal vessels; and the cut edge of the aneurysmal wall. These may result from technical oversight or residual intraoperative anticoagulation.

MYOCARDIAL INFARCTION. The most common cause of early and late postoperative death following abdominal aortic aneurysm resection is myocardial infarction. Routine preoperative coronary artery angiography and selective revascularization have been advocated in patients with aortic aneurysms as a means of reducing the rate of operative mortality.[35] Excellent results in reducing myocardial complications have been reported with the maintenance of optimal cardiac performance through the use of a thermistor-tipped pulmonary artery balloon catheter. This catheter, placed the evening before surgery, can be used to construct a myocardial performance curve that can be used to monitor pre-, intra-, and postoperative fluid requirements.[85] Routine postoperative intensive care and arterial blood gas monitoring are probably also important to reduce the incidence of myocardial infarction. Fatal myocardial infarction can be expected in around 3% of elective aneurysms, 10% of symptomatic intact aneurysms, and 16% of ruptured aneurysms.

RESPIRATORY INSUFFICIENCY. Acute respiratory failure is another important complication of aortic surgery, particularly ruptured abdominal aortic aneurysm resection. Death secondary to pulmonary failure can be expected in 2% of elective aneurysm resections and in 5% or greater of ruptured aneurysms. The etiology of the pulmonary insufficiency following aortic surgery is probably multifactorial. A long upper abdominal incision, multiple blood transfusions, release of microaggregates from the lower extremities after aortic clamping, as well as pancreatitis and ischemic colon injury may all contribute to the development of acute respiratory failure.[59] Preexisting pulmonary disease and pulmonary sepsis also contribute to respiratory morbidity. Detailed respiratory assessment, appropriate preoperative preparation, and careful postoperative pulmonary monitoring can decrease the risk of aortic surgery in patients with severe preexisting lung disease.[70]

RENAL INSUFFICIENCY. Renal function following abdominal aortic surgery may be altered by a variety of mechanisms. Hypotension, as may be experienced with a ruptured abdominal aortic aneurysm, can be implicated in acute renal failure. There is evidence that infrarenal clamping of the abdominal aorta results in decreased renal blood flow, although the clinical importance of this experimental finding is unknown. Aortic clamping in close proximity to the renal arteries may result in embolization of atheromatous debris or deformation of the renal artery ostia, which will result in impaired renal blood flow and function. Intraoperative mannitol may be a useful adjunct in the maintenance of normal renal function during aortic surgery.[4] However, some authors have shown that adequate hydration affords similar protection.[6]

Acute renal failure is seen in less than 3% of elective resections and in greater than 20% of ruptured abdominal aortic aneurysms.[46] Acute renal failure is much less frequently seen in aortic occlusive disease.

The mortality rate of patients who develop renal failure is about 50%, and if coexisting respiratory insufficiency is present, the mortality rate is greater than 90%. Patients are supported by hemodialysis during the postoperative period while awaiting return of renal function.

PARAPLEGIA. The spinal cord is supplied by the anterior spinal artery formed high in the neck by branches from the vertebrals. It descends with the spinal cord gathering radicular arterial branches from the vertebral, intercostal, and lumbar arteries. The most distal radicular artery supplying the anterior spinal is usually the largest and best developed. This arteria radicular magna anterior (or artery of Adamkiewicz) usually arises fom T8 to L1 and therefore is not disturbed by surgery of the infrarenal aorta. However, an occasional low origin will be obliterated by aortic surgery, resulting in paraplegia. This complication can be expected in 0.5% of abdominal aortic resections. Other factors that contribute to cord damage are the necessity of high aortic clamping during the course of ruptured aneurysm surgery, hypotension associated with arteriosclerotic stenosis of the spinal arteries or their collaterals, and the rare embolization of atheromatous debris.[76] Treatment of this neurologic deficit is limited to rehabilitation. Unfortunately, there is no sure way to identify a low-lying arteria radicularis magna preoperatively. Retrospective examination of abdominal aortograms in patients who have developed postoperative paraplegia fail to identify a large predominant lumbar artery supplying the spinal cord. In contrast, patients with one or two quite large lumbar arteries have tolerated their sacrifice without developing this complication. Prevention, for all practical purposes, must be limited to avoidance of hypotension and clamping above the renal arteries, as well as adequate heparinization.

CHYLOUS ASCITES. Usually a result of malignancy, inflammation, trauma, or congenital abnormality, chylous ascites has been reported associated with abdominal aortic surgery. Careful control of lymphatics surrounding the infrarenal aorta is important in the prevention of this complication. Treatment can be surgical, or total parenteral nutrition may be used.[50]

MESENTERIC ISCHEMIA. Colon ischemia may be expected in 1% to 2% of patients undergoing aortic surgery. Small bowel ischemia is even rarer, but they are significant complications, for the mortality rates are 40% for colon ischemia and 90% for small bowel ischemia. Detection of patients at risk for ischemia and its prevention are most important. Any history suggestive of mesenteric ischemia is an important consideration prior to aortic surgery. Aortic angiography, especially lateral films to visualize the superior mesenteric and celiac origins, are needed to establish the importance of the inferior mesenteric artery to mesenteric perfusion. Additionally, a large meandering mesenteric artery is an indication of occlusive disease of a major mesenteric vessel, requiring collateral circulation.[39]

Measurement of the inferior mesenteric stump pressure has been advocated by Ernst and colleagues as an index of the safety of ligation of this vessel during aortic surgery. These researchers did not find ischemic colitis if the stump pressure was greater than 40 torr, if the inferior mesenteric artery/systemic ratio was greater than 0.40, or if the vessel was thrombosed.[26] The inferior mesenteric artery should be ligated carefully and as close to the aorta as possible, usually from within the aneurysmal sac so as not to disrupt collaterals. The indications for implantation of the inferior mesenteric artery into the aortic graft are listed below:

- Stenotic or occluded SMA with meandering artery
- IMA patent; occluded or stenotic iliac arteries
- Bypass procedure proximal to patent IMA
- IMA patent, intraoperative evidence of bowel ischemia
- IMA patent, poor or absent back bleeding
- IMA patent, stump pressure < 40 torr
- IMA patent, stump pressure/systemic ratio < 0.40
- IMA occluded, evidence of mesenteric ischemia

This implantation should be performed in an end-to-side manner by excising a button or cuff of aortic wall surrounding the inferior mesenteric artery orifice to allow an easier anastomosis.

PERIPHERAL ISCHEMIA. Ischemia of the extremities following aortic surgery may be the result of macro- or microembolization from dislodgment of clot from an aneurysmal sac, mural thrombosis, or atheromatous debris showered during mobilization or clamping of the aorta. This complication may be recognized intraoperatively or in the early postoperative period. Intraoperative angiography will reveal macroemboli that can be retrieved using a Fogarty catheter from a groin exposure. However, signs of acute arterial occlusion associated with normal angiograms are the hallmark of microembolization of atheromatous debris. Unfortunately, such embolization cannot be cleared with Fogarty catheters and only rarely is the anatomy favorable for bypass to relieve ischemia. Usually such microembolization is worse in the extremity with the better blood flow; thus, the "better limb" prior to revascularization is noted to be the "worse limb" after surgery.

Late Complications of Aortic Surgery

The late complications of infected grafts and anastomotic aneurysms have been discussed previously.

AORTOENTERIC FISTULA. Secondary aortoenteric fistula is noted in 1% to 4% of aortic prostheses and is thought to occur from erosion of a rigid graft into the overlying gut, usually the duodenum. However, some experimental evidence suggests that this complication may be the result of an unrecognized graft infection.[15] Aortoenteric fistulas can be divided into two groups. The first, true aortoenteric fistulas, originate in an infected vascular suture line either as a result of primary contamination or secondary to intestinal operative trauma. This complication ultimately leads to massive exsanguinating hemorrhage. The second group, paraprosthetic-enteric fistulas, is characterized by erosion of the gastrointestinal tract by the underlying prosthesis without true fistulous connection. Once such necrosis occurs, the patient may experience abdominal pain and gastrointestinal bleeding (usually not massive) and show evidence of sepsis. If this paraprosthetic fistula is not recognized at this time, the perigraft sepsis will proceed to involve the suture line and to develop a true aortoenteric fistula and accompanying hemorrhage.[57]

Such fistulas have been noted to occur between a prosthetic graft (aortic, renal, iliac) and the duodenum, colon, small intestine, appendix, stomach, and esophagus.

The diagnosis is often difficult to establish securely but must be considered in any patient with a prosthetic graft who manifests gastrointestinal bleeding. Urgent evaluation in such patients is required to prevent massive exsanguinating hemorrhage. Warning signs that may help with the diagnosis are fever, back pain, anemia, and positive blood cultures. Emergent endoscopy should identify another source of gastrointestinal bleeding and identify the fistula from inspection, if possible, of the third and fourth portions of the duodenum. Arteriography is usually not helpful, for it will not identify paraprosthetic fistulas and will only delineate a true fistula if it is actively bleeding, at which time it is better to be in the operating room. CT scanning and gallium-67 citrate scanning may prove helpful.[60]

At the time of the operation, the aortic graft must be totally removed. The aorta is oversewn using monofilament suture material. If the aorta at this point has lost some integrity and tensile strength secondary to the septic process, reinforcement with fascia or omentum may prevent secondary hemorrhage, which is always fatal. Duodenal closure should rigorously follow the principles of tension-free anastomosis and decompression by means of nasogastric, gastrostomy, or jejunostomy suction. Drainage and continuous antibiotic irrigation of the aortic stump and the retroperitoneum are important. After the abdomen is closed, the extremities are inspected for viability. If they are viable, vascular reconstruction may be delayed. Otherwise the patient should be reprepped and draped for axillobifemoral bypass.

Techniques to prevent the development of aortoduodenal fistulas are designed to separate the graft from the duodenum physically. The graft should be covered by the aneurysmal wall. A type of Z-plasty can be used to rotate one wall of the aneurysm upward to cover the proximal anastomosis. The graft can be covered again with peritoneum so as to leave the third and fourth portions of the duodenum within the peritoneal cavity and not in contact with the prosthesis.[52]

LATE GRAFT THROMBOSIS. Thrombosis of at least one limb of aortofemoral and aortoiliac bypass grafts (Fig. 27-4) will occur in from 4% to 7.5% of patients.[18, 54] This complication is more frequent in patients whose aortic operation was for occlusive disease and in whom the distal anastomosis was not carried to the femoral arteries. Obstruction of the run-off bed, usually progressive profunda femoris stenosis associated with superficial femoral occlusion, is the most common cause of graft limb thrombosis. Other causes include kinked grafts, defective grafts, and false aneurysms, although the etiology may be indeterminate. After graft limb thrombosis, the patient will usually present with evidence of recurrent claudication, rest pain, or tissue loss. An aortogram is needed to help delineate the cause of graft failure as well as to plan the secondary procedure. Usually these operations can be limited to the groin.

Thrombectomy of the graft is best done as soon as possible after the occlusion, although thrombectomy may be feasible several months after the occlusion. To remove all remnants of thrombus and adherent pseudointima, a strong silicone-rubber Foley catheter may be used as a Fogarty catheter would be. At the conclusion of the thrombectomy, an intraoperative arteriogram is performed to assure that no kinks exist and no thrombus is retained. Attention is then directed to improvement of outflow, usually by profundoplasty.[7] The excellent results that have been reported following reoperation for aortofemoral graft thrombosis emphasize the need for an aggressive approach to these late failures.[40]

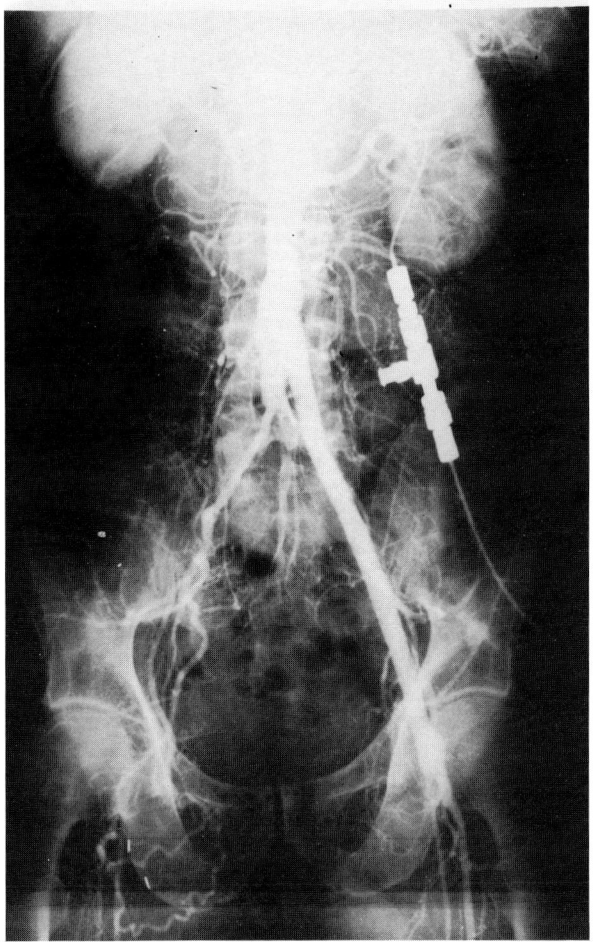

FIG. 27-4. Occlusion of the right limb of an aortobifemoral graft.

SEXUAL DYSFUNCTION. Sexual dysfunction after aortic surgery is noted in from 56% to 58% of men and takes two forms, inability to attain or maintain erection and the inability to ejaculate (retrograde ejaculation).[48, 74] Both of these complications occur as a result of damage to the sympathetic nervous plexus surrounding the infrarenal aorta and the left common iliac artery. A vascular etiology of sexual dysfunction following aortic surgery is less common but can occur if perfusion to the internal iliacs is not preserved. This may happen when an aortobifemoral bypass graft is constructed end-to-end proximally, thus depriving the internal iliacs of the perfusion for which retrograde flow through severely stenotic or occluded external arteries does not compensate.[62] The sympathetic plexus lies over the left anterior surface of the aorta and over the left common iliac artery, extending down to the hypogastric plexus formed in front of the left common iliac vein. To prevent such sexual dysfunction, aortic dissection should be limited as much as possible and confined to the right anterior aorta. The area from the aortic bifurcation to the left iliac bifurcation should be disturbed as little as possible.[83] Adherence to these principles can preserve both erectile and ejaculatory function following aortic surgery.[22]

COMPLICATIONS OF AORTIC TRAUMA

Aortic injuries comprise about 1% of civilian arterial trauma. The patient usually presents with massive intraperitoneal hemorrhage and profound shock. But the absence of shock does not preclude the presence of aortic trauma. Concomitant injuries are the usual rule, including small bowel, colon, vena cava, and liver trauma. Complications are usually seen intraoperatively and in the early postoperative period and are in large part related to the degree and duration of hypotension as well as the extent of concomitant injuries. Late complications have been quite infrequent.[63]

Complications of Lower Extremity Vascular Surgery and Trauma

Many of the complications seen after arterial reconstruction distal to the inguinal ligament can be prevented. The patient's skin, especially the groin, should be free of superficial infection. Distal infection should be under control. Prophylactic antibiotics should be administered before surgery if use of a prosthetic graft is anticipated. Plastic adherent drapes should cover the expanse of skin to be exposed during these procedures. Incisions should be made directly over the femoral artery and the saphenous vein. Flaps that predispose patients to seroma, hematoma, and wound edge necrosis should be avoided. Lymph nodes and lymphatics encountered in the groin should be reflected medially to avoid their disruption. Such care will prevent the spillage of bacterially contaminated lymph as well as the development of postoperative lymph fistula and leg edema.

The saphenous vein should be harvested with great care. Excessive traction will result in a tear of venous side branches where repair is difficult, resulting in stenosis of the vein graft. Experimental studies have shown that saphenous veins are best prepared by avoiding high distention pressure and using a cold irrigation solution, preferably blood rather than saline.[8, 34] To be considered suitable for use the vein must be at least 4 mm in diameter. Gentle occlusion clamps should be used in the groin and avoided if possible in the popliteal fossae. Clamps should not be used during tibial vessel anastomosis; silicone-rubber loops or soft internal occluders are better. The vein should be drawn through a tunneling device designed to ensure that the graft does not twist. Care should be exercised that the graft is of the proper length and is not compressed by muscle or tendon. At the conclusion of the final anastomosis, an intraoperative angiogram should be performed to detect technical errors that might result in early graft failure.

Femoropopliteal and femorotibial bypasses have many complications in common with arterial surgery elsewhere, but there are several problems unique to this location.

The approach to early thrombosis was discussed in detail previously. Because the majority of bypass grafts in this area are performed using autologous reversed saphenous vein, the routine Fogarty method of thrombectomy is impossible because of the venous valves. Several techniques have been suggested to accomplish this thrombectomy. The thrombus may be pushed rather than pulled through the vein graft, the Fogarty catheter may be modified to allow introduction and withdrawal in the same direction, or a newly designed double balloon catheter may be used.[27, 38, 51]

Early postoperative bleeding may be the result of residual heparinization but most often is seen when a vein graft side branch tie comes loose. Anastomotic bleeding and wound oozing may also occur. All are best treated by early reoperation, not only to control the source of bleeding but also to remove the accumulated hematoma to prevent early tamponade and late infection. False anastomotic aneurysms are rarely seen involving saphenous vein grafts, and their presence should arouse the suspicion of infection.

Sepsis involving a femoropopliteal vein graft may result in hemorrhage or graft thrombosis. An autologous vein graft may tolerate an infection, providing drainage is adequate and local and systemic antibiotics are employed. Such a favorable outcome from infection could not be expected from a prosthetic graft.

Edema following femoropopliteal or femorotibial bypass grafting is common. It may resolve quickly or be present for months. Edema is probably related to multiple factors, including lymphatic disruption, increased perfusion pressure, and increased permeability of the distal capillary bed.

A lymph leak from a groin incision is infrequently seen. A small amount of lymphorrhea may be observed for 48 hours. If the leak does not stop, the patient should be returned to the operating room for suture ligation of the damaged lymphatic. Prolonged groin lymphorrhea predisposes the patient to infection.

The saphenous nerve, purely sensory, is often injured during vein harvesting. The section of this nerve results in numbness of the medial aspect of the thigh and leg. Entrapment of this nerve with a suture or scar will produce an uncomfortable paresthesia.

Several complications are the result of the use of the saphenous vein itself. Spontaneous necrosis, arteriosclerotic aneurysm, and simple aneurysmal dilatation and stenosis have been noted.[30, 31, 81] Fibrous intimal hyperplasia is a common cause of late graft failure.[32]

Vascular trauma below the inguinal ligament is complicated by massive hemorrhage and concomitant nerve injury and long bone fracture. Venous repair, especially at the popliteal level, is important to maintain early patency of the reconstructed arterial segment. Amputation is a significant complication of lower extremity vascular trauma.

Complications of Arterial Embolectomy

Since its introduction in 1963, the Fogarty embolectomy balloon-tipped catheter has revolutionized the approach to arterial embolic disease.[29] The simplicity and ease of use and the need for minimal anesthesia are important advantages of this technique. The complications observed through the use of this embolectomy catheter include:[68]

Perforation of artery by catheter
Rupture of artery by inflated balloon
Arteriovenous fistula
Balloon rupture and embolization
Intimal disruption
Anterior compartment syndrome
Brachial plexus neuropraxia

Gentleness and the awareness that these complications may occur are important parts of balloon catheter embolectomy. At the conclusion of embolectomy, an on-the-table postoperative angiogram should be performed to identify any residual embolus as well as to rule out, or to identify, any complications of the procedure.

Revascularization of an acute, severely ischemic extremity may result in severe metabolic abnormalities as products of muscle ischemia are released into the systemic circulation. The limb will release severely acidic blood with a high potassium concentration and myoglobin. Acidosis and hyperkalemia must be recognized and corrected. High urine volumes and alkalization help to avoid precipitation of myoglobin in the renal tubules, a cause of renal failure.

Reperfusion in an acutely, severely ischemic limb may result in severe muscle swelling that may progress to ischemia as a result of a compartment syndrome. In such patients fasciotomy is indicated. Usually this can be achieved through small incisions over the involved compartments. However, occasionally fibulectomy and decompression of all four lower leg compartments are indicated.[58]

Complications of Carotid Surgery and Trauma

COMPLICATIONS OF CAROTID DISEASE

The complications of arteriosclerotic disease and fibromuscular dysplasia of the carotid arteries are mainly neurologic, including transient ischemia attacks (TIAs), stroke, and chronic cerebral ischemia. The uncommon carotid body tumors and carotid aneurysms usually present as asymptomatic masses, but they may enlarge to produce dysphagia as well as cranial nerve compression, resulting in facial pain from the facial nerve, hoarseness through the vagus, and fifth and sixth nerve palsies. Carotid aneurysm may also produce neurologic deficit by embolization and rarely may rupture with bleeding from the nose, mouth, or ear (Fig. 27-5). The complications of carotid disease surgery and trauma are summarized below.

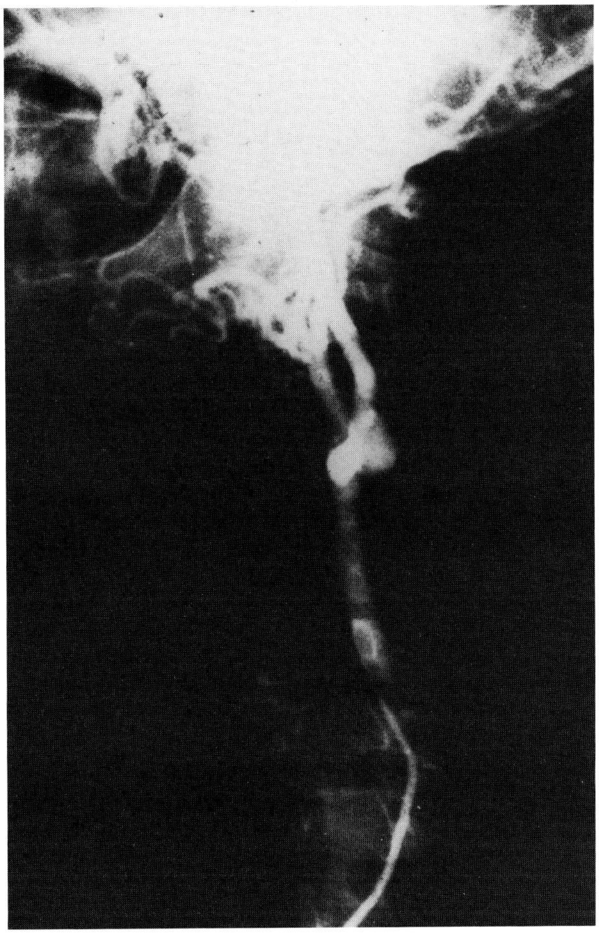

FIG. 27-5. Carotid aneurysm.

Complications of Occlusive and Aneurysmal Disease
Stroke
TIA
Chronic cerebral ischemia
Dysphagia
Cranial nerve compression
Nose, ear, mouth hemorrhage

Early Complications of Carotid Surgery and Trauma
Neurological
  Stroke; TIA; hypoglossal, vagus, facial, superior laryngeal, glossopharyngeal, and superficial sensory nerve injury; convulsions; Horner's syndrome
Myocardial infarction
Hypertension
Hypotension
Carotid body dysfunction
Parotitis
Tracheal obstruction
Wound infection

TABLE 27-2. NERVE INJURIES DURING CAROTID SURGERY

Nerve	Unilateral Injury	Bilateral Injury
Hypoglossal	Tongue biting, speech problems, swallowing difficulties	Upper airway obstruction
Vagus	Hoarseness, ineffective cough mechanism	Upper airway obstruction
Superior laryngeal	Loss of vocal range, easy voice fatigue	Exacerbation of unilateral problem
Facial, marginal, mandibular branch	Weakness, drooping lower lip	Bilateral weakness
Glossopharyngeal	Rarely clinically evident	Swallowing difficulty, pulmonary aspiration, loss of gag reflex
Greater auricular nerve	Numbness over parotid, lower ear	Bilateral numbness
Transverse cervical nerve	Numbness anterior in triangle of neck	Bilateral numbness

Late Complications of Carotid Surgery and Trauma
False aneurysm
Recurrent stenosis
Arteriovenous fistula

Early Complications of Carotid Surgery

The incidence of neurologic deficits following carotid endarterectomy is less than 2% in the best series. The presence of contralateral carotid obstruction or vertebral disease is associated with an increased risk of stroke.[17] These neurologic deficits are usually the result of a technical error. General anesthesia with continuous monitoring of intra-arterial pressure and the electroencephalogram are preferred. The carotid artery should be dissected very carefully without disturbing the carotid bulb until the proximal common and distal internal and external carotids have been isolated and clamps applied. Then the carotid bulb may be expeditiously freed from its bed.

If a shunt is used, it should be inserted very gently into the internal carotid without force that may cause intimal damage. Taking 15 to 30 seconds to introduce vessel dilators sequentially into the internal carotid artery may facilitate shunt introduction. Use of a sterile Doppler probe will confirm flow through the shunt. Careful and meticulous endarterectomy is important to remove any debris and adherent intima. The endarterectomy should proceed distally with care and recognition of the transition zone that usually exists as the arteriosclerotic plaque tapers into the internal carotid. This transition should be recognized and the endarterectomy plane terminated or the plaque sculpted to yield an adherent intima without flap. Heparinized saline irrigation should be used to identify debris or intimal flaps. If a distal intimal flap does exist, very fine longitudinally placed simple sutures using monofilament material are important to prevent intimal dissection and internal carotid occlusion.

The arteriotomy should be closed using 6-0 or 7-0 monofilament polypropylene suture taking 1-mm bites 1 mm apart. Before the suture line is completed, each clamp should be released to flush any debris. A patch graft is rarely needed. The clamps should be released in a definite, established sequence. First the internal carotid should be released to allow back bleeding to flush air through the suture line. This clamp is then reapplied. Flow then should be established from the common carotid sequentially into the superior thyroid artery, the external carotid artery, and finally the internal carotid artery. A sterile Doppler probe is again used to confirm normal flow through the internal and external carotid. Not infrequently this maneuver reveals an occluded external carotid as a result of an intimal flap. A separate external carotid arteriotomy and endarterectomy are performed in this important collateral.

After hemostasis is achieved, the wound is closed in only two layers, the platysma and the skin. If continued ooze is possible, continuous suction closed drainage should be used. The nerves that may be injured during carotid surgery and the sequelae of such injury are listed in Table 27-2.

The hypoglossal nerve crosses both the internal and external carotid arteries above the carotid bifurcation and may be injured. This nerve's intimate relationship with the internal carotid poses a special danger during distal exposure of the artery. The division of the artery and the vein to the sternocleidomastoid muscle frees the hypoglossal nerve, allowing easy retraction.[37] The superior laryngeal nerve may be injured during dissection of the external carotid artery especially near the superior thyroid artery. The vagus nerve travels in the carotid sheath and can be easily protected by identifying it throughout the carotid dissection. Details of the anatomy of the marginal mandibular branch of the facial nerve, glossopharyngeal nerve, and the other cranial nerves encountered in carotid surgery should be reviewed to avoid injury.[23, 36, 37, 82] Injury to the superficial sensory nerves, the greater auricular nerve, or the transverse cervical nerve may result in numbness in their innervated areas.

Myocardial infarction is the second most common cause of operative death and the leading cause of death in the long-term follow-up period of patients who undergo carotid surgery. A patient with symptomatic coronary artery disease has a much greater chance of sustaining a fatal myocardial infarction (14%) during the perioperative period than does an asymptomatic patient (< 1%).[25] The risk of myocardial infarction is increased with the use of vasopressors during carotid endarterectomy.[65] Patients who are candidates for carotid endarterectomy should be thoroughly evaluated for coronary artery disease. Simultaneous or staged carotid and coronary surgery should be considered when severe coronary arteriosclerotic disease coexists with symptomatic çerebrovascular disease.

Both systemic hypotension and hypertension have been noted following carotid endarterectomy. Hypotension may be secondary to increased stimulation of the carotid sinus baroreceptors after removal of the rigid atheromatous plaque that dampened the arterial pressure wave. Hypertension is more difficult to explain but may be secondary to decreased baroreceptor impulses secondary to carotid sinus nerve trauma.[10, 79] Postoperative hypertension following carotid endarterectomy is associated with a significant increase in neurologic deficits and death.[80] Rarely carotid surgery may cause injury to the parotid gland resulting in postoperative parotitis.

Upper airway obstruction secondary to tracheal and laryngeal edema or as a result of an expanding wound hematoma occurs infrequently following carotid surgery This complication should be suspected if the patient develops respiratory stridor. The first step is to open the wound rapidly to drain any possible hematoma. If this does not eliminate the stridor and respiratory difficulty, then an endotracheal tube should be promptly inserted.

Late Complications of Carotid Surgery

False aneurysm of the carotid artery has been noted following carotid endarterectomy. This complication may be associated with a wound infection or with the use of a synthetic prosthetic graft or jugular vein patch. Repair should be performed using saphenous vein. Occasionally lateral sutures can be used if the anastomotic defect is easily identified.[24]

Recurrent symptomatic stenosis of the carotid after endarterectomy occurs in less than 2% of cases. Prospective follow-up using noninvasive diagnostic techniques suggests that recurrent stenosis is more frequent, from 15% to 40%. There are two distinct categories of this complication. One occurs quite early (within a year) and is secondary to intimal fibrosis. The late presentation (after 2 years) is caused by progressive arteriosclerosis of the endarterectomized artery. These lesions usually produce recurrent symptoms and are best treated by patch grafting using either a Dacron or saphenous vein to enlarge the lumen.[73]

COMPLICATIONS OF CAROTID TRAUMA

Early complications that may suggest carotid injury, especially after blunt trauma, are neck hematoma, Horner's syndrome, TIAs, and hemiplegia. Penetrating neck wounds that bleed briskly or are in proximity to the carotid should suggest carotid injury. Death secondary to hemorrhage and major neurologic ischemic injury are common complications of carotid trauma. Less frequent complications include arteriovenous fistula and false aneurysm.

References

1. Adair HM: Duodenal obstruction due to abdominal aortic aneurysm. Br Med J 95:727–728, 1975
2. Alpert JR, Ring EJ, Freiman DB et al: Treatment of stenosis of the iliac artery by balloon catheter dilatation. Surg Gynecol Obstet 150:481–485, 1980
3. Babu SC, Bole P, Sharma P et al: Pathological fibrinolysis secondary to pseudoaneurysm. Surgery 87:202–204, 1980
4. Barry KG, Malloy JP: Oliguric renal failure. JAMA 179:510–513, 1962
5. Beall AC, Cooley DA, Morris GC, BeBakey ME: Perforation of arteriosclerotic aneurysm into inferior vena cava. Arch Surg 86:809–818, 1963
6. Berman LB, Smith LL, Chisholm GD, Weston RE: Mannitol and renal function in cardiovascular surgery. Arch Surg 88:239–243, 1964
7. Bernhard VM, Rory LI, Towne JB: The reoperation of choice for aortofemoral graft occlusion. Surgery 82:867–874, 1977
8. Bonchek LI: Prevention of endothelial damage during preparation of saphenous veins for bypass grafting. J Thorac Cardiovasc Surg 79:911–915, 1980
9. Bone GW, Hayes AC, Slaymaker EE: Value of segmental limb blood pressure in predicting results of aortofemoral bypass. Am J Surg 132:733–738, 1976
10. Bove EL, Fry WJ, Gross WS, Stanley JC: Hypotension and hypertension as consequences of baroreceptor dysfunction following carotid endarterectomy. Surgery 85:633–637, 1979

11. Brener BJ, Darling RC, Frederick PL, Linton RR: Major venous anomalies complicating abdominal aortic surgery. Arch Surg 108:159–165, 1974
12. Brewster DC, Ottinger LW, Darling RC: Hematuria as a sign of aortocaval fistula. Ann Surg 186:766–771, 1977
13. Bush HL, Logerfo FW, Weisel RD et al: Assessment of myocardial performance and optimal volume loading during elective aortic aneurysm resection. Arch Surg 112:1301–1306, 1977
14. Busuttil RW, Abou–Zamzam AM, Machleder HI: Collagenase activity of the human aorta. Arch Surg 115:1373–1378, 1980
15. Busuttil RW, Rees W, Baker JD, Wilson SE: Pathogenesis of aortoduodenal fistula: Experimental and clinical correlates. Surgery 85:1–13, 1979
16. Carmichael D, Barnes W: Obstruction of the ureter due to a false aneurysm. Surgery 86:769–771, 1979
17. Collins GJ, Rich NM, Andersen CA, McDonald PT: Stroke associated with carotid endarterectomy Am J Surg 135:221–225, 1978
18. Crawford ES, Manning LG, Kelly TF: "Re-do" surgery after operations for aneurysm and occlusion of the abdominal aorta. Surgery 81:41–52, 1977
19. Dardik H, Dardik I, Strom MG et al: Intravenous rupture of the arteriosclerotic aneurysm of the abdominal aorta. Surgery 80:647–651, 1976
20. Darke SG, Glass RE, Eadie DGA: Abdominal aortic aneurysm: Perianeurysmal fibrosis and ureteric obstruction and deviation. Br J Surg 64:649–652, 1977
21. Daugherty MM, Shearer GR, Ernst CB: Primary aortoduodenal fistula: Extra-anatomic vascular reconstruction not required for successful management. Surgery 86:399–401, 1979
22. DePalma RG, Levine SB, Feldman S: Preservation of erectile function after aortoiliac reconstruction. Arch Surg 113:958–962, 1978
23. Durham CF, Harrison TS: The surgical anatomy of the superior laryngeal nerve. Surg Gynecol Obstet 118:38–44, 1964
24. Ehrenfeld WK, Hays RJ: False aneurysm after carotid endarterectomy. Arch Surg 104:288–291, 1972
25. Ennix CL, Lawrie GM, Morris GC et al: Improved results of carotid endarterectomy in patients with symptomatic coronary disease: An analysis of 1546 consecutive carotid operations. Stroke 10:122–125, 1979
26. Ernst CB, Hagihara PF, Daugherty ME, Griffen WO: Inferior mesenteric artery stump pressure. Ann Surg 187:641–646, 1978
27. Flannigan DP, Goodreau JJ, Burnham SJ: Technique for thrombectomy of reversed saphenous vein arterial bypass grafts. Am J Surg 138:334–335, 1979
28. Fletchner HS, Frankel J: Ruptured abdominal aneurysms presenting with unilateral peripheral neuropathy. Surgery 79:120–121, 1976
29. Fogarty TV, Cranely JJ, Krause RJ et al: A method of extraction of arterial emboli and thrombi. Surg Gynecol Obstet 116:241–244, 1963
30. Friedman S, Cerruti MM, Amadeo B: Spontaneous necrosis of a functioning saphenous vein graft. Surgery 66:1022–1025, 1969
31. Friedman SA, Cerruti MM, Gerstmann KE, Washor H: Aneurysm formation: A late complication of venous bypass grafting. Am Heart J 89:366–368, 1975
32. Fush JCA, Mitchner JS, Hagen P: Postoperative changes in autologous vein grafts. Ann Surg 188:1–15, 1978
33. Guba AM, Collins GJ, Rich NM: Coverage of exposed vascular conduits. Am J Surg 137:263–266, 1979
34. Gundrey SR, Jones M, Ishihara T, Ferrans VJ: Optimal preparatory techniques for human saphenous vein grafts. Surgery 88:785–794, 1980
35. Hertzer NR: Fatal myocardial infarction following abdominal aortic aneurysm resection. Ann Surg 192:667–673, 1980
36. Hertzer N, Feldman BJ, Beven EG, Tucker HM: A prospective study of the incidence of injury to cranial nerves during carotid endarterectomy. Surg Gynecol Obstet 151:781–784, 1980
37. Imparato AM, Bracco A, Kim GE, Bergmann L: The hypoglossal nerve in carotid arterial reconstructions. Stroke 3:576–578, 1972
38. Jacobson JH, Cohen WB: A bidirectional embolectomy catheter. Surgery 85:761–763, 1979
39. Johnson WC, Nabseth DC: Visceral infarction following aortic surgery. Ann Surg 180:312–318, 1974
40. Kanaly PJ, Dilling EW, Robinson HB, Elkins RC: Discussion and management of late failure in reconstructive procedures involving the abdominal aorta. Am J Surg 136:709-713, 1978
41. Lewis RT, Allan CM: Spontaneous aortoduodenal fistula: Successful treatment by extra-anatomic vascular bypass. Can J Surg 22:234-236, 1979
42. Liebman PR, Menzoian JO, Mannick JA: Intraoperative arteriography in femoropopliteal and femorotibial bypass grafting. Arch Surg (in press)
43. Liekweg WG, Greenfield LJ: Vascular prosthetic infections: Collected experience and results of treatment. Surgery 81:335-342, 1977
44. Lord JW, Rossi G, Daliana M et al: Unsuspected abdominal aortic aneurysms as the cause of peripheral arterial occlusive disease. Ann Surg 177:767-771, 1973
45. Mashiah A, Thompson JM, Poller L, Charlesworth D: Changes in the coagulation of blood during resection of the abdominal aorta. Surg Gynecol Obstet 149:214-216, 1979
46. McCombs PR, Roberts B: Acute renal failure following resection of abdominal aortic aneurysm. Surg Gynecol Obstet 148:175-178, 1979
47. McLoughlin GA, Grindlinger GA, Manny J et al: Intrapulmonary clotting and fibrinolysis during abdominal aortic aneurysm surgery. Ann Surg 190:623-630, 1979
48. May AG, DeWeese JA, Rob CG: Changes in sexual function following operation in the abdominal aorta. Surgery 65:41-46, 1969
49. Medical and Surgical History of the War of the Rebellion, vol. 2, part 3, Surgical Volume. Washington, DC, Government Printing Office, 1883
50. Meinke AH, Estes NC, Ernst CB: Chylous ascites following abdominal aortic aneurysmectomy. Ann Surg 190:631-633, 1979
51. Meredith J, Walley B, Meredith JW: A simple technique for thrombectomy of vein grafts in the arterial system. Surg Gynecol Obstet 151:424-425, 1980
52. Miller DR: Prevention of aortoduodenal fistula by duodenal reflection. Am J Surg 138:332-333, 1979
53. Moore WS, Rosson CT, Hall AD, Thomas AN: Transient bacteremia: A cause of infection in prosthetic vascular grafts. Am J Surg 117:342-343, 1969
54. Najafi H, Dye WS, Javid H et al: Late thrombosis affecting one limb of aortic bifurcation graft. Arch Surg 110:409-412, 1975

55. O'Donnell TF, McBride KA, Callow AD et al: Management of combined segment disease. Am J Surg 141:452-459, 1981
56. Olcott C, Holcroft JW, Stoney R, Wylie EJ: Unusual problems of abdominal aortic aneurysms. Am J Surg 135:426-431, 1978
57. O'Mara C, Imbembo AL: Paraprosthetic-enteric fistula. Surgery 81:556-566, 1977
58. Pathman RD, Thompson JE: Fasciotomy in peripheral vascular surgery. Arch Surg 101:663-672, 1970
59. Patten MT: In Hechtman HB (ed): Acute Respiratory Failure, pp 140-142. Boca Raton, FL, CRC Press, 1979
60. Perdue GD, Smith RB, Ansley JD, Costantino MJ: Impending aortoenteric hemorrhage. Ann Surg 192:237-243, 1980
61. Pitt HA, Postier RG, MacGowan WAL et al: Prophylactic antibiotics in vascular surgery. Ann Surg 192:356-363, 1980
62. Queral LA, Whitehouse WM, Flinn WR et al: Pelvic hemodynamics after aortoiliac reconstruction. Surgery 86:799-809, 1979
63. Rich NM, Spencer FC: In Vascular Trauma, pp 441-456. Philadelphia, WB Saunders, 1978
64. Rhodes GR, Cox C, Silver D: Arteriovenous fistula and false aneurysm as the cause of consumption coagulopathy. Surgery 73:535-540, 1973
65. Riles TS, Kopelman I, Imparato AM: Myocardial infarction following carotid endarterectomy: A review of 683 operations. Surgery 85:249-252, 1979
66. Schaberg FJ, Wong R, Phillips MR et al: Management of draining wounds in vascular surgery. Arch Surg (in press)
67. Schechter DC: Atheromatous embolization to lower limbs. NY State J Med 79:1180-1186, 1979
68. Schweitzer DL, Aquam AB, Wilder JR: Complications encountered during arterial embolectomy with Fogarty balloon catheter. Vascular Surgery 10:144-156, 1976
69. Siebert WT, Natelson EA: Chronic consumption coagulopathy accompanying abdominal aortic aneurysm. Arch Surg 111:539-541, 1976
70. Smith PK, Fuchs JCA, Sabiston DC: Surgical management of aortic abdominal aneurysms in patients with severe pulmonary insufficiency. Surg Gynecol Obstet 151:407-411, 1980
71. Snider RL, Porter JM, Eidermiller LR: Inferior vena cava obstruction caused by expansion of an abdominal aortic aneurysm. Report of a case and review of the literature. Surgery 75:613-616, 1974
72. Starr DS, Foster WJ, Morris GC: Resection of abdominal aortic aneurysm in the presence of horseshoe kidney. Surgery 89:387-389, 1981
73. Stoney RJ, String ST: Recurrent carotid stenosis. Surgery 80:705-710, 1966
74. Subi S, Colton L: Sexual function following aortoiliac reconstruction. Lancet 2:1218-1219, 1971
75. Swanson RJ, Littooy FN, Hunt TK: Laparotomy as a precipitating factor in rupture of intraabdominal aneurysms. Arch Surg 115:299-304, 1980
76. Szilagyi DE, Hageman JH, Smith RF, Elliott JP: Spinal cord damage in surgery of the abdominal aorta. Surgery 83:38-56, 1978
77. Szilagyi DE, Smith RF, DeRusso FJ et al: Contribution of abdominal aortic aneurysmectomy to prolongation of life. Ann Surg 164:678-699, 1966
78. Szilagyi DE, Smith RF, Elliott JP et al: Anastomotic aneurysm after vascular reconstruction: Problems and incidence, etiology and treatment. Surgery 78:800-816, 1975
79. Tarlow E, Schmidek H, Scott RM et al: Reflex hypotension following carotid endarterectomy: Mechanism and management. J Neurosurg 39:323-327, 1973
80. Towne J, Bernhard V: The relationship of postoperative hypertension to complications following carotid endarterectomy. Surgery 88:575-580, 1980
81. Vanttinen E: Postoperative changes in bypass vein grafts and collateral arteries after femoropopliteal arterial reconstructive surgery. Acta Chir Scand 141:731-738, 1975
82. Verta MJ, Applebaum EL, McClusky DA et al: Cranial nerve injury during carotid endarterectomy. Ann Surg 185:192-195, 1977
83. Weinstein MH, Machleder HI: Sexual function after aortoiliac surgery. Ann Surg 181:787-790, 1975
84. Whittemore AD, Clowes AW, Couch NP, Mannick JA: Secondary femoropopliteal reconstruction. Ann Surg 193:35-42, 1981
85. Whittemore AD, Clowes AW, Hechtman HB, Mannick JA: Aortic aneurysm repair. Ann Surg 192:414-421, 1980
86. Zarins CK, Lu C, McDonnell AE, Whitehouse WM: Limb salvage by percutaneous transluminal recanalization of the occluded superficial femoral artery. Surgery 87:701-708, 1980

28
Complications of Cardiac Surgery and Trauma

H. Newland Oldham, Jr.

OVERVIEW

As a result of advances in cardiac surgery, the incidence of major postoperative complications has decreased at the same time that other previously unrecognized difficulties have arisen. The widespread performance of coronary bypass surgery has been responsible in part for the simplification and standardization of many aspects of intraoperative and postoperative management. It is now not only possible but also quite probable for an elective cardiac operation to be followed by a short, largely complication-free hospital course. This may be contrasted with Williams's description in 1965 of 197 complications in 107 patients undergoing cardiac procedures.[189] Prior to the era of the coronary bypass, such events as perioperative myocardial infarction and complex postoperative dysrhythmias received little emphasis. It is therefore possible that the incidence of complications following heart surgery has not decreased but only that the names have been changed. In the broadest sense every cardiac patient will have postoperative events requiring specific treatment, and the distinction between an anticipated finding and a complication may be rather arbitrary. The postoperative course may be predicted with reasonable accuracy based on a combined assessment of (1) the patient's preoperative cardiopulmonary, renal, and nutritional reserves; (2) the elective or urgent indications for surgery; (3) the curative or palliative design of the procedure; and (4) the degree of technical or hemodynamic completeness and success achieved during the operation.

The changing incidence and nature of cardiac surgical complications have also been influenced by improved technical results. Patients with previously fatal complications of myocardial infarction are now successfully operated upon during cardiogenic shock, although they require intensive treatment for multiple postoperative problems formerly considered insurmountable. Changes in techniques have directly influenced certain problems: for example, the incidence of serum hepatitis has decreased with changes in laboratory identification and also blood conservation techniques. Certain complications such as those following pulmonary artery banding have become almost historical curiosities as the indications for operations have changed. Longer survival of patients operated on at an earlier time in the progression of their disease has produced long-term problems such as the late complications of prosthetic valves or the problems encountered during re-operations. Finally, some complications have either vanished or changed before they were ever completely understood, such as the so-called pump-lung, which was probably a nonspecific form of what we now consider the adult respiratory distress syndrome.

The principles of managment of the major complications encountered after cardiac surgery are presented in the following section with emphasis on the causative factors, preventive measures, and steps in diagnosis and treatment. Thromboembolic, pulmonary, renal, and nutritional complications are described in separate chapters of this text, although each of these complications occurring after cardiac surgery may present major problems in management. The discussion is not oriented toward the large numbers of anatomical diagnoses encountered or the many specific operative procedures utilized in treating patients with valvular, coronary artery, and congenital heart disease. Instead, complications that may be shared by all postoperative cardiac patients are presented, with appropriate reference to specific disease- or procedure-related problems. Additional information on this subject is presented in excellent specialty texts, including the handbook by Behrendt, the inclusive volume edited by Cordell, and the personal recollections of Roe.[7, 31, 157]

Major Complications of Cardiac Surgery and Trauma

LOW CARDIAC OUTPUT

By the simplest definition, low cardiac output syndrome is synonymous with cardiogenic shock and represents cardiac output insufficient to meet the metabolic demands of the patient. This condition may occur in the operating room or recovery room following any cardiac operation and in its final state can be diagnosed by an experienced glance. This end stage is rare today and is usually preceded by a state of depressed function that will progressively deteriorate if untreated. Reduced cardiac function requires recognition before the onset of intense peripheral constriction, oliguria, pulmonary edema, or metabolic acidosis and is indicated by one or more of the following measurements: cardiac index less than 2.0 L/min/m^2, mean intra-arterial blood pressure below 70 torr, and pulmonary capillary wedge pressure greater than 18 torr.

Incidence and Cause

Most cardiac operations are associated with some degree of transient cardiac insufficiency, but a persistent reduction in cardiac performance fortunately is uncommon. A recent review of over 14,000 adult patients undergoing cardiac surgery reported that 10.6% required pharmacologic support and volume loading to wean them from cardiopulmonary bypass.[107] Two percent of patients required additional intra-aortic balloon support, which led to a satisfactory response in two thirds of them. In most patients this insufficiency can be explained by a combination of the preexisting level of cardiopulmonary function, the demands imposed by anesthesia and surgery, and the balance between induced ischemia and myocardial protection against this insult. It is assumed that the operation will improve overall myocardial function even in the presence of hypertrophy, fibrosis, and ischemia by eliminating valvular dysfunction, excising dyskinetic regions of myocardium, revascularizing areas of ischemia, and correcting congenital defects. It is likewise assumed that temporary myocardial dysfunction following a properly designed and executed procedure will improve within hours to days if the patients can be adequately supported during this transitional period.

Preventive Measures

Prevention of reduced cardiac function is based primarily upon maintaining the proper relationships between myocardial oxygen consumption and myocardial blood supply. Myocardial oxygen consumption is determined by heart rate, left ventricular wall tension, and the level of intrinsic contractility and can be estimated by the tension time index of the left ventricle or the heart rate–systolic blood pressure product. This simple determination has been reported to be a valid correlate of myocardial oxygen consumption during anesthesia and surgery in patients with ischemic heart disease.[188] Coronary blood flow is influenced by the length of diastole and the diastolic difference between coronary ostial and coronary sinus pressures. Indices and ratios of these variables have been proposed and can be electronically calculated and displayed in the operating room, but the main emphasis should be on individual control of each of these variables.[16, 138]

Methods of prevention differ during the successive stages of the operation and are the combined responsibility of the surgeon and the anesthesiologist. For most patients it is helpful to monitor the electrocardiogram, intra-arterial blood pressure, pulmonary capillary wedge or pulmonary artery diastolic pressure, and cardiac output. Aided by these measurements the initial aim is to provide adequate anesthesia with a minimal disturbance of the myocardial oxygen supply-and-demand relationships. It is often advantageous to supplement anesthetic agents with the intravenous infusion of drugs to control appropriate variables. Thus hypertension during the initial part of the procedure may be controlled by infusion of sodium nitroprusside rather than by changing anesthetic levels, which might depress myocardial function. By means of similar approaches toward control of heart rate, blood pressure, and myocardial contractility, it is unusual to encounter major difficulties during anesthetic induction and the initial portion of the operation. This has drastically reduced the need for intra-aortic balloon support of patients with lesions such as left main coronary obstruction and has confined its use primarily to the treatment of preexisting cardiogenic shock.[29, 46]

During cardiopulmonary bypass the basic determinants of myocardial oxygen supply remain valid, but their relationships are altered. The beating, nonworking (vented) heart utilizes less oxygen while coronary perfusion continues. This state may be appropriate for certain procedures such as pulmonary valvulotomy, but most operations are facilitated by the presence of a relaxed heart produced by a combination of ischemia, hypothermia, and cardioplegia. Extensive basic and clinical investigations on optimal myocardial preservation have established several important principles.[8, 44, 47, 61, 70, 84, 111, 152, 159] Myocardial preservation is necessary only because of the demands for operative conditions that are harmful to the myocardium. Simply stated, the less myocardial ischemia, the less need there is for myocardial protection. The hypertrophied, ischemic heart is more susceptible to damage than is normal myocardium.[167] It should finally be emphasized that myocardial oxygen consumption is highest during normothermic ischemia and induced ventricular fibrillation and lowest with a hypothermic nonbeating heart. Thus the basic components of myocardial preservation are a reduction of oxygen consumption by hypothermia and rapid elimination of contraction by chemical arrest. Suggested modifications include the addition of oxygen-carrying capacity and metabolic substrates to the solution and pharmacologic manipulation of the cellular energy requirements. With this approach, clinical cardioplegia may be easily achieved with effective reduction of myocardial oxygen consumption, and the acceptable period of ischemia can be extended from minutes to hours.

Myocardial preservation techniques, though still evolving, are presently credited with a reduction in both mortality and moribidy rates following major cardiac surgery. In spite of the almost universal acceptance of these approaches toward myocardial preservation, human confirmation of these largely experimental and theoretical techniques remains incomplete. A recent clinical report by Roberts failed to show a difference in either perioperative myocardial damage or changes in left ventricular peformance when comparing the use of hypothermic intermittent ischemic arrest and hypothermic potassium cardioplegia.[153] If these techniques have been effective, cardiac function promptly returns after normothermic coronary blood flow has been reestablished. A period of bypass under normothermic, beating, nonworking conditions is recommended to offset the oxygen debt incurred; this should be discontinued only when satisfactory left ventricular function is achieved.[97]

Diagnosis and Management

If all abnormalities of cardiac function could be determined by measurement of the heart rate and blood pressure and by clinical assessment of peripheral perfusion, determinations of filling pressure and cardiac output would not be needed. These measurements, however, improve assessment of myocardial performance and provide helpful documentation of response to therapy. Treatment consists of sequential manipulation of the determinants of cardiac output, heart rate and rhythm, left ventricular preload and afterload, and the level of myocardial contractility. These maneuvers may be considered in the order of their influence on myocardial oxygen consumption. If AV dissociation or heart block occurs after conduction system trauma or as a temporary consequence of potassium cardioplegia, sequential atrioventricular pacing will increase the cardiac output by 10% to 25%.[74, 131, 168] Heart rate should be increased to 100 to 110 beats per minute by atrial pacing if sinus or nodal bradycardia is present, as may occur in patients who are taking large doses of propranolol.[100] Depending on the compliance of the ventricle, stroke volume may be limited, and a substantial improvement in cardiac output may follow the simple maneuver of atrial pacing.[191] Temporary transthoracic epicardial pacing wires should be left in place in any patient with less than ideal rate or rhythm.[184] Other arrhythmias that reduce cardiac output, including tachycardia, atrial fibrillation, and ventricular irritability, should be controlled at this time by a combination of pacing, cardioversion, and drugs, discussed later.

If hypertension is present and is associated with reduced cardiac output and elevated filling pressure, systemic vascular resistance should be decreased by afterload reduction. Vasoconstriction may also be present following cardiopulmonary bypass without an elevated blood pressure, and calculation of peripheral vascular resistance may be helpful in assessing treatment of this condition.[176] A variety of drugs are useful, but continuous intravenous infusion of a rapid-acting agent is preferred. Sodium nitroprusside produces both arterial and venous dilatation and is the recommended first drug.[23, 122, 175] Intravenous nitroglycerin produces more venodilatation with reduction of preload, and hydralazine selectively decreased arterial resistance.[72] A reduction in both blood pressure and filling pressure occurs after nitroprusside treatment is begun, and this usually requires volume infusion to maintain an adequate preload. This combination of reduction of vascular resistance plus volume infusion has been shown to produce a significant increase in cardiac output in almost all patients.[122, 175]

A condition not characterized by low cardiac output is occasionally encountered after cardiopulmonary bypass and should be considered in the differential diagnosis. This state is one of inappropriate vasodilatation and is characterized by hypotension and an elevated cardiac output, often as high as 8 to 10 L/min. The etiology of this condition is unclear, but it may be associated with minor platelet or granulocytic transfusion reactions. The diagnosis of an elevated cardiac output may be confirmed by a low arteriovenous oxygen difference. Treatment consists of increasing the systemic vascular resistance by drugs such as phenylephrine, methoxamine, or norepinephrine.

Hypovolemia is characterized by reduced cardiac output, arterial pressure, and filling pressure. The filling pressure should be increased to 15 to 18 torr by volume infusion and the results reassessed. If ventricular compliance is abnormal or if the preoperative filling pressure was abnormally high, it may be necessary to continue volume infusion until a filling pressure of 20 to 22 torr is reached. In most situations reduced cardiac output is due to left ventricular dysfunction, and treatment is therefore guided by left-sided filling pressures. Correction of certain congenital defects, elevated pulmonary vascular resistance, or right ventricular infarction may all produce right ventricular failure, and treatment should be based on right-sided filling pressures. The manipulation of filling pressures is intended to use the Frank–Starling relationship to increase stroke volume in response to an increase in ventricular diastolic volume.[113] This relationship may not consistently apply to critically ill patients, and the pressure to volume relationships may be better characterized by a group of compliance curves.[20] The critical determination, left ventricular end diastolic volume, is not readily measured by current clinical techniques and is estimated from the left ventricular filling pressure. With abnormal compliance, pulmonary capillary wedge pressure may not accurately reflect either left ventricular filling pressure or volume. In most situations, however, this estimate has been clinically helpful, and the use of pulmonary capillary wedge pressures has been a major advance in the management of the postoperative cardiac patient.

These measures—that is, control of rate and rhythm, establishment of adequate preload, and afterload reduction—improve cardiac output with minimal adverse effects on myocardial oxygen consumption. It may also be necessary to increase the level of myocardial contractility by administering inotropic drugs, which increase the stroke volume. These effective drugs may additionally produce adverse effects on both the heart and the peripheral circulation. An increase in contractility is accompanied by an increase in oxygen utilization. This is further increased by the associated elevation in heart rate and left ventricular wall tension. In order that the net influence of these drugs be beneficial, there must be an adequate increase in myocardial oxygen supply or ischemia will result, especially in the vulnerable subendocardium. Dose-related peripheral side-effects of these agents include alterations of peripheral vascular resistance, pulmonary vascular resistance, and renal blood flow. Naturally occurring and synthetic drugs most often used include dopamine, dobutamine, epinephrine, norepinephrine, and isoproterenol.

Improved results from these agents are based on three factors. First, there is a better understanding of the relative pharmacologic effects of these agents on the cardiac, peripheral, pulmonary, and renal circulations, allowing the use of these agents to be individualized to the specific needs of the patient. Second, the use of controlled dosage ranges by continuous infusion has decreased the incidence of adverse dose-related side-effects. Third, the utilization of drugs in combination allows a blocking of some of the less desirable effects of catecholamines. Thus the use of low-to-medium-dosage infusion of a catecholamine plus the concomitant infusion of sodium nitroprusside permits an increase in contractility without an increase in peripheral vascular resistance.[122, 170, 175] The success of this treatment depends upon experience with several agents and careful maintenance within the proper dosage range. The combination of dopamine and nitroprusside is usually effective, but comparable results have been achieved by the combination of norepinephrine and phentolamine. Finally, if the desired response is not achieved by one agent, it may follow empirical substitution of an alternate drug for reasons that are not always clear. It also may be beneficial to use the additive effect of two inotropic drugs at low to medium dosage rather than to increase the dosage of a single agent to inordinate levels. The usual pharmacologic effects of these drugs on regional blood flow (systemic, pulmonary, renal, and coronary) are presented in Table 28-1, which is reproduced from Roe.[157] It should again be noted that these changes are dose dependent, and not all of the pharmacologic effects have been confirmed in humans.

With the addition of inotropic agents to the previously described steps, a substantial improvement in cardiac performance is usually achieved. If this does not occur, support should be reassessed before reaching an unacceptable balance between improved

TABLE 28-1. RESPONSES OF DRUGS USED TO SUPPORT CIRCULATION

Agent	CO	HR	SVR	PVR	CBF	SBF	MBF	dp/dt
Catecholamines								
Epinephrine	**↑**	**↑**	↑↓	**↑**	↑	**↓**	**↓**	**↑**
Norepinephrine	**↑**	0–neg	**↑**	**↓**	↑	**↓**	**↓**	**↑**
Dopamine	**↑**	0–pos	**↓**	**↑**	**↑**	↑	↑↓	↑
Dobutamine	**↑**	↑	↓		↑	↑	**↓**	**↑**
Isoproterenol	**↑**	**↑**	**↓**		↑	↑↓	↑	↑
Vasodilator-inotrope combinations								
Phentolamine-norepinephrine	**↑**	↑	↓	**↓**		↑		**↑**
Nitroprusside-norepinephrine	**↑**	**↑**	**↓**	**↓**		↑		**↑**
Miscellaneous								
Glucagon	↑	**↑**	**↓**		**↑**	**↑**	**↓**	↑
Salbutamol	**↑**	**↑**	**↓**	**↓**		↑		↑

Key: CO = cardiac output; HR = heart rate; SVR = systemic vascular resistance; PVR = pulmonary vascular resistance; CBF = coronary blood flow; SBF = splanchnic and renal blood flow; MBF = muscle and skin (peripheral) blood flow; dp/dt = pressure velocity; ↑ = increase, slight, or moderate; ↓ = decrease, slight, or moderate; **↑** = increase, marked, or pronounced; **↓** = decrease, marked, or pronounced; ↑↓ = either decrease or increase

(Roe BB: Perioperative Management in Cardiothoracic Surgey, p 75. Boston, Little, Brown & Co, 1981)

cardiac function and increasing myocardial energy requirements. With the availability of intra-aortic balloon support, the acceptable level of pharmacologic treatment has decreased over the past few years.[10, 17, 46, 175, 176] The unique feature of the intra-aortic balloon is its ability to improve myocardial function without adverse cardiac side-effects, as long as proper synchronization is maintained. Thus it is possible with this mechanical support system both to increase myocardial blood flow by diastolic augmentation (increase supply) and to reduce left ventricular work by afterload reduction (decrease demand). Complications of insertion including aortic dissection may occur, and there may be local effects at the insertion site including an increased risk of infection and compromise of extremity perfusion. Design changes permitting rapid percutaneous balloon insertion have been helpful, but a significant complication rate is still reported.[69, 106] In situations with associated lower extremity vascular occlusion, the balloon can be inserted in the ascending aorta or the subclavian artery. In most patients this device is needed for only a period of hours to a few days, although prolonged use with success has been reported.[152] With adequate myocardial protection, the need for intra-aortic balloon pumping has decreased. Its success, however, in the treatment of that small group of patients unable to be safely weaned from cardiopulmonary bypass has been impressive.[10, 17, 46] Certain patients with marked preoperative reduction of ventricular function should still be considered for the preoperative insertion of a balloon. This includes patients with preexisting cardiogenic shock and certain patients with very unstable conditions secondary to coronary artery disease. In the event that cardiac function cannot be adequately supported by the combination of drugs and balloon pumping, other means of treatment have been proposed. The use of a left ventricular assist device, an artificial heart, and cardiac transplantation are options currently being evaluated.[80, 107, 139, 148]

This discussion of treatment of low cardiac output syndrome has emphasized serial hemodynamic measurements as a guide to both diagnosis and response to therapy. It is recognized that the skilled physician can make reasonable decisions based on the skin temperature, the palpable volume of the pedal pulse, the urine output, and the general appearance of the patient. Further clinical judgment is required to know when these observations are inadequate and should be supplemented by additional measurements. Not all patients require extensive invasive monitoring, but this approach on a short-term basis provides helpful documentation of the patient's condition. This may improve patient care, particularly in an active cardiac service involving surgeons, anesthesiologists, resident physicians, and recovery-room nurses.

PERIOPERATIVE MYOCARDIAL INFARCTION

Incidence and Cause

Perioperative myocardial infarction has become a recognized but controversial entity since the introduction of coronary bypass surgery. It should be recalled, however, that both electrocardiographic (EKG) and clinical findings of myocardial infarction may follow any type of cardiac surgery as a result of unrecognized or untreated associated coronary artery disease, intraoperative difficulties, or ischemia induced as a technical step in the operation. Since one of the proposed benefits of coronary bypass surgery is prevention of myocardial infarction, the not uncommon occurrence of a perioperative myocardial infarction (PMI) has been a source of concern and confusion. The incidence of PMI following coronary bypass surgery is reported to be between 1% and 36%.[5, 6, 25, 77] This wide variation in incidence depends primarily upon the diagnostic criteria utilized and has been a major obstacle both in interpretation of the significance of PMI and in attempts to minimize its occurrence.[169] There is no doubt that in the few patients who die after coronary surgery, myocardial infarction is a common cause or effect of the events leading to death. The causes and significance of PMI are more difficult to interpret in the vast majority of surviving patients. The predictors of PMI are generally agreed to be the descriptors of severe coronary disease or reduced ventricular function, including left main or diffuse three vessel disease, a very low ejection fraction, and a significantly elevated left ventricular end diastolic pressure. Baur reported that 50% of patients with three or more such risk factors experienced a PMI, contrasted to 7% with fewer risk factors.[6] Most authors note a relationship between PMI and the length of cardiopulmonary bypass time or the length of aortic cross-clamp time, both of which are indirect measurements of the extent of vascular or myocardial disease, or the occurrence of difficulties. It is not unusual for the patient with findings of a PMI to have an entirely uneventful postoperative course. Although some reports indicate a reduction in late graft patency and ejection fraction in these patients, Codd could not establish any adverse influence of PMI on late survival, relief of angina, treadmill performance, or ventricular function, and he concluded that PMI is a benign electrophysiologic event.[11, 25, 99] Others strongly disagree with this conclusion and would interpret PMI as a major complication followed by a 12% to 64% mortality rate.[22, 109]

Diagnosis

Diagnosis of PMI is based on a combination of EKG changes, serum enzyme determinations, and isotopic imaging. Levels of sensitivity and specificity will vary widely according to the criteria used to interpret these three tests. Postoperative changes in the EKG appearance of ST and T waves are inconclusive. The appearance of new Q waves has been more helpful, although both false-positive Q waves and the disappearance of previous Q waves are known to occur.[5, 178] The isoenzyme CPK-MB is thought to be specific for irreversible myocardial damage, but it is so sensitive that falsely positive results occur, and some have reported its presence in all postoperative cardiac patients.[55] Arbitrary levels of CPK-MB considered to indicate significant myocardial necrosis vary among institutions. It has not been established whether these levels indicate death of a few grams of tissue or a large mass of left ventricular myocardium. Myocardial imaging, usually with technetium-99m pyrophosphate, is reported to be more specific for irreversible myocardial damage, but it may be positive preoperatively in up to 40% of unstable angina patients, is weakly positive in up to 14% of normal patients, and may be falsely positive owing to surgically induced artifacts.[5, 75] The present expense of preoperative and early and late postoperative imaging prohibits its routine use. Balderman concluded that myocardial imaging was the most predictable test and reported that positive results from two of these three tests (EKG, CPK-MB, ^{99m}Tc) were considered diagnostic for PMI and occurred in 8% of his patients.[5]

Preventive Measures and Management

Coronary bypass grafting is undertaken to prevent myocardial damage, among other reasons, but varying degrees of damage are common sequelae of the procedure. Thus efforts to reduce intraoperative damage should logically improve not only operative survival but also late functional results. Results of these efforts have not been conclusive, largely owing to the difficulties just described in accurately diagnosing PMI. Nonetheless, utilizing the appearance of new Q waves to diagnose PMI, Loop reported a decrease in incidence from 7.1% to 1.2% and attributed this change to improved intraoperative myocardial preservation.[103] Most current reports indicate that the incidence of PMI has been reduced, but it is not clear how this change relates to other factors such as the extent of vascular and myocardial disease, surgical techniques, and the trend toward more complete revascularization. Baur was not able to demonstrate any change in incidence of PMI from the use of hypothermic cardioplegic protection compared with intermittent aortic cross-clamping under moderate systemic hypothermia.[6] In contrast, the Coronary Artery Surgery Study reported a significant difference in PMI with the use of hypothermia alone over hypothermia plus potassium.[8] Thus the current claims that cardioplegic myocardial protection, better surgical techniques, and more complete revascularization have reduced the incidence of PMI are attractive but not completely established.

If PMI is accompanied by arrhythmias or alterations in cardiac function, treatment is directed toward these associated complications. If the diagnosis is based on laboratory results without clinical findings, no specific treatment is recommended, progressive activity is permitted, hospitalization is not extended, and a satisfactory functional symptomatic result is anticipated. This approach may be permissible because of the ability of patients with good left ventricular function to tolerate small amounts of myocardial damage remarkably well if the operation has been successful in providing improved myocardial blood flow.

DISTURBANCES OF CARDIAC RATE AND RHYTHM

Some type of rhythm disturbance, either as a result of a planned portion of the operation or as a consequence of manipulation of the heart, occurs with almost every open-heart operation. Skill in management begins with distinguishing transient, benign disturbances from those that require treatment. Most cardiac surgeons have witnessed as many dysrhythmias as have their cardiology consultants and have probably spent more time focused on the oscilloscope; thus they should have acquired the appropriate knowledge to manage successfully most perioperative dysrhythmias. Current understanding of complex rhythm disturbances has, however, dramatically increased over the past decade owing in part to the introduction of new drugs, the recognition of the limitations of the surface EKG, and the introduction of invasive electrophysiologic evaluation. The appearance of recurrent or refractory rhythm disturbances implies ineffective treatment or diagnosis, which necessitates close cooperation with the proper consultants.

Incidence and Cause

Perioperative arrhythmias constitute the most common postoperative complication, occurring in one half of all major cardiac procedures.[7, 31] Fortunately many of these are transient and are expected sequelae of the procedure rather than significant complications. The numerous causes are often interrelated and can be categorized according to the time of occurrence.

PRIOR TO OPERATION. Arrhythmias prior to operation may be inherent in the patient's pathologic process. Examples include atrial fibrillation with rheumatic heart disease and coronary artery disease; ventricular dysrhythmias ranging from premature contractions to cardiac arrest with coronary artery disease, ventricular aneurysms, and cardiomyopathies; and conduction difficulties secondary to myocardial fibrosis, alterations in coronary blood flow, and intrinsic or even congenital disorders of the conduction system.[187] Treatment of these disturbances may have been only partially successful and may have been complicated by other manifestations of the patient's disease. A common pattern is the presence of atrial fibrillation and heart failure, treated with digitalis and diuretics with inadequate replacement of total body potassium. More complex, life-threatening ventricular dysrhythmias require multiple drugs, each with its own side-effects and interactions with other agents.

DURING THE OPERATION. Rhythm disturbances may recur during the operation from the stress of anesthetic induction and surgical manipulation. Hypoxemia, hypertension, tracheal irritation, and endogenous catecholamine secretion may be transiently associated with anesthetic induction and intubation and produce direct or reflex rhythm changes. Placement of a monitoring catheter may cause mechanical irritation or may be a source of coronary emboli and subsequent arrhythmias in patients with intracardiac communications. Anesthetic agents may predispose the patient to intrinsic myocardial irritability or may interact with other drugs or conditions to cause a dysrhythmia. Cardiopulmonary bypass may dilute the serum concentration of digoxin, and the myocardium may also be more sensitive to this agent after bypass.[123] This, coupled with the frequent use of cardioversion after bypass, makes digitalis toxicity possible. Operative dissection may cause ventricular irritability or may damage specific structures such as the sinus node. Rhythm changes predictably follow myocardial cooling, but they are rare above 30° C. Each step of the surgical manipulation may be a direct or indirect cause of dysrhythmias: cardiac incision or resection of myocardium may produce an irritable focus; débridement of a calcified valve may traumatize the conduction tissue; cannulation may injure the sinus node; and traction or suturing of communications in the low atrium or upper ventricle may produce complete heart block. Ventricular distention not only alters ventricular performance but may also produce myocardial irritability. Incomplete removal of intracardiac air or calcium may lead to coronary embolization followed by ventricular dysrhythmias. Valve-replacement sutures may damage adjacent coronary arteries or conduction tissue, and mechanical irritation of the left ventricle may follow insertion of a high-profile valve in a small ventricle. Infusion of hypothermic potassium cardioplegic solution may be followed by temporary conduction abnormalities, but this is more likely related to the amount of potassium administered than to the effect of cooling.[48] Intraoperative diuretic therapy following hemodilution predisposes the patient to a large urinary loss of potassium, which contributes to postoperative myocardial irritability. This partial listing of operative causes of dysrhythmias emphasizes the hazards all patients confront, but most cardiac procedures fortunately are followed by a stable cardiac rhythm.

FOLLOWING THE OPERATION. Electrolyte imbalance, acidosis, and hypoxemia may be present. Drugs used to increase myocardial performance including isoproterenol, epinephrine, and dopamine have a chronotropic effect and also may increase myocardial irritability. Less common drug effects include sinus arrest after lidocaine infusion and sinus dysfunction following high dosages of sodium nitroprusside.[19, 26]

Untreated hypertension may produce reflex changes, and endogenous catecholamine secretion is increased when the patient experiences anxiety and pain. Additional drugs or resumption of preoperative medications may be indicated, including digoxin, diuretics, and antiarrhythmic agents, each with its own risk-to-benefit ratio.

Preventive Measures

Prevention begins with the recognition of each of the hazards just enumerated and the principles that they illustrate. Preoperatively certain drugs should be discontinued. Unless essential, digoxin should be stopped at least 1 or 2 days before the operation, if renal clearance is normal. Dosage of diuretics should be reduced and efforts made to restore serum potassium toward normal, although total body potassium may still be depleted. Quinidine and propranolol may be continued, but drugs such as reserpine should be discontinued.[185] Anesthetic agents, such as halothane, known to produce myocardial irritability, have generally been replaced by safer drugs. Control of hypertension and blocking of reflexes during tracheal intubation are usually possible. Insertion of intracardiac monitoring lines may cause irritability, which should be treated with lidocaine before proceeding. All cardiac incisions, sutures, and cannulation sites should be placed carefully in light of a complete understanding of the normal and abnormal anatomy of the conduction system and the position of the coronary arteries. In most procedures for congenital abnormalities, the location of conduction tissue in relation to known landmarks can be anticipated and avoided.[41] Intraoperative conduction mapping may be helpful with defects such as corrected transposition and atrioventricular canal. Avoidance of injury to the sinus node and the AV node is probably more important in surgery for transposition than are the incisions and suture lines between the two nodes. Following cardiopulmonary bypass, serial potassium determinations are necessary to monitor replacement therapy of potassium losses. If multiple, coupled, or multifocal premature ventricular contractions occur, a lidocaine infusion should be started; it is considered preventive for subsequent ventricular tachycardia or fibrillation. Adequate myocardial protection and appropriate recovery time following an ischemic insult are important preventive measures. Prophylactic digitalization has been recommended for coronary bypass patients, owing to an incidence as high as 20% of postoperative atrial flutter–fibrillation.[18] This practice may actually increase the incidence of dysrhythmias, and a recent study reports that low-dose propranolol begun immediately after the operation reduces the incidence of atrial fibrillation.[36, 158]

Diagnosis and Management

At present, patients usually do not die from an undiagnosed or undocumented postoperative dysrhythmia. Several factors have contributed to this change. Advances in monitoring have made it both possible and practical to provide a continual EKG recording by telemetry with capability of visual display, central surveillance, and recording of abnormalities. Twenty-four-hour tape recordings of rhythm aid in the identification of low-incidence disturbances. These advances, which originated in the cardiac-care unit, are now available both in the surgical recovery units and in the ambulatory wards. A second factor has been the introduction of new antiarrhythmic drugs, more reliable pumps for the continuous intravenous infusion of these agents, and the available measurements of serum drug levels.

A third contribution has been the use of temporary transthoracic atrial and ventricular electrodes and the development of reliable, versatile external pacemakers for use with these electrodes. This approach is elegantly presented and documented in the recent monograph by Waldo and MacLean, which describes the uses of these electrodes in over 9000 patients.[184] The diagnosis of tachyarrhythmias is greatly facilitated by the simultaneous recording of the atrial electrogram and the surface EKG. Recordings of ventricular electrograms are less helpful, but they may aid in timing mechanical assist devices. Therapeutic applications of these electrodes have been even more beneficial. Atrial pacing may be used to overdrive ectopic atrial or ventricular foci and also to increase cardiac output secondary to bradycardia. Temporary ventricular pacing is used for the various types of heart block, and it is possible sequentially to pace the atria and ventricles to achieve synchronized atrioventricular contraction. Rapid atrial pacing may capture the atrium in flutter, or it may capture paroxysmal atrial tachycardia, with resumption of sinus rhythm on termination of pacing.[21] Cardiac pacing is a safe, rapid, versatile treatment with no side-effects or interactions with other drugs. It should be strongly considered as the first choice of treatment prior to utilizing the two other traditional approaches to dysrhythmias—drug therapy and cardioversion. In view of their safety and potential utility, a strong argument can be made for leaving temporary electrodes on most if not all patients following major cardiac procedures.[184]

In most patients, serial tracings of the surface EKG plus recordings of atrial and ventricular electrograms will lead to an accurate diagnosis, which can then be followed by a rational plan of treatment: a combination of pacing, drugs, and cardioversion. Initial control of heart rate and rhythm is often possible by pacing, reserving drugs for conditions that either persist or recur. The primary goals of dysrhythmia therapy are first to correct whatever sustained situation might cause an inadequate cardiac output and, second, to control irritability, which might precipitate life-threatening ventricular tachycardia or fibrillation. Underlying causes and specific etiologies should at the same time be identified and treated. Occasionally a complete intracavitary electrophysiologic study will need to be performed to diagnose and localize a complex arrhythmia properly.

Specific treatment may be approached from the viewpoint of individual dysrhythmias, drugs, or, as noted here, therapeutic objectives. It is essential that the dosages, rates of administration, metabolism, and adverse side-effects of each of the drugs listed in Table 28-2 be completely understood and that drug interactions and additive effects be considered before using multiple agents. The three specific steps of treatment are control of heart rate, suppression of irritability, and synchronization of rhythm. A slow heart rate from sinus or nodal bradycardia may be treated by atrial pacing or isoproterenol infusion. If heart block is present, ventricular pacing or, preferably, AV sequential pacing is temporarily utilized, followed if necessary by insertion of a permanent pacemaker. Supraventricular tachyarrhythmias may be captured and slowed by rapid atrial pacing, or the rate may be decreased by intravenous propranolol. Simultaneous slowing of AV conduction is achieved by digoxin, but this requires several hours to achieve therapeutic concentrations. If the tachycardia produces rapid hemodynamic decompensation, electrical cardioversion should be performed,

TABLE 28-2. ANTIARRHYTHMIC DRUGS

Drug	Dosage	Indication	Organ Responsible for Metabolism	Effective Concentration
Lidocaine	50–200 mg, IV bolus; 1–4 mg/min, IV infusion	Ventricular irritability	Liver	2–5 mcg/ml
Procainamide	1–4 mg/min, IV infusion; 100–200 mg, q3h IM; 250 mg, q3h oral	Ventricular irritability	Liver, 50%; kidney, 50%	4–8 mg/L
Quinidine	300 mg, q8h IM; 300 mg, q8h oral	Atrial irritability	Liver, 50%; kidney, 50%	4–8 mg/L
Diphenylhydantoin	100 mg × q5min up to 1000 mg, IV; maintenance, 100 mg, q4-8h IM or oral	Ventricular irritability Digitalis toxicity	Liver	10–20 mg/L
Disopyramide	150 mg, q6h oral	Ventricular irritability	Kidney, 70%; liver 30%	2–4 mg/ml
Propranolol	0.5–1 mg, q5min, up to 5 mg, IV; 10–120 mg, q6h oral	Ventricular irritability, atrial irritability	Liver; kidney	< 100 ng/L
Bretylium tosylate	5 mg/kg over 10–20 min; q6h IV	Ventricular irritability	Kidney	
Digoxin	Loading, 1–2 mg in divided doses, IV or oral; maintenance, 0.125–0.5 mg, qd IV or oral	Atrial fibrillation or flutter	Kidney	0.8–1.6 ng/ml
Verapamil	5–10 mg over 5 min, IV	Supraventricular tachycardia	Liver	

(Modified after Behrendt DM, Austen WG: Patient Care in Cardiac Surgery, 3rd ed. Boston, Little, Brown & Co, 1980)

in full knowledge that the tachycardia may recur and that cardioversion may predispose the patient to digitalis toxicity. Recurrence of the tachycardia after initial control requires the addition of drugs such as quinidine or propranolol. The recent approval of several calcium blocking agents may alter these recommendations. Verapamil effectively slows AV conduction and may also aid in conversion of supraventricular rhythms to normal sinus rhythm. Persistent sinus tachycardia rarely requires treatment, but heart rate may be decreased with low dosages of oral propranolol.

Premature ventricular contractions are the most common disorder of myocardial irritability. Treatment is indicated when a frequency of 6 to 10 beats a minute suddenly occurs or when coupled or multifocal beats occur. Suppression by overdrive pacing is often possible if the underlying heart rate permits. Hypokalemia should be corrected and an initial bolus of lidocaine should be followed by a continuous intravenous infusion if the problem persists. Lidocaine produces minimal depression of ventricular contractility and is the established drug of choice. On the basis of its safety and effectiveness in treating patients recovered from myocardial infarction, lidocaine is recommended for the first 24 to 48 hours after coronary artery surgery at the initial sign of ventricular irritability. Persisting irritability may be treated by oral agents such as procainamide, quinidine, diphenylhydantoin, or disopyramide, with careful monitoring of drug levels and observation of the patient for depression of myocardial function. Progression to ventricular tachycardia must be treated immediately by a lidocaine bolus, followed by countershock if control is not achieved within minutes. Recurrence of ventricular tachycardia while the patient receives a lidocaine infusion requires the addition of other drugs such as procainamide or bretylium tosylate. Ventricular fibrillation may be an initial arrhythmia, or it may be precipitated by premature beats or ventricular tachycardia. Treatment consists of cardiopulmonary resuscitation with artificial maintenance of ventilation and circulation until an effective cardiac rhythm can be restored by a combination of drugs and countershock. Proficiency in resuscitation is mandatory for all personnel involved in any stage of the perioperative care of the cardiac surgical patient. Cardiac surgeons and anesthesiologists should additionally be aware of the changing understanding of the physiologic mechanisms of resuscitation and the resultant introduction of new techniques for more effective maintenance of artificial circulation.[105, 131]

The final step in treatment is synchronization of conduction. This is initially achieved in the presence of heart block by sequential AV pacing, particularly important for patients with a fixed strike volume secondary to altered ventricular compliance.

For these patients, proper timing of the atrial contraction may produce a substantial increase in cardiac output.[39, 132] If asynchronous contraction is the result of atrial fibrillation or flutter, the rhythm must be converted by the use of digoxin, quinidine, propranolol, and cardioversion in various combinations. If this condition has been chronic, perioperative conversion is unwise because its success will be temporary at best. Multiple drugs should be administered cautiously because digitalis toxicity is not uncommon and may be more difficult to manage than was the initial arrhythmia. The addition of propranolol has been helpful in this regard in patients with refractory atrial flutter or recurrent atrial fibrillation.

The role of surgical treatment in the control of preexcitation arrhythmias and malignant ventricular tachyarrhythmias has recently been established.[34, 57, 77, 130, 131, 160] The techniques and indications for these disorders are applied differently but share the need for complete pre- and intraoperative electrophysiologic mapping and specialized knowledge of the cardiac conduction system. Centers with experienced personnel have had remarkable success in controlling these life-threatening arrhythmias.

Occasional arrhythmias will continue to be an inevitable consequence of major cardiac surgery. The incidence, however, has decreased with careful planning of the perioperative management and the technical steps of the procedure, plus a better understanding of underlying causes. Advances in proper diagnosis and treatment of serious arrhythmias have allowed successful control of previously life-threatening complications of cardiac operations.

MECHANICAL BLEEDING

Excessive bleeding in the operating room or in the postoperative period continues to be a vexing problem following cardiac surgery and may be the cause of considerable illness and even an occasional death. Systemic bleeding problems related to transfusion of blood products and the use of cardiopulmonary bypass are described in additional chapters of this text. The diagnosis and management of mechanical or localized bleeding and its differentiation from a diffuse coagulation disorder are discussed in this section.

Incidence and Cause

Excessive bleeding associated with cardiac operations may be due to a preexisting coagulation disorder, an imbalance between heparin and protamine sulfate, an alteration of clotting factors by cardiopulmonary bypass, a transfusion reaction, and mechanical bleeding due to inadequate hemostasis. Of these, the last is the most common and most closely related to the technical aspects of the procedure. The incidence of bleeding from each of these causes has decreased over the past few years, but reexploration for bleeding still occurs in between 1% and 10% of large series of patients.[103] Our reoperation rate for bleeding has averaged 2.9% in 2000 coronary bypass patients, with an incidence under 1% for the most recent 500 patients. Although a specific abnormality has not clearly been identified, the incidence of diffuse bleeding has long been recognized to be increased in cyanotic congenital heart disease. Diffuse and localized bleeding has decreased since the introduction of hemodilution and blood conservation techniques.[32, 181]

Preventive Measures

The current practice of preoperative screening for coagulation disorders and modern cross-matching techniques should minimize formerly unrecognized problems. The surgeon's primary responsibility to minimize operative hemorrhage is precise technique. The liberal use of electrocautery while opening the chest is recommended and has not been documented to produce problems with healing.

Several technical developments have been helpful in reducing mechanical bleeding. Proper construction of suture lines has been aided by the excellent exposure and visualization possible with a quiet, bloodless operative field afforded by cardioplegic arrest and circulatory arrest or low-flow perfusion. Polypropylene suture material allows a continuous suture line to be pulled up tightly with an even distribution of tension and less tendency for bleeding between sutures. The additional use of felt bolsters or pledgets is at times helpful. Bleeding from prosthetic grafts is minimized by a variety of preclotting techniques and the use of low porosity materials.[28, 64] With these techniques, all anastomoses and suture lines are remarkably hemostatic after the reversal of heparin. Administration of autologous blood, platelet concentrate, and fresh frozen plasma and the use of autotransfusion have been recommended but have not conclusively been shown to be necessary.[32, 181] Accurate neutralization of heparin has been improved by the use of activated clotting time, although a recent report indicates that this determination may be misleading.[37, 81, 140] Prostacyclin infusion during experimental cardiopulmonary bypass has been reported to preserve platelet function, but clinical studies have not yet confirmed a reduced blood loss.[30, 146]

Diagnosis and Management

Prior to chest closure, suture-line bleeding and diffuse bleeding can usually be differentiated easily.

With diffuse bleeding, chest closure should be delayed, and specific treatment of the clotting abnormalities should be instituted after appropriate diagnostic tests. If the bleeding persists after the combined efforts of the surgeon, anesthesiologist, hematologist, and blood bank personnel, the chest may be closed, although reexploration may be required for continued bleeding or tamponade. If the usual methods of controlling mechanical bleeding are unsuccessful, rarely a variety of innovative techniques, including external wrapping of vascular anastomoses, application of external onlay patches over bleeding areas, balloon tamponade of inaccessible bleeding points, diversion of adjacent bleeding into the right atrium as a controlled fistula, and topical application of various thrombogenic agents, may help. Only in extreme instances of mechanical bleeding has packing of the area, with subsequent reexploration for pack removal, been effective.

Once the chest is closed, differentiating localized and diffuse bleeding is more difficult. If the field was completely dry and the patient bleeds in the recovery room, the bleeding is most probably mechanical. Specific treatment of clotting abnormalities is begun and reexploration is indicated for continued volume loss that requires repeated transfusions. The use of positive end-expiratory pressure has been reported to reduce postoperative bleeding, allowing avoidance of reoperation in 73% of patients so treated, but this finding was not confirmed by a subsequent study.[78, 193] A variety of formulas for excessive bleeding have been proposed, but reexploration is usually necessary after several hours of 200 to 300 ml of blood loss per hour. If during this time, persistent hypotension or mediastinal tamponade occurs, expeditious reexploration is necessary. The risk of a controlled exploration is minimal, and this approach is safer than is waiting until the patient is unstable. If acute tamponade or massive bleeding occurs, the chest should be opened in the recovery room, and the patient then returned to the operating room. A report of 74 such emergency procedures indicated four patients out of five with tamponade and nine out of fifteen with massive bleeding who survived, with a 6% incidence of wound infection.[53]

Life-threatening hemorrhage continues to be an important complication of cardiac surgery, though less common than it was in the past. The current approach to this problem is based on a logical evaluation and treatment of the causative factors, coupled with newer methods of prevention. As a result, it is currently rare to encounter uncontrollable perioperative bleeding. Perhaps the major error in management is failure to return a postoperative patient to the operating room prior to the onset of secondary complications.

INFECTIOUS COMPLICATIONS

Infectious complications common to any surgical procedure may occur after cardiac operations. The principles of antibiotic administration, septic shock, and general wound infections are described in separate chapters. Two specific problems following cardiac surgery—infections of the mediastinum and sternum and intravascular sepsis and endocarditis—are discussed in this section.

Infections of the Sternum and Mediastinum

INCIDENCE AND CAUSE. The most common incision utilized in cardiac surgery is the median sternotomy. The rate of primary healing of this incision is generally high and is comparable to that of most clean incisions used in other surgical procedures. The rate of sternotomy wound complications ranges between 0.5% to 5.9% but is under 2% in most series.[83] Serry reported that 54 of 74 sternotomy complications were localized wound infections without sternal or mediastinal involvement.[163] Extension to the sternum or mediastinum requires prolonged treatment and additional operations and produces significant rates of morbidity, mortality, and lengthy hospitalization. A secondary involvement of these regions may follow either a superficial infection or separation of an initially sterile wound. Antibiotic prophylaxis has been assumed, but not proven, to reduce the incidence of these complications. Factors that have been reported to increase the incidence of sternal wound complications include the technique of closure, prolonged operative time, postoperative low cardiac output, reexploration for bleeding, external cardiac massage, prolonged mechanical ventilation, and the use of a tracheostomy.[163] Age, sex, diabetes, thickness of the sternum, prolonged hiccoughs, and chronic bronchitis have been implicated but probably are not significant contributing factors.

PREVENTIVE MEASURES. All principles of wound and tissue healing should be observed, and elective procedures should be postponed if the skin is infected in the region of incisions. Thorough skin preparation and draping, midline placement of the sternotomy, preservation of one internal mammary artery, and the minimal use of bone wax have been advocated.[155, 156] Secure approximation of the sternal edges during closure is essential because any initial instability will usually worsen during the postoperative period. A variety of suture materials and bands have been recommended, but the method of placement is probably more important than is the type of material. Sutures placed around the sternum medial to the internal mammary vessels achieve a more secure closure than transsternal sutures. If the sternum has been fractured or opened off center, additional figure-of-eight or peristernal enforcing sutures are advisable.[154] If prolonged respiratory support is needed, tracheostomy should be delayed until the wound is well healed. Finally, the maintenance of adequate postoperative nutrition is recognized as an important factor in wound healing and host defense against infection.[66]

DIAGNOSIS AND MANAGEMENT. Principles of management of sternal wound complications are directed toward early control and selective need for open treatment. Any sterile defect in the skin closure, subcutaneous fluid collection, or instability of the sternum requires reoperation before secondary contamination occurs. A minor clicking of the sternal periosteum with no other wound difficulty may be observed, but major instability is an indication of improper sternal closure and should be followed by rewiring. Localized infections of the skin and subcutaneous tissue should be opened and treated by wound dressings if the sternum is stable and there is no evidence of communication with the mediastinum. Primary or secondary sternal or mediastinal involvement requires immediate reoperation with débridement, irrigation, and evaluation of the extent of the infection. At reoperation considerable judgment is required to decide which patients are best treated open or closed. The use of débridement, reclosure of the sternum, continuous irrigation and drainage of the mediastinum with povidine-iodine or antibiotic solution, and appropriate systemic antibiotics has significantly reduced the mortality and morbidity rates associated with this complication.[83, 163] This method should be considered in all patients with mediastinitis, but approximately one half of patients will require additional operative procedures. Certain patients with deep mediastinal infections or extensive sternal involvement should initially be treated with open packing. If the closed method is chosen, further wound complications should be considered an indication to convert to the open method. Once the open wound has begun to granulate and local infection is under control, time to ultimate wound closure can be reduced by the use of muscle and tissue flaps, as described by Jurkiwicz.[83] Infection of the sternum, ribs, or costal cartilages requires débridement of all involved tissue, systemic antibiotics, and open wound care. With the application of these techniques, Jurkiewicz reported a decrease in mortality from 18% in 50 of 3239 patients prior to 1978 to no deaths in the 12 infections in the most recent 1052 patients.[83]

Special mention should be made of the difficult problems of mediastinitis in the presence of essential foreign material used for reconstruction of the aorta or closure of cardiac incisions. Fatal bleeding from suture-line infection may occur, but long-term survival has also been reported.[124] Late infection may occur with fatal hemorrhage, chronically draining sinuses, or false aneurysms with late rupture. This problem is also an indication for pedicle flaps, including omentum, to cover the prosthetic material. Any problem with sternal closure unrelated to the initial infection should be noted. After certain prolonged and difficult procedures, it may be impossible to close the sternum without producing cardiac compression and low cardiac output. This may be related to diffuse mediastinal edema or compression of reconstructions used for complex congenital defects. Closure of the skin and subcutaneous tissue or the temporary interposition of prosthetic material with secondary closure of the sternum after several days has been successful.[58, 62]

Intravascular Sepsis and Postoperative Endocarditis

INCIDENCE AND CAUSE. Persistent bacterial or fungal infections of the bloodstream are of particular concern in patients with cardiac and vascular suture lines and implanted prosthetic patches, grafts, or valves. Once an infection is established at these sites, the chance of antibiotic sterilization is generally low, and the probability of local abscess formation, mycotic aneurysm, suture-line disruption, or prosthetic dysfunction is high. Most postoperative bacteremias are transient but almost always require aggressive therapy because of the serious consequences of seeding of foreign material. The incidence of persistent sepsis following cardiac operations is fortunately quite low, especially considering the many opportunities for introduction of organisms in this type of relatively lengthy surgery, including exposure of the blood to multiple interfaces, invasion of the bloodstream with various cannulas and infusion lines, instrumentation of most orifices of the body, and exposure to a large number of personnel. The epidemiology is obvious for each of these levels of exposure. The low incidence of sepsis has not been clearly attributable to the almost uniform use of short-term prophylactic antibiotics, but the risk of withholding antibiotics in these patients has been considered so high that it has been difficult to perform an acceptable clinical study of this problem. Of particular concern are the multiple opportunities in these complex procedures for breaks in technique at each level, ranging from contamination during insertion of the monitoring line to use of improper technique for endotracheal suctioning.

Sepsis associated with intravascular catheters is particularly noteworthy. Two recent studies have emphasized the following conclusions: Positive cultures have been obtained from betwen 9% and 34% of catheters removed; the incidence is greater in infants and older adults whose catheters have been in place for over 3 to 4 days—and in cut-down as contrasted with percutaneous catheters; the incidence of sepsis is reduced when either dilute heparin or an inotropic drug containing the antioxidant sodium metabisulfate is infused.[56, 119]

A numerical value for the incidence of transient sepsis is not available, but the incidence of endocarditis following prosthetic valve insertion has decreased from 10% to the current reports of between 1% and 5% in both clinical and autopsy series.[82, 91, 115, 137] The incidence of endocarditis is between four and seven times more frequent following valve replacement than it is after other types of open heart surgery.[54] A recent multicenter study reported that 63 of 278 patients (23%) treated for infectious endocarditis during a 1-year period had undergone previous cardiovascular surgery.[85] Over one half of these patients had prosthetic valves, and in the remaining patients the most common disorder was cyanotic congenital heart disease with a previous systemic-pulmonary shunt. Of interest was the finding that only 14% developed endocarditis within 90 days of surgery, and none of this early group had congenital heart disease. In the third of patients with a probable predisposing event, dental procedures were most common, followed by respiratory, gastrointestinal, and genitourinary procedures or infections.

PREVENTIVE MEASURES. All patients scheduled for elective cardiac surgery should be free of any infections or potentially infectious conditions. Recurrent respiratory or urinary infections should have been treated and be in a quiescent phase. Significant dental problems should have been treated under antibiotic coverage prior to cardiac surgery, especially in patients requiring prosthetic materials. If the patient has an unexplained fever the day before elective surgery, the operation should be postponed. Short-term intravenous antibiotics are indicated for endocarditis prophylaxis in patients with valvular or congenital heart disease, according to the 1977 American Heart Association recommendations.[27] This is supported by the known incidence of bacteremia of 16% during nasotracheal intubation or nasotracheal suctioning and 8% following uretheral catheterization, both methods of which are commonly employed with major cardiac surgery.[45] Prophylactic antibiotics for prosthetic valve insertion have been recommended in retrospective studies reporting a significant reduction of endocarditis.[82, 91] Prospective attempts to confirm this finding have been inconclusive, and the currently accepted practice is not based on controlled data. It is agreed, however, that prolonged prophylaxis is not acceptable because of the risk of additional infections and the emergence of resistant organisms. Perioperative antibiotic administration should be directed toward prevention of the most common causes of early prosthetic endocarditis, *Staphylococcus aureus* and *epidermidis*, and gram-negative bacilli.[4, 59] During the operation constant attention must be directed toward prevention of contamination because reports of cultures from the operative field and equipment have demonstrated an inordinately high incidence of contamination by these very organisms.[91] Routine cultures of the pump oxygenator contents have been positive in between 7.5% and 75% of procedures.[3, 9]

Late infection in the patient with a prosthetic valve is primarily prevented by proper antibiotic coverage for bacteremias known to be associated with dental, respiratory, gastrointestinal, and genitourinary procedures or infections. The pathogenesis and therefore prophylaxis of late infections caused by fungi or less common bacteria unassociated with known predisposing events are not clearly understood. The possibility has been raised that these infections may have been present from the initial operation and delayed in clinical emergence for unknown reasons. That the prosthesis might be contaminated at the time of insertion has led to the policy of culturing specimens from the valve container, especially with biologic valves. This has produced reports of positive cultures, often of multiple slow-growing exotic organisms of uncertain clinical significance.[96] In my experience this has been associated with a clinical infection by the same organisms on only one occasion and then that resulted in a late infection, after several months.

During the postoperative period any infectious complications should be treated with appropriate antibiotics to aid in local control of the process and prevention of secondary bacteremia. Meticulous care of all indwelling lines and catheters is necessary, and these should be removed as soon as possible. If long-term intravascular catheters are essential, their use should observe the principles developed by parenteral nutrition services.[66] At the earliest sign of sepsis, catheters should be removed, or at least changed.

DIAGNOSIS AND MANAGEMENT. The presence of a persistent or recurrent fever in a postoperative cardiac patient is adequate indication for multiple blood cultures with simultaneous search for the cause of the fever. One particularly vexing problem is the differential diagnosis of the patient with either the postcardiotomy or postperfusion syndrome, as discussed in a following section. The presence of a positive blood culture raises the possibility of either contamination or transient bacteremia without seeding of prosthetic material. Contamination is ruled out by obtaining multiple cultures, correlating with the patient's clinical course, and often by initiating a course of treatment while waiting for culture results. The clinical and laboratory features of primary endocarditis are less helpful in the patient recovering from cardiac surgery because these associated findings can be explained in several ways. The report of two or more positive cultures of the same organism is a definite indication for antibiotic treatment. If an extracardiac cause for the bacteremia is established and a rapid response of this problem follows, then there may not be persistent infection of the cardiovascular system. Without prosthetic dysfunction and with a strong alternate etiology, a short course of antibiotics has been successful. Other authors have assumed that prosthetic material is infected in this setting and that short course treatment is inadequate.[137] Positive blood cultures are readily obtained in prosthetic endocarditis, and the finding of multiple sterile aerobic and anaerobic cultures after several weeks' incubation is strong evidence against infection.[1, 108] Blind therapy should be avoided (except for extreme clinical instability consisting of prosthetic dysfunction or systemic embolization), because the spectrum of organisms is wide, ranging from diphtheroids to fungi, and bactericidal concentrations cannot be determined without identification of the agent.

Endocarditis in the late period after cardiac surgery may be difficult to diagnose because of the gradual onset of a low-grade fever and vague symptoms and because partial antibiotic treatment may have been undertaken as a result of an improper diagnosis. The presence of a new murmur, changing prosthetic sounds, excessive motion of the valve ring on fluoroscopy, and systemic embolization may all be associated with late-onset endocarditis. All patients with culture-proven early or late prosthetic endocarditis require intensive intravenous treatment with a synergistic combination of two bactericidal antibiotics chosen according to appropriate sensitivity testing and serum bactericidal assays.[59] It was initially thought that antibiotic treatment for 6 to 8 weeks was the preferred method for all patients with prosthetic endocarditis, but this has been associated with an overall mortality rate of 61%.[82] The mortality rate for antibiotic treatment alone is reported as 81% in infections occurring within 60 days of valve insertion, compared to 41% in the late-onset group.[59] In this same review, the mortality rate for surgical replacement of the infected prosthesis was 63% for the early-onset group and 30% for the late group. The results of antibiotics alone *versus* surgery are not statistically different, but the surgical patients were characterized by greater prosthetic dysfunction, hemodynamic instability, and uncontrolled infection. These results coupled with improved results from prompt surgical treatment, have led to the recommendation that antibiotic therapy alone should be reserved for that specific group of patients with late-onset, highly sensitive, nonfungal infections, with no evidence of uncontrolled infection, paravalvular leak, prosthetic dysfunction, systemic embolization, or congestive heart failure. This aggressive surgical treatment has been extended recently with the recommendation that medical treatment be reserved for patients with uncomplicated streptococcal infections involving the mitral valve only.[115] These recommendations are in part supported by the improved results obtained by early valve replacement in patients with active nonprosthetic infectious endocarditis.[190] It should be recognized that early surgical treatment during active infection may necessitate radical surgical débridement followed by demanding and innovative surgical reconstruction of the infected area.[149] The higher incidence of residual paravalvular leaks in these patients is not surprising, but the low incidence of either early or late recurrence of the original infection when operating on culture-positive patients has been reassuring.[151]

NEUROLOGIC COMPLICATIONS

Neurologic and psychological disturbances following cardiac operations have decreased in recent years but have not vanished. Air and particulate embolic problems related to extracorporeal circulation and the behavioral complications following surgery are discussed in additional chapters of this text. Attention is focused here on some of the additional problems that are occasionally encountered.

Ischemia

Permanent ischemic changes of the central nervous system or spinal cord are infrequent but devastating complications of cardiac surgery. Many of the more common transient alterations of central nervous system function are thought to have a multifactorial etiology, but ischemia undoubtedly contributes. Systemic blood pressure, systemic blood flow, congenital or occlusive changes in blood vessels, and local autoregulatory responses are but a few of the influences on adequate regional blood supply. The utilization of oxygen by the brain, however, is rather constant, is almost completely derived from aerobic metabolism, and may be clinically reduced only by a decrease in temperature or deep anesthetic depression. Three specific concerns about blood supply to the nervous tissue merit discussion, although they remain largely problematic.

CEREBRAL BLOOD FLOW DURING CARDIOPULMONARY BYPASS. In spite of considerable clinical and experimental evaluation, the safe level of cerebral blood flow during the period of extracorporeal circulation has not been established, nor is it known how this should best be achieved. Most perfusion systems deliver mean arterial pressure, and it has been recommended that a normothermic flow rate of 2 L to 2.5 L/min/m^2 at a mean arterial pressure greater than 60 torr will avoid cerebral hypoperfusion.[14, 98] Others have emphasized pressure dependence rather than flow and recommend pressures of at least 70 torr.[172, 173] It has also been noted that the incidence of CNS dysfunction increases with bypass time, independent of the perfusion pressure.[14, 93] It is not clear how these recommendations should be altered in the presence of cerebral vascular disease or preoperative hypertension. Two recent clinical reports challenge these findings; they conclude that a reduction in pump flow to less than 40 ml/kg/min with a mean arterial pressure below 60 torr at 28° C produces no long-term cerebral dysfunction.[47, 93] A higher than usual incidence of transient cerebral dysfunction in these patients was noted, however, during the first postoperative week. Regardless of the pressure chosen as safe, data are inadequate to recommend the proper treatment when pressure drops below this level. Whether to increase the flow rate or to increase pressure by drug-induced vasoconstriction is not known.

These considerations become even more pertinent when treating a patient with combined cerebrovascular and cardiac disease. Various approaches ranging from a simultaneous correction of both problems almost independent of symptoms to an individualized approach have been advocated.[71, 117, 129, 179] Myocardial infarction may be a complication of carotid endarterectomy, and stroke may follow coronary bypass surgery in the absence of either carotid or cardiac symptoms. The incidence of simultaneous symptomatic carotid and coronary occlusive disease is under 2%.[71] My current approach to these patients is as follows:

- Cerebral angiography is performed only in symptomatic patients.
- In the absence of left main coronary artery occlusion or unstable angina, a staged approach is recommended, beginning with endarterectomy for significant symptomatic carotid occlusive disease.
- Stable coronary patients are operated on without preceding carotid surgery if ulcerated plaques are responsible for cerebral symptoms.
- Simultaneous carotid and coronary surgery is reserved for symptomatic patients with significant carotid occlusions and left main or unstable coronary artery disease.

HYPOTHERMIC CIRCULATORY ARREST. The reintroduction of profound hypothermic circulatory arrest has been one of the major advances of cardiac surgery during the past decade. Initial reports indicated minimal cerebral dysfunction in children subjected to 60 minutes of circulatory arrest at temperatures below 20° C. With experience came the recognition that many of the same technical advantages may be achieved with low-flow hypothermic perfusion, regional myocardial ischemia, and adjuncts to protect the myocardium. At present, total circulatory arrest is considered less essential for the successful treatment of complex neonatal cardiac malformations. In spite of continuing concern over possible late cerebral dysfunction in patients so treated, the neurologic evaluation and the testing of psychomotor development and intelligence quotient for several years following surgery have been encouraging.[24, 68]

As a result of early experience with adults in whom excessive cerebral dysfunction was reported, these techniques were initially reserved for pediatric patients. These initial impressions must be reevaluated in light of the experience of Griep and of Crawford, who successfully utilized hypothermic cerebral circulatory arrest in adults undergoing reconstruction of aneurysms of the transverse aortic arch.[35, 67] Crawford produced cerebral ischemia for 25 to 55 minutes at a temperature of 15° C and reported no immediate ischemic cerebral complication in 17 patients. The associated anesthetic and perfusion techniques he utilized may have contributed to this remarkable success.

SPINAL CORD ISCHEMIA AFTER THORACIC AORTIC OPERATIONS. Paraplegia from spinal ischemia occurs in less than 1% of patients following resection of coarctation, in approximately 5% to 10% of patients after resection of a descending thoracic artery aneurysm, and in up to 21% of patients having repair of a transected thoracic aorta.[15, 86, 125, 161, 192] Anatomical variations in the major blood supply to the spinal cord, the presence of collateral blood supply to the spinal cord, the extent of collateral flow to the lower body, the duration of aortic cross clamping, and the blood pressure during the operation are the most important variables influencing the incidence of this complication. In most patients with coarctation of the aorta, extensive collaterals around the coarctation provide an adequate blood flow beyond the point of aortic clamping and thus prevent spinal cord ischemia. No correlation among the incidence of paraplegia in these patients and the length of aortic clamping, the length of aorta resected, or the number of intercostal arteries divided has been demonstrated.[15] The most important factor is probably avoiding intraoperative hypotension. It has been recommended that if collaterals are inadequate to provide a mean pressure greater than 50 torr distal to the coarctation, further protection should be provided by the use of a shunt or partial cardiopulmonary bypass.[76] This inadequacy is rare, and the need for additional protective measures is not clearly established in these patients.

In patients with thoracic aortic aneurysm, occlusion of primary and collateral sources of blood flow to the spinal cord may be a part of the atherosclerotic process. This partially explains the rare spontaneous paraplegia and the variable incidence of postoperative paraplegia. The use of shunts or bypass support was formerly considered essential in the management of these patients, but recent reports have demonstrated no increase in the incidence of paraplegia without those protective adjuncts.[35, 42, 125] Remarkably short cross-clamp times and effective control of intraoperative blood pressure may have partially allowed this success. It is not certain that this change in technique should be adopted by all thoracic surgeons for all thoracic aneurysm resections. An individualized application of both shunting and bypass techniques should be considered for patients with complicated lesions requiring extended operations.

The increased incidence of paraplegia following traumatic thoracic aortic transection may be due to a combination of injury to spinal blood supply, hypotension associated with the trauma, and the absence of collateral blood flow to the lower body or the spinal cord. Many such patients have been treated without the use of shunts or bypass with a low incidence of paraplegia. I concur with Katz's recent recommendation that a shunt should still be considered if a cross-clamp time exceeding 30 minutes is anticipated.[86]

Peripheral Nerve Injuries

BRACHIAL PLEXUS INJURY. Injury to the brachial plexus was found in 34 of 180 adult patients undergoing cardiac operations through a median sternotomy.[182] This is usually manifest by transient sensory and motor involvement in the C8–T1 distribution, but the deficit may occasionally be prolonged and severe.[89] The cause of this injury was formerly thought to be stretching secondary to abduction of the arm. A recent report did not support this etiology and found no relationship to the position of the arm. The cause of injury was shown to be pressure from the first rib, which may be fractured by wide opening of the sternal retractor. It was also shown in a companion autopsy study that this problem could be reduced significantly by placing the sternal retractor as low as possible. These precautions should decrease the incidence of this troublesome complication.

PHRENIC NERVE INJURY. Complete transection of the phrenic nerve should be avoidable, but injuries due to traction, cold, or electrocautery may be more difficult to avoid consistently. Phrenic trauma due to retraction on the adjacent pericardium is a recognized complication of operations such as systemic-pulmonary shunt, patent ductus ligation, and pulmonary artery banding. Although a recent report indicates only seven such injuries following operations on 1500 patients with congenital cardiac defects, six of these were under 5 months of age so that the age-adjusted incidence was therefore considerably higher.[165] A second series of 1891 procedures performed in children between 1 month and 14 years of age reported an overall incidence of 1.7% with the highest incidence being 7% following Blalock–Taussig shunts.[120] Although minor episodes of direct or indirect operative trauma are the primary cause, phrenic paralysis has been reported following internal jugular vein cannulation, which may explain the occasional paralysis of the contralateral nerve.[183] Operative trauma in small infants undergoing patent ductus ligation may be reduced by utilizing a short lateral thoracotomy and approaching the ductus posteriorly and avoiding proximity to the phrenic nerve. The respiratory deficit following unilateral diaphragmatic paralysis is usually tolerated well in the older child or adult. Infants whose cardiac condition is complicated by varying degrees of respiratory distress may suffer respirator dependence and even death. Transthoracic diaphragmatic plication has been a simple and very effective aid in improving respiratory function in these infants, and most can be extubated within a few days of plication.[165]

During a reoperation, dissection of adhesions may injure one or both phrenic nerves by direct trauma or by the adjunct use of the electrocautery. If the nerve has not been transected, function should return within 1 to 3 months. Following complete unilateral transection, the injury is well tolerated in most patients with stable cardiac function. In the case of bilateral injury, respiratory support is necessary until function returns at least on one side. If permanent phrenic injury is the final result, an implantable nerve stimulator is not an option because neither the distal end of the transected nerve nor the diaphragm can be effectively paced on a chronic basis.[63]

Cold injury to the left phrenic nerve may follow intrapericardial instillation of iced saline utilized for myocardial hypothermia. Prolonged cooling of the dependent pericardium adjacent to the phrenic nerve should be avoided, or attempts should be made to insulate this region by interposition of a pack or a specially designed insulated pad. This cold injury is usually transient with return of function by 6 weeks. In patients with chronic pulmonary disease this complication can be significant enough to require prolonged ventilatory assistance. Minor degrees of cold injury may be a contributing factor to the uncomfortable complication of prolonged postoperative hiccoughs.

RECURRENT LARYNGEAL NERVE INJURY. Injury to the recurrent laryngeal nerve is due to direct trauma in operations on upper mediastinal great vessels. The most common operations associated with this injury are ligation of patent ductus arteriosus, resection of coarctation of the aorta, anastomosis between the subclavian and pulmonary artery, and resection of a thoracic aortic aneurysm. The injury usually is due to traction, and the nerve rarely is completely transected. This should not cause respiratory problems unless there is preexisting severe pulmonary disease or an associated glottic or subglottic abnormality following prolonged intubation. Hoarseness is the primary finding and is disturbing to the patient. This symptom may also be secondary to direct vocal cord trauma related to intubation. Vocal cord paralysis or paresis may be confirmed by laryngoscopy. If the nerve is intact, function should return within several months. Persistent dysfunction after 6 to 9 months may be treated successfully by injection of the affected vocal cord.

INJURY OF CARDIOTHORACIC SYMPATHETIC NERVES. Cardiothoracic sympathetic nerve injury is most often heralded by the appearance of Horner's syndrome. This has been reported following first rib fracture and after excessive opening of the sternal retractor.[182] The most common cause of postoperative Horner's syndrome is injury to the ansa subclavia during performance of a subclavian-pulmonary anastomosis. This nerve should be preserved by removing the transected subclavian artery from the surrounding nerve. This injury produces a temporary Horner's syndrome in almost all instances, but a permanent deficit is rare. The syndrome usually is first recognized by the parents and may be upsetting if it has not been properly anticipated.

PLEURAL AND PERICARDIAL COMPLICATIONS

Pericardial Tamponade

Pericardial tamponade is a well-known entity with classical physical findings and established pathophysiologic mechanisms. When it follows open-heart procedures, its clinical presentation is less clear, but it should be considered in the differential diagnosis in every patient with the low cardiac output syndrome.

INCIDENCE AND CAUSE. Following cardiac surgery, drainage tubes are positioned inside the pericardium, and then the pericardium may or may not be closed. Wide opening of both the mediastinal pleura and the pericardium was thought to provide better postoperative drainage and to lessen the possibility of tamponade. With the recognition that reoperation for a subsequent valve replacement or coronary bypass is facilitated by an intact pericardium, it is now common practice to close the pericardium at the end of the procedure. It has been reported that this policy also reduces the incidence of tamponade and the amount of postoperative bleeding, but this is not completely established.[38] The mediastinal pleura is known to be functionally sealed within several hours in most patients, and mediastinal tamponade may occur even after removal of the pericardium. Early postoperative tamponade within the first few days after surgery was reported to follow as many as 15% of operations but is presently less common.[50, 126] This reduced incidence corresponds to a decrease in the amount of postoperative bleeding over the past few years: most tamponade is seen in patients with increased bleeding. As blood clots accumulate within the pericardium or mediastinum, tamponade may occur with or without a change in the volume of chest tube drainage. This increased mediastinal blood may produce a localized alteration in cardiac performance, depending on the position of the clot, or it may cause a uniform increase in mediastinal pressure with the classical changes in hemodynamics, such as an increase in filling pressures, a decrease in the volume of cardiac filling, a decrease in stroke volume, and a reduction in myocardial contractility.[43, 147, 164]

Late pericardial tamponade more than 1 week postoperatively has been reported to follow from 0.1% to 6% of cardiac operations.[12, 73, 143] Earlier articles indicated the problem primarily to follow valvular operations and to be associated with anticoagulation. A recent review of 1290 adult patients found a 0.8% incidence with the presentation ranging from 15 to 180 days following surgery.[128] In this series there was no association with the type of surgery performed or the use of anticoagulants, but all the patients were noted to have had the postcardiotomy syndrome. A second recent series reported that 28 (4.7%) of 596 adult patients developed a late pericardial effusion, but only 1.3% of these progressed to tamponade.[12]

PREVENTIVE MEASURES. Early tamponade is exceedingly rare in the absence of postoperative bleeding, and measures ranging from hemodilution to effective heparin neutralization have been helpful. Closure of the pericardium may be beneficial and at least has not increased the incidence. Proper positioning and maintenance of patency of drainage tubes should be routine, and the tubes should not be removed until drainage has become negligible. Care in the use of postoperative anticoagulation will decrease, but not eliminate, the occurrence of late cardiac tamponande.

DIAGNOSIS AND MANAGEMENT. Diagnosis may be difficult because the extent of tamponade may vary and may produce localized cardiac compression. A larger mediastinal volume is necessary for tamponade if the pericardium is open. These patients also may have other reasons for compromised cardiac function. A patient with a good initial hemodynamic course following operation who then has excessive bleeding, a widened mediastinal silhouette on x-ray examination, elevated and equalized left and right heart filling pressures, hypotension, paradoxical pulse, and an otherwise unexplained low cardiac output may be obviously diagnosed as having tamponade. The presentation is rarely so straightforward, and most of these classical findings are often absent. Waiting for a definitive diagnosis usually results in a severe reduction in cardiac output, the need for excessive inotropic support, cardiac dysrhythmias, and cardiac arrest. Once the problem of reduced cardiac output has been identified, tamponade should be considered as a primary or contributing cause. With the performance of sequential manipulations to improve the hemodynamic state, the diagnosis becomes more certain as any of the above findings plus an inadequate improvement of cardiac function in response to treatment appear. Proper treatment consists of mediastinal exploration in the operating room with evacuation of blood and clots and control of any bleeding. If done before the end stages, the procedure is safe and is followed by a dramatic improvement in cardiac function. In extreme situations it may be advisable to open the subxiphoid portion of the incision in the recovery room. Under sterile conditions clots may be broken with an inserted finger or suction tip, with effective relief of tamponade.[88] If bleeding continues, the patient should then be returned to the operating room for completion of the procedure. Otherwise, an additional drainage tube may be positioned and the incision reclosed. In the absence of bleeding, this simple exploration may be indicated in the patient with severe low cardiac output, with few if any indications of tamponade, to ensure that occult tamponade has not been overlooked. However, partial tamponade can produce significant cardiovascular compromise when it is added to the effects of postoperative decreased cardiac function, and a recent study presents the additive effects of tamponade and pulmonic insufficiency and speculates that following tetralogy of Fallot repair with resultant pulmonic insufficiency, otherwise minor degrees of tamponade may be life threatening.[121]

If the onset of tamponade occurs over an extended period of time or in the case of late cardiac tamponade, additional diagnostic maneuvers may be helpful. Serial chest x-ray films and echocardiograms will document the widened mediastinum and demonstrate the increase in extracardiac volume. In late tamponade the mediastinal contents are liquefied and diagnosis may be confirmed by pericardiocentesis. In the recent series of such patients, most had pericardial pain and low-grade fever in the period immediately before diagnosis.[128] These patients were treated successfully by pericardiocentesis with only one requiring subsequent pericardial stripping. An alternate simple and effective technique is the insertion of a subxiphoid drainage tube under local anesthesia.[177, 186] In patients with either acute or late cardiac tamponade, the cardinal principle of management is to establish an accurate, early diagnosis, which can then be followed by prompt and effective treatment.

Postpericardiotomy Syndrome

Postpericardiotomy syndrome is important primarily because of its common occurrence and its confusion with postoperative infectious complications.

INCIDENCE AND CAUSE. The postpericardiotomy syndrome (PPS) has been reported in one recent series in only 1.6% of 1290 patients.[128] This is in sharp contrast to the ongoing clinical studies of Engle and coauthors who report an incidence of 17.6% in adults and 27% in children.[51, 52] Forty percent of patients in the latter series were considered mildly afflicted, and differing diagnostic criteria are probably responsible for these divergent incidence reports. The syndrome may follow all operations involving the pericardium and blunt or penetrating chest trauma and is similar to postmyocardial infarction pericarditis.[88] The etiology of this syndrome is not definite, but the two most probable causes are a viral infection and an autoimmune process. Engle has identified heart reactive antibody in all patients with the clinical syndrome and an increase in antiviral antibody titer to one or more of eight viruses tested in 68% of patients. She noted an almost total absence of the syndrome in patients under the age of 2 years and a decreased incidence in patients older than 60 years. She related these observations to immunologic immaturity in the young and protective previous viral exposure in older patients. She concluded that the syndrome is caused by a recent or reactivated viral illness, which triggers an autoimmune response.[51, 52]

PREVENTIVE MEASURES. Early attempts to prevent or limit the syndrome by bedrest have been largely abandoned. It has been suggested that viral exposure can be minimized by limited public contact for 2 weeks prior to elective surgery and by more effective masks for operating-room personnel, but these hypotheses have not been tested.[51] Pericardial closure has also been reported to decrease the incidence of PPS.[38]

DIAGNOSIS AND MANAGEMENT. PPS classically occurs approximately 1 week after surgery but has been reported between the third day and sixth month. PPS presents as fever, malaise, and pericardial pain with a pericardial or pleural friction rub. Laboratory findings include an elevated sedimentation rate, leukocytosis, pleural or pericardial effusions, and electrocardiographic evidence of pericarditis, but all of these findings may be inconsistent. The syndrome is largely self limited and resolves over several weeks. Antibiotics are not indicated, and symptomatic relief usually follows salicylate treatment in mild cases and a short tapering course of steroids in more disabled patients. Reported late complications include recurrence of the syndrome, recurrent effusions requiring drainage, constriction requiring pericardiectomy, and reduced patency of aortocoronary grafts.[116, 150, 180] These complications are infrequent, and evidence has not yet shown that aggressive drug treatment of the initial syndrome will reduce their incidence or severity. Whether the syndrome occurs more often after a repeated operation or whether prophylactic drug treatment is indicated in a patient with a previous severe syndrome undergoing a second operation has not been answered.

A particularly important problem presented by this common syndrome is its differential diagnosis in the evaluation of the febrile postoperative patient. Overzealous diagnosis and treatment with steroids may hamper the proper diagnosis and management of more severe complications ranging from localized infections to prosthetic endocarditis. Unless the diagnosis of PPS is highly probable, observation should be continued for several days before steroids are initiated, or at the least, multiple cultures should be obtained prior to beginning therapy.

The Postperfusion Syndrome

The postperfusion syndrome is mentioned here for completeness although this syndrome is less common than PPS and has received less emphasis in recent years. Postperfusion syndrome follows approximately 5% of cardiac cases involving the use of blood. It is seasonal and most probably viral in origin.[88] With the recent reduction in amount of blood utilized in cardiac operations and the decrease in the use of fresh blood, this syndrome is rarely seen today. The appearance of fever several weeks following surgery followed by atypical lymphocytosis and splenomegaly is diagnostic. Treatment of this benign self-limited condition consists of symptomatic control of fever by salicylates.

Pericardial and Pleural Effusions

Small accumulations of fluid in the pericardium, mediastinum, and pleural cavities are commonly seen following major cardiac operations and usually resolve without treatment if the patient has achieved a satisfactory hemodynamic status. Significant effusions may, however, recur and require specific treatment.

INCIDENCE AND CAUSE. Effusions may be infectious, inflammatory, hemodynamic, or traumatic. Mediastinitis or empyema may first present as increasing fluid accumulation, seen on the chest film, before fever and systemic symptoms appear. Inflammatory pleuropericardial effusions often accompany the postpericardiotomy syndrome. Postoperative heart failure, especially with right-heart dysfunction, is commonly accompanied by pleural effusions. Pulmonary embolism is often associated with a bloody pleural effusion. Following correction of congenital cardiac abnormalities accompanied by elevated right atrial pressure, pleural effusions may be present for weeks to years. This is most common following atriopulmonary shunting for tricuspid atresia. The chronic elevation of atrial pressure is accompanied by an elevation of lymphatic pressure above its usual value of 15 torr and an increase in the formation of pleural fluid. This same hemodynamic cause may explain the recurrent effusions following unresolved tricuspid insufficiency, excision of the tricuspid valve for endocarditis, or stenosis of the superior vena cava after operation for transposition of the great vessels. Chylous effusion of the pleural space or pericardium may follow operative disruption of the thoracic duct or one of its tributaries. This has been reported to occur in approximately 0.5% of operations on the great vessels in the upper mediastinum, including pulmonary systemic anastomosis, coarctation resection, correction of patent ductus arteriosus, and resection of thoracic aortic aneurysm or transections.[112, 141] Chylopericardium is rare but may follow traumatic disruption of the thoracic duct while encircling the vena cava. It has also been caused by thrombosis of the left subclavian and jugular veins by intravascular catheters, with resultant obstruction of thoracic duct flow.[141] Chylous effusion, even if prolonged, is rarely complicated by secondary infection, owing to the poorly understood bactericidal properties of chyle. A rare but confusing cause of continually recurring effusion is perforation of a venous catheter into the pleural cavity, mediastinum, or pericardium with infusion of the intended intravenous solution into these spaces.

PREVENTIVE MEASURES. Prevention is based on a knowledge of these causes, achievement of satisfactory hemodynamic state for the procedure, and recognition of disruption of major lymphatic tributaries. After operations in the superior mediastinum, control of bleeding should be followed by a second inspection for lymphatic fluid. In the fasting state even thoracic duct drainage will be clear and should not be misinterpreted as pericardial fluid. The incidence of chylous effusion secondary to venous thrombosis is not frequent enough to warrant avoiding the left subclavian or jugular routes for venous access when they are needed.

DIAGNOSIS AND MANAGEMENT. Diagnosis of an effusion is usually first made by the chest x-ray film. Confirmation of a pleural effusion is aided by the lateral decubitus film, and mediastinal or pericardial effusion is established by echocardiography. If the initial volume of fluid is large, aspiration or tube drainage is indicated. The fluid should be inspected for the typical milky appearance of chyle, the presence of blood, or the appearance of infection. Specimens should always be submitted for culture and sensitivity, and aliquots may be sent for additional laboratory analysis ranging from lipoprotein content to cytomegalous viral cultures, depending on the clinical circumstances. If the effusion is secondary to inflammation or infection, it will respond to proper treatment of the condition. If the effusion results from hemodynamic alterations, treatment consists of diuretics, digoxin, and afterload reduction. If recurrent effusions are disabling in this setting, cardiac catheterization and a second operation may be necessary, as is seen with superior vena caval obstruction following correction of transposition. After the Fontan procedure, chronic diuretics may be required for a prolonged period of time, although this has been less of a problem with better selection of patients and recent modifications of the techniques of the operation.

Chylous effusion is diagnosed by the typical appearance of the fluid, staining by Sudan III, or the biochemical composition of the fluid. Thoracic duct flow can approach 2 L to 3 L per day and contains 2 g to 6 g of protein per 100 ml. Although drainage of the fluid is the initial treatment, drainage should not be prolonged because serum protein and fat-soluble vitamins become depleted and the immune system depressed.[136] Chyle formation may be reduced and nutrition improved by a low-fat diet, the addition of medium-chain triglycerides, or parenteral nutrition.[94] Recent reports of successful surgical control of the leakage have emphasized the decrease in rates of morbidity and length of hospital stay.[136, 162] Lymphangiography may be helpful in preoperative identification of the location of lymphatic disruption. Surgery may consist of ligation of the fistula if it is accessible or ligation of the thoracic duct below the level of leakage or as it penetrates the diaphragm.[136, 174]

Constrictive Pericarditis

INCIDENCE AND CAUSE. By 1980, only 20 patients had been reported with constrictive pericarditis following cardiac surgery severe enough to require pericardiectomy.[87, 150] This condition, although rare, is undoubtedly under reported because most busy cardiac surgical groups have seen several such patients. Although constriction has been described as a consequence of retained pericardial blood, this etiology is not consistent; most postoperative patients resolve any residual mediastinal blood with no late difficulties. Engle's large experience with postpericardiotomy syndrome has resulted in only one patient with late constriction, in contrast to a recent report of five patients with late constriction, four of whom had postpericardiotomy syndrome after their initial surgery.[51, 52, 150] Irrigation of the pericardium with povidone-iodine has been suggested but not confirmed as a possible cause.[114]

PREVENTIVE MEASURES. There are no maneuvers established to decrease the incidence of this poorly understood but serious complication. If the association with postpericardiotomy syndrome is valid, then early treatment of this syndrome with salicylates or steroids might reduce late constriction. The low incidence of the phenomenon almost prohibits the design of a clinical evaluation of this relationship.

DIAGNOSIS AND MANAGEMENT. Unexplained heart failure in the late period following any cardiac surgery may be due to cardiac constriction. Late cardiac tamponade may be differentiated by echocardiography. Once the diagnosis is considered, cardiac catheterization must be performed to demonstrate the equalization of right- and left-sided filling pressures, the typical contour of the pressure tracings, and also to rule out primary or secondary myocardial dysfunction. Treatment consists of pericardial resection by a median sternotomy. Constricting bands that require localized resection have been encountered, but in most patients the process diffusely involves the visceral and parietal pericardium and requires extensive removal. If the original procedure was a coronary bypass, the location and patency of all grafts and the status of the remaining coronary arteries must be documented before pericardiectomy. Cardiopulmonary bypass may be required to reinfuse blood loss, to facilitate complete pericardial resection, to repair transected grafts, to simultaneously replace occluded grafts or to revascularize new coronary artery occlusions. In the few reported cases, the mortality rate has been low, and the relief of symptoms has been usual. Recurrence of postoperative constrictive pericarditis has not yet been reported.

MYOCARDIAL CONTUSION FOLLOWING CARDIAC TRAUMA

The management of patients with blunt and penetrating injuries of the heart and intrathoracic vessels is extensively described in three recent books.[13, 40, 90] Every structure in the mediastinum has been involved by blunt or penetrating trauma, producing immediate or delayed injury. Thus the major complication of cardiac trauma is primarily the specific damage produced by the injury. Treatment of these disorders ranging from early thoracotomy to replacement of damaged cardiac valves is thoroughly presented by the authors of these books, and this information is essential for the successful management of these critically ill patients. Several secondary complications of trauma are discussed earlier in this chapter, including pericardial tamponade and paraplegia related to aortic transection. Myocardial contusion is a confusing and commonly unrecognized complication of all forms of cardiac trauma, which merits special emphasis.

Incidence and Cause

The incidence of the often overlooked myocardial contusion is proportional to efforts expended to diagnose it. Parmley reviewed 546 fatal instances of nonpenetrating cardiac trauma in which 129 instances of contusion did not produce myocardial rupture.[134] Contusion is associated with other cardiac injuries, and the finding has been reported in three fourths of patients with blunt cardiac trauma.[166] Clinical series indicate an incidence of 25% in patients with nonpenetrating injuries that range from minor blows to the chest to steering-wheel injuries.[90] Myocardial contusion may be caused by any of the established etiologic mechanisms of blunt cardiac trauma, including direct and transmitted blows, compression injuries, deceleration forces, and blast injuries.[79] The resultant injury to the myocardium is due to the forces involved and not to a decrease in coronary flow. Experimental evaluation by Anderson confirmed that the primary process was one of contusion and intramyocardial hemorrhage without disruption of the adjacent coronary vessels.[2] In this model, resorption of hemorrhage occurred by 3 weeks, at which time histologic evidence of fibrosis was documented. The process may therefore be similar to a myocardial infarction in its variable extent and ultimate damage, although the underlying pathologic mechanism is quite different. Delayed rupture of the heart is the ultimate sequel of myocardial contusion, although survival to 7 days is reported in less than 1% of patients with cardiac rupture.[134] The second delayed complication of contusion is late ventricular aneurysm formation. This is an equally unusual occurrence, but both true and false aneurysms requiring resection have been reported.[133, 144]

Diagnosis and Management

The diagnosis of myocardial contusion should be considered in all patients with major or minor chest trauma. In the presence of other major injuries, contusion is difficult to diagnose and may present as nonspecific EKG changes. Changes consistent with a transmural infarction are rare but may evolve over several days. The most common EKG abnormalities are ST and T-wave changes consistent with ischemia, although recurrent atrial and ventricular dysrhythmias and conduction abnormalities have been reported.[79] Reduced cardiac function is not uncommon, and Pomerantz reported a significant reduction in cardiac output in the majority of patients with myocardial contusion.[142] The clinical findings of reduced output may be masked by other injuries and by the occurrence of varying degrees of right or left ventricular dysfunction. Noninvasive evaluation of these patients by two-dimensional echocardiography or myocardial imaging is currently recommended.[65] These tests are most helpful in patients with other major injuries and should be performed on all patients with chest trauma severe enough to require hospitalization. Serum enzyme determinations have not been helpful owing to the associated soft tissue damage. Diagnosis of myocardial contusion is therefore based on a high suspicion followed by serial noninvasive testing in the patient with EKG changes or unexplained changes in cardiac function. Management is similar to that for a patient with a myocardial infarction with the same expected time course and similar immediate and late complications. Anesthetic and surgical risks are increased in these patients, and if surgery is indicated, the patient may require invasive monitoring and support of depressed myocardial function.

COMPLICATIONS OF REPEAT CARDIAC OPERATION

Incidence and Cause

Several factors combine to influence the incidence of repeated cardiac operations. The improved results following single-stage correction of congenital defects during infancy has decreased the need for a second operation. Patients requiring valve replacement are undergoing surgery at an earlier time in their functional course and hence at a younger age and with a myocardial reserve consistent with a longer rate of survival. These policies plus the acknowledged limited longevity of tissue valves and the ever present possibility of mechanical valve dysfunction have significantly increased the number of repeated valve replacements performed in recent years. Coronary bypass surgery is now in its second decade and the 10-year reoperation rate is approaching 10%, in spite of more complete revascularization and improved graft patency.[101] Thus the total number of repeated operations will inevitably increase during this decade. The two major technical problems during elective second operations are injury to the underlying heart while reopening the sternum and trauma to the heart, great vessels, or adjacent mediastinal structures during dissection of mediastinal and pericardial adhesions.

Preventive Measures

Early recommendations for maneuvers during the initial operation designed to minimize these subsequent difficulties are now being offered, but the results of these attempts are not yet established. Approximation of tissue behind the sternum should prevent adherence of the right ventricle, aorta, coronary graft, or prosthetic conduit to the back of the sternum and allow safer reopening. This may be accomplished by closure of the pericardium, approximation of thymic and mediastinal tissue, or the interposition of autologous or prosthetic material as an anterior pericardial substitute.[38, 92, 95] Following coronary bypass grafting or positioning of a graft or conduit, distortion of these structures must be avoided by a loose closure, adequate amount of interposed material or the use of a lateral pericardial relaxing incision.[118] Although these techniques may be helpful during a repeated sternotomy, they do not decrease intrapericardial adhesion formation. It has been claimed that closure of the pericardium decreases the incidence of the postpericardiotomy syndrome, but the relationship between this syndrome and late adhesions is unknown.[38] Virtually no information exists on safe and practical methods of decreasing mediastinal and pericardial adhesions. The finding of dense adhesions following a simple initial procedure is as unexplained as is the almost total absence of adhesions in a patient with prior excessive bleeding or severe postpericardiotomy syndrome.

Diagnosis and Management

Diagnosis of major cardiac injury during sternal opening is obvious and is usually manifested by hemorrhage. Transection of a patent and essential coronary bypass graft adherent to the posterior sternum may cause severe myocardial ischemia or even cardiac arrest. It is therefore advisable to expose the femoral artery prior to sternotomy for inflow perfusion in case rapid institution of cardiopulmonary bypass is necessary. Technical maneuvers found beneficial in reoperation have been described and are only summarized briefly.[104, 110, 145, 171] If the retrosternal space is free, a reciprocating saw is safe, but, if not, the oscillating saw may be helpful. Each side of the sternum is dissected freely along the posterior periosteum with electrocautery prior to inserting and opening the sternal retractor. The extent of adhesions and the nature of the repeated operation determine whether the heart is completely or partially freed. This dissection may be safer after beginning bypass or even after the heart is cold and relaxed. Lateral dissection toward the lungs or phrenic nerves should be as limited as possible. Complete mobility of the heart is preferred for repeated coronary operations but may be an unnecessary hazard in situations such as replacement of an outflow tract conduit. If only minimal exposure is required, sufficient myocardium should be exposed for effective and safe defibrillation. The actual performance of the repeated operation is usually no more difficult than is the initial procedure. Following the procedure, diffuse bleeding may occur from the multiple areas of dissection. Average blood loss is usually higher after reoperation although this has been improved with blood-conservation techniques.[33] Loop has reported excellent results in 500 patients undergoing repeat coronary bypass surgery with a 4% mortality rate, effective relief of symptoms, and an 89% 5-year survival rate.[102] Parr has reported equally good results following re-replacement of the aortic valve, with a 3.7% mortality rate in 81 elective patients.[135]

The Changing Spectrum of Late Postoperative Complications

This chapter focused on the major complications of cardiac surgery that are encountered during the perioperative period, emphasizing the principles involved in their management. An equally important subject is the recognition and treatment of late postoperative complications. The long-term evaluation of patients who have undergone cardiac surgery is a continuing responsibility of cardiologists and cardiac surgeons. With the exception of defects such as patent ductus arteriosus and secundum atrial septal defect, surgical treatment of congenital, valvular, and coronary artery lesions should not be considered curative but rather corrective, or even palliative. Patients may more appropriately be considered to have exchanged one disease for another, as with the conversion of rheumatic heart disease to prosthetic heart disease. This is anticipated to improve survival and functional status but usually commits the patient to life-long follow-up. Computer technology has made the storage, retrieval, and evaluation of descriptors of chronic disease feasible, and this approach has aided in documentation of known complications and identification of previously unrecognized complications. This information is especially important when the success of cardiac surgery is no longer determined by survival, but by a technically complete operation producing late functional improvement.

Late problems that were not completely anticipated are now recognized after almost all cardiac procedures. Residual hypertension has been identified with increasing frequency following elective resection of coarctation. Both ventricular dysfunction and late dysrhythmias are seen after repair of tetralogy of Fallot, and their incidence and significance are currently influencing recommendations for single- *versus* multiple-stage repair, the proper age for repair, and the effects of pulmonary insufficiency. The late complications of ventricular dysfunction, dysrhythmias, and baffle obstruction have been recognized and reduced following the atrial repair of transposition, but the complications following arterial repair await clarification. The long-term significance of chronic venous hypertension following repair of tricuspid atresia is now being evaluated.

The continuing design changes in both mechanical and tissue valves are a response to late evaluations of thromboembolism, durability, and hemodynamic function. The unexpected finding of early calcific degeneration of tissue valves in children is a recent unsolved problem. The late functional effects of myocardial ischemia induced during coronary bypass surgery are not adequately documented, nor is the influence of current myocardial preservation techniques on this problem completely established. The proper role of complete revascularization, including grafting of coronary arteries with 25% to 50% occlusions, in the treatment of a chronic disease process is a subject presently being debated.

References

1. Amoury RA, Bowman FO Jr, Malm JR: Endocarditis associated with intracardiac prostheses. J Thorac Cardiovasc Surg 51:36, 1066
2. Anderson AE, Doty DB: Cardiac trauma: An experimental model of isolated myocardial contusion. J Trauma 15:237, 1975
3. Ankeney JL, Parker RF: Staphylococcal endocarditis following open-heart surgery related to positive intraoperative blood cultures. In Brewer LA III (ed): Prosthetic Heart Valves, pp 719-730. Springfield, IL, Charles C Thomas, 1969
4. Arnett EN, Roberts WC: Prosthetic valve endocarditis. Am J Cardiol 38:281, 1976
5. Balderman SC, Bhayana JN, Steinbach JT et al: Perioperative myocardial infarction: A diagnostic dilemma. Ann Thorac Surg 30:370, 1980
6. Baur HR, Peterson TA, Arnar O et al: Predictors of perioperative myocardial infarction in coronary artery operation. Ann Thorac Surg 31:36, 1981
7. Behrendt DM, Austen WG: Patient Care in Cardiac Surgery, 3rd ed. Boston, Little, Brown & Co, 1980
8. Berger RL, Davis KB, Kaiser GC et al: Preservation of the myocardium during coronary artery bypass grafting. Circulation (Suppl II) 64:61, 1981
9. Blakemore WS, McGarrity GJ, Thurer RJ et al: Infection by air-borne bacteria with cardiopulmonary bypass. Surgery 70:830, 1971
10. Bolooki H, Thuren R, Vargas A et al: Intra-aortic balloon pumping for heart failure in cardiac surgery. Circulation (Suppl II) 52:162, 1975
11. Bonchek LI, Rahimtoola SH, Chaitman BR et al: Vein graft occlusion: Immediate and late consequences and therapeutic implications. Circulation (Suppl II) 49,50:84, 1974
12. Borkon AM, Schaff HV, Gardner TJ et al: Diagnosis and management of postoperative pericardial effusions and late cardiac tamponade following open-heart surgery. Ann Thorac Surg 31:512, 1981
13. Borrie J: Management of Thoracic Emergencies, 3rd ed. New York, Appleton-Century-Crofts, 1980
14. Branthwaite MA: Prevention of neurological damage during open-heart surgery. Thorax 30:285, 1975
15. Brewer LA III, Fosburg RG, Mulder GA et al: Spinal cord complications following surgery for coarctation of the aorta. J Thorac Cardiovasc Surg 50:166, 1972
16. Buckberg GD, Towers B, Paglia DE et al: Subendocardial ischemia after cardiopulmonary bypass. J Thorac Cardiovasc Surg 64:669, 1972
17. Buckley MJ, Craver JM, Gold HK et al: Intra-aortic balloon pump assist for cardiogenic shock after cardiopulmonary bypass. Circulation (Suppl III) 47:90, 1973
18. Buxton AE, Josephson ME: The role of P wave duration as a predictor of postoperative atrial arrhythmias. Chest 80:68, 1981
19. Cacace L: Sinus standstill from lidocaine. JAMA 224:1428, 1973
20. Calvin JE, Driedger AA, Sibbald WJ: The hemodynamic effect of rapid fluid infusion in critically ill patients. Surgery 90:61, 1981
21. Camm J, Ward D, Spurrell R: Response of atrial flutter to overdrive atrial pacing and intravenous disopyramide phosphate, singly or in combination. Br Heart J 44:240, 1980
22. Cannom DS, Miller DC, Shumway NE et al: The long-term follow-up of patients undergoing saphenous vein bypass surgery. Circulation 49:77, 1974
23. Chatterjee K, Parmley W: The role of vasodilator therapy in heart failure. Prog Cardiovasc Dis 19:301, 1977
24. Clarkson PM, MacArthur BA, Barrate–Boyes BG et al: Developmental progress after cardiac surgery in infancy using hypothermia and circulatory arrest. Circulation 62:855, 1980
25. Codd JE, Wiens RD, Kaiser GC et al: Late sequelae of perioperative myocardial infarction. Ann Thorac Surg 26:208, 1978
26. Come PC, Pitt B: Nitroglycerin-induced severe hypotension and bradycardia in patients with acute myocardial infarction. Circulation 54:624, 1976
27. Committee on Prevention of Rheumatic Fever and Bacterial Endocarditis of the American Heart Association.

Prevention of bacterial endocarditis. Circulation 56:139A, 1977
28. Cooley DA, Romagnoli A, Milam JD et al: A method of preparing woven Dacron aortic grafts to prevent interstitial hemorrhage. Bulletin of the Texas Heart Institute. Cardiovascular Diseases 8:48, 1981
29. Cooper GN, Singh AK, Christian FC: Preoperative intraaortic balloon pump support in surgery for left main coronary stenosis. Ann Surg 185:242, 1977
30. Coppe D, Sobel M, Seamans L et al: Preservation of platelet function and number by prostacyclin during cardiopulmonary bypass. J Thorac Cardiovasc Surg 81:274, 1981
31. Cordell AR, Ellison RG: Complications of Intrathoracic Surgery. Boston, Little, Brown & Co, 1979
32. Cordell AR, Lavender SW: An appraisal of blood salvage techniques in vascular and cardiac operations. Ann Thorac Surg 31:421, 1981
33. Cosgrove DM et al: Blood conservation during myocardial revascularization. Ann Thorac Surg 28:184, 1979
34. Cox JL: The surgical management of cardiac arrhythmias. In Gibbon's Surgery of the Chest. Philadelphia, WB Saunders (in press)
35. Crawford ES, Saleh SA: Transverse aortic arch aneurysm. Ann Surg 194:180, 1981
36. Csicsko JF, Schatzlein MH, King RD: Immediate postoperative digitalization in the prophylaxis of supraventricular arrhythmias following coronary artery bypass. J Thorac Cardiovasc Surg 81:419, 1981
37. Culliford AT, Gitel SN, Starr N et al: Lack of correlation between activated clotting time and plasma heparin during cardiopulmonary bypass. Ann Surg 193:105, 1981
38. Cunningham JN, Spencer FC, Zeff JR et al: Influence of primary closure of the pericardium after open-heart surgery on the frequency of tamponade, postcardiotomy syndrome, and pulmonary complications. J Thorac Cardiovasc Surg 70:119, 1975
39. Curtis JJ, Madigan NP, Whiting RB et al: Clinical experience with permanent atrioventricular sequential pacing. Ann Thorac Surg 32:180, 1981
40. Daughtry DC: Thoracic Trauma. Boston, Little, Brown & Co, 1980
41. Deanfield JE, McKenna WJ, Hallidie–Smith KA: Detection of late arrhythmia and conduction disturbance after correction of tetralogy of Fallot. Br Heart J 44:248, 1980
42. DeBakey MD: Commentary on an update of treatment of aneurysms of the descending thoracic aorta by Najafi. World J Surg 4:553, 1980
43. DeCristofaro D, Kiu CK: The haemodynamics of cardiac tamponade and blood volume overload in dogs. Cardiovasc Res 3:292, 1969
44. Digerness SB, Vanini V, Wideman FE: In vitro comparison of oxygen availability from asanguinous and sanguinous cardioplegic media. Circulation (Suppl II) 64:80, 1981
45. Dismukes WE: Who needs endocarditis prophylaxis. J Cardiovasc Med 6:347, 1981
46. Downing TP, Miller DC, Stinson EB et al: Therapeutic efficacy of intraaortic balloon pump counterpulsation. Analysis with concurrent "control" subjects. Circulation (Suppl II) 64:108, 1981
47. Ellis RJ, Mangano D, Vandyke D et al: Protection of myocardial function not enhanced by high concentrations of potassium during cardioplegic arrest. J Thorac Cardiovasc Surg 78:698, 1979
48. Ellis RJ, Mavroudis C, Gardner C et al: Relationship between atrioventricular arrhythmias and the concentration of K^+ ion in cardioplegic solution. J Thorac Cardiovasc Surg 80:517, 1980
49. Ellis RJ, Wisniewski A, Potts R et al: Reduction of flow rate and arterial pressure at moderate hypothermia does not result in cerebral dysfunction. J Thorac Cardiovasc Surg 79:173, 1980
50. Engelman RM, Spencer FC, Reed GE, Tice DA: Cardiac tamponade following open-heart surgery. Circulation (Suppl II) 41:165, 1970
51. Engle MA, Gay WA, McCabe J et al: Postpericardiotomy syndrome in adults: Incidence, autoimmunity and virology. Circulation (Suppl II) 64:58, 1981
52. Engle MA, Zabriskie JB, Senterfit LB et al: Viral illness and the postpericardiotomy syndrome. A prospective study in children. Circulation 62:1151, 1980
53. Fairman RM, Edmunds LH Jr: Emergency thoracotomy in the surgical intensive care unit after open cardiac surgery. Presented at the 17th Annual Meeting of the Society of Thoracic Surgeons, January, 1981
54. Finland M: Current problems in infective endocarditis. Mod Concepts Cardiovasc Dis. 41:53, 1972
55. Flemma RJ, Torpy SD: Complications of aortocoronary bypass grafting. In Complications of Intrathoracic Surgery. Boston, Little, Brown & Co, 1979
56. Freeman R, Hjersing N, Burridge A: Catheter tip cultures on open-heart surgery patients: Associations with site of catheter and age of patients. Thorax 36:355, 1981
57. Gallagher JJ, Cox JL: Status of surgery for ventricular arrhythmias. Circulation 60:1440, 1979
58. Gangahar DM, McGough EC, Synhorst D: Secondary sternal closure: A method of preventing cardiac compression. Ann Thorac Surg 31:282, 1981
59. Gardner P, Saffle JR, Schoenbaum SC: Infections of Prosthetic Heart Valves and Vascular Grafts. Baltimore, University Park Press, 1977
60. Garson A, Gillette PC, Gutgesell HP, McNamara DG: Stress-induced ventricular arrhythmia after repair of tetralogy of Fallot. Am J Cardiol 46:1006, 1980
61. Gay WA Jr, Ebert PA: Functional, metabolic, and morphologic effects of potassium-induced cardioplegia. Surgery 74:284, 1973
62. Gielchinsky I, Silidker M, Krishnan B, Parsonnet V: Secondary sternal closure following open heart surgery. Presented at the 17th Annual Meeting of the Society of Thoracic Surgeons, January, 1981
63. Glenn WWL: Discussion of clinical implications of postoperative unilateral phrenic nerve paralysis by Mickell. J Thorac Cardiovasc Surg 76:303, 1978
64. Glynn MFX, Gay WA: A technique for pre-clotting vascular grafts. Ann Thorac Surg 29:182, 1980
65. Go RT, Doty DB, Chiu CI, Christie JH: New method of diagnosing myocardial contusion in man by radionuclide imaging. Radiology 116:110, 1975
66. Grant JP: Handbook of Total Parenteral Nutrition. Philadelphia, WB Saunders, 1980
67. Griepp RB, Stinson EB, Hollingsworth JF, Beuhler D: Prosthetic replacement of the aortic arch. J Thorac Cardiovasc Surg 70:1051, 1975
68. Haka–Ikse K, Blackwood JA, Steward DJ: Psychomotor development of infants and children after profound hypothermia during surgery for congenital heart disease. Dev Med Child Neurol 20:62, 1978
69. Harvey JC, Goldstein JE, McCabe JC et al: Complications of percutaneous intraaortic balloon pumping. Circulation (Suppl II) 64:114, 1981

70. Hearse DJ, O'Brien K, Braimbridge MV: Protection of the myocardium during ischemic arrest. J Thorac Cardiovasc Surg 81:873, 1981
71. Hertzer NR, Loop FD, Taylor PC, Beven EG: Staged and combined surgical approach to simultaneous carotid and coronary vascular disease. Surgery 84:803, 1978
72. Hill NS, Antman EM, Green LH, Alpert JS: Intravenous nitroglycerin. A review of pharmacology, indications, therapeutic effects and complications. Chest 79:69, 1981
73. Hill JD, Johnson DC, Miller GE et al: Latent mediastinal tamponade after open-heart surgery. Arch Surg 99:808, 1969
74. Hilton JD, Weisel RD, Baird RJ et al: The hemodynamic and metabolic response to pacing after aortocoronary bypass. Circulation (Suppl II) 64:48, 1981
75. Howe WR, Goodrich JK, Bruno FP et al: Technetium-99m pyrophosphate detection of perioperative myocardial infarction in cardiac surgery patients (abstr). J Nucl Med 17(6):524, 1976
76. Hughes RK, Reemtsma K: Correction of coarctation of the aorta. Manometric determination of safety during test occlusion. J Thorac Cardiovasc Surg 62:31, 1971
77. Hultgren HN, Shettigar UR, Pfeifer JF et al: Acute myocardial infarction and ischemic injury during surgery for coronary artery disease. Am Heart J 94:146, 1977
78. Ilabaca PA, Ochsner JL, Mill NL: Positive end-expiratory pressure in the management of the patient with a postoperative bleeding heart. Ann Surg 30:281, 1980
79. Jackson DH, Murphy GW: Nonpenetrating cardiac trauma. Mod Concepts Cardiovasc Dis 45:123, 1976
80. Jarvik RK, Smith LM, Lawson JH et al: Comparison of pneumatic and electrically powered total artificial heart in vivo. Transactions of the American Society of Artificial Internal Organs 24:593, 1978
81. Jobes DR, Schwartz AJ, Ellison N et al: Monitoring heparin anticoagulation and its neutralization. Ann Thorac Surg 31:161, 1981
82. Johnson WD Jr: Prosthetic valve endocarditis. In Infective Endocarditis, Chap 9. Baltimore, University Park Press, 1976
83. Jurkiewicz MJ, Bostwick J, Hester R et al: Infected median sternotomy wound. Successful treatment by muscle flaps. Ann Surg 191:738, 1980
84. Kanter KR, Flaherty JT, Bulkley BH et al: Beneficial effects of adding propranolol to multidose potassium cardioplegia. Circulation (Suppl II) 64:84, 1981
85. Kaplan EL, Rich H, Gersony W, Manning J: A collaborative study of infective endocarditis in the 1970's. Circulation 59:327, 1979
86. Katz NM, Blackstone EH, Kirklin JW, Karp RB: Incremental risk factors for spinal cord injury following operation for acute traumatic aortic transection. J Thorac Cardiovasc Surg 81:669, 1981
87. Kendall ME, Rhodes GR, Wolfe W: Cardiac constriction following aorta to coronary bypass surgery. J Thorac Cardiovasc Surg 65:142, 1972
88. Kirsh MM, McIntosh K, Kahn DR et al: Postpericardiotomy syndromes. Ann Thorac Surg 9:158, 1970
89. Kirsh MM, Magee KR, Gagot O et al: Brachial plexus injury following median sternotomy incision. Ann Thorac Surg 11:315, 1971
90. Kirsh MM, Sloan H: Closed injuries of the heart and pericardium. In Blunt Chest Trauma, Chap 7. Boston, Little, Brown & Co, 1977
91. Kloster FE: Infective prosthetic valve endocarditis. In Infective Endocarditis, Chap 8. New York, Grune & Stratton, 1978
92. Kohanna FH, Adams PX, Cunningham JN, Spencer FC: Use of autologous fascia lata as a pericardial substitute following open-heart surgery. J Thorac Cardiovasc Surg 74:14, 1977
93. Kolkka R, Hilberman M: Neurologic dysfunction following cardiac operation with low flow, low pressure cardiopulmonary bypass. J Thorac Cardiovasc Surg 79:432, 1980
94. Kosloske AM, Martin LW, Schubert WK: Management of chylothorax in children by thoracentesis and medium-chain triglyceride feedings. J Pediatr Surg 9:365, 1974
95. Laks H, Hammon G, Geha A: Use of silicone rubber as a pericardial substitute to facilitate reoperation in cardiac surgery. J Thorac Cardiovasc Surg 82:88, 1981
96. Laskowski LF, Marr JJ, Spernoga JF et al: Fastidious mycobacteria grown from porcine prosthetic heart valve cultures. N Engl J Med 297:101, 1977
97. Lazar HL, Buckberg GD, Foglia RP et al: Detrimental effects of premature use of inotropic drugs to discontinue cardiopulmonary bypass. J Thorac Surg 82:18, 1981
98. Lee WH Jr, Brady MP, Rowe JM et al: Effects of extracorporeal circulation upon behavior, personality, and brain function. Part II. Hemodynamic, metabolic, and psychometric correlations. Ann Surg 173:1013, 1971
99. Lim JS et al: Perioperative myocardial infarction related to coronary bypass surgery. Am Heart J 96:463, 1978
100. Litwak RS, Kuhn LA, Gadboys HL et al: Support of myocardial performance after open cardiac operation by rate augmentation. J Thorac Cardiovasc Surg 56:484, 1968
101. Loop FD: Editorial. On reoperations. Ann Thorac Surg 32:4, 1981
102. Loop FD, Cosgrove DM, Kramer JR et al: Late clinical and arteriographic results in 500 coronary artery reoperations. J Thorac Cardiovasc Surg 81:675, 1981
103. Loop FD, Cosgrove DM, Lytle BW et al: An 11 year evolution of coronary arterial surgery (1967–1978). Ann Surg 190:444, 1979
104. Loop FD, Thurer RL, Lytle BW, Cosgrove DM: Reoperation for myocardial revascularization. World J Surg 2:719, 1978
105. Luce JM, Cary JM, Ross BK et al: New developments in cardiopulmonary resuscitation. JAMA 244:1366, 1980
106. McCabe JC, Abel RM, Subramanian VA, Gay WA Jr: Complications of intra-aortic balloon insertion and counterpulsation. Circulation 57:769, 1978
107. McGee MG, Zillgitt SL, Trono R et al: Retrospective analyses of the need for mechanical circulatory support (intraaortic balloon pump/abdominal left ventricular assist device or partial artificial heart) after cardiopulmonary bypass. Am J Cardiol 46:135, 1980
108. McGoon DC, Ellis FJ Jr, Kirklin JW: Late results of operation for acquired aortic valvular disease. Circulation 31:1, 1965
109. McIntosh HD, Garcia JA: The first decade of aortocoronary bypass grafting, 1967–1977. Circulation 57:405, 1978
110. Macmanus Q, Okies E, Philipps SJ, Starr A: Surgical considerations in patients undergoing repeat median sternotomy. J Thorac Cardiovasc Surg 69:138, 1975
111. Magovern GJ, Dixon CM, Burkholder JA: Improved myocardial protection with nifedipine and potassium-based cardioplegia. J Thorac Cardiovasc Surg 82:239, 1981
112. Maloney JV Jr, Spencer FC: The nonoperative treatment of traumatic chylothorax. Surgery 40:121, 1956
113. Mangano DT, Van Dyke DC, Ellis RJ: The effect of increasing preload on ventricular output and ejection in man. Circulation 62:535, 1980

114. Marsa R, Mehta S, Willis W, Bailey L: Constrictive pericarditis after myocardial revascularization. Am J Cardiol 44:177, 1979
115. Masur H, Johnson WD Jr: Prosthetic valve endocarditis. J Thorac Cardiovasc Surg 80:31, 1980
116. McCabe JC et al: Chronic pericardial effusion requiring pericardiectomy in the postopericardiotomy syndrome. J Thorac Cardiovasc Surg 67:814, 1974
117. Mehigan JT, Buch WS, Pipkin RD, Fogarty TJ: A planned approach to coexistent cerebrovascular disease in coronary artery bypass candidates. Arch Surg 112:1403, 1977
118. Merav AD, Brodman R, Attai LA, Robinson G: A simple technique for tension-free pericardial closure. Ann Thorac Surg 28:399, 1979
119. Michel L, Marsh HM, McMichan JC et al: Infection of pulmonary artery catheters in critically ill patients. JAMA 245:1032, 1981
120. Mickell JJ, Oh KS, Siewers RD et al: Clinical improvement of postoperative unilateral phrenic nerve paralysis. J Thorac Cardiovasc Surg 76:297, 1978
121. Milo S, Salem G, David I et al: Pericardial tamponade and its effect on cardiac performance in absence of the pulmonic valve. J Thorac Cardiovasc Surg 81:787, 1981
122. Miller CD, Stinson EB, Oyer PE et al: Postoperative enhancement of left ventricular performance by combined inotropic-vasodilator therapy with preload control. Surgery 88:108, 1980
123. Morrison J, Killip T: Serum digitalis and arrhythmias in patients undergoing cardiopulmonary bypass. Circulation 47:341, 1973
124. Moseley PW, Oshsner JL, Mills NL, Chapman J: Management of an infected Hancock prosthesis after repair of truncus arteriosus. J Thorac Cardiovasc Surg 73:306, 1977
125. Najafi H, Javid H, Hunter JA et al: An update of treatment of aneurysms of the descending thoracic aorta. World J Surg 4:553, 1980
126. Nelson RM, Jenson CB, Smoot WM III: Pericardial tamponade following open-heart surgery. J Thorac Cardiovasc Surg 58:510, 1969
127. Oakes DD, Wilmot CB, Halverson D, Hamilton RD: Neurogenic respiratory failure: A 5-year experience using implantable phrenic nerve stimulators. Ann Thorac Surg 30:118, 1980
128. Ofori–Krakye S, Tybert TI, Geha AS et al: Late cardiac tamponade after open heart surgery: Incidence, role of anticoagulants in its pathogenesis and its relationship to the postpericardiotomy syndrome. Circulation 63:1323, 1981
129. Okies JE, MacManus Q, Starr A: Myocardial revascularization and carotid endarterectomy: A combined approach. Ann Thorac Surg 23:560, 1977
130. Oldham HN Jr: Surgical interventions for sudden cardiac death. In Electrophysiological Mechanisms Underlying Sudden Cardiac Death, Chap 19. Mt. Kisko, Futura Publishing, 1982
131. Oldham HN Jr: Cardiopulmonary arrest and resuscitation. In Gibbon's Surgery of the Chest. Philadelphia, WB Saunders (in press)
132. Oldham HN Jr, Vasko JS, Brawley RK et al: The hemodynamic effects of atrial fibrillation. J Surg Res 7:587, 1967
133. O'Reilly RJ, Kazenelson G, Spellberg RD: Traumatic pseudo-aneurysm of the left ventricle. Am J Dis Child 120:252, 1970
134. Parmley LF, Manion WC, Mattingly TW: Nonpenetrating traumatic injury of the heart. Circulation 18:371, 1958
135. Parr GVS, Kirklin JW, Blackstone EH: The early risk of re-replacement of aortic valves. Ann Thorac Surg 23:319, 1977
136. Patterson GA, Todd TRJ, Delarue NC et al: Supradiaphragmatic ligation of the thoracic duct in intractable chylous fistula. Ann Thorac Surg 32:44, 1981
137. Petheram IS, Boyce JMH: Prosthetic valve endocarditis: A review of 24 cases. Thorax 32:478, 1977
138. Phillips PA, Marty AT, Miyamoto AM: A clinical method for detecting subendocardial ischemia after cardiopulmonary bypass. J Thorac Cardiovasc Surg 69:30, 1975
139. Pierce WS, Myers JL Donachy JH et al: Approaches to the artificial heart. Surgery 90:137, 1981
140. Pifarre R, Babka R, Sullivan HJ et al: Management of postoperative heparin rebound following cardiopulmonary bypass. J Thorac Cardiovasc Surg 81:378, 1981
141. Pollard WM, Schuchmann GF, Bowen TE: Isolated chylopericardium after cardiac operations. J Thorac Cardiovasc Surg 81:943, 1981
142. Pomerantz M, Delgado F, Eiseman B: Unsuspected depressed cardiac output following blunt thoracic or abdominal trauma. Surgery 70:865, 1971
143. Prewitt TA, Rackley CE, Wilcox BR et al: Cardiac tamponade as a late complication of open heart surgery. Am Heart J 76:139, 1968
144. Pupello DF, Daily PO, Stinson EB, Shumway NE: Successful repair of left ventricular aneurysms due to trauma. JAMA 211:826, 1970
145. Qazi A, Garcia JM, Mispireta LA, Corso PJ: Reoperation for coronary artery disease. Ann Thorac Surg 32:16, 1981
146. Radegran K, Papaconsantinou C: Prostacyclin infusion during cardiopulmonary bypass—Clinical experiences. Presented at the 61st Annual Meeting of the American Association for Thoracic Surgery, May, 1981
147. Reddy PS, Curtiss EI, O'Toole JD, Shaver JA: Cardiac tamponade: Hemodynamic observations in man. Circulation 58:266, 1978
148. Reemtsma K, Drusin R, Bregman ER et al: Cardiac transplantation for patients requiring mechanical circulatory support. N Engl J Med 238:680, 1978
149. Reitz BA, Stinson EB, Watson DC et al: Translocation of the aortic valve for prosthetic valve endocarditis. J Thorac Cardiovasc Surg 81:212, 1981
150. Rice PL, Pifarre R, Montoya A: Constrictive pericarditis following cardiac surgery. Ann Thorac Surg 31:450, 1981
151. Richardson JV, Karp RB, Kirkin JW, Dismukes WE: Treatment of infective endocarditis: A 10-year comparative analysis. Circulation 58:589, 1978
152. Roberts AJ, Hoover EL, Alonso DR et al: Prolonged intraaortic balloon pumping in Klebsiella-induced hypodynamic shock: Cardiopulmonary, hematologic, metabolic, and pathologic observations. Ann Thorac Surg 128:73, 1979
153. Roberts AJ, Sanders JH Jr, Moran JM et al: Nonrandomized matched pair analysis of intermittent ischemia arrest versus potassium crystalloid cardioplegia during myocardial revascularization. Ann Thorac Surg 31:502, 1981
154. Robicsek F, Daugherty HK, Cook JW: The prevention and treatment of sternum separation following open-heart surgery. J Thorac Cardiovasc Surg 73:267, 1977
155. Robicsek F, Daughertry HK, Cook JW et al: Mycobacterium fortuitum epidemics after open-heart surgery. J Thorac Cardiovasc Surg 75:91, 1978
156. Robicsek F, Masters TN, Littman L, Born GVR: The embolization of bone wax from sternotomy incisions. Ann Thorac Surg 31:357, 1981

157. Roe BB: Perioperative Management in Cardiothoracic Surgery. Boston, Little, Brown & Co, 1981
158. Roffman JA, Fieldman A: Digoxin and propranolol in the prophylaxis of supraventricular tachydysrhythmias after coronary artery bypass surgery. Ann Thorac Surg 31:496, 1981
159. Rousou JH, Engelman RM, Dobbs WA, Lemeshow S: The optimal potassium concentration in cardioplegic solutions. Ann Thorac Surg 32:75, 1981
160. Sealy WC: Complications following repair of coarctation of the aorta. In Complications of Intrathoracic Surgery, Chap 21. Boston, Little, Brown & Co, 1979
161. Sealy WC, Wallace AJ, Ramming KP et al: An improved operation for the definitive treatment of the Wolff–Parkinson–White syndrome. Ann Thorac Surg 17:107, 1974
162. Selle JG, Snyder WH III, Schreiber JT: Chylothorax: Indications for surgery. Ann Surg 177:245 1973
163. Serry C, Bleck PC, Javid H et al: Sternal wound complications. Management and results. J Thorac Cardiovasc Surg 80:861, 1980
164. Shabetai R, Meney E: Proceedings: Haemodynamics of cardiac restriction and tamponade. Br Heart J 37:780, 1975
165. Shoemaker R, Palmer G, Brown JW, King H: Aggressive treatment of acquired phrenic nerve paralysis in infants and small children. Presented at the 17th Meeting of the Society of Thoracic Surgeons, January, 1981
166. Sigler LH: Traumatic injury of the heart. Am Heart J 30:459, 1945
167. Sink JD, Pellom GL, Currie WD et al: Response of hypertrophied myocardium to ischemia. J Thorac Cardiovasc Surg 81:865, 1981
168. Skinner NS Jr, Mitchell JH, Wallace AG, Sarnoff SJ: Hemodynamic consequences of atrial flutter at constant ventricular rates. Am J Med 36:342, 1964
169. Spencer FC: The significance of myocardial preservation and subclinical myocardial infarction following coronary bypass. Ann Thorac Surg 26:197, 1978
170. Stephenson LW, Edmunds LH Jr, Raphaely R et al: Effects of nitroprusside and dopamine on pulmonary arterial vasculature in children after cardiac surgery. Circulation (Suppl I) 60:104, 1979
171. Stiles QR, Lindesmith GG, Tucker BL et al: Experience with fifty repeat procedures for myocardial revascularization. J Thorac Cardiovasc Surg 72:849, 1976
172. Stockard JJ et al: Pressure-dependent cerebral ischemia during cardiopulmonary bypass. Neurology 23:521, 1973
173. Stockard JJ et al: Hypotension induced changes in cerebral function during cardiac surgery. Stroke 5:730, 1974
174. Strausser JL, Flye MW: Management of nontraumatic chylothorax. Ann Thorac Surg 31:520, 1981
175. Strum JT, Fuhrman TM, Sterling R et al: Combined use of dopamine and nitroprusside therapy in conjunction with intra-aortic balloon pumping for the treatment of postcardiotomy low-output syndrome. J Thorac Cardiovasc Surg 82:13, 1981
176. Strum JT, McGee MG, Fuhrman TM et al: Treatment of postoperative low output syndrome with intra-aortic balloon pumping: Experience with 419 patients. Am J Cardiol 45:1033, 1980
177. Thomas TV: Emergency evacuation of acute pericardial tamponade. Ann Thorac Surg 10:566, 1970
178. Ullyot DJ, Wisneski J, Sullivan RW et al: The impact of coronary artery bypass on late myocardial infarction. J Thorac Cardiovasc Surg 73:165, 1976
179. Urschel HC Jr, Razzuk MA, Gardner MA: Management of concomitant occlusive disease of the carotid and coronary arteries. J Thorac Cardiovasc Surg 72:829, 1976
180. Urschel HC Jr, Razzuk MA, Gardner M: Coronary artery bypass occlusion secondary to postcardiotomy syndrome. Ann Thorac Surg 22:528, 1976
181. Utley JR, Moores WY, Stephens DB: Blood conservation techniques. Ann Thorac Surg 31:482, 1981
182. Vander Salm TJ, Cereda J–M, Cutler BS: Brachial plexus injury following median sternotomy. J Thorac Cardiovasc Surg 80:447, 1980
183. Vest JV, Pereira MB, Senior RM: Phrenic nerve injury associated with venipuncture of the internal jugular vein. Chest 78:777, 1980
184. Waldo AL, MacLean WAH: Diagnosis and Treatment of Cardiac Arrhythmias Following Open Heart Surgery. Mount Kisco, New York, Futura Publishing, 1980
185. Wechsler AS: Assessment of prospectively randomized patients receiving propranolol therapy before coronary bypass operation. Ann Thorac Surg 30:128, 1980
186. Wei JY, Taylor GJ, and Achuff SC: Recurrent cardiac tamponade and large pericardial effusions: Management with an indwelling pericardial catheter. Am J Cardiol 42:281, 1978
187. Wessel HU, Bastanier CK, Paul MH et al: Prognostic significance of arrhythmia in tetralogy of Fallot after intracardiac repair. Am J Cardiol 46:843, 1980
188. Wilkinson PL, Moyers JR, Ports T et al: Rate-pressure product and myocardial oxygen consumption during surgery for coronary artery bypass. Circulation (Suppl I) 60:170, 1978
189. Williams JF, Morrow AG, Braunwald E: The incidence and management of "medical" complications following cardiac operations. Circulation 32:608, 1965
190. Wilson WR, Danielson GK, Giuliani ER et al: Valve replacement in patients with active infective endocarditis. Circulation 58:585, 1978
191. Wisheart JD, Kirklin JW: The effect of rate augmentation on myocardial blood flow and oxygen consumption following extra-corporeal circulation. J Cardiovasc Surg 16:291, 1975
192. Wolfe WG, Kleinman LH, Wechsler AS, Sabiston DC Jr: Heparin-coated shunts for lesions of the descending thoracic aorta. Arch Surg 112:1481, 1977
193. Zurick A, Urzua J, Ghattas M, Cosgrove D: Decreased bleeding with PEEP. Ann Thoracic Surg 32:216, 1981

29 Complications of Extracorporeal Circulation

Timothy Wolfgang

OVERVIEW

Extracorporeal circulation (ECC) is a technique in which the venous return blood is shunted away from the heart and the gas exchange functions of the lung by a machine that controls the blood temperature, allows gas exchange, and maintains adequate circulation to the rest of the body (Fig. 29-1). For most cardiac procedures the venous return to the machine, or pump oxygenator, is by one or two cannulas in the right atrium with the arterial return cannula inserted in the ascending aorta (most commonly) or the femoral artery.

FIG. 29-1. An ECC apparatus with a right atrial cannula for venous drainage and an arterial cannula to the ascending aorta for blood return to the patient. The heart and lungs are thus bypassed.

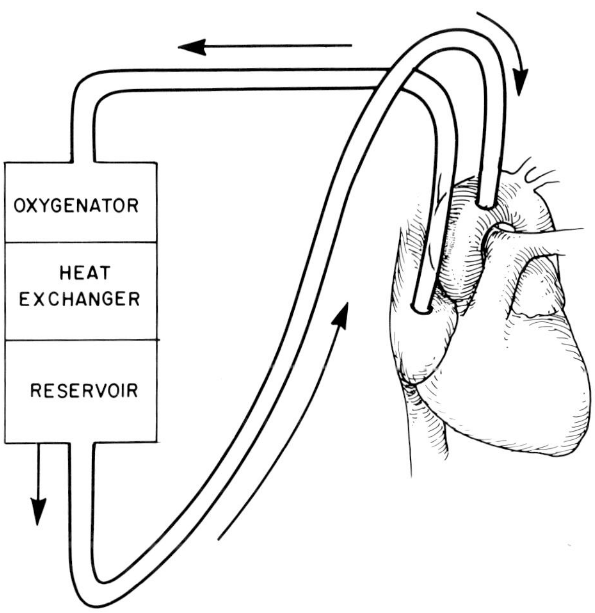

The intra-aortic balloon pump (IABP) is an internal counterpulsation system. This method of circulatory support uses a balloon (usually 40 cc) that is introduced through the femoral artery and is passed retrograde into the descending thoracic aorta (Fig. 29-2).

The balloon cycle of inflation and deflation is synchronized with the patient's EKG or arterial pressure curve. The balloon is inflated during early dias-

FIG. 29-2. The intra-aortic balloon positioned in the descending aorta, with inflation and deflation synchronized with diastole and systole.

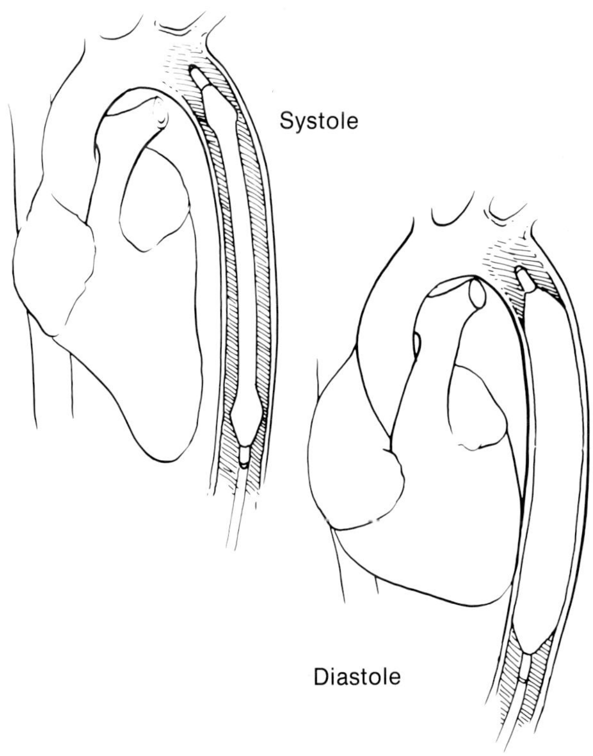

tole and deflated before systole. This results in an increased diastolic pressure and also reduces the afterload on systolic ejection. The compromised left ventricle is able to eject a greater quantity of blood against a decreased afterload. This form of support has been highly effective in treating a damaged left ventricle with potential for recovery after subsequent weaning and removal of the support device.

Hematologic Complications

Both ECC and the IABP have well-described adverse effects on the circulating blood components due primarily to mechnical trauma. The most sensitive of the blood components are the platelets. Changes in platelet concentrations during and after cardiopulmonary bypass have been well documented.[21, 29, 33]

It has been suggested that the mechanism for this decrease in platelet counts could be platelet destruction, aggregation, or trapping within the oxygenator circuit.[33] There are two types of oxygenators available—the bubble oxygenator and the membrane oxygenator (MO). Due to the differences in the method of oxygenation, superior function of the MO has been demonstrated in carefully controlled animal experiments in relation to having fewer adverse effects on the blood elements. However, clinically no definite benefits have been demonstrated between the two types of oxygenators. Both types have equally adverse effects on platelet function and hemolysis during cardiopulmonary bypass that lasts up to 2 to 3 hours.

Other blood components destroyed are leukocytes and erythrocytes. The destruction of the white blood cells releases fibrinolytic activators, and the destruction of the red cells releases a thromboplastinlike material. These can lead to the development of disseminated intravascular coagulation and secondary fibrinolysis.

All of these factors contribute to the complication of excessive bleeding following ECC. The red cell destruction can lead to hemolysis with jaundice and secondary damage to the kidneys.

Patients with cyanotic congenital heart disease and secondary polycythemia have an increased red cell mass with impairment of clot retraction, alteration in blood clotting factors, and increased fibrinolysis. These are all felt to be compensatory mechanisms to prevent intravascular clotting. In clinical studies, it has been shown that this group of patients has a greater likelihood of excessive bleeding postoperatively. A striking example is a study by Gomes and McGoon comparing repair for tetralogy of Fallot in acyanotic *versus* cyanotic patients.[10] Cyanotic patients lost 982 ml/m² of blood in the first 24 hours postoperatively compared to 350 ml/m² in acyanotic patients.

Another important factor in blood destruction is the use of cardiotomy suction.[8, 26, 29] This is a suction system to return the blood that collects within the pericardial sac to the oxygenator. The blood/air interface in cardiotomy suction produces mechanical trauma in excess of any other component of the extracorporeal system. DeJong and colleagues have shown that controlled low-vacuum suction has less cellular trauma than does high-vacuum suction.[8]

Anticoagulation is necessary for ECC, and heparin is the drug of choice, owing to its rapid action and its quick reversal with protamine sulfate. This drug, however, can also contribute to excessive bleeding if the level is not monitored properly. There are individual variations in the heparin response curve. At the end of perfusion, the hypocoagulable state may be further accentuated by improper neutralization of the heparin.[3] The heparin levels must be monitored throughout bypass and after reversal with protamine sulfate.[15, 28] In addition, there are other drugs that affect the coagulation mechanism such as warfarin, aspirin, amitriptyline, diphenhydramine, dipyridamole, imipramine, indomethacin, papaverine, phenoxybenzamine, phenylbutazone, propoxyphene, and sulfinpyrazone.[7]

When excessive bleeding after extracorporeal circulation is encountered and inadequate surgical hemostasis has been ruled out, other methods must be used to identify the problem. Heparin levels can be measured directly with a Hepcon unit.* This same unit is used to monitor heparin levels throughout bypass. Appropriate screening tests include:[2, 18, 24]

- Examination of the peripheral smear
- Clot retraction
- Bleeding time
- Prothrombin time
- Partial thromboplastin time
- Platelet count and platelet aggregation
- Fibrinogen
- Tri-F filter[19]
- Fibrin–fibrinogen split products

Using the results of these studies, the following bleeding disorders can be identified:

- Excessive or hyperfibrinolytic activating time that is compensated
- Excessive or hyperfibrinolytic activating time that is uncompensated
- Unneutralized heparin or heparin rebound
- Surgical bleeding

Platelets can be administered empirically since it is well known that all these patients have a de-

* Hemotec Inc., Englewood, Colorado

crease in absolute platelet count as well as platelet function. Usually, 6 to 8 units are given. Excessive heparin is reversed with protamine sulfate. Fresh frozen plasma (FFP) can be given empirically to replete the clotting factors depleted by ECC. Usually two units of FFP are given initially with clinical results and effects on the coagulation studies observed.

A useful adjunct to decrease blood loss is the use of positive end expiratory pressure to levels of 10 cm to 15 cm of water, as described by Ilabaca.[13]

With definite evidence of primary hyperfibrinolysis in a patient not responsive to these measures, epsilon-aminocaproic acid (EACA) should be administered.[20] In our experience the drug is rarely needed, however, and there are some dangerous side-effects. Absolute laboratory confirmation of hyperfibrinolysis without evidence of disseminated intravascular coagulation is needed to use the drug.

If postbypass bleeding does not respond to these measures, the patient should be returned to the operating room to recheck surgical hemostasis and evacuate clots. Frequently this maneuver will halt excessive bleeding even if no definite bleeding site is identified.

The following points are important in preventing postoperative hemorrhage:

Screen all patients for preexisting coagulation disorders and for drugs that affect coagulation.

Control heparin levels during bypass with a device such as the Hepcon unit.

Use cardiotomy suckers sparingly and at low vacuum.

Treat patients with polycythemia and cyanotic heart disease preoperatively to reduce the hematocrit.

The IABP is much less traumatic to the blood components. Red cell destruction with an increase in plasma hemoglobin to 20 mg/dl to 25 mg/dl may be seen. Thrombocytopenia may also occur, but it rarely reaches a level sufficient to cause a clinical bleeding diathesis.

Renal Complications

Renal failure is an ominous prognostic sign following extracorporeal circulation, carrying a mortality rate of 65%.[1, 5] Patients can be classified in different groups ranging from those who develop mild azotemia to those who develop severe acute renal failure and require dialysis. The causes of renal complications range from intraoperative insults to the kidney to postoperative dysfunction secondary to low cardiac output.

Preexisting renal disease may render the kidneys more susceptible to injury, especially in older patients with diffuse atherosclerotic disease and narrowing of the renal vessels. The kidneys might also be damaged from hypertensive disease or glomerulonephritis.

During extracorporeal circulation, it is necessary to maintain adequate renal blood flow with an adequate perfusion rate and pressure. However, Hilberman and colleagues have recently demonstrated that low-flow, low-pressure cardiopulmonary bypass has no outward effect on renal function.[11]

Renal perfusion during ECC may also be improved by using pulsatile blood flow.[25] Although pulsatile flow is not widely used, there are many devices available.

One important intraoperative cause of renal damage is hemolysis with excessive production of free hemoglobin and subsequent renal tubular obstruction and renal failure. The cardiotomy suction is perhaps the major culprit in producing excessive hemolysis.

Embolism during ECC is always a concern. In patients with valvular disease, calcific emboli can occur after débridement of the valve. Cholesterol emboli also may result from manipulation and clamping of an atherosclerotic aorta. Intracardiac thrombus either from valvular disease or infarction may also embolize at the time of surgery.

The major factor that affects renal function in the postoperative period is left ventricular function.[5, 23] It is extremely important that adequate renal perfusion be maintained postoperatively. Intraoperatively urine output can be maintained with adequate perfusion pressures and flows. Occasionally mannitol or lasix can be given to maintain adequate urine flow. Alkaline urine output must be sought because an acid urine makes the deposition of hemoglobin in the renal tubules more likely. Low-vacuum cardiotomy suction is preferable, although its use should be limited.

Since oliguria is usually not recognized until after the operation, any patient who develops it to the extent of 1 ml/kg/hour should be managed initially with improvement of cardiac output. This is most easily monitored by the readings from a thermodilution Swan–Ganz catheter. Left ventricular performance usually can be improved by adjusting preload and afterload. If this fails to augment cardiac output, then the use of the IABP to restore adequate renal blood flow must be considered.

Acute renal failure may also have a mechanical cause. This is rare, but it can occur with a retrograde unrecognized aortic dissection if femoral cannulation has been used. If a patient has had the IABP inserted in the femoral artery at the time of surgery, this can also cause a retrograde dissection.

Low Cardiac Output Syndrome

One of the most serious problems following extracorporeal bypass is the low cardiac output state. This syndrome is manifested by the inability to wean the patient from cardiopulmonary bypass successfully. Preexisting cardiac damage may be an important contributing factor, but some form of intraoperative or perioperative damage may also contribute to the syndrome since the patient usually has an adequate cardiac output prior to the initiation of bypass.

This damage may be mechanical from emboli obstructing a major coronary artery. Cholesterol or calcium emboli may originate from a diseased aorta after cross clamping or the application of a partial occlusion clamp. Calcium emboli also can result from débridement of a heavily calcified aortic valve. Air embolism may occur and is more likely with an open cardiac procedure, but it may also result from the use of a left ventricular vent if aspiration of air into the left ventricular chamber occurs.

Intraoperative damage most commonly comes from inadequate myocardial protection with cardioplegic solution. This solution is administered after aortic cross clamping by way of the aortic root or by direct coronary infusion. The solution is hyperkalemic and hyperosmolar and is maintained at 4° C to 8° C; the myocardial protection results from the low myocardial temperature with total electrical arrest. The solution is administered intermittently during the operative procedure using a myocardial temperature probe as an indicator of adequate hypothermia. However, in the presence of multiple coronary lesions, the cardioplegia may not produce uniform cooling of the myocardium. Also, myocardium in contact with the pericardium posteriorly and laterally may have a tendency to warm more quickly than other areas. The use of a cooling pad beneath the heart helps to prevent some of the heat transfer.

Despite satisfactory cardioplegic protection, the length of cross clamping that the myocardium will accept is limited by the risk of irreversible cellular damage. With longer, more complicated surgical procedures, the limit may be exceeded with subsequent myocardial damage.

The most common level of myocardial damage is the subendocardium, which is highly susceptible to injury. This is now thought to be secondary to redistribution of blood flow from this area during ventricular fibrillation with subsequent ischemia and necrosis.

Other causes of myocardial damage are technical errors. For example, endarterectomies of coronary arteries have a higher incidence of perioperative infarction, and a well-described complication of mitral valve replacement comes from the inadvertent placement of a posterior suture too deeply through the annulus with occlusion of the circumflex coronary artery (Fig. 29-3).

Intraoperative prevention of myocardial damage is provided by uniform cooling of the myocardium with total electrical arrest. Ventricular fibrillation should be avoided and great care taken to avoid air emboli or emboli from other debris. Left ventricular distension is avoided to prevent subsequent subendocardial perfusion imbalance. This is most easily achieved by the use of a left ventricular vent.

Despite all of these precautions, patients still

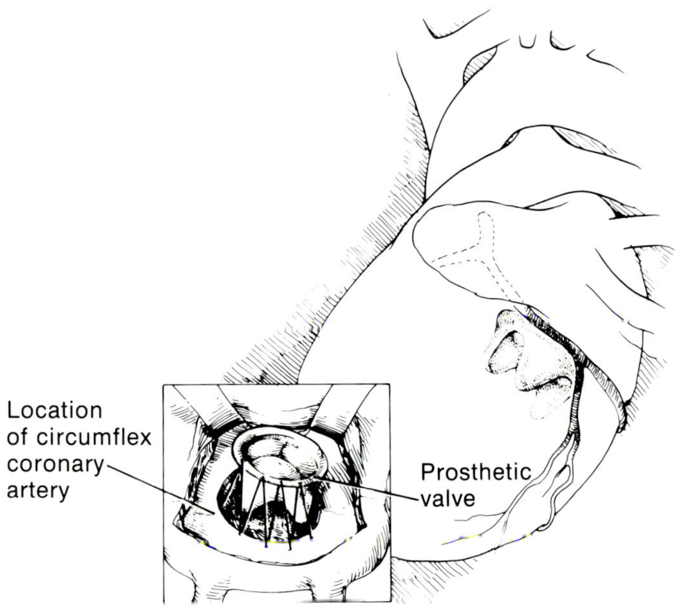

FIG. 29-3. The relationship of the circumflex coronary artery to the sutures used for mitral valve insertion. (*Inset*) Sutures placed too deeply can injure or occlude this vessel.

develop low cardiac output syndrome, most commonly during the weaning from bypass, but it can be manifested later by arrhythmias, hypotension, low urinary output, and so on. Patients at a higher risk to exhibit this syndrome usually can be identified prior to surgery. Those with diminished left ventricular function preoperatively are more likely to need additional support postoperatively. Patients at increased risk should have a Swan–Ganz catheter inserted at the beginning of the surgical procedure to facilitate induction and to guide the surgeon in weaning from bypass. The ability to measure cardiac output by thermodilution is very helpful postoperatively in evaluating the patient's recovery and to assess response to therapy.

If a patient does not have a Swan–Ganz catheter and has difficulty in weaning from bypass, then a left atrial line is needed to monitor preload accurately.

Another important step in managing an unstable patient is the insertion of two atrial and two ventricular pacing lines. These can be used to diagnose arrhythmias as well as to pace the patient. The paired atrial lines can also be used to treat atrial tachyarrhythmias with the use of a rapid atrial pacemaker.

Once adequate monitoring lines are in place and an adequate A-V synchronous heart rate is established, the patient can frequently be weaned from bypass with careful monitoring. Many patients require some form of inotropic support. We commonly use dopamine or isoproterenol (Isuprel), but others prefer epinephrine. All these drugs have positive inotropic action with varying chronotropic actions. Dopamine has the added advantage of producing renal vascular dilatation. The addition of nitroprusside to this regimen can reduce central venous pressure and pulmonary vascular pressures by vasodilatation. The combined use of an inotropic drug along with the afterload reduction from nitroprusside can markedly improve cardiac output.

An important concept to appreciate is that diastolic pressure is important for coronary blood flow. It is also important to prevent tachycardia by the judicious use of propranolol. Slowing the rate will improve coronary flow and oxygenation by prolonging the diastolic phase.

If these actions still do not allow successful weaning from bypass, then the intra-aortic balloon is needed. The balloon is introduced either from the femoral artery or ascending aorta. The balloon is positioned in the descending aorta just distal to the left subclavian artery. The balloon is then inflated during diastole and deflated before systole (see Fig. 29-2). This increases the diastolic-pressure-time index, improving coronary flow and subsequent myocardial oxygenation. With deflation in systole there is decreased resistance to ejection of the left ventricle and more effective emptying.

With the combined use of drug therapy and IABP, most patients can be successfully weaned from bypass. Over the subsequent days in the recovery room, the drug therapy is weaned as the ventricular function improves. Once drug therapy is stopped, the IABP can be weaned by changing from 1:1 to 2:1, then to a 4:1 ratio between the heart rate and the inflation cycle of the balloon.

Vascular Complications

Circulatory support with either cardiopulmonary bypass or the intra-aortic balloon pump requires vascular access to the arterial circulation through a major artery or the aorta. The site chosen for the arterial inflow cannula for extracorporeal circulation is usually the ascending aorta. A cross clamp is then applied to the aorta proximal to the cannula in order to administer cardioplegic solution to the aortic root. Both of these events (*i.e.*, the cannulation and the clamping) can disrupt the intima and media of the aorta and allow the wall to dissect (Fig. 29-4). The event can be recognized almost immediately at the time of surgery by the progression of a hemorrhagic false lumen either proximally or distally beneath the remaining adventitia and media. If the complication arises, it must be recognized immediately and repaired. This is accomplished by opening the aorta

FIG. 29-4. Cannulation of the ascending aorta or femoral artery can cause elevation of an intimal flap and a subsequent dissecting hematoma as blood accumulates beneath the flap.

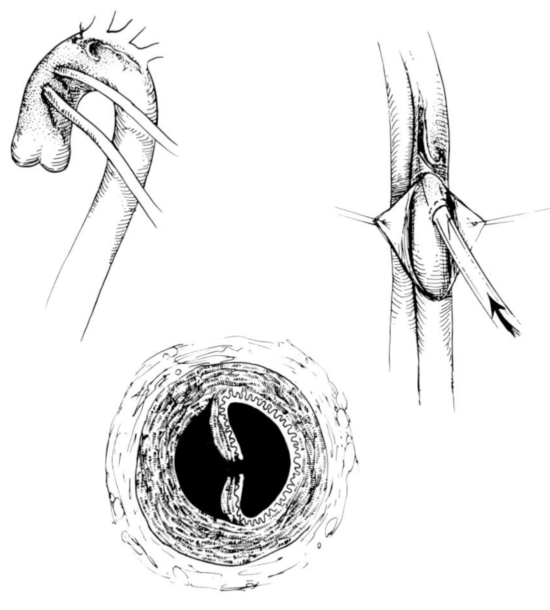

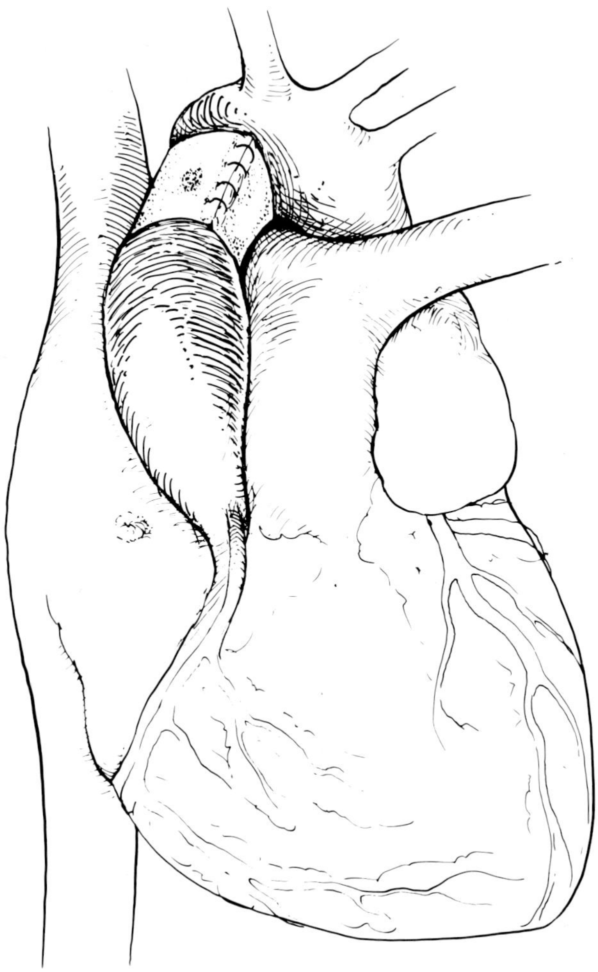

FIG. 29-5. The technique for reinforcing the cannulation site of the ascending aorta with a Teflon "cuff" to prevent hemorrhage from lateral expansile forces disrupting the site.

and reattaching the intima and adventitia to obliterate the false lumen.[22] The aortic cannula must be moved—most commonly to a femoral artery—to allow proper exposure.

In some patients the site of initial arterial cannulation is a femoral artery. This site may be chosen because of abnormalities of the ascending aorta that make cannulation more difficult. A retrograde dissection may develop from the site of cannulation, but this complication is more difficult to recognize than is acute ascending aortic dissections (see Fig. 29-4). The etiology is either direct injury to the vessel by the cannula or the creation of a dissection by the hemodynamic changes induced by extracorporeal circulation. There may be increased pressure in the arterial perfusion line, or the pressure in the ascending aorta may be relatively low despite a good pressure in the arterial perfusion line.

The initial manifestation of retrograde dissection may be sudden oliguria. Once the dissection is recognized, treatment is directed toward reestablishing forward arterial flow.[9] This can be done by either discontinuing bypass and reestablishing normal cardiac function and output *or* by switching the arterial cannula to a site on the ascending aorta. The change in the flow will obliterate the false lumen and prevent further progression of the dissection.

The site of aortic cannulation on the ascending aorta may be through friable, nonelastic tissue. This is usually not recognized until after the cannula has been inserted. The complication that can arise is disruption of the aorta at this site. Usually upon termination of cardiopulmonary bypass, the aortic cannula is removed and the opening closed with a pursestring or mattress suture reinforced with Teflon pledgets. With a tenuous aorta, bleeding at the cannulation site continues despite reinforcement with additional suture material. To prevent further disruption of this area by additional ineffectual suturing, the aorta is wrapped with a heavy piece of Teflon, usually ½-inch wide, which is sutured firmly over the site (Fig. 29-5). This puts direct pressure on the Teflon pieces already in place and prevents further disruption by restricting the lateral expansile stresses on the previous sutures.

The intra-aortic balloon is a necessary adjunct in the management of low cardiac output. The balloon is most commonly inserted by way of the common femoral artery and is threaded into the descending thoracic aorta. One possible complication is aortic dissection.[4, 6, 12] As with femoral artery cannulation, this event is difficult to recognize, and frequently the intra-aortic balloon can function properly despite its location within a false lumen. Recognition of the complication necessitates the removal of the balloon; this will reestablish antegrade flow that should obliterate the false lumen. This complication can be prevented by avoiding forceful insertion of the balloon and by using one of the newly designed balloons that are introduced over a guide wire.

Ischemia of the leg secondary to impaired inflow due to the balloon catheter is the most common complication of the use of the balloon.[2, 4, 6] This can be partially avoided by using the common femoral artery for the insertion site and by choosing the femoral artery with the stronger pulse. At the time of cardiac catheterization, dye can be injected into the femoral and iliac arteries to identify vascular disease prior to any procedure that may require the use of the intra-aortic balloon.

After the insertion of the balloon, the circulation of the leg must be carefully monitored. If leg ischemia occurs, the treatment is removal of the balloon and insertion through the opposite common femoral artery. If the opposite vessel cannot be used, an alternative is to perform a crossover graft from the opposite femoral or iliac artery to the femoral artery distal to the site of the balloon insertion.[2]

An alternative site for introduction of the intra-aortic balloon is the ascending aorta. Recently a case of small bowel infarction was reported as a complication of this approach when the tip of the catheter entered the superior mesenteric artery.[14] The complication can be avoided by obtaining a lateral chest film to assess the direction of the catheter tip.

Neurologic Complications

Neurologic dysfunction persists as a major complication following extracorporeal circulation. This either can be secondary to overt brain damage or can be a manifestation of a severe stress-induced decompensation. The causes of overt brain damage are embolism or inadequate cerebral perfusion. There may be large emboli from the aorta or a calcified valve or, during intraoperative manipulations, a piece of cholesterol or calcium may embolize. Another source of embolism is an intracardiac clot that is secondary to valvular disease such as mitral stenosis; or clots may form in the left ventricle at areas of infarction.

Air embolism is a well-described cause of neurologic dysfunction.[31] This can be secondary to a massive air embolus from the arterial perfusion line or from air trapped within a cardiac chamber, which is ejected into the cerebral circulation when cardiac function returns. Air embolism occurs more commonly with open cardiac procedures. With coronary artery bypass grafting, the heart is rarely opened except to insert a left ventricular vent. Therefore large volumes of air are less likely to enter the heart. The vent, however, can create enough of a negative pressure that air can be sucked into the heart from any opening in the aorta or around the vent insertion site itself. When using a vent, the amount of suction must be regulated, and the likelihood of this complication must be appreciated.

Other sources of embolism are microemboli from foreign particles, platelet and fibrin aggregates, and so on, that come from the pump. Micropore filters aid in removing much of this debris.

Inadequate cerebral perfusion can be due to a major obstruction to cerebral flow secondary to significant carotid or vertebral artery disease. It may also occur from hypotension during extracorporeal circulation.[16]

There are many other factors that contribute and are related to the development of postcardiotomy delerium.[17, 32] These are preoperative organic brain disease, severity of the heart disease, age, cardiopulmonary bypass time, severity of recovery room illness, unexpressed anxiety, sensory isolation, and sleep deprivation. Many of these factors are aggravated by the nature of intensive-care units and thus can be eliminated by having patients leave recovery areas as soon as they are stable.

Prevention consists of recognizing patients that are at high risk for neurologic dysfunction. Patients can be screened for vascular disease by Doppler examinations of the carotid artery. If significant disease is identified, then a cerebral angiogram can help determine the need for cerebral revascularization in relation to cardiac surgery.

Intraoperative prevention consists of providing adequate perfusion and pressure. Emboli are prevented by the use of micropore filters. Air emboli are carefully avoided by aspiration of each cardiac chamber at the termination of the procedure.

Treatment of massive air embolism consists of stopping cardiopulmonary bypass and removing all air from the aorta.[27] The patient's head should be lowered. Air is aspirated from all chambers of the heart. Bypass is then resumed. The use of hyperbaric treatment at this point is the most promising modality for this complication. The personnel of each institution using cardiopulmonary bypass should be familiar with the nearest suitable hyperbaric chamber and have a protocol developed to manage a patient with massive air embolism.

Despite all preventive measures, neurologic dysfunction still follows cardiac surgery. Once this is recognized, satisfactory perfusion and oxygenation of the brain must be assured. Cerebral edema can be prevented by careful management of fluids. Anticoagulation does not usually play a role in postoperative cerebral infarction since it can produce a hemorrhagic infarct. Seizures can be prevented by adequate anticonvulsant medication. Steroids probably do not have any significant effect once a defect has occurred.

The prognosis depends upon the etiology and extent of the damage. EEGs are helpful along with computed tomography (CT) scans to help assess these variables and to follow a patient's course. In many instances, the neurologic dysfunction is reversible.

Respiratory Complications

With refinements in extracorporeal circulation and in postoperative pulmonary management, the incidence of postoperative pulmonary complications following cardiac surgery has markedly diminished from earlier studies that showed a 15% to 25% pulmonary complication rate.

Patients with preexisting lung disease have a higher incidence of complications.[30] This is especially the case with patients with chronic bronchitis and copious sputum production. Other patients that appear to be more susceptible are those with pulmonary change secondary to their underlying cardiac disease, that is, pulmonary venous congestion or hypertension secondary to valvular disease or diminished left ventricular function.

There are two major areas of extracorporeal management that can affect lung function. The first is the limitation of pulmonary venous congestion and the second is the limitation of microparticles delivered to the patient's circulation. Pulmonary venous congestion is brought on by elevation of the left atrial pressure to the point at which interstitial pulmonary edema develops. Other important contributing factors are the osmolality of the perfusate and the amount of damage done to the capillary network by microparticle matter sequestered in the lung.

The left atrial pressure is controlled intraoperatively by the use of a left ventricular vent that is usually inserted by way of the right superior pulmonary vein. By controlling the amount of blood returning to the left ventricle by way of bronchial collaterals or through an insufficient aortic valve, pulmonary venous engorgement can be prevented and need not contribute to interstitial changes.

Most patients are managed with a hyperosmolar pump prime solution and hemodilution. The oxygenator is primed with a crystalloid solution containing various amounts of albumin to create a slightly hyperosmolar solution. During bypass the patient's hemocrit drops to 20% to 25% from the dilution. Upon the termination of bypass, the fluid retained in the oxygenator is returned to the patient as tolerated by left atrial pressure measurements, thus partially restoring the preoperative blood volume. During extracorporeal circulation, fluids are sequestered in the interstitial spaces, and during the days following surgery, these fluids are mobilized back into the intravascular space and then excreted. This process partially explains the interstitial and alveolar edema noted postoperatively following cardiopulmonary bypass.

Particulate matter in the circulation is filtered by the microcirculation of the lungs. This can contribute to capillary damage and resulting interstitial edema. The major sources of the particulate matter are homologous blood and material suctioned back to the pump by the cardiotomy suckers. As discussed previously, the bypass apparatus causes moderately severe trauma to the blood elements. These damaged cells and platelets are also filtered by the lungs, and they can release histamine, serotonin, and fibrinopeptides that cause further lung damage.

The diagnosis of respiratory failure following extracorporeal circulation is made immediately because of a relative hypoxemia. Cardiac surgical patients are maintained on a respirator with controlled ventilation until they are stable both from the cardiac as well as from the respiratory standpoint. Postoperatively, all patients are placed initially on an F_IO_2 of 0.8 until a set of blood gases and chest x-ray film are obtained. This allows a margin of safety in oxygenation. The majority of patients have a PaO_2 >200 torr. The F_IO_2 is then adjusted to maintain a PaO_2 of 70 to 100 torr. Patients with interstitial edema may have a clear chest x-ray film, but the PO_2 will be disproportionately low. These patients are treated with diuretics to remove excess free water along with the addition of positive end-expiratory pressure (PEEP). With the use of PEEP care must be taken not to increase it to the extent that cardiac output is diminished. This is best monitored by using a Swan–Ganz catheter to measure cardiac output and left atrial pressure. Usually with these maneuvers, the patient's PO_2 will rise quickly over the next few hours to allow the F_IO_2 to be decreased. It is important to manage the fluids in these patients carefully. Free water and sodium should be restricted, and the effective hydrostatic–osmotic pressure relationship should be maintained by salt-free albumin or plasma.

The prevention of postoperative respiratory problems depends upon recognizing preoperatively patients with preexisting lung disease and placing them in optimal condition for surgery with such measures as pulmonary toilet, antibiotics, and the cessation of smoking. Intraoperatively postoperative problems can be minimized by the use of micropore filters to remove all particulate matter before it can be recirculated to the patient. Pulmonary congestion can also be prevented by controlling the left atrial pressure and carefully monitoring the fluid volumes while coming off bypass. Postoperatively patients with interstitial edema must be recognized early and an aggressive approach taken to reverse respiratory difficulties with the use of PEEP, diuretics, and fluid management.

References

1. Abel RM, Buckley MH, Austin WG et al: Etiology, incidence, and prognosis of renal failure following cardiac operations. J Thorac Cardiovasc Surg 71:323–333, 1976
2. Albert J, Parsonnet V, Goldenkrantz RJ et al: Limb ischemia during intra-aortic balloon pumping: Indication for femorofemoral crossover graft. J Thorac Cardiovasc Surg 79:729–734, 1980
3. Bachmann F, McKenna R, Cole E, Najafi H: The hemostatic mechanism after open heart surgery. J Thorac Cardiovasc Surg 70(1):76–85, 1975
4. Beckman CB, Geha AS, Hammond GL, Baue AE: Results and complications of intra-aortic balloon counterpulsation. Ann Thorac Surg 24(6):550–559, 1977.
5. Bhat JG, Gluck MG, Lowenstein J, Baldwin DS: Renal failure after open heart surgery. Ann Intern Med 84:677–682, 1977
6. Bolooki H: Complications of intra-aortic balloon pumps

and their treatment. In Clinical Application of Intra-Aortic Balloon Pumps, pp 125–132. Mt. Kisko, Futura Publishing Company, 1977

7. Cordell AR: Hematological complications of extracorporeal circulation. In Complications of Intrathoracic Surgery, pp 27–34. Boston, Little, Brown & Co, 1977
8. de Jong JCF, ten Duis HJ, Sibinga C et al: Hematologic aspects of cardiotomy suction in cardiac operations. J Thorac Cardiovasc Surg 79(2):227–236, 1980
9. Elliott DP: Aortic dissection during cardiopulmonary bypass. J Thorac Cardiovasc Surg 50:357–363, 1965
10. Gomes MMR, McGoon DC: Bleeding patterns after open-heart surgery. J Thorac Cardiovasc Surg 60(1):87–97, 1970
11. Hilberman M, Myers B, Carrie B et al: Acute renal failure following cardiac surgery. J Thorac Cardiovasc Surg 77(6):880–888, 1979
12. Hines GL, Delaney TB, Goodman M, Mohtashemi M: Intra-aortic balloon pumping. J Thorac Cardiovasc Surg 78(1):140–146, 1979
13. Ilabaca PA, Ochsner JL, Mills NL: Positive end-expiratory pressure in the management of the patient with a postoperative bleeding heart. Ann Thorac Surg 30(3):281–4, 1980
14. Jarmolowski CR, Poirier RL: Small bowel infarction complication intra-aortic balloon counterpulsation via the ascending aorta. J Thorac Cardiovasc Surg 79:735–737, 1980
15. Kaul TK, Crow MJ, Somasundram MR et al: Heparin administration during extracorporeal circulation. J Thorac Cardiovasc Surg 78(1):95–102, 1979
16. Kolka R, Hilberman M: Neurological dysfunction following cardiac operation with low-flow, low-pressure cardiopulmonary bypass. J Cardiothor and Cardiovasc Sur 79(3):432–437, 1980
17. Kornfield DS, Heller SS, Frank KA et al: Delirium after coronary artery bypass surgery. J Thorac Cardiovasc Surg 76(1):93–96, 1978
18. Lambert CJ, Marengo–Rowe AJ: The management of postperfusion bleeding after cardiopulmonary bypass. Monograph, Pearl River, NY, Lederle Laboratories
19. Lambert CJ, Marengo–Rowe AJ, Levenson J et al: The Tri-F Titer. Ann Thorac Surg 18(4):357–363, 1974
20. Lambert CJ, Marengo–Rowe AJ, Levenson JE et al: The treatment of postperfusion bleeding using epsilon-amino caproic acid, cryo-precipitate, fresh-frozen plasma, and protanine sulfate. Ann Thorac Surg 28(5):440–444, 1979
21. Laufer N, Merin G, Grover NB et al: The influence of cardiopulmonary bypass on the size of human platelets. J Thorac Cardiovasc Surg 70(4):727–731, 1975
22. Litchford B, Okies JE, Sugimura S, Starr A: Acute aortic dissection from cross-clamp injury. J Thorac Cardiovasc Surg 72:709, 1977
23. McLeish KR, Luft KC, Klein SA: Factors affecting prognosis in acute renal failure following cardiac operations. Surg Gynecol Obstet 145:28–32, 1977
24. Marengo–Rowe AJ, Lambert CJ, Levenson JE et al: The evaluation of hemorrhage in cardiac patients who have undergone extracorporeal circulation. Transfusion 19(4):426–433, 1979
25. Mavroudis C: To pulse or not to pulse. Ann Thorac Surg 25(3):259–271, 1978
26. Okies JE, Goodnight SH, Litchford B et al: Effects of infusion of cardiotomy suction blood during extracorporeal circulation for coronary artery bypass surgery. J Thorac Cardiovasc Surg 74:440–444, 1977
27. Pierce EC: Specific therapy for arterial air embolism. Ann Thorac Surg 29(4):300–303, 1980
28. Ponai O, Corsi M, Manotti C et al: Predictive value of preoperative in vitro and in vivo studies for correct individual heparinization in cardiac surgery. J Thorac Cardiovasc Surg 78(1):87–94, 1979
29. Siderys H, Herod GT, Halbrook H et al: A comparison of membrane and bubble oxygenation as used in cardiopulmonary bypass in patients. J Thorac Cardiovasc Surg 69(5):708–712, 1975
30. Stein M, Cassara E: Preoperative pulmonary evaluation and therapy for surgery patients. JAMA 211(5):787–790, 1970
31. Stoney AS, Alford WC, Burrus GR et al: Air embolism and other accidents using pump oxygenators. Ann Thorac Surg 29(4):337–340, 1980
32. Sweinsson IS: Postoperative psychosis after heart surgery. J Thorac Cardiovasc Surg 70:717–726, 1975
33. Trumbull HR, Howe J, Mottl J, Nicoloff DM: A comparison of the effects of membrane and bubble oxygenators on platelet counts and platelet size in elective cardiac operations. Ann Thorac Surg 30(1):52–57, 1980

30
Complications of Venous Thrombosis and Pulmonary Embolism

Lazar J. Greenfield

OVERVIEW

The development of a deep vein thrombosis in a postoperative or posttraumatic patient is a most serious complication requiring expeditious diagnosis and management to prevent the potentially lethal complication of pulmonary embolism. Our present level of understanding of venous thrombosis evolved from very limited autopsy data in contrast to in vivo *studies of the dynamics of the venous circulation by means of radiographic contrast injections and noninvasive flow studies. When contrast medium is injected into the feet of supine immobilized patients, it may remain in venous valve sinuses for as long as an hour, confirming the stasis in the soleal sinuses. This is the favored location for the formation of a nidus of thrombus. Successive layering of platelets, fibrin, and leukocytes produces an organized white thrombus that is more adherent to the vein wall than is the propagating red thrombus, which extends into the venous stream (Fig. 30-1) and is more likely to embolize. The original thrombus may become attached to the opposite wall, causing interruption of flow, retrograde thrombosis, and signs of venous stasis in the extremity. Subsequent edema formation within the confines of the deep muscular fascia produces pain and the characteristic Homans' sign elicited by forcible dorsiflexion of the foot. More common, however, in about 60% of patients the thrombus propagates without interrupting flow and develops a long floating "tail" that is highly susceptible to breaking loose from its tenuous anchor within the valvular sinus. It is this sequence of events that is the most dangerous aspect of the disorder, since major pulmonary embolism can and does occur without premonitory signs or symptoms at its point of origin.*

The site of venous obstruction determines the level at which swelling is observed clinically. Swelling at the thigh level always implies obstruction at the level of the iliofemoral system, while swelling of the calf or foot suggests obstruction at the femoropopliteal level. Autopsies suggest that it is more common for thrombi to originate in the veins of the soleus and then propagate proximally, but there is also evidence of primary thrombosis of femoral and iliac venous tributaries as well.

In addition to stasis, hypercoagulability must be considered as a causative factor with the recognition that women who use oral contraceptive anovulatory agents develop thrombotic disorders three to six times more frequently than those who do not take these agents. Earlier efforts to find differences in coagulation factors among patients with or without deep venous thrombosis were unrewarding, but it was possible to identify a naturally occurring inhibitor of activated factor X called antithrombin III. *This factor was thought to be reduced by oral contraceptives, but subsequent studies have shown that the increased susceptibility is more likely to be related to a reduction in factor Xa inhibitory activity. Congenital deficiency in antithrombin III levels has been found to predispose patients to venous thrombosis and pulmonary embolism. Other unexplained hypercoagulable states seem to be associated with recent trauma, major surgical procedures, and sepsis. When stasis develops, the substances that promote platelet aggregation, including activated factor X, thrombin, fibrin, and catecholamines, remain at high concentration in a particular area. This leads to platelet aggregation, which initiates coagulation and thrombin generation with release of ADP, which further aggregates platelets as the fibrin complex propagates. Opposing this process is the fibrinolytic system of the blood and vein walls. The endothelium of the vein wall contains an activator that converts plasminogen to plasmin, which lyses fibrin. As might be expected, however, the fibrinolytic system is inhibited after surgery and trauma, and there is less activity in the veins of the lower extremity than in the upper extremity.*[17] *The third major causative factor of Virchow's triad is vessel wall damage, which usually is not demonstrable in areas of thrombosis. Obesity, aging, and malignancy also increase the risk of developing deep vein thrombosis by mechanisms that are not well understood.*

Resolution of deep venous thrombosis will affect the competence of the valves within the veins and can result in the postphlebitic syndrome, which is discussed in Chapter 27.

Diagnosis

Major venous thrombosis involving the deep venous system of the thigh and pelvis produces a characteristic clinical picture of pain, extensive pitting edema, and blanching that has been termed phlegmasia alba dolens, or "milk leg." Association with pregnancy may derive from hormonal effects on blood, relaxation of vessel walls, or mechanical compression of the left iliac vein at the pelvic brim, resulting in the term "milk leg of pregnancy." It was originally believed that the blanching was due to spasm and compromise of arterial flow, but arteriograms fail to confirm this. Efforts to achieve sympatholysis to overcome "vasospasm" are ill advised, since it is the subcutaneous edema that is responsible for the blanching. In addition to pregnancy, mechanical factors that can affect the left iliac vein include compression from the right iliac artery or an overdistended bladder and congenital webs within the vein. These factors are responsible for the observed 4:1 preponderance of left versus right iliac vein involvement.

With further progression of venous thrombosis to impede most of the venous return from the extremity, there is danger of limb loss from cessation of arterial flow. The clinical picture is characteristic, with sufficient congestion to produce phlegmasia cerulea dolens, or a blue leg. With the loss of sensory or motor function, clinical grounds can be diagnostic and treatment started. Venous gangrene is likely unless the approach is aggressive to remove the thrombus and restore blood flow. A variant of this disorder occurs peripherally in the leg and is associated with concurrent malignant disease and a high mortality rate.

As indicated earlier, these major complications represent less than 10% of the patients with venous thrombosis. In fact, only 40% of patients with venous thrombosis have any clinical signs of the disorder. In addition, false-positive clinical signs occur in up to 50% of patients studied.[16] Because of this a great deal of interest in the development of screening tests that could reveal thrombi before they became evident clinically has arisen. Of course, contrast venography provides direct evidence of both occlusive and nonocclusive thrombi, but it is invasive and requires movement of the patient to a radiographic suite. Ideally, the screening test would be accurate, noninvasive, and performed at the bedside. Although the ideal has not been achieved, there are a number of tests that have proved useful.

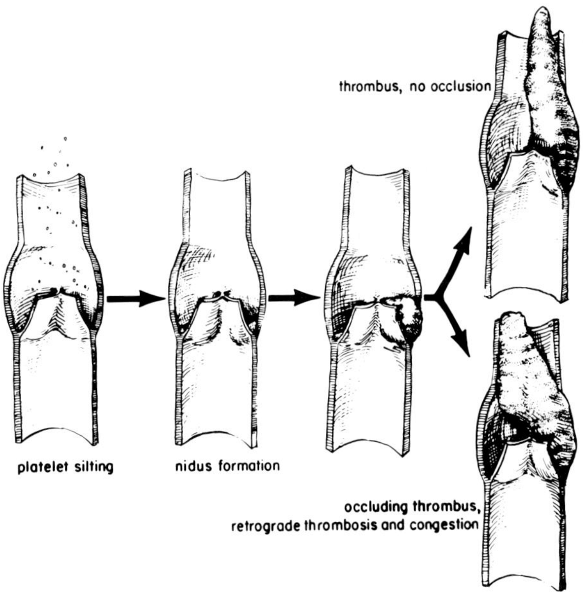

FIG. 30-1. The evolution of venous thrombosis begins with stagnant flow that permits silting of platelets, which form a nidus in the venous valvular sinus. The cycle of fibrin retraction and thrombin release aggregates more platelets as the thrombus enlarges and usually extends into the stream without occlusion, or it may occlude the vein with retrograde thrombosis. (Greenfield LJ: Acute venous thrombosis and pulmonary embolism. In Hardy JD [Ed]: Hardy's Textbook of Surgery. Philadelphia, JB Lippincott, 1983)

ULTRASOUND

The Doppler probe can be used to advantage to detect major venous thrombi with a high degree of accuracy, but it is a subjective form of testing dependent on the examiner's experience. The principle is straightforward and is based on the impairment of an accelerated flow signal produced by intraluminal thrombi.[22] The examination begins at the ankle with identification of the posterior tibial vein signal adjacent to the artery. The flow signal should be altered by distal and proximal compression producing, respectively, augmentation and interruption of flow, which also can be produced by the Valsalva maneuver. The same maneuvers are repeated over the superficial and deep femoral veins and can be done over the popliteal vein (Fig. 30-2). Failure to augment flow on compression below or release of interruption of flow above the probe suggests venous

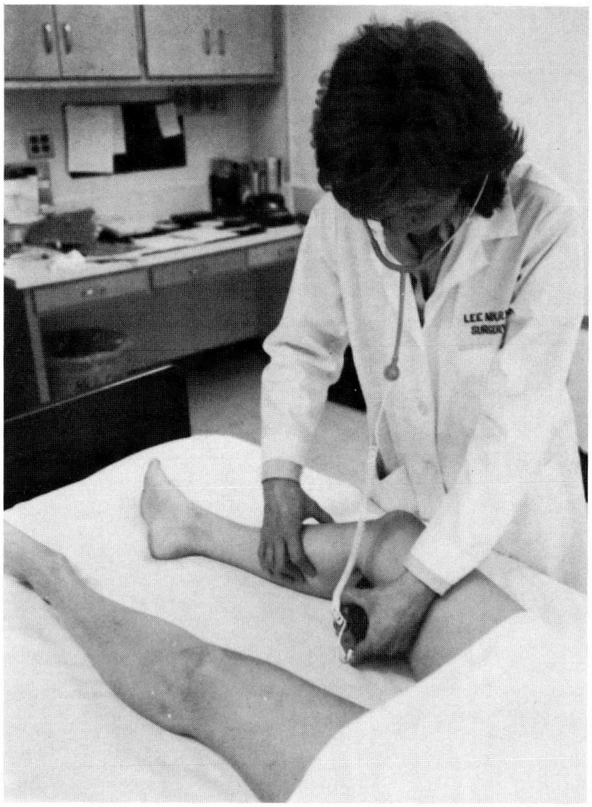

FIG. 30-2. Use of the Doppler probe to examine the politeal vein. The technician is compressing the calf to detect the increased velocity signal that indicates absence of an intraluminal thrombus.

thrombi. The sensitivity of the test exceeds 90%, but the specificity is 5% to 10% lower owing to the interference of other mechanical problems (Baker's cyst, hematoma, etc.) with venous flow. A negative Doppler ultrasound examination is reassuring, but a positive or equivocal test should be confirmed by contrast venography. A negative test is *not* reassuring when thromboembolism is suspected, since the thrombus may have been evacuated from the extremity. The test is also less sensitive to calf vein thrombi, but it can be used in patients in traction or who are wearing a plaster cast.

IMPEDANCE PLETHYSMOGRAPHY

Impedance plethysmography (IPG) measures the volume response of the extremity to temporary occlusion of the venous system. The diagnosis of venous thrombosis depends on the changes in venous capacitance and rate of emptying after release of the occlusion.[25] A proximal thigh cuff is inflated to 40- to 50-torr pressure for 30 to 120 seconds or until maximum filling has occurred by plateau of the electrical signal. The inflation cuff is then rapidly deflated, allowing rapid outflow and reduction of volume in a normal limb. Prolongation of the outflow wave suggests major venous thrombosis with 95% accuracy and is much more reliable than any voluntary technique of venous occlusion (Fig. 30-3). The deficiency with this technique, as with all of the noninvasive methods, is in its detection of calf vein thrombosis or definition of new pathology in patients with old postthrombotic sequelae. The strain gauge plethysmograph can be used in a similar fashion. A positive IPG test can be used to make therapeutic decisions in the absence of clinical conditions that can produce false-positive tests such as cardiac failure, constrictive pericarditis, hypotension, arterial insufficiency, or external compression of veins.

RADIOACTIVE-LABELED FIBRINOGEN

Clinical application of labeled fibrinogen has been facilitated by the development of portable scintillation counters for bedside use. After iodine blockage of the thyroid gland, the counts are obtained from marked locations on the lower extremities and expressed as a percentage of the radioactivity measured by counting over the heart. An increase of 20% or more in one area indicates the presence of an underlying thrombus. The test permits sequential scanning of the extremities over a period of days and is most sensitive to thrombi forming in the veins of the calves shortly after an operative procedure.[7] Thrombi in pelvic veins cannot be detected, and it cannot be used in an extremity with a healing wound, fracture, cellulitis, arthritis, edema, ulceration, or superficial thrombophlebitis in which false-positive results are likely. It is also contraindicated in patients under 30 years of age and in women of childbearing age. Otherwise, it is quite accurate, however, showing 90% positive correlation with contrast venograms. A negative correlation usually is explained by cessation of active thrombosis and failure to incorporate the tagged fibrinogen, making the test useful in discriminating between old and new venous thrombi.

VENOGRAPHY

The injection of contrast material for direct visualization of the venous system of the extremity is the most accurate method of confirming the diagnosis of venous thrombosis and the extent of the involvement. Injection is usually made into the foot while the superficial veins are occluded by tourniquet. A supplementary injection into the femoral veins may be required to visualize the iliofemoral system. Both

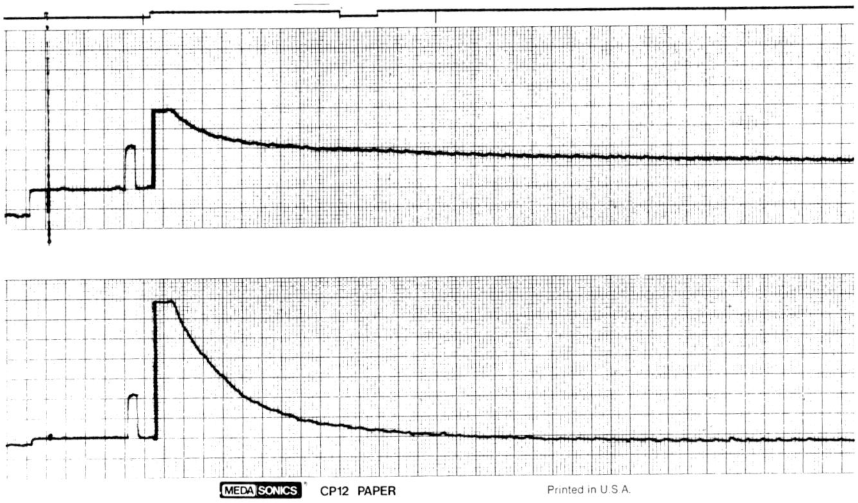

FIG. 30-3. Plethysmographic tracing shows normal response (*below*) to proximal thigh occlusion by pneumatic cuff. In contrast, the presence of an obstructing thrombus limits the volume increase after occlusion and prolongs the drainage downslope when the cuff is released (*above*).

filling defects and nonvisualization can be found and provide an assessment of the threat of a thrombus, such as from one seen to be floating free and extending into the iliofemoral system (Fig. 30-4). Potential false-positive examinations may result from external compression of a vein or washout of the contrast material from collateral veins. The procedure can also be performed with isotope injection using a gamma scintillation counter to record flow of the isotope. Delayed imaging of persistent "hot spots" may also reflect isotope retention at the sites of thrombus formation. A perfusion lung scan can also be obtained for baseline comparison and to detect silent embolism. Deep vein thrombi are less well defined with isotope injection than with contrast venography, but it is a valuable technique for sequential study of patients and avoids the potential thrombogenesis of the injection of contrast medium.

FIG. 30-4. Large free-floating thrombus within the femoral vein seen on contrast venogram (*arrow*). Such a thrombus can become detached during movement to produce pulmonary embolism.

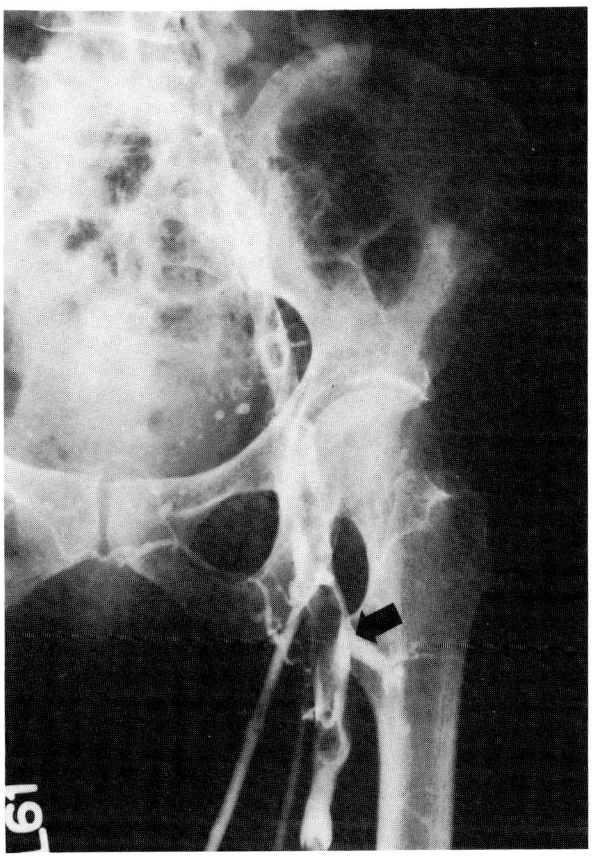

ASSAY OF FIBRIN/FIBRINOGEN PRODUCTS

The degradation of intravascular fibrin can be detected by measuring the plasma products of the lysis of fibrin or fibrinogen. Both fibrinopeptide A and fibrin fragment E can be detected by radioimmunoassay, but these are not specific for acute venous thrombosis. A negative test could conceivably have some value in excluding the diagnosis, but the tests are difficult and will require more investigation and simplification.

Prophylaxis

In theory the formation of venous thrombi should be prevented either by eliminating or reducing venous stasis or by altering blood coagulability. The belief that early ambulation prevents stasis and reduces the formation of thrombi has been controversial and not supported by studies using tagged fibrinogen. One explanation for this is that early ambulation often consists of having the patient walk to a chair and sit, whereupon the legs are subjected to even more stasis. Other efforts, including electrical stimulation of calf muscles and passive motor-driven flexion of the foot, are under investigation, but discomfort, type of operative procedure, and cost remain obvious limitations.

There has been considerably more interest in the prophylactic use of anticoagulant drugs and, more recent, drugs that inhibit platelets such as aspirin and dipyridamole. These two drugs are under evaluation for this role, but preliminary reports have not shown much protection from their use. However, there are strong data to support the use of preoperative oral anticoagulant therapy with coumarin derivatives in high-risk patients. Unfortunately, this increases the risk of hemorrhage, and with the added difficulties of laboratory control of prothrombin time, the approach has not been widely accepted. The administration of dextran 40, which produces a variety of effects on platelets and clotting factors, has been demonstrated to reduce the incidence of thrombi that can be detected, but it too can produce hemorrhagic problems as well as allergic reaction, and, in older patients, congestive failure.

In an effort to minimize the problems associated with anticoagulant prophylaxis, renewed interest in administration of heparin prior to and following surgery in low ("mini") doses that do not alter the laboratory clotting profile has arisen. Generally, a 5000-μ dose is given subcutaneously 2 hours preoperatively and then every 8 or 12 hours postoperatively for 6 days. This has appeared to provide protection for most high-risk patients with the exception of those undergoing orthopaedic procedures. The beneficial effect may be due to the enhancement of heparin cofactor (antithrombin III) as a natural inhibitor of activated factor X. Although some studies have failed to show protection, Kakkar and colleagues showed protection against fatal pulmonary embolism in a randomized series of 4121 patients as well as against deep venous thrombosis.[18] There is a higher incidence of bleeding and wound complications associated with heparin prophylaxis three times daily, and since its major benefit appears to be reducing the incidence of calf vein thrombosis, which is of questionable clinical significance, the choice of optimal prophylaxis remains unresolved.

For the general population of surgical patients under age 40 years, the risk of deep vein thrombosis is low, and prophylaxis can be limited to early ambulation with or without graduated compression stockings. For patients over age 40 undergoing major surgical procedures, the risk is moderate, and prophylaxis, such as intermittent pneumatic compression or low-dose heparin administered subcutaneously, twice daily, should be considered. The patients at highest risk, aged over 40 and obese, with malignant disease, history of deep vein thrombosis, or major trauma, need more protection, which might include low-dose heparin, intermittent pneumatic compression, oral anticoagulants, or dextran.[3] Low-dose heparin should not be used in neurosurgical patients because of the consequences of any intracranial bleeding. For these patients, external pneumatic compression is the prophylaxis of choice.

Treatment

Management of the patient with deep venous thrombosis must attempt to minimize the risk of pulmonary embolism, limit further thrombosis, and facilitate resolution of existing thrombi to avoid the postphlebitic syndrome.

Initially, the patient is placed on bed rest with the foot of the bed elevated 8 to 10 inches. Generally, pain, swelling, and tenderness resolve over a 5- to 7-day period, when ambulation with continued elastic stocking support can be permitted. Warm, moist compresses also have been used to improve blood flow and can provide symptomatic improvement. Standing still and sitting should be prohibited in order to avoid the increased venous pressure and stasis.

ANTICOAGULATION

The foundation of therapy for deep venous thrombosis is adequate anticoagulation, initially with heparin and then with coumarin derivatives for prolonged protection against recurrent thrombosis. Unless there are specific contraindications, heparin should be administered in an initial dose of 100 u to 150 u/kg intravenously. Heparin is an acid mucopolysaccharide that neutralizes thrombin, inhibits thromboplastin, and reduces the platelet release reaction. It may be administered by continuous or intermittent intravenous doses regulated by whole blood clotting time. Bleeding complications can be minimized by doses of heparin that prolong the laboratory clotting determinations in the range of twice normal with no loss of effectiveness. Continuous intravenous infusion regulated by an infusion pump seems to minimize the total dose required for control and is associated with a lower incidence of complications.

The side-effects associated with heparin treatment include bleeding, thrombocytopenia, hypersensitivity, arterial thromboembolism, and osteoporosis. Bleeding is more likely to occur in elderly females, in patients treated with aspirin, or in patients after recent surgery or trauma. It has been well demonstrated that bleeding can occur when the results of laboratory monitoring tests are within the therapeutic range, which may be due to the effect of heparin on platelets. Some evidence suggests that the risk of bleeding is proportional to the dose administered and that the risk is lessened by continuous rather than intermittent intravenous infusion.

Arterial thromboembolism can complicate heparin administration by any route and is more common in the elderly. It tends to occur after 7 to 10 days of therapy and is associated with thrombocytopenia. This complication carries high morbidity and mortality rates and requires immediate cessation of heparin treatment. Thrombocytopenia as a complication may be due to an immune reaction but is rapidly reversed when heparin is stopped, usually within 2 days. Hypersensitivity to heparin may take the form of a skin rash or, rarely, may produce anaphylaxis. Subcutaneous injections that show urticaria may become necrotic as an unusual form of sensitivity. Osteoporosis has been seen in patients on long-term heparin therapy in excess of 6 months. It is probably due to a direct effect on bone resorption and can be avoided by shorter periods of treatment and dosage less than 15,000 u/day.

Oral administration of anticoagulants is begun shortly after initiation of heparin therapy, since several days usually are required to bring the prothrombin time within the therapeutic range of two to two and a half times the control value and to provide the maximal antithrombotic effect. The coumarin derivatives block the synthesis of several clotting factors, and prolongation of the prothrombin time beyond the range suggested is associated with a high incidence of bleeding complications. The nonhemorrhagic side-effects are uncommon but include skin necrosis, dermatitis, and a syndrome of painful blue toes. Skin necrosis is heralded by painful erythema in areas of large amounts of subcutaneous fat and is reversible if the drug is stopped. Fortunately, the administration of vitamin K usually can rapidly restore the prothrombin time. After an episode of acute deep venous thrombosis, anticoagulation should be maintained for a minimum of 3 months; some investigators favor 6 months for thrombi in the larger veins. There are many drugs that interact with the coumarin derivatives (e.g., barbiturates), and therefore a routine for regular monitoring of prothrombin time is essential after the patient leaves the hospital. Oral anticoagulants are teratogenic and should not be used during established or planned pregnancy. In the pregnant patient, heparin is the drug of choice, and for long-term management, subcutaneous self-administration should be taught. This regimen allows a normal delivery and can be continued postpartum.

FIBRINOLYSIS

There has been great interest in the use of fibrinolytic agents to activate the intrinsic plasmin system. Both streptokinase and urokinase have been used and found to be effective although associated with a high incidence of hemorrhagic complications. Streptokinase is also associated in 10% of patients with allergic reactions, which vary from urticaria to anaphylaxis. In addition, it offers no advantage over heparin in the treatment of recurrent venous thrombosis or when thrombosis has existed for over 72 hours, and the lytic agents are contraindicated in the postoperative or posttraumatic patient. Rarely, the fibrinolytic agent has apparently lysed the attachment of the thrombus, allowing it to embolize.

SURGICAL APPROACHES

Operative Thrombectomy

A direct surgical approach to remove thrombi from the deep veins of the leg by way of the common femoral vein has been employed and facilitated by the use of Fogarty venous balloon catheters and an elastic wrap for milking the extremity. Although the operative results are impressive, venograms obtained prior to discharge from the hospital show rethrombosis in the majority of patients, and there does not seem to be any lesser incidence of the postphlebitic syndrome. Consequently, the procedure is now usually reserved for limb salvage in the presence of phlegmasia cerulea dolens and impending venous gangrene.

Vena Cava Interruption

Adequate anticoagulation usually is effective in managing deep venous thrombosis, but if recurrent pulmonary embolism occurs during anticoagulant therapy or if there is a contraindication to anticoagulation, then a surgical approach is necessary. Operation is also indicated as prophylaxis against recurrence of embolism for the patient who has required pulmonary embolectomy and in some high-risk patients who could not tolerate recurrence.

Indications for Insertion of a Vena Caval Filter

- Recurrent thromboembolism in spite of adequate anticoagulation
- Documented thromboembolism in a patient who has a contraindication to anticoagulation
- Complication of anticoagulation forcing therapy to be discontinued

Chronic pulmonary embolism with associated pulmonary hypertension and cor pulmonale (class V patient)
Immediately following pulmonary embolectomy
Septic pulmonary embolism
Relative indications: patient with more than 50% of the pulmonary vascular bed occluded (class III) who would not tolerate any additional embolism; patient with a propagating iliofemoral thrombus despite anticoagulation; patient with a large free-floating iliofemoral thrombus on venogram

Early surgical efforts to prevent recurrence of pulmonary embolism were directed to the common femoral vein, which was ligated bilaterally. This resulted in a high incidence of sequelae owing to stasis in the lower extremities and an unacceptable rate of recurrent pulmonary embolism. The next approach was ligation of the inferior vena cava below the renal veins, which added the adverse effect of a sudden reduction in cardiac output. This effect, coupled with stasis sequelae and recurrent embolism through dilated collateral veins, led to efforts to compartmentalize the vena cava by means of sutures, staples, and external clips in order to provide filtration without occlusion.

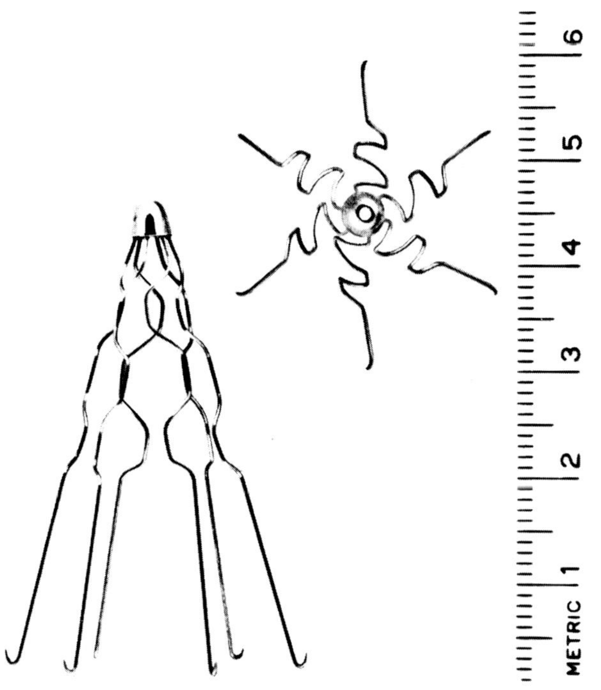

FIG. 30-5. The Greenfield filter permits trapping of emboli without loss of patency because of the geometry of the cone. If a thrombus is trapped in the filter, flow can continue around it to facilitate lysis and avoid the stasis sequelae of complete vena caval occlusion.

Since these procedures required general anesthesia and laparotomy, the next logical step was to devise a transvenous approach that could be performed under local anesthesia. The Mobin–Uddin "umbrella" unit was the first to be inserted from the jugular vein and positioned under fluoroscopy below the renal veins, where it usually produced thrombosis of the vena cava (70% of cases).[6] It also has been associated with complications of proximal thrombus formation and lethal migration into the pulmonary artery.

The Greenfield cone-shaped filter was developed to maintain patency after trapping emboli and to permit continued flow to avoid stasis and facilitate lysis of the embolus (Fig. 30-5). It can be inserted from either the jugular vein or the femoral vein, the femoral reserved for inadequate size of the jugular vein or open wound of the neck.[10] The recurrent embolism rate with this device has been 2% to 4%, and its long-term patency rate of 95% allows it to be placed above the renal veins when necessary for embolism control, such as thrombus within the renal veins or vena cava.[14] Another device, the Hunter balloon, occludes the vena cava after positioning below the renal veins and contributes to stasis sequelae. Additional indications for vena caval filter placement can be found in the management section of Pulmonary Embolism.

The complications of filter insertion range in severity from minor wound hematomas due to early resumption of anticoagulation to potentially lethal migration of the device into the pulmonary artery, as documented with the Mobin–Uddin umbrella. The most common complication with the Greenfield filter has been misplacement in 7% of cases.[10] When the filter is misplaced below the diaphragm, the patient has inadequate protection but the location (renal or iliac vein) poses no regional problem. A second filter can be placed in the appropriate location, or the misplaced filter can be retrieved using a guidewire, which is always advocated if there has been misplacement into the right heart (Fig. 30-6).[11] Air embolism can occur during jugular insertion, but the risk is minimized by having the patient hold his breath while the vein is open. In some patients the veins may be too small or fragile to permit insertion of the carrier catheter, and rarely the patient may be too obese to permit fluoroscopy.

Recurrent embolism after filter placement has been seen in 2% to 4% of cases and may be due to a source of thrombus outside of the filtered flow,

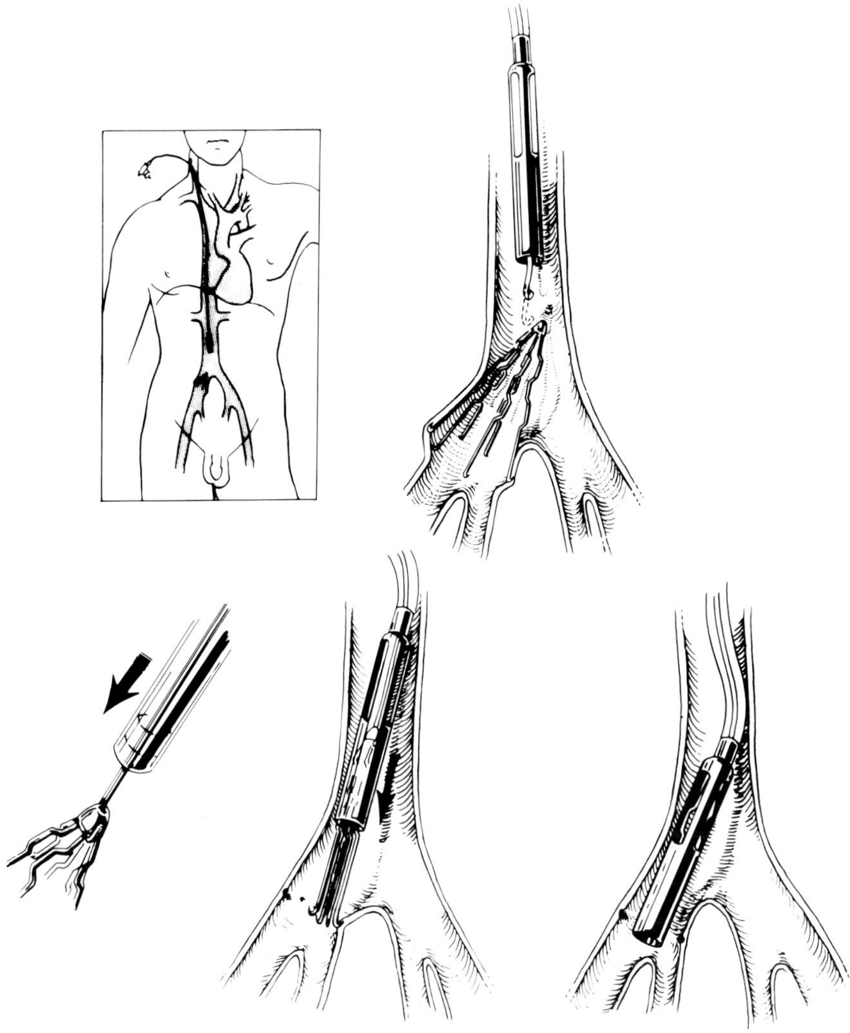

FIG. 30-6. Retrieval of a misplaced filter is possible with a guidewire bent to a J shape and used to hook the apex of the filter (*lower left*). The cylinder is advanced as the guidewire is held to fold the limbs in the cylinder (*middle*). The hooks can be disengaged by advancing the cylinder, but they may protrude from it, preventing proximal removal. (Greenfield LJ et al: Transvenous management of pulmonary embolic disease. Ann Surg 180:461, 1974)

such as the upper extremities or the right atrium. In one case a tilted filter was found to have allowed proximal thrombus formation, but this responded to treatment with urokinase and oral anticoagulation.[14]

Secondary infection of the Mobin–Uddin umbrella has been reported and required removal of the device. Secondary infection of captured thrombus within a Greenfield filter has been produced in the laboratory, but it was possible to sterilize the stainless steel filter and thrombus with antibiotic therapy. The capture of a very large embolus within a filter may suddenly occlude the vena cava with a precipitous fall in blood pressure. In a patient with known prior pulmonary embolism, this event can be mistaken for recurrent pulmonary embolism with disastrous results from vasopressor therapy. The basic distinction between functional hypovolemia and right ventricular overload can be made by the measurement of central venous pressure and PaO_2. The response to volume resuscitation for the patient with sudden vena caval occlusion should be dramatic.

There is one circumstance in which migration of a Greenfield filter is possible after discharge, that is, when heparinized saline is not flushed through the cylindrical carrier and a thrombus forms within it during the period of positioning under fluoroscopy. The thrombus can then tether the limbs of the filter, preventing their expansion and fixation to the wall of the vena cava. Only one such episode has been reported to me, and it remains a complication that can be completely avoided. For optimal protection a continuous drip of heparinized saline can be attached by intravenous tubing directly to the insertion catheter. An improved technique of insertion over a guide wire should minimize this complication.[15a]

Other Types of Venous Thrombosis

The term *thrombophlebitis* should be restricted to the disorder of the superficial veins characterized by a local inflammatory process that is usually aseptic. The cause in the upper limb is usually acidic fluid infusion or prolonged cannulation. In the lower extremities, it is usually associated with varicose veins and may coexist with deep vein thrombosis. The association with the injection of contrast material can be minimized by washout of the contrast material with heparinized saline.

THROMBOPHLEBITIS MIGRANS

Thrombophlebitis migrans, a condition of recurrent episodes of superficial thrombophlebitis, has been associated with visceral malignancy, systemic collagen vascular disease, and blood dyscrasias. Involvement of the deep veins and the visceral veins has also been described.

SUBCLAVIAN VEIN THROMBOSIS

Subclavian vein thrombosis is most likely to be secondary to an indwelling catheter and can occur in children. It may also occur as a primary event in a young, athletic person ("effort thrombosis"), presumably as a result of injury at the thoracic inlet. There is usually a satisfactory response to elevation and anticoagulation, although some venous insufficiency and discomfort with exercise may persist.

ABDOMINAL VEIN THROMBOSIS

Thrombosis of the inferior vena cava can result from tumor invasion or propagating thrombus from the iliac veins. Most common, however, it results from ligation, plication, or insertion of partially occluding caval devices such as the Mobin–Uddin umbrella. Any caval filtration device can become totally occluded by a trapped massive thrombus with sudden reduction in venous return and cardiac output, as described previously. Thrombosis of the renal vein is most likely to be associated with the nephrotic syndrome. It can be a source of thromboembolism and has been treated successfully by suprarenal placement of the Greenfield filter.[13]

Portal vein thrombosis may occur in the neonate, usually secondary to propagating septic thrombophlebitis of the umbilical vein. Collateral development leads to the occurrence of esophageal varices. Thrombosis of the portal, hepatic, splenic, or superior mesenteric vein in the adult can occur spontaneously, but usually it is associated with hepatic cirrhosis. Thrombosis of mesenteric or omental veins can simulate an acute abdomen but usually results in prolonged ileus rather than intestinal infarction.

Hepatic vein thrombosis (Budd–Chiari syndrome) usually produces massive hepatomegaly, ascites, and liver failure. It can be associated with a congenital web, endophlebitis, or polycythemia vera. Although some success has been reported using a direct approach to the congenital webs, the usual treatment is a side-to-side portacaval shunt to allow decompression of the liver. The development of pelvic sepsis after abortion, tubal infection, or puerperal sepsis can lead to septic thrombophlebitis of the pelvic veins and septic thromboembolism. Ovarian vein and caval ligation have been the traditional treatment, but the emphasis should be on drainage or excision of the abscesses and appropriate antibiotic therapy. We have also used the Greenfield filter for this thrombosis since the filter is inert stainless steel and does not lead to the development of an intraluminal abscess, which could occur after the traditional approach of ligation of the vena cava.

Pulmonary Thromboembolism

The clinical significance of major pulmonary embolism can be appreciated from the annual rate of mortality attributed to it, which has been estimated to be 90,000 deaths in the United States alone. It is estimated that 5 of every 1000 adults undergoing major surgery will die from massive pulmonary embolism. Since it represents the most important complication of deep vein thrombosis, it is of particular concern to surgeons whose patients are prone to develop deep vein thrombosis in the immediate postoperative period. The full spectrum of the disorder ranges from asymptomatic minor embolism to sudden death from massive embolism.

DIAGNOSIS

The signs and symptoms of an embolic episode obviously depend primarily on the quantity of embolus involved and to a lesser extent on the cardiopulmonary status of the patient. In the classic presentation, the patient suddenly develops chest pain, cough, dyspnea, tachypnea, and marked anxiety. Although hemoptysis has traditionally been associated with pulmonary embolism, it is actually an uncommon sign; when present it usually occurs late in the course and probably represents pulmonary infarction. Objectively, the patient with major embolism usually shows tachycardia, an increased pulmonary second sound, cyanosis, prominent jugular veins, and varying degrees of collapse. Less common, there may be wheezing, a pleural friction rub, splinting of the chest wall, rales, low-grade fever, ventricular gallop, and wide splitting of the pulmonic second sound. The incidence of these findings is shown in Table 30-1.

The differential diagnosis includes esophageal perforation, pneumonia, septic shock, and myocardial infarction. Since all of these entities are life threatening, it is mandatory that an orderly approach be formulated to confirm or reject the working diagnosis. Laboratory studies in general are not very helpful in the differential diagnosis, although a white blood cell count of less than 15,000 per ml may help to rule out pneumonitis when a pulmonary infiltrate is present.[3] The following determinations are particularly useful in the evaluation of suspected major embolism.

TABLE 30-1. CLINICAL MANIFESTATIONS OF MAJOR PULMONARY EMBOLISM

Symptoms	Incidence (%)	Signs	Incidence (%)
Dyspnea	80	Tachypnea	88
Apprehension	60	Tachycardia	63
Pleural pain	60	Accentuated P_2	60
Cough	50	Rales	51
Hemoptysis	27	S_3 or S_4	47
Syncope	22	Pleural rub	17

(Data from the Urokinase Pulmonary Embolism Trial: A national cooperative study. Circulation [Suppl] 2:47, 1973)

Electrocardiography

The most common electrocardiographic change associated with pulmonary embolism is nonspecific ST- and T-wave changes (66% of patients). More specific signs of right ventricular overload such as the often quoted S_1, Q_3, T_3 pattern are seldom seen. Consequently, the primary value of the electrocardiogram is to exclude the presence of a myocardial infarction. Unfortunately, the finding of a myocardial infarction does not exclude the diagnosis of pulmonary embolism, and in some cases a pulmonary angiogram may be required to clarify the problem.

Chest Radiography

Although the chest radiograph may suggest the diagnosis of pulmonary embolism because of central vascular enlargement, asymmetry of the vascular markings with segmental or lobar ischemia (Westermark's sign), or pleural effusion, these signs are nonspecific. The chest radiograph then serves to exclude other diagnostic possibilities such as pneumonia, pneumothorax, esophageal perforation, or congestive heart failure. It also is essential in the interpretation of a lung scan, since any radiographic density or evidence of chronic lung disease makes a perfusion defect in that area less likely to represent pulmonary embolism. Chronic lung disease also reduces the applicability of lung scanning to the diagnosis.

Arterial Blood Gases

The more widespread availability of blood gas and pH determinations has improved the assessment of all critically ill patients and provides important support for the diagnosis of pulmonary embolism. Hypoxemia with PaO_2 less than 60 torr is found in the majority of patients and is thought to be due to shunting by overperfusion of nonembolized lung and widened alveolar–arterial oxygen gradient due to reduced cardiac output. The reduction in arterial PCO_2 that follows major embolism is the most discriminating finding, since hypoxemia can be seen in several disorders likely to be misdiagnosed as massive embolism (*e.g.*, septic shock).[8] In the absence of hypoxemia and hypocarbia, the diagnosis of major embolism in the severely ill patient can be excluded with a high level of confidence, and an alternate diagnosis should be sought.

Central Venous Pressure

In the patient with systemic hypotension, the central venous pressure line can provide valuable information as well as access for administration of drugs and fluids. Low central venous pressure virtually excludes pulmonary embolism as the primary cause of the hypotension, since massive embolism almost always is accompanied by right ventricular overload and elevated right atrial pressures. Elevated right ventricular filling pressures may be transient, however, as hemodynamic accommodation occurs, and in subacute or chronic embolism the central venous pressure may be normal.

Lung Scan

Availability and widespread usage of lung photoscanning has led to overemphasis on this test and a tendency to overdiagnosis of pulmonary embolism. In the presence of a normal chest radiograph and in a nonhypotensive patient, the lung scan is a valuable screening test that has increasing validity as the size of the perfusion defect approaches lobar distribution. Smaller peripheral perfusion defects are much more difficult to interpret, since pneumonitis, atelectasis, or other ventilation abnormalities alter pulmonary perfusion. A normal lung scan, on the other hand, usually excludes the diagnosis of pulmonary embolism. Adding a ventilation scan for combined ventilation–perfusion imaging increases the accuracy of the diagnosis of thromboembolism, provided that there are at least two moderate-size or one large area of ventilation–perfusion mismatch. The assumption that the underperfused regions of the lung after embolism will remain normally ventilated, producing the mismatch in the scans, is clouded by the known physiologic effect of bronchoconstriction produced by embolism. Adding the additional variable of wide variance in scan interpretation among observers makes the diagnosis much more reliable when it is based on arteriography.[2]

Pulmonary Arteriography

Selective pulmonary arteriography is the most accurate method of confirming the presence, size, and distribution of pulmonary emboli. The procedure is inavasive, requiring passage of a cardiac catheter into the main pulmonary artery for injection of a bolus of contrast medium. A rapid film changer produces a series of radiographs that outline areas of decreased perfusion and usually show filling defects or the rounded trailing edge of impacted emboli. Straight cutoffs of the smaller pulmonary arteries are more difficult to interpret, particularly if there is associated chronic lung disease that tends to obliterate pulmonary vessels. The procedure can be performed with low risk, although this is the most hazardous group of patients for this type of study, which usually carries a 0.5% mortality rate.[2] Avoidance of main pulmonary artery injection of contrast minimizes the complication rate. Additional useful information is obtained prior to contrast injection by measurement of pulmonary arterial pressures. A normal pulmonary angiogram excludes the diagnosis of pulmonary embolism in acutely ill patients. Although the resolution rate for pulmonary emboli is unpredictable, it is unrealistic to assume that a negative arteriogram within a week of the clinical event might miss the diagnosis because of rapid fibrinolysis. In the Urokinase Pulmonary Embolism Trial report, the earliest complete resolution was not seen before 14 days.[24]

PATHOPHYSIOLOGY

Although deep vein thrombosis precedes pulmonary embolism, less than 33% of patients with documented pulmonary embolism show signs of venous thrombosis. Despite this, it is estimated that 85% to 90% of all pulmonary emboli originate from the veins of the lower extremity, while the remainder arise from the right side of the heart or other veins. In fact, the lower incidence of deep vein thrombosis after embolism may reflect the evacuation of the thrombus from the lower extremity. In addition, the emboli tend to be multiple, fragmenting either in the right side of the heart or during impaction into the pulmonary vascular bed. Older thrombi, however, contain laminated fibrin layers that make them more solid and more difficult to lyse.

Once the embolus has lodged and interrupted pulmonary blood flow, the ratio of regional ventilation to perfusion increases and the lung responds by bronchoconstriction to reduce wasted ventilation. This response is mediated by local reduction in CO_2 output, since it can be prevented by ventilation with increased concentration of CO_2. Some experimental studies also suggest a generalized neural reflex vasoconstriction, but even if this occurs in humans, it is not likely to be as significant a factor in survival as the mechanical effect of major vascular occlusion. Similarly, the effects of vasoactive humoral agents can be demonstrated in animals, and there is strong documentation that serotonin is elaborated from platelets adherent to the embolus, which also contributes to the bronchoconstriction observed. The ability of heparin to inhibit the release of serotonin adds further weight to the early use of this drug. Other vasoactive agents such as histamine and prostaglandins may play a role in humans, but the net effect is a reduction in size of peripheral airways, reduced lung volume, and reduced static pulmonary compliance.

The hypoxemia that characterizes major embolism is thought to be due to a ventilation–perfusion imbalance secondary to the ventilation changes described above, although the findings in some patients resemble true arteriovenous shunting. The latter becomes anatomically possible if there is an unobliterated foramen ovale that opens in the presence of elevated right atrial pressures. Such an opening may allow passage of a venous embolus into the systemic circulation, which then is termed *paradoxical embolism.* Although there may be some improvement in PaO_2 after supplemental oxygen is administered, the effects usually are minimal. The return of pulmonary blood flow effected by embolectomy restores respiratory gas exchange, but the ischemia appears to result in some loss of capillary integrity, causing interstitial pulmonary edema or overt pulmonary hemorrhage.

Pulmonary infarction as a consequence of embolism is relatively rare and is associated clinically with problems of poor systemic perfusion such as shock or congestive heart failure. In these patients the symptoms include pleuritic chest pain, dyspnea, cough, and hemoptysis. The signs include fever, tachycardia, splinting, and occasionally friction rub. There is usually prominent leukocytosis, an elevated lactic dehydrogenase level, and bilirubinemia. A wedge-shaped density usually is seen on chest radiography.

The pulmonary vascular and cardiac effects of embolism are a direct consequence of the degree of obstruction of the pulmonary vascular bed. Occlusion of more than 30% of the vascular tree is required to begin to elevate mean pulmonary artery pressure, and usually more than 50% occlusion is required to

TABLE 30-2. CLASSIFICATION OF PULMONARY THROMBOEMBOLISM

Class	Symptoms	Gases (torr)	PA Occlusion (%)	Hemodynamics
I	None	Normal	<20	Normal
II	Anxiety, hyperventilation	PaO_2 <80 $PaCO_2$ <35	20–30	Tachycardia
III	Dyspnea, collapse	PaO_2 <65 $PaCO_2$ <30	30–50	CVP elevated, $\overline{PA}$ >20 torr
IV	Shock, dyspnea	PaO_2 <50 $PaCO_2$ <30	>50	CVP elevated, $\overline{PA}$ >25 torr BP <100 torr
V	Dyspnea, syncope	PaO_2 <50 $PaCO_2$ 30–40	>50	PA >40 torr, CVP elevated, CO_2 low, no shock

PA, pulmonary artery; CVP, central venous pressure; $\overline{PA}$, pulmonary artery pressure; BP, blood pressure.

reduce systemic pressure. The degree of pulmonary hypertension produced is proportional to the extent of angiographic vascular occlusion, but in a previously normal patient, the limit of pressure generated by the right ventricle is approximately 40 torr.

The fate of pulmonary emboli in human patients is not easy to predict, although a great deal of experimental work in animals has been reported. Injection of autologous thrombi into the pulmonary circulation of dogs is followed by relatively rapid recovery of pulmonary function and objective evidence of lysis over a period of weeks. Activation of plasminogen to plasmin, which is found in high concentration in the pulmonary circulation, promotes this fibrinolytic effect. Unfortunately, the resolution of aged thrombi proceeds more slowly and is hampered further by impaction of the embolus and isolation from pulmonary blood flow. Consequently, resolution after massive embolism in patients is unpredictable and often incomplete. It is not unusual at autopsy to find residual fibrin strands or webs in the pulmonary arteries as remnants of prior embolism.

CLASSIFICATION AND MANAGEMENT

The hemodynamic variables mentioned above provide a means of classification of patients that employs five grades of severity and is a useful guide to therapy and prognosis (Table 30-2). The minor degrees of embolism (class I and II) usually can be managed by anticoagulants alone. Heparin is selected for initial treatment in a dose range designed to prolong the partial thromboplastin time to at least twice normal. At this dosage of approximately 150 u/kg there is adequate protection against further attachment of thrombi and platelets to the embolus. The heparin should be administered intravenously by pump-regulated continuous infusion. Many clinicians also begin oral anticoagulation therapy with coumarin derivatives shortly after starting heparin administration in order to allow several days' overlap of the drugs while prothrombin time is extended into the therapeutic range.

In some patients, however, anticoagulants cannot be used because of associated problems (e.g., peptic ulcer disease), and management must be directed to a mechanical means of protection against recurrent embolism, as outlined previously (see list on pp. 411–412). Other patients, in whom anticoagulation appears to be adequate, sustain recurrent embolism and become candidates for surgical intervention. The third indication for a surgical procedure is to protect against recurrent embolism in a patient who has sustained massive pulmonary embolism requiring open or catheter embolectomy. In these patients, even though a satisfactory embolectomy of the pulmonary circulation has been performed, the original focus of venous thrombosis remains untreated and is very likely to promote recurrent embolism, usually of major sze.

There are additional relative indications for vena caval procedures to prevent embolism. One is in the high-risk patient over 40 years of age who is obese, has a serious associated medical illness (e.g., heart disease or malignant disease), has a history of recent deep vein thrombosis, and is about to undergo major surgery. Another relative indication is a long, free-floating thrombus at the groin level. The final relative indication is in the patient in whom 40% to 50% of the vascular bed has been occluded by embolism (class III) and who would most likely not be able to tolerate an additional embolus, particularly if there is associated cardiac or pulmonary disease.

Pulmonary emboli may accumulate gradually over a prolonged period if they are small enough to produce microembolism rather than macroembolism. The clinical picture in this case is then one of chronic cor pulmonale because significant pulmonary hypertension results from changes in the pulmonary vascular bed (class V). The presentation may be subtle, with only dyspnea or syncope on exertion,

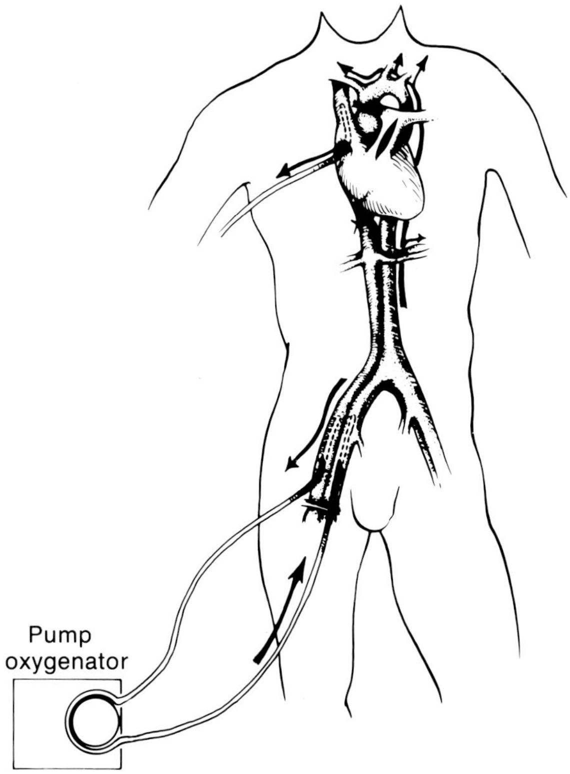

FIG. 30-7. The patient who sustains massive pulmonary embolism with shock (class IV) and fails to respond to resuscitation must be supported by partial bypass and considered for open pulmonary embolectomy. The partial bypass is accomplished by cannulation of the femoral artery and vein under local anesthesia. After general anesthesia and median sternotomy, insertion of a cannula into the superior vena cava and connection to the pump permit conversion to total bypass by snare of the inferior vena cava. The main pulmonary artery is opened, and the emboli are extracted by forceps and suction.

but there is a loud P_2 and right ventricular strain on the EKG. The sequence may also not be accompanied by significant respiratory symptoms and may explain the etiology in some of the patients considered to have primary pulmonary hypertension. When the diagnosis is made, there is a very limited life expectancy and the patient may benefit from a vena caval procedure to prevent further embolism even if the disorder is primary pulmonary hypertension.[15] The rationale is that these patients develop right heart failure predisposing them to deep vein thrombosis and pulmonary embolism, which is lethal even if it is small. When acute cardiopulmonary decompensation occurs in these patients after embolism, they are not good candidates for embolectomy because of fixation of the older thrombi to the pulmonary arterial wall. They should be classified separately (class V) and managed by long-term anticoagulation and filter placement.

When the emboli originate from a septic focus, usually the pelvis in a female, the classic treatment has been vena caval ligation with ligation of the ovarian or spermatic veins. It must be recognized, however, that large collateral veins develop as a consequence of vena caval occlusion and may then become the avenues of recurrent embolism. For this reason, we have used the Greenfield filter at either suprarenal or infrarenal levels in conjunction with antibiotic therapy, which can sterilize the stainless steel device.

The methods of vena caval protection are reviewed in the preceding section on acute deep venous thrombosis. It is worth repeating that the present transvenous methods of permanent implantation of devices in the inferior vena cava will probably be greatly enhanced by further technological improvements.

Pulmonary Embolectomy

For patients who sustain massive embolism (class III and IV), management must be coordinated and rapidly responsive, since survival may be only a matter of minutes. As indicated earlier, it is critical to document the presence of massive pulmonary embolism by pulmonary arteriography, since the clinical diagnosis, regardless of the "classic" appearance, often is in error. The initial approach to patients who have either transient collapse (class III) or persistent systemic hypotension (class IV) should include full heparinization and administration of inotropic drugs, if necessary, to support the circulation while the diagnosis is confirmed. Isoproterenol (4 mg in 1000 ml 5% dextrose in water) is useful initially because of its bronchodilator and vasodilator effects as well as its positive inotropic cardiac effect. It may provoke arrhythmias, however, and necessitate use of dopamine. For the class II patient who responds to heparin and does not require vasopressors for maintenance of systemic pressure or urine output, careful monitoring is essential to determine whether anticoagulation alone will control the disorder. Under most circumstances the spontaneous lysis of pulmonary emboli will proceed over a period of days and can be documented by serial lung scans performed at weekly intervals. The rate of clearing may be prolonged for weeks, particularly after a sizeable embolism, and may be incomplete, as indicated previously. The incomplete condition has been observed in association with persistent pulmonary hypertension even after additional lytic drugs were administered (e.g., urokinase). Lytic agents, however, may become a useful adjunct in the future.

The direct surgical approach to pulmonary embolism can be traced back to Trendelenburg (1908), who advocated a direct approach to the pulmonary artery at thoracotomy.[23] Without circulatory support, the number of survivors of these efforts was very small, and the first successful case in the United States was not reported until 1958, by Steenberg and colleagues.[21] A modification of this technique using hypothermia to occlude the circulation temporarily was reported by Allison and colleagues in 1960.[1] The very high mortality rate associated with the Trendelenburg procedure prompted the use of extracorporeal circulation to bypass the impacted pulmonary circulation. Embolectomy during cardiopulmonary bypass was reported first by Sharp in 1962.[20] Since then, partial bypass support has also been utilized; under local anesthesia, the femoral artery and vein are cannulated for venoarterial bypass (Fig. 30-7). The equipment is fully portable, and the patient can be supported during the performance of pulmonary arteriography, then transported to the operating room where he can tolerate general anesthesia and thoracotomy much better while being maintained on partial cardiopulmonary bypass. Once the sternotomy is performed, the partial bypass can be converted to total bypass by insertion of a superior vena caval catheter; the pulmonary emboli are then removed through a pulmonary arteriotomy.

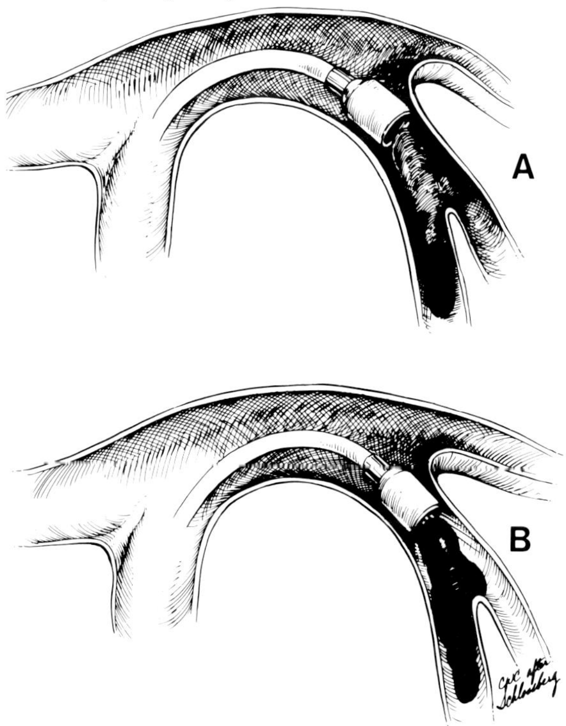

FIG. 30-8. After insertion under local anesthesia, the cup device is attached to a steerable catheter that permits entry into branches of the pulmonary artery through either the femoral or jugular vein. The catheter is positioned under fluoroscopy near the embolus identified by angiography (*A*). After injection of contrast medium to verify proximity to the embolus (*B*), the embolus is aspirated into the cup and held there by syringe vacuum as the entire catheter and embolus are withdrawn (see Fig. 30-9).

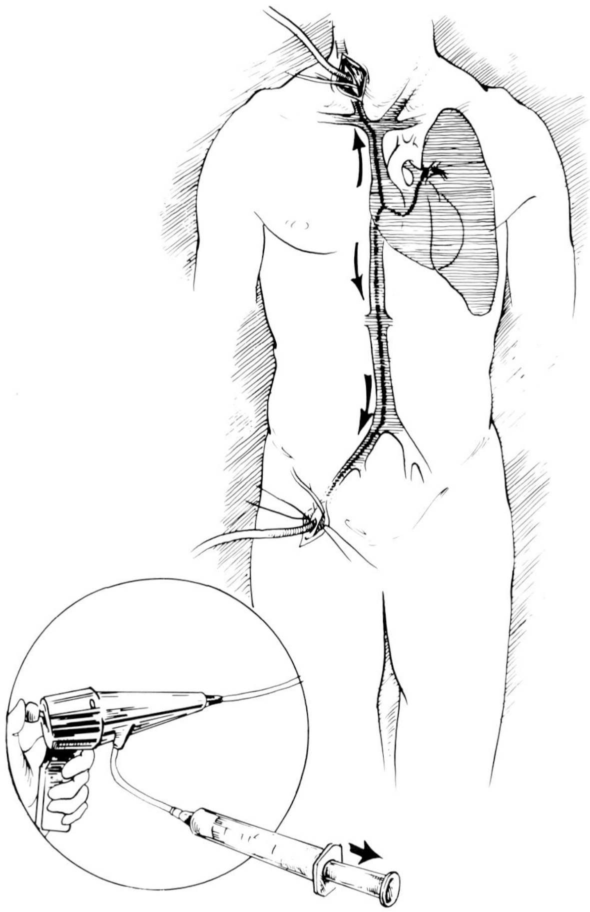

FIG. 30-9. Either the femoral or jugular veins provide access for the embolectomy catheter. The steerable cup is directed under fluoroscopy to the region of the pulmonary artery in which the embolus was identified.

Open pulmonary embolectomy still carries a high mortality rate, however, and the most serious complication is uncontrollable pulmonary hemorrhage, which may follow restoration of pulmonary perfusion.[4] Consequently, an alternative approach utilizing local anesthesia has been suggested by Greenfield and co-workers for transvenous removal of pulmonary emboli.[12] A cup device attached to a steerable catheter (Figs. 30-8 and 30-9) is inserted in the femoral or jugular vein, and the cup is positioned adjacent to the embolus seen on arteriography. The position is verified by injection of contrast medium through the catheter. Then syringe suction is applied to aspirate the embolus into the cup, where it is held by suction as the catheter and captured embolus are withdrawn (Fig. 30-10). Clinical experience with the technique, reported in 1978, in 15 patients showed that emboli could be extracted in 13 of them (87%) with an overall survival of 73%.[9] Emboli could not be removed when they had been impacted for more

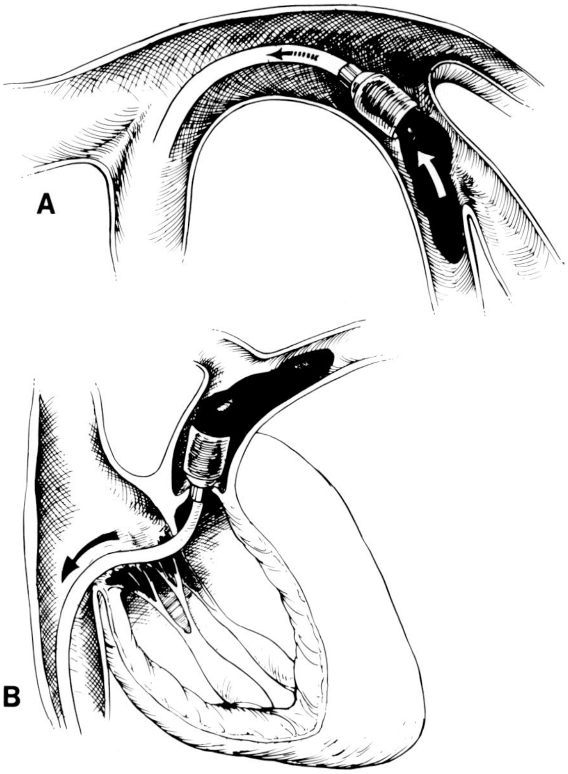

FIG. 30-10. Continuation from Figure 30-8 after positioning of the cup catheter. Syringe suction is applied, which aspirates the embolus into the cup (*A*). Maintaining suction to hold the embolus within the cup, the entire catheter is withdrawn through the right heart (*B*) and out the femoral or jugular venotomy.

than 72 hours or if the patient arrested at the time of angiography, in which case open embolectomy was required. Placement of the Greenfield vena caval filter after removal of sufficient emboli to produce nearly normal hemodynamics protected the patients from recurrent embolism.

Chronic Pulmonary Embolism and Pulmonary Hypertension

Recurrent thromboembolism may lead to progressive oblitoration of the pulmonary vascular bed if the thrombi fail to undergo lysis. The resultant pulmonary hypertension produces exertional dyspnea and signs of right heart strain with cor pulmonale. With further progression of right heart overload, tricuspid insufficiency may develop. This disorder may be difficult to distinguish from primary pulmonary hypertension, although the hypertension is more likely to be found in women under 20 years of age without a history of deep venous thrombosis. Severe pulmonary hypertension is a serious problem, usually limiting the life expectancy to less than 2 years from diagnosis.

Open thrombectomy for chronic occlusion was first performed by Allison and colleagues in 1958, and remains a possibility for improving pulmonary blood flow.[1] Unfortunately, to be eligible for this procedure, the occlusion must involve the proximal portion of the pulmonary arterial tree and the distal bed must be patent. The physiologic basis for continued distal patency after proximal occlusion is by way of the bronchial arterial collateral flow. The procedure also has a significant mortality rate, reported at 38% by Cabrol and colleagues in a series of 16 patients.[5] The complications of the procedure reported by these authors include hemorrhagic pneumonitis, cardiac failure, persistent pulmonary hypertension, pulmonary edema, hemothorax, empyema, and pulmonary infarction. The long-term results in surviving patients have been favorable, with improved respiratory function and relief of pulmonary hypertension.[19] For the majority of patients with severe pulmonary hypertension, however, the outlook is poor unless they receive maximum protection from recurrent embolism, which in our experience has required both anticoagulation and vena caval filter placement.[15]

References

1. Allison PR, Dunhill MS, Marshall R: Pulmonary embolism. Thorax 15:273, 1960
2. Bell WR, Simon TL: A comparative analysis of pulmonary perfusion scans with pulmonary angiograms—From a national cooperative study. Am Heart J 92:700, 1976
3. Bonnar J, Walsh J: Prevention of thrombosis after pelvic surgery by British dextran 70. Lancet 1:614, 1972
4. Brown S, Muller D, Buckberg G: Massive pulmonary hemorrhagic infarction following revascularization of ischemic lungs. Arch Surg 108:795, 1974
5. Cabrol C, Cabrol A, Acar J et al: Surgical correction of chronic postembolic obstruction of the pulmonary arteries. J Thorac Cardiovasc Surg 76:742, 1968
6. Cimochowski GE, Evans RH, Zarius CK et al: Greenfield filter versus Mobin–Uddin umbrella: The continuing quest for the ideal method of vena caval interruption. J Thorac Cardiovasc Surg 79:358, 1980
7. Flanc C, Kakker VV, Clarke MB: The detection of venous thrombosis of the legs using ^{125}I-labeled fibrinogen. Br J Surg 55:742, 1968
8. Goodall RJR, Greenfield LJ: Clinical correlations in the diagnosis of pulmonary embolism. Ann Surg 191(2):219, 1980
9. Greenfield LJ: Intraluminal techniques for vena caval interruption and pulmonary embolectomy. World J Surg 2:4559, 1978
10. Greenfield LJ: Technical considerations for insertion of vena caval filters. Surg Gynecol Obstet 148:422, 1979
11. Greenfield LJ, Crute SL: Retrieval of the Kimray-Greenfield[R] vena caval filter. Surgory 88(5):719, 1900
12. Greenfield LJ, Peyton MD, Brown PP, Elkins RC: Trans-

venous management of pulmonary embolic disease. Ann Surg 180:461, 1974
13. Greenfield LJ, Peyton R, Crute S: Hemodynamics and renal function following experimental suprarenal vena caval occlusion. Surg Gynecol Obstet 155:37, 1982
14. Greenfield LJ, Peyton R, Crute S, Barnes R: Greenfield vena caval filter experience: Late results in 156 patients. Arch Surg 116:1451, 1981
15. Greenfield LJ, Scher LA, Elkins RC: KMA-Greenfield[R] filter placement for chronic pulmonary hypertension. Ann Surg 189:560, 1979
15a. Greenfield LS, Stewart JR, Crute S: Improved technique for Greenfield vena caval filter insertion. Surg Gynecol Obstet 156:217, 1983
16. Hirsh J, Hull R: Comparative value of tests for the diagnosis of venous thrombosis. World J Surg 2:27, 1978
17. Innes D, Sevitt S: Coagulation and fibrinolysis in injured patients. J Clin Pathol 17:1, 1964
18. Kakkar VV, Carrigan TP, Spindler JR et al: Efficacy of low doses of heparin in prevention of deep vein thrombosis after major surgery: A double-blind, randomized trial. Lancet 2:101, 1972
19. Sabiston DC Jr, Wolfe WG, Oldham HN Jr et al: Surgical management of chronic pulmonary embolism. Ann Surg 185:699, 1977
20. Sharp EH: Pulmonary embolectomy: Successful removal of a massive pulmonary embolus with the support of cardiopulmonary bypass: A case report. Ann Surg 156:1, 1962
21. Steenburg RW, Warren R, Wilson RE, Rudolf LE: A new look at pulmonary embolectomy. Surg Gynecol Obstet 107:214, 1958
22. Strandness DE, Schultz RD, Sumner DA, Rushmer RF: Ultrasonic flow detection. A useful technique in the evaluation of peripheral vascular disease. Am J Surg 113:311, 1967
23. Trendelenburg F: Uber die operative behandlung der embolie der lungenarterie. Arch Klin Chir 86:686, 1908
24. Urokinase Pulmonary Embolism Trial: A national cooperative study. Circulation (Suppl) 2:47, 1973
25. Wheeler HB, Mullick SC: Detection of venous obstruction in the leg by measurement of electrical impedance. Ann NY Acad Sci 170:804, 1970

Part Five

Complications of Alimentary Tract Surgery and Trauma

31 Complications of Gastric Surgery

Frank G. Moody | James M. McGreevy

OVERVIEW

Operations on the stomach can be performed with minimal risk if potential complications are appreciated and steps are taken to avoid them. The stomach, in contrast to the colon, has a rich blood supply and is usually free of enteric organisms. Most complications, therefore, are not infectious in nature but rather derive from a technical error or from the extent and type of disease encountered at operation. This chapter emphasizes the importance of these factors and provides a framework whereby complications can be anticipated and thereby avoided.

Pathophysiology of Peptic Ulcer

MECHANISMS OF ACID SECRETION

The exact etiology of peptic ulcer disease remains unknown in spite of two centuries of clinical observation and intense study. Gastric acid secretion, however, is known to be a major contributing factor in duodenal ulcer.[7]

The secretion of hydrochloric acid by the parietal cells of the epithelial lining of the proximal stomach is a unique biologic process. Precisely how this occurs is not known, but current thought involves a K^+ for H^+ exchange at a critical site along the secretory canaliculus.[19] This is an energy-requiring process, for the H^+ ions must be transported against a millionfold concentration gradient. There are three well-known endogenous substances capable of initiating the secretory process: gastrin, acetylcholine, and histamine. Each, in fact, enhances the secretory potency of the other. Soll and his colleagues, working with isolated parietal cells, developed the concept that each of these substances activates a receptor on the parietal cell surface.[30] Histamine, a classic secretagogue, acts as a modulator of the secretory response and may be essential to the action of gastrin, the secretory hormone, and acetylcholine, the secretory neurotransmitter.

The key to understanding the pathogenesis and treatment of pepic ulcer disease resides in a familiarity with the mechanisms of neurohumoral control of acid secretion.[12] Pavlov appropriately emphasized the importance of cephalic factors in his early studies of acid secretion from canine gastric pouches. From his studies and those of others, we now know that the sight and smell of food activate the vagal centers within the hypothalamus, which, in turn, transmit a signal to the stomach by way of the vagus nerves. Acetylcholine is released at the terminal ends of the vagi within the gastric wall, which, in turn, leads to a release of gastrin and a sensitization of the parietal cell to both histamine and gastrin. Within minutes, acid secretion flows from gastric glands. Acetylcholine may also have a direct action on the parietal and chief cells, the latter containing pepsinogen, a proteolytic enzyme that is activated at low *p*H (3.5 or less), which derives from the active secretion of hydrochloric acid.

The stomach has numerous checks and balances against the indiscriminate secretion of hydrochloric acid. For example, the central release of gastrin is modulated by intraluminal *p*H. As antral *p*H decreases during acid secretion, the rate of gastrin release also decreases. The sympathetic nervous system also plays an as yet undefined role in modifying the acid secretory process. It may influence the delivery of gastrin to the parietal cells through its control of the microcirculation within the secretory mucosa. Prostaglandins may also impose a regulatory influence on parietal cell function, since they are potent inhibitors of acid secretion and present in high concentrations within the secretory mucosa.

Our understanding of how acid and pepsin cause a peptic ulcer is at best tentative and is based upon several loosely related observations. Patients with duodenal ulcer have rates of acid secretion increased over those of the normal population, while patients with gastric ulcer are on the low side of normal. Duodenal ulcer is accompanied by an augmented cumulative release of gastrin following a meal. In addition, duodenal ulcer patients appear to be more responsive to exogenous gastrin, suggesting a vagally primed parietal cell mass. Finally, patients with hypergastrinemia and high levels of acid secretion (Zollinger–Ellison syndrome) have a flagrant ulcer diathesis in the late stages of their disease. These clinical observations, along with the fact that inhibition or neutralization of H^+ ions leads to ulcer healing, clearly links the lesion to gastric acid. Less is known about the role of pepsin. Possibly it contributes to the chronicity of the disease through its ability to digest devitalized tissue at the margin of an ulcer. The role of blood supply is also obscure, although it is now known that mucosal microcirculation plays an important role in the pathogenesis and prevention of stress erosive gastritis.

SIGNIFICANCE OF ULCER LOCATION

The complications of peptic ulcer disease and the morbidity of their treatment by operation are directly related to the location and depth of penetration of the lesion. Superficial erosive gastritis, for example, is associated with only a minor disruption of the outer layers of the gastric epithelium. Deeper lesions may lead to free perforation into the peritoneal cavity or penetration into adjacent viscera. Posterior duodenal ulcers, for example, are notorious for producing both life-threatening hemorrhage from the gastroduodenal artery and enlargement of the head of the pancreas from acute pancreatitis. Long-standing, deeply penetrating ulcers may also contribute to a marked distortion of the gastric or duodenal wall. Repeated episodes of inflammation and repair lead to extensive fibrosis of the duodenal bulb or distal stomach with subsequent gastric outlet obstruction. These anatomical defects greatly enhance the risk of operative therapy and provide a rationale for early surgical intervention when medical therapy fails to control the disease.

FIG. 31-1. Regional gastric anatomy. The stomach occupies a position in the upper abdomen which is directly in contact with the spleen and the pancreas.

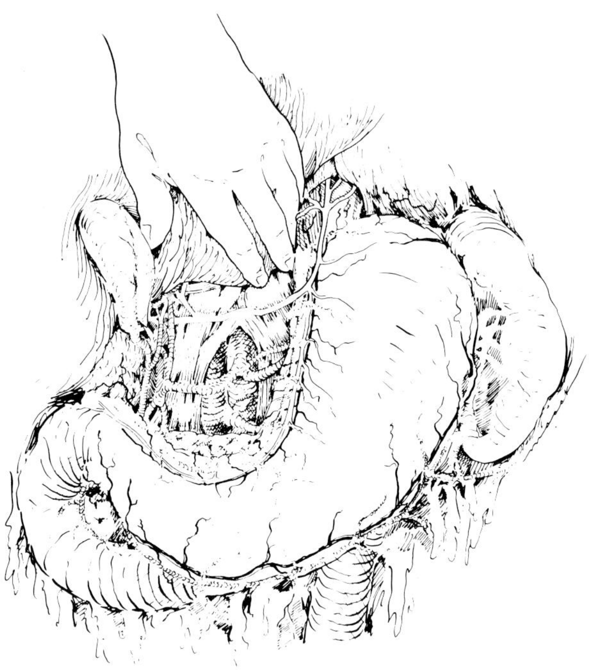

DISEASE-RELATED ANATOMICAL DIFFICULTIES

There are several specific anatomical distortions created by acid-peptic disease that deserve special consideration. The first, and most common, is the extensive scarring and inflammation associated with a long-standing posterior duodenal ulcer. It is almost predictable that such an ulcer will be associated with a marked inflammatory response within the adjacent pancreas and structures within the free edge of the gastrohepatic ligament, especially the bile duct. More distal ulcers within the second part of the duodenum may infringe upon the papilla of Vater.

Gastric lesions present a unique problem in that one cannot be sure of their origin, especially when they are large and located on the greater curve of the stomach. In this location they may be in close proximity to the middle colic artery. Their resection, therefore, regardless of their origin, may be associated with ischemic injury to the colon. High lesser-curvature lesions, while usually of acid-peptic origin, also present special considerations because of their proximity to the esophagus. It is usually desirable to leave such lesions in place and promote their resolution by decreasing gastric acid secretion by techniques described below.

This discussion would be remiss if the gastrosplenic and gastropancreatic relationships were not recognized (Fig. 31-1). There is now general agreement that the spleen should be left in place when gastric operations are performed for either peptic ulcer or gastric cancer, except for proximal lesions of gastric cancer. The days of inadvertent splenectomy are past, and every effort should be made to avoid splenic injury. This can be accomplished by appreciating the intimate vascular relationships between the stomach and spleen at the level of the upper short gastric vessels. Furthermore, adhesions between the gastrocolic omentum and the lower tip of the spleen are the rule rather than the exception and should be sought early in the course of a gastric procedure. They can be divided if they are in a position where added exposure cannot be obtained without placing undue tension upon them. Otherwise, they can be protected by avoiding tension on the omentum and by gentle, precise division of the vessels along the greater curve during gastrectomy.

Gastropancreatic relationships are equally important to recognize during operations upon the stomach. Remind yourself that even mild blunt trauma to the pancreas by your hand or an instrument may initiate an episode of acute pancreatitis. Disruption of the pancreatic capsule can lead to the extravasation of pancreatic juice into the peritoneal cavity (pancreatic ascites). The pancreas is especially vulnerable during the dissection of an inflamed duodenal bulb or the separation of an ulcer in the stomach or duodenum from its point of penetration into the pancreas. A worthwhile rule of thumb is to avoid dissection of peptic ulcers that involve the pancreas.

CONSEQUENCES OF DISEASE PROGRESSION

The consequences of disease progression can best be summarized by relating an example of how uncontrolled peptic ulcer may lead to serious complications both from the disease and its therapy. Let us consider the potential consequences of a posterior duodenal ulcer that has penetrated into the gastroduodenal artery. This lesion usually is associated with massive upper gastrointestinal bleeding (in excess of 1500 ml of blood loss) that, if not immediately treated by volume replacement, may lead to cardiovascular decompensation, arterial hypotension (shock), and tissue hypoxia. The consequences of this course of events can be severe, especially if the bleeding persists and requires operative intervention. The low perfusion state, if prolonged, has several serious sequelae. Tissue hypoxia is associated with anaerobic metabolism and the release of acid metabolites that contribute to an existing impairment of cardiac, pulmonary, and renal function. The immunologic system is compromised, thereby rendering the patient more susceptible to infectious complications. The ability to resist intravascular coagulation is disturbed, and thromboembolic complications are common. The tracheobronchial tree and alveolar function are also disturbed, contributing to a high incidence of atelectasis and pneumonitis. Finally, prolonged shock may contribute to acute tubular necrosis and renal failure, further complicating the patient's condition after therapy. It is for these reasons that peptic ulcer disease should be treated early, before serious complications occur.

Persistent or recurrent bleeding from a posterior penetrating ulcer requires surgical control. By definition, the operative risk in this situation is high for reasons outlined above. Massive hemorrhage can be lethal, especially when it occurs in the age group over 65. Once recognizing this fact, the operating surgeon should minimize intraoperative and postoperative complications by preparing both himself and the patient for an optimal outcome. Therapeutic steps would include volume and red cell replacement, correction of hematologic defects, perioperative antibiotics, detailed management of associated disease (chronic pulmonary disease, congestive heart failure, and diabetes), and an appropriate surgical intervention done well. This approach is expanded upon below for the various complications of peptic ulcer that are amenable to surgical therapy. The principles of safe operative management are extended to include gastric cancer. A discussion of the complications of gastric procedures for chronic morbid obesity is also included, since operations of this type are gradually replacing procedures for peptic ulcer and gastric cancer in their frequency. Surgical decision making and technique are emphasized, since therein lies the best possibility for a safe and effective operation.

Specific Risk Factors of Disease

Surgical diseases of the stomach may present as specific complications that in and of themselves increase the risk of operative intervention. Ulcer penetration into the pancreas, free perforation with peritonitis, gastric outlet obstruction, massive hemorrhage, and cancer each place the patient at risk for unique postoperative complications. The surgeon who is familiar with these risk factors can influence these complications with appropriate diagnostic testing, adequate preoperative preparation, and proper operative management.

PENETRATION WITHOUT HEMORRHAGE

A duodenal ulcer that penetrates into the pancreas can be suspected from a history of back pain, jaundice, or pain that is incompletely alleviated with antacids. Hyperamylasemia may be present, but it can also occur in patients with active duodenal ulcer disease without penetration. Duodenoscopy is the most reliable way to identify this complication, although it can be suspected when a large ulcer crater is identified on a barium upper gastrointestinal series (Fig. 31-2). This type of ulcer heals slowly. A medical trial is indicated with its first occurrence,

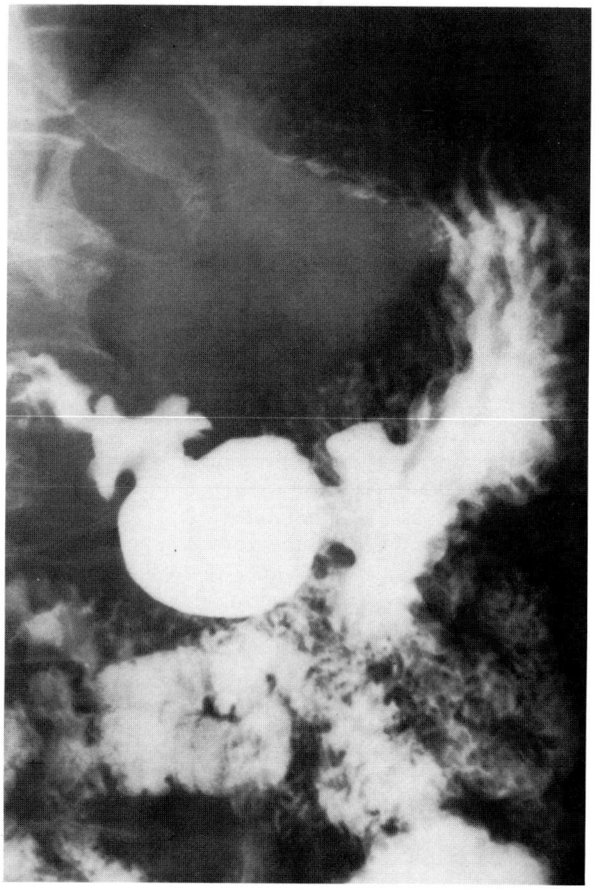

FIG. 31-2. Barium upper gastrointestinal examination. This pylorus is deformed from active ulcer disease.

but if symptoms persist or recur, surgical therapy should be undertaken.

A penetrating ulcer presents an unusual surgical challenge. In the past, such ulcers have accounted for the majority of complications and deaths from ulcer surgery. The lethality of penetrating ulcers relates to the extensive inflammatory response that may involve the pancreas, bile duct, duodenum, and other structures in the area. The procedures of choice in the past have been partial gastrectomy or antrectomy and vagotomy. Both of these operations unfortunately require dissection of the duodenum and its contained ulcer from adjacent structures. Complications from this approach include bile duct injury, acute pancreatitis, pancreatic fistula, gastroduodenal leak if a gastroduodenostomy is performed, and a blown duodenal stump if a gastrojejunostomy is employed for reconstruction of intestinal continuity.

It is now known that even deeply penetrating duodenal ulcers will heal following a complete gastric vagotomy. Furthermore, it is not necessary to bypass the deformed duodenal bulb or the ulcer crater. All that is required is an adequate drainage procedure (pyloroplasty or gastroenterostomy) at the gastric outlet. The choices for surgical therapy of this are therefore as follows:[17]

Selective vagotomy and drainage
Truncal vagotomy and drainage
Selective vagotomy and antrectomy
Truncal vagotomy and antrectomy
Partial gastrectomy

We do not recommend a proximal gastric vagotomy (highly selective) for deeply penetrating duodenal ulcer disease.

The technical features of these procedures are described below. Their rationale, however, is as follows. A selective vagotomy performed as described by Griffith and employed so successfully with antrectomy by Sawyers and Scott at Vanderbilt provides the most secure way to denervate the stomach from its central vagal connections.[11, 28] A *selective vagotomy* coupled with antrectomy offers the surest way to prevent ulcer recurrence and is the procedure of choice in patients with a long-standing chronic peptic ulcer who are at risk for recurrence but do not have an active ulcer or deep penetration at the time of operation. A gastroduodenostomy should always be performed in this circumstance in order to avoid the complications associated with a gastrojejunostomy (Billroth II reconstruction).

Why then should a *selective vagotomy* and antrectomy not be employed for a deeply penetrating active duodenal ulcer? Clearly, the risks associated with a difficult dissection in performing an antrectomy are too high. A *selective vagotomy,* with drainage either by pyloroplasty or gastrojejunostomy, provides immediate relief of symptoms and adequate protection from recurrence in 90% of patients so treated, unless they have undetected Zollinger–Ellison syndrome.

In practice, we employ a carefully performed truncal vagotomy and an appropriate pyloroplasty, depending upon the extent of duodenal deformity. Recall that with a posterior ulcer, the anterior surface of the duodenum is usually available for a standard Heineke–Mikulicz pyloroplasty. If there is marked deformity of the bulb or extensive inflammation, then a Finney pyloroplasty should be employed, since it provides for a wider opening at the gastric outlet. A gastrojejunostomy is readily accepted as an alternative drainage procedure when there is extensive inflammation or a mass in the region of the gastroduodenal junction.

When then should resection be employed? We perform an antrectomy with vagotomy in the patient in whom the ulcer is healed, but who is at risk for recurrence because of personality, smoking, drinking, or severity of past recurrences of the ulcer diathesis. Careful attention must be given during the dissection of the duodenum away from the pancreatic bed and the structures within the gastrohepatic ligament. If a residual ulcer crater is present, it should be left in place and the duodenal wall resected from it. Enough of the posterior wall of the duodenum must be mobilized to allow the performance of a gastroduodenostomy. This will prevent the most lethal complication of ulcer surgery, a blown duodenal stump. Drainage of the pancreatic bed is always required by an active drain when this approach is employed.

PERFORATION

Perforation remains one of the most serious complications of duodenal ulcer. The clinical presentation is usually dramatic and unmistakable when the patient has severe peritonitis of sudden onset associated with free intra-abdominal air on erect chest x-ray film. There may be no antecedent history of peptic ulcer complaints (⅓ of patients). However, in more subtle cases, the diagnosis can be elusive. In an autopsy series of 126 deaths from perforated ulcer, 25% were unrecognized prior to postmortem examination.[6] The diagnosis in these subtle cases may be made by air insufflation through a nasogastric tube followed by erect chest x-ray film. The extravasation of water-soluble contrast material instilled into the stomach may also indicate a perforation. A neglected or unrecognized perforation can result in intra-abdominal sepsis or may be associated with bleeding from the ulcer or obstruction from an inflammatory mass.

Even though some surgeons have successfully treated gastroduodenal perforation nonoperatively, we prefer to operate on all patients with evidence of a perforated viscus and peritonitis.[20] The 6- to 12-hour delay while waiting to see if nonoperative measures will be successful may be harmful to patients who will eventually require exploration. At operation, we prefer simple plication of the ulcer with an omental patch, as originally used by Graham, when perforation is the initial manifestation of the patient's ulcer disease. A definitive ulcer procedure is used when the patient presents with well-established symptoms or prior complications of ulcer disease, and there is not extensive soilage at the time of exploration. Highly selective vagotomy done at the time of ulcer plication may be an acceptable compromise between plication alone and a definitive ulcer operation.[27] The highly selective vagotomy does not create an anastomotic line and therefore should be safe in the face of peritonitis. In addition, the operation has few side-effects and an acceptably low recurrent ulcer rate. It is important to remember that the goal of therapy is closure of the perforation (*i.e.*, a life-saving procedure). One should not impose the burden of a complex procedure on patients who may be metabolically disturbed or septic from their complication.

OBSTRUCTION

Obstruction of the gastric outlet is usually caused by many years of active peptic ulcer disease that leads to fibrosis and narrowing of the pyloroduodenal channel. Eighty percent of patients suffering from obstruction will have had previous symptoms of ulcer disease. Those who present with obstruction and no history of ulcer pain or vomiting may have acid peptic disease but must be suspected of having cancer. The diagnosis of obstruction can be made by contrast radiography. This will show a large atonic stomach, which retains most of the barium meal 4 hours after its ingestion. The upper GI tract may appear normal in cases of partial obstruction, however, and in these cases the diagnosis of ulcer can be made by gastroduodenoscopy. The saline load test is a simple, bedside physiologic test of gastric emptying, which can confirm the diagnosis of obstruction and follow its progress during nonoperative management.[2] Seven hundred fifty milliliters of normal saline is instilled by way of the nasogastric tube, then aspirated with syringe 30 minutes later. If the gastric residual is greater than 400 ml, obstruction is present. A patent pylorus will give residuals of less than 200 ml.

The problems associated with gastric outlet obstruction are weight loss, malnutrition, hypochloremic alkalosis, gastric atony, uremia, and anemia. Each of these factors can predispose the patient to complications if it is not corrected in the preoperative period. The amount of weight loss correlates with the rates of operative mortality. Those patients with severe weight loss should be given 2 to 3 weeks of parenteral nutrition prior to operation. Correction of the nutritional deficit will decrease the risk of mortality, improve wound healing, diminish septic complications, and improve anemia. The uremia and metabolic consequences of pyloric obstruction are corrected with normal saline infusions to restore water and chloride losses. The potassium deficit may be as high as 300 mEq. Once the total body chloride and potassium concentrations are corrected, the kidney can excrete bicarbonate and restore the proper acid–base balance. During this period of preoperative preparation, the stomach is decompressed with a nasogastric tube to improve gastric tone and prevent pulmonary aspiration. Prior to operation, a dose of broad-spectrum antibiotic is given with the preoperative medications.

The choice of operation is influenced by the status of the patient. An elderly, fragile patient is best treated with a gastroenterostomy and truncal vagotomy. In fact, we tend toward this procedure in most patients with this complication, since they have "burned out" indolent ulcer disease that has a low incidence of recurrence. Others, however, prefer a partial gastrectomy with gastroduodenostomy, since this allows for reduction of the gastric mass and avoids the motility disturbances associated with truncal vagotomy. Recently we have adopted the procedure of proximal gastric vagotomy and gastrojejunostomy. Although this is an experimental approach, it has a rationale. The highly selective vagotomy should provide adequate protection from this type of low-grade ulcer disease often encountered in the older patient, while maintaining the function of the central pump, thereby reducing the complications of total vagotomy. The gastrojejunostomy provides a way to bypass the point of chronic obstruction, thereby obviating the need for dissection of the scarred duodenal bulb. An adequate pyloroplasty is also an acceptable drainage procedure.

MASSIVE HEMORRHAGE

Massive hemorrhage from duodenal ulcer disease is infrequent, but when it occurs, treatment must be swift and appropriate to avert a fatality. Hemorrhage from the upper alimentary tract, which results in hypotension that cannot be controlled by volume infusion, requires immediate laparotomy. Diagnostic tests that prolong the period of shock prior to operative control of the bleeding point cannot be justified when the risks are weighed against the information likely to be obtained. Prolonged shock can result in renal failure, myocardial infarction, pulmonary failure, and coagulopathy from massive transfusion.

Endoscopy should be performed after the stomach has been washed free of blood through the use of a large orogastric tube (Ewald). This should be done during the period of resuscitation and blood replacement in the emergency room. Identification of an actively bleeding posterior penetrating ulcer that has eroded into the gastroduodenal artery or one of its branches requires immediate operation.[1] The bleeding point within the artery should be controlled with figure-of-eight suture ligatures using 2-0 silk swedged on a stout needle. If the individual bleeding vessel cannot be identified, the ulcer base is plicated with several interrupted sutures of 2-0 silk. Once the bleeding has been controlled, a truncal vagotomy is performed and the opening through the pylorus is closed with a pyloroplasty. There is no indication for resectional therapy, since the complication implies the presence of an active ulcer the resection of which might lead to all the complications discussed above.

The incidence of rebleeding depends critically upon the care with which the bleeding points within the ulcer bed are secured. Again, we emphasize the seriousness of the complication and its shock-rendering hemorrhage. The simplest procedure with the lowest potential for operative complications should be selected. Gaining the ultimate in protection from ulcer recurrence is a secondary consideration in this situation.

If the gastroduodenostomy fails to reveal a bleeding duodenal ulcer, then a second gastrostomy should be made in the body of the stomach. This may show a bleeding gastric ulcer, diffusely bleeding gastritis, or bleeding esophageal varices. A gastric ulcer is managed by wedge excision or partial gastrectomy with gastroduodenostomy if the patient is otherwise stable. Diffusely bleeding gastritis is treated by plication of deeply penetrating lesions and a vagotomy and pyloroplasty. Esophageal varices are treated with a nonshunt procedure (vasopressin, Blakemore tube, esophageal interruption with the EEA Stapler, sclerotherapy, or oversewing) so that the patient may be prepared for an elective portasystemic shunt at a later date.

CANCER

The treatment of carcinoma of the stomach can be complicated by errors in judgment about two questions: which cancers should be resected and which type of gastrectomy should be used for the resection? Advanced gastric malignancy (stage III and stage IV) is a highly lethal disease with no long-term survivorship in spite of radical operations.[25, 29] Since the majority of gastric cancers present as advanced lesions, the overall survival rate has not changed in the past 60 years.[3] Operation has proven ineffective in the control of advanced disease, and heroic resections will result in high rates of mortality and morbidity.

Treatment of stage III and IV gastric cancer should involve simple measures if this is possible (e.g., gastrojejunostomy). Bypass operations for gastric cancer do not provide good palliation; however, the alternative of extended gastrectomy and reconstruction with jejunal loop is likely to fail owing to rapid local recurrence.[3] Early lesions are not fixed to the adjacent organs, with no disease in lymph nodes beyond 3 cm from the tumor (stages I and II). This type of early gastric malignancy is best managed with a subtotal gastrectomy that provides a 10-cm margin. While total gastrectomy for early cancer may provide a longer term of survival than would subtotal gastrectomy, it is associated with a higher rate of morbidity and should be used only where large numbers of such procedures are performed.[25, 29]

The complications of operations for gastric cancer, therefore, relate to a variety of technical problems, the extent of the disease, and the nutritional status of the patient at the time of surgery. Patients who are nutritionally depleted suffer a variety of metabolic defects. Hypoproteinemia may compromise their ability to contain fluid within the intravascular compartment of their extracellular space. Furthermore, severe protein deficiency may compromise the healing of their anastomosis and wound. Probably more important is the immunodeficiency state that accompanies advanced cancer and malnutrition. There is, therefore, a need to consider a preoperative course of parenteral hyperalimentation in this population of patients. They may also need repletion of their red cell mass.

Patients with gastric cancer are in one important way different from those with acid peptic disease. They may be achlorhydric and often have a stomach that is populated with enteric organisms. They should be prepared by a modified chemical bowel preparation in which the stomach is washed three times at 6-hour intervals by a nasogastric tube with 200 ml of a 1% neomycin solution on the day prior to operation. Broad-spectrum antibiotics should be used preoperatively and continued in the recovery room only.

Subtotal gastrectomy with omentectomy and ligation of the right and left gastric arteries and the right gastroepiploic artery at their base is the procedure of choice. With distal lesions, at least 4 cm of the first part of the duodenum should be resected. A gastrojejunostomy is always performed in reconstruction in order to minimize the chances of recurrence that might accompany a gastroduodenostomy. A splenectomy in continuity will sometimes facilitate removal of a high-lying cancer. Total gastrectomy is also indicated in bulky tumors that have not spread, high-lying lesions, and in linitis plastica confined to the gastric wall. A well-trained surgeon who is willing to take the time and care to perform a careful operation can offer considerable palliation in this dismal disease. The complication rate is high, but so is the suffering associated with unoperated advanced gastric cancer.

Endoscopic Complications

Modern gastroduodenoscopy has developed into a safe diagnostic procedure. Complications are rare and basically derive from perforation at the gastroesophageal junction or bleeding from a biopsy site. There is an occasional adverse reaction to the sedative employed for the procedure or aspiration of gastric contents during its performance.

Perforation of the esophagus or stomach is suspected when the patient complains of chest or abdominal pain. A chest x-ray film may show signs of perforation with mediastinal air, pleural fluid, or free air under the diaphragm. Confirmation should be obtained with a water-soluble contrast swallow. Once the diagnosis of perforation has been established, we believe that exploratory thoracotomy or laparotomy is indicated. Early, small perforations can be treated with primary closure and drainage, supplemented with parenteral nutrition and antibiotics. Late perforation with collections of infected fluid requires drainage with the possibility that a later reconstruction may be required if stricture or fistula results. Major perforations with sepsis and esophageal necrosis are best treated with esophageal exclusion and later reconstruction with gastric transposition or colon interposition. Nonoperative treatment with total parenteral nutrition and antibiotics may be successful with small esophageal perforations. Operative delay, however, may preclude the chance for primary closure of the esophageal wound. Gastric and duodenal perforations are usually apparent early and respond to simple plication.

Bleeding from a biopsy site may present as hematemesis following the endoscopy or a gradual drop in hematocrit with melena. Persistent blood loss that requires transfusion is an indication for endoscopy and electrocautery or photocoagulation of the biopsy site. If this fails, celiotomy with suture ligature of the biopsy site may be required.

Technique and Intraoperative Complications

Some complications can be avoided by proper selection and preparation of the patient upon whom a procedure is to be performed. For example, young, tall, healthy people at their ideal weight, without associated disease, who neither drink nor smoke make excellent candidates for operation. But, unfortunately, people with stomach diseases usually do not present that way in our country. The thrust of surgical therapy, therefore, must be related to early diagnosis, matching of the patient to the safest and most effective operation for the problem to be treated, and the careful performance of the procedure.[24] Gastric operations require attention to fine details of technique. The following suggestions may help to avoid intraoperative problems that may prolong the recovery period and avoid serious long-term sequelae.

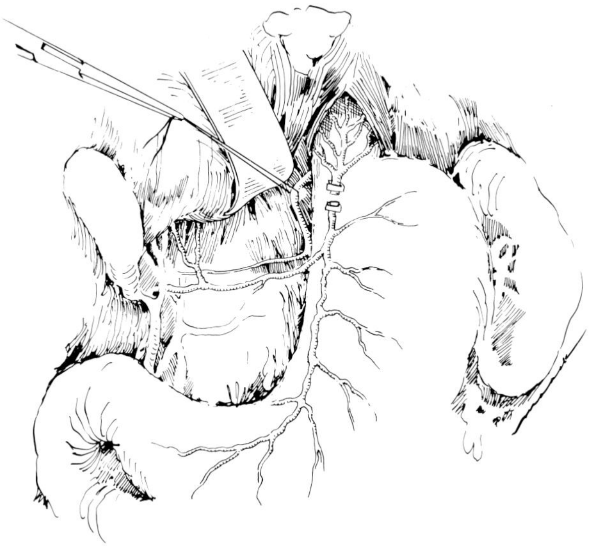

FIG. 31-3. Truncal vagotomy. The anterior vagus nerve has been severed by removing a centimeter of it between metallic clips. The posterior nerve has been isolated in preparation for vagectomy.

Operations within the peritoneal cavity require good exposure, and procedures on the stomach and the vagus nerves are not without exception to this important surgical principle. A midline incision from xiphoid to umbilicus is usually adequate for this purpose. It is direct, bloodless, and provides easy access to the upper abdomen. A retractor placed beneath the costal confluence at the xiphoid and attached to a fixed frame provides a full view of the contents of the upper abdomen. Exploration of the peritoneal cavity should be carried out during elective procedures.

Care must be taken when applying traction to the gastrocolic omentum housed within the left upper abdomen, since this may lead to a capsular tear of the spleen. We prefer to leave the colon and gastrocolic omentum within the abdomen during gastric procedures. This keeps loops of small bowel from wandering into the field and reduces heat loss and drying of the serosal surfaces of intra-abdominal viscera.

A headlight is useful for operations within the abdominal cavity. This device provides for maximal illumination wherever the surgeon's eyes are directed, thereby obviating the need for constant changes of the overhead light.

Finally, be precise. Always see what you are cutting. Use fine clamps, fine sutures for ties, sharp dissection, and good judgment. Avoid blunt dissection, rough maneuvers, and short cuts that present an incalculable or identifiable risk. Modern anesthesia precludes the need for rapid surgery. Proceed at a steady, efficient pace, which insures a safe outcome every time.

VAGOTOMY

The vagus nerves have been conveniently placed within the abdomen where they can be easily identified as they course through the esophageal hiatus. Recall that the left vagus lies anterior, and it usually branches high into two or more trunks. It gives off its anterior branch before it terminates within the anterior nerve of Laterjet. The right vagus is a stout trunk that lies posterior to the esophagus. It may, in 20% of cases, provide a small branch to the left called the "criminal nerve" of Grassi, since it is commonly overlooked. The celiac branch, which goes posteriorly, is its major extragastric communication. It then terminates within the posterior nerve of Laterjet. The major complications with vagotomy are threefold:

Esophageal or gastric perforation
Splenic injury
Incomplete vagotomy

These are considered in the context of the three types of vagotomy currently in use: truncal, selective, and proximal gastric vagotomy.

Truncal Vagotomy

We prefer to perform truncal vagotomy under direct vision, without mobilizing the esophagus from its bed within the lower part of the mediastinum (Fig. 31-3). This is accomplished by first incising the peritoneum overlying the esophagogastric junction. Downward traction on the anterior surface of the upper part of the stomach and elevation of the left lobe of the liver by a Herrington retractor provide a full view of the branches of the anterior vagus. They are elevated with a right-angled clamp under direct vision, clipped, and divided, providing a 2-cm interruption of the nerve. The dissection is then carried to the right side of the esophagus, and with the operator's middle finger of the left hand inserted between the esophagus and right side of the right crus, the index finger can feel the position of the posterior vagal trunk as downward traction is exerted. A 2-cm segment of the nerve is divided between clips. Accessory nerves are sought. Finding none, the operation is complete. Note that the nerves and their branches have been identified, and there has been no blunt dissection behind the esophagus. There is no possibility for esophageal or gastric injury. Splenic injury is another matter. It may result from excessive traction on the gastrosplenic ligament, capsular tear from an adhesion, or trauma from drift of the retractor elevating the left lobe of

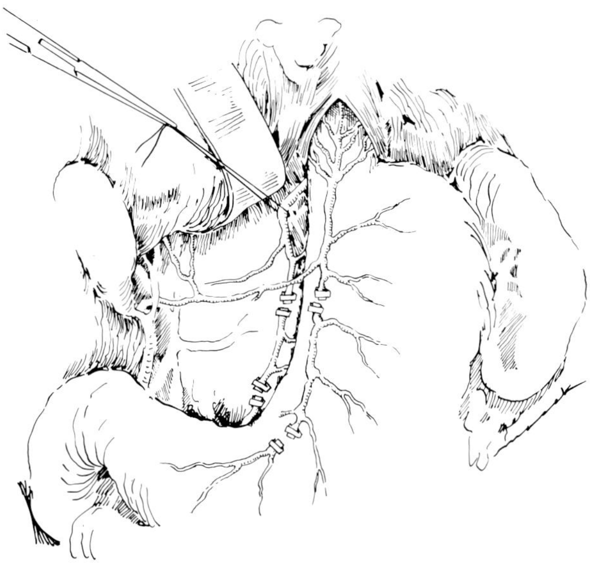

FIG. 31-4. Selective vagotomy. The anterior and posterior nerves of Latarjet have been divided below the branches to the hepatic and celiac ganglia.

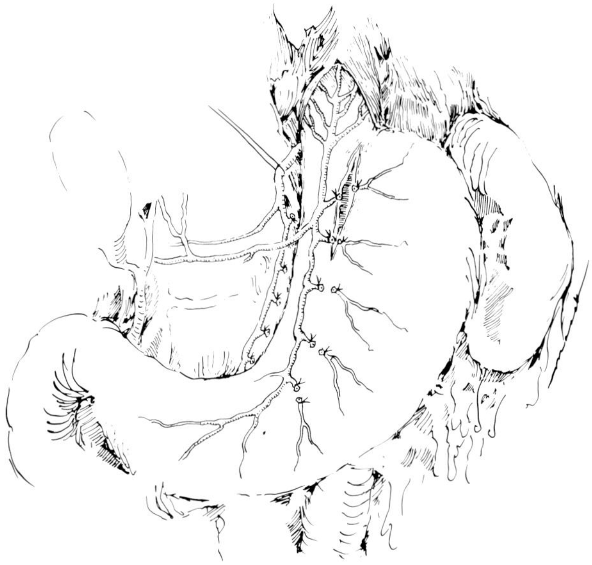

FIG. 31-5. Proximal gastric vagotomy. The branches from the nerve of Latarjet to the parietal cell-bearing stomach have been severed. The innervation to the antrum is spared.

the liver. The only way to avoid splenic injury is gentle moves and constant vigilance.

Selective Vagotomy

The technique of selective vagotomy is of necessity a blind procedure (Fig. 31-4). We prefer the technique of Burge wherein a window is made from the angle of His to the right side of the esophagogastric junction.[4] A second window is made to the bare area below the hepatic branch of the left anterior vagus. A third window is made close to the incisura of the lesser curve of the stomach. All the tissues between these points are divided and secured by silk ligatures. It is safe, but not as easy as it sounds. We imagine that this is why selective vagotomy, while representing a superior way to gain total gastric vagotomy, has not become popular in America. Furthermore, it places the esophagus at risk because of the blind finger dissection behind it.

Highly Selective Proximal Gastric Vagotomy

Proximal gastric vagotomy, a newer form, is emerging as the procedure of choice because of its low mortality (0.3%) and minimal side-effects (Fig. 31-5). The recurrence rate from the hands of those who are expert in its performance is about 10%. Its safety relates to the fact that the procedure is carried out with a high degree of precision, with division of the blood vessels and branches of the nerves of Laterjet close to the gastric wall, as described by Goligher.[8] There is no rapid or blunt way to perform the procedure. The low mortality rate likely relates to the fact that the operation is only performed by careful surgeons who are willing to take the time it requires. Furthermore, no openings are made in the stomach or duodenum. Perforation of the lesser curve has been reported, possibly as a consequence of devascularization. It is for this reason that we advise approximation of the anterior and posterior walls of the stomach in order to reperitonealize the portion of the lesser curve that has been stripped of its blood supply. Dissection of the lesser curve too distally can lead to antropyloric dysfunction and gastric retention. The upper angle of the crow's foot formed by the antral branches of the nerve of Laterjet must be respected. This is a relatively constant landmark that lies about 7 cm from the pylorus in most cases. It is important to carry the proximal dissection well up on the esophagus, as pointed out by Hallenbeck and his colleagues.[13]

PARTIAL GASTRECTOMY

The incision for removal of all or portions of the stomach is the same as that used for vagotomy, an upper midline incision from xiphoid to umbilicus (Fig. 31-6). Gastric resections can best be considered for peptic ulcer disease, with or without vagotomy, and for gastric cancer. In a partial gastrectomy for peptic ulcer, approximately 60% to 65% of the distal stomach is removed. A hemigastrectomy comprises removal of 50% of the stomach, and in an antrectomy

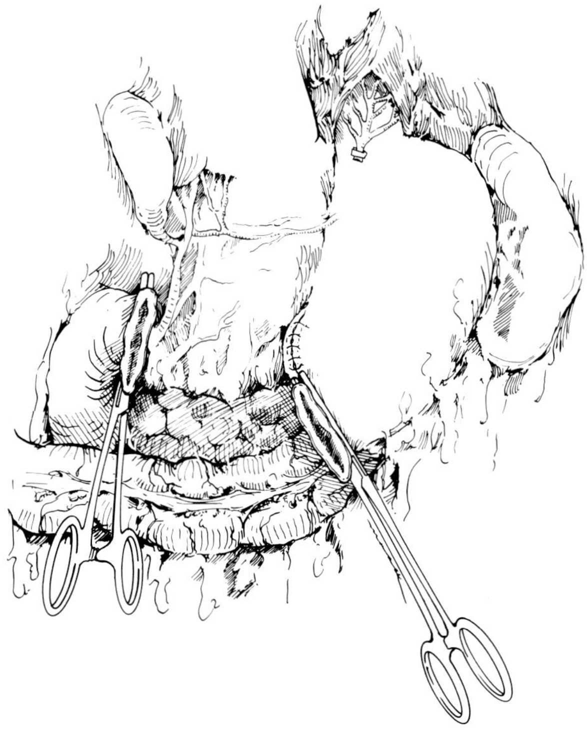

FIG. 31-6. Partial gastrectomy. The antrum has been removed. The lesser curvature has been closed so that the gastric opening matches the diameter of the duodenum.

somewhere between 30% to 50% of the stomach is removed. The initial phases of all these operations are the same. If a truncal vagotomy is to be performed, then this is carried out before the gastric resection, as described above. Once this is completed, the lesser sac is entered through the gastrocolic omentum by dividing the vessels in this area outside of the gastroepiploic vascular bundle. The lesser sac should be entered at a point opposite from the incisura, usually 5 cm to 6 cm from the pylorus. Further division of the gastrocolic omentum can then be carried out orad by dividing the vessels to the stomach with fine clamps and then, after division, suturing them by ligature. We prefer fine silk suture for this purpose because of its tying quality. Large bites should be avoided.

It is important early in the procedure of division of vessels along the greater curvature to identify the course of the middle colic artery. This artery can be avoided by brushing the transverse mesocolon away from the antrum and dividing the filmy adhesions that are often present in the lesser sac in this area. Excessive traction on the stomach should be avoided since this can result in a splenic capsular tear or an avulsion of the vessels along the greater curvature from the gastric wall. Division of the right gastric artery can be facilitated by placing the right hand behind the antrum and placing tension on the lesser curve. The passage of a clamp close to the lesser curve, just above the pylorus, will allow clamping of the right gastric artery close to the stomach, thereby avoiding any possible compromise of the gastrohepatic artery or the bile duct. The artery should be doubly clamped and doubly tied in order to gain secure ligature. An opening is then made in the gastrohepatic ligament, and the left gastric artery is divided in its descending portion.

It is at this point that one decides how much stomach to remove. This is determined by how high the dissection is carried out on the lesser curvature. The left gastric artery is usually divided just as it joins the lesser curvature of the stomach just above the incisura. This is best accomplished by placing two clamps proximal on the vessel and one distal before division. It is important to gain two secure ligatures on this artery. The mesenteric attachment should be cleared for a distance of about 10 cm on the lesser curve and about 6 cm on the greater curve before transection. We prefer to divide the stomach by first placing two vascular clamps across the stomach at right angles on the greater curve for a distance of about 4 cm. This will be the point of anastomosis to the duodenum. Larger clamps are placed along the lesser curve and angled high to ensure that all of the antrum is removed. Attention is then turned to the duodenum.

Billroth I

Once the stomach is divided, it is a simple matter to dissect the posterior duodenal wall from the head of the pancreas (Billroth I, Fig. 3-7). The duodenum should be mobilized for a distance of at least 2 cm or even farther if there is extensive scarring and an ulcer in the area. As mentioned above, we try to avoid having to dissect in the region of marked inflammation. It is necessary only to mobilize enough duodenum so that a posterior row of fine seromuscular silk sutures can be placed between the greater curvature side of the gastric remnant and the duodenum. We prefer a two-layer closure in which the inner layer consists of 3-0 vicryl placed in continuing running fashion on the posterior wall of the anastomosis and in Connell fashion anteriorly. It is important to take fine small bites in order to minimize the formation of a cuff at the point of anastomosis. The anterior row is then completed with fine silk sutures placed in Lembert fashion. The lesser curvature of the stomach has previously been closed by undersewing the proximal clamp with fine vicryl, which is sewn back on itself in a running-lock fashion. This ensures that the blood vessels within the submucosa are entrapped in the hemostatic stitch. The lesser curvature is then closed upon itself with

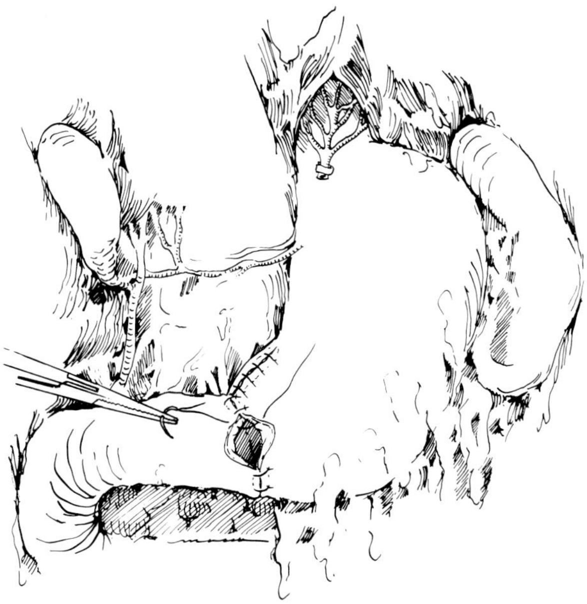

FIG. 31-7. Billroth I. The gastroduodenostomy is completed with an outer row of silk sutures.

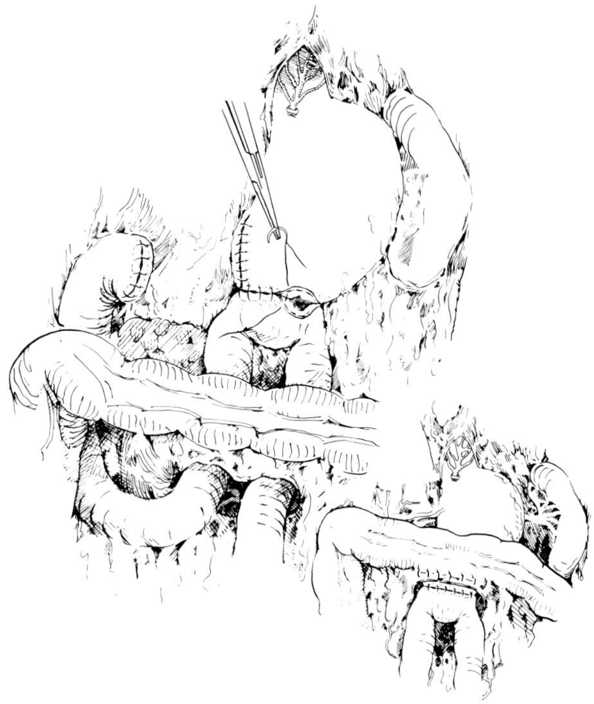

FIG. 31-8. Billroth II. The gastrojejunostomy may be completed above or below the colon. However, the finished anastomosis should be secured below the colon with interrupted silk sutures into the mesocolon (*lower-right-hand inset*).

fine silk. The lesser curvature portion of the gastroduodenostomy must be completely closed. This is best accomplished by placing a stitch through the anterior and posterior walls of the stomach as well as through the superior angle of the duodenum. This triangulating stitch closes this area securely. It is also important to guard against a narrow anastomosis. At its completion, it should be at least 4 cm in diameter with a minimal ridge from the inverted gastroduodenal wall.

Billroth II

The performance of a Billroth II gastrojejunostomy requires closure of the duodenal stump (Fig. 31-8). We prefer to do this by first dividing the duodenum just below the point of deformity and ulceration with a GIA stapler. The staple line is then inverted with fine silk sutures, and the stump of the duodenum is then secured to the fibrotic tissues in this area with fine silk sutures. Occasionally it is necessary to place a small Foley catheter into the duodenum for decompression, but more common, if we are concerned about the duodenal closure, we place an active drain to the area.

The gastrojejunostomy is always carried out in a retrocolic fashion for peptic ulcer disease. For this purpose, the afferent limb is usually about 5 cm in length and is attached to the stomach in an isoperistaltic fashion, which is with the proximal jejunum attached to the greater curvature side of the gastric remnant and the efferent loop to the lesser curvature side. In practice, the loop should be placed however it seems to lie best. Again, the anastomosis is carried out with an inner row of fine vicryl placed in continuous running lock fashion on the posterior row and Connell fashion anteriorly. The external layer consists of fine silk sutures placed in Lembert fashion. This provides an anastomosis that should allow at least three fingers' room after its completion. The major problem against which to guard is that of kinking of the efferent loop. In addition, it is important to sew the stomach to the transverse mesocolon so that there is no possibility for the small bowel to herniate into the lesser sac.

DRAINAGE PROCEDURES

There are several ways to provide for an enlargement of the gastric outlet when the stomach is not resected for ulcer surgery (Fig. 31-9). Total gastric vagotomy, whether truncal or selective, requires a drainage procedure if gastric stasis is to be prevented. Proximal gastric vagotomy does not require alteration of the gastric outlet if injury to the nerves of Laterjet and their antral branches is avoided.

Pyloroplasty is the most popular way to enlarge the gastric outlet. There are three types in common usage that have been associated with the names of the surgeons who have popularized them. The Heineke–Mikulicz pyloroplasty is accomplished by dividing the gastroduodenal junction on its anterior surface in a longitudinal fashion and closing the opening horizontally with a single layer of fine silk sutures placed in Lembert (seromuscular) fashion (Fig. 31-9*A*). The closure may be difficult when there is extensive scarring or inflammation from an ulcer. In this situation, it is best to make a longer incision along the stomach and duodenum and close the opening as is done in a Finney pyloroplasty (Fig. 31-9*B*). This procedure requires a two-layer closure, the inner of a fine absorbable suture and the outer of fine silk.

When duodenal deformity is severe, the gastric outlet may be refashioned by a gastroduodenostomy (Jaboulay pyloroplasty, Fig. 31-9*C*) or a posterior gastrojejunostomy (Fig. 31-9*D*). We prefer the latter, since it is easier to perform and less complicated to resect if the ulcer disease persists or recurs. A word of caution: Take care to place the gastrojejunostomy close to the pylorus in the distal antrum. High gastrojejunostomies may divert acid from the antrum and contribute to excessive release of gastrin and a subsequent stomal ulcer. In addition, it is important to attach the opening through the transverse mesocolon to the posterior gastric wall in order to prevent herniation of small bowel into the lesser sac. A short afferent limb will reduce the possibility of torsion or volvulus. A carefully performed posterior gastroenterostomy in combination with a complete truncal vagotomy is an excellent operation for a penetrating duodenal ulcer that is associated with marked deformity of the duodenal bulb or an inflammatory mass. Again, we emphasize the importance of opting for a lesser procedure when there is a risk of a pancreatic leak, bile duct injury, or a blown duodenal stump that might accompany gastric resection. Truncal vagotomy and pyloroplasty has been shown by Goligher and his colleagues to give results that are not too different from those obtained by operations that require gastric resection.[9, 10]

FIG. 31-9. Drainage procedures. The Heineke–Mikulicz procedure (*A*) is a genuine pyloroplasty in that the pyloric channel is refashioned. The Finney and the Jaboulay procedures (*B* and *C*) are gastroduodenostomies. A posterior gastrojejunostomy (*D*) is placed close to the pylorus for drainage in difficult cases of gastric-outlet obstruction.

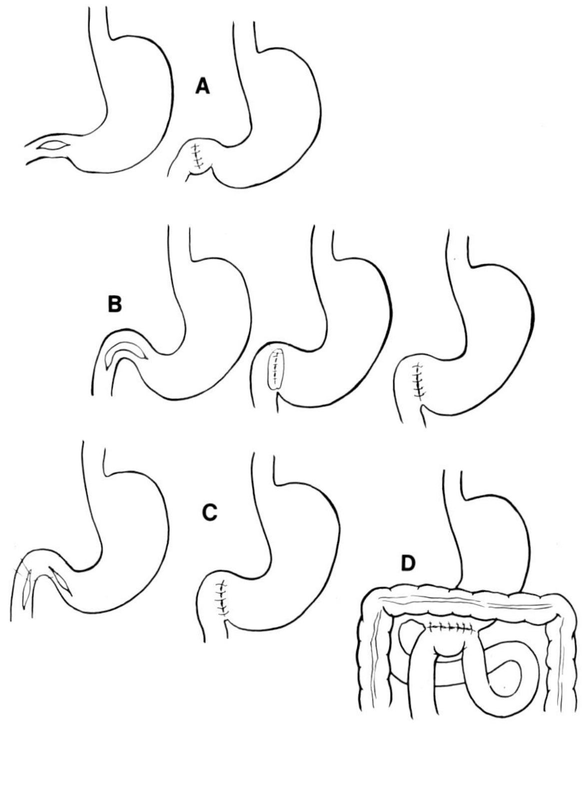

SUBTOTAL GASTRECTOMY FOR CANCER

Gastric resections for cancers that lie within the lower half of the stomach should be initiated by first removing the gastrocolic omentum from the transverse mesocolon (Fig. 31-10). This operation differs from that for peptic ulcer disease in that the blood

FIG. 31-10. Subtotal gastrectomy. A proximal cuff of stomach makes reconstruction after gastrectomy safer and easier.

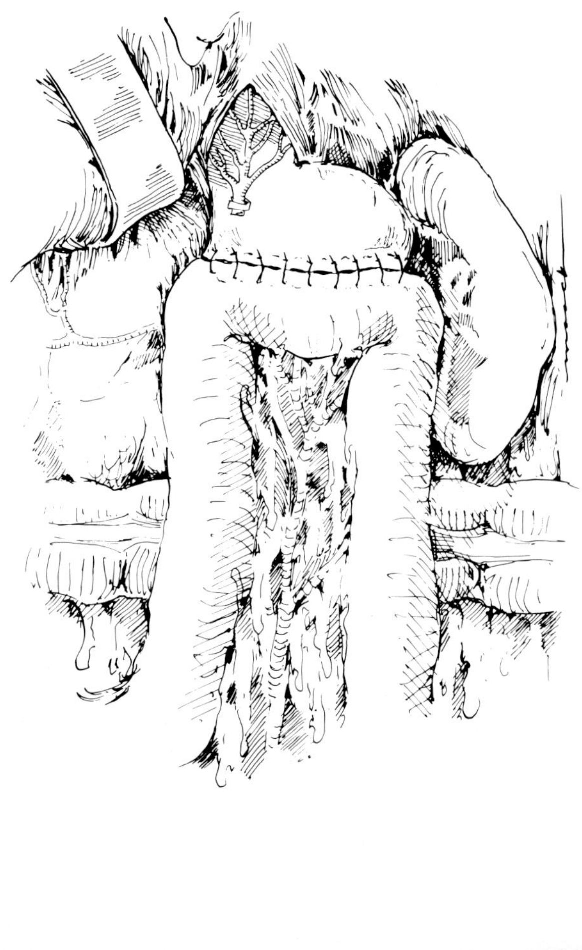

vessels are secured at their origins. We usually prefer first to divide the right gastroepiploic vessel at its origin from the gastroduodenal artery. The right gastric and, in turn, left gastric vessels are then divided at their origins, and a wide sweep of the gastrohepatic ligament is included with the resected specimen. Finally, the greater curvature vessels are divided high up on the greater curve so that approximately 80% of the stomach is removed. It is also important to mobilize at least 4 cm of duodenum in order to prevent recurrence in this area. The duodenal stump is closed as described above, and a gastrojejunostomy is performed usually in antecolic manner in order to keep the anastomosis out of the lesser sac where recurrence usually first occurs.

TOTAL GASTRECTOMY FOR CANCER

For high-laying lesions, the operation includes omentectomy as well as ligation of vessels close to their origin, splenectomy, and total gastrectomy (Fig. 31-11). This can also be carried out with relatively low rates of morbidity. We prefer to leave the stomach attached to the esophagus, bring a Roux limb of jejunum up to the esophagus, and place a posterior row before gradual division of the esophagus. This reconstruction is usually not associated with leak if the end of the esophagus is sewn to the side of jejunum (see Fig. 31-11), thereby providing adequate tissue for performance of the anastomosis as well as a good blood supply to all of its margins. We prefer to use an inner row of 2-0 vicryl placed in interrupted fashion through all layers of the jejunal wall and esophagus and an outer row of 2-0 silk placed in such a manner that the jejunum is rolled over the inner row for further protection. We always place two medium-size Penrose drains to the lesser sac area and remove them after the fifth postoperative day when a water-soluble contrast swallow confirms integrity of the anastomosis.

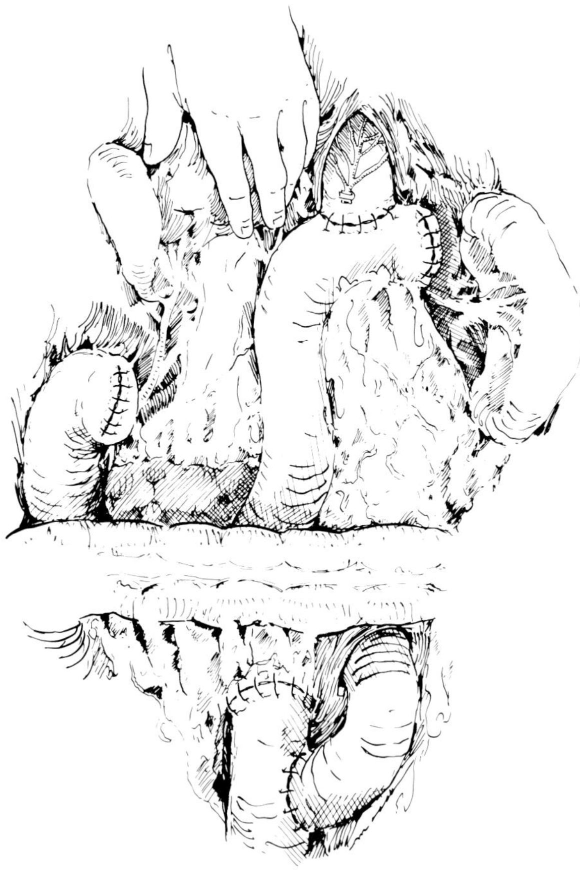

FIG. 31-11. Total gastrectomy. Sewing the esophagus to the side of the jejunum is safer than an end-to-end anastomosis.

Diagnosis and Treatment of Postoperative Complications

INTRALUMINAL BLEEDING

Intraluminal bleeding occurs in 5% of all postgastrectomy patients. One third bleed from the source that originally prompted operation; one third bleed from an anastomotic line; and one third bleed from an unknown source. This complication is heralded by signs of hypovolemia (oliguria, hypotension, tachycardia, respiratory distress), bloody nasogastric drainage, falling hematocrit, and, much later, melena. Endoscopy is usually the only diagnostic test that should be performed. Arteriography will localize the bleeding to the stomach but will not be able to differentiate between an operative problem (suture-line bleeding, bleeding ulcer) and a nonoperative problem (esophageal varices, gastritis). Management of postoperative intraluminal hemorrhage requires the following steps:

1. Support and monitoring systems: Insert several large-bore intravenous catheters, central venous pressure line, Foley catheter, arterial catheter, and Swan–Ganz catheter (if there is cardiopulmonary disease).
2. Correction of coagulation: If the clotting profile is abnormal, the necessary factors are infused, including fresh frozen plasma, aquamephyton, platelets, or cryoprecipitate.
3. Restoration of circulating volume: Shock should be aggressively managed with packed red blood cells, plasma products, and Ringer's lactate solution.
4. Iced saline lavage: This will quantitate the speed of bleeding and will signal re-bleeding once it has stopped. If bleeding does not cease or if brisk bleeding recurs, endoscopy is indicated.

5. Endoscopy: The stomach should be evacuated of blood and clots with an Ewald tube. The endoscopist may be able to correct a bleeding site with electrocoagulation or laser photocoagulation. If the source of bleeding cannot be identified, operative exploration is indicated. If the bleeding site is identified, the lesion will dictate whether operation will be required.
6. Nonoperative management of postoperative bleeding: Esophageal varices should be managed by nonshunt procedures (Blakemore tube, pitressin, sclerotherapy). If the variceal bleeding is stopped, the patient's nutritional status is then improved for 3 months prior to selective or nonselective shunting. Esophageal varices that do not quit bleeding must be approached operatively. Portacaval shunt is done unless this is not technically possible. The esophageal interruption with the EEA stapler or variceal ligation is tried. Diffuse gastritis should be managed with cimetidine and antacids.
7. Operative management of postoperative bleeding: Bleeding from the lesser curve closure or anastomosis may be secured by suture ligature through a gastrotomy proximal to the anastomosis or may require re-resection and a second anastomosis. If the bleeding site is not known, a gastrotomy is made above the anastomosis and the stoma (Billroth I or II) is inspected for bleeding. Blood may be seen coming from the duodenum (Billroth I) or afferent limb (Billroth II). Both conditions suggest bleeding from an ulcer bed left behind. This may require opening of the duodenal stump (B-II) or gastroduodenostomy (B-I) for control. Finally, if no source of bleeding is identified, the cardia and esophagus are inspected through the gastrotomy for ulcer, mucosal tears, or varices. Bleeding from these lesions should be controlled by suture ligature.

INTRA-ABDOMINAL BLEEDING

Postoperative intra-abdominal bleeding will present as hypovolemic signs and a falling hematocrit similar to that of intraluminal bleeding. In contrast, however, there will be little or no blood in the nasogastric tube, more abdominal distension, more peritoneal irritation, and a more prolonged ileus. Diagnostic studies are not very specific for this complication. Endoscopy can help by excluding an intraluminal source for the postoperative blood loss. Ultrasound and the CT scanner can identify an intra-abdominal fluid (blood) collection. Paracentesis and lavage may identify blood in the peritoneum, but this result is equivocal for the postoperative patient. Angiography may pinpoint the origin of the hemorrhage if the bleeding rate is fast enough. Postoperative hemorrhage is usually related to the operation, so exploratory laparotomy should not be delayed for diagnostic studies that may yield equivocal information. Bleeding into the abdomen after gastric surgery can be from one of many possible sources: a torn spleen, an anastomosis (more common with stapled than sewn anastomoses), a bleeding mesenteric vessel, an excluded ulcer crater, the vagotomy site on the esophagus, the gastrotomy site, or hemorrhagic pancreatitis. The management of this problem is similar to that for intraluminal bleeding:

1. Support and monitoring systems
2. Correction of coagulation
3. Restoration of circulatory volume
4. Iced saline lavage: This will produce a small amount of blood, which is usual for the postoperative stomach. Then, if bleeding continues, endoscopy is indicated.
5. Endoscopy: If the endoscopist is unable to identify significant bleeding, intra-abdominal bleeding is suspected. If the patient has suffered hemorrhagic shock, laparotomy should be the next step. Slower bleeding may allow confirmatory studies prior to operation (sonogram or paracentesis).
6. Operation: At exploration for postoperative bleeding, a systematic search for technical errors is conducted. The spleen is examined for capsular tear. If the bleeding spleen cannot be corrected with hemostatic agents (Surgicel, Avitene), it should be removed. Anastomotic lines are inspected for bleeding vessels. These are controlled with 4-0 silk suture ligatures. The mesenteric margins, which had been freed from the stomach, are searched. Uncontrolled arteries are ligated. If the original operation was done for a bleeding ulcer, there is a greater chance that rebleeding in the postoperative period will be from that ulcer.[15] If an excluded ulcer is bleeding, it is controlled with suture ligatures of 4-0 silk. The esophagus, which had been dissected for the vagotomy, is examined for bleeding arterial branches, including injured short gastrics. The "upper hand" retractor helps this exposure, yet control of these vessels might best be accomplished with hemoclips if ligature is awkward. A gastrostomy site is taken down from its peritoneal attachments and examined for an intramural artery that may have been severed. This problem is best fixed by stapling off the

old gastrostomy, using the TA 55 and 4.5 staples, then creating a new gastrostomy. If hemorrhagic pancreatitis is found, the common duct is drained with a t-tube, a gastrostomy inserted, large sump drains placed in the lesser sac, and a peritoneal dialysis catheter is inserted in the lower midline for peritoneal lavage.

DELAYED GASTRIC EMPTYING

Delayed gastric emptying will occur in approximately 4% of patients who have had gastric procedures.[5] It is more frequent after operation for pyloric obstruction, especially if this condition is managed by vagotomy and pyloroplasty. This problem begins as vomiting and inability to take fluids after the nasogastric tube has been removed. The patient may complain of continuous hiccups caused by gastric bloating. When the nasogastric tube is replaced, the amount of drainage will be greater than 600 ml per day. The saline load test will be positive (*i.e.*, greater than 400 ml of saline will be recovered from the stomach after 30 min). This simple test can be repeated daily to monitor emptying. If the saline load test remains positive 14 days after operation, radiographic contrast studies should be done. Ninety-five percent of patients who do not pass contrast out of their stomachs at this time will have a mechanical obstruction.[16] On the other hand, 95% of patients whose delayed emptying is due to gastric atony will pass some contrast out of the stomach at the 14th postoperative day. Endoscopy can confirm the radiographic diagnosis or discriminate between mechanical obstruction and atony where x-ray findings were equivocal.

The management of this complication should actually begin before the diagnosis. Any patient who still requires nasogastric decompression 7 days after a gastric procedure should be treated for metabolic causes of delayed emptying. Parenteral nutrition is begun, electrolytes corrected, and any septic sources (pulmonary, urinary, wound, etc.) eliminated. If the patient is still obstructed 14 days after operation, upper GI studies and endoscopy are done. If no mechanical obstruction is demonstrated, parenteral nutrition is continued for several more weeks. Gastroduodenostomy and pyloroplasty may open up very late, especially with a history of obstruction. The saline load test is done regularly to determine the proper time to remove the nasogastric tube. During this waiting period, Urecholine stimulation can be tried. Bushkind and Woodward described a successful technique of treatment that consisted of successive doses of Urecholine (2.5 mg, subcutaneously), every 10 minutes.[5] They watched the stomach under fluoroscopy until peristalsis ensued or the patient developed side-effects. The drug was then given orally (15 mg before meals) and parenterally (5 mg, subcutaneously, every hour from 7 A.M. to midnight) in gradually decreasing doses over the next week.

If the patient with gastric atony had not responded to 4 weeks of parenteral nutrition, operative intervention was indicated. A Billroth I or pyloroplasty would be converted to a Billroth II. If the patient had previously had a Billroth II, it was to be redone. A gastrostomy tube would be inserted and TPN continued until the stomach emptied. If the x-ray and endoscopy results suggested mechanical obstruction, immediate operation was indicated.

A common cause for postoperative obstruction is inflammatory adhesions about the anastomosis, presumably caused by leakage.[15] When this is found, the anastomosis should be redone in clean, healthy tissue. The edematous, inflamed stomach and small bowel must be removed prior to creating the new stoma. The anastomosis may be obstructed by excessive tissue that had been turned in during the two-layer closure. The old stoma must be completely excised so that the new one can be constructed more carefully in normal tissue. Retroanastomotic hernia and volvulus (afferent or efferent loop) occur more commonly in an antecolic Billroth II that has a long afferent limb. When these conditions are found, the new anastomosis should be made retrocolic with a 5-cm efferent limb. If a retrocolic gastrojejunostomy herniates above the mesocolon, it can obstruct the gastric outlet. This condition can be managed by reducing the stoma below the mesocolon and securing it there with interrupted 4-0 silk sutures. Infrequently, a small bowel obstruction may result from an internal hernia behind the gastrojejunostomy or through the opening in the mesocolon. Once the hernia has been reduced, it is closed with interrupted silk sutures. Intussusception of a Billroth II limb (afferent or efferent) into the stomach is rare, but occurs usually after an antecolic Polya B-II with the efferent limb as the intussusceptum.[21, 31] Approximately two thirds of these cases have been treated nonoperatively, especially in the early postoperative period. Shock, hematemesis, peritonitis, or prolonged obstruction is an indication for operation. Correction of jejunogastric intussusception consists of conversion of a B-II to a B-I, or recreation of a Hofmeister B-II with an efferent limb that is sutured to the mesocolon.

PANCREATITIS

Postoperative pancreatitis is twice as fatal as pancreatitis that does not follow an operation; the incidence of serious complications that accompany postoperative pancreatitis is five times greater.[26] When this complication is associated with renal or hepatic failure, the mortality rate approaches 100%. Over 90% of cases of postoperative pancreatitis follow operations that are directly related to the pancreas, such as gastric resection. The incidence of this complication following gastric procedures is 1% to 2%; the mortality rate approaches 50%.

The diagnosis of this complication may be difficult unless the level of serum amylase is markedly elevated. But modest amylase elevations after gastric surgery are indiscriminate and not helpful. Postoperative pancreatitis can be mild, with epigastric pain, vomiting, prolonged ileus, leukocytosis, oliguria, and icterus, or it can be severe with fever, hypotension, falling hematocrit, and an epigastric mass. The diagnosis can be suggested by ultrasound or CT scan. But frequently, the diagnosis must be made at laparotomy because the patient with severe pancreatitis usually cannot be distinguished from one with a serious complication that requires operative correction (stump leak, anastomotic dehiscence, intestinal obstruction, intestinal infarction, or afferent loop syndrome).

The patient with mild postoperative pancreatitis found at laparotomy or suggested by ultrasound (pancreatic swelling, phlegmon, or pseudocyst) can be treated with parenteral nutrition, nasogastric decompression, antibiotics, and vigorous rehydration. If the clinical condition deteriorates with this treatment, operation is undertaken. At laparotomy, if no other technical problem is found and the pancreas is inflamed, the drainage technique described by Ranson may be of value.[18] Large sump drains are placed in the lesser sac. The common duct is opened, patency to the duodenum is established with an 8-Fr red rubber catheter, then a T-tube is inserted. If a stone is lodged in the ampulla, it must be removed. If the common duct is small, obstruction is unlikely, and a cholecystectomy can be done. A decompression gastrostomy and feeding jejunostomy complete the treatment. A Tenckhoff catheter can be inserted for peritoneal lavage. This complication may be induced by excessive trauma to the pancreas, especially during the dissection of a difficult ulcer, so great care must be exercised during duodenal dissection and stump closure.

BLOWN DUODENAL STUMP

The incidence of duodenal stump leak is approximately 3%.[22] The mortality rate has been high from this complication, up to 50%; recent advances in medical management (e.g., parenteral nutrition) may be decreasing it, however. Harrison, White, and Heimbach quote no deaths in a series of 11 stump leaks managed at the University of Washington.[15] A blown duodenal stump is usually due to an error in technique or judgment, most commonly extensive duodenal dissection. The duodenum should be mobilized only enough for a technically sound closure (1 cm of posterior wall covered with peritoneum). The posterior duodenal wall can be left on the pancreas in a difficult ulcer if the anterior wall is healthy and mobile (Nissen–Cooper closure). When this technique is used, a Kocher maneuver should be done to lift tension from the stump suture line. Minimal duodenal dissection preserves the blood supply and ensures against stump leak. Another common cause of duodenal blowout is afferent limb obstruction.

A leaking duodenal stump usually becomes evident on the fifth postoperative day. If the leak is confined to the right upper quadrant, it is heralded by signs of localized sepsis: fever, pain, leukocytosis, oliguria, prolonged ileus, respiratory failure, pancreatitis, or a mass in the right upper quadrant. If the leak is not confined, it presents as prostration, shock, peritonitis, and abdominal rigidity. If a drain has been left in the area of the duodenal closure, stump leak is evident by an increase in bilious drainage, which is high in amylase. This diagnosis is simple. Contrast placed into the drain will visualize the duodenum. If there is no drain to facilitate the diagnosis, several other diagnostic studies may be helpful. An erect abdominal film may show free air. Ultrasound can identify a fluid collection in the right upper quadrant, which can then be aspirated to show typical small bowel juice. Contrast upper GI studies may show the leak, but endoscopy is not helpful. The management of this problem is nonoperative if a drain was placed at the original operation and is controlling sepsis. If the diagnosis has been confirmed with a sinogram, a larger sump drain is placed in the drain tract, total parenteral nutrition is begun, and nasogastric decompression reinstituted. If no drain is present, the patient with a stump leak must be explored.

At laparotomy, a small clean hole can be closed primarily and drained. If the hole is large, a controlled fistula is created by closing the stump around a drain, total parenteral nutrition is begun, and a gastrostomy is inserted. If the fistula has not closed after 6 weeks of hyperalimentation, it should be treated operatively. The duodenal hole, which is left, is best managed with a Roux-en-Y.[15]

ANASTOMOTIC LEAK

The incidence of leaking anastomosis is less than 2% after gastric operations. This rate is much higher for the esophageal anastomosis after total gastrectomy; drains are placed routinely after this operation in anticipation of an anastomotic leak. The presentation of an anastomotic leak after a gastric procedure may be dramatic, with peritonitis and shock.

More common, it becomes manifest by one or more of the following subtle signs: pain, ileus, outlet obstruction, vomiting, intraluminal bleeding, leukocytosis, fever, hyperbilirubinemia, hyperamylasemia, pulmonary insufficiency, or oliguria. The diagnosis is first pursued radiographically with supine and erect abdominal x-ray films. These films may show free air, the "soap bubble" sign of abdominal abscess, or a distended afferent loop. If a drain is in place and actively producing fluid, a sinogram may demonstrate the leak. An upper GI series will usually confirm the diagnosis by demonstrating the actual leak or outlining the inflammatory mass near the anastomosis caused by the leak.

Very small leaks may be confined by the omentum and well tolerated without operation. Leaks that had been anticipated by placing drainage tubes at the original operation also can be managed without operation. If the drainage is adequate, sepsis from the leak will be controlled. The patient is given parenteral nutrition, nasogastric decompression, and broad-spectrum antibiotics. Unless there is distal obstruction or carcinoma in the suture line, the fistula created by the drains will close. If no drainage has been provided for an anastomotic disruption, then an operation is needed once the leak has been demonstrated. At operation, a small suture line hole may be closed primarily if there is minimal inflammatory reaction and if the tissues are healthy. After placing two or three simple silk sutures, the area is covered with omentum. Leaks that require more than three sutures are large enough to require revision.

LEAKING PYLOROPLASTY. If there is minimal contamination, the anastomotic margins can be trimmed back to healthy tissue and a new pyloroplasty done. A larger opening should be made by converting the Heineke–Mikulicz to a Finney pyloroplasty. If the patient is stable, conversion of the pyloroplasty to a Billroth II with stump drainage is safer and avoids postoperative outlet obstruction. If the patient is unstable, drains may be placed to create a controlled fistula with a gastrostomy for gastric decompression. This may heal or result in outlet obstruction with the later need for a gastrojejunostomy.

LEAKING BILLROTH I. The treatment for leaking Billroth I is identical to that outlined above for pyloroplasty if the dehiscence is in the gastroduodenostomy. If the leak is in the reconstructed lesser curvature, this usually requires additional gastric resection back to healthy stomach wall and reanastomosis with a Billroth II or a Roux-en-Y reconstruction. In the rare case, gastric necrosis or intra-abdominal contamination may be so severe that re-anastomosis is dangerous. In this situation, White recommends placing a gastrostomy and jejunostomy only with later reconstruction when sepsis has subsided.[7]

LEAKING BILLROTH II. Duodenal stump leak is controlled with a duodenostomy tube, as discussed earlier. The leaking gastrojejunostomy will usually require resection and reconstruction. Refashioning a Billroth II with unhealthy jejunum is not wise. The entire old anastomosis should be removed. The reconstruction occasionally can be carried out as a Billroth I and jejunojejunostomy where the old anastomosis had been. More often, the best reconstruction will be a Roux-Y limb, once the jejunum has been divided by removing the leaking gastrojejunostomy. All operations for anastomotic dehiscence are supplemented with wide abdominal drainage, gastrostomy for decompression, antibiotics, and parenteral nutrition.

Postgastrectomy Sequelae

The risk of morbidity from gastric surgery and division of the vagal trunks can extend far beyond the perioperative period.[18] Some of the so-called postgastrectomy syndromes can be devastating to the patient's well-being and functional role in society. The major incapacitating syndromes are discussed in the context of their prevention, since their treatment is only palliative.[14]

In order to simplify prevention, it is important to understand three common, easily avoidable problems. First, the small-capacity syndrome is usually associated with a feeling of early satiety. It is related to a small proximal pouch and therefore can be avoided by limiting the extent of distal gastric resection to no more than 60% of the stomach in benign ulcer disease. A second less common but more serious problem, recurrent ulcer, can be minimized by adequate gastric vagotomy. Although *selective vagotomy* is best for this purpose, it is difficult to perform. A carefully executed truncal vagotomy is almost as effective when all of the branches to the proximal stomach are sought and divided. Finally, it is of the utmost importance to be sure that the patient to be treated surgically in fact has ulcer disease. Indiscriminate procedures that include vagal section or gastrectomy are almost always followed by undesirable side-effects.

AFFERENT LOOP SYNDROME

Reconstruction of the gastrointestinal tract after a gastrectomy that employs a gastroenterostomy (Billroth II) must ensure that the jejunal limb coming from the duodenum (afferent loop) empties freely into the limb that drains the gastric remnant (efferent loop). When this is not true, bile, pancreatic juice, and duodenal succus regurgitate into the stomach and can lead to bilious vomiting. The usual history is one of the onset of severe epigastric pain an hour or so after eating, which is relieved by the emesis of copious amounts of bile without food. The food has passed down the efferent limb after stimulation of the secretion of bile and pancreatic juice. These secretions cause distention of the afferent loop and the severe pain associated with the syndrome.

Afferent loop problems are almost always mechanical and a consequence of obstruction at the point of entrance into the stomach. The obstruction may be due to a faulty anastomosis, intussusception, stomal ulcer, volvulus or kinking at the stoma, or efferent loop deformity. Preventive measures include the use of a short afferent loop placed in a retrocolic position, the careful fashioning of the gastrojejunostomy, and the assurance of avoiding ulcerogenic situations such as an overlooked antrum, incomplete vagotomy, or unsuspected Zollinger–Ellison syndrome.

The diagnosis of an afferent loop problem is usually made from the history. Barium roentgenogram may reveal a dilated afferent loop. Endoscopy is mandatory, for it often will reveal the pathologic anatomy at the gastrojejunal stoma. We prefer to correct this mechanical problem by converting the stoma to a long limb (60 cm) Roux-en-Y gastrojejunostomy. When ulcer disease is present, it is usually necessary to resect the stoma and look for an undivided vagal trunk. Otherwise, the obstructed afferent limb can be displaced to the appropriate point on the jejunal limb. Corrective surgery enjoys a high success rate in this syndrome.

BILE GASTRITIS

A small number of patients following gastric procedures for peptic ulcer complain of a burning discomfort in their epigastrium. They usually complain of bile-stained emesis of undigested food. Curiously, weight loss is not a prominent feature of the syndrome. Barium roentgenograms are usually nondiagnostic, but endoscopy reveals an erythematous, bile-stained mucosa, with superficial gastric erosions. The presence of inflammation can be established by mucosal biopsy in about half the patients suspected of the disease.

Unfortunately, the syndrome of bile gastritis remains poorly defined; therefore, its therapy remains empirical. Prevention may relate to selection of an appropriate surgical procedure for ulcer therapy. Highly selective vagotomy appears to be immune to this complication, which occurs with about equal frequency following all the other procedures. The common denominator is division or bypass of the pylorus. Surgical correction is directed toward diversion of bile from the gastric remnant by a long Roux-en-Y gastrojejunostomy (60 cm). The importance of a complete gastric vagotomy must be stressed, since in this arrangement the gastrojejunal stoma lies unprotected from the alkaline secretions of the liver and pancreas. The results of this therapy are only modest (in the range of 50% of total relief of symptoms) and will remain so until more is known about the pathogenesis of this curious entity.

DUMPING SYNDROME

Much has been written but little is known about the dumping syndrome. It is convenient to identify two phases of the illness, each with distinct features. Early dumping is a clinical entity whereby the patient experiences light-headedness, palpitations, nervousness, and a sensation of fullness during or immediately after eating. This is usually followed by intestinal cramps and diarrhea. The symptom complex relates to the rapid passage of food of high osmolarity from the stomach into the upper intestine. This draws water rapidly into the intestinal lumen to provoke an autonomic response from the distention that follows. Late dumping, when similar neurologic symptoms occur 3 to 4 hours after a meal, is related to a delayed reactive hypoglycemia. Gastric procedures in some patients are followed by a disturbance in the usually finely modulated response to a carbohydrate load. This is a rare syndrome and as yet unexplained.

Early dumping is common after all gastric procedures except highly selective vagotomy. Again, the common denominator is division or bypass of the pylorus. It is for this reason that we prefer proximal gastric vagotomy as the treatment for the intractable pain of peptic ulcer.

The early dumping syndrome can be treated in most patients by simple measures such as avoidance of sweets, separation of liquids from solids during a meal, and lying down when the symptoms occur. Occasionally, when symptoms persist and are severe, relief will follow the placement of a short (10 cm), reversed jejunal limb at the gastric outlet. The diarrhea may or may not be affected by this maneuver, since it may be a consequence of a truncal vagotomy or the blind loop syndrome. Postvagotomy diarrhea is difficult to distinguish from the dumping syndrome. Usually it occurs in an unpredictable, episodic, explosive manner, unrelated to meals. It is a most distressing complication for social reasons and may be associated with profound weight loss. Some patients are helped by a reversal of a 10-cm loop of small bowel, 90 cm from the ligament of Treitz. The results from this simple approach can be dramatic for reasons as yet not understood.

STOMAL STENOSIS

Some patients following a gastroduodenal or gastrojejunal anastomosis after gastric resection for peptic ulcer develop a delayed cicatricial stenosis of their stoma. This is a variant of persistent acid peptic disease. Unfortunately, revision of the stoma may be accompanied by a recurrence of the process. Patients with this complication should be assessed for evidence of incomplete vagotomoy (pentagastrin-stimulated gastric analysis), retained antrum (serum gastrin), or Zollinger–Ellison syndrome (basal gastric analysis, serum gastrin). Patients with stomal stenosis should be explored for an overlooked nerve or retained antrum and receive a long anastomosis between the gastric remnant and duodenum on its anterior surface, if possible, or otherwise to the jejunum.

It is important to remember that almost all of the above delayed complications of gastric surgery for peptic ulcer can be obviated by the performance of a proximal gastric vagotomy. This operation will offer long-term relief from ulcer complications in about 85% to 90% of patients so treated. (The remainder may have mild, symptomatic recurrences that respond to medical therapy.) Candidates for surgery can be offered a more aggressive surgical approach to their ulcer disease with its attendant sequelae.

Complications of Gastric Procedures for Morbid Obesity

Gastric procedures have gradually replaced jejunoileal bypass for morbid obesity and now are being performed in great numbers in this country. Our discussion is limited to operations that create a small proximal gastric pouch, gastric bypass, and gastric partition with or without division between staple lines. These procedures have a variety of modifications, but in essence they share in a proximal pouch made by the TA-90 stapling device. The proximal stomach is completely stapled when gastrointestinal continuity is to be established by a loop or Roux-en-Y gastrojejunostomy. Three or more staples are removed from the cartridge when the proximal pouch is to be allowed to empty into the distal stomach. The opening may be at either end or in the middle of the staple line.

The complications of these procedures have recently been reviewed by Mason, a pioneer of this surgical approach to obesity.[21] Morbidly obese patients and their surgeons are indebted to Mason for his imaginative approach to their problem and the honesty with which he has related his results. The incidence of complications reported from his large experience with gastric bypass are shown in Table 31-1. The mortality rate, while high (about 5%) during the early experience at Iowa, is now in the range of 2%. The main causes of death have been pulmonary embolus and peritonitis from gastric leaks. Others have also reported deaths from these problems, as well as early postoperative complications including wound infections, nonfatal gastric leaks, nonfatal pulmonary emboli, pneumonia, atelectasis, iatrogenic splenic injury, subphrenic abscess without gastric leak, and wound herniation discovered at a later date. This is quite a litany of serious problems for a procedure usually performed on well-nourished, relatively healthy people. Furthermore, since the procedures are primarily prophylactic and are designed to prevent the medical complications of the morbidly obese state, they should have a low risk-to-gain ratio.[23] With safety foremost in mind, we have utilized the gastric partition as our procedure of choice for chronic morbid obesity. Our technique and results to date with complications are described below.

TABLE 31-1. MAJOR COMPLICATIONS OF GASTRIC BYPASS

Complication	Incidence (%)
Wound infection	14
Wound hernia	6
Splenectomy	2
Subphrenic abscess	2
Gastric leak	5
Pouch ulcer	3
Pouch obstruction	5
Bile gastritis	1
Pneumonia	2
Atelectasis	3
Embolism	1
Early reoperation	7
Readmission for vomiting	5
Postoperative death	
Pulmonary embolus	0.6
Peritonitis	2

(Data from Mason EE: Surgical treatment of obesity. In Ebert PA [ed]: Major Problems in Clinical Surgery, vol XXVI, pp 154-155. Philadelphia, WB Saunders, 1981).

PATIENT SELECTION AND PREPARATION

The morbidity of gastric procedures for obesity, as with other operative interventions, relates directly to patient selection, operative technique, and pre- and postoperative care. We have limited our bariatric surgery to patients between the ages of 18 and 65. The older patients (over 55) are very carefully screened for associated disease and brought to an optimal state of health prior to operation. Patients with advanced cardiopulmonary disease, long-standing hypertension, and diabetes present a significant risk, but often have the most to gain from surgical weight loss and control.

The majority of patients with chronic morbid obesity are middle aged and healthy. We perform a superficial endocrine screen that includes a plasma cortisol, T_3 and T_4, and fasting blood sugar analysis. An ultrasound of the gallbladder is obtained because of the high incidence of gallstones. Barium studies of the upper gastrointestinal tract are performed to delineate the anatomy of the esophagus, stomach, and duodenum.

We employ mini-heparin in a dose schedule of 5000 units, subcutaneously, on call to the operating room, and 5000 units, three times a day, for 4 days thereafter. Preoperative antibiotics are also utilized in a dose schedule of 1 g of cefazolin (Ancef), on call to the operating room, with two additional doses at 6-hour intervals. A trial with pneumatic boots was unsuccessful because of the large size and unusual contour of the obese patient's legs.

Intraoperative monitoring has included a urinary catheter and an arterial line. The latter has been of great help in monitoring oxygenation by blood gas analysis within the operating and recovery rooms.

TECHNIQUE OF DOUBLE-STAPLE LINE GASTRIC PARTITION

The abdomen is entered through an upper midline incision, with the fat teased apart by blunt dissection to the linea alba (Fig. 31-12). The fascia is divided in the midline from xiphoid to umbilicus, and the peritoneal cavity is entered to the left of the round ligament. Following exploration, the wound edges are covered with moist pads, and the upper abdomen, is elevated at the costal margins by a frame retractor. The vessels along the upper half of the greater curve are divided between ligatures of 2-0 silk tied in continuity, with care being taken to avoid tension on the gastrosplenic ligament. It is usually not necessary to divide the upper short gastric vessels. A 3-cm window is then developed into the lesser sac high on the lesser curve of the stomach by dividing the anterior and posterior leaves of the gastrohepatic ligament close to the gastric wall, similar in technique to a highly selective vagotomy. The dissection should not be carried up onto the esophagus. Adhesions between the stomach and pancreas are divided by sharp dissection, with care being taken to avoid disruption of the capsule of the pancreas.

FIG. 31-12. Double-staple line gastric partitioning. Two rows of staples from the TA-90 produce a proximal pouch that holds 50 ml of saline at 25 cm of water pressure. The opening to the lower portion of the stomach is 10 mm as measured with a Hegar dilator.

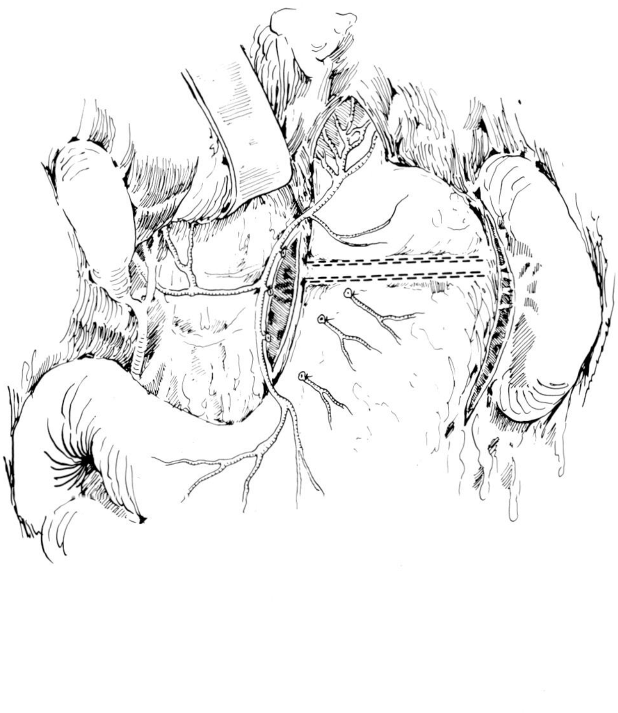

The staple cartridges are prepared by removing three staples from the greater curvature end. The hammer is removed from these empty staple sites, and the cartridge is amputated from this area. This should reduce injury due to compression at the opening between the upper and lower compartments of the stomach.

The TA-90 stapling device with its contained cartridge is passed from left to right, and the greater curve pin is secured. Prior to this maneuver, a 16 Fr nasogastric tube is curled up into the cardia of the stomach. The staple device is then maneuvered into place. This is accomplished by placing tension on the lesser and greater curves of the upper portion of the stomach. It is most important to bring the greater curve to the pin and pinch its farthest extent into a flattened position. The staple arm is then screwed down slowly to a snug but not a crushingly tight position. Fifty milliliters of saline is then instilled through the nasogastric tube into the proximal pouch. The pressure generated by this maneuver is measured by a manometer attached to the nasogastric tube. This pressure should be greater than 25 cm of water. After aspiration of the fluid from the proximal pouch, the staple line is fired. We place a second staple line approximately 5 mm to 10 mm below the first, care being taken to line up precisely the openings on the greater curve. This opening is then checked by inserting a No. 10 Hegar dilator from below through a small gastrotomy. The fit must be snug, so four vertical seromuscular sutures can be placed anteriorly and posteriorly. Circumferential sutures are not used, since we purposely have avoided maneuvers that might contribute to a fixed area of stenosis.

The gastrotomy is closed with an inner row of a fine absorbable suture and an outer row of fine silk. The gallbladder is removed if stones are present.

Wound closure is performed in layers, the falciform ligament being approximated with a polyglycolic stitch placed in running fashion. The linea alba is closed with interrupted synthetic nonabsorbable sutures. The skin edges are secured with a subcuticular stitch of fine Prolene and Steri-strips.

Postoperative care emphasizes early ambulation, pulmonary exercises, and adequate hydration by the parenteral route until oral feedings are adequate. The nasogastric tube and Foley catheter are removed the next morning. On the following day, a water-soluble contrast radiograph of the pouch is obtained to ascertain its ability to empty without leak. Liquids, 30 ml per hour, are then offered by mouth and increased in 30-ml increments over the next 3 days. Patients are usually discharged on the fifth postoperative day after a barium roentgenogram has been taken of the stomach for future reference. They remain on a progressive liquid diet for 6 weeks and are counseled by a nutritionist during their period of rapid weight loss.

TABLE 31-2. COMPLICATIONS OF 225 GASTRIC PARTITIONS AT THE UNIVERSITY OF UTAH MEDICAL CENTER (1979–1981)

Complication	Incidence (Number)
Mortality	0
Atelectasis	17
Seroma	4
Wound infection	3
Gastric leak	3
Pulmonary embolus	3
Phlebitis (IV)	3
Hepatitis	3
Cardiac irregularities	3
Splenectomy	2
Pneumothorax	2
Pneumonia	1
Deep vein thromboses	1

COMPLICATIONS OF GASTRIC PARTITION

We have had no deaths in our experience with 225 patients who have undergone gastric partition in the last 3 years at the University of Utah Medical Center. The postoperative complications encountered are listed in Table 31-2. There were six life-threatening complications, three pulmonary emboli, and three gastric leaks. The pulmonary emboli were in each instance associated with hypoxia that required oxygen therapy but no cardiovascular dysfunction. The three leaks occurred at the point of vessel division on the greater curvature and were not at the staple lines. They were treated by early exploration, suture of the small opening, and drainage of the area. We have not encountered this complication since we recognized that it relates to a weakness in the gastric wall at the point where it is entered by the short gastric vessels. It is important to secure these vessels at a point distant from the wall in order to minimize this serious complication.

Stomal stenosis (five cases) was a significant problem in our early experience prior to removal of the portion of cartridge that would crush the greater curve opening. Care must be taken not to form a valve if vertical suturing is required. This was done in two cases by suturing above the first staple line. One patient was relieved of his obstruction by division of the septum by electrocautery through the endoscope. The second required a gastrogastrostomy. Two additional cases required gastrogastrostomy for late stomal stenosis that occurred without vertical suture. An additional patient required dilatation through the endoscope. The remaining patients (219) have been relatively symptom-free except three suffered chronic heartburn and regurgitation.

Stomal enlargement has been a common problem in all reported series. We have reoperated upon five patients with this problem and were surprised to find that their staple lines were intact. In fact, we have not as yet identified staple-line disruption. Possibly the early reports of staple-line disruption were related to inadequate use of the device or failure to monitor the size of the neostoma. It must be precisely 1 cm or less in size to be effective. Reoperations are difficult and risky. We would prefer to attempt restapling but currently believe that the chances of success with a second gastric procedure are limited in patients who eat through their initial procedure.

Procedures to Prevent Complications

Gastric procedures for peptic ulcer, neoplasms, and chronic morbid obesity are associated with well defined, and for the most part avoidable, complications. There is no substitute for appropriate selection of an effective and safe procedure. If the operation is performed with care on a patient who is well prepared for it, the risks of morbidity should be minimal and mortality, nil. We have enumerated several well-established surgical principles:

- Adequate exposure
- Appropriate procedure
- Good lighting
- Gentle handling of tissues
- Plenty of time
- A well-trained surgeon
- A competent anesthesiologist
- No extraneous distractions

Under these conditions, the operative procedure will be successful, and the postoperative recovery will be smooth. To avoid late sequelae, we cannot overemphasize the importance of choosing operations that are associated with the least disturbance of the normal physiology. For example, a highly selective vagotomy will offer long-term relief of ulcer symptoms in 90% of patients with almost no risk of mortality and minimal chances for late morbidity. The risk-to-gain ratio is low, and those who develop recurrence can be offered a more aggressive surgical approach. The same principle applies for prophylaxis against the medical complications of morbid obesity. Gastric partition is a safe way to offer 85% to 90% of such patients significant weight control. Remind yourself as you operate that the risk incurred in the procedure is in your hands but borne in its entirety by your patient.

References

1. Berne CJ, Rosoff L: Peptic ulcer perforation of the gastroduodenal artery complex: Clinical features and operative controls. Ann Surg 169:141-144, 1969
2. Boyle JD, Goldstein H: Management of pyloric obstruction. Med Clin North Am 52(6):1329-1337, 1968
3. Buchholtz TW, Welch CE, Malt RA: Clinical correlates of resectability and survival in gastric carcinoma. Ann Surg 188:711-715, 1978
4. Burge H, Frohn MJN: The technique of bilateral selective vagotomy with the electrical stimulation test. Br J Surg 56:452-460, 1969
5. Bushkind FL, Woodward ER: Delayed gastric emptying. In Bushkind FL, Woodward ER (eds): Major Problems in Clinical Surgery, vol XX, Postgastrectomy Syndromes, chap 7, pp 72-82. Philadelphia, WB Saunders, 1976
6. Felix WR, Stahlgren LH: Death by undiagnosed perforated peptic ulcer. Ann Surg 177:344-351, 1973
7. Fisher RS (ed): Peptic Ulcer Disease: An Update. New York, Biomedical Information Corporation Publication, 1979
8. Goligher JC: A technique for highly selective (parietal cell or proximal gastric) vagotomy for duodenal ulcer. Br J Surg 61:337-345, 1974
9. Goligher JC, Pulvertaft CN: Comparison of different operations. In Williams JA, Cox AG (eds): After Vagotomy, chap 8, pp 93-118. New York, Appleton-Century-Crofts, 1969
10. Goligher JC, Pulvertaft CN, Irvin TT et al: Five- to eight-year results of truncal vagotomy and pyloroplasty for duodenal ulcer. Br Med J 1:7-13, 1972
11. Griffith CA: Selective gastric vagotomy. In Nyhus LM, Wastell C (eds): Surgery of the Stomach and Duodenum, 3rd ed, chap 12, pp 275-305. Boston, Little, Brown & Co, 1977
12. Grossman MI: Control of gastric secretion. In Sleisenger MH, Fordtran JS (eds): Gastrointestinal Disease, chap 36, pp 640-659. Philadelphia, WB Saunders, 1978
13. Hallenbeck GA, Gleysteen JJ, Aldrete JS, Slaughter RL: Proximal gastric vagotomy: Effects of two operative techniques on clinical and gastric secretory results. Ann Surg 184:435-442, 1976
14. Halpern NB, Hirschowitz BL, Moody FG: Failure to achieve success with remedial gastric surgery. Am J Surg 125:108-115, 1973
15. Harrison RC, White TT, Heimbach DM: Early reoperations in gastroduodenal surgery. In White TT, Harrison RC (eds): Reoperative Gastrointestinal Surgery, 2nd ed, chap 5, pp 45-87. Boston, Little, Brown & Co, 1979
16. Hermann G, Johnson V: Management of prolonged gastric retention after vagotomy and drainage. Surg Gynecol Obstet 130:1044-1048, 1970
17. Herrington JL Jr: Current operations for duodenal ulcer. In Ravitch MM (ed): Current Problems in Surgery. Chicago, Year Book Medical Publishers, 1972
18. Herrington JL Jr: Remedial operations for postgastrectomy syndromes. In Ravitch MM (ed): Current Problems in Surgery. Chicago, Year Book Medical Publishers, 1970
19. Koelz HR, Sachs G, Berglindh T: Cation effects on acid secretion in rabbit gastric glands. Am J Physiol 241:G431-442, 1981
20. Kurzweg FT, Danna SJ, Daron PB, Williamson JW: The management of perforated duodenal ulcer. Surg Gynecol Obstet 135:365-368, 1972
21. McClelland RN: Peptic ulcer surgery: Postoperative care and immediate complications. In Sleisenger MH, Fordtran JS (eds): Gastrointestinal Disease: Pathophysiology–Diagnosis–Management, chap 61, pp 791-821. Philadelphia, WB Saunders, 1973
22. Mason EE: Surgical treatment of obesity. In Ebert PA (ed): Major Problems in Clinical Surgery, vol XXVI. Philadelphia, WB Saunders, 1981
23. Moody FG: An ounce of surgery for a pound of cure. The Pharos of Alpha Omega Alpha 43:19-21, 1980
24. Moody FG, Steichen FM: Gastric Operation. In Schwartz SI (ed): Modern Techniques in Surgery, Abdominal Surgery, pp I-1–I-58. New York, Futura Publishing, 1980
25. Papachristou DN, Fortner JG: Adenocarcinoma of the gastric cardia. Ann Surg 192:58-64, 1980
26. Peterson LM, Collins JJ, Wilson RE: Acute pancreatitis occurring after operation. Surg Gynecol Obstet 127:23-28, 1968
27. Sawyers JL, Herrington JL: Perforated duodenal ulcer managed by proximal gastric vagotomy and suture plication. Ann Surg 185: 656-660, 1977
28. Sawyers JL, Scott HW Jr: Selective gastric vagotomy with antrectomy or pyloroplasty. Ann Surg 174:541-547, 1971
29. Shiu MH, Papachristou DN, Kosloff C, Epiopoulous G: Selection of operative procedure for adenocarcinoma of the midstomach. Ann Surg 192:730-737, 1980
30. Soll AH et al: The actions of secretagogues on oxygen uptake by isolated mammalian parietal cells. J Clin Invest 61:370-380, 1978
31. Waits JO, Beart RW Jr, Charboneau W: Jejunogastric intussusception. Arch Surg 115:1449-1452, 1980

32 Complications of Intestinal Surgery

Hunter H. McGuire, Jr.

OVERVIEW

Paralytic ileus and incisional pain are inevitable effects of every laparotomy. A surgeon must anticipate their normal intensity and duration in order to recognize abnormal variations and complications of postoperative convalescence. A surgeon must also instruct his patients to expect ileus and pain in order to minimize postoperative anxiety. A patient who confidently recognizes ileus and pain as normal will require fewer analgesic drugs, be more active, and recover more quickly than one alarmed by unexpected events.

Paralytic Ileus

Paralytic ileus is a reflex caused by excitation of splanchnic sympathetic nerves during surgical manipulation of viscera. It can be prevented by splanchnic denervation and reversed by spinal anesthesia, but no pharmacologic or electrical device has yet proven safe and effective for overriding the sympathetic reflex that inhibits peristalsis.

During laparotomy splanchnic inhibition affects the entire gut from stomach to rectum. The stomach recovers in a few hours, small bowel within a day, and colon in 2 to 3 days. Intuition and experience lead most surgeons to believe that the severity and duration of ileus are increased by more extensive and prolonged dissection of viscera or by retroperitoneal dissection, which irritates splanchnic nerves. Thus we expect only brief ileus after cholecystectomy or hysterectomy but prolonged ileus after total proctocolectomy or pancreaticoduodenectomy. There is, however, no experimental evidence to support this bias. Ileus lasting longer than 72 hours is probably prolonged by continuing splanchnic stimulation, owing to peritonitis, hemoperitoneum, or mesenteric or retroperitoneal hematoma.[7]

Following operations in which there is virtually no risk of intra-abdominal infection or bleeding, most patients will tolerate oral feeding as soon as the small bowel has recovered, or within 24 hours of the operation. By the time the first meal reaches the colon, it too will have recovered. Such is the experience after hysterectomy, proximal gastric vagotomy, cholecystectomy, and appendectomy without peritonitis. Even after gastric resection without vagotomy, most patients tolerate solid food within 24 hours.[10]

PROLONGED ILEUS

After operations for preexisting peritonitis and operations liable to produce peritonitis or mesenteric or retroperitoneal hematoma, feeding must be delayed until the ileus is clearly resolved. Clues to resolution of ileus are resumption of appetite and audible peristalsis, but the only reliable evidence of colonic motion is passage of flatus. Until patients prone to prolonged ileus pass flatus, they should have nothing by mouth and have continuous gastric drainage, intravenous fluid maintenance, and replacement of electrolytes. Failure to keep the paralyzed gut empty will result in gaseous distention, which, in turn, will further delay resumption of effective peristalsis. Gut distended by gas loses rather than absorbs potassium, and hypokalemia prolongs ileus.

RECURRENT ILEUS

Ileus does not resolve instantaneously. Strength and effectiveness of peristalsis recover segmentally and gradually over several days, and recovery may be reversed by ingestion of certain substances, by overeating, or by constipating opiates. Best tolerated are hot clear liquids, which must be sipped gingerly with minimal air swallowing, and solid foods containing little or no fat. Least tolerable during recovery from ileus are citrus juices and milk. These should be avoided so that any recurrence of ileus cannot be blamed on them but instead promptly recognized as manifestations of peritonitis, abscess, or obstruction.

PARALYTIC ILEUS *VERSUS* OBSTRUCTION

Prolonged or recurrent ileus typically produces silent, painless distention, while mechanical obstruction usually causes colic with tinkling peristalsis. In the second week after laparotomy, however, these two complications may coexist in varying degrees and be impossible to distinguish by symptoms and physical signs. Complete obstruction requires laparotomy. Ileus should not be operated upon unless it is caused by an abscess that needs drainage. In this quandary Gastrografin should be introduced by nasogastric tube and followed by serial x-ray films. If complete obstruction is found, the patient should be reexplored. If not, a gallium or CT scan should be obtained to search for abscess. Sonography is ineffective when gaseous distention impairs the acuity of its images.

PREVENTION OF PROLONGED ILEUS

Normal paralytic ileus cannot be prevented, and it might even be desirable to rest the wounded gut during its inflammatory phase of healing. Prolonged ileus, however, can be prevented or its intensity reduced by intraoperative measures to minimize peritonitis. These measures include washing powder from surgical gloves, gentle handling of gut and omentum, covering them with moist pads or bags to prevent drying, avoidance of retractor trauma, scrupulous prevention of spillage from enterotomies, careful hemostasis, and making ostomies of gut ends that cannot be anastomosed with dependable safety.

Pain

NORMAL INCISIONAL PAIN

Incisional pain is normally severe and constant during the initial 36- to 48-hour inflammatory phase of wound healing. During this time skin edges should be swollen, pink, and tender. The inflammation is sterile and causes neither fever nor leukocytosis. It is confined to the incision and affects its entire length uniformly. Pain, tenderness, or swelling affecting one segment of the wound more than another is a signal of infection or hematoma. Pain or tenderness apart from the incision suggests peritonitis.

Symptoms and signs of normal wound inflammation should reach maximum intensity within a few hours of wound closure, remain constant for a day or two, and then subside. An increase in pain or tenderness after the first day is a signal of some complication, usually infection, and requires immediate examination. After the second day pain should be felt only transiently when coughing, turning in bed, or rising to walk. A return of constant incisional pain after the second day suggests wound infection. Development of constant pain elsewhere in the abdomen indicates some visceral complication.

INTERPRETATION OF ABNORMAL POSTOPERATIVE PAIN

When exacerbation or recurrence of wound pain coincides with incisional erythema, swelling, tenderness, fever, or leukocytosis, skin sutures should be removed, infection drained, and the wound allowed to heal secondarily. Failure to drain an abdominal wound abscess invites fascial destruction, subfascial abscess, and enteric fistula. When examination of an infected wound reveals dusky skin, crepitus, or "dish water" drainage, the wound should be opened in the operating room under anesthesia to permit extensive débridement of necrotic fascia (see Chap. 3).

When abdominal pain becomes worse or constant but the incision appears healthy, visceral complications must be suspected, especially if the pain is associated with fever or leukocytosis. Interpretation and management depend on the risks known to be inherent in the original operation. For instance, sudden right upper quadrant peritonitis a week after Billroth II gastrectomy would require immediate reexploration without further studies. Any abdominal catastrophe after mesenteric endarterectomy would require immediate angiography and surgery. When the need for reoperation is less clear and urgent, imaging studies often help determine what has happened and whether surgery is required. An upright or lateral decubitus x-ray film of the abdomen may normally show air in the peritoneal cavity for 3 to 5 weeks after laparotomy and is thus of no value in detecting early postoperative perforations. Perforation of an upper intestinal anastomosis may be shown by Gastrografin swallow and of a colon anastomosis, by Gastrografin enema. Such studies may not obviate the need for reoperation but may facilitate finding a leak amid postoperative adhesions.

Postoperative Fever

Uncomplicated laparotomy causes no fever. When fever appears in the first 48 hours, it is most often due to atelectasis caused by refusal to turn, cough, or breathe deeply for fear of incisional pain. It is best prevented by instructing patients in how to cough effectively before the operation and by frequent encouragement after surgery. Chest x-ray films often fail to show atelectasis, which is best diagnosed and cured by rapid defervescence after coughing, using endotracheal suction when necessary.

Another extra-abdominal cause of fever after laparotomy is phlebitis around intravenous catheters. The problem is usually obvious on inspection of peripheral catheter sites. Central venous catheters need removing and culturing to prove them sources of sepsis. Urinary and choledochal catheters, if properly tended, rarely produce sepsis but if present should be examined and cultures obtained.

While attending to pulmonary toilet and catheter sites, the surgeon must frequently and carefully examine the patient's wounds, inquiring about progress of pain, tenderness, and bowel function. Diarrhea is a symptom of pelvic abscess; paralytic ileus with nausea and vomiting indicates abscesses elsewhere in the abdomen. It is essential to examine the entire abdomen, including motion of the diaphragm by percussion and the pelvic cul-de-sac by rectal or vaginal examination. All findings must be carefully recorded on progress notes. They are far more significant than most x-ray and laboratory reports, which are often more carefully transcribed.

INTRA-ABDOMINAL ABSCESSES

Spontaneous abscesses may develop before surgery, often before admission, as a result of diseases such as diverticulitis, appendicitis, salpingitis, Crohn's disease, pancreatitis, cholecystitis, and perforations of ulcers, cancers, or foreign bodies. The diagnosis, suggested by fever, leukocytosis, tender mass, and a history of the disease-producing abscess, is easily confirmed by contrast studies or scans. Suppuration is usually advanced, and the need for surgical drainage is clear. Appropriate antibiotics are begun at once and the abdomen opened through whatever incision gives safest exposure of the organ causing the abscess. For stomach and intestines, midline incisions give the safest exposure and provide space for any enterostomies that may be needed. Appendiceal abscess is best approached and drained through McBurney's incision. Biliary and liver abscesses are best exposed through subcostal incisions. Pancreatic abscesses tend to recur, owing to their depth, their tendency to invade adjacent tissues, and the hazards of débriding a diseased pancreas. Pancreatic abscesses are therefore best exposed through midline incisions and drained through flanks, leaving room for enterostomies when needed.

POSTOPERATIVE INTRA-ABDOMINAL ABSCESSES

Most postoperative abscesses are caused by technical errors such as spillage of enteric contents, contamination of hematoma or devitalized tissue, anastomotic leakage, or contamination of an unneeded or poorly tended drain. Except occasionally when overwhelming preoperative contamination exceeds the cleansing capacity of omentum and peritoneum (such as in trauma, perforated colon, or advanced gut gangrene), postoperative abscesses can be prevented by perfect technique and appropriate antibiotics. Abscesses may occur beneath the diaphragm, beneath the liver, in the pelvic cul-de-sac, between leaves of mesentery or loops of bowel, or beneath the repaired fascia of an abdominal incision. About 15% of patients have more than one abscess. If abscesses are not completely drained, their victims will die of sepsis with multiple organ failure.[5]

Diagnosis

Detection of a postoperative intra-abdominal abscess is difficult. The diagnosis is confused by other sources of sepsis such as pulmonary, catheter, and wound infections. The location is obscured by incisional tenderness, ileus, distention, and by the paucity or even absence of pus when fever and leukocytosis are first noticed. One of the best guides, then, to diagnosis is the surgeon's knowledge of risks inherent in his original operation. For instance, the surgeon who has hastily removed a shattered spleen and bruised the tail of the pancreas should anticipate and be quick to detect a left subphrenic abscess.

When intra-abdominal abscess is suspected, other sources of sepsis eliminated, and blood cultures drawn, intravenous antibiotics appropriate for enteric bacteria should be started. Our current preference is a combination of gentamicin, 1 mg/kg, clindamycin, 600 mg, and ampicillin, 500 mg, administered intravenously every 8 hours. Infrequently, these appear to sterilize and cure an area of cellulitis before enough pus is generated or tissue destroyed to require surgical drainage. At the same time antibiotics are started, a gallium scan should be ordered. Any area of abnormal uptake should be studied by sonography. If gaseous distention interferes with the sonographic image, a CT scan may be necessary to define the abscess. A CT scan usually shows cavities over 2 cm in diameter, but in rare instances all these techniques fail to show an existing abscess. Negative reports should therefore not be deterrents to draining clinically obvious pus.

Routes of Access

A clearly palpable and fluctuant cul-de-sac abscess is most safely and effectively drained transanally by simple incision through the anterior rectal wall. A solitary right posterior subphrenic abscess is best drained through the bed of the 12th rib, the incision being long enough to admit the surgeon's entire hand and wrist. All other intra-abdominal abscesses are best approached by reopening the incision of the antecedent operation. Reopening the old incision often reveals an unsuspected subcutaneous or subfascial abscess, and if that incision gave safest exposure of the diseased organ in the first operation, it will also be safest for coping with its complication.

Before approaching an abscess near an anastomosis, one needs to know whether the anastomosis has leaked or is intact. Gentle contrast studies by nasogastric tube, T tube, or enema may prove this point. If an anastomosis is proven intact, a nearby abscess may be drained without disrupting its suture line and creating an unnecessary fistula. If a contrast study shows an anastomosis has leaked, the risks of morbidity and mortality are minimized by enterostomies or drains, which assure a controlled fistula.

Techniques of Drainage

There is no perfect technique, route, or material for draining an intra-abdominal abscess. The theoretical ideals of wide open and dependent drainage are precluded by the threat of evisceration and by thoracic and pelvic bones, the spine, and paraspinal muscles. Suction catheters threaten adjacent viscera with pressure necrosis and fistula if they are large and stiff enough to remain patent and overcome gravity for many days. Compensating for these obstacles are the cleansing power of peritoneum and omentum and the contractile power of collagen. Thus most intra-abdominal abscesses heal if all pus is evacuated and all spaces within them connected by Penrose drains to the outside through the nearest soft part of abdominal wall other than the initial incision. For capillary action at least two adjacent Penrose drains are required. Addition of a small soft multiperforated suction catheter provides still better drainage, plus a means for sterile irrigations and sinograms.

When drains or suction catheters exit the abdomen, they must be fixed to skin sutures with sterile safety pins. They must be dressed with scrupulously aseptic technique and preferably enclosed in sterile ostomy bags. Suction catheters require sterile connections. A drain may be irrigated to assure or restore patency, but when drainage ceases and sinogram shows a cavity has contracted to the size of its drain, the drain must be removed. A drain should be advanced in stages, such as 2 cm per day, permitting the tract to close from within, while always refixing the drain to a skin suture to prevent accidental loss of the drain into the abdomen or into the bandage.

When a suspected intra-abdominal abscess cannot be confirmed by scans and contrast studies, the antibiotics already begun should be continued for a week after fever and leukocytosis have resolved, and scans should be repeated before the patient is declared well. When an abscess is thoroughly drained, antibiotics may be stopped when temperature and blood counts are normal. With adequate drainage a patient's health should flourish. If not, other abscesses must be suspected and sought.

ENTEROCUTANEOUS FISTULA

Enterocutaneous fistula follows drainage of an intra-abdominal abscess adjacent to injured, diseased, or perforated bowel. Although a few fistulas develop spontaneously from Crohn's disease or diverticulitis, the vast majority follow laparotomy in which the bowel is accidentally injured or an anastomosis leaks or is invaded and destroyed by adjacent abscess. A fistula is manifest by an abrupt increase in the volume of drainage with a change in its character from thick pus to thin green liquid.

Skin about a fistula must immediately be protected from excoriation by karaya gum and suction catheter or ostomy bag to collect its output. The volume must be measured to guide fluid and electrolyte replacement and to plot progress toward healing. X-ray contrast studies, by fistula, mouth, or enema, should define the fistula's level and size, whether the distal bowel is obstructed, and whether any cavity between bowel and skin is adequately drained. Such information will determine the optimal method of nutrition and predict the chance of spontaneous closure.

Fistulas arising from cancer, Crohn's, diverticulitis, foreign bodies, or obstructed or irradiated bowel and those with very short tracts (less than 2 cm long) do not close spontaneously. The goal of nutritional therapy for these is merely to restore strength required for safe elective surgery.[14] When such fistulas arise from the jejunum, total parenteral nutrition (TPN) will be required. Patients with fistulas from distal ileum or colon are best prepared for surgery with oral feeding if they can tolerate it. A patient with a low fistula who is intolerant of oral feeding may have an intra-abdominal infection, which must be cured before elective repair is undertaken.

When none of the foregoing features prohibits spontaneous closure, healing may be encouraged by diverting enteric juices through nasogastric suction, by assuring ample drainage of any cavity between bowel and skin, by protecting skin from excoriation, and by TPN. Low fistulas with modest outputs may be treated with an elemental diet rather than by gastric suction and TPN. With such regimens, over 50% of fistulas have healed spontaneously, even on specialized services populated by refractory cases referred from other hospitals.[14] Success rates are probably higher in community hospitals. Of fistulas that close spontaneously, 90% do so within 1 month. Reoperation on those who fail to heal, however, should not be perfunctorily scheduled at the end of

1 month because still more patients will heal spontaneously and many who ultimately require surgery will become safer candidates after additional nutrition and maturation of wounds. The ultimate mortality of nonmalignant fistulas is about 10%, much of which is caused by complications of premature operations for fistula closure. Fistulas should not be resected and repaired until patients have regained acceptable weight and serum albumin levels, are without antibiotics, and are free of any evidence of sepsis.[11]

Complications in Specific Intestinal Operations

From complications in surgery we learn many of our most valuable lessons. To learn, however, each complication must be honestly attributed to one of four basic causes. Following our last 10,000 operations, mostly elective procedures with few admissions for acute trauma, over 600 resulted in complications that prolonged hospital stay, increased the morbidity, or were fatal. The causes that we identified are shown in Table 32-1. Because of these findings the remainder of this chapter emphasizes technical complications, their prevention and management.

TABLE 32-1. CAUSES OF COMPLICATIONS IN INTESTINAL SURGERY*

Cause	Percentage of Occurrence
Technical or judgmental error	60
Progression of disease despite hope of cure or palliation by correctly performed operation	15
Inherent risk of necessary and correctly performed operation (e.g., pulmonary embolus)	10
Deficient equipment or nursing support	3
Unrelated coincidence	7

* Based on 600 complications in a series of 10,000 operations. Complications that prolonged hospital stay, increased morbidity, or were fatal are included.

LYSIS OF OBSTRUCTING ADHESIONS

Bowel Injury

The most common complication of adhesion lysis is caused first by incising too deeply an abdominal scar to which the bowel is adherent. When entry through an old scar is necessary, safety requires superficial strokes with a sharp blade in a bloodless, well-lit field where the bowel can be instantly recognized.

The bowel is also injured when a fibrous band under traction is cut close to the bowel wall. Because the bowel wall is more elastic than is scar tissue, traction creates diverticula, which are easily entered. This accident is avoided by sharp dissection, which leaves abdominal wall scar on bowel. When the bowel is adherent to a more precious structure, such as the ureter, traction must be minimized and efforts directed toward the side of tissue the sacrifice of which will be least costly. Fresh fibrin and young disorganized collagen may be bluntly separated, but mature collagen is stronger than is serosa or smooth muscle. It must not be blindly and bluntly kneaded through a small abdominal incision. Ample exposure is necessary for sharply incising mature adhesions (Fig. 32-1).

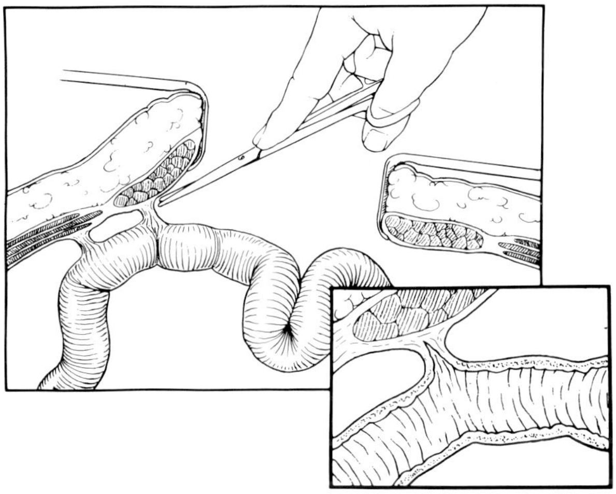

FIG. 32-1. Traction on a fibrous adhesion creates a diverticulum vulnerable to accidental incision and spillage of feces.

Bowel injuries occur at various depths. Injuries of peritoneum are inevitable, but they need no repair because sutures cause more inflammation and scar than does the spontaneous regrowth of peritoneum. Defects through the muscle must be repaired to restore strength and minimize the contracture of the healing bowel. Accidental enterotomy requires immediate repair while spilled feces are recovered with suction and controlled with atraumatic intestinal clamps. The worst complication of adhesion lysis is an overlooked or forgotten hole in the bowel. Its best outcome is an enterocutaneous fistula. Its worst and more likely outcome is peritonitis, abscess, and fatal sepsis.

Shock

Hypotension is often reported by an anesthesiologist as loops of massively distended bowel are delivered through a laparotomy incision. The dominant cause

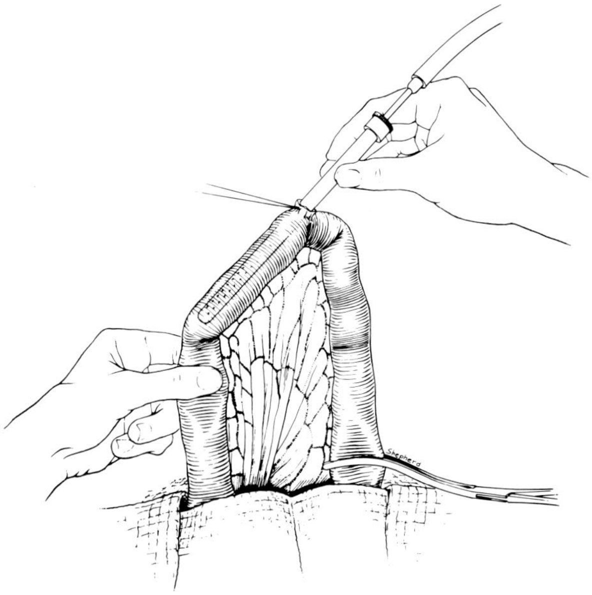

FIG. 32-2. Suction enterostomy facilitates abdominal closure after operation for intestinal obstruction. It also enhances the likelihood of wound infection unless the wound is protected with dry towels; the ends of bowel not being suctioned are occluded with atraumatic clamps; the entered bowel is kept elevated so gravity will deter spillage; and the suction apparatus is kept patent and functional.

is usually a blood volume deficit, which should have been replaced before the induction of anesthesia. Adequate replacement with Ringer's lactate should have been proven by urine output and serum electrolyte determination. In long-standing obstruction, an intracellular potassium deficit may be greater than serum potassium measurements suggest. During preoperative hydration, serial *p*H and bicarbonate levels may suggest the need for additional intravenous potassium. This problem is fortunately rare in acute strangulated obstruction, which permits little or no time for preoperative resuscitation. If sequestered fluid has been replaced before surgery, it need not be replaced again when the enteric contents are removed by suction enterostomy; doing so invites pulmonary edema.

Dead Bowel

Bowel that is infarcted by thrombosis, strangulation, volvulus, or intussusception will, if not resected, perforate and produce fatal peritonitis during the early convalescence when the abdomen is difficult to evaluate. This disaster must be prevented by being certain no bowel that does not regain its color, mesenteric pulse, and peristalsis is left in the abdomen. Doubtful segments may be gently covered with warm moist packs and reevaluated after 15 minutes for evidence of recovery. If recovery is not certain, the doubtful segment must be resected. If the segment is so long that resection might produce a short bowel syndrome, viability may be tested by intravenous injection of an ampule of sodium fluorescein and observation under a Wood's lamp. Any segment that fails to fluoresce must be resected.

Irradiated Bowel

Irradiated bowel, most often found in the pelvis after treatment of uterine, bladder, or prostate cancer, is already injured and unable to heal. If its adhesions are lysed, even small superficial wounds carefully sutured are liable to spontaneous perforation, fistulization, or fatal sepsis. For this reason adhesions in an irradiated pelvis should not be lysed. If they cause obstruction, the side of proximal unirradiated bowel should be anastomosed to the side of the unirradiated transverse colon as long as the distal colon is patent. If the rectum is also injured by irradiation or obstructed by a tumor, obstructing pelvic adhesions are best treated by proximal ileostomy.

Incomplete Lysis

Persistent mechanical obstruction due to incomplete lysis is extremely costly, not only in prolonged hospital care but in the danger and difficulty of a soon repeated laparotomy for more adhesion lysis. In view of these costs, one must, before closing an abdomen, be completely certain that the obstruction has been relieved. When a single distinct band occludes a small bowel that is proximally distended and distally collapsed and when division of that band allows immediate passage of fluid from proximal to distal bowel, relief is sure. If the passage of fluid does not prove patency, however, it must be proved by passing a long intestinal tube beyond the most distant small bowel adhesion. Hours of tedious but safe dissection are far better than are days of gastric suction for unrelieved obstruction.

Difficult Abdominal Closure

Difficult abdominal closure may result from intestinal distention. Rather than force wound edges together with necrotizing sutures, which invite evisceration or hernia, the risk of morbidity is reduced and time saved by intraoperative evacuation of the bowel (Fig. 32-2). The safest and cleanest method is to massage through the bowel a long suction tube introduced through the nose and stomach. When this fails, a sheathed metal sucker may be introduced through a small enterotomy in mid bowel, exercising great care not to spill intestinal contents. This requires covering the field with dry towels, elevating the enterotomy site so gravity will keep contents in the bowel, and placing an atraumatic clamp on the side of the enterotomy not being suctioned. The possible need for enterotomy must be anticipated before every operation for intestinal obstruction, and antibiotics appropriate for intestinal flora must be given preoperatively.

Wound Infection

Antibiotics appropriate for enteric bacteria should be given preoperatively. Without accidental or intentional enterotomy, the wound will be clean and the likelihood of infection less than 2%. Enterotomy without fecal spillage creates a "clean contaminated" wound, but with antibiotic protection, the infection rate is only about 6%. This is sufficiently low to justify primary closure of subcutaneous fat and skin. Gross spillage creates a "contaminated" wound with a probability of infection of about 20%, despite the use of antibiotics. In this circumstance some surgeons might choose only antibiotic irrigation and primary skin closure, but it is safer to pack the skin open in a patient who is also at risk for intra-abdominal abscess.

Recurrent Obstruction

Although most adhesions re-form, recurrent obstruction is remarkably uncommon. Adhesions from upper abdominal surgery and from right and left colectomies rarely obstruct. The procedures most often responsible for subsequent obstruction are those in the pelvis. Total proctocolectomy and ileostomy are followed by obstruction in 9% of cases. Certain patients for unknown reasons appear more likely than others to form adhesions. Some require many laparotomies for obstruction. Procedures such as Noble's plication are not uniformly successful in maintaining patency, and, when followed by recurrent obstruction, lysis is extremely difficult. A more popular method of directing new adhesions that will not interfere with bowel function is to pass a long tube through the entire small bowel; replace the intestine in its normal, left upper to right lower orientation; and leave the tube in place for a week until effective peristalsis and fixation have occurred. No drugs administered parenterally in safe doses have been shown to affect adhesions.

Both injured parietal and visceral peritoneum normally regenerate without adhesion to healthy surfaces. When two injured surfaces are left in apposition, however, their shared fibrin and collagen mature as a permanent bond. A surgeon must reduce this likelihood by minimizing the number and size of peritoneal injuries and by placing omentum between the small bowel and injured parietal peritoneum.

SMALL BOWEL RESECTION AND REPAIR

The failure of resection is accompanied by dismal complications. When the purpose was to remove infarcted bowel, residual gangrene will perforate and cause peritonitis and fatal sepsis at a time when the abdomen is most difficult to evaluate. Sometimes the only clues to this complication are shock and acidosis with a high cardiac output. Residual or recurrent infarct requires instant reexploration if there is any hope of survival. The complication is prevented by leaving no bowel in the abdomen that does not regain its color, pulse, and peristalsis. A doubtful bowel may be evaluated with intravenous fluorescein and Wood's lamp. Unless both ends of the resected bowel are clearly healthy, anastomosis should be deferred, cutaneous enterostomies performed, and their viability assured by frequent postoperative inspection. When an elderly patient with proximal superior mesenteric artery obstruction is found to have gangrene of the right colon and 80% of his small bowel, resection may prolong his hospital survival but his prospects of discharge are negligible. Whether to remove any bowel in such a case must be answered individually on social, economic, or theological grounds.

When the purpose of the surgery was to remove neoplastic or inflammatory obstructions, arrest bleeding, or close perforations, one must be certain that all lesions are identified, that margins of resection are appropriate to the disease at hand, and that anastomoses are made with healthy tissue. Failure to follow these rules may result in persistent obstruction, continued bleeding, or prompt reperforation. The rules, however, are modified in Crohn's disease in which the probability of recurrent obstruction, perforation, abscess, or fistula is about 9% per year regardless of the extent of resection. Anticipating future complications of Crohn's disease, one must preserve as much bowel as possible. Only segments that are obstructed or involved in abscesses or disabling fistulas should be removed; others should be left untouched. Margins of resection need not be histologically normal but only thin and pliable enough to heal.

When the purpose of section and anastomosis is to make a Roux-en-Y limb for draining another organ, one must be certain the limb conducts its contents toward the distal bowel and is 45 cm in length. A rare but catastrophic error of Roux-en-Y drainage is anastomosis of the wrong end of the jejunum to the esophagus, stomach, bile duct, or pancreas. A similar error is the accidental reversal of an intermediate segment when two or more portions of bowel are resected. If a reversed segment is over 8 cm long, its orally directed peristalsis causes obstruction. This complication is best prevented by

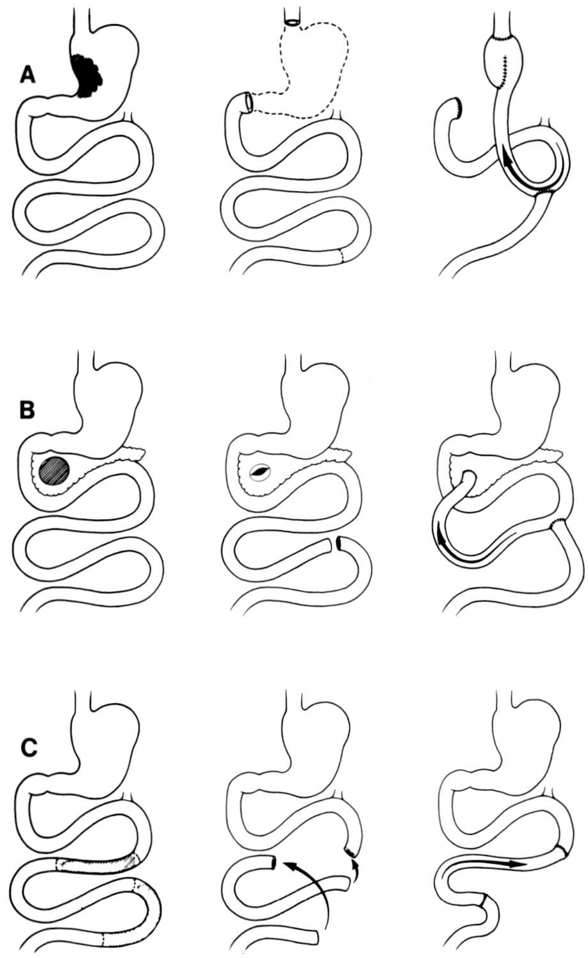

FIG. 32-3. Three devastating errors that can be made in repairing loops of small intestine. (*A* and *B*) Roux-Y limbs for total gastrectomy, pseudocyst, or biliary drainage, where proximal end of jejunum is used for drainage. Sure orientation to ligament of Treitz (not an adhesion) prevents these errors. (*C*) Multiple resections for trauma or necrosis with reversal of intervening segment, can be prevented by anastomosis after each segment is excised.

making each anastomosis as soon as its intervening segment is removed (Fig. 32-3).

Spilled Feces

Although the upper small bowel is sterile in most normal persons and in others contains only a small fraction of the colon's bacterial concentration, even the most careful enterotomy is a clean contaminated operation and merits prophylactic antibiotics. Gross spillage from the small bowel contaminates the operation and invites peritonitis, prolonged ileus, intraperitoneal abscess, fistula, and wound infection. These complications, already described as common denominators of intestinal surgery, must be prevented by applying gentle atraumatic intestinal clamps to both sides of every planned division of small bowel.

Anastomotic Leakage

Peritonitis, abscess, and fistula due to postoperative anastomotic leaks are extremely rare, owing to the small bowel's rich circulation, fast growing epithelium, abundant collagen, and low bacterial content. The small bowel heals so well, in fact, that it is difficult to prove the superiority of inverted serosa to serosa anastomoses. Nevertheless, technical errors can cause leakage.

Anastomoses may be made ischemic by ligating peripheral mesenteric vessels more than 5 mm from the bowel ends. Ischemia may be produced by injuring vessels deep in the mesentery during attempts to recapture accidental bleeders, where original ligatures were too broad and short. Ischemia may also be produced during development of a Roux-en-Y or isolated limb if the arcade supplying straight vessels is not carefully protected or if rotation of the limb occludes its venous drainage.

Other technical errors that promote anastomotic leaks are poorly placed sutures tied too tight or too loose and failure of EEA staple devices to excise complete "doughnuts" of purse-stringed tissue. During convalescence, healing may be impaired if the fibrin and collagen seal of an anastomosis is removed by an adjacent drain, abscess, or ascites. Anastomoses may be separated from these threats by covering them with omentum.

Obstruction

An anastomosis may be transiently occluded by a hematoma from incorporation of an open artery or from needle penetration of an unseen artery. It may be permanently occluded by inverting too much tissue, by anastomosis with continuous, unlocked purse-string suture, or by catching the opposite wall with a closing stitch. These errors, impossible with EEA staple devices, can be completely avoided with meticulous hand-suture technique and palpation of finished stomata. Obstruction may also be caused by internal hernia if a mesenteric defect is not closed, but the closing suture must be placed superficially to avoid mesenteric vessels, the injury of which would produce hematoma or bowel ischemia.

Blind Loop Syndrome

Blind loop syndrome is characterized by diarrhea, macrocytic anemia, and hypocalcemia. It may be caused by bacterial overgrowth in a partially obstructed surgically bypassed segment of the bowel. It is surely produced by accidental creation of a limb the peristalsis of which fills rather than empties itself. Because the syndrome is extremely rare and because diarrhea and anemia have many more common causes, blind loop should not be treated by reoperation until its diagnosis is confirmed by studies of fecal fat, Schiller's test, and the response to broad-spectrum antibiotics.

Diarrhea

Removing 100 cm of terminal ileum may produce diarrhea from colonic irritation by unabsorbed bile salts. Concomitant failure to absorb vitamin B_{12} may produce macrocytic anemia. Anemia is easily treated with intramuscular B_{12}, 1000 μg every 3 months, but cholestyramine administered orally to bind salts may be more disagreeable than is the diarrhea. Cholestyramine, however, is worth trying, especially after resection for Crohn's disease. A satisfactory response to cholestyramine suggests that the diarrhea is caused by ileum loss rather than by residual Crohn's disease.

Short Bowel Syndrome

Short bowel syndrome is manifested by very rapid transit; profuse diarrhea; deficits of all nutrients, vitamins, minerals, and water; and production of renal calculi due to excessive colonic absorption of oxalate. It is inevitably produced by resecting over 75% of the small bowel. Loss of terminal ileum renders the syndrome more likely and more severe. Loss of jejunum may cause hypergastrinemia and might predispose the patient to duodenal ulcer.

As soon as it is clear that a patient has lost so much small bowel that recovery by oral nutrition is impossible, TPN must be started with meticulous technique, in anticipation of possible lifetime dependence. The patient is allowed nothing by mouth while gastric secretion is controlled with cimetidine and the transit time prolonged with opiates. The volume of diarrhea will diminish. When less than 2.5 L per day, a dilute, isotonic elemental diet is begun by continuous nasogastric-tube feeding. Diet stimulates the remaining intestine to adapt by dilatation of its lumen and lengthening of its villi. Diet is advanced as tolerated, and within 6 months patients with 100 cm or more of healthy bowel should be free of all parenteral treatment except B_{12}. Patients learn to control their own diets, using opiates as needed, but they must be continually followed for vitamin and mineral deficiencies and for renal stones. They may require parenteral fluids during acute illnesses.

Operations that create reversed limbs or recirculating loops have failed to control diarrhea or caused obstruction and sacrifice of precious remaining bowel. Any benefits thought to have been observed were more likely attributable to spontaneous adaptation, which may unpredictably prove adequate even in some patients with less than 100 cm of small bowel. This hope, however, must never license a surgeon to sacrifice more small bowel than is necessary. Every centimeter of healthy terminal ileum must always be preserved, and in Crohn's disease all functioning bowel must be saved in anticipation of the probable need for future resection.

COLOTOMY

Colotomy is an ineffective way to locate active bleeding. When it is used for this purpose, recurrent or persistent bleeding yields a mortality rate of about 20%. Bleeding is more safely controlled by resecting angiographically proven bleeding segments or by resecting all the intra-abdominal colon.

Colotomy may miss small polyps. They are more dependably found and more safely removed by colonoscopy. When colotomy is required to remove a very large polyp, preparations, precautions, and complications are identical to those associated with colon resection.

CECOSTOMY

Tube cecostomy may be effective for fixation of a mobile cecum to prevent recurrent volvulus, but cecopexy appears more effective and has far less risk of morbidity. Ogilvie's cecal paralysis is more safely deflated by colonoscopy. Tube cecostomy is effective for decompressing obstructed colon only when a large 30-Fr mushroom catheter is used and irrigated every 8 hours with 50 ml of water. Smaller catheters are quickly plugged and ineffective and allow feces to leak about the catheter and into the abdomen.

The leading intraoperative complication of tube cecostomy is accidental spillage of feces, prevented by very gentle handling and trocar decompression of the dilated cecum before purse-string sutures are placed. The laparotomy incision is inevitably contaminated, and skin closure must be delayed. When tubes are removed, 6% of cecostomies result in persistent cecocutaneous fistulas in which skin irritation is severe and difficult to control. This unavoidable complication should be a deterrent to tube cecostomy except for emergency decompression before a right colectomy.

LOOP COLOSTOMY

Loop colostomy is effective and safe for temporarily enteriorizing a perforation or for decompressing obstruction. It is ineffective for diverting feces from distal disease. The only advantage a loop bestows over end colostomy is that, if the loop is opened longitudinally, it may be closed without resecting the bowel. When a colostomy will not be closed, stomal problems make loop a poor technique for prolonged colon evacuation.

Retraction

If a loop is held out by a bridge of fascia or skin sewn beneath it, the bridge may separate and the loop disappear into the abdomen. If an opened loop vanishes prematurely, it must be recovered by laparotomy. This is prevented by passing a 5-cm section of heavy rubber tube through mesentery beneath the loop and sewing its ends to skin with nonabsorbable sutures. A collecting device may be cumbersome to apply while the tube is in place, but it may be removed after a week if wound healing and peristalsis are normal.

Evisceration

Evisceration of the small bowel around an adult loop colostomy occurs when its opening through the abdominal wall is made larger than two fingerbreadths. It is prevented by making small openings. In struggling infants, evisceration must be prevented by sewing colon wall to adjacent parietal peritoneum and fascia. Most loop colostomies are closed before peristoma hernia can occur. If hernia does occur and colostomy is still needed, it should be converted to an end colostomy at a fresh site.

FIG. 32-4. Imperfect closure of loop colostomy invites life-threatening peritonitis, abscesses, fistula, and obstruction. The safest technique keeps the posterior wall of the loop intact and simply repairs anterior wall. (*A*) A mature stoma with posterior wall intact. (*B*) Eliptical skin incision 3 mm from mucosa, carried through fat to fascia. (*C*) Colon wall carefully freed from fascia about entire circumference. (*D*) Skin and scar excised from stoma. (*E*) Opening in colon closed transversely with interrupted inverting nonabsorbable sutures. (*F*) Colon returned to abdominal cavity so suture line does not abut fascial repair. (*G*) Fascia repaired with interrupted steel wire.

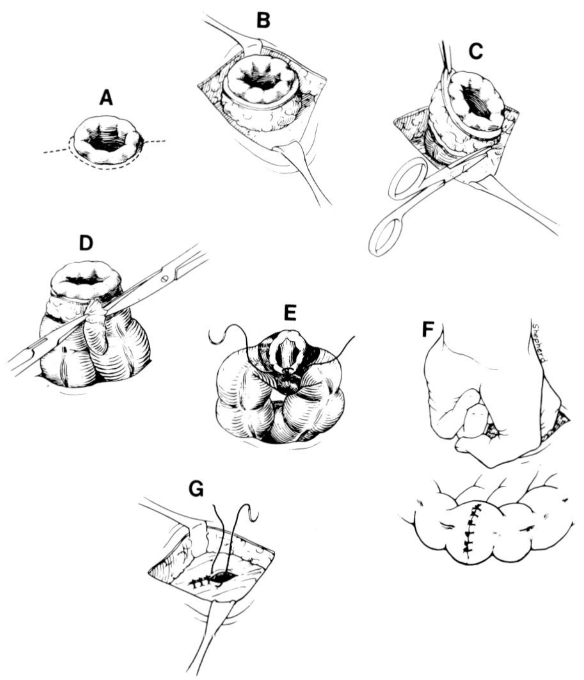

Prolapse

Prolapse complicates one quarter of adults' and most of children's loop colostomies. Distal ends prolapse more often and in greater length. Colostomies made of right colon prolapse more often than those of left, perhaps because they require larger openings. Making small openings and using the most distal colon feasible may reduce but not eliminate the risk of prolapse.

Prolapses are easily reduced, immediately recur, fill stoma appliances, and are unsightly nuisances. They are, however, no threat to life or bowel function. When colostomy closure is anticipated, it should not be hastened on account of prolapse. Instead the prolapse should be tolerated until the patient's underlying condition permits safe resection, repair, and elimination of the colostomy.

Severe prolapse in a loop designed for several months' use but subsequently shown necessary for years, should be treated surgically. The only reliable technique is to resect all the colon involved in the stoma, to make a single matured stoma of the proximal end through a fresh small opening, to close the distal end, and to leave it in the abdomen. If the distal colon is or may become completely obstructed, the distal side of the loop should not be closed but made a small mucous fistula well away from the functioning proximal stoma.

CLOSURE OF LOOP COLOSTOMY

Obstruction

Postoperative obstruction at the site of closure may be caused by either hematoma or inversion of too much tissue. Both errors must be scrupulously avoided, especially in the narrow and powerful sigmoid colon. Both are more likely after resection and anastomosis but may occur after simple repair of a loop's anterior wall. Thus in mobilizing a loop for closure, care must be taken not to enlarge its opening or injure any part of the colon or its mesentery. A narrow ellipse of skin is left attached to mucosa until the loop is clearly free of abdominal wall and all layers are ready for repair. Then only enough skin and scar are débrided from healthy pliable colon to permit repair with inverting, interrupted, nonabsorbable sutures. This semicircumferential repair allows a more ample lumen than does complete circumferential anastomosis (Fig. 32-4). It also avoids scarred or edematous mesocolon where bleeding may predispose the patient to hematoma.

Obstruction is manifested by constipation, distention, and pain after resolution of ileus. In the absence of peritonitis, the symptoms should be evaluated by gentle barium enema. Usually the narrowed segment will be found sufficiently large to function satisfactorily and will enlarge as its scar matures. If cecal distention progresses, however, the patient must have a new colostomy.

Abscesses

If skin is closed, subcutaneous abscess will complicate a third of colostomy closures despite optimal cleansing and the use of antibiotics. Such a complication may be considered a technical error because these small wounds heal very rapidly when packed open and allowed to close spontaneously.

Intra-abdominal abscesses after colostomy closure have three sources. One is contaminated hematoma, prevented only by meticulous hemostasis but discouraged by cleansing the colon and giving prophylactic antibiotics. A second source is an anastomotic leak, prevented by meticulous suture technique. An abscess from either of these sources will occur adjacent to the colon repair, cause its dissolution, feculent peritonitis, or colocutaneous fistula. A third source of intra-abdominal abscess is residual infection from the event for which colostomy was originally performed. To obviate this possibility one must be certain a patient is well before a colostomy is closed.

END COLOSTOMY

Necrosis

A new colostomy must be inspected daily through its clear plastic collecting bag. Some venous congestion and superficial slough of mucosa are tolerable, but if the entire stoma appears necrotic, its circulation should be tested with cautious débridement of one edge. If there is no bleeding, the patient should be returned to surgery and the colon advanced and resutured to skin to prevent retraction and stenosis. Although shock and arteriosclerosis may contribute to stomal necrosis, more common and easily controlled causes are removal of too much mesentery and strangulating the stoma by too tight an opening in the abdominal wall. Mesentery must be preserved to within 1 cm of the stoma, fascia opened with a cruciate incision, and the opening made large enough to accommodate mesentery and colon so that the stoma bleeds when it is sutured to skin.

Retraction

Retraction of an end colostomy is normally prevented by sewing its viable edges under minimal tension to adjacent skin with eight chromic or Dexon sutures. In very obese patients, however, long segments of colon and mesentery are required to reach skin, and tension that seems tolerable in the supine position may be intolerable when the patient turns in bed. In such patients the colon must be mobilized with great care to protect its mesentery. The length of colon necessary to traverse abdominal wall may be minimized by locating a colostomy in the umbilicus where the wall is thinnest. When retraction occurs, the patient should be immediately returned to surgery and the wound explored in hopes of drawing out enough viable colon to be resutured to skin. If this fails, repeated laparotomy and mobilization of more colon is necessary to prevent intraperitoneal spillage of feces and late stomal stenosis.

Stenosis

When necrosis or retraction leaves a gap of granulating wound between mucosa and skin, contracture causes stenosis, which may lead to fecal impaction. In diagnosing fecal impaction, one must be careful not to overlook small bowel obstruction, which occurs after 1% of end colostomies. The small bowel may be obstructed by distant adhesions or by internal hernia, which should have been prevented by sewing colon to the lateral abdominal wall.

For urgent relief of impaction, stomal dilatation is acceptable, but fractured scar will heal by renewed contraction. A stenotic stoma must be revised by circumferential excision of just enough skin and scar so that pliable colon easily expands to fill the enlarged opening.

Peristomal Hernia

Peristomal hernias may follow up to 25% of permanent end colostomies. Conditions that favor hernia are obesity, openings that admit over two fingers, and openings through oblique muscles or muscles weakened by adjacent laparotomy scars. The strongest and most convenient site for a colostomy is in the lateral third of the rectus muscle just far enough below the waist to permit wearing a belt above a collecting device. The laparotomy incision that least interferes with a colostomy is through the midline.

Most peristomal hernias are little bother to patients who often refuse repair for fear of jeopardizing functioning stomas. When a hernia is painful or irreducible or impairs stoma care, local repair may be attempted but recurrence is probable. Dependable cure requires laparotomy and relocation of the colostomy in another part of the abdominal wall.

Colostomy Care

Problems with stomal hygiene are rare after a properly located, well-constructed end colostomy of the sigmoid or descending colon. Patients who are capable of safely irrigating their colostomies should be trained to do so in hopes of regulating output. Instruction, however, must be flexible and individualized so that patients with intrinsically unpredictable colonic motility will not feel ashamed of always having to wear appliances. More proximal colostomies, especially in the right transverse colon, require continuous collection of liquid or semisolid feces. These patients must not be misled to expect continence. Their peristomal skin must be protected as carefully as it is with ileostomy. Optimal adaptation to colostomy is not acquired by rigid compliance with published instructions, but rather by highly individualized, flexible, and imaginative manipulation of diet, deodorants, and appliances. Satisfactory adaptation is most rapidly achieved with the advice of an experienced enterostomal therapist.

Depression

Despondency and social and sexual disability must not be attributed to the colostomy. When profound and inappropriate depression occurs despite optimal instruction in stomal care, its cause is either a psychiatric disorder present but undiscovered before surgery or some factor unrelated to colostomy, such as fear of recurrent cancer. To minimize emotional disability and eliminate the risk of suicide, coincidental psychiatric disorders must be recognized promptly and treated expertly.

COLON RESECTION AND REPAIR

The most common and costly complications of colectomy are persistence and progression of diseases that surgery fails to control. To cite the peculiar shortcomings of colectomy for cancer, diverticulitis, infarction, granulomatous and ulcerative colitis, volvulus and a dozen other disorders is beyond the scope of this text. It must be recognized, however, that to perform an uncomplicated colectomy, one must be thoroughly familiar with the pathology and natural history of the disease being treated and must know how it may respond to resection.

Injuries of Adjacent Organs

Vital structures adjacent to the colon or its mesentery include ureters, kidneys, duodenum, gallbladder, pancreas, stomach, spleen, ovaries, tubes, bladder, and iliac and superior mesenteric vessels. Unless they are involved in colonic disease, they should be easily identified and protected. When an accidental injury occurs, it is usually attributable to too short an abdominal incision, too little assistance, or too much haste.

Colonic cancer invading genitourinary organs, gallbladder, stomach, or spleen may be resected *en bloc* if other metastases do not prevail. For resection of the kidney, however, preoperative intravenous pyelogram must have shown function in the opposite kidney.

Inflammatory diseases of the colon may be cautiously peeled from adherent but innocent organs, dissecting with a sucker tip under clear vision, and leaving granulation tissue or even colon mucosa on the organ being protected. If, despite optimal caution, a small hole is left in the bladder, it may be closed with chromic catgut and drained with a urethral catheter. A small injury to the ureter may be delicately repaired with chromic catgut and drained through the flank. Ureter divided within 4 cm of the bladder is best repaired by ureteroneocystostomy. An injured gallbladder should be removed, pancreas drained through the flank, and stomach simply repaired. A duodenal perforation may be difficult to repair while maintaining patency. One too large to close by simple inverting sutures should be covered by attaching the unopened wall of the jejunum as a "serosal patch" to the duodenal defect, with interrupted sutures about its entire circumference.

Delayed Hemorrhage

Postoperative hemorrhage requiring reexploration and mesenteric hematoma evolving to abscess may complicate resection of colon, the mesentery of which is too edematous or inflamed to hold secure ligatures. Diverticular abscess, Crohn's colitis, and perforated cancer create such conditions. When inflamed bowel is resected, stumps of edematous mesentery must be doubly ligated. Hemorrhagic shock after resection, unless caused by coincidental upper gastrointestinal bleeding, requires immediate reexploration. An unexpected fall in the hematocrit is a harbinger of intra-abdominal hematoma, which is probably contaminated by enteric bacteria and will probably require drainage.

Anastomotic Leak

Colonic anastomoses are more prone to leak than are those of the stomach and small bowel. Among features that predispose patients to leakage are a high concentration of virulent bacteria, single thin layer of circular muscle, liability to distention, slow recovery from ileus, and contractions that are more segmental than directional. The more distal an anastomosis, the greater is its tendency to leak. Ileotransverse colostomy is usually safe even in emergency, unprepared right colectomy, but rectal anastomoses show radiologic leakage in about 20% and clinical leak in about 5% of cases. Although the rectum has two muscular layers, it is difficult to expose it for hemostasis and suturing, and it lacks the protection of peritoneum.

Anastomotic leaks are clinically manifested, usually in the second postoperative week, by signs of intra-abdominal or pelvic abscess, which were discussed as the common denominators of intestinal surgery. A leak within the peritoneal cavity is best treated by dismantling the anastomosis, making a proximal end colostomy and distal mucous fistula or Hartman's pouch. Leak from a rectal anastomosis is best treated by proximal loop colostomy and pelvic drainage. When it appears that a rectal anastomosis may be precarious, many surgeons add prophylactic loop colostomy and suction drains in the pelvis.

To prevent leakage requires optimal preparation and perfect technique. The colon must be cleansed with cathartics, enemas, and oral antibiotics. Intraperitoneal spillage of its contents must be scrupulously prevented to avoid destruction of an anastomosis by an adjacent abscess. Ends must meet without tension. Marginal arteries and mesentery must be preserved to within 5 mm of bowel ends. Ischemia of apposed tissues is minimized by interrupted sutures or staples. Sutures must be perfectly placed and tied without excessive force. When poor exposure of the lower rectum prohibits a perfect manual suture, an EEA-stapled anastomosis is safer if care is taken to avoid injury to the distal rectum, to be certain a complete "doughnut" of tissue is excised, to inspect the anastomosis, and to reinforce it with sutures if necessary.[1] All colon and rectal anastomoses must be inverted. Eversion is an unsafe compromise.

Obstruction

Stomal obstruction is manifested by gaseous distention any time after the resolution of paralytic ileus. Early incomplete obstruction may be caused by inversion of too much tissue, by the purse-string effect of continuous unlocked sutures, or by intramural hematoma. Although these errors are impossible with EEA staple devices, membranes and strictures have been reported after stapled anastomoses.[3] Strictures are probably caused by contracture of excessive scar associated with healing of leaked anastomoses.

When contrast studies show early partial obstruction of an intact anastomosis, subsequent x-ray films usually show progressive improvement while distention subsides. Complete or persistent obstruction requires resection and reanastomosis, except in the low rectum where a mature stricture may be manually dilated. Late obstruction requires colonoscopy and biopsy to detect recurrence of the disease, such as cancer or Crohn's, for which the colon was originally resected.

Small bowel obstruction by adhesions cannot be totally prevented, but internal hernia through a mesenteric defect must be avoided by repair of such defects. When proximal transverse colon is anastomosed to distal sigmoid or rectum, mesenteric repair is impossible, but the likelihood of internal hernia can be minimized by drawing the proximal end through a window in the right mesocolon and behind the ileum to the rectum.

Subcutaneous Wound Infection

The threat of wound abscess, a common denominator of all intestinal surgery, is greatest following colon resection. Without bowel preparation and antibiotics, skin must never be closed, for the probability of infection exceeds 50%. With optimal preparation, antibiotics, and avoidance of any fecal spillage, a 6% incidence of infection permits primary wound closure. On our own service the incidence of infection after elective colectomy is less than 4%. Our preparation includes 2 days of clear liquid diet, magnesium sulfate catharsis (30 ml, three times a day), and saline enemas until clear. Neomycin, 1 g, and erythromycin, 500 mg, are given by mouth on the day before surgery at 1, 2, and 11 P.M. The laparotomy incision is protected with a plastic barrier, but no antibiotic irrigations are used. Whether an intravenous antibiotic can further reduce this rate of infection has not been proven.

Diarrhea

Loss of absorptive and storage capacity can produce diarrhea, especially if terminal ileum is also resected. Severe diarrhea upon recovery from ileus always improves spontaneously. An ileorectal anastomosis may at first produce a dozen liquid stools per day, but within 3 months patients on no medication will have three or four soft stools daily. Diarrhea may be controlled with loperamide, but this must not be prescribed in the first week after surgery because residual ileus may compound its effect and cause distention.[12]

The likelihood of diarrhea must be minimized by removing only enough bowel to cure the disease at hand. Length of resection for cancer is dictated by lymphatic drainage and by knowing that intramural microscopic disease is rarely found over 5 cm from the palpable tumor. In ulcerative colitis and diverticulitis, all but 1 cm of terminal ileum must be preserved. In Crohn's disease of terminal ileum involving the cecum, some ascending colon can usually be preserved.

Fecal Incontinence

Incontinence may complicate rectal resection when anastomosis is made within 5 cm of the anus. It is more likely to occur in elderly patients with weak sphincters already incontinent of flatus, and more often after operations that involve anal dilatation, such as anal pull-through procedures. While transacral anastomosis avoids injury to sphincters, its advantage may be lost in retrorectal abscess and rectocutaneous fistula requiring colostomy. Sphincter strength is perhaps best protected by an EEA-stapled anastomosis. After low anterior resection, incontinence usually improves in the first 3 months of convalescence. During this time, it may be controlled by constipating drugs and diet, anal pads, and, if the suture line is proven intact, gentle irrigations at convenient times of the day.

TOTAL PERINEAL PROCTECTOMY

When treating cancers, three mistakes may be made in selecting patients for perineal proctectomy. The first is to assume wrongly that a tumor is too low for partial proctectomy and rectal anastomosis. After lateral attachments of the lower rectum are divided from within the abdomen, the rectum often stretches to provide an adequate, 5-cm margin distal to the tumor. This possibility must not be lost by premature destruction of the anus. In a two-team approach, the perineal team must wait patiently until the abdominal team has determined a tumor's mobility and possible margin.

The second mistake is to assume a tumor cannot be resected when it feels large and fixed on rectal palpation. Unless pelvic wall invasion is proven by CT scan, abdominal exploration should be done because extension of a mass may consist of inflamed lymph nodes. Preoperative irradiation may reduce the size and increase mobility of a mass initially thought to be unresectable.

The third mistake is to attempt proctectomy for relief of pain or obstruction in a tumor that cannot be totally resected. Incomplete removal is ineffective for palliation because a locally persistent tumor is often more disabling than was the original tumor. For palliation, proximal end colostomy and radiation or chemotherapy are more effective.

For chronic ulcerative colitis total proctocolectomy always effects a cure. Subsequent disease in the small bowel proves the initial diagnosis should have been Crohn's colitis. Crohn's proctitis is very effectively palliated by proctocolectomy. When the small bowel is normal, the probability of needing small bowel resection in the future is only 3% to 4% per year. Even when the small bowel is involved, over 90% of patients with severe disabling Crohn's proctitis are rehabilitated by and grateful for proctocolectomy and ileostomy.

For ulcerative colitis, familial polyposis and radiation proctitis, procedures have been recently described for preserving the lower rectum and anus.[2, 13] Because the risk of complications after these operations is great, a surgeon undertaking them must be thoroughly up-to-date with the literature.

Leg Injuries

Deep vein thromboses, tibial or peroneal nerve injuries, and gastrocnemius muscle necrosis may occur if an anesthetized patient is held in the lithotomy position by unpadded supports. These complications are prevented by bearing most weight of the legs on padded stirrups so that calves and knees need only light suspension. The feet must be high to favor venous drainage. Legs must be positioned simultaneously to prevent hip dislocation. Before radical perineal proctectomy in a patient without femoral pulses, one must consider the risk of leg ischemia from loss of collateral circulation.

Bleeding

Bleeding should not occur from superior or inferior hemorrhoidal vessels because they are easily seen and ligated through abdominal and perineal approaches. Bleeding from middle hemorrhoidal arteries is prevented by bluntly developing the lateral attachments to the lower rectum and clamping them before they are cut. There should be no other sources of bleeding unless a large tumor has invaded sacral or iliac veins, circumstances in which resection should be abandoned. After the rectum is out, time is well spent stopping hemorrhage from any visible vessels because a pelvic hematoma is liable to become an abscess.

Ureteral Injury

Ureteral injury is caused by failure to identify ureters, by inadequate exposure, or by operating in a bloody field. In a synchronous, two-team abdominoperineal proctectomy, the perineal surgeon must stop work on the prostate gland or upper vagina because his exposure of ureters is unsafe. The abdominal surgeon must expose both ureters from iliac vessels to bladder, watch them as he clamps and cuts middle hemorrhoidal vessels and as he divides Denonvilliers' fascia, and check their integrity as he repairs pelvic peritoneum. If a ureter is adherent to an inflammatory mass, the bowel should be carefully peeled away so that granulation tissue or scar is left on the ureter. If a lower ureter must be resected with cancer, its proximal end may be anastomosed to the side of the opposite ureter with 5-0 chromic catgut. A ureter accidentally divided in its distal 4 cm should be reimplanted by ureteroneocystostomy. Simple ligation would stop urine excretion and cause acute renal atrophy. Unrecognized division of a ureter during proctectomy results at first in urinary fistula through the perineum, later in partial obstruction, hydronephrosis, and pyelonephritis. During proctectomy for cancer, seminal vesicles may be sacrificed, but membranous and prostatic urethra must be preserved unless one is prepared for pelvic exenteration.

Pelvic Abscess and Perineal Sinus

Pelvic abscess complicates about 5% of elective proctectomies despite preoperative cathartics, enemas, and antibiotics. Urgent unprepared proctectomy for inflammatory disease yields pelvic abscess in about 30% of cases. Abscess is manifested by fever, leukocytosis, and recurrent ileus after pelvic drains have been removed, usually in the second week after surgery. When these signs appear, the perineal wound must be immediately reopened, packed, and irrigated. Three of four wounds that are packed open will completely heal spontaneously. One quarter will form persistent sinus tracts. Such sinuses are rarely disabling to patients, but if they are, they may be filled and healed by pedicle grafts of gracilis muscle. Coccygectomy is ineffective for facilitating closure.

Although pelvic abscess and perineal sinus cannot be completely prevented, their frequency must be minimized. Fecal contamination must be prevented by suture ligation of the anus. Care must be taken not to perforate the rectum. Hematoma must not be allowed to collect in the inevitably contaminated pelvic space. It is prevented by careful hemostasis and by suction drainage through the loosely closed perineal wound. Many surgeons also use Penrose drains for 2 to 3 days, leaving the suction catheter until its output is less than 50 ml per day.

Urinary Retention

Several factors contribute to urinary retention after proctectomy. Among them are bladder denervation, posterior angulation of bladder, incisional pain, narcotics, and bladder outlet obstruction by prostatic hypertrophy. These factors are so often combined in elderly men that most cannot void for 7 to 10 days after proctectomy. Catheters should be left in all patients until they are free of pain and no longer need narcotics and intravenous fluids. Residual volume should be tested by instilling 200 ml of sterile water just before a catheter is withdrawn. A residual volume of 100 ml or more 2 weeks after surgery warrants cystoscopy and cystometric examination to determine the need for transurethral resection or continuous or intermittent catheterization.

Impotence

Afferent pudendal nerves vital to erection and pelvic sympathetics that direct ejaculation must often be sacrificed to remove rectal cancer. When erectile capacity is lost, a patient may be grateful for a penile prosthesis. In proctectomy for ulcerative colitis or Crohn's disease, neither erection nor ejaculation should be impaired. By cutting peritoneum close to the rectal wall, sympathetic nerves are spared. From the perineal approach, dissection should stay close to the anus and rectum, preserving external sphincter, levator muscles, seminal vesicles, and Denonvilliers' fascia.

ILEOSTOMY

Until Brooke's technique was combined in the 1960s with improved skin adhesives, karaya gum, and plastic-collecting devices, simple ileostomy bore a forbidding reputation for complications. Now most complications can be prevented. Patients with ileostomies enjoy normal activities, restricted only by the need to empty bags four or five times each day, to wash or change bags daily, and to change adhesive wafers about every 5 days. Having never observed this experience, many physicians and patients still dread simple ileostomy and seek continent ileostomy pouches. Continent ileostomy holds great promise but in its present state of evolution requires surgical revision in over 20% of cases for complications that cannot yet be avoided. The following complications of simple ileostomy can be prevented.

Excoriation

If more than a 3-mm to 4-mm rim of skin is exposed to feces, severe excoriation will occur. The problem is caused either by applying too large a protective ring or by placing an ileostomy where a crease, scar, iliac crest, or umbilicus prevents perfect adhesion of the plate or wafer to the underlying skin. Excoriation will heal under careful and constant karaya gum protection.

Prevention of excoriation must begin before the operation by using an adhesive wafer to select the ideal site for ileostomy while the patient is standing or sitting and clothed. Once an ileostomy is formed, excoriation must be prevented by applying well-fitted karaya gum rings and adhesive wafers. Ring size must often be reduced during the 3 months after surgery because an ileostomy contracts as it matures. Excoriation is best prevented and cured with directions from an enterostomal therapist. A surgeon who must direct ileostomy hygiene without help from an enterostomal therapist needs advice from a text that treats the problem in great detail.[6]

Stenosis

Ileostomy stenosis is manifested as partial small bowel obstruction. X-ray study with retrograde contrast injection is necessary to prove that the obstruction is in the stoma and not in more proximal small bowel. Forceful dilatation may give temporary relief, but stricture will recur. Successful treatment requires laparotomy and construction of a new ileostomy using fresh, pliable ileum.

In the absence of Crohn's disease, the cause of stenosis is either ischemic necrosis of the ileum or exposure of ileal serosa to fecal irritants. Ischemia must be prevented by preserving mesentery at least to skin level, preferably to within 2 cm of the bowel's cut end. Serosal exposure must be prevented by

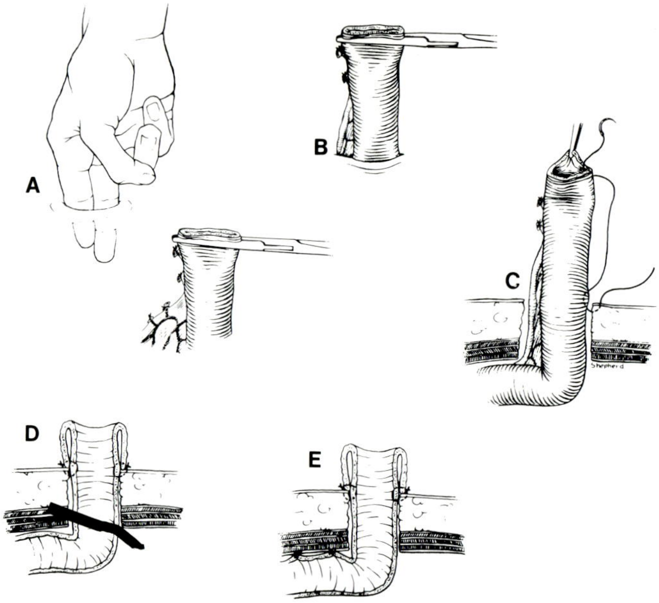

FIG. 32-5. Technical perfection is prerequisite to easy, complication-free management of an ileostomy. (*A*) The abdominal opening must admit only two fingers, and mesentery must be preserved to within 2 cm of bowel end. (*B*) Ileum must be drawn 5 cm beyond skin. (*C*) Chromic or Dexon sutures must grasp skin edge, adjacent seromuscular wall of bowel, and bowel edge. Placement of six to eight sutures at equal intervals about circumference must avoid injury to mesentery. (*D*) When sutures are tied, the nipple must project 2 cm beyond skin. (*E*) Unless terminal ileum is drawn up between peritoneum and abdominal wall, it must be sutured to peritoneum to prevent internal hernia.

turning back 2 cm of ileum on itself and suturing cut edges to the underlying bowel wall as well as to adjacent skin (Fig. 32-5).

Prolapse and Hernia

Ileal prolapse and hernia beside an ileostomy are prevented by making the cruciate incision in the rectus sheath only large enough to admit two fingers tightly and by fixing the distal ileum to the lateral abdominal wall. Fixation may be accomplished either by tunneling the ileum beneath the peritoneum from the right gutter to the ileostomy site or more simply by sewing the ileum to the wall with interrupted, nonabsorbable sutures. Immediate prolapse or hernia should be treated by laparotomy and reconstruction of the ileostomy. Later it requires relocation of the ileostomy, a procedure most patients may safely decline unless these complications are painful or interfere with stomal hygiene.

CONTINENT ILEOSTOMY

A continent ileostomy should consist of a pouch that accommodates up to 500 ml of liquid feces, a valve that retains liquid and gas under pressure, and a stoma that can be easily catheterized three to five times each day. Since first performed by Nils Koch, in 1967, the effectiveness and durability of pouches have been enhanced by technical modifications that yield 75% perfect continence, 93% freedom from appliances, and 95% patient satisfaction. Whether the remaining failures are inevitable risks or technical flaws must yet be learned. The technique is still evolving, so that a surgeon preparing to create an ileal pouch must study critically the latest publications of its most experienced investigators.[4, 6]

Suture-Line Leakage

The greatest danger from continent ileostomy is manifested by signs of peritonitis or intra-abdominal abscess. It is proven by Gastrografin instillation and treated by immediate laparotomy and repair or excision of the pouch. The complication is rare and can be prevented by using inverted, interrupted, nonabsorbable sutures, by continuous catheter drainage for the first 4 weeks, and by frequent intubation in the next 4 weeks.

Stenosis

Contraction of the cutaneous stoma may prevent intubation. Its cause is imperfect approximation of mucosa to skin. For perfect approximation and primary healing, one must preserve the stoma's mesentery to prevent ischemia and make the efferent limb long enough to minimize tension and prevent retraction.

Protrusion

Protrusion of an ileal bud above the skin requires bag or bandage to protect mucosa and clothing. This is prevented by pulling the efferent limb through the abdominal opening until the pouch is apposed to abdominal wall, by sewing the pouch to the wall, and by amputating any excess efferent limb so it is only long enough to reach from peritoneum to skin.

Incontinence

Incontinence may be caused by a valve that is too short or by spontaneous disruption, extrusion, and effacement of the valve. The valve must protrude into the pouch for at least 5 cm. It may be kept intact by rows of staples through opposite sides of the valve (avoiding mesentery) and by interrupted, non-absorbable seromuscular sutures between pouch and efferent limb where the latter emerges from the pouch, but even these techniques have not achieved perfect continence.

Intestinal Obstruction

Obstruction by adhesions elsewhere in the abdomen cannot completely be prevented, but an internal hernia around the pouch can be prevented by sewing the pouch and ileum to the lateral parietal peritoneum. Obstruction caused by the pressure of pregnancy may be relieved by induction of early delivery.

Diarrhea

Diarrhea, reported in 7.5% of continent ileostomies, is caused by overgrowth of anaerobic bacteria in the pouch or in the ileum proximal to it. Like blind loop syndrome, it responds to oral broad-spectrum antibiotics, recurs after treatment, but responds to repeated treatment.

OPERATIONS FOR RECTAL PROLAPSE

Transient rectal prolapse of infancy is cured by simple manual reduction and external compression. Mucosal prolapse in adults is easily cured by excision and continuous suture of each of three or four groups of internal hemorrhoids. Complete adult prolapse, however, requires fixation of rectum to sacrum, perineal repair, or a combination of fixation and repair. The most experienced advocates of these techniques report curing up to 97% of prolapses, but complications are frequent and discouraging.

Ureters or sympathetic nerves that control ejaculation may be injured during the dissection of the rectum. Pelvic abscess may follow low rectal anastomosis, sewing Marlex to the rectum, or implanting an Ivalon sponge to incite inflammatory adhesions to sacrum. The most common complications, however, are fecal impaction and fecal incontinence. Any procedure that avoids one is liable to produce the other.

Fecal Impaction

Impaction often complicates minor procedures that simply encircle anal sphincters with wire or Marlex ribbon. Following these operations, patients require stool softeners, lubricants, frequent digital examinations, irrigations or suppositories, and sometimes laxatives. If severe impactions recur despite these measures, the anal ligature must be released, which may cause recurrent prolapse. The same dilemma may be created by abdominal operations that suspend the rectum with a complete anterior apron of Marlex sewn to sacrum.

Fecal Incontinence

When the operation is not complicated by impaction, 50% to 60% of patients will suffer fecal incontinence. It is probably caused not by surgery but by whatever neuromuscular disorder allowed the prolapse. Like idiopathic megacolon, prolapse is often associated with psychiatric disability, and complications of impaction or incontinence may prove as difficult to manage as is prolapse.

HEMORRHOIDECTOMY

Pain

Pain after anorectal surgery is caused either by anal sphincter spasm or by sutures in sensitive squamous epithelium. Gentle, four-finger anal dilatation before hemorrhoidectomy prevents spasm. Sutures or rubber bands must be confined to columnar epithelium above the pectinate line. Squamous epithelial wounds left open will heal quickly and painlessly.

Bleeding

Postoperative bleeding sufficient to require a transfusion also requires reoperation. Suture ligating a bleeder in an edematous, friable rectum narrowed by recent surgery is as difficult as it is embarrassing, so every effort must be made to secure the hemostasis in the original operation. Two maneuvers help. The first is through a well-dilated anus initially to excise the most dependent hemorrhoid so that blood running down will not obscure a site of subsequent incision. The second is to clamp all tissue to be excised, under-run the clamp with to-and-fro continuous 0 chromic catgut, excise tissue beyond the clamp, remove the clamp, continuously oversew crushed tissue by running the same suture back to the point it began, and then tie it to its original tail.

Stricture

Stricture of the anus or distal rectum may result from excising such broad strips of mucosa that none is left to repair or reepithelialize the rectum. Most strictures, however, are not complications of surgical technique but of faulty postoperative care. Prescriptions and advice must make stools sufficiently bulky, malleable, and well-lubricated to produce daily spontaneous anal dilatation. Patients must be strictly warned not to use laxatives that produce liquid stools and promote stricture. Instead, they should begin taking twice daily a bulk-softener, such as psyllium mucilloid, and mineral oil as a lubricant. Patients must be advised to evacuate quickly, to avoid prolonged straining, and to return at least once for a follow-up examination to be certain that this advice is followed and effective.

Persistence or Recurrence

Hemorrhoids are often found coincidental to colorectal cancer or to ulcerative, granulomatous, and infectious colitides. It is imperative that these more dangerous conditions be ruled out before any hemorrhoidectomy is performed. After the surgical cure of hemorrhoids, any recurrent bleeding, mass, or pain requires another complete evaluation.

DRAINAGE OF PERIRECTAL ABSCESS

Persistent Cellulitis

Persistent or progressive cellulitis is caused by inadequate drainage or débridement. It may be caused by any of three errors.[9] The first error is to delay drainage until fluctuance is palpable. Any patient with pain, tenderness, and induration on one side of the anus or rectum has pus that must be drained promptly before it spreads to areas where drainage is less effective. The second error is to attempt drainage with a needle or under local anesthesia. The volume of pus is always greater than expected. Complete evacuation requires general or spinal anesthesia and a radial incision long enough for digital exploration. The third error is failure to recognize synergistic necrotizing cellulitis. Its hallmarks are toxicity and dishwater drainage, often in an obese, diabetic, or uremic patient.[15] Survival of this rare but devastating infection requires immediate radical débridement; intravenous gentamicin, chloramphenicol, and cephalosporin; and daily redébridement under anesthesia until the cellulitis is controlled.

Recurrent Abscess and Fistula

After the cellulitis has subsided, the prompt recurrence of an abscess in the same spot may be caused by allowing too small a skin incision to heal before contraction has closed the cavity beneath it. Although most patients may be discharged from the hospital without packs after 1 or 2 days, they must be reexamined regularly until closure from within is assured.

Anal fistula is caused by the persistence of the connection of an abscess to the gland and crypt from which it arose and by persistence of the opening created for external drainage. When abscess that is clearly connected to a diseased crypt by a superficial tract is drained, coincidental fistulotomy should be performed. When the connection is not obvious and superficial, fistolotomy must be deferred, in the hope that the internal opening will be obliterated by scar. Anticipating the possibility of fistula and the likelihood that a fistula will produce recurrent abscess, one must instruct each patient to return for elective fistulotomy if drainage persists from a perianal dimple.

ANAL FISTULOTOMY

Incontinence

Permanent fecal incontinence will result if anal sphincters are divided in two places at the same operation. To prevent this complication, the course of a fistula must be clearly identified before any muscle is cut. With knowledge of Goodsall's rule most fistulas are easily traced. When two or more coincidental fistulas traverse the sphincter at separate points, only one may be laid open at the first operation. A second fistulotomy must be delayed until the first wound is soundly healed. In a patient rendered incontinent by simultaneous separate sphincterotomies, continence can usually be restored by carefully exposing and reapproximating the muscle at the single point where its gap is greatest.

Recurrence

Recurrent fistula is rare if its entire tract is laid open and all epithelium lining is excised or destroyed with cautery. Any tissue in a fistula having extraordinary firmness or mass over 2 mm in thickness must be excised and labeled for histologic examination to rule out carcinoma. When fistulas treated properly fail to heal or recur, one must suspect cancer, Crohn's disease, tuberculosis, or lymphopathia venereum.

DILATATION FOR ANAL FISSURE

An anal fissure is a superficial vertical tear of posterior squamous epithelium caught between forces of hard feces and tight anal sphincters. Inflammation causes sphincter spasm, which then perpetuates the fissure. Adults manifest acute fissure by intense sphincter pain, refusal of rectal examination, and reluctance to defecate. Gentle, four-finger dilatation under brief general anesthesia immediately relieves spasm and pain, allowing the fissure to heal.

The worst complication of treating a fissure is to overlook epidermoid cancer. Cancer usually presents as more bleeding than pain, but its appearance may at first be grossly indistinguishable from chronic fissure. A biopsy must be taken from every chronic fissure and any acute fissure with thickness in its edge or base.

Persistent Pain

Persistent pain after dilatation suggests another diagnosis such as pararectal abscess. Abscess is usually distinguished from fissure preoperatively by tenderness confined to one side of the anus. Because of coincidental spasm, however, some abscesses may be detected only after dilatation under anesthesia. Even then a few may be missed and diagnosed only after dilatation fails to relieve pain. Venereal infections may cause painful fissures not cured by dilatation. They must be suspected and cultured in effeminate men with multiple or lateral fissures, proctitis, and inguinal lymphadenopathy.

Fecal Incontinence

Although dilatation may cause incontinence in elderly patients with weak sphincters, such patients do not develop fissures and are not subject to this risk. Incontinence may, however, be a complication of lateral internal sphincterotomy. If only 5 mm thickness of sphincter is cut and the incision left open, lateral internal sphincterotomy is harmless. It may also be useless. Performed under local anesthesia, the results of sphincterotomy are inferior to those of simple dilatation.[8] Improvement attributed to general anesthesia may be due only to wider dilatation.

Bacteremia

Patients in whom transient bacteremia may produce infection of heart valves, prostheses, or hematomas should be given antibiotics for enteric organisms during anal dilatation. I produced an *E. coli* median sternotomy infection by dilating an anal fissure 10 days after a heart transplantation. Happily, the patient has survived 8 years without recurrence of the fissure or infection.

References

1. Beart RW Jr, Kelly KA: Randomized prospective evaluation of the EEA stapler for colorectal anastomoses. Am J Surg 141:143-147, 1981
2. Bricker EM, Johnston WD, Patwardhan RV: Repair of postirradiation damage to colorectum: A progress report. Ann Surg 193:555-564, 1981
3. Brain J, Lorber M, Fiddian–Green RG: Rectal membrane: An unusual complication following use of the circular stapling instrument for colorectal anastomosis. Surgery 89:271-274, 1981
4. Dozois RR, Kelly KA, Beart RW Jr et al: Improved results with continent ileostomy. Ann Surg 192:319-324, 1980
5. Fry DE, Garrison RN, Heitsch RC et al: Determinants of death in patients with intraabdominal abscess. Surgery 88:517-530, 1980
6. Goligher JC: Surgery of the Anus, Rectum and Colon, 4th ed. London, Bailliere Tindall, 1980
7. Graber JN, Schulte WJ, Condon RE et al: Duration of postoperative ileus related to extent and site of operative dissection. Surgical Forum 31:141-143, 1980
8. Keighley MRB, Arabi Y, Gatehouse D et al: A clinical trial to compare manual dilatation of the anus and lateral subcutaneous sphincterotomy for anal fissure. Br J Surg 65:371, 1978
9. Kovalcik PJ, Peniston RL, Cross GH: Anorectal abscess. Surg Gynecol Obstet 149:884-886, 1979
10. McDonald RF, Byrd CW: Early postoperative oral feeding. Surg Gynecol Obstet 110:510-513, 1960
11. Mullen JL, Buzby GP, Matthews DC et al: Reduction of operative morbidity and mortality by combined preoperative and postoperative nutritional support. Ann Surg 192:602-613, 1980
12. Palmer KR, Corbett CL, Holdsworth CD: Double-blind cross-over study comparing loperamine, codeine and diphenoxylate in the treatment of chronic diarrhea. Gastroenterology 79:1272-1275, 1980
13. Peck DA: Rectal mucosal replacement. Ann Surg 191:294-303, 1979
14. Reber HA, Roberts C, Way LW et al: Management of external gastrointestinal fistulas. Ann Surg 188:460-467, 1978
15. Stone HH, Martin JD: Synergistic necrotizing cellulitis. Ann Surg 175:702-711, 1972

33 Complications of Abdominal Wall Surgery

Hunter H. McGuire, Jr.

Complications of Laparotomy Incisions

ACCIDENTAL INJURY OF VISCERA

Viscera may be accidentally injured when the peritoneum is opened. Where there are no scars, adhesions, or distended viscera, injury is prevented by clearly exposing the peritoneum, elevating the abdominal wall with retractors, elevating the peritoneum with forceps, and incising the peritoneum superficially until an influx of air lets the viscera fall away. When an abdomen must be entered at a site to which bowel may be adherent, safety depends on highly cautious, sharp dissection in a bloodless field where potential planes and the smooth muscle of bowel or bladder are instantly recognizable.

Viscera may be injured when retractors are placed. They must be protected by placing moist gauze pads beneath retractor blades. Retractor injury is not always visible at the time of abdominal closure and may be first manifested by intestinal perforation or obstruction during convalescence.

During closure of the peritoneum and fascia, sutures may penetrate the intestine. The costs of this accident (peritonitis, fistula, and bowel obstruction) are so great as to mandate patience on the part of both surgeon and anesthesiologist during laparotomy closure. When a patient is "light" and struggling, closure should be delayed until anesthetic relaxation is restored. Edges of peritoneum and fascia must be so clearly exposed that needles can be advanced with absolute assurance that the viscera are out of danger. Retention sutures that bridge more than 2 cm of peritoneal cavity may cut through the wall of adjacent bowel. The longer the distance bridged, the greater the likelihood of this complication. It is prevented by far-near, near-far sutures. Far bites are 1.5 cm from edges, near bites 0.5 cm from edges, and sutures placed 1 cm apart.

POOR EXPOSURE

The primary goal of every laparotomy incision is exposure sufficient for safe examination, excision, or repair of viscera. This goal must never be compromised for speed, comfort, or cosmetic reasons. The worst complications of laparotomy may result from an incision's being misplaced or too short. Examples are ureteral injuries through incisions that are too high; bile duct, esophageal, and splenic injuries through incisions that are too low; and accidental enterotomies through incisions that are too short.

To suggest the best incision for every procedure is beyond the scope of this text. Nevertheless some general principles can be offered because violating them invites complications. Emergency laparotomy for blunt or penetrating trauma must always begin through a midline incision because it is most versatile for coping with unpredictable injuries. Elective procedures on the small bowel and colon are best performed through the midline to leave room for possible ileostomies or colostomies, either in the same operation or in the future. Procedures deep in the pelvis near both ureters are exposed safely only through the midline. The liver, biliary tract, pancreas, and spleen are most easily and safely exposed through subcostal incisions. For the stomach, proximal duodenum, and intra-abdominal esophagus, most surgeons prefer a midline incision, although a subcostal incision with vertical or intrathoracic extension can provide safe exposure.

No matter what the direction of an incision, its length must be ample. Each extra inch requires only a minute to open and close, while lack of a needed inch may cause death or years of disability.

RETAINED SPONGE OR INSTRUMENT

A retained sponge, instrument, or needle is a technical error to which laparotomy is peculiarly prone. The danger is greatest when procedures are performed in two or more widely separated parts of the cavity, especially when they are performed rapidly, using packs for hemostasis. Laparotomy for trauma would seem the most likely setting for this error, but it has occurred too often in elective pelvic procedures and even in simple ventral herniorrhaphies. Retained gauze usually harbors bacteria and causes abscess formation. Retained instruments or needles may penetrate viscera and cause peritonitis, abscess, fistula, or obstruction.

Retention of needles is best prevented by the surgeon's compulsive reapplication of needle holders to needles and by the technician's demand for a needle with every returned needle holder. Since this practice is not feasible in some procedures, such as vascular anastomoses, it must in every case be reinforced by the nurse's needle count. Small instruments such as bull-dog clamps must also be counted. In some hospitals all instruments are counted, but in most communities a high standard of safety is sustained by the practice of immediately returning to the technician all hardware that is not in use.

Retained gauze is first prevented by not using small, free sponges during laparotomy. Gauze must never be removed from "sponge sticks" or "peanut" dissectors. In the rare instance when a free sponge is required, such as to tamponade oozing from a venous anastomosis, its presence in the abdomen must be kept acutely in mind by the operating team.

Large gauze pads should be easily palpable during careful manual search of the peritoneal cavity, but their complete removal must be assured in three ways. First, the surgeon must always know where he intended to place pads, where he did place them, and where he removed them. Second, the surgeon must explore all areas where pads might have been left. Third, the nurse's sponge count must be correct. An incomplete count requires reexploration and retrieval of the missing sponge, or an x-ray film must prove without any doubt that no radioopaque marker remains in the abdomen.

Rarely, as a result of both the surgeon's oversight and the nurse's miscount, a gauze pad is left, despite announcement of "sponge count correct." This error, usually detected on x-ray film for a postoperative complication, is the surgeon's responsibility. His first duty is to inform the patient or patient's family of the presence and risk of the foreign body and to recommend its removal at the safest moment. That moment is usually as soon as the patient can be prepared for reoperation. Patients, insurance companies, and courts are remarkably sympathetic to surgeons who quickly acknowledge responsibility for this error.

PAIN

Two days of constant pain and a week of pain on motion are inevitable effects of every laparotomy incision. Some incisions are more painful than others, require more narcotics, and thus predispose the patient to atelectasis, urinary retention, and venous thromboses. Pain is greatest in the vertical midline and paramedian incisions because they are most mobile and subject to traction by oblique muscles from both sides. Pain is least in transverse and oblique incisions, especially those stabilized by costal margins. In a patient with pulmonary disease a transverse incision is preferred so long as it assures ample exposure.

INFECTION

Three types of infections complicate abdominal incisions (see also Chap. 3). The rarest type is invasive infection that destroys healthy tissue. Bacteria that have this capacity include hemolytic streptococci and staphylococci, clostridia, and synergistic combinations of gram-negative rods and anaerobes (streptococci or bacteroides). These infections are manifested by intense pain, tenderness, toxemia, and sometimes crepitus, often as early as the second day after surgery. Only streptococcal erysipelas and clostridial cellulitis respond to antibiotic (penicillin) alone. All other invasive infections require immediate radical débridement of destroyed tissue as well as immediate intravenous antibiotics for all potential pathogens. Débridement must be repeated daily under anesthesia until the cellulitis is eliminated. Such débridement of the abdominal wall usually leaves defects that must be bridged with Prolene mesh and subsequently covered with split thickness skin grafts.[4] Nomenclature of invasive infections is sometimes confusing and clinical differences among synergistic cellulitis, Meleney's cellulitis, and necrotizing fasciitis are not always clear. What must be clear, however, is the need instantly to recognize and treat any infection that invades and destroys healthy, unwounded tissue.

Most infections are confined to subcutaneous fat, but after contaminated laparotomy a local infection may involve fascia and muscle. Sutures tied very tightly render fascia vulnerable to infection, and inflammatory edema makes sutures too tight. Sutures then cut through friable fascia, predisposing the patient to dehiscence. In such dehiscences, evisceration is rare because inflammatory adhesions

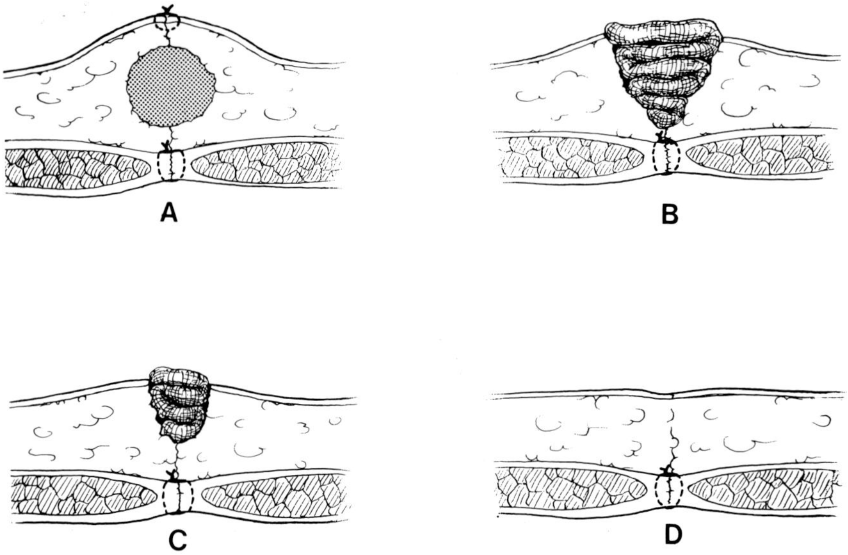

FIG. 33-1. Evolution of a subcutaneous wound abscess shown in cross section. (*A*) Pus confined by healthy adjacent tissues. (*B*) Sutures removed and wound packed open with moist gauze. (*C*) Spontaneous closure from within as daily cleansing and gentle packing prevents premature skin closure. (*D*) Complete healing. When intraoperative contamination makes abscess probable, healing will occur more safely and quickly if skin and fat are packed open (step *B*) at initial operation.

tend to hold the bowel in the abdomen. When escape of the bowel appears imminent, however, the defect should be bridged with Prolene mesh. Mesh must be sewn with great care to avoid bowel injury, which leads to enterocutaneous fistula.

Subcutaneous abscesses occur in patients whose fascia is healthy and resistant to infection but whose subcutaneous fat is made vulnerable to minimal contamination as a result of hematoma, seroma, excess cautery, mass ligatures, or strangulating sutures. Because the ideal balance between perfect hemostasis and no devitalized tissue is unattainable in every case, a 1% to 2% incidence of subcutaneous abscess is an inherent risk of laparotomy. The incidence is higher in obese patients and in contaminated procedures. As an impetus to self-criticism and to technical excellence, our service attributes all subcutaneous infections to technical error. All can be prevented by packing wounds open.

Subcutaneous abscess is manifested by increasing wound pain and tenderness, usually on the fifth to seventh days when normal inflammation should have subsided. Fever and leukocytosis are usually present and are cured by amply opening the skin and draining all pus. Antibiotics are unnecessary unless there is also evidence of invasive infection or a prosthesis needing protection. The wound should be irrigated and packed several times each day until lined with healthy granulation tissue, then allowed to close spontaneously (Fig. 33-1).

Any multifilament, nonabsorbable suture material other than stainless steel may harbor bacteria and produce recurrent stitch abscess or sinus. When a stitch abscess appears months or years after its original wound has healed, an effort should be made to grasp and extract the infected suture by probing its sinus with a fine hemostat. If that fails, the patient may be offered the safe choices of either waiting for spontaneous expulsion of the suture or having the wound reexplored. Most patients prefer to wait.

DEHISCENCE AND EVISCERATION

Dehiscence occurs in two forms. One is the grossly infected wound in which sutures cut through friable fascia, allowing edges to separate gradually. When small, evisceration may not occur because inflamed viscera adhere to one another and to parietal peritoneum. Débridement may produce enterocutaneous fistula. Small dehiscence without evisceration is best treated by gentle irrigations and nonadherent dressings until covered with healthy granulation, then closed or covered with split-thickness skin graft, if needed. When completely healed, the inevitable hernia may be repaired. When the infected dehiscence is large enough to threaten evisceration, the defect must be bridged with Prolene mesh and subsequently covered with skin (Fig. 33-2).

The second form of dehiscence occurs without infection. On the fifth to tenth days, often just after skin sutures are removed, dressings or sheets are suddenly soaked with serosanguineous fluid. Shortly thereafter, any remaining skin sutures break or cut through the skin, allowing the small bowel and omentum to eviscerate. This unhappy event complicates about 0.5% of major laparotomy incisions. The subsequent mortality of 15% is caused by factors that predispose patients to evisceration.

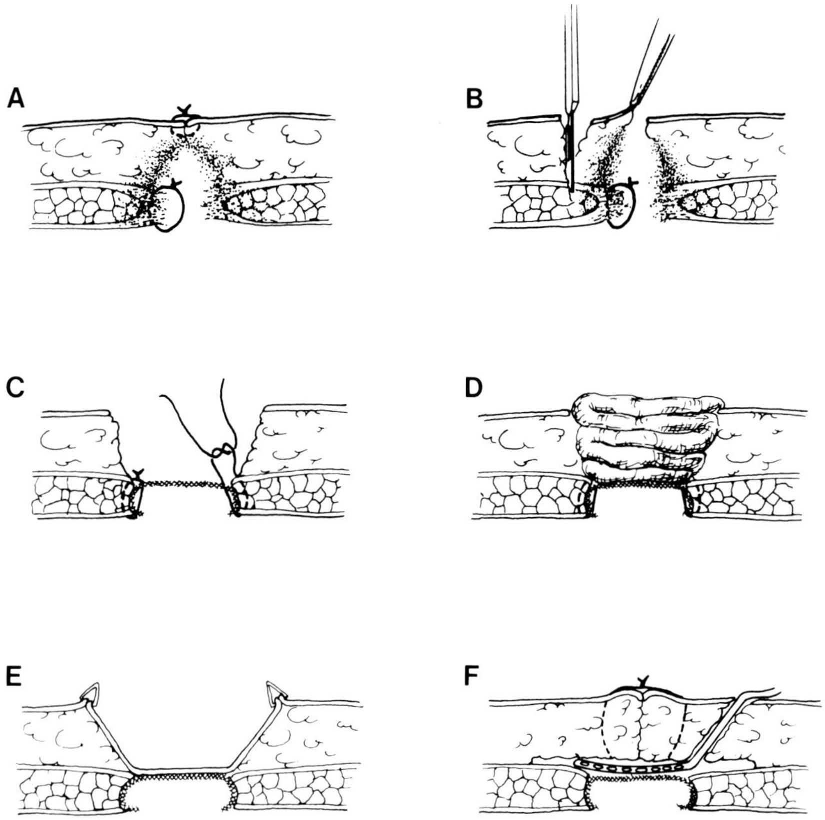

FIG. 33-2. Invasive infection with fascial dehiscence shown in cross section. (*A*) Suture tears through necrotic fascia. (*B*) Wound opened and necrotic tissue débrided. (*C*) To prevent evisceration while permitting drainage of intraperitoneal infection, a bridge of Prolene mesh is sewn to fascia with Prolene sutures. (*D*) Wound is gently washed and dressed until mesh is covered with granulation tissue. (*E*) Broad defects are healed temporarily in most patients and permanently in a few by application of split-thickness skin graft. (*F*) In narrow defects and in those in which grafts have failed, skin flaps are mobilized and closed over soft suction catheters.

Studies from which these figures and subsequent opinions are derived share two common faults. One is the failure to discriminate between dehiscence caused by infection and those that occurred without infection. The other fault is inclusion in many studies of large numbers of patients who are at little or no risk of dehiscence.[2]

Predisposing systemic factors appear to be starvation, uremia, anemia, shock, liver failure, obesity, and advanced age. Local factors are distention by ileus or ascites and disruptive forces of coughing, vomiting, convulsions, or delirium tremens. Infants whose struggling is uninhibited by pain appear prone to dehiscence. For this reason multilayer transverse and paramedian incisions are preferred to midline incisions in infants.

Although most eviscerations occur through midline incisions, there is no proof that a midline incision in an adult is more liable to eviscerate than are other incisions. The association between midline incision and evisceration is probably explained by the frequent need for midline incision in severely injured, starved, septic, and cancer-ridden patients. Most surgeons have seen at least one simple, elective subcostal incision eviscerate. We have seen dehiscence of a McBurney incision closed with chromic catgut in the presence of acute pancreatitis. Sutures were probably dissolved by intraperitoneal enzymes and disrupted by distention.

Fascial repair with nonabsorbable suture results in fewer dehiscences than closure with any absorbable suture, but no technique gives perfect protection.[1] In theory, circulation and healing should be best between interrupted, nonreactive sutures that incorporate about 1 cm of fascia on each side of an incision, are placed 1 cm apart, and tied to approximate but not strangulate tissue. In fact, dehiscence has not been shown to be more frequent with continuous-suture technique, and the only proven disadvantage of a single continuous suture is that if it breaks, the whole wound will separate at once. Some surgeons use retention sutures through all layers of abdominal wall to prevent evisceration in selected patients who are prone to dehiscence. Such sutures do not prevent dehiscence but do prevent evisceration. Most surgeons believe that the ischemic and skin cutting effects of retention sutures outweigh their rare and limited prophylactic value.

When a dresssing is found soaked with salmon-pink fluid, the wound must be immediately examined with sterile gloves, pads, and binder ready for application. Sometimes bowel or omentum will be found already protruding through skin. More often skin will be still intact, but a fascial defect or a loop of bowel will be palpable just beneath the skin. In either case, dressing and binder must be applied and the patient sent promptly to the operating room. In a few cases the subcutaneous wound may feel hard, sound dull to percussion, and suggest delayed hematoma rather than dehiscence as the cause of sudden drainage. In such cases, one may remove a few skin sutures and very cautiously probe the wound with sterile gloves. If the fascia is clearly intact, the wound merely needs packing. If fascia has parted, it must be immediately repaired. Delay of reclosure is acceptable only when a patient's cardiovascular status is too precarious for transportation to the operating room. A patient who has eaten within 8 hours before dehiscence must either be intubated awake or have gastric aspiration prior to induction of anesthesia.

Failure to repair dehiscence results in evisceration in most cases and in disabling hernia in the few who do not eviscerate. Reclosure, in contrast, is strikingly successful. For some reason the factors that cause dehiscence of a first repair rarely delay healing after a second repair. In the second repair, tissues are always unfit for closure in separate layers. The wound must be closed with strong, nonabsorbable, nonreactive sutures placed 2 cm apart, each stitch incorporating at least 2 cm of fascia on each side of the incision. Near-far, far-near placement prevents long intraperitoneal bridges of suture that would threaten to erode the viscera. Skin may be closed loosely if there is no evidence of infection.

INCISIONAL HERNIA

Causes of incisional hernia already discussed are infection and dehiscence. Another cause of wound hernia in the midline is diastasis of the linea alba, usually in obese patients. When possible, a diastasis should be repaired during closure of its original incision. Other hernias are caused by stresses that exceed the tensile strengths of the wounds. Surgeons must advise patients how much stress their incisions can safely bear, but scientific validation for such advice is vague. A common practice is to advise healthy patients with strong tissues to resume in 2 weeks all planned stresses that comfort permits, but to avoid circumstances in which unforeseen stress may be required, such as walking on ice or on rough ground in the dark. Sudden stresses are best deferred for 9 months or undertaken sooner at the patient's own risk. A patient whose livelihood depends on heavy lifting should seek light duties during the first 6 weeks when tensile strength grows most rapidly and collagen begins maturation and realignment.

CHRONIC COMPLAINTS

After complete recovery from laparotomy, some patients return regularly to their surgeons' offices with complaints of incisional pain, protrusion, numbness, or unsightly appearance. Such complaints must not be attributed to incisions until one is sure from history, examination, and needed tests that complaints do not arise from recurrent or new visceral disorders. Assurance that viscera are healthy often makes a complaint tolerable. When it is still not tolerable, one must ask whether a patient's threshold for discomfort has been lowered by his dependence on an excuse for disability. Through appropriate questions, many patients can be helped to understand that their wounds are not abnormal, that remedies must be social or emotional, and that a search for surgical cures will be fruitless.

Patients are often anxious about the color or mass of their scars. During the proliferative phase of healing, this anxiety can be resolved or prevented by explaining that redness and thickness of scar normally increase for 6 weeks after the operation and require 9 months for maturation. If the complaint comes after 2 months and the scar is still growing and superficially painful, one must be concerned about keloid formation (see Chap. 1). Other cosmetic complaints are of excessive breadth and of cicatricial contracture. They are caused by cutting across skin lines and by delayed healing, which requires epithelial migration. Some can be prevented. Most are amenable to plastic revision.

After transverse and oblique incisions, patients sometimes complain of numbness distal to transections of spinal nerves. Patients may be reassured that numbness usually becomes unnoticeable after several months. So few patients are truly annoyed by numbness that it is not a contraindication to transverse incision.

Chronic pain in a scar is often difficult to explain and frustrating to treat, perhaps because it is so often amplified by psychosocial factors. Incisional hernia must be ruled out by palpation. A visceral disorder is unlikely when pain is aggravated by straining and when tenderness is worse with muscles tensed. In some cases pain is caused by ossification of the scar and relieved by excision of bone. An upper midline scar may be painfully jabbed by an everted xiphoid process, which should have been excised at the initial laparotomy. Any scar may be painful if large suture knots are close to the overlying skin. In thin patients this complaint is prevented by using simple square knots of steel or silk rather than the plastic sutures that require large knots.

Eccentric bulging of the abdominal wall may be caused by weakness of muscle the nerve or arterial supply of which has been divided by surgical incision. Accidental division of the 12th intercostal nerve during rib resection in a flank incision will produce this complication. It may occur where a long subcostal incision is superimposed on a previous midline incision and will occur between any two parallel incisions. Laparotomy incisions must therefore be selected and made with this complication in mind. In the absence of hernia, bulging cannot be corrected surgically, but the disability may be reduced by a tailored corset.

Ventral Hernia Repair

In addition to risks common in all laparotomies, repair of large ventral hernias is especially prone to subcutaneous hematoma, pulmonary failure, and recurrent hernia. The best way to minimize these complications is to repair incisional and umbilical hernias before they become very large.

HEMATOMA

Wound hematomas are prone to occur where fascia is broadly exposed and where relaxing incisions are made. These procedures require meticulous hemostasis and suction drainage for 3 days or longer until drainage has ceased. A hematoma may also fill dead space created in the repair of an infant's umbilical hernia. This is prevented by hemostasis, by obliterating dead space insofar as possible, and by applying a pressure dressing over the umbilicus for 2 days.

PULMONARY COMPLICATIONS

Repair of a large hernia under great tension impairs cough due to pain and impairs ventilation due to elevation of diaphragms. If a reducible hernia can be contained preoperatively by a corset without dyspnea, postoperative ventilation should be no problem. Repair of a huge irreducible hernia, however, may make a patient ventilator-dependent for many days until the pain has subsided and the abdominal cavity has become accommodated to its new contents. Rather than inviting this complication, one may prefer staged interposition of plastic mesh for a less tight repair, or perhaps no repair at all. Large hernias are often disabling but rarely lethal. Before undertaking what may be a life-threatening repair, pulmonary function must be critically evaluated.

RECURRENT HERNIA

There are four causes of ventral hernia recurrence. One is infection that prolongs inflammation, delays collagen deposition, and extrudes suture material. Because hernia recurrence is almost inevitable after infection, elective repair must never be undertaken in the presence of stitch abscess or sinus or skin excoriation. Infected foreign material must be removed and skin healed before any repair is attempted. When the repair is done, care and closure of tissues must be perfect.

A second cause of recurrence is approximation of tissues that are too thin and weak to bear the force of abdominal muscle contractions. A clear example is recurrence of a small umbilical or epigastric hernia after repair of linea alba attenuated by diastasis. In repairing such a hernia, strong tissue can always be obtained for complete diastasis repair. When there is a question whether a small procedure to close the thin fascia will succeed or whether major abdominal wall repair is necessary, one is justified in trying the minor operation first if the patient understands that there is some risk of recurrence.

A third cause of recurrence is premature stress on a repair due to vomiting, coughing, ascites, or gaseous distention. This risk should be minimized by preoperative control of any ascites or bronchial secretions, by catharsis and gastric suction before the repairs that are expected to be most difficult, and by delaying postoperative feeding until peristalsis is clearly effective. Any postoperative vomiting or distention signals the need for immediate nasogastric decompression.

The fourth and most common cause of ventral hernia recurrence is closure under intolerable tension. The problem is difficult when scars of several old wounds compete for mobility. It is worst when a large hernia defect is adjacent to completely immobile costal margin or iliac crest. A technique for overcoming immobility that must be categorically condemned is simply pulling very hard on sutures too heavy to break. The inevitable result is ischemic necrosis of fascia and a new hernia worse than its predecessor. As in all surgical wounds, sutures must simply approximate edges while allowing blood to circulate through tissues between each stitch. In this regard it should be mentioned that incisional hernias, the tissues of which have already shown their disposition to failure, must never be repaired with continuous running sutures because they maximally impair circulation. Repair must always be made with interrupted, nonabsorbable sutures.

In repairing midline hernias up to 5 cm wide, tension can usually be reduced to an acceptable level by long relaxing incisions in both rectus sheaths.

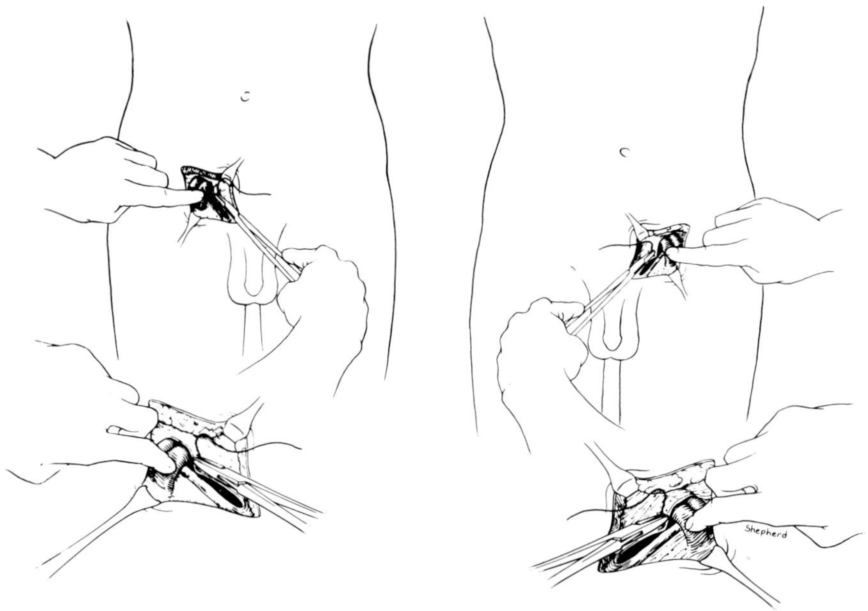

FIG. 33-3. To many surgeons, a deterrent to Cooper's ligament repair is the technical difficulty of avoiding injury to the femoral vein. This difficulty is overcome by positioning the needle holder parallel to Cooper's ligament, a maneuver best achieved on the left side by sewing with the left hand.

When relaxing incisions are impossible or ineffective, defects are best bridged with Prolene mesh sewn to strong fascia with Prolene sutures.

Groin Hernia Repair

ANESTHETIC RISKS

Direct and easily reducible indirect hernias in adults may be disabling but are not life threatening. Their repairs are justified only when anesthetic risk is negligible. For most adults the safest anesthetic is infiltrated locally after moderate sedation or narcosis.

The maximum recommended dose of 1% lidocaine with epinephrine for a healthy adult is 50 ml (500 mg). After premedication with 100 mg of meperidine, our residents are able to perform most Cooper's ligament repairs with 10 ml to 20 ml. A practiced and confident surgeon needs less. Prerequisites to successful local anesthesia are a relaxed cooperative patient and a perfectly placed incision. Perfect placement is unpredictable in recurrent hernias and in obese patients. They require general or spinal anesthesia to avoid the dangers of lidocaine and narcotic overdosage.

VISCERAL INJURIES

The bowel may be injured during the opening or during high ligation of an indirect sac. This error is prevented by very cautious entry into tissue presumed to be peritoneum, by warily exposing sliding hernias (best exposed through LaRoque's approach), and by exposing the inside of a hernia sac during its suture ligation. The bladder may be injured if a suture in the medial corner of an indirect sac penetrates any tissue other than peritoneum. The bladder may also be injured by an unnecessary opening of a direct sac. When the bladder is entered, it must be repaired with chromic catgut and continuously drained with an indwelling catheter until healing is proven by cystogram.

VASCULAR INJURIES

Ample exposure in a bloodless field is necessary to prevent needles from penetrating aberrant obturator or inferior epigastric vessels. Penetration of the femoral vein during Cooper's ligament repair is best prevented by sewing from the opposite side with the needle holder parallel to Cooper's ligament so that the needle's arc does not threaten the vein (Fig. 33-3). If a needle should accidentally penetrate a vessel, its suture should be removed and hemostasis secured before a new stitch is placed.

NERVE INJURIES

Three nerves are exposed to injury. They are the ilioinguinal, genitofemoral (both on or in the cord), and the iliohypogastric (on the internal oblique muscle). Nerve division may cause groin anesthesia, which is transiently bothersome. Nerve injury presumably accounts for a few cases of disabling postoperative pain. For this reason care must be taken not to include nerves in sutures through oblique muscles and fascia. When, after initial recovery, a patient develops worse pain, one must suspect an abscess if the incision is tender, dehiscence if it is nontender. If neither of these complications evolves, pain usually subsides. When it persists with no explanation, there is often a psychosocial reason for dependence on disability.

TESTICULAR INFARCT

Severe testicular pain, swelling, tenderness, and fever may occur after repair in which the spermatic cord is either divided or stripped of muscle and fat. If in the same or a previous operation the testicle has been delivered from the scrotum, infarction is almost certain to occur. Orchiectomy is sometimes necessary to cure this complication, and the pain, disability, and cost of infarction outweigh the value of the maneuvers that produce it. When it appears that cure of a recurrent hernia may require obliteration of the internal ring, a surgeon should seek permission for orchiectomy and testicular prosthesis at the time of repair. When debulking a thick cord, fat and muscle may be removed with great care to protect artery and veins, but overly tight closure should be avoided because the hernia rarely recurs through the internal ring.

HEMATOMAS

Subcutaneous and subfascial hematomas are most prone to develop following repairs under local anesthesia with epinephrine. A vessel occluded by vasoconstriction may not appear to need ligature until after the wound has been closed. Meticulous care must therefore be taken to ligate all visibly transected vessels.

A hematoma in the scrotum arises from vessels in cremasteric muscle that are so small they would be occluded by pressure in any anatomical area other than the loose unsupported scrotum. This complication is best prevented by leaving most of an indirect scrotal sac attached to cord structures and by freeing only enough of the upper end of the sac to permit its high ligation in the internal ring. When a long sac must be completely removed from the scrotum, as in a large sliding hernia, the risk of scrotal hematoma may be reduced by scrotal support and bed rest for 2 days after surgery. Prophylactic drainage does not prevent scrotal hematoma.

When hematoma develops, it is usually dispersed between several layers of repair or of spermatic cord. Needle aspiration is useless. Effective evacuation requires complete reopening of the wound. This should be done only for very tense and progressively enlarging hematomas that appear immediately after surgery and indicate the need for another ligature. Stable hematomas should be treated with rest, warm compresses, and observation in the hospital until one can be certain that absorption has begun without secondary infection.

RECURRENT HERNIA

One cause of recurrence is a hernia that was incompletely repaired or overlooked in the first operation. Indirect sacs must be circumferentially ligated high in the internal ring. In every case all three potential hernia sites must be carefully explored. During indirect repair, the posterior wall and femoral canal must be palpated from within. During direct repair the proximal cord must be carefully explored and the femoral sheath inspected.

Another cause of recurrence is wound infection. The probability of recurrence after infection is so great that, unless a hernia is strangulated, the operation must not be performed when any source of infection is present in the patient, surgeons, or operating theater. When infection occurs, it must be amply drained, infected sutures removed, and wound healing completed before another repair is attempted. A truss may prevent and occasionally cures recurrence as scar contracts.

A third cause of recurrence is intolerable stress on a fascial repair. Such stress may be applied in the operating room by a surgeon who fails to make a needed relaxing incision or by an anesthesiologist who permits a patient to cough or retch violently. For a week or two after the operation, wound pain protects a repair from disruptive forces. After that, patients with strong tissues may resume all activities except those liable to produce sudden, unpredicted stresses. Very heavy lifting should be deferred for 6 weeks. When tissues are weak or difficult to approximate, heavy lifting should be avoided for the 9 months of wound maturation and the patient advised that recurrence may be produced by heavy lifting anytime thereafter.

A fourth cause of recurrent hernia is intrinsic weakness of inguinal fascia. Recurrence for this reason occurring shortly after repair is an indictment of the technique employed, because in almost every inguinal hernia there is some strong native tissue to sew to Cooper's ligament. Recurrence many years after initial repair is probably caused by progressive collagen depletion. This is usually seen as a direct recurrence years after indirect repair. McVay's results suggest that late recurrences might be reduced from 3.2% to 0.85% if all repairs included Cooper's ligament.[3] Most surgeons, however, refrain from using Cooper's ligament in the repair of small indirect hernias where exposure of the ligament would require destruction of healthy transversalis fascia.

References

1. Bucknall TE, Ellis H: Abdominal wound closure—A comparison of monofilament nylon and polyglycolic acid. Surgery 89:672-677, 1981
2. Ellis H: Management of the wound. In Maingot's Abdominal Operations, vol 1, pp 62-72. New York, Appleton-Century-Crofts, 1980
3. McVay CB, Chapp JD: Inguinal and femoral hernioplasty. Ann Surg 148:499-512, 1958
4. Stone HH, Fabian TC, Turkleson ML et al: Management of acute full thickness losses of the abdominal wall. Ann Surg 193:612-618, 1981

34 Complications of Appendectomy

Kimball I. Maull

OVERVIEW

Most appendectomies in the United States are performed to treat or prevent inflammation of the appendix. Complications following appendectomy are largely a function of the state of the diseased appendix; that is, the timing of the operation, the choice of antibiotic therapy, and numerous technical considerations depend entirely upon whether the appendix is intact or perforated. An understanding of the natural history of acute appendicitis, therefore, is essential to the prevention, recognition, and treatment of postoperative complications.

Most authorities agree that appendicitis arises from luminal obstruction, usually from inspissated feces, but occasionally from a foreign body, stenosis, external bands or adhesions, lymphoid hyperplasia, or, rarely, tumors. Appendicitis is caused by bacterial invasion of the appendiceal wall. The inciting obstruction leads to stasis, bacterial overgrowth, damage to the appendiceal mucosa, and invasion of the wall by organisms and their toxins. With bacterial invasion, the appendix swells; the vascular supply is impaired; and the course is set for eventual gangrene or perforation. This initial distention of the appendiceal lumen is responsible for the first pain of appendicitis, and the progression of pathologic events can be correlated predictably with the concurrent progression of clinical findings.

Acute appendicitis may be classified pathophysiologically into catarrhal, *an early inflammation limited to the mucosa;* interstitial, *a transmural process that evokes a sterile peritoneal reaction;* suppurative, *a partial-thickness necrosis of the appendiceal wall with surrounding inflammatory exudate, peritoneal reaction, and outpouring of cloudy peritoneal fluid; and* gangrenous, *a full-thickness necrosis of the appendix in which bacteria seep through to the periappendiceal environs, producing bacteria-rich peritoneal fluid. Since the microbial flora of the normal and diseased appendix are similar, the final arbiter is the ability of the appendix to resist invasive infection.*

DIAGNOSIS OF ACUTE APPENDICITIS

Because the timing of the appendectomy and the progression of the inflammatory process are interdependent variables in the occurrence of postoperative complications, early diagnosis offers the best chance of avoiding serious complications. The diagnosis of appendicitis must be seriously considered for any patient with abdominal pain in whom the appendix is still present, regardless of other symptoms. The difficulty in establishing acute appendicitis as the most likely explanation for a patient's condition is usually the result of a lack of understanding of the pathophysiology of the disease and a failure to appreciate that the classic cluster of signs and symptoms of appendicitis actually occurs in only 50% of adults and children and in significantly less than 50% of infants and the elderly. Since a large number of patients with appendicitis present with either an atypical history or atypical physical findings or both, the clinician must maintain a high index of suspicion in order to avoid missing the diagnosis.

An intelligent layman can usually diagnose classic appendicitis. These are not the patients who create problems for the clinician. The sequence of generalized abdominal pain, vomiting, and localized right lower quadrant pain is almost pathognomonic of acute appendicitis. Rather, the patient with an atypical history and inconsistent physical findings taxes the most astute surgeon's acumen. The prodrome of poorly localized epigastric pain may not occur at all. A small number of patients, especially children, may actually be hungry. Depending on the position of the appendix, the pain may localize to the right lumbar area, right groin, pelvis, or other quadrants. Left-sided pain from appendicitis is rare but can be caused by situs inversus, nonrotation of the midgut, the hypermobile or wandering cecum, or an extremely long appendix that crosses the midline.[42] In many instances, the appendix lies lateral to or behind the cecum; in about a third it is located in the pelvis; and in about 10% it is along the medial side of the ascending colon, posterior to the mesentery of the terminal ileum. Because of the variation in the position of the cecum and in the position of the appendix relative to the cecum, pain is not always localized to McBurney's point. A retrocolic appendix with an inflamed tip pointing upward may cause pain in the loin, back, or pararenal area. If the appendix rests on the psoas muscle or pelvis, the pain may be perceived in the groin or thigh.

Abdominal tenderness, the most common objective physical finding in early appendicitis, precedes signs of peritoneal irritation. The proximity of the inflamed parietal peritoneum to the anterior abdominal wall is the major determinant of whether peritoneal signs appear early, late, or not at all. In contrast, when the appendix lies retrocecal or in the pelvis, abdominal signs may be obscure. Rebound tenderness, an often described but gross estimate of peritonitis, is very uncomfortable to the patient, who tends toward voluntary guarding during subsequent examination. Referred rebound tenderness from the left to the right lower quadrants is more informative and is extremely helpful in distinguishing localized right lower quadrant inflammation from pelvic inflammation (Fig. 34-1). Tenderness confined to the right lower quadrant with gentle percussion of the abdomen is also a highly reliable sign of underlying localized peritonitis.

FIG. 34-1. To elicit referred rebound tenderness, the left lower quadrant is deeply palpated and quickly released. Pain perceived only in the right lower quadrant constitutes positive referred rebound tenderness.

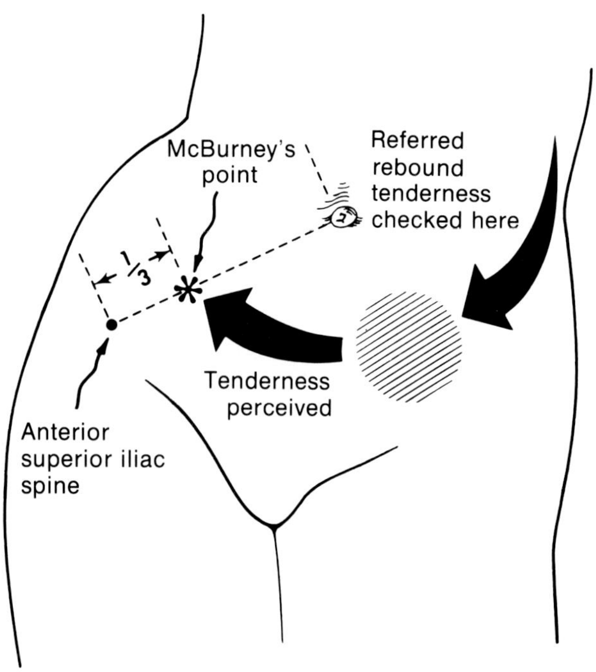

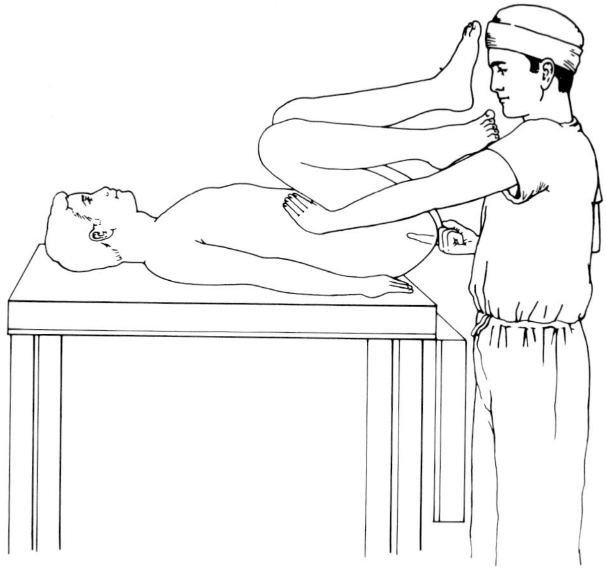

FIG. 34-2. The supine knee–chest position affords the most informative rectal examination, especially in patients with acute abdominal conditions.

Examination of the abdomen is incomplete without a rectal examination. The patient, whether male or female, is best examined supine in the knee–chest position because a higher examination of the pelvis is possible, the intrapelvic structures are low and in their normal anatomical relationship to one another, and the examiner can bimanually feel for a mass (Fig. 34-2). Rectal findings, including tenderness or tenderness with induration limited to the right side, suggest appendicitis in 40% to 50% of patients. A mass suggests perforation with pelvic abscess. Pelvic examination is essential in women and helps exclude common gynecologic causes for abdominal pain.[8] Common gynecologic causes of acute abdominal pain include the following:

Ectopic pregnancy
Septic abortion
Acute salpingitis
Hemorrhagic corpus luteum ("mittelschmerz")
Torsion, ovarian cyst
Endometriosis
Fibroid infarction

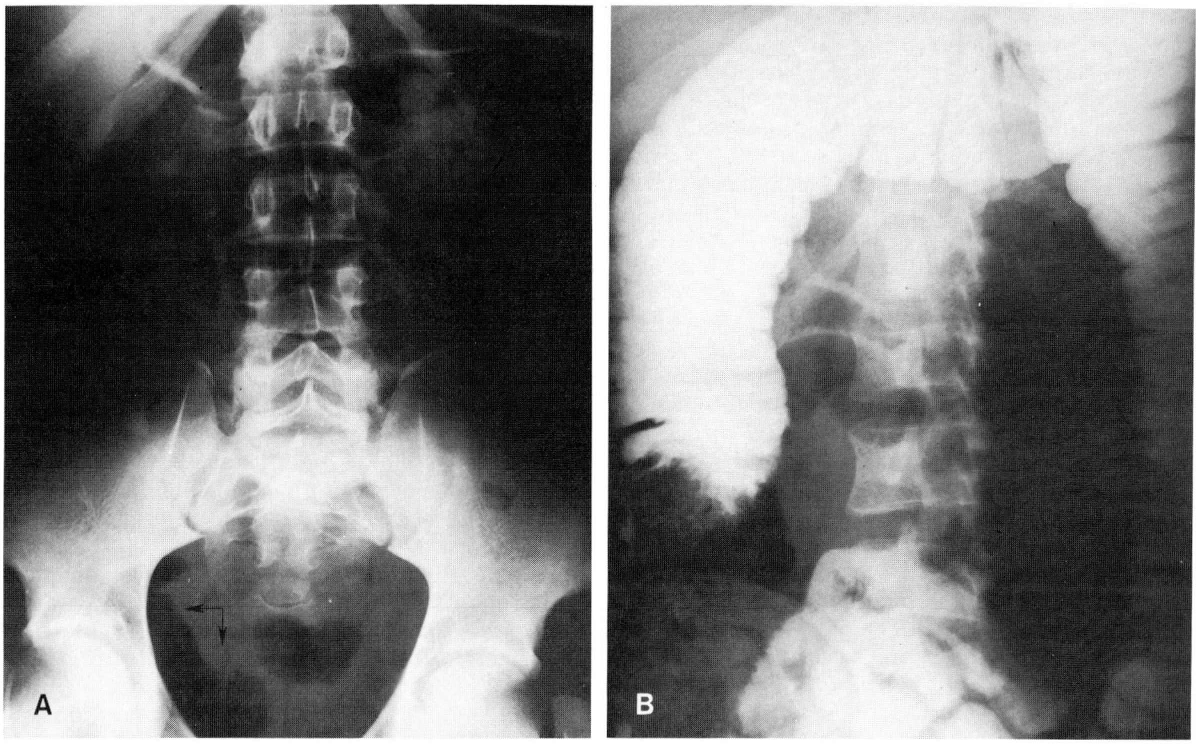

FIG. 34-3. (*A*) Plain abdominal roentgenogram of an 18-year-old youth with acute appendicitis demonstrating multiple appendicoliths (*single arrow*) and localized pelvic ileus (*double arrows*). (*B*) Barium enema in a 31-year-old man with acute appendicitis with perforation. Note effacement of cecum and nonfilling of the appendix. Cecal spasm was apparent during fluoroscopy.

Despite the lack of absolute correlation between leukocyte counts and the duration or severity of appendicitis, leukocyte and differential cell counts should routinely be obtained in all patients as a diagnostic adjunct but not as the definitive factor for recommending or deferring an operation. If undue reliance is placed on the white cell count when it is at variance with the history and physical findings, operative management is likely to be delayed unduly. Although Ackerman found that all patients with perforated appendicitis, even those with normal or low leukocyte counts, had increased neutrophils and band forms, the differential count is only slightly more reliable than the total leukocyte count in indicating the presence of acute infection.[1] Therefore, leukocyte and differential counts must be interpreted in light of the total clinical picture. Indeed, a low white blood count in the presence of significant clinical findings may be a grave sign. Urinalysis is important, and modest numbers of red or white cells are consistent with appendicitis. Serum amylase, often drawn as an added guide in the differential diagnosis, can be a real pitfall if it is not recognized that elevation of serum or urine amylase occurs in 10% of patients with acute appendicitis.[45]

The routine use of roentgenographic studies is probably not indicated in acute appendicitis since the diagnosis of appendicitis may often be confidently established without them. In difficult cases, however, flat and upright abdominal films and posterior–anterior and lateral chest films should be obtained. Findings on plain roentgenographs suggesting appendicitis include appendicolith, sentinel loop of distal ileum, gas-fluid interface or edema in the cecum, soft tissue density in the right lower quadrant, and, rarely, pneumoperitoneum (Fig. 34-3). The last is much more common with perforated gastric or duodenal ulcers, but it occurs in 0.5% to 7% of patients with acute appendicitis and usually leads to misdiagnosis but early operation.[40] Fecalith, though visible in a minority of patients, is a very specific finding. Wilkinson described the x-ray features in the diagnosis of appendicitis in infants and reported a fecalith in 33% of the cases.[49] The incidence in adults is lower, but a patient with abdominal pain and a detectable calcified fecalith has a 90% chance of having appendicitis. Appendiceal calculi are probably a more serious threat than is an asymptomatic gallstone. Copeland and Long assert that the asymptomatic appendix containing a typical calculus should be removed as a prophylactic measure, particularly in the young age group.[10]

The chest film is an important baseline measure in difficult cases, especially in view of the tendency for basilar pneumonia to mimic acute appendicitis.[22] Barium enema examination is also helpful. Sakover and Del Fava were able to fill 85% of normal appendices in a large series and believe that nonfilling of the appendix is strong supportive evidence for appendicitis.[41] Other authors cite cecal spasm, incomplete appendiceal filling, and edema of the cecal wall as corroborative.[38] With a false-negative rate of 7%, barium enema may now be considered a useful adjunct in difficult cases.

According to Lewis, the median interval between onset of symptoms and hospital admission for patients with acute appendicitis without perforation is 16 hours.[25] This increases to 34 and 72 hours for perforated appendicitis and appendicitis with abscess, respectively. Appendicitis in childhood is much more likely to result in perforation because of its insidious onset and rapid progression to gangrene and perforation. Approximately 2% of appendicitis occurs in infants under the age of 2 years. Parents usually note irritability, poor feeding, and vomiting. Meaningful abdominal examination requires sedation and usually yields localized tenderness in the right lower quadrant or an abdominal mass. Rectal tenderness is demonstrable in over 50% of such infants. The white count is usually elevated with a marked shift to the left, and roentgenographic studies are often helpful, the most common abnormalities being lumbar scoliosis, intestinal obstruction, and fecalith. Rupture occurs in over 80% of infants and accounts for the significant rate of complications.[4] A similarly high incidence of perforation is found in the elderly. Although the appendix is fibrosed, the lumen obliterated, and the likelihood of appendicitis is reduced in the elderly, perforation is the rule. Owens and Hamit confirmed that the high incidence of appendiceal perforation in the elderly is invariably related to delay in seeking medical treatment.[35]

COMPLICATIONS OF APPENDICITIS

Early diagnosis promotes early operation. Therefore, when the diagnosis is delayed, the operation is withheld, and complications increase.

The most common complication of acute appendicitis is peritonitis, which represents extension of the infectious process beyond the confines of the appendix. Peritonitis most often either follows perforation in which bacteria-rich fluid suddenly spills into the peritoneal cavity or from gangrene of the appendix, which allows a slow leak of contaminated contents from the organ. Peritonitis may be localized or generalized. As a rule, localized peritonitis follows gangrene in which the slow extravasation of contaminated fluid evokes a protective response from the surrounding peritoneum, and the process is walled off from the general peritoneal cavity. Occasionally, this is seen when the appendix has ruptured shortly before the operation. Generalized peritonitis follows free perforation of the appendix or when the host cannot adequately contain the infectious process. The latter is characteristic of appendicitis in children in whom perforation occurs rapidly; omental tissues are sparse; and containment fails. Generalized peritonitis is characterized by minimal adhesions and profuse pus, in which the intestines freely float. Perforation at the base of the appendix causes generalized peritonitis because of the continued release of contaminated cecal contents and the inability of the body's defenses to prevent the spread of infection. Generalized peritonitis may also follow rupture of a periappendiceal abscess. In most instances, clinical examination can distinguish localized from generalized peritonitis. This distinction is important since every attempt to prevent contamination of the generalized peritoneal cavity should be made if the peritonitis is localized.

Synergistic effects from aerobic and anaerobic microorganisms play a major role in the progression of appendiceal sepsis in both adults and children. The most common aerobic organisms cultured include *E. coli* and enteric streptococci, whereas the anaerobic group are predominantly bacteroids and gram-positive anaerobic cocci.[7] The appearance of a chill during the course of appendicitis suggests gangrene of the appendix, perforation, or septic thrombosis of the appendiceal veins. If the inflammatory process extends to the pelvis, pelvic thrombophlebitis may result and lead to significant circulatory disturbance and septic pulmonary embolism.[17]

Periappendiceal abscess is another serious complication following acute appendicitis. When the initial bolus of contamination is small and the body's response prevails, localized peritonitis is controlled, and an abscess, usually located lateral to or inferior to the cecum, results. The omentum plays an important role in containing collections of intraperitoneal pus. If the perforation is retrocolic, a retroperitoneal abscess that is not as readily contained may develop. Periappendiceal retroperitoneal abscess may extend superiorly to and through the diaphragm, inferiorly to the iliac fossa, or pass through the femoral canal to a point in the thigh.

Intestinal obstruction may follow acute appendicitis, although mechanical obstruction is far less frequent than the paralytic ileus complicating acute appendicitis. Obstruction is usually caused by adhesions or encirclement of the base of the ileum and kinking of the intestine as it is involved in the attempt to localize the inflammatory process. Intestinal necrosis occurs less commonly following appendicitis than does obstruction and usually follows perforation of the appendix directly into the cecum or some adjacent part of the intestinal tract. In certain instances, the periappendiceal abscess may rupture into the intestine or compromise blood supply to an adjacent intestinal segment, leading to ischemia and localized gangrene of the segment.

Extension of the inflammatory process or abscess to the perimesenteric area is the most common setting for pylephlebitis, fortunately a rare complication of appendicitis. Pylephlebitis results from septic thrombosis of the intestinal veins with extension to the portal vein and eventually to multiple intrahepatic abscesses. This condition most commonly follows delay in the institution of appropriate surgical therapy.

Complications of Operation

PREOPERATIVE CONSIDERATIONS

The ideal time to operate in acute appendicitis is early, before perforation or gangrene can develop. Surgery offers the best chance for cure, and, once the diagnosis is reasonably certain, there is little reason to delay operative intervention. Since 15% of appendices rupture within 24 hours of the onset of symptoms and 40% rupture within 48 hours, the need to proceed promptly is obvious.

An operation undertaken for perforated or gangrenous appendicitis, by definition, means that the optimal time for the operation has passed. However, if the operation is undertaken within a few hours of perforation, the results are generally favorable.

When the operation is considerably delayed (*i.e.*, by days), opinions differ on the timing of operative intervention.[48] If the operation is withheld, the goal of treatment is to promote resolution of the infection by bowel rest, intensive antibiotic therapy, and close observation.[15] Appendectomy is deferred to a later time. One of the difficulties involved in nonoperative therapy of appendiceal abscesses is determining whether the abscess is developing into diffuse peritonitis. If infection spreads while the patient is being treated nonoperatively, the patient is in jeopardy, and the operation should proceed forthwith. In children, rapid changes can occur, and the child may relapse following release from the hospital. This recurrence rate varies from 8% to 65%.[16] If nonoperative treatment is chosen, it is essential to perform delayed elective appendectomy because the rate of recurrence is high, and elective appendectomy is safe.

Most surgeons employ preoperative antibiotic prophylaxis in patients in whom perforation, peritonitis, or abscess is suspected. This approach is well supported in the literature, although some controversy continues.[12] Antibiotic prophylaxis for nonperforated appendicitis is less clear, although Foster and O'Toole demonstrated a tenfold reduction in the rate of wound infection with preoperative prophylactic cephaloridine.[13]

INTRAOPERATIVE DECISIONS

The time-honored incision is the right lower quadrant muscle splitting (McBurney) incision. The Rockey–Davis incision is a transverse muscle splitting incision that, additionally, can be extended across the lower abdomen; it is the incision of choice in women. Both incisions provide direct and safe access to the site of inflammation, minimize the possibility of extending the inflammatory process to uninvolved portions of the peritoneal cavity, are inherently strong, and have a low incidence of postoperative herniation. Because of variations in the location of the cecum, the incision may be shifted slightly with respect to the area of maximal tenderness. The Fowler–Wier modification adds incision of the anterior and posterior rectus sheaths with retraction of the rectus muscle and affords additional medial and pelvic exposure.[3] Occasionally, the incision is off target and the appendix is located aberrantly. The cecum should be identified and the tinea followed to the base of the appendix. Once the appendiceal base is identified, the remainder of the organ can be located, dissected, and brought into view. Occasionally, more extensive mobilization of the cecum is necessary to reach a long retrocolic appendix,

When the peritoneal cavity is entered, peritoneal fluid cultures should be secured for both aerobic and anaerobic organisms, the cecum identified, and the status of the appendix determined. A limited local exploration of adjacent viscera should be done, as indicated. If the inflammatory process is limited to the pericecal and the periappendiceal area, the cecum should be gently delivered into the wound, the base of the appendix identified, and the appendix mobilized. If the cecum is tightly bound to the iliac fossa, the fibrous attachments may be divided under direct vision to allow adequate cecal mobilization to accomplish appendectomy. Following control of the appendiceal artery and adjacent mesoappendix, a seromuscular purse-string suture is placed around the base of the appendix. The wound is protected by moistened gauze pads and the appendix clamped, ligated, and amputated. The stump is inspected, cauterized, and inverted through the purse-string suture, which is tied securely about the base of the appendix. The cecum is then replaced, the protective gauze pads removed, and the mesoappen-

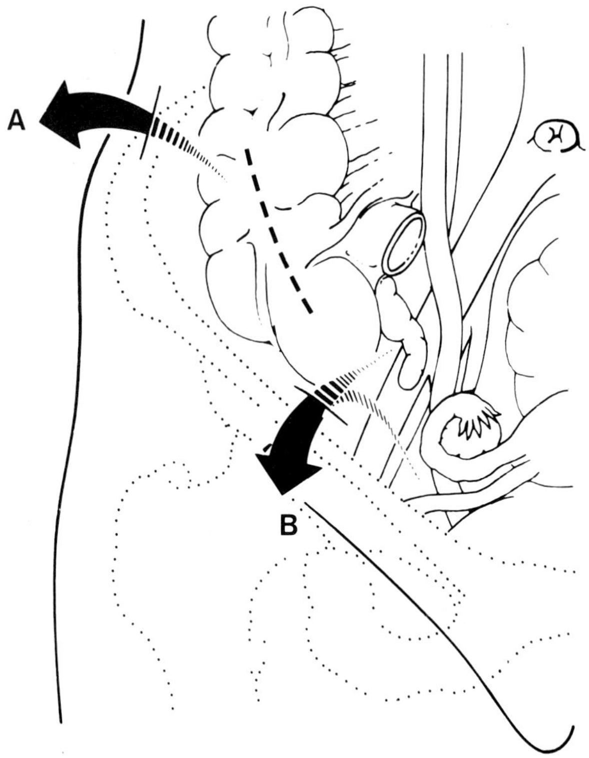

FIG. 34-4. Routes of drainage for periappendiceal abscess include (*A*) for collections lateral to the cecum and (*B*) for pelvic abscess and collections medial to the cecum.

dix is reinspected to assure hemostasis. In uncomplicated acute appendicitis in which the viability and pliability of the cecal wall is intact, inversion of the stump is preferred. The wound is subsequently closed anatomically in layers using absorbable suture material. Irrigation of the wound with antibiotic solution appears to offer some additional benefit in the prevention of wound infections.[2] The skin should be closed primarily.

The operative approach is the same for perforation or gangrene. If the appendix is perforated, gangrenous, or perforated with localized peritonitis, appendectomy should be performed whenever possible because continued soilage of the peritoneum will likely result in additional complications. If an abscess is encountered, the remaining loops of intestine, omentum, and pelvic viscera should be packed out of the operative field with moistened gauze pads and the abscess dealt with definitively. This is best accomplished by entering the cavity, evacuating the pus, and identifying and removing the appendix. If the appendix is necrotic, it is safer to ligate the stump doubly with absorbable suture and omit stump inversion. The presence of cloudy peritoneal fluid alone or in combination with an exudate over the appendix or adjacent cecum is not an indication for drainage. Therefore, in uncomplicated acute appendicitis, drainage is not indicated. Localized accumulations of pus, however, may require drainage, which is most effectively accomplished using sump drains brought out of a site separate from the incision.[30] Sump drains are preferred because the pelvis will not drain dependently through the anterior abdominal wall. Drains should be placed within the abscess cavity, lateral to the cecum or along the wall of the iliac fossa and away from the appendiceal stump (Fig. 34-4). Abscesses that occur medial to the cecum usually involve the cecum, appendix, mesentery, omentum, and small intestine in their wall and are the most difficult to drain safely because medial drains encourage the formation of adhesions and, if placed close to the appendiceal stump, also promote fecal fistula.

Periappendiceal abscesses that occur posterior to the cecum may be approached extraperitoneally. After transperitoneal exploration and identification of the process, the peritoneal cavity should be closed and a counter incision made in the right flank. When the retrocecal appendiceal abscess is drained, the appendix can often be identified and removed. If viable adjacent colon may be damaged, however, the appendix should be left for a later appendectomy.

Pelvic abscess from appendicitis presents a different problem and may require transperitoneal drainage or may be drained through the vagina or rectum, depending on the location of the abscess. When transperitoneal drainage is required, the intestines should be packed cephalad and the pelvis completely isolated. The abscess cavity is opened, pus aspirated and cultured, and the appendix removed, as previously described. Sump drains are placed in the abscess cavity and brought out through separate incisions. Occasionally, the pelvic abscess may be juxtaposed to the vagina or rectum; in such instances, transvaginal or transrectal drainage is safe and effective. Interval appendectomy is required. Wound closure in all instances of perforated or gangrenous appendicitis requires the use of absorbable synthetic suture and delayed primary closure of the skin and subcutaneous tissue. The latter is most conveniently accomplished 3 to 5 days postoperatively with skin tapes.

In neglected or far advanced appendicitis with perforation and gangrene, the necrotic process often involves the wall of the cecum in close proximity to the base of the appendix. Such circumstances carry a high risk of fecal fistula. If cecal viability is questionable, the area may be turned in with inverting sutures, provided healthy tissue can be brought over the closure. Often, a tag of omentum can be secured to the closure to aid in the healing process. Prophylactic drains should be used but should be located dependently and not left in contact with the repair. A frankly necrotic wall is one of the few indications for the use of a cecostomy. Again, drains should be employed.

POSTOPERATIVE PROBLEMS

The complications of appendectomy closely resemble the complications of appendicitis itself. The incidence, nature, and severity of postoperative problems are directly proportional to the time from onset of symptoms to the operation and operative findings.

Wound infection is the most common complication following appendectomy, and its frequency varies with the state of appendiceal disease. Kazarian found an incidence less than 1% in negative appendices, approximately 7% in acute nonperforated appendicitis, 16% in perforated appendicitis, and 35% if the perforation was associated with generalized peritonitis.[23] Proliferation of bacteria in the surgical wound can best be controlled by careful handling of tissues, selection of the appropriate operative procedure, and meticulous intraoperative wound hygiene. Selection of the antibiotic specific for the offending organism is also important. Preoperative use of an aminoglycoside and clindamycin is indicated in all cases of suspected perforation, peritonitis, and abscess because of the polymicrobial nature of appendiceal infection and the relative overgrowth of anaerobic organisms. Berger demonstrated high therapeutic levels of clindamycin in appendiceal tissue following a single 600-mg intravenous bolus.[5] The new third-generation cephalosporins hold promise for effective prophylaxis and therapy. Stewart and Matheson, in a review of 189 children with peritonitis secondary to appendiceal perforation, demonstrated a reduced incidence of septic and adhesive complications and wound infection after antibiotic peritoneal wound lavage.[43]

In a controlled clinical trial on the prophylactic use of topical ampicillin in nonperforated appendicitis, Anderson and associates demonstrated a statistically significant reduction in the frequency of wound infections after operations for nonperforated appendicitis.[2] However, they could not demonstrate a similar beneficial effect in perforated appendicitis.

Fever is the usual harbinger of septic complications following appendectomy. If wound infection and the other causes of postoperative fever are excluded, intra-abdominal abscess should be suspected. Paracecal, iliac fossa, and pelvic abscesses are the most common, followed by interloop, subhepatic, and subphrenic abscesses. Postoperative intra-abdominal abscesses are uncommon following appendectomy for nonperforated appendicitis but their incidence increases following perforation, especially when it is associated with generalized peritonitis. Elevation of the head of the bed postoperatively significantly reduces the occurrence of postoperative abscesses outside the pelvis.[44] Physical examination may disclose localized tenderness or a mass on abdominal or rectal examination. Impingement on the ureter on intravenous pyelography or on the colon on barium enema examination may suggest an extrinsic process. Ultrasonography and abdominal computed tomography (CT) are accurate methods of identifying intraperitoneal and retroperitoneal collections, which can be aspirated and cultured prior to surgical drainage. Successful evacuation of small collections of pus followed by CT-guided catheter placement has been reported.[18]

Breakdown of the appendiceal stump or necrosis of adjacent cecum leads to fecal fistula, intra-abdominal abscess, and generalized sepsis if it is not recognized promptly. If effective local drainage can be established, most fistulas will close. The colon distal to the fistula must be studied to rule out a distal obstructing lesion.

Fever, shaking chills, and jaundice associated with rapid clinical deterioration of the patient's condition suggest pylephlebitis with septic thrombosis of the portal vein and disseminated intrahepatic abscesses. Identification and surgical drainage of intra-abdominal suppuration, high-dose antibiotic therapy, and intensive supportive care are warranted. The multiplicity of intrahepatic abscesses usually precludes therapeutic drainage, although sonography should be performed to diagnose the occasional large intrahepatic abscess that can be drained.

Special Considerations in Surgery of the Appendix

THE NEGATIVE APPENDIX

Unnecessary operation is in itself a complication. In order to avoid missing acute appendicitis and the inevitable perforation that follows, however, a certain number of normal appendices will invariably be removed. The literature is filled with considerable discussion on what constitutes an appropriate rate for the removal of normal appendices, ranging from 9% to 45%, with young women having the highest rate because of their potential for gynecologic problems.

It has been feared that any attempt to lessen the percentage of negative explorations would appreciably add to the risk of missing perforations. Yet,

Chang showed that the "negative appendix" is accompanied by a significant complication rate of 17%.[9] Jerman described six patients with intestinal obstruction from adhesions that followed the removal of a normal appendix.[21] Gentle handling of the bowel and minimal traction to prevent serosal injury were recommended to reduce the likelihood of postoperative adhesions. Limiting the number of appendectomies performed for nonsurgical conditions, therefore, still remains a clinical challenge. White and colleagues have been able to reduce unnecessary appendectomy to less than 10% by using intensive in-hospital observation.[48] In their experience, most children whose appendices ruptured did so prior to the time of presentation. By observing questionable cases in-hospital, surgical decisions were more likely to be appropriate.

If a normal appendix is encountered, it is important to evaluate the uterus and both ovaries carefully and examine systematically the terminal ileum and its mesentery for at least 3 feet to exclude Meckel's diverticulitis and mesenteric adenitis. The retroperitoneum should be palpated in the area of the ureter, gonadal vessels, psoas muscle, and iliac fossa.[31] With unexplained evidence of peritonitis or hemoperitoneum that cannot be treated by a right lower quadrant incision, the incision should be closed and a generous midline incision employed to correct the problem. In contrast, if local exploration is negative and there is little evidence for a surgical problem, an appendectomy should be performed and the patient closed. In at least 50% of patients, no surgical problem will be found.

CHRONIC APPENDICITIS

The hallmark of chronic appendicitis is recurrent pain in the right lower quadrant that resolves without an operation. The pathogenesis of chronic (recurrent) appendicitis is inflammation in the absence of total lumenal obstruction. The appendix decompresses spontaneously without perforation, and the inflammation subsides only to recur. Leigh found histologic evidence of chronic inflammation in 30% of 1777 appendectomy specimens, which correlated well with the clinical history of right lower quadrant pain in a third of the patients.[24]

In a review of pathologic changes in 1000 appendices, Dymock defined chronic appendicitis by the infiltration of lymphocytes and eosinophils, fibrosis, and change of the epithelium to a simple cuboidal form.[11] More advanced examples demonstrated the total loss of epithelial lining and fibrous replacement of the lumen. McLennan and Watts studied a group of 286 patients with symptoms of right lower quadrant pain of at least 1-year duration.[28] Following elective appendectomy, 85% had complete relief, and similar changes were found in 75% of the appendices.

APPENDICITIS DURING PREGNANCY

Appendicitis occurs once in every 1600 pregnancies. Diagnosis of appendicitis in pregnancy is often clouded by the presence of significant pyuria in about 25% of pregnant women. In a review of 50,000 pregnancies during a 14-year period, Frisenda noted that the rate of misdiagnosis of appendicitis in pregnancy was comparable to that of the general female population, that fetal mortality was minimal, and that clinical judgment rather than laboratory data was most reliable in determining the need for an operation.[14] The presenting symptoms are similar to those of the nonpregnant patient, except during the last trimester when the pain is located higher on the right side. The likelihood of appendiceal perforation also appears to be highest during the third trimester.[27] The natural leukocystosis during pregnancy reduces the value of this parameter. The diagnostic error during pregnancy is 40% or greater in most series, but the diagnostic error in the nonpregnant woman of child-bearing age is also high, ranging from 30% to 45%. Reported fetal mortality is from 12% to 37%, but the risk of negative exploration on the fetus is probably no more than is the risk of spontaneous abortion in the population at large.

When the pregnant patient is operated on for appendicitis, especially during the second and third trimesters, placing the patient obliquely on her left side displaces the enlarging gravid uterus out of the operative field, minimizes uterine manipulation, and improves placental perfusion.

INCIDENTAL APPENDECTOMY

Incidental appendectomy may be justified only if the risk of future appendicitis exceeds the risk of complications resulting from the appendectomy itself. The overall annual incidence of appendicitis is 0.1% in the general population, and although the overall risk of undergoing appendectomy for appendicitis during one's lifetime is approximately 20%, appendicitis most commonly occurs between the ages of 10 and 30 years.[26] Several studies indicate that the risk of appendicitis is significant until the age of 50.[26, 34]

In potentially contaminated primary operations, the addition of incidental appendectomy does not appear to increase the risks of operative morbidity or mortality, provided the appendix can be readily located and removed through the existing incision. However, opening a contaminated organ during a clean procedure may represent an unwarranted risk and should not be practiced indiscriminately.[32]

TUMORS

Tumors of the appendix are uncommon. Carcinoid, the most common, is typically encountered as an incidental finding at appendectomy. No further therapy is required if the entire lesion is removed with the appendix. Mucous cystadenocarcinoma, although malignant, does not usually metastasize but does lead to mucocele and, with rupture of the appendix, to pseudomyxoma peritonei. Large amounts of gelatinous material within the peritoneal cavity may lead to mechanical obstruction. Therefore, all of the gelatinous material should be removed and submitted for cytologic study.[39] Qizilbash believes that this lesion is similar to villous adenoma and that the most common histologic lesion in a mucocele is a mucinous cystadenoma.[37] Mucocele may also occur following obstruction of the appendix, causing mucous distention and rupture.

Primary adenocarcinoma of the appendix is rare with fewer than 200 cases reported. Primary adenocarcinoma is virtually never diagnosed preoperatively but presents either as appendicitis or, following rupture, as disseminated disease. Since the lymphatics of the appendix drain into the regional nodes of the terminal ileum and cecum, either the upper or lower ileocolic chain may constitute the primary drainage and contain metastases. Right hemicolectomy to include the node-bearing drainage is the treatment of choice for adenocarcinoma and cystic mucinous cystadenocarcinoma. For carcinoid tumors, appendectomy is usually adequate unless the tumor involves the base of the appendix or wall of the adjacent cecum, which mandates wider resection.[19]

Whether appendectomy predisposes patients to carcinoma of the colon and other malignancies has been raised by several authors.[29] Moertel, in a controlled prospective study of a large patient population, demonstrated no evidence that any patient who underwent an appendectomy was predisposed to cancer, regardless of the age at which the appendectomy was performed.[33] Increased risk of malignancy does not appear to be a complication of appendectomy.

CROHN'S DISEASE

Involvement of the appendix in Crohn's disease has been reported.[47] Occasionally, it may be the initial target of the disease and, only later, involve other parts of the intestinal tract. The clinical pattern of the disease of the appendix cannot be distinguished from that of acute appendicitis. Appendectomy is indicated in Crohn's disease of the appendix and in patients with terminal ileal involvement operated upon for acute Crohn's disease, unless the cecum is diseased. Appendectomy in patients with Crohn's disease is of obvious benefit in the subsequent management of patients subject to recurrent attacks of right lower quadrant pain.

DIVERTICULOSIS OF THE APPENDIX

Diverticulosis of the appendix is rare and may be congenital or acquired. The congenital form is usually found as an isolated lesion in young persons. Acquired diverticula are multiple and probably relate to obstruction of the appendix. Because of their etiology, diverticula may be clinically significant in early perforation of the appendix.[46]

INTUSSUSCEPTION OF THE APPENDIX

Intussusception of the appendix may mimic appendicitis, cause recurrent right lower quadrant pain from intestinal obstruction, or present as a mass. Since a healthy appendix is capable of peristalsis and not fixed by inflammatory adhesions, the appendix may slip into the cecal lumen and intussuscept. Contributing factors to the development of appendiceal intussusception are the fetal-type appendix with a wide proximal lumen and a thin narrow mesoappendix.

TRAUMA

Injury to the appendix is rare. Diagnosis is usually made only at laparotomy, and the treatment is appendectomy. Penetrating injuries produce clinical signs early and allow a prompt operation, during which the injury to the appendix is usually discovered. Blunt trauma often results in a delayed diagnosis. The mechanism of injury to the appendix after blunt trauma is thought to be a direct force compressing the appendix and its mesentery against the spine. The presence of a fixed cecum aids in the avulsion of the appendix if a decelerating force is applied to the area.[36]

MEDICOLEGAL CONSIDERATIONS IN APPENDECTOMY

The physician and surgeon have two major concerns about appendicitis: missing the diagnosis and performing an unnecessary operation. Missing the diagnosis of the appendicitis does not, in and of itself, indicate negligence on the part of the physician, provided the evaluation of the patient meets the standard of practice. However, when the diagnosis of appendicitis appears likely or at least probable, surgical intervention is justified, both medically and legally. Since appendectomy is used as a diagnostic as well as therapeutic measure and is, as such, a standard of care, as long as there is no negligence during the procedure, it is highly unlikely that a physician would be found negligent for performing an appendectomy on a patient who does not have appendicitis. At the same time, if the physician fails to diagnose appendicitis, he is not likely to be held liable, provided there are grounds for a diagnosis other than that of appendicitis.[20] For the practicing emergency physician, surgical consultation is strongly recommended whenever the possibility of appendicitis is considered.

References

1. Ackerman NB: The continuing problems of perforated appendicitis. Surg Gynecol Obstet 139:29, 1974
2. Andersen B, Bendtsen A, Holbraad L et al: Wound infections after appendectomy. Acta Chir Scand 138:531, 1972
3. Askew AR: The Fowler–Weir approach to appendectomy. Br J Surg 62:303, 1975
4. Bartlett RH, Eraklis AJ, Wilkinson RH: Appendicitis in infancy. Surg Gynecol Obstet 130:99, 1970
5. Berger SA, Barza M, Leslie SW et al: Penetration of clindamycin into the human appendix. Arch Surg 113:1094, 1978
6. Bierman HR: Human appendix and neoplasm. Cancer 21:109, 1968
7. Brook I: Bacterial studies of peritoneal cavity and postoperative surgical wound drainage following perforated appendix in children. Ann Surg 192:208, 1980
8. Cameron M: Gynaecology and general surgery. Ann R Coll Surg Engl 56:115, 1975
9. Chang FC, Hogle HH, Welling DR: The fate of the negative appendix. Am J Surg 126:752, 1973
10. Copeland EM, Long JM: Elective appendectomy for appendiceal calculus. Surg Gynecol Obstet 130:435, 1970
11. Dymock RB: Pathological changes in the appendix: A review of 1,000 cases. Pathology 9:334, 1977
12. Fine M, Busuttil RW: Acute appendicitis: Efficacy of prophylactic preoperative antibiotics in the reduction of septic morbidity. Am J Surg 135:210, 1978
13. Foster PD, O'Toole RD: Primary appendectomy—The effect of prophylactic cephaloridine on postoperative wound infection. JAMA 239:1411, 1978
14. Frisenda R, Roty AR, Kilway JB et al: Acute appendicitis during pregnancy. Am Surg 45:503, 1979
15. Gastrin U, Josephson S: Appendiceal abscess—Acute appendectomy or conservative treatment. Acta Chir Scand 155:539, 1969
16. Gierup J, Karpe B: Aspects on appendiceal abscess in children with special reference to delayed appendectomy. Acta Chir Scand 141:801, 1976
17. Griffith GL, Maull KI, Sachatello CR: Septic pulmonary embolization. Surg Gynecol Obstet 144:105, 1977
18. Haaga JR, Weinstein AJ: CT-guided percutaneous aspiration and drainage of abscesses. AJR 135:1187, 1980
19. Herczeg E, Winter S, Weissberg D: Primary carcinoma of the appendix. JAMA 238:51, 1977
20. Holder AR: Misdiagnosis of appendicitis. JAMA 212:1763, 1970
21. Jerman RR: Removal of the normal appendix: The cause of serious complications. Br J Clin Pract 23:466, 1969
22. Jona JZ, Belin RP: Basilar pneumonia simulating acute appendicitis in children. Arch Surg 111:552, 1976
23. Kazarian KK, Roeder WJ, Meisheimer WL: Decreasing mortality and increasing morbidity from acute appendicitis. Am J Surg 119:681, 1970
24. Leigh PG: Appendicitis—Still a considerable problem. S Afr Med J 43:700, 1969
25. Lewis FR, Holcroft JW, Boey J et al: Appendicitis—A critical review of diagnosis and treatment in 1,000 cases. Arch Surg 110:677, 1975
26. Ludbrook J, Spears GF: The risk of developing appendicitis. Br J Surg 52:856, 1965
27. McComb P, Laimon H: Appendicitis complicating pregnancy. Can J Surg 23:92, 1980
28. McLennan K, Watts JK: Justification for appendectomy in chronic appendicitis. Br Med J 2:736, 1954
29. McVay JR: The appendix in relation to neoplastic disease. Cancer 17:929, 1964
30. Mason JH, Byrne MP, Gau FC: Surgery of the vermiform appendix. Surg Clin North Am 57:1303, 1977
31. Maull KI, van Nagell JR, Greenfield LJ: Surgical implications of ovarian vein thrombosis. Am Surg 44:727, 1978
32. Miranda R, Johnston AD, O'Leary JP: Incidental appendectomy: Frequency of pathologic abnormalities. Am Surg 43:355, 1977
33. Moertel CC, Nobrega FT, Elveback LR et al: A prospective study of appendectomy and predisposition to cancer. Surg Gynecol Obstet 138:549, 1974
34. Norton LW, Sweeney M, Eiseman B: Incidental appendectomy with laparotomy for trauma. Br J Surg 62:487, 1975
35. Owens BJ, Hamit HF: Appendicitis in the elderly. Ann Surg 187:392, 1978
36. Pillary SP, Baker LW: Appendiceal injuries. S Afr Med J 51:900, 1977
37. Qizilbash AH: Mucoceles of the appendix. Arch Pathol 99:548, 1975
38. Rajagopalan AE, Mason JH, Kennedy M et al: The value of the barium enema in the diagnosis of acute appendicitis. Arch Surg 112:531, 1977
39. Rosato FE, Seltzer MH: Pseudomyxoma peritonei: Case report including in vitro mucolysis. Surgery 68:301, 1970
40. Saebo A: Pneumoperitoneum associated with perforated appendicitis. Acta Chir Scand 144:115, 1978
41. Sakover RP, Del Fava RL: Frequency of visualization of the normal appendix with the barium enema examination. AJR 121:312, 1974
42. Smith DE, Jacquet JM, Virgilio RW: Left upper quadrant appendicitis. Arch Surg 109:443, 1974
43. Stewart DJ, Matheson NA: Peritoneal lavage in appendicular peritonitis. Br J Surg 65:54, 1978
44. Stone HH, Sanders SL, Martin JD: Perforated appendicitis in children. Surgery 69:673, 1971
45. Swensson EE, Maull KI: Clinical significance of elevated serum and urine amylase in patients with acute appendicitis. Am J Surg 142:667, 1981
46. Trollope ML, Lindenauer SM: Diverticulosis of the appendix. Dis Colon Rectum 17:200, 1974
47. Wang TK, Tolnai G, Campbell JS et al: Crohn's disease of the appendix. Can Med Assoc J 106:233, 1972
48. White JJ, Santillana M, Haller JA: Intensive in-hospital observation: A safe way to decrease unnecessary appendectomy. Am Surg 41:793, 1975
49. Wilkinson RH, Bartlett RH, Eraklis AI: Diagnosis of appendicitis in infancy: The value of abdominal radiographs. Am J Dis Child 118:687, 1969

35 Complications of Pediatric Surgery and Trauma

Martin R. Eichelberger | Judson G. Randolph

OVERVIEW

Surgery is performed on patients to reverse anatomical and physiologic derangements. Surgical procedures evolve with the development of technical methods that reduce postoperative complications. Safe surgery depends on the selection of an appropriate operation that minimizes both the physiologic stress to the patient and the potential for complications. When performing surgery on children, especially the neonate, the surgeon must be cognizant of a variety of unique physiologic and anatomical factors that will improve outcome and minimize predictable complications.

Infants and childen manifest predictable complications following surgery. Knowledge of their unique physiology and injury patterns provides the opportunity to anticipate and prevent complications. Appropriate surgical technique and judgment are essential in guaranteeing a successful outcome for the child with congenital anomalies or trauma. The mechanical ventilator, total parenteral nutrition (TPN), specific antibiotics, neonatology, and improved surgical technique are the major factors contributing to the continued improvement in outcome following surgical treatment of the child.

General Physiology Unique to the Child

The neonate is an organism who is adapting to extrauterine life. This patient is extremely sensitive to changes in the internal and external environment. Intelligent care of the surgical neonate requires an understanding of fluid and electrolytes, renal function, glucose metabolism, calcium metabolism, blood volume, thermoregulation, and host defenses.

The size of the patient makes one "think small." The child must not be treated as a "small adult" by using miniaturized adult guidelines. The size of the patient affects blood volume, which is 7% to 8% of the body weight.[14] Blood volume is small in relation to size, which accounts for shock following a small amount of blood loss or third-space fluid shift. Underestimation of fluid hydration leads to oliguria, metabolic acidosis, hypoxia, and possible cardiac arrest, while overestimates of fluid hydration can result in pulmonary edema.

Maintenance of the neonate's fluid and electrolyte requirements must also provide adequate kilocalories for metabolic activity. A rapid and efficient method is based on body weight, which is correlated with calories expended in 24 hours under basal conditions (Table 35-1).[13a, 41, 85, 101] Fluid requirements for infants who weigh between 1 kg and 10 kg are 100 ml/kg/day. The infant requires 3 mEq Na^+/kg/day and 2 mEq K^+/kg/day. A solution of D10 1/4 NSS provides 3.8 mEq NaCl/dl, which represents adequate Na^+ at maintenance rates. Neonates with surgical diseases of the abdomen frequently experience large third-space losses.[39] To prepare the infant for surgery adequately, this sequestered fluid must be replaced. Fluid resuscitation in the immediate preoperative and postoperative period is accomplished by utilizing a solution of D10 1/2 NSS calculated to infuse at a rate equal to one and a half times maintenance. A bolus infusion ("pump priming") of 20 ml/kg of a Ringer's lactated solution or 1/2 NSS is effective in establishing urine output and improved tissue perfusion. Adequacy of fluid hydration is ascertained, as in the adult patient, by measuring urine output.

The renal function in the child less than a year of age is different from that of the adult. Imbalance in the maturation of glomeruli is reflected by a glomerular filtration rate that provides only one half of the osmolar concentrating capacity of the adult kidney.[18] The neonate or child concentrates urine to a

TABLE 35-1. Maintenance Fluid Requirements in Children (D5¼ NSS)*

Weight (kg)	Amount of Fluid
0–10	100 ml/kg/day
11–20	1000 ml + 50 ml/kg/day over 10 kg
21–40	1500 ml + 20 ml/kg/day over 20 kg
>40	2500 ml/day (adult requirements)

* D10¼ NSS for neonate

level of 450 to 700 mOsm/L, while the adult level is 1200 to 1400 mOsm. The newborn kidney has limited ability to concentrate urine during fluid loss and to dilute urine when excess fluid is present.[46] Hypovolemia in the neonate is manifested by poor tissue perfusion (pale, cool, mottled extremities), hypoxia, acidosis, and a decreased urine output. Adequacy of hydration is ascertained by urine output, urine specific gravity, serum electrolytes, change in body weight, vital signs, and serum osmolality. Calculated urine output for the neonate is 1 ml to 2 ml/kg/hour, or 40 ml/kg/day.[101] Urine specific gravity below 1.015 indicates adequate hydration.

Glucose metabolism in the neonate is extremely labile and dependent on endogenous stores.[100] The neonate must adjust to extrauterine life in which energy demands are met during the postnatal period by metabolism of glycogen and depletion of the hepatic reserves. The neonate has an inefficient system of gluconeogenesis, which is reflected by precipitous drops in glucose level during the first days of life, leading to seizures, apnea, jitteriness, and cyanosis. Consequently, the neonate must maintain a serum glucose level of 45 mg/dl. During the initial evaluation of the surgical neonate, a rapid determination of blood glucose obtained by heelstick with a Dextrostix reagent strip is helpful. A glucose level above 45 mg/dl is maintained by infusing a 10% glucose solution. With symptoms of hypoglycemia or a glucose level below 45 mg/dl, administration of 4 ml/kg of 25% D5W intravenously over a 5-minute period is indicated. The neonate is subject to a variety of stresses, which increase the metabolic demand for energy supplied by the glucose substrate. Postoperatively, a variable response to stress is reflected in the inability of the infant to handle a glucose load. Glucose infusion should be adjusted by following the serum glucose level with Dextrostix.

Calcium metabolism is also important in the management of the surgical newborn.[79] Calcium stores are transferred from the mother to the newborn during gestation. At birth the newborn has a low production of parathormone and a kidney that cannot excrete phosphate, resulting in a decrease in the serum calcium level. The symptoms of hypocalcemia are nonspecific and similar to those of hypoglycemia. In contrast to hypoglycemia, in which residual central nervous system deficits can occur, adequately treated hypocalcemia has minimal long-term residual effects.[50] The symptoms of hypocalcemia are seizures, jitteriness, twitching, and occasional cyanosis. Serum calcium levels below 7 mg/dl are abnormal and require treatment. Most patients are maintained with an intravenous infusion of calcium gluconate, which is added to a maintenance solution that provides 1 g to 2 g per day. Rapid adjustment of the calcium level is accomplished by infusing 1 ml to 2 ml/kg of a 10% calcium gluconate solution over a 5-minute period.

In summary, the surgical neonate is safely managed in the pre- and postoperative period by infusing a solution of 250 ml of D10 1/2 NSS with 5 miliequivalents of potassium chloride, 500 mg of calcium gluconate, 1 ml of MVI, and 250 units of heparin. This solution is infused at a rate of one and a half times maintenance (1-1/2 M). The urine output is followed and a rate of 1 ml to 2 ml/kg/hour or 40 ml/kg/day is optimal. A 20-ml/kg infusion over 20 minutes of crystalloid, as Ringer's lactated solution or 1/2 NSS, is safe since this approximates one quarter of the patient's blood volume.

Thermal regulation of the child is affected by the relatively large surface area to body mass ratio. The lack of substantial subcutaneous tissue and a thin skin contribute to evaporative heat loss in a child. Caloric expenditure results in higher energy requirements. This is especially likely in a child under 6 months of age who maintains body temperature by a metabolic process whereby catecholamines act upon brown fat in the intrascapular region and mediastinum to generate energy.[15] This nonshivering thermogenesis requires energy expenditure that leads to acidosis if consumption continues unabated. As the patient strives to maintain thermal neutrality with the environment, energy expenditure is directed toward heat production by utilizing available calories.[86] Consequently, energy stores are depleted; products of metabolism accumulate; and acidosis develops.[81] Hypothermia causes a release of catecholamines that also affect the pulmonary vasculature, resulting in pulmonary hypertension and leading to hypoxia, metabolic acidosis, and anaerobic metabolism. Optimal care of the neonate requires that resuscitation occur in an environment where heat loss is minimized. This is guaranteed if external heating devices are available and temperature is monitored from the outset. The core temperature should be maintained at 36° C to 37° C.

The final general consideration for the neonate is the intrinsic immaturity of the host defenses.[80] White blood cell function and opsonization are thought to be functional, but complement activity is decreased. IgG is present in normal amounts; however, IgM is absent.[81] Therefore, the serum factors required for host defense are depressed in the neonate. Septicemia places an overwhelming burden on the immune system of the immature neonate. Patients with sepsis from intestinal surgical diseases usually have a large third-space loss that requires vigorous fluid resuscitation. The resuscitation of the infant requires that supplemental factors be administered to assist in combating sepsis after blood cultures are obtained. This is accomplished by infusing 20 ml/kg of fresh whole blood or fresh frozen plasma. The surgical neonate is treated prophylactically with ampicillin, 150 mg to 400 mg/kg per day in four doses, and gentamicin, 5 mg to 7 mg/kg/day in two divided doses, to assist the newborn in his fight for life. The antibiotic regimen is continued for 7 to 10 days under surveillance for ongoing sepsis. Blood cultures, platelet count, and thermal stability are monitored throughout the neonate's course.

Anticipation of the physiologic requirements of the neonate prevents perioperative physiologic complications, which are treated as outlined below. The neonate requires close monitoring and clinical evaluation every few hours in the immediate postoperative period. The newborn is physiologically labile but exceedingly responsive to appropriate therapy.

SUMMARY—TREATMENT OF PHYSIOLOGIC COMPLICATIONS

HYPOGLYCEMIA

4 ml/kg of D25%, IV push over 5 minutes

HYPOKALEMIA

Standard replacement is 2 to 3 mEq/kg/day, which is equal to 5 mEq KCl/250 ml solution at 4 ml/kg/hr.
For K+ = 2.5 to 3.5 add 1 mEq KCl to 50 ml of standard solution (*i.e.,* 2 mEq KCl/50 ml) to run at 4 ml/kg/hr.
For K+ less than 2.5 add 2 mEq KCl to 50 ml of standard solution (*i.e.,* 3 mEq KCl/50 ml) to run at 4 ml/kg/hr.
Repeat lytes in 3 hours.

HYPOCALCEMIA

2 ml/kg of 10% calcium gluconate IV push over 5 minutes—monitoring heart rate for bradycardia

METABOLIC ACIDOSIS (treat base deficit greater than 5)

mEq $NaHCO_3$ required = (-B.E.) × (wt. in kg) × (Factor). Factor = 0.5 for newborn, 0.4 for small child, 0.3 for others. Correct with ½ mEq/ml and give half of the corrective dose.

BRADYCARDIA

Atropine 0.01 mg/kg

CARDIAC ARREST	*Frequency of Dose*
$NaHCO_3$, 2 to 4 mEq/kg	5–10 min
Epinephrine, 1:10,000 0.01 mg/kg	5–10 min
Isoproterenol, 1:10,000 0.01 mg/kg	Single dose
Dopamine, 2.0 to 20.0 mg/kg/min	Continuous infusion
Atropine sulfate, 0.01 to 0.02 mg	30 min
Calcium chloride 10%, 20 mg (2 ml)/kg	10 min
Calcium gluconate, 10% 60 mg (6ml)/kg	10 min
Defibrillation—2 to 5 watts-seconds/kg	(external)

ELECTROLYTES

Sodium and chloride,
3 mEq/kg/day (up to 45 mEq/day)
Potassium,
2 mEq/kg/day
Calcium,
20 mEq/kg (elemental) infants
200 mg/kg (calcium gluconate)

GASTRIC LOSS

Fluid management should be reevaluated every 3 to 12 hours. Replacement of losses milliliter for milliliter every 4 hours
Gastric suction or vomitus: Approximate composition is NA −60 to 75 mEq/liter; chloride 100–150 mEq/liter, K −5 to 20 mEq/liter. *Replace with* D5 1/2NS + 5 mEq K/250 ml.

BLOOD PRODUCTS	
Whole blood	20 ml/kg
Plasma	20 ml/kg
5% albumin	20 ml/kg
Packed RBCs	10 ml/kg
25% albumin	4 ml/kg
Platelets	1 unit 20–35 ml

Complications of Stomach Surgery

GASTROSTOMY

Gastrostomy is a procedure used frequently in the care of the pediatric surgical patient (Fig. 35-1). Complications that ensue from utilizing this technique are best avoided.[36] Bleeding from the gastros-

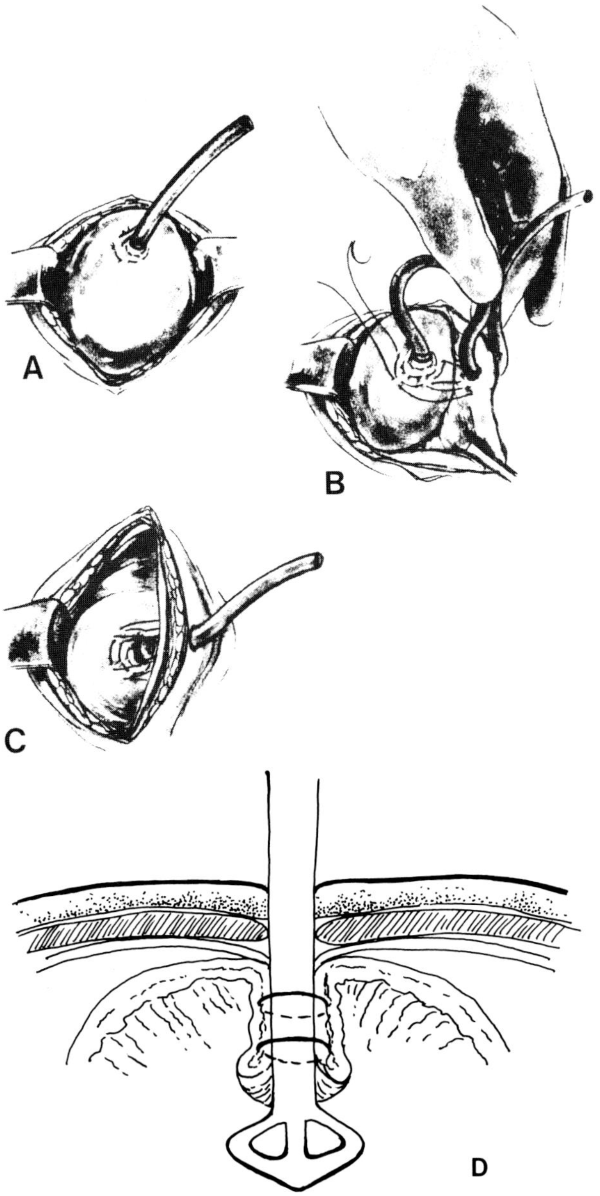

FIG. 35-1. Gastrostomy. (*A*) Use of a concentric purse-string suture (3-0 silk) minimizes bleeding from the gastrotomy incision. (*B*) Attachment of the gastric seromuscular layer to the anterior abdominal wall. (*C*) Catheter pulled up and secured with sutures at three points. (*D*) The sagittal section shows an inverted Stamm gastrostomy secured to the anterior abdominal wall. The Malecot catheter is pulled up against the wall. (*A*, *B*, and *C* from Redo FS: Atlas of Surgery in the First Six Months of Life, p 17. Hagerstown, MD, Harper & Row, 1978. *D* reproduced with permission from Welch CE: Surgery of the Stomach and Duodenum, 5th ed. Copyright © 1973 by Year Book Medical Publishers, Inc, Chicago)

tomy incision is minimized by use of a double "purse-string" suture. The inner purse-string suture is hemostatic. The second purse-string suture is used to invert the gastrostomy site, which includes a Malecot catheter (14–16 Fr) to establish a serosa-to-peritoneum approximation to the abdominal wall. Location of the gastrostomy tube on the abdominal wall is important and requires planning. The gastrostomy tube is managed more easily if it is placed in the center of a triangle formed by the umbilicus, the left costal margin, and the xiphoid. Inadvertent placement of the gastrostomy tube through the lower portion of the thorax and diaphragm can occur with imprecise attention to location. It is best to bring the gastrostomy tube out through a separate stab wound, which is made slightly smaller in diameter than the gastrostomy tube. This allows a tight seal between the skin and the catheter, to minimize leakage. Once the catheter is pulled through this tight opening, the seromuscular layer of the stomach is secured to the anterior peritoneal wall by three separate 3-0 silk sutures. The tube is secured to the skin by a nylon suture.

The after-care of the gastrostomy tube is important to prevent long-term complications. The catheter is kept at a 90° angle to the skin for at least a 5- to 7-day period, which allows formation of a tract and maintenance of the small orifice through the abdominal wall that minimizes leakage of gastric material. On the second postoperative day, the gastrostomy tube is elevated. Small feedings are begun the third day. To avoid overdistention of the stomach, the gastrostomy tube is left unclamped for at least a week postoperatively. Gastric dilatation can result in the stomach tearing loose from its attachment to the abdominal wall, with intraperitoneal soilage by gastric contents.

A common complication of gastrostomy is inadvertent removal by either the patient or the attending medical personnel. This is prevented by adequate taping of the gastrostomy to the patient's anterior abdominal wall in the postoperative period. Nevertheless, should the tube dislodge in the first week after gastrostomy, reoperation and placement of a new tube is usually necessary. After the first week the gastrostomy site is mature enough to permit replacement of the gastrostomy tube. A Foley catheter is placed more easily and safely than a Malecot catheter.

The gastrostomy catheter should be replaced within a 4- to 6-hour period following inadvertent discontinuation, since the stoma closes quickly. The tract of the gastrostomy site is gently probed with a hemostat or thin dilator to establish the course of the tract. The tract is usually directed medially toward the vertebral spine at a 45° angle. Adequate lubrication of the Foley catheter allows easy inser tion. The Foley balloon is inflated to 4 cm to 5 cm of water and pulled gently up against the abdominal wall. The Foley balloon has a tendency to migrate through the pylorus into the small bowel, with subsequent obstruction. The balloon catheter can also migrate into the esophagus with symptoms of lower esophageal obstruction. These complications are avoided by securing the Foley gastrostomy tube, as demonstrated in Figure 35-2. A large red rubber catheter is cut at its largest end and two holes placed in the catheter. The Foley catheter is pulled through the opening to form a bridge that prevents migration of the catheter and maintains the 90° exit of the catheter from the abdominal wall. The red rubber catheter can then be rotated 360° for care of the skin.

The second method of replacing the gastrostomy tube involves insertion of a Malecot catheter, which has a flanged distal end. This requires a delicate touch, knowledge of the direction of the tract, and adequate lubrication of the tube. A thin metal dilator or the end of a Q-tip applicator is used to stretch the Malecot to allow its insertion through the gastrostomy opening. This technique requires adequate pressure to the abdominal wall and may be associated with traumatic separation of the stomach from the abdominal wall.

Accurate reinsertion of the gastrostomy tube into the stomach is confirmed by one of several methods: (1) Instillation of 30 cc of air through the gastrostomy tube, which is then clamped, followed by a radiograph of the abdomen to document the absence of pneumoperitoneum. (2) Infusion of one-quarter-strength Gastrografin into the gastrostomy tube for x-ray confirmation of the intraluminal position of the catheter. (3) This method is exclusively employed in those patients who have had long-term gastrostomy: The tube is reinserted, and aspiration of obvious gastric content provides confirmation of appropriate placement.

Chronic complications of gastrostomy tube include leak around the tube or prolapse of gastric mucosa. Leak from an enlarged gastrostomy site is managed by discontinuation of the tube for 24 hours to allow the stoma to close partially. If this is not effective, then a Foley catheter with a balloon is inserted and pulled against the abdominal wall to seal the orifice. Application of Stoma-adhesive around the catheter minimizes excoriation and allows reepithelialization of the skin.

Patients with excessive dilatation of the gastrocutaneous tract will develop prolapse of the gastric mucosa, leading to bleeding or leakage from the site. Leaking from the gastrostomy site or chronic prolapse with gastric fluid loss can result in inadequate caloric intake with failure to thrive. Such instances require surgical repair to reconstitute the gastrostomy. The stomach is detached from the abdominal wall, the old gastrostomy site oversewn, and a new gastrostomy created.

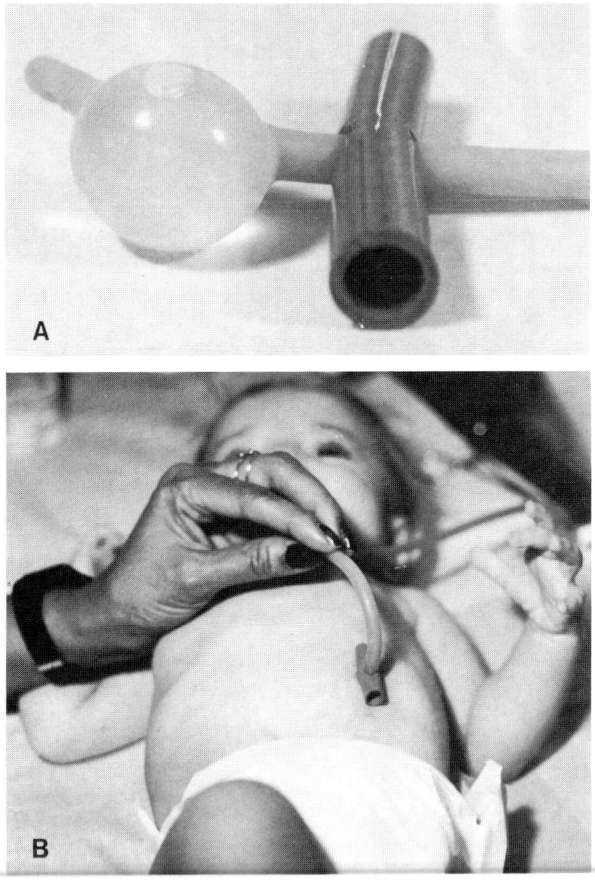

FIG. 35-2. (*A*) Foley catheter gastrostomy system. A 36-Fr red rubber catheter is cut at the widest end (3–4 cm), and two holes are cut in the middle of this piece on opposite sides. The Foley catheter is pulled through these holes by hemostat, and the catheter is inserted into the gastrostomy orifice. The balloon is inflated with 3 ml to 4 ml saline and the red rubber bolster advanced to the skin for a snug fit. In this system the catheter exits the stoma at a 90° angle, skin care at the stoma is facilitated, and migration of the catheter is prevented. (*B*) A Foley catheter gastrostomy in place.

Once the patient no longer requires a gastrostomy, the tube is discontinued. Within several days the gastrostomy site closes spontaneously. If the gastrocutaneous tract epithelializes, the stoma will persist. This is treated with local silver nitrate cautery and the orifice sealed with Stoma-adhesive. Cautery of the tract with silver nitrate should be frequent until gastric mucosa, granulation tissue, or epithelium is adequately traumatized to allow fusion of the layers. A Steri-strip is helpful in approximating the skin edges. If the stoma site persists and continues to leak, a formal surgical closure is required.

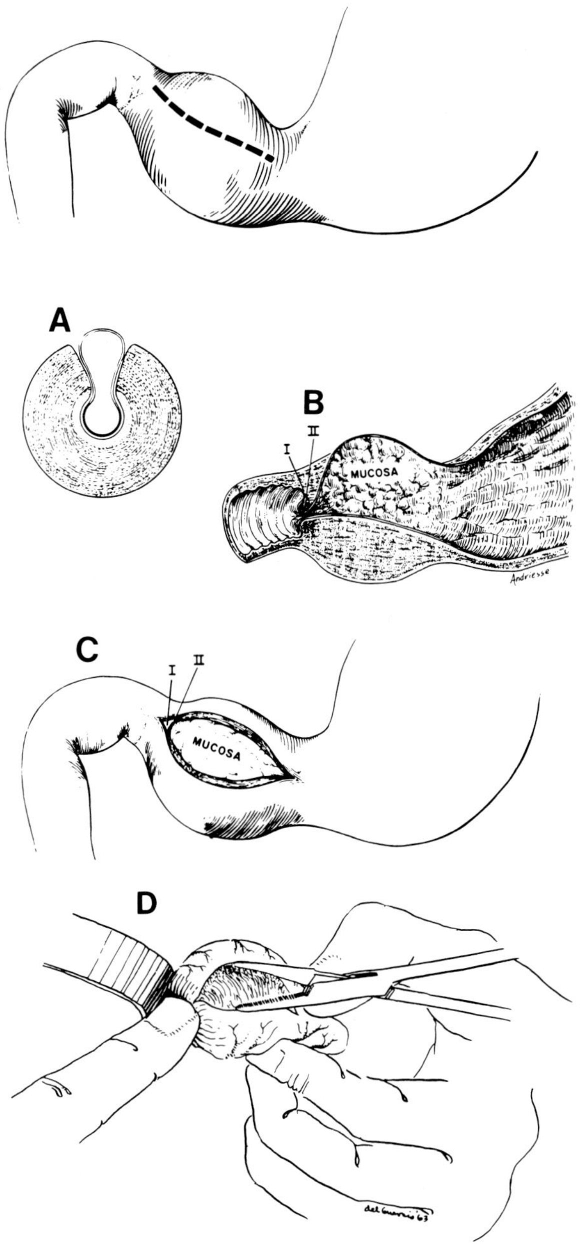

FIG. 35-3. Pyloromyotomy. (*A*) The mucusa bulging through the myotomy. (*B* and *C*) The pyloroduodenal junction—the point of usual injury. *I* indicates duodenal mucosa; *II*, gastric mucosa. (*D*) With the left index finger indenting the duodenal mucosa to reduce the likelihood of injury to the duodenal mucosa, a hemostat is used to spread the circular muscle fibers of the pylorus after incision of the serosa. (*A*, *B*, *C* from Sieber WK: The Stomach. In Holder TM, Ashcraft KW [eds]: Pediatric Surgery, p 320. Philadelphia, WB Saunders, 1980. *D* from Koop CE: Pyloromyotomy for pyloric stenosis. In Cooper P [ed]: The Craft of Surgery, 2nd ed, vol. 3, p 1639. Copyright © 1971 by Little, Brown & Co, Boston)

PYLORIC STENOSIS

Hypertrophic pyloric stenosis is a disease of infants who experience recurrent projectile vomiting.[5] A common metabolic complication of the disease is metabolic hypochloremic hypokalemic alkalosis. Infants developing this triad require a period of hydration and electrolyte management before induction of anesthesia. This is essential because of a contracted intravascular volume, depletion of total body potassium, and decreased chloride levels. Infants with severe metabolic derangements may require nasogastric suction and intravenous hydration for several days before undergoing pyloromyotomy.

For pyloric stenosis the Ramstedt pyloromyotomy is used almost exclusively (Fig. 35-3).[49, 73, 84] The operative procedure is performed through a right upper quadrant transverse incision, which minimizes dehiscence in these nutritionally depleted infants. The hypertrophied muscle of the pylorus is incised and spread so that the pyloric mucosa is visualized, and all fibrous bands are gently separated. The incision of the pylorus is extended onto the stomach for a centimeter to guarantee that the incision of the pyloric muscle is complete. The incision on the pylorus is carried up to the region of the pyloroduodenal junction (Fig. 35-3*B* and *C*), which is identified by invagination of the duodenum into the pylorus with the left index finger (Fig. 35-3*D*). This junction is also identified by a color change from the pale hypertrophied muscle to the pink of the thin duodenal wall. All bands of muscle are gently separated without tearing the mucosa. Completeness of the pyloromyotomy is evaluated by demonstrating mobility of the separated muscle in the longitudinal plane.

Inadvertent duodenal penetration, a common technical error, must be recognized during the operative procedure. Milking of gastric or duodenal content into the region of the pylorus will demonstrate a bilious effluent through any tear. This complication is managed in one of several ways (Fig. 35-4). A 5-0 nonabsorbable silk suture can be utilized to close the mucosa transversely with omentum applied as a buttress at the site of the perforation. Thereafter the patient is maintained on nasogastric suction for 48 hours before beginning oral alimentation.

Another method of repairing inadvertent mucosal penetration is to utilize a Gambee stitch, which begins on the pyloric side, passes horizontally through the duodenum, and is brought back through the pyloric mucosa. This pulls the duodenal mucosa up into the region of the pylorus. If omentum is available, it is placed over this region for reinforcement. The third method of repair involves closing the pyloromyotomy with interrupted 5-0 silk sutures and rotating the pylorus 90°. The pyloromyotomy is recreated with an incision parallel to the first. Nasogastric suction for a 48-hour period is sufficient.

During the operative procedure, bleeding from the edges of the pyloromyotomy site usually reflects venous obstruction caused by the muscles of the abdominal wall through which the pylorus is pulled. This bleeding does not require ligature or cautery, since it ceases when the pylorus is returned to the abdomen. The surgeon can check hemostasis by visualizing the pylorus or by inserting a dry sponge into the abdominal cavity just before closure of the abdomen.

Wound infection is another complication in patients undergoing pyloromyotomy. The infection is usually caused by *Staphylococcus aureus* and is probably a result of trauma to the local tissues of the wound in the infant with impaired host defense as a consequence of malnutrition.

Vomiting postoperatively is also common, for which the parents should be prepared, since the infant may vomit several times in the immediate postoperative period. If vomiting persists beyond 3 to 4 days and is constant, one should suspect an incomplete pyloromyotomy or local edema. Upper gastrointestinal series at this time is not useful, since an abnormal configuration is seen in postoperative pyloromyotomy patients in spite of an adequate procedure. These patients are treated with intravenous support and nothing by mouth for up to 2 weeks. Gastric saline lavage is occasionally helpful. In most cases the patient will begin to pass material through the pylorus without requiring reoperation. After 2 weeks of conservative therapy, one should evaluate the pylorus with a barium swallow. If gastric outlet obstruction persists, reoperation is required.

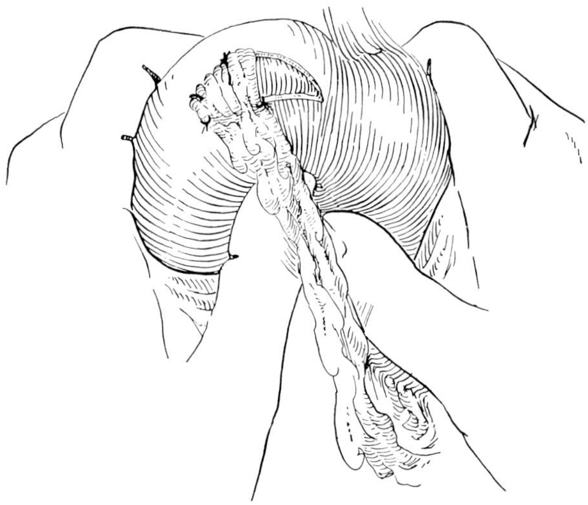

FIG. 35-4. Repair of duodenal perforation following pyloromyotomy. A nonabsorbable suture of 5-0 silk approximates the mucosa. Available omentum is sutured over the injury. Nasogastric decompression is applied for 24 to 48 hours. (Reproduced with permission from Welch CE: Surgery of the Stomach and Duodenum [A Handbook of Operative Surgery], 5th ed. Copyright © 1973 by Year Book Medical Publishers, Inc, Chicago)

NISSEN FUNDOPLICATION

Gastroesophageal reflux in the child less than a year of age is common. Complications of the gastroesophageal reflux are treated by performing surgical procedures to establish competence at the gastroesophageal junction. The most commonly performed procedure for the correction of gastroesophageal reflux is the Nissen fundoplication (Fig. 35-5).[74] The ease of construction and low morbidity in the very young patient is appealing; nonetheless, complications occur.

After mobilizing the left lobe of the liver, an incision is made in the peritoneum that invests the upper stomach and lower portion of the intra-abdominal esophagus. The esophagus is circumferentially isolated with care not to enter the posterior wall of the esophagus or damage the vagus nerves inadvertently. Mobilization of the stomach begins with division of the gastrocolic omentum and the

FIG. 35-5. Nissen fundoplication. (*A*) The first suture is placed to draw the fundus around the gastroesophageal junction. The suture is passed through esophageal muscle. (*B*) Completed fundoplication. (Reproduced with permission from Randolph JG: Hiatal hernia and gastroesophageal reflux. In Ravitch MM et al [eds]: Pediatric Surgery, 3rd ed, vol 1. Copyright © 1979 by Year Book Medical Publishers, Inc, Chicago)

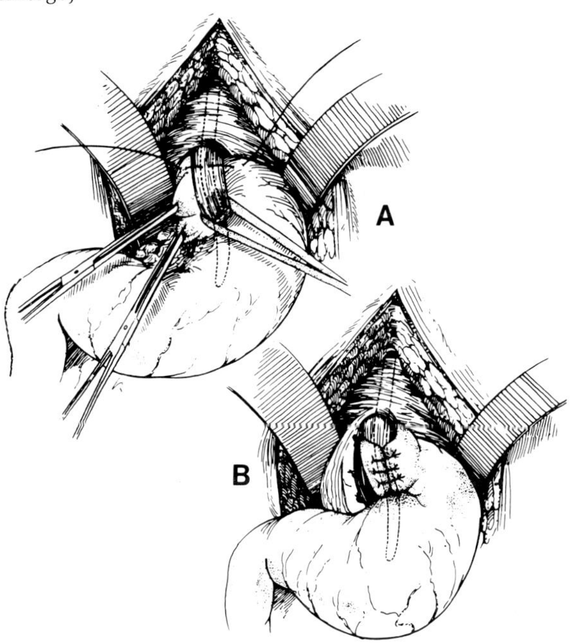

short gastric vessels, thus avoiding trauma to the spleen. Careless ligation of the short gastric vessels to include a portion of the gastric wall can lead to necrosis. The left gastric artery is ligated, since it limits the ability to wrap the fundus of the stomach 360° around the esophagus loosely, without tension. Tension at the wrap may lead to a failed fundoplication. The recurrence of gastroesophageal reflux from breakdown of the fundic wrap occurs in 13% of the patients.[74]

FIG. 35-6. The reversed gastric tube. The blood supply is from the left gastroepiploic artery. (Anderson KD, Randolph JG: The gastric tube for esophageal replacement in children. J Thorac Cardiovasc Surg 66:333, 1973)

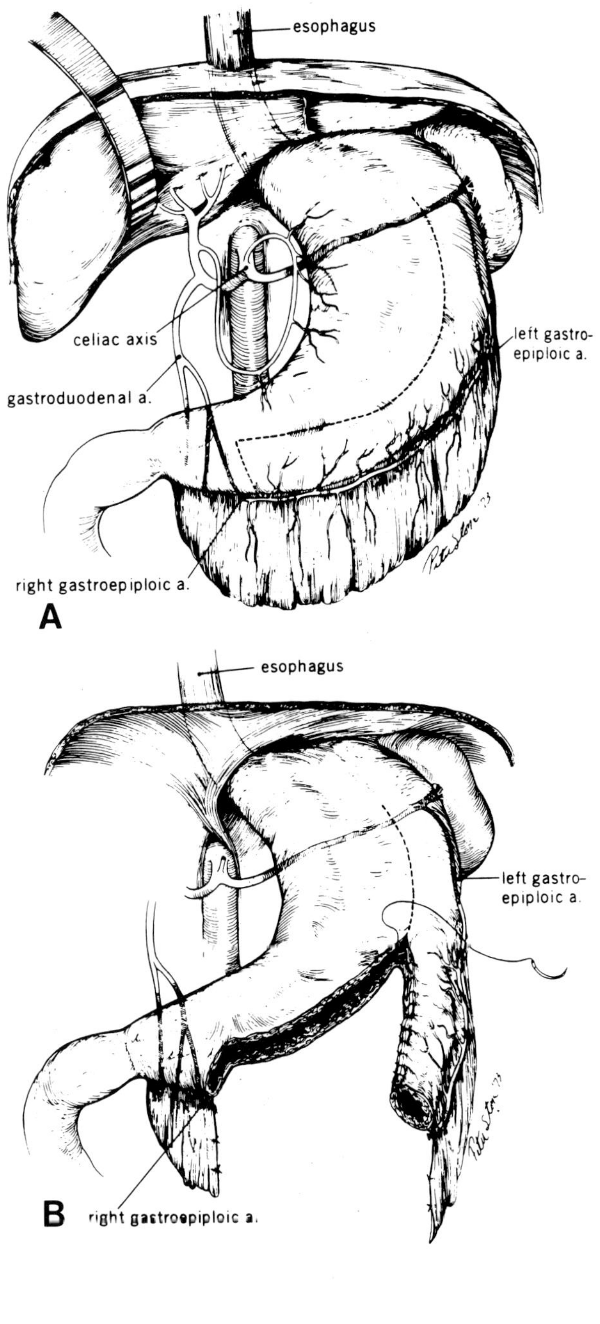

Once the stomach is mobilized, the nasogastric tube is removed and a well-lubricated Maloney dilator is inserted into the esophagus. The largest dilator than can easily pass into the infant's esophagus is used as the stent around which the fundoplication is constructed. Usually the neonate and small infant require between a 28-Fr and 32-Fr dilator. Before accomplishing the fundic wrap, the hiatus of the diaphragm is tightened around the dilator with a 2-0 silk suture. The fundus of the stomach is wrapped 360° loosely around the dilator (see Fig. 35-5). It is important to place the lowest suture at the apparent gastroesohageal junction. The three-point suture that holds the wrap in place should be in the seromuscular layer on the stomach and pass just through the muscular layer of the esophagus, thus preventing the wrap from slipping distally and producing an "hourglass" gastric obstruction.

Infants less than a year of age have a propensity to swallow air. A loosely wrapped fundoplication usually allows the infant to burp while preventing gastroesophageal reflux. The "gas-bloat syndrome" is observed when the fundoplication is too tight. A gastrostomy left in place for 6 to 8 weeks allows decompression of air. If the wrap is too tight, it is managed by antegrade dilatation with Maloney dilators. The fundic wrap that is too loose results in persistent gastroesophageal reflux.

The patient with an unrecognized laceration of the posterior esophagus sutained during isolation of the esophagus usually becomes febrile with tachycardia in the immediate postoperative period. A chest x-ray examination demonstrates air in the mediastinum, and dilute Gastrografin swallow demonstrates the perforation. This requires laparotomy and reconstruction of the esophagus using a Thal technique combined with a Nissen fundoplication.

Long-term complications of fundoplication may include the inability to vomit and occasionally diarrhea as a consequence of trauma to the vagus nerves. (Children who undergo the Nissen fundoplication must not receive ipecac to induce vomiting.) Another complication, attributed to injury to the nerves of Laterje, is pyloric dysfunction with gastric outlet obstruction. Pyloroplasty may be required to treat this condition.

GASTRIC TUBE

Esophageal replacement by gastric tube interposition is reliable but associated with predictable complications (Fig. 35-6).[3, 10, 24] To avoid these complications, certain technical considerations are imperative.[2] After ligating and transecting the right gastroepiploic artery, an "oblique" incision in the anterior and posterior gastric walls 2 cm proximal to the pylorus is created. This guarantees that there will be an adequate blood supply to the antimesenteric side of the distal tube, which reduces the potential for leak at the cervical anastomosis. It is important that the incision be far enough proximal to the pylorus to avoid gastric outlet obstruction.

Another consideration is the junction of the right and left gastroepiploic arteries, which occasionally lies within the gastric wall. While establishing the gastric tube along the greater curvature of the stomach, the midportion is made slightly wider to avoid damage to the gastroepiploic arcade. The short gastric arteries can usually be spared, allowing preservation of the spleen. Finally, retrohilar placement of the gastric tube is preferred, since this allows a straighter route between the pharynx and stomach.

Complications of the gastric tube are a result of technical errors. Salivary leaks at the cervical anastomosis occur in one half of patients. This leak rate is a consequence of the confluence of three anastomotic lines, compromise of the distal gastric mucosa from an insufficient gastroepiploic artery, or an inadequate oblique incision in the distal gastric wall. The cervical esophageal anastomosis is staged if the blood supply to the distal portion of the gastric tube is in doubt. Salivary leak at the cervical anastomosis is managed conservatively with enteric nutrition by a gastrostomy tube. Surgical closure of a persistent leak of the proximal anastomosis is rarely necessary but is effective. Ischemia of the proximal anastomosis also may lead to stricture, which is adequately managed by antegrade dilatation. The gastric tube may perforate during dilatations of the anastomosis and, depending on their location, may require cervical drainage or thoracotomy. Ulceration of the muscosa of the gastric tube with gastrointestinal bleeding occurs infrequently and is usually responsive to antacids. Unfortunately, reflux into the gastric tube may also occur. One solution to gastroesophageal reflux is to leave 3 cm to 4 cm of gastric tube intra-abdominally.

Complications of Duodenum Surgery

DUODENAL OBSTRUCTION

Duodenal obstruction in the newborn period is a consequence of atresia, stenosis, annular pancreas, intrinsic web, or malrotation of the midgut.[25] Complications of duodenal surgery in the newborn are delayed emptying of the anastomosis, obstruction of the efferent loop, obstruction of the extrahepatic biliary tree, and small bowel herniation through the colonic mesentery.

For operations on the second portion of the duodenum, the right colon is mobilized from its peritoneal attachments and reflected medially. Identification of the type of duodenal obstruction determines which anastomosis is best suited for the local anatomy. The patient with an "in-continuity" atresia can be treated by duodenoduodenostomy. The patient with a large-gap atresia or an annular pancreas requires duodenojejunostomy to establish intestinal continuity. Malrotation of the intestine requires the Ladd procedure.

The most common surgical procedure performed is the retrocolic duodenojejunostomy. In this procedure, the duodenum is mobilized from the retroperitoneal attachments, avoiding trauma to the pancreas. It is important to mobilize the dependent portion of the duodenum through the mesentery of the colon. A rubber catheter is placed through the pylorus to assist localization of the dependent aspect of the duodenum. The duodenum is secured to the mesenteric leaf to prevent postoperative mesenteric herniation of the small bowel. After identifying the ligament of Treitz, a proximal segment of jejunum is selected for an isoperistaltic anastomosis. The loop of the proximal jejunum should easily sweep to the duodenal bulb. Proper establishment of the duodenojejunostomy is exceedingly important, since function is associated with appropriate dependent placement of the efferent loop.[6] The duodenojejunostomy is constructed end-to-side with a length of 1½ cm to 2 cm. The efferent loop of jejunum is placed along the mesentery of the right colon so that there is a gradual exit from the region of the anastomosis. A kink of the efferent jejunum or malposition of the anastomosis will delay or prevent emptying of the duodenal content. A "bypass phenomenon" can occur with the intestinal content proceeding to the most dependent portion of the duodenum, passing by the malpositioned anastomosis with reflux into the upper intestinal tract. Obstruction of the efferent loop also occurs if the mesentery of the transverse colon is not secured to the duodenum; in such instances, the jejunum slips into the retrocolic position with a "pantaloon" obstruction of the two limbs of the anastomosis. Appropriate identification of the ligament of Treitz is essential to avoid inadvertent construction of a duodenoileostomy.

Duodenoduodenostomy is a procedure employed for "in-continuity" atresia or intrinsic web (Fig. 35-7). Delayed emptying can occur with angulation of the anastomosis or excessive "turning-in" of duodenal mucosa. The pancreas is in the region of the posterior wall of the anastomosis, which can lead to pancreatitis if sutures are placed inadvertently through its substance.

The patients with obstruction from a duodenal web may manifest the "Windsock" phenomenon

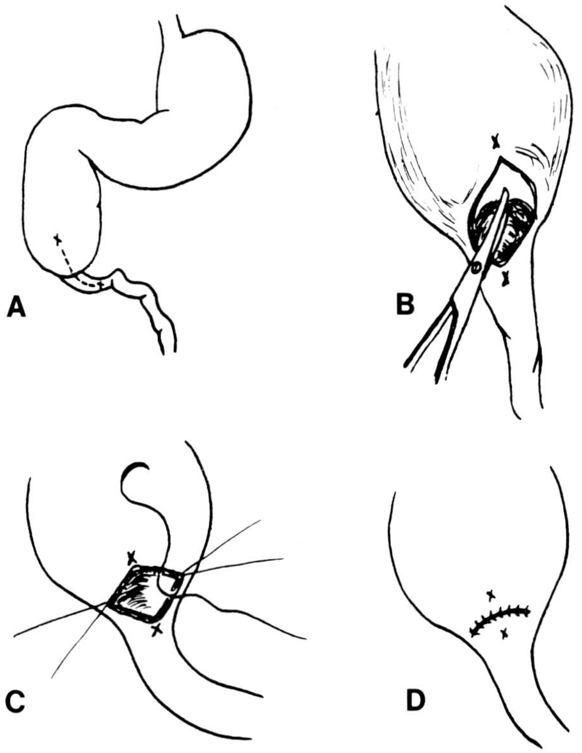

FIG. 35-7. Duodenoduodenostomy. (Bishop HC: Small bowel obstruction in the newborn. Surg Clin North Am 56:331, 1976)

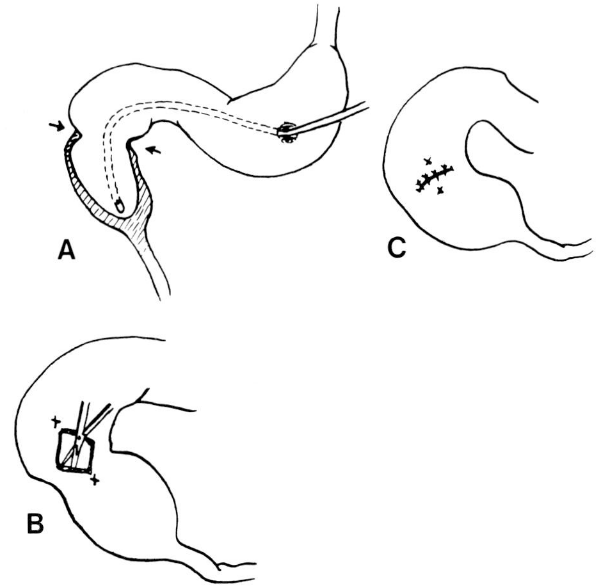

FIG. 35-8. "Windsock" deformity. (*A*) The catheter demonstrates the proximal attachment of the membrane. Traction sutures are applied at this point. (*B*) A longitudinal incision is made and the membrane resected. (*C*) The incision is closed transversely. (Bishop HC: Small bowel obstruction in the newborn. Surg Clin North Am 56:336, 1976)

(Fig. 35-8).[43, 82] The web is identified by placement of an 8 F rubber tube through a gastrotomy. Pressure from the tube against the distal duodenal web creates a dimpling of the duodenum at its proximal attachment. Traction sutures for a longitudinal incision are inserted at the point of dimpling. The web is excised carefully so as not to injure an aberrant common duct in the posterior wall of the web. Incision of the web should be on the anterior–lateral wall to minimize inadvertent trauma to such a duct. A lacrimal probe occasionally can be placed into the common duct and an excision undertaken with the probe in place. A running chromic suture (5-0) provides hemostasis at the site of the excised mucosal web. Postoperative hyperbilirubinemia may occur in patients with duodenal atresia, and concern for extrabiliary obstruction is minimized by compressing the gallbladder while observing the duodenal mucosa for bile during surgery.

Patients with duodenal obstruction require a gastrostomy. Infants with congenital duodenal atresia have such a dilated duodenum that the function of the anastomosis may be delayed for up to 3 weeks. During this period of delayed function, the patient requires total parenteral nutrition to maintain adequate caloric intake. An upper gastrointestinal tract barium contrast study is appropriate after 3 weeks to document malposition, stricture, or anatomy of the anastomosis before surgical revision.

Complications of Small Bowel Surgery

JEJUNOILEO ATRESIA

Patients with jejunoileo atresia develop postoperative complications from excessive small bowel resection, dysfunction of the anastomosis, concomitant atresia, or malabsorption.[37, 56]

Massive dilatation of the proximal small intestine at the point of obstruction is common. The bulbous end of the dilated small bowel is incapable of normal peristalsis and must be resected to avoid anastomotic dysfunction.[29] Resection of the bulbous tip permits anastomosis of the bowel ends of more equal diameter. The distal collapsed small bowel is opened along the antimesenteric border, creating an oblique "fish-mouth" incision that is fashioned into an "end-to-back" anastomosis (Fig. 35-9).[55, 68] Interrupted 5-0 silk, full-thickness sutures with purchase on the seromuscular portion of the bowel wall and the edge of the mucosa are best for creation of the anastomosis. If properly placed, a simple, full-thickness suture offers a safe closure and avoids

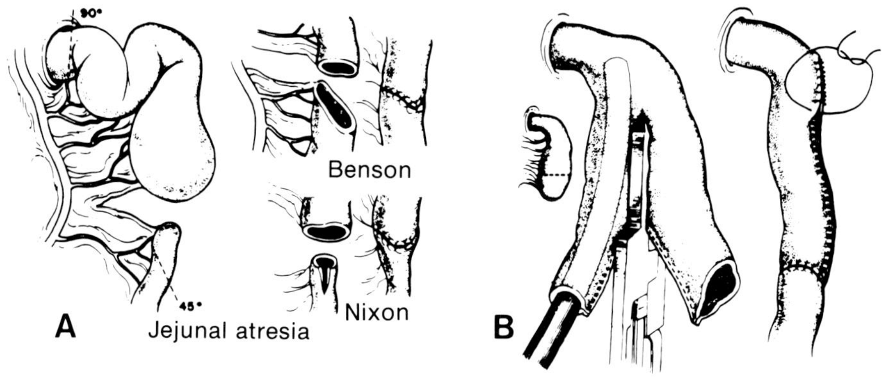

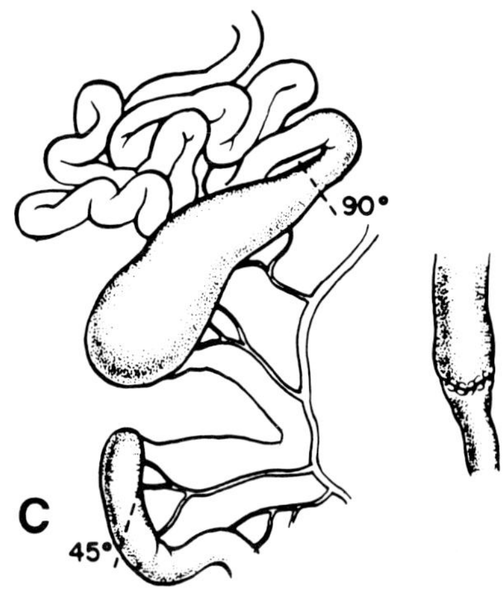

FIG. 35-9. (*A*) Method of anastomosis in high jejunal atresia. The ligament of Treitz limits wide proximal resection:end-to-back anastomosis. The Benson technique of preparing the distal lumen is preferred. (*B*) Modified Thomas taper. An enteroplasty using a 22- or 24-Fr catheter stent and staples is used for high jejunal atresia. (*C*) For ilealatresia, a similar procedure is performed end to back, assuring mucosa-to-mucosa mesenteric approximation. The anastomosis is accomplished with 5-0 silk on an atraumatic curved swedge needle. Impregnation of the suture with mineral oil decreases friction. A 5-0 chromic suture on an atraumatic curved swedge needle is used for the inner layer connel stitch. (Grosfeld JL, Ballantine TVN, Shoemaker R: Operative management of intestinal atresia and stenosis based on pathologic findings. J Pediatr Surg 14:368–375, 1979, by permission)

turning excess mucosa into the lumen of the small distal bowel. It is necessary to instill saline into the distal small bowel to identify other areas of atresia.

High proximal jejunal atresia creates technical difficulty in anastomosis, since resection of the dilated segment is not feasible. Either a Bishop–Koop Roux-en-Y anastomosis (Fig. 35-10) or tapering (see Fig. 35-9*B*) of the proximal jejunum is recommended.[7, 97] Proximal jejunostomy and mucous fistula are not optimal but can be managed with adjunctive TPN if necessary.

Another anomaly encountered during operation for jejunoileo atresia is the "Christmas-tree," or "apple-peel" mesenteric deformity. The ileocelic artery supplies blood to the entire small bowel. A carefully placed anastomosis is essential to avoid ischemia resulting from a twist of the mesentery.

Delayed function of a jejunal or ileal anastomosis in an infant can occur as a result of adhesions, sharp angulation, or a leak. Consequently, TPN is essential for nutritional support of these debilitated infants. After 3 weeks of anastomotic dysfunction, a small amount of barium is instilled in the upper intestinal tract and followed through the intestine. Reoperation is indicated if there is no evidence of patency of the anastomosis. At laparotomy the anastomosis may appear normal and patent, which suggests that an inadequate amount of small bowel was resected. The anastomosis is resected with several centimeters of proximal and distal bowel.

Anastomotic leak is suggested when intra-abdominal air persists postoperatively for longer than 24 hours. If the leak is localized and drains externally as an enterocutaneous fistula, then nutritional support with TPN is instituted to avoid reoperation with further small bowel resection. However, the patient who is clinically septic and unstable requires exteriorization of the anastomosis as a stoma and mucous fistula.

For congenital intestinal atresia, appropriate resection of dilated proximal small bowel is important. However, when extended resection is necessary, malabsorption and malnutrition can result in the short gut syndrome. Wilmore has shown that 15 cm of small bowel with an intact ileocecal valve is adequate for oral enteric support of a newborn infant.[103] A baby with no ileocecal valve must have at least 40 cm to survive. Vitamin deficiency is com-

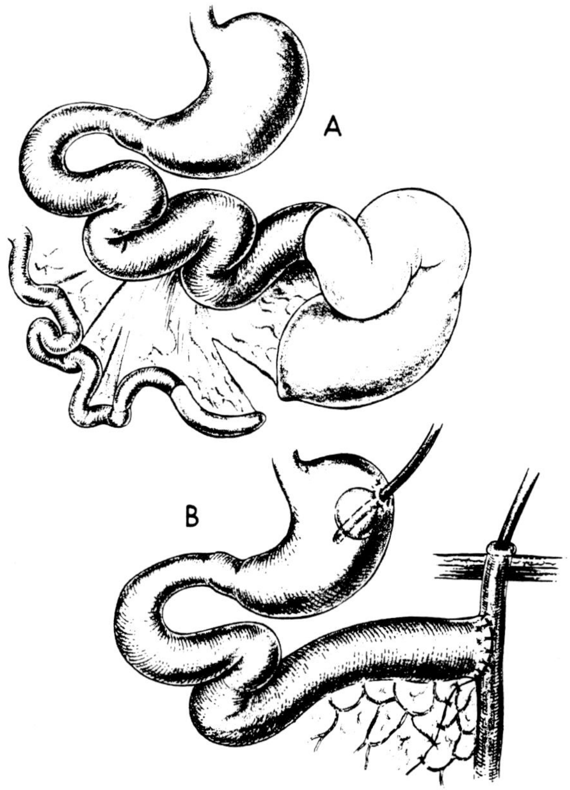

FIG. 35-10. Alternate method of anastomosis in proximal jejunal atresia. (*A*) Lines of resection. (*B*) Bishop-Koop Roux-en-Y anastomosis. The end of the proximal intestine and the side of the distal intestine undergo anastomosis. The distal intestine is exteriorized through the abdominal wall as a vent. 5-0 silk impregnated with mineral oil and 5-0 chromic are used for the anastomosis. The intralumened tube is used if one is treating meconium ileus or for refeeding. A gastrostomy should be used because of the potential for delayed emptying. (Becker JM et al: Jejunal and ileal atresia in the newborn. In Cooper P [ed]: The Craft of Surgery, 2nd ed, vol 3, p 1649. Copyright © 1971 by Little, Brown & Co, Boston)

mon in the infant with a short bowel. The patient can develop vitamin D deficiency, rickets, folic acid deficiency, vitamin B_{12} deficiency, and prolonged bleeding time from abnormal vitamin K absorption.

MALROTATION

Malrotation of the intestinal tract during the 6th to 10th week of gestation leads to abnormal retroperitoneal fixation of the intestine.[93] Fibrous bands from the cecum to the retroperitoneum (Ladd's bands) or malposition of the ligament of Trietz leads to duodenal obstruction. The free swinging mesentery permits volvulus of the midgut, which leads to infarction. The Ladd procedure was designed to widen the base of the mesentery, thereby eliminating the possibility of volvulus, and to sever the obstructing duodenal bands.[51] The duodenum is mobilized from the abnormal retroperitoneal attachment so that it lies along the right gutter in a straightened fashion. Injury to the pancreas must be avoided during this dissection to prevent postoperative pancreatitis. The cecum is mobilized so that it can easily be placed in the left lower quadrant without fixation. Inversion appendectomy is part of the operative procedure to avoid the future potential of a left-sided appendicitis.

The patient with volvulus and ischemia undergoes untwisting of the small bowel to allow improvement of the blood flow to the midgut. The ischemic intestine must be given every opportunity to recover after the volvulus is reduced. Initial judgments of viability are extremely unreliable; therefore, ischemic bowel is packed in warm moist gauze for at least 30 minutes and resection avoided at the initial surgery unless portions of the bowel are perforated or necrotic.

In far advanced ischemia, reduction of the volvulus and gastrostomy only should be performed. Reexploration 36 to 48 hours later permits identification of obvious areas of infarction. Conservative practice limits resection to bowel judged absolutely unrecoverable (e.g., perforated or necrotic). Anastomosis should not be attempted in this ischemic bowel; rather, the ends of the resected bowel are exteriorized and the patient resuscitated. If these principles are ignored, the patient will develop a leak at the intestinal anastomosis since the surgery is performed in compromised, ischemic bowel. Several laparotomies may be necessary to allow maximum recovery of the small intestine and permit the most conservative resection.

The short-gut syndrome is a long-term complication that ensues from excessive resection of small intestine.[103] Occasionally patients with malrotation and volvulus develop malabsorption as a consequence of ischemic injury to the mucosa. This is treated by TPN for 2 to 3 weeks or utilization of predigested formulas with a casein base (e.g., Pregestimil).

Patients who undergo the Ladd procedure for malrotation risk developing postoperative adhesions that may cause chronic abdominal pain, constipation, or partial bowel obstruction. Many of these patients can be treated by nasogastric decompression or, for older children, long-tube decompression in conjunction with TPN. Complete or recurrent bowel obstruction requires laparotomy for lysis of adhesions. Recurrent volvulus following the Ladd procedure is uncommon but possible.

MECONIUM ILEUS

Meconium ileus is an obturator obstruction of the lumen of the small intestine in the newborn that is caused by persistence of tenacious meconium in the distal ileum.[70] Noblett showed the efficacy of a nonoperative method using Gastrografin (diatrizoate meglumine) enema to relieve the obstruction in approximately 80% of patients.[69] Complications from this technique are minimized by employing the following steps:[70]

1. Perform diagnostic barium enema to rule out anatomical colonic obstruction
2. Exclude volvulus, atresia, perforation, or peritonitis by clinical and radiologic assessment
3. Provide adequate intravenous fluid and electrolyte replacement in the form of 20 ml/kg, IV, over a 20-minute period with half normal saline or Ringer's lactate solution
4. Administer prophylactic antibiotics (ampicillin, 150–400 mg/kg/day in four doses and gentamicin, 5–7 mg/kg/day in two doses)
5. Perform enema with fluoroscopic control
6. Obtain surgical consultation before the hyperosmolar enema is administered
7. Dilution of the Gastrografin 4:1 to minimize fluid shifts caused by the hyperosmolarity (1900 mOsm) of Gastrografin, which can lead to hypovolemic shock in the neonate
8. Undertake nasogastric decompression
9. Guarantee temperature control of the neonate

Perforation of the bowel during the enema requires prompt laparotomy, resection of the dilated proximal bowel and exteriorization of the proximal ileum, and creation of a mucous fistula.

Operative intervention is required if nonoperative management of meconium ileus is unsuccessful.[71] The large dilated ileum (6–8 cm) is resected, and no attempt is made to extract the meconium mechanically from the bowel lumen, since excessive trauma to the mucosa with denudation and perforation may be a complication. The Bishop–Koop Roux-en-Y anastomosis is performed by bringing the distal small bowel to the abdominal wall as a chimney with anastomosis of the proximal ileum to the side of the distal small bowel (Fig. 35-11).[7, 85] The distal ileum must be irrigated clear with N-acetylcysteine (Mucomyst) or Gastrografin before creating the end-to-side anastomosis. An 8-Fr rubber catheter is placed through the chimney in the abdominal wall into the distal ileum past the anastomosis. The distal ileum is irrigated with a solution that dissolves the tenacious meconium, such as N-acetylcysteine (Mucomyst), dilute Gastrografin (4:1), or Viokase.[7]

A complication of the Bishop–Koop Roux-en-Y anastomosis is anastomotic leak on the antimesenteric aspect of the proximal small bowel. A second complication is persistence of the chimney stoma after adequate distal decompression of the bowel occurs. This requires formal closure of the stoma, which is a limited procedure.

A second operative approach to meconium ileus is the construction of the double-barreled Mikulicz enterostomy, popularized by Ladd and Gross.[32] The double-barrel anastomosis offers a simple method of exteriorization of the bowel and extraperitoneal closure. The Mikulicz enterostomy may be complicated with misplacement of the crushing clamp, which can lead to perforation and peritonitis. Finally, an ileostomy and distal mucous fistula are an adequate treatment for the patient with meconium ileus since the nutritional status of these youngsters can be maintained for prolonged periods with TPN; however, this approach requires a second formal laparotomy in infants with known pulmonary compromise. Pulmonary infections are minimized by attention to pulmonary hygiene and vigorous prophylactic antibiotics. Parenteral nutritional support of these youngsters is usually protracted, then enteric feedings are begun with a predigested formula (Pregestimil). Pancreatic malfunction, another result of mucoviscidosis, requires replacement of pancreatic enzymes in the form of Viokase or Cotazym.

Chronic or recurrent complications occur throughout the lifetime of any child with meconium ileus. The early complications are seen in the form of obstruction due to persistent inspissated meconium or postoperative adhesions, breakdown of the anastomosis, or pulmonary complications. Later complications are malabsorption, pulmonary pathology peculiar to cystic fibrosis, constipation, cirrhosis with hepatic failure, or esophageal varices. Meconium ileus equivalent is an obstruction in older patients with cystic fibrosis due to abnormal composition of the intestinal contents associated with the discontinuation of pancreatic enzymes or dehydration.[13]

MECKEL'S DIVERTICULUM

Meckel's diverticulum is a structure representing a remnant of the omphalomesenteric duct.[90] Complications of Meckel's diverticulum are obstruction, inflammation, perforation, or hemorrhage.[61] If a Meckel's diverticulum is encountered during laparotomy for other intra-abdominal pathology, a closed technique of diverticulectomy should be carried out. It is important that the clamp be placed in an oblique fashion to avoid compromise of the lumen. Lumen of the bowel may be obstructed postoperatively if inversion of the bowel wall is excessive.

Patients undergoing resection of a Meckel's diverticulum for diverticulitis are at risk for developing an anastomotic leak if anastomosis is performed in inflamed bowel. Segmental resection of the ileum is performed in such patients with inflammation or perforation of the diverticulum. In exceptional circumstances, when the integrity of the bowel wall is

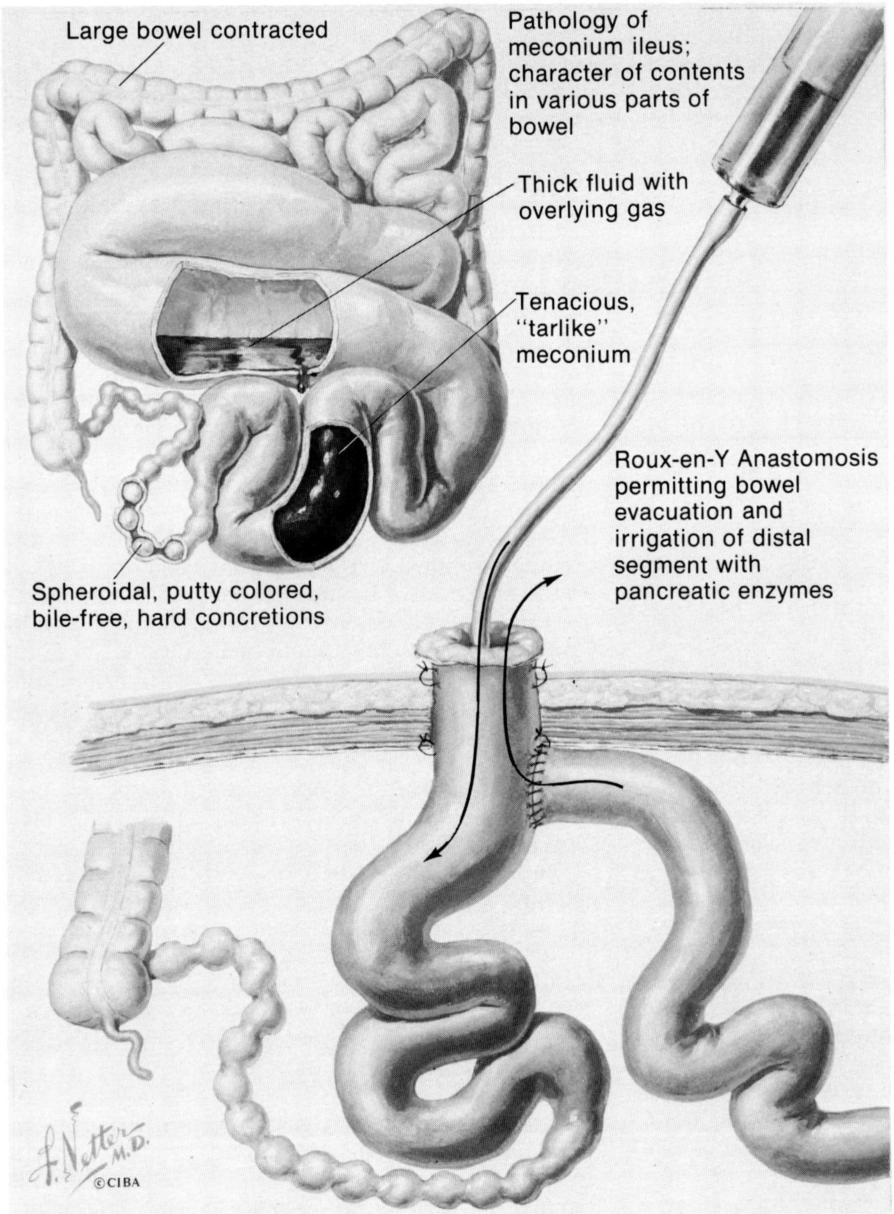

FIG. 35-11. Meconium ileus. Surgical pathology and Bishop–Koop Roux-en-Y anastomosis following resection of the massively dilated small bowel. (© copyright 1962, 1979, CIBA Pharmaceutical Company, Division of CIBA–GEIGY Corporation. Reprinted with permission from The CIBA Collection of Medical Illustrations, illustrated by Frank H. Netter, M.D. All rights reserved)

in doubt, then ileostomy and mucous fistula are the safest alternative. This avoids postoperative peritonitis from leak at the anastomosis.

Bleeding Meckel's diverticulum is treated by a wedge resection of the ileum or a segmental resection of the small bowel. A wedge resection of the ileum is performed if the base of the Meckel's diverticulum is narrow and resection will not compromise the integrity of the lumen of the small bowel. The bowel is opened so that the ulcer that is usually found at the junction between the ileum and the diverticulum can be identified and resected. If the base of the Meckel's diverticulum is broad or the bleeding site not obvious, a segmental resection with anastomosis is required. Postoperative bleeding may occur if the ulcer is not excised or oversewn. Since the ectopic gastric mucosa is resected in the diverticulum, the bleeding will cease as the ulcer heals. In the patient who has persistent bleeding postoperatively, an air contrast enema should be accomplished to investigate the potential of a concomitant juvenile polyp.

INTUSSUSCEPTION

Intussusception of the intestine occurs in children between the ages of 6 and 24 months and is usually ileocolic in position.[59, 75] The diagnosis is often unsuspected and confused with other entities. Frequently the infant is evaluated for sepsis or meningitis since the patient presents with obtundation, lethargy, and nonspecific complaints. A high index of suspicion for intussusception in this age group should lead to a correct diagnosis. Uncommonly, the youngster is severely dehydrated as a consequence of intestinal obstruction and ischemia. Before diagnostic evaluation begins, nasogastric decompression and intravenous fluid hydration with Ringer's lactate solution (20 ml/kg, IV, bolus) are essential. Intravenous antibiotics (ampicillin and gentamicin) are administered because of the risk of perforation with ischemic bowel. If the patient is critically ill with peritonitis, radiologic evaluation or attempts at hydrostatic reduction are contraindicated, and the patient should be taken promptly to the operating suite.

Diagnostic barium enema is performed when evidence of peritonitis is absent. Hydrostatic barium enema reduction of the intussusception under fluoroscopic control is successful in one half to two thirds of the patients.[63] Perforation can occur at the site of intussusception in the region of the ischemic bowel if excessive hydrostatic pressure is applied. Elevation of the barium column above the patient is limited to 1 m. This hydrostatic force is usually adequate to move the intussusceptum retrograde toward the ileocecal valve to accomplish reduction. Perforation of the colon during the barium enema requires immediate operative intervention; therefore, the operating room is prepared before beginning nonoperative reduction. Retrograde flow of barium into the distal ileum must always be demonstrated to be certain that the "ileo-ileo" component of the intussusception is reduced.

If the diagnosis is established but hydrostatic barium reduction is unsuccessful, surgical reduction is necessary. The intussusception is usually noted in the region of the transverse colon and can be manipulated into an incision in the right lower quadrant. The technique for reduction of the intussusception should minimize trauma to the compromised bowel. The intussusception is never pulled apart; rather, gentle, retrograde pressure is applied (Fig. 35-12).[75] Mineral oil placed in the interface between the two bowel walls helps decrease friction and improves the potential for reduction. If the bowel is pulled apart, the likelihood for trauma to the seromuscular layer with perforation is significant. Appendectomy is performed if the cecum is healthy in appearance or if the appendix has become ischemic as a result of the intussusception. The intussusception that cannot be manually reduced is resected and an end-to-end anastomosis performed while recognizing that the mesentery of the small bowel is involved in the process. The mesentery is divided close to the bowel, thus preventing compromise of the remaining major vessels of the small bowel mesentery. Surgical judgment is essential for determining whether primary anastomosis should be performed. If the bowel is compromised, then ileostomy and mucous fistula are the safest treatment.

Recurrent intussusception may occur if a lead point is present. The immediate postoperative recurrence of the intussusception is unusual, although the incidence of long-term recurrence is 4% to 6%.[21] If the intussusception recurs in the immediate postoperative period, a barium enema is obtained to delineate the lesion and to apply hydrostatic pressure. An ileo-ileo intussusception is most common in the immediate postoperative phase. Should hydrostatic reduction be unsuccessful, then laparotomy and resection of the lesion are indicated.

A common postoperative complication is oliguria from inadequate fluid resuscitation. The third-space losses are unusually great in these patients. Scrutiny of the urine output, urine specific gravity, and BUN levels guides the fluid management of the patient. In such circumstances, a bolus infusion of crystalloid solution at 20 ml/kg helps establish the appropriate level of hydration.

FIG. 35-12. Manual reduction of intussusception. (Reproduced with permission from Ravitch MM: Intussusception. In Ravitch MM et al [eds]: Pediatric Surgery, 3rd ed, vol 2, p 994. Copyright © 1979 by Year Book Medical Publishers, Inc, Chicago)

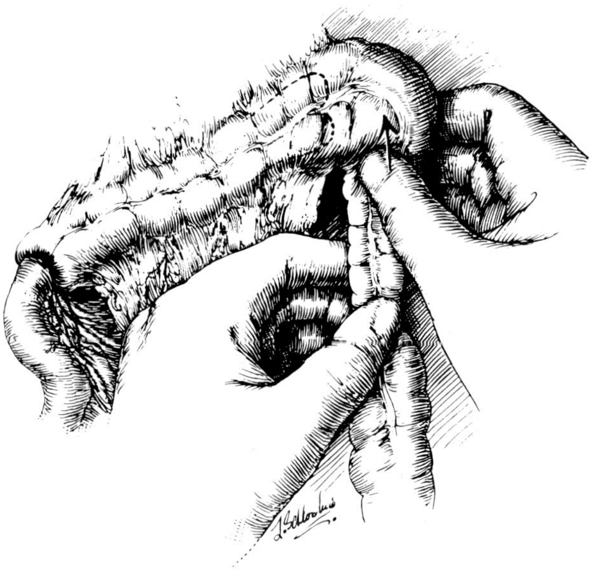

NECROTIZING ENTEROCOLITIS

Mechanical ventilators, improved nutritional support, antibiotics, monitoring devices, and skilled neonatologists have created an environment that saves or prolongs the lives of many premature infants. Necrotizing enterocolitis has appeared as an entity affecting stressed premature neonates.[42] The pathophysiology of necrotizing enterocolitis is poorly understood; however, hypoperfusion of the mesenteric blood supply is a necessary component.[35] Stress of the premature neonate leads to ischemia of the intestinal mucosa with bacterial invasion. The ischemia and bacteria combine to produce a transmural process resulting in perforation and peritonitis. Recognition that the intestinal tract sustains an ischemic insult is imperative if operative management is to minimize subsequent complications.

The patient who develops peritonitis, refractory metabolic acidosis, pneumoperitoneum, thrombocytopenia, or abdominal wall erythema should undergo laparotomy.[98] The most common areas affected by the disease process are the ileocecal region, sigmoid colon, and small bowel. Resection is limited to irretrievably infarcted bowel. Primary anastomosis in the face of ischemic disease risks anastomotic leak; therefore, enterostomy and mucous fistula are the procedures of choice.

If the ischemia involves a major portion of the intestinal tract without definite areas of necrosis, then resection is deferred. As in the surgical technique for volvulus, the intestine is returned to the abdominal cavity without resection and the infant treated vigorously for 36 to 48 hours after which a second operation is performed. Bowel that appeared irreversible at the first operation many times is viable, and a more limited resection of bowel can be undertaken.

Infants developing necrotizing enterocolitis are usually premature with a predilection for malnutrition, leading inevitably to poor healing and wound dehiscence. Dehiscence of the wound is minimized if a transverse incision is employed and the layers closed separately. If the abdominal closure is difficult because of distention of the intestines or fusion of the muscle layers, then retention sutures should be used. TPN is essential to the survival of these infants.

Use of drains in the abdominal cavity is unusual since resection of the affected bowel and diversion, complemented by broad-spectrum antibiotics, will usually control the infected region.[22] Occasionally, a patient who has undergone resection continues to deteriorate with signs of peritonitis. Reexploration of these infants may demonstrate localized areas of infected fluid, which are drained.

Formation of the stoma is important, since the exteriorized bowel is often compromised. The stoma, which is usually the distal ileum, is brought out through the wound or a separate opening in the abdominal wall in such a fashion that the mesenteric blood supply is uncompromised. If the blood supply to the distal stoma is insufficient, the stoma becomes dusky and progresses to infarction with eventual stenosis of the stoma. The stoma should be secured with several superficial seromuscular sutures. If the sutures are placed through all layers of the intestine, a cutaneous fistula develops, making application of a stoma appliance difficult. Prolapse of the stoma or peristomal evisceration is unusual since the intestines are bound down by the intra-abdominal inflammatory process.

The late complications of necrotizing enterocolitis are malabsorption, short-gut syndrome, or intestinal stricture.[83] Patients sustaining ischemia to the intestinal mucosa develop malabsorption with intolerance to carbohydrates and inability to digest proteins. Predigested formulas such as Pregestimil are used for these infants. The short-bowel syndrome is a consequence of excessive resection of the intestine. These youngsters require protracted TPN and component diets to survive while the intestine adapts by hypertrophy of the villi. These infants are at risk to develop recurrent sepsis. Stricture occurs in the region of the ischemia and is commonly found in the left colon. Infants in whom operative treatment is not necessary may manifest these strictures as a large bowel obstruction. Barium enema is obtained only on infants who develop abdominal signs such as distention following treatment for necrotizing enterocolitis. The strictures are resected and a colostomy with mucous fistula created. The infant is allowed to gain weight and to achieve improved nutritional status before intestinal continuity is reestablished.

Complications of Colon Surgery

APPENDICITIS

One of the most common procedures performed in children is appendectomy. Acute appendicitis has a mortality rate of 0.1% in children over 2 years of age, is approximately 10% in infants, and may reach 80% in neonates.[9, 31] Although the mortality from appendicitis has been significantly reduced with early diagnosis and appendectomy, complications after surgery still occur.

The most common complication in the patient undergoing appendectomy is infection. Infection is noted in 10% to 30% of the patients with the wound being the most common site affected.[42] Infection in the wound is manifest as tenderness and erythema. Separation of the wound edge and drainage of the wound abscess (usually gram-negative organisms) are adequate treatment. In smaller infants or neonates, the patient should be treated with systemic antibiotics chosen according to wound cultures.

The child with gangrenous, perforated appendicitis is at high risk to develop an intraperitoneal abscess. The common location for abscess formation is the pelvis, right gutter and subhepatic and subphrenic spaces. During the operative procedure, drains can be placed in the pelvis and along the right gutter if these regions are soiled with purulent material. If drainage is not provided and abscess develops, the patient will develop a fever and a palpable mass on rectal examination. Galium scan, ultrasonography, or CT scan can aid in localizing the mass.[9, 104] Surgical drainage is not always necessary since intravenous antibiotics (clindamycin and gentamicin) are effective in treating the septic focus. If a well-localized intra-abdominal abscess persists, surgical drainage is required.

Paralytic ileus is encountered commonly in patients with peritoneal infections. For these patients, nasogastric decompression and nutritional support are required for varying periods of time. These children are candidates for TPN, which hastens the return of an anabolic state.

Obstruction of the intestinal tract can occur early in the postoperative course of ruptured appendicitis. If obstruction is partial, the patient is treated with nasogastric decompression; intravenous antibiotics are added if fever persists. Occasionally, reexploration is required to treat complete intestinal obstruction, but conservative treatment is warranted in the first 2 weeks after appendectomy if no signs of intestinal infarction are present.

An infrequent complication is the breakdown of the appendiceal stump with localized abscess or enterocutaneous fistula. A localized abscess should be drained after adequate antibiotic therapy and enterocutaneous fistula treated with TPN. If distal obstruction is absent, the enterocutaneous fistula will close spontaneously. Reoperation is required in the early postoperative period when an abscess is identified and the intestinal tract is completely obstructed. If the appendiceal stump is leaking and is the cause of the abscess, then a tube cecostomy is created to establish a controlled fistula. The tube is left in place until distal continuity of the intestinal tract is demonstrated. Removal of the tube is followed by spontaneous closure of the fistula, as seen in patients with gastrostomy.

Many surgeons believe that young girls with right lower quadrant pain and tenderness should undergo early appendectomy since perforated appendicitis and pelvic sepsis may place the young female at risk for compromise of the ovary and fallopian tube.

HIRSCHSPRUNG'S DISEASE

Hirschsprung's disease or congenital megacolon occurs as a consequence of the absence of parasympathetic innervation of the distal intestine. Absence of ganglion cells creates a segment of bowel that prevents the propulsion of the fecal stream. The aganglionic segment usually involves the rectum and rectosigmoid. Complications of the management of this disease begin during the initial diagnostic evaluation.

The definitive method for diagnosis of Hirschsprung's disease is rectal biopsy. The aganglionic segment begins at the anorectal junction and extends proximally; therefore, the biopsy is obtained 1 cm above the pectinate line. If suction biopsy of the superficial layers of the bowel demonstrates ganglion cells, then the disease is excluded. The patient in whom no ganglion cells are demonstrated should still be suspected of having Hirschsprung's disease, and a full-thickness rectal biopsy is then performed to establish the diagnosis. During the full-thickness rectal biopsy, the muscular layers of the posterior wall of the rectum are closed to prevent formation of a presacral abscess. If an abscess does occur low in the rectum, transrectal drainage is satisfactory and safe. Occasionally, punch biopsy may result in a full-thickness defect with contamination in the presacral space or pelvis. These patients require a proximal diverting colostomy and drainage of the presacral space through a dependent stab wound. Drainage is accomplished by excision of the coccyx and drainage with rubber drains from below. Intravenous broad-spectrum antibiotics (clindamycin and gentamicin) are begun immediately.

Once the diagnosis of Hirschsprung's disease is established, the patient undergoes a loop colostomy and transabdominal biopsy. The initial intraperitoneal biopsy is performed at the peritoneal reflection and encompasses the seromuscular layers without violation of the mucosa. Sequential biopsies are performed in the transition zone until ganglion cells are identified.

A complication of surgery in Hirschsprung's disease is colostomy dysfunction from placement in aganglionic bowel. Such an oversight resulting in physiologic obstruction can lead to acute enterocolitis with ulceration and ischemic necrosis of the mucosa of the proximal bowel.[96] Profuse diarrhea with abdominal distention, perforation, septicemia, and intra-abdominal abscess may develop in these children. In the acute stages of acute enterocolitis of Hirschsprung's disease, a tube passed through the stoma or rectum into the bowel with saline enemas

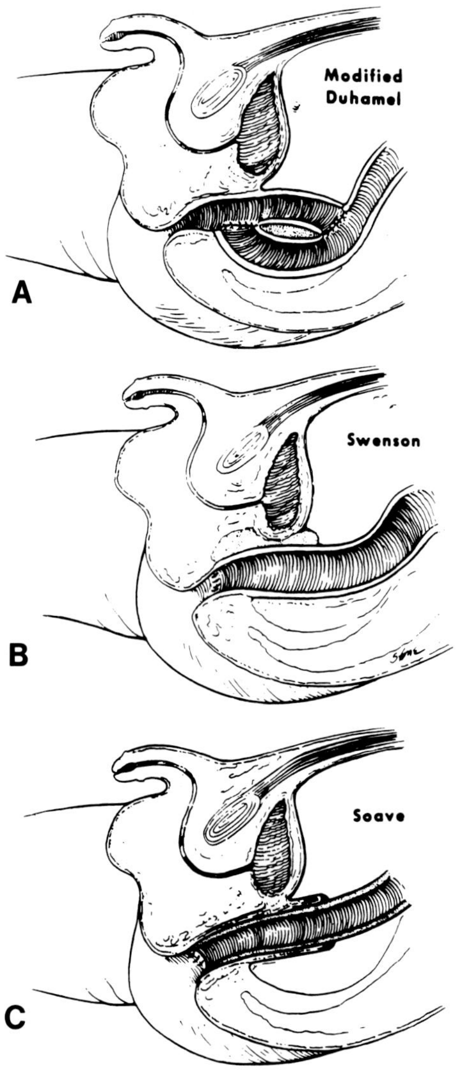

FIG. 35-13. Operative procedures for Hirschsprung's disease. *A*, The Duhamel procedure. The rectum is left in place with ganglionic bowel brought into the retrosecal space. *B*, The Swenson procedure. A low anterior resection of the rectum with end-to-end anastomosis. A segment of bowel with Hirschsprung's disease is left in site. *C*, The Soave procedure. The rectal mucosa is excised leaving a seromuscular cuff intact. The ganglionic proximal bowel is pulled through the cuff and endoanal anastomosis performed. (From Altman RP, Randolph JC, Anderson KD: Pediatric surgery. In Schwartz SI et al [eds]: Principles of Surgery, vol 2, p 1650. Copyright © 1969 by McGraw-Hill Book Company. Used with the permission of McGraw-Hill Book Company)

and rectal dilatation may effectively decompress the colon. Fluid and electrolyte support are mandatory, as is administration of antibiotics. Patients who do not respond to nonoperative measures must undergo laparotomy with establishment of a colostomy in a segment of bowel that contains ganglion cells. Close communication with a competent pathologist is important to establish the level of aganglionic bowel so that this complication can be avoided.

A variety of operative procedures are performed to reestablish anal continence in patients with Hirschsprung's disease. The patient usually undergoes a pull-through operation at a year of age.[76] This delay allows growth of the pelvis and nutritional development of the infant. The three operative procedures employed are those described by Swenson, Duhamel, and Soave (Fig. 35-13).[17, 88, 96]

The *Swenson operation* is a low anterior resection of the dilated aganglionic colon and rectum with a primary anastomosis low in the pelvis.[96] A complication observed with this operation is distal obstruction as a consequence of a small remaining segment of aganglionic rectum. These youngsters are treated with dietary manipulation and enemas by the uninitiated pediatrician or surgeon. The Swenson operation requires that the anus be dilated to traumatize the remnant aganglionic segment effectively in the low rectum. Dilatation can be done with bouginage or finger dilatation under general anesthesia. If a considerable segment of aganglionic rectum persists, an anorectal myectomy or internal sphincterotomy is performed.[58, 67] The patient not responding to local transanal repair of aganglionic segment should undergo a repeated operative procedure to establish a functional anus. This procedure is also associated with urinary retention following the extensive pelvic dissection. Some have abandoned the procedure because of the potential for damage to the nervi erigentes.

Duhamel's operation is a pull-through procedure requiring a more limited retrorectal dissection.[17] The ganglionic bowel is brought to the anus behind the aganglionic rectum. The common wall thus created is resected using the GIA stapler, which allows anastomosis transanally with minimal effort. The most annoying complication of this procedure has been the accumulation of fecal material in the rectal spur that is created in the aganglionic segment. The resulting fecaloma dilates the rectum with impingement on the urinary tract, resulting in urgency and frequency. Constipation from obstruction of the innervated colon can occur with compression by the fecaloma. The patient with a large fecaloma should undergo disimpaction under general anesthesia. Subsequently, the patient is managed with stool softeners (Colace, prune juice, or mineral oil) to minimize the likelihood of impaction of stool in the rectal spur. Surgical modifications were developed to obliterate the rectal spur.[65, 91] By obliterating the spur between the two segments of colon, a large rectal ampulla results, which effectively prevents the formation of the fecaloma.

The anastomosis with the GIA stapler occasionally results in bleeding from the staple line. This is managed transanally by dilating the anus and oversewing the staple line with a running 2-0 chromic suture. The irritation of the anastomosis can produce a localized proctitis with persistent bleeding. Steroid enemas and a low-residue diet are effective in treating the inflammatory process.

A third operative procedure for Hirschsprung's disease described by *Soave* is designed to avoid the complications of the Swenson and Duhamel operations.[88] In this procedure the dilated, aganglionic segment is resected, leaving the distal rectum *in situ*. The mucosa is dissected free from the muscular layer to the anal verge, creating a seromuscular tunnel. The innervated colon is pulled through this cuff with anastomosis to the anus.[4] A unique complication is a cuff abscess between the remnant seromuscular layer and the pull-through colon. Drainage of the cuff with a Penrose drain through the endoanal anastomosis minimizes this complication. Some surgeons criticize the procedure for preservation of the seromuscular layer, which lacks innervation and may cause the symptoms of obstruction. To avoid the symptoms of obstipation and allow the colon mesentery access to the pelvis, the posterior layer of the seromuscular tunnel can be incised.

Although least frequent with the Duhamel operation, all of these procedures can allow stricture to develop at the lower anal portion of the anastomosis. The aftercare of the patient requires attention to dilatation of the anus until the anastomosis is supple. Enterocolitis may ensue if anal stricture causes partial or intermittent obstruction, simulating the original pathology of Hirschsprung's disease.

A small percentage of patients will manifest total colonic aganglionosis. These patients require ileostomy, which some infants tolerate poorly. Total aganglionosis coli is probably best managed by using the Duhamel operation with the Martin modification, creating a long, beveled ileorectal anastomosis.[64] This procedure attempts to provide a larger surface area of colonic mucosa for absorption. A second operative procedure is a low anterior anastomosis of ileum to a small segment of aganglionic rectum. This procedure is functional, and the level of continence is acceptable. The common complications are malnutrition and diarrhea, which are a consequence of malabsorption. Treatment is similar to that employed for the short-gut syndrome.

After performing the endoanal anastomosis, any manipulation should be deferred for 2 weeks. A sign by the child's bedside should read "No Rectal Temperatures" and the nursing staff informed of its importance. A thermometer is easily passed through the newly formed anastomosis, resulting in a perirectal or pelvic abscess.

IMPERFORATE ANUS

The surgical correction of imperforate anus may be accompanied by a variety of complications. Operative repair is technically demanding and requires precise knowledge of the anatomy of the pelvis and anorectal canal. The mortality rate from this anomaly approximates 20% as a result of the associated anomalies of the genitourinary tract, heart, and intestine.[47]

Patients with a low imperforate anus are treated with anoplasty, while intermediate or high imperforate anus is best handled by diverting colostomy. Two complications observed following establishment of a loop colostomy are hyperchloremic acidosis and urinary tract infection. Patients with a high imperforate anus have a rectourethral or rectovesicle fistula. This connection permits reflux of urine into the distal rectal pouch with absorption of the chloride ion, elevation of the BUN level, tachypnea, and lethargy. The resulting hyperchloremic acidosis requires adequate fluid and electrolyte resuscitation with bicarbonate infusions. Occasionally, refractory metabolic acidosis with hyperchloremia develops, and division of the fistula becomes imperative. Similarly, bacteria from the colon may contaminate the urinary tract with resultant infection. During the interval between colostomy formation and definitive repair, treatment with prophylactic sulfonamide antibiotics is indicated to protect the infant from urinary tract infection.

Complications occurring during the operative procedure for imperforate anus are trauma to the urethra, malposition of the pull-through colon, and ischemia of the distal colon (Fig. 35-14). Urethral trauma can be avoided in the boy by inserting a sound in the urethral tract during the pelvic dissection. The urethral sound permits identification of the urethra, localization of the puborectalis sling, and accurate ligation of the rectourethral fistula. Improper fistula closure can compromise the urethra and result in stricture. A Foley catheter or suprapubic cystostomy is left in the bladder for 7 to 10 days to protect the ligated urethral fistula and prevent extravasation of urine into the abdominal cavity from the seromuscular cuff.

The major technical error committed during a pull-through procedure for high imperforate anus is to miss the puborectalis sling, thus placing the colon outside the sling with inevitable incontinence. This complication is avoided by assuring retrourethral placement of the mobilized colon: If the colon is properly placed within the puborectalis sling, the status of fecal continence is greatly improved. Some surgeons use a sacral dissection to visualize the fibers of the sling to assure proper colonic placement.[47]

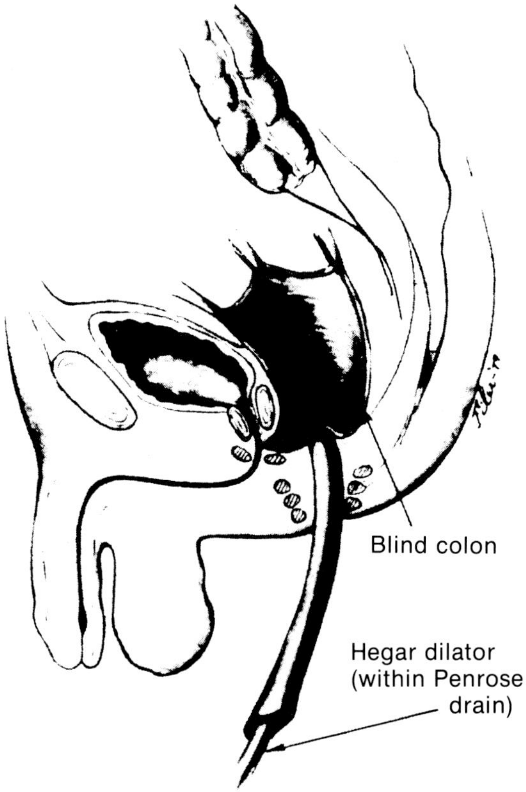

FIG. 35-14. Sacroabdominoperineal pull-through procedure for high imperforate anus. A fistula between the rectum and urethra is demonstrated. The pull-through of the colon must be precise to be within the puborectalis sling. (Kiesewetter WB: Imperforate anus. In Holder TM, Ashcraft KW [eds]: Pediatric Surgery, p 413. Philadelphia, WB Saunders, 1980)

Another complication from the operative procedure is ischemia of the distal colon. This results from compression or tension of the mesenteric blood supply to the pulled-through colonic segment. To avoid this complication, 3 cm to 4 cm of colon are allowed to remain outside the anus for 4 to 5 days. The delay in performing an anoplasty allows delineation of the ischemic segment and guarantees construction of the anus in viable tissue. Ischemic distal colon will heal imperfectly with resulting stenosis.

Several late complications can occur after anal pull-through procedures. The first is formation of a urethral diverticulum at the site of the divided rectourinary fistula. Excision and closure of the diverticulum is hazardous because it must be accomplished transperineally. A second complication is retraction of the colon at the mucocutaneous junction secondary to excessive tension at the anastomosis. This creates a deformed, stenotic, inelastic, poorly functioning anus. A third complication is postoperative diarrhea, which occurs when the anus is stenotic from retraction or ischemia. If the anal opening is narrow, then the stool collects behind the obstruction and loose watery stools pass around the impacted feces. Another complication from obstruction is enterocolitis in the proximal bowel, which causes a paradoxical diarrhea. Patients with diarrhea require urgent evaluation and treatment.

Fecal incontinence is most commonly associated with a high imperforate anus since the operative procedure is more demanding with greater risk for complications. Fecal continence can be expected to improve with age and reach a plateau in adolescence. The long-term satisfactory functional result of surgery for imperforate anus is approaching 75%.[47] Twelve percent of the patients require regular enemas, reoperation, or permanent colostomy.

Complications of Abdominal Wall Defect Surgery

Integrity of the abdominal wall is dependent on fusion of the abdominal wall somites that meet at the umbilicus during fetal development. Between the 4th and 10th week of gestation, the intestinal tract elongates and returns to the abdominal cavity. Abnormalities in the abdominal wall are correlated with embryologic arrest of the normal formation of the body wall and rotation of the intestinal tract. The two major abdominal wall defects are omphalocele and gastroschisis.

OMPHALOCELE

Neonates with omphalocele have a high incidence (67%) of associated anomalies involving the cardiac, neurologic, genitourinary, skeletal, and chromosomal systems.[66] These infants are at high risk of death because of the associated conditions. Children with large omphalocele frequently have the liver as part of the contents of the large hernia sac and a small chest cavity. This creates a technical problem since reducing the abdominal contents leads to impingement of the diaphragms.

Nonoperative treatment of omphalocele can sometimes be accomplished by daily application of a 2% aqueous mercurochrome solution. An eschar forms over the sac with eventual epithelialization. These patients may develop a pink urine, which is indicative of mercury poisoning.[92] Other alternative methods of nonoperative therapy are the application of Silvadene and, more recently, Op-site. Nonoperative treatment bears the disadvantages of local infections, sepsis, rupture of the sac, overlooked intestinal anomalies, and prolonged hospitalization. Nevertheless, in the patients with massive hernia, a period of nonoperative support and growth improves the patient's chances for survival.

A variety of operative techniques are available to treat patients with omphalocele. Surgical repair of the small omphalocele can be accomplished by primary closure after stretching of the abdominal wall. Skin-flap mobilization and application of a silastic pouch are the methods used for large omphaloceles. During closure of the omphalocele, the liver is vulnerable to rupture or laceration with uncontrollable hemorrhage and exsanguination. The dorsal aspect of the liver is closely adherent to the omphalocele sac, and no effort should be made to resect the sac at this junction. In the event hemorrhage ensues, application of direct pressure and the application of topical Avitene along with the infusion of fresh whole blood or fresh frozen plasma may provide hemostasis.

Application of a silastic pouch and too rapid closure of the chimney may result in respiratory embarrassment requiring ventilatory support. With the sequential application of pressure to the abdominal contents, the vena cava may be compressed with development of decreased blood return to the heart and edema of the lower extremities. Elevation or wrapping of the lower extremities minimizes the peripheral edema. If venous return to the right side of the heart is compromised, then partial release of the pouch is necessary. Finally, reduction of the silastic pouch may lead to partial obstruction of the duodenum by the liver as it is forced into the abdominal cavity. This phenomenon is particularly evident in older infants who are undergoing ventral hernia repair for omphalocele.

In the past sepsis was a major cause of death of these patients. With appropriate antibiotic coverage, usually ampicillin and gentamicin, the incidence of sepsis is greatly diminished. TPN provides support for infants whose gastrointestinal tract is not functional. With specific antibiotics and good nutrition, the survival rate has increased significantly over the past decade.[17]

Omphalocele, macroglossia, and gigantism constitute the Beckwith–Wiedemann syndrome.[102] Infants with these findings may develop hypoglycemia secondary to pancreatic hypoplasia or nesidioblastosis. Close monitoring of their blood glucose levels is essential. The macroglossia may obstruct the airway or prevent swallowing. Gastrostomy may be necessary for feeding, and, rarely, tracheostomy may be necessary.

GASTROSCHISIS

The infant with gastroschisis is born with eviscerated intestines without a visible hernia sac and the umbilical cord attached immediately to the left of the defect.[66] The midgut comprises the herniation, while the liver is usually intra-abdominal. These patients inevitably develop hypothermia from exposure of the intestinal tract and hypovolemia from large third-space losses. Intestinal atresia may be associated with gastroschisis and is usually the only associated anomaly. No attempt is made to separate the adherent loops of bowel when reducing the eviscerated midgut, since any trauma to the serosa can lead to perforation and fistula formation. Consequently, primary anastomosis of an associated atresia is delayed. Since a prolonged ileus lasting 4 to 6 weeks is anticipated in these youngsters, nutrition is provided by TPN. Similarly, sepsis is minimized by administration of antibiotics (ampicillin and an aminoglycoside) until the abdominal wall is closed.

Primary closure is possible in infants with gastroschisis after stretching the abdominal wall. It is extremely important to stretch the abdominal wall enough to allow comfortable reduction of the midgut. The defect in the abdominal wall is extended longitudinally to allow easy reduction of the intestines. Pressure on the small bowel from effort at primary closure can lead to ischemia of the intestinal tract with infarction. If a silastic pouch is required, it should be applied so the lower portion of the chimney diameter is larger than the upper portion. This assures that the intestinal contents can be manually reduced.

The silastic pouch may separate from the fascia after pressure is applied for reduction of the intestine. If the separation is localized, then infection is prevented by applying Silvadene, povidone-iodine (Betadine) ointment, pigskin xenograft, or Op-site. Major separation of the pouch from the abdominal wall is best treated by resuturing the silastic pouch to the fascia, if possible. Covering the defect with Betadine gauze, pigskin, homograft, or Op-site until a pseudoperitoneum forms avoids second application of silastic. The incidence of sepsis in patients requiring the silastic pouch has been reduced by the application of topical antibiotics and skin substitutes for coverage. These maneuvers may leave a sizable ventral hernia that requires later secondary closure.

The survival rate with gastroschisis has improved significantly as a result of better technical management, topical and systemic antibiotics, and parenteral nutritional support.[60] Enteric feedings are begun gradually to minimize postoperative necrotizing enterocolitis.

UMBILICAL HERNIA

Umbilical herniorrhaphy has a low complication rate.[52] The most common complication experienced by patients undergoing this procedure is subcutaneous hematoma from inadequate hemostasis during the operative procedure. A pressure dressing applied for 24 to 48 hours can minimize the incidence of this complication. If hematoma occurs within the first 24 to 48 hours, prompt evacuation is important. The hematoma that is not recognized for several days is allowed to resolve without surgery unless the collection of blood is extremely large.

A second complication is paralytic ileus, which is occasionally noted in patients who undergo repair of a large umbilical hernia. Postoperatively the patient develops abdominal distention with vomiting. Management consists of nasogastric decompression and intravenous fluid hydration. The ileus is self limiting and resolves in 3 to 4 days.

Care during umbilical herniorrhaphy is taken to identify any intestinal contents in the hernia sac such as a Meckel's diverticulum. If encountered, then the diverticulum should be removed by a closed technique.

Finally, a hernia may recur in patients who have undergone repair of an umbilical hernia, particularly with attenuated tissues. This requires reoperation and an effort made to close the defect, incorporating strong fascial layers.

INGUINAL HERNIA

The most common operation performed in infants and children is inguinal herniorrhaphy. The complication rate is low when it is performed by skilled surgeons. The most common type of pediatric hernia is the indirect inguinal hernia. Direct inguinal hernia or femoral hernia is rare.

Infants undergoing inguinal herniorrhaphy are commonly treated as ambulatory surgical patients. With the improved care given in neonatal nurseries, high-risk infants require inguinal herniorrhaphy. These infants may have respiratory distress syndrome, Ehlers–Danlos syndrome, cystic fibrosis, hydrocephalus, or congenital heart disease. The patient with cystic fibrosis may demonstrate atrophy or absence of the vas deferens; therefore one need not identify this structure if the diagnosis of cystic fibrosis is established.[57] The infant with Ehlers–Danlos syndrome has a connective tissue abnormality and poor healing, which leads to a high recurrence rate.[60] A deficiency in platelet function, which can result in a bleeding diathesis, may also be present. The third association is the patient with hydrocephalus and ventriculoperitoneal shunt whose inguinal hernia can be large since the increased abdominal fluid dilates the sac.[30] Routine inguinal herniorrhaphy with prophylactic antibiotics is curative.

Most complications associated with inguinal herniorrhaphy are related to the size of the structures of the infant inguinal canal. Recurrent inguinal hernia usually results from not identifying the processus vaginalis during the initial operative procedure or improper ligation of the sac. Meticulous ligation of the sac with a nonabsorbable suture minimizes the potential for this complication.

Transection of the vas deferens may occur if this small structure is mistaken for a redundant hernia sac or fibrous tissue. Repair is accomplished by placing a single 6-0 chromic suture through the lumen of each end of the transsected vas to assure approximation. The chromic stitch absorbs, and the vas deferens will either recannulate or the ends will remain in proximity for later repair. Techniques of microvascular anastomosis should be deferred until the youngster has achieved full growth.

Injury to the bladder can occur during mobilization of the cord structures when dissection is carried medially through the rectus muscle. The abdominal wall is extremely thin in infants and the bladder, being mistaken for a hernia sac, can be mobilized in error. If the bladder is entered, the defect should be repaired with a two-layer closure of chromic sutures and the bladder decompressed with a suprapubic cystostomy.

At the termination of the inguinal herniorrhaphy, it is routine to palpate the testicles in the scrotum. Oversight of this maneuver can lead to iatrogenic retracted testicle, requiring orchiopexy. Traction on the testicle should be gentle, since laryngospasm can ensue while the patient is emerging from anesthesia.

Another postoperative complication is a reactive hydrocele, which is a consequence of the trauma of surgery. Fluid accumulation commonly occurs when a moderate to large hydrocele is associated with an inguinal hernia. A hydrocelectomy that does not provide an adequate opening of the hydrocele sac leads to chronic accumulation of fluid. It is inadvisable in the early postoperative period to aspirate this hydrocele, since reaccumulation of fluid is common and the potential for scrotal abscess is significant. The postoperative, reactive hydrocele should be left alone for at least 6 months so that resorption can occur. After this period aspiration is indicated, but reoperation is often necessary. Aspiration of any presumed hydrocele in the preoperative period is condemned, since the intestinal tract may reside in this inguinal hydrocele and inadvertent penetration will contaminate the tissue planes, leading to sepsis and abscess.

Another complication is inadvertent trauma to bowel or ovary in the lumen of the sac. This is avoided by opening the sac and inspecting the contents before performing transection and ligation if it is not absolutely clear that the sac is empty.

Wound infection in an inguinal hernia is exceedingly uncommon but can be seen when circum cision is performed in conjunction with the herniorrhaphy. The potential for this infection is minimized if inguinal herniorrhaphy is accomplished with application of collodion before circumcision is performed.

The inexperienced surgeon often mistakenly transfers principles of repair from the adult to the infant. Flaps and translocation of the cord have no place in the uncomplicated inguinal hernia of infants and children.

Complications of Liver Surgery

BILIARY ATRESIA

Biliary atresia is a disease entity that has recently become amenable to surgical correction. The procedure utilized today is the hepatic portoenterostomy described by Kasai (Fig. 35-15).[45] The complications associated with this procedure are related to the technical procedure or the disease process. Technical complications in the creation of the portoenterostomy are frequent. Anastomosis between the intestinal tract and the porta hepatis to encompass the minute ductules is difficult. Stricture of the anastomosis leads to obstruction of biliary flow, necessitating reexploration and reconstruction of the portoenterostomy. A leak at the site of the portoenterostomy yields a collection of bile in the right upper quadrant, which also requires surgical correction and drainage.

The most significant complication in patients undergoing the Kasai procedure is development of ascending cholangitis. Cholangitis accounts for more than 50% of the deaths of patients who become jaundice-free after hepatic portoenterostomy. The Kasai technique was modified by exteriorizing part of the Roux-en-Y limb of jejunum to decrease the continuing incidence of cholangitis.[95] Exteriorization of bile flow has allowed early recognition of cholangitis and facilitated culture of the responsible organism. All patients undergoing portoenterostomy must be maintained on long-term prophylactic antibiotics, usually Septra.

A complication of the disease process itself is hepatic fibrosis, occurring in many patients in spite of adequate drainage. With resulting portal hypertension, bleeding from esophageal varices may become a major problem. Every conservative medical effort should be made to treat these children. The medical management involves replacement of blood, vitamin K to return the prothrombin time to normal, fresh frozen plasma, and platelets. Occasionally, a patient requires a Sengstacken–Blakemore tube to effect compression of the varices. In young patients the potential for gastric and esophageal perforation by the tube is significant. Surgical decompression of the portal system in a young patient is limited by the small size of the portosystemic shunt, resulting in a high failure rate. Mesocaval shunt using autogenous vein has been used successfully in these patients.[1] Lilly has used sclerosis by injection of the varices with some success.[54]

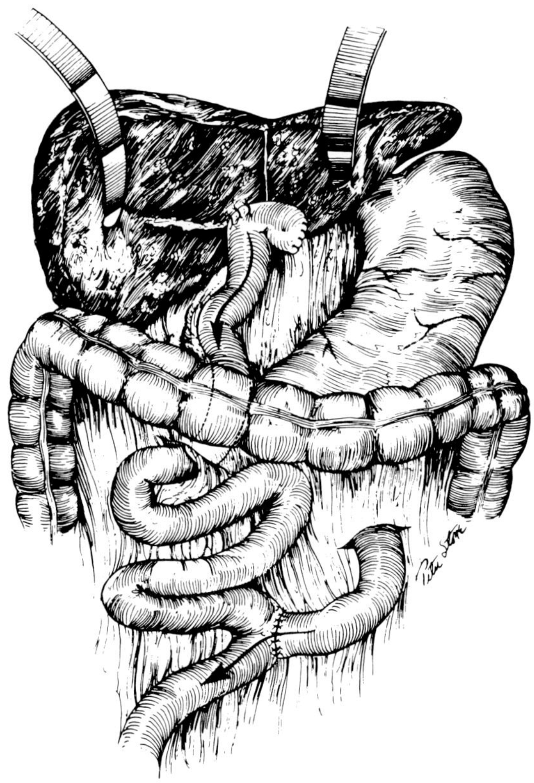

FIG. 35-15. Kasai Portoenterostomy for biliary atresia. (From Altman RP, Randolph JC, Anderson KD: Pediatric surgery. In Schwartz SI et al [eds]: Principles of Surgery, vol 2, p 1652. Copyright © 1969 by McGraw-Hill Book Company. Used with permission of McGraw-Hill Book Company)

Patients with bilary atresia develop ascites as their cirrhosis progresses. This complication can sometimes be controlled by dietary restriction of salt and water, while maintaining the patient on spironolactone (Aldactone). The small infant's stoma in the right upper quadrant can prolapse if ascites and intra-abdominal pressure are excessive. This is avoided by oversewing the distal limb, creating a single stoma, or securing the peritoneum and fascia about the intestinal stoma. Should prolapse persist, surgical correction is required if ischemia occurs or bile flow is restricted.

The patient with biliary atresia develops difficulties with absorption of fat-soluble vitamins. The most significant vitamin deficiency is that of vitamin D. The use of long-term synthetic vitamin D to avoid the postoperative complications of vitamin-D deficient rickets is indicated. Similarly, the levels of vitamin K must be monitored in these patients to avoid a bleeding diathesis, especially in patients with esophageal varices.

CHOLEDOCHAL CYST

Excision of the cyst and establishing a Roux-en-Y anastomosis is the therapy for idiopathic cystic dilatation of the extrahepatic or intrahepatic biliary ductal system.[53] A complication observed after this procedure is acute pancreatitis as a result of trauma to the pancreatic duct or parenchyma of the pancreas. Anastomotic stricture is uncommon if an adequate hepatojejunal anastomosis is created. Ascending colangitis can occur, but long-term antibiotic prophylaxis is not required. Episodes of acute cholangitis are treated with intermittent antibiotic therapy. Retention of a segment of cyst has been associated with a reported incidence of 3% to 5% of biliary carcinoma. This has caused surgeons to favor complete resection of the cyst. Also, the Roux-en-Y cystjejunostomy and cystduodenostomy have resulted in gallbladder calculi, ineffective cyst decompression, and progressive hepatic fibrosis.[28]

LIVER TUMOR

Technical complications during resection of tumors of the liver can usually be avoided. Hemorrhage during dissection of the hepatic venous branches avulsed from the vena cava or from venocaval injury is minimized if dissection and suture ligation are accomplished with meticulous surgical technique. During liver surgery, intraoperative hypovolemia occurs when blood loss and third-space losses have been underestimated in the small patient. This, coupled with decreased right heart venous return from angulation of the vena cava during manipulation of the tumor, can lead to cardiac arrest. During resuscitation of the patient with intraoperative cardiac arrest, the aorta can be cross clamped at the diaphragmatic hiatus. This permits perfusion of the myocardium through the coronary arteries and maintenance of cerebral blood flow. Intermittent unclamping of the aorta allows perfusion of the organs distal to the hiatus. This maneuver may lead to an ischemic insult to the kidney, which is manifested portoperatively as renal insufficiency and azotemia. Air embolism can occur during the operative procedure if the portal system is opened inadvertently with access of air into the right heart.

After massive hepatic resection, the patient is always at risk to develop infection. Infection typically occurs from accumulation of blood in the subphrenic or subhepatic space. Meticulous intraoperative hemostasis and adequate drainage minimize this complication. Gallium scan, sonography, and CT scan are utilized to demonstrate such loculations, which may require drainage. Antibiotic therapy during the operation will help avoid contamination of the perihepatic region. With resection of large amounts of liver, the patient will require administration of glucose and albumin in the perioperative phase to treat hypoglycemia and hypoalbuminemia.[94]

Complications of Pancreas Surgery

ACUTE PANCREATITIS

Acute pancreatitis in children was thought to be rare.[20] Nevertheless with increased intensive-care capabilities and expanding surgical efforts, particularly for the trauma patient, the number of children developing acute pancreatitis has increased.[19] Postoperative acute pancreatitis occurs after dissection in the region of the porta hepatis, mesentery of the small bowel, and lesser sac. Patients with hematologic disorders requiring splenectomy may develop acute pancreatitis if the tail of the pancreas is damaged in the hilus of the spleen. Similarly, young patients undergoing common duct exploration for cholelithiasis, associated with sickle cell disease, can develop acute pancreatitis. Treatment of acute pancreatitis requires long-term decompression of the intestinal tract. Support with TPN is required for 4 to 6 weeks until the inflammatory process in the pancreas subsides and enteric feedings can be resumed.

Following acute pancreatitis, pseudocyst of the pancreas can result from ductal disruption within the pancreas. The diagnosis of pseudocyst of the pancreas is made by physical examination, sonography, or CT scan. The pseudocyst is allowed to mature for 3 to 6 weeks before surgical decompression is undertaken. The surgical procedure most commonly employed is cystgastrostomy with an anastomosis created between the posterior wall of the stomach and the pancreatic pseudocyst.[12] Roux-en-Y cystjejunostomy may be appropriate in pancreatic pseudocysts that cannot be approached through the stomach. A complication following cystgastrostomy is bleeding from the anastomosis. This is best avoided by using a running, locking sutured nonabsorbable material. If postoperative bleeding occurs, the patient should undergo arteriography to delineate the site of bleeding, which is either the suture line or the pancreaticoduodenal artery in the cyst. Embolization of autologous clot or Gelfoam may effect nonoperative hemostasis. If embolization is unsuccessful, exploratory laparotomy is necessary for suture ligation of the bleeding vessel.

SUBTOTAL PANCREATECTOMY FOR HYPOGLYCEMIA

The entities encountered in infants that lead to hypoglycemia and seizures immediately after birth are islet cell adenoma and nesidioblastosis.[89, 105] If the infant has refractory hypoglycemia in spite of all efforts at medical management, abdominal exploration is mandatory. The pancreas is evaluated intraoperatively for an islet cell adenoma, which would be enucleated. If no adenoma is found, a subtotal pancreatectomy encompassing 85% of the pancreas is indicated.[33] In this operation the spleen should be preserved. Hypoglycemia can recur in the postoperative period. Treatment is conservative medical management with intravenous glucose, glucagon, and diazoxide (10–15 mg/kg/day). If medical management is ineffective, then a near-total pancreatectomy of the remaining pancreatic tissue is indicated.[34] Meticulous dissection in the region of the head of the pancreas and ampulla of Vater helps avoid a common duct injury. Should the common duct be injured, a decompression of the biliary tree can be accomplished by cholecystojejunostomy. Care is also taken to minimize trauma to the duodenum. Inadvertent splenic injury should be treated by splenorrhaphy if that is technically feasible.

Complications of Spleen Surgery

SPLENECTOMY

Splenectomy is a surgical procedure that is employed for a variety of hematologic disorders and, occasionally, trauma. The complications of splenectomy result from improper management of the splenic hilus during dissection. During mobilization of the hilus of the spleen, the tail of the pancreas is especially vulnerable to injury leading to postoperative pancreatitis and pseudocyst. During the immediate postoperative period, patients must be protected from acute gastric dilatation to avoid bleeding from the short gastric vessels, which are ligated during the mobilization of the spleen from the greater curvature of the stomach. Necrosis and perforation of the greater curvature of the stomach can occur if overzealous ligation of the gastric vessels incorporates part of the wall in the ligature.

The most lethal complication of splenectomy is postsplenectomy sepsis caused by encapsulated organisms such as pneumococci, *Hemophilus influenzae*, or meningococci.[26, 87] Following splenectomy the child is at a much greater risk to develop pneumonia, meningitis, and overwhelming sepsis, which leads rapidly to death. The incidence of postsplenectomy sepsis in asplenic children is 85 times the rate of normal population and develops in 4.25% of splenectomy patients, with a mortality rate exceeding 50%.[87] The onset of the sepsis is usually within the first 2 years postoperatively and occurs more commonly in youngsters less than five years of age. Children undergoing splenectomy are treated with pneumococcal vaccine and long-term penicillin prophylaxis. The penicillin prophylaxis takes the form of Bicillin monthly or Pen-Vee-K orally at one half the therapeutic dose.

Subphrenic abscess can follow splenectomy, especially in patients who undergo the procedure for a massively enlarged spleen. Most surgeons do not advocate drainage of the left upper quadrant in the patient undergoing splenectomy, but closed drainage may be indicated when a large dead space persists. Meticulous hemostasis during the left upper quadrant dissection will minimize bleeding and the potential for abscess formation. Any child with an intermittent spiking temperature is suspected of having subphrenic abscess. Subphrenic abscess is diagnosed by sonography or CT scan. Drainage of the left subphrenic abscess should be deferred for at least 14 days so that the abscess can mature and drainage accomplished extraperitoneally by excising the 12th rib.

Complications of Trauma

The leading cause of death in children aged 1 year to 14 years is accidental death. The most common mechanism of injury is blunt trauma to the torso with a concomitant injury to the head. The mortality of blunt abdominal trauma is 4% to 12%. Care for the child with multiple injuries requires that diagnosis and therapy be accomplished simultaneously. Improvement in diagnosis results from peritoneal lavage, CT scan of the head, and liver–spleen scan.

The patient sustaining abdominal trauma frequently manifests hemorrhagic shock. In the initial triage of the patient, an effort is made to improve tissue perfusion with infusion of crystalloid solutions and O positive blood. The decision making during the initial evaluation of the pediatric trauma patient depends on an awareness of the injuries common to blunt abdominal trauma.

GASTROINTESTINAL INJURY

The patient with blunt abdominal trauma is always evaluated for gastrointestinal tract injury. A common organ involved in pediatric trauma is the stomach. The usual response of patients to blunt abdominal trauma is aerophagia with subsequent gastric dilatation. On physical examination the dilatation of the stomach produces a left upper quadrant mass, which can lead to erroneous diagnosis of splenic injury.

Gastric dilatation in small infants and children can impair the function of the left diaphragm, leading to respiratory insufficiency and arrest. Therefore, any patient sustaining blunt abdominal trauma requires insertion of a nasogastric tube to decompress the air from the stomach, to prevent respiratory insufficiency, to minimize the potential of gastric rupture, and to facilitate physical examination of the abdomen without gastric dilatation. Penetrating injuries to the abdomen can lead to significant gastric hemorrhage.

Blunt trauma to the abdomen with rapid deceleration or a direct blow may result in a duodenal hematoma.[40] Bleeding into the submucosa of the duodenum produces a hematoma that causes luminal obstruction. The patient presents a clinical picture of gastric outlet obstruction with gastric dilatation and vomiting. This injury is evident on a limited upper gastrointestinal tract contrast study by observing the diagnostic "coiled spring" sign.[62] Management of the lesion is usually nonoperative, employing TPN and nasogastric decompression. Surgical evacuation of the hematoma is avoided because of the likelihood of a duodenal leak and enterocutaneous fistula.

A deceleration injury may lead to partial or complete transection of the jejunum and occurs commonly at or just below the ligament of Trietz, where the small bowel is fixed to the retroperitoneum.[44] Children with this injury present with varying degrees of pneumoperitoneum, which may lead to massive abdominal distention and subsequent respiratory arrest from impingement of the diaphragms. If nasogastric tube decompression is unsuccessful, insertion of an 18-gauge needle transabdominally midway between the xiphoid and the umbilicus in the midline temporarily relieves the pressure on the diaphragms. Occasionally, the laceration of the proximal jejunum is unnoticed, and peritonitis develops in the ensuing 4 to 6 hours. This injury can be recognized if peritoneal lavage fluid shows bacteria, bile, or an elevated amylase level. Repair is accomplished by débridement of the perforation with transverse closure or end-to-end anastomosis, following mobilization of the ligament of Treitz.

The second common area of perforation secondary to blunt trauma is the distal ileum on the antimesenteric border. This usually is a blowout in the ileocecal region. The injury commonly presents as peritonitis in the right lower quadrant 6 to 12 hours following injury. Management involves débridement and transverse closure or a local segmental resection with end-to-end anastomosis. Postoperative complications from either of these injuries are minimized by broad-spectrum antibiotics since the intestine involved is the small bowel.

The colon is uncommonly involved in blunt abdominal trauma in children but can be impaired by a knife or bullet.[16] The colonic trauma is best managed by colostomy and mucous fistula with resection of the involved segment. Some advocate primary closure if the wound to the colon is inflicted by a knife so that a clean laceration occurs with minimal soilage.[48] However, diversion of the fecal stream with a staged anastomosis is always the safest method of management. Rectal injuries are treated by proximal, diverting colostomy and mucous fistula with drainage of the presacral area through the region of the coccyx. This method allows dependent drainage of the retrorectal area, minimizing formation of a supralevator, perirectal abscess.

A final complication in trauma to the gastrointestinal tract is postoperative adhesions with partial and complete obstruction of the intestinal tract. Partial obstruction of the intestinal tract is managed by nasogastric decompression or long-tube decompression. With the advent of TPN, these patients can be maintained in an anabolic state without enteral nutrition. Patients who develop complete obstruction require laparotomy and lysis of adhesions. When multiple laparotomies are required for recurrent intestinal obstruction, the patient can develop the short-bowel syndrome with malabsorption. Therefore, every effort is made to preserve as much of the intestinal tract as possible.

SPLEEN INJURY

The most common organ sustaining injury from blunt abdominal trauma is the spleen. Nonoperative management of the spleen is a prime consideration whenever possible in the child with stable vital signs. The asplenic young patient is at risk of developing postsplenectomy sepsis and death. A liver–spleen scan or CT scan can determine the integrity of this organ.[99] In cases of demonstrated splenic injury, nonoperative therapy is advocated if the patient maintains stable vital signs, does not require replacement of more than one third of the blood volume, and is free of concomitant intra-abdominal injury requiring surgery.[23] If clinical deterioration occurs, laparotomy is undertaken. Splenectomy for pediatric trauma is unusual today because of technical alternatives to splenectomy.[8] The patient must be in an intensive-care unit for monitoring during the first 24 to 48 hours. If the patient remains stable, he is discharged on the 10th day to limited activity.

LIVER INJURY

The liver is the second most commonly injured organ in the abdominal cavity.[16] The injury usually consists of a laceration with bleeding. Subcapsular hematoma of the liver is managed nonoperatively in the stable patient if sonography and CT scan are available to follow the resolution of this hematoma.[77] Hemorrhage is managed by direct ligation of the hepatic vessels and drainage of the hepatic space. Rarely, massive injury to the liver requires hepatic lobectomy to control bleeding. Right hepatic artery ligation is a reasonable alternative for management of uncontrolled hepatic hemorrhage when other methods fail.[11] With massive hemorrhage from the liver, the patient can develop bleeding diathesis as a consequence of dilution of the clotting factors. This risk is minimized by infusing fresh whole blood, platelets, and fresh frozen plasma every fourth unit of banked blood.

Hematoma in the parenchyma of the liver or the subcapsular region can lead to abscess formation, requiring drainage. Hematobilia may develop as a consequence of pressure necrosis from a hematoma in the liver parenchyma, which is manifested by upper gastrointestinal bleeding.[38] Angiography documents the bleeding site, and embolization of an autologous clot or Gelfoam can lead to adequate cessation of bleeding. If this maneuver fails, then hepatic resection is indicated for hemostasis.

Resection of the liver for trauma may be followed in 2 to 3 weeks by subphrenic or subhepatic abscess. This complication is minimized by adequate broad-spectrum antibiotic coverage, effective drainage, and intraoperative hemostasis. Drainage is best accomplished by resecting the bed of the 12th rib and placing several Penrose drains and a sump catheter through this dependent location. Adequate drainage will allow evacuation of hematoma and egress of infected debris.

PANCREAS INJURY

The pancreas is vulnerable during blunt trauma to the abdomen.[20] The most common injury observed in the pediatric age group is posttraumatic acute pancreatitis. Elevation of the amylase level is a variable sign of acute pancreatitis. The amylase-creatinine ratio in children is difficult to interpret and is not specific for pancreatic injury. A trauma patient who develops a protracted ileus is suspected of developing acute pancreatitis. Any patient with hyperamylasemia and a sonogram or CT scan that shows edema of the pancreas is presumed to have acute pancreatitis. These patients can develop hyperbilirubinemia since the edema of the pancreas may partially obstruct the common duct. Effusion in the left hemithorax with a transudate that contains an elevated amylase level has been observed during this disease process. The patient requires TPN for 4 to 6 weeks with nasogastric decompression during the initial phase of therapy. Attention to volume resuscitation of the patient is important to minimize renal hypoperfusion and oliguria, as a consequence of third-space losses. Renal failure associated with acute pancreatitis is difficult to manage and requires the capability for hemodialysis.

The patient with acute pancreatitis is at risk to develop a pseudocyst of the pancreas, which may be a consequence of the inflammatory process or the result of direct trauma to a major duct system.[12] Pseudocyst of the pancreas is diagnosed by sonography or CT scan. The complications of traumatic pseudocyst are gastric outlet obstruction, perforation into the abdominal cavity, hemorrhage from the wall, and abscess formation. Spontaneous perforation in the first 3 weeks is treated with adequate internal drainage or tube decompression. An infected pseudocyst requires drainage of the abscess and exteriorization through the flank by soft rubber drains and sump catheters. The patient with hemorrhage into the pseudocyst requires arteriography and laparotomy. Hypertension has been observed in patients with pseudocyst of the pancreas as a consequence of compression of the renal artery. Medical control of the hypertension is indicated until adequate maturation of the cyst (3–6 weeks) allows adequate internal decompression.

Injury to the head of the pancreas is rare but may require pancreaticoduodenectomy. This maneuver is usually required in patients sustaining penetrating trauma to the pancreas and duodenum. Total pancreatectomy may also be employed for the patient with pancreatic injury if the duodenum is viable. Another method of management is diverticulization of the duodenum, which requires a Billroth II operative decompression and vagotomy. Injury to the tail of the pancreas requires limited resection, ligation of the pancreatic duct with a nonabsorbable suture, and sump drainage without splenectomy if possible. Inadequate ligation of the pancreatic duct leads to pancreaticocutaneous fistula. This is treated with TPN, electrolyte management, and skin care of the abdominal wall.

PELVIC FRACTURE

Patients who sustain major fractures to the pelvis can develop massive bleeding into the retroperitoneum.[27, 78] Retroperitoneal hematoma and hemorrhage are difficult to control if the retroperitoneum is opened. Immobilization and replacement of blood is usually adequate to stop bleeding from a pelvic fracture. The patient with pelvic fracture and massive bleeding is initially managed by application of a MAST suit to increase the abdominal pressure in the pelvis. Operative intervention is the last method employed to control pelvic fracture hemorrhage in the absence of concomitant intra-abdominal injury. Angiography can localize the bleeding artery, and hemostasis can be accomplished by embolization. Operative approach to the retroperitoneal bleeding is to ligate the internal iliac arteries, avoiding injury to the ureter on either side. An operation to stop bleeding may infect a retroperitoneal hematoma, leading to sepsis and death. Neural injury to the sciatic, obturator, or femoral nerves can occur and should be documented early in the management of these patients.

References

1. Altman RP: Portal decompression by interposition mesocaval shunt in patients with biliary atresia. J Pediatr Surg 11:809, 1976
2. Anderson KD: Esophageal substitution. In Holder TM, Ashcraft KW (eds): Pediatric Surgery, p 284. Philadelphia, WB Saunders, 1980
3. Anderson KD, Randolph JG: The gastric tube for esophageal replacement in children. J Thorac Cardiovasc Surg 66:333, 1973
4. Baley SJ, Lafer DJ, Kleinhause BD et al: Endorectal pull-through procedure for Hirschsprung's disease with and without primary anastomosis. J Pediatr Surg 3:258, 1968
5. Benson CD: Infantile pyloric stenosis. Progr Pediatr Surg 1:63, 1970
6. Bishop HC: Small bowel obstructions in the newborn. Surg Clin North Am 56:329, 1976
7. Bishop HC, Koop CE: Management of meconium ileus. Resection, Roux-en-Y anastomosis and ileostomy irrigation with pancreatic enzymes. Ann Surg 145:410, 1957
8. Buntain WL, Lynn HB: Splenorrhaphy: Changing concepts for the traumatized spleen. Surgery 86:748, 1979
9. Cloud DT: Appendicitis. In Holder TM, Ashcraft KW (eds): Pediatric Surgery, p 498. Philadelphia, WB Saunders, 1980
10. Cohen DH, Middleton AW, Fletcher J: Gastric tube esophagoplasty. J Pediatr Surg 9:451, 1974
11. Conty TG, Aaron WS: Hepatic artery ligation for exsanguinating liver injuries in children. J Pediatr Surg 10:693, 1975
12. Cooney DR, Grosfeld JL: Operative management of pancreatic pseudocysts in infants and children. A review of 75 cases. Ann Surg 182:590, 1975
13. Cordomier SK, Izant RJ: Meconium ileus equivalent. Surgery 54:667, 1963

13a. Downes JJ, Raphaely RC: Anesthesia and intensive care. In Ravitch MM, Welch KJ, Benson CD et al: Pediatric Surgery, p 16. Chicago, Year Book Medical Publishers, 1979

14. Crumrine RS: Postoperative hypoxia in infants and children. Int Anesthesiol Clin 9:83, 1971
15. Dawkins MJR, Scopes JW: Nonshivering thermogenesis and brown adipose tissue in the human newborn infant. Nature 206:201, 1965
16. Drew R, Perry JF, Fischer R: The expediency of peritoneal lavage for blunt trauma in children. Surg Gynecol Obstet 145:885, 1977
17. Duhamel B: Retrorectal and trans and pull-through procedure for the treatment of Hirschsprung's disease. Dis Colon Rectum 7:455, 1964
18. Edelmann CM, Spitzer A: The maturing kidney. J Pediatr 75:509, 1969
19. Eichelberger MR, Chatten DA, Bruce DA et al: Acute pancreatitis and increased intracranial pressure. J Pediatr Surg 16:562, 1981
20. Eichelberger MR, Hoelzer DJ, Koop CE: Acute pancreatitis: The difficulties of diagnosis and therapy. J Pediatr Surg 17:244, 1982
21. Ein SH: Recurrent intussusception in children. J Pediatr Surg 10:751, 1975
22. Ein SH, Marshall DG, Girvan D: Peritoneal drainage under local anesthesia for perforations from neonatal necrotizing enterocolitis. J Pediatr Surg 12:963, 1977
23. Ein SH, Shandling B, Simpson JS, Stephans CA: Nonoperative management of traumatized spleen in children: How and why. J Pediatr Surg 13:117, 1978
24. Ein SH, Shandling B, Simpson JJ et al: Fourteen years of gastric tubes. J Pediatr Surg 13:638, 1978
25. Fonkalsrud EW, DeLorimer AA, Hays DM: Congenital atresia and stenosis of the duodenum. A review compiled from the members of the Surgical Section of the American Academy of Pediatrics. Pediatrics 43:79, 1969
26. Francke EL, Neu HC: Post-splenectomy infection. Surg Clin North Am 61:135, 1981
27. Garcia V, Eichelberger M, Ziegler M et al: Use of military antishock trouser in child. J Pediatr Surg 16:544, 1981
28. Glenn F, McSherry CK: Congenital segmental dilatation of the biliary ductal system. Ann Surg 177:705, 1973
29. Grosfeld JL, Ballantine TVN, Shoemaker R: Operative management of intestinal atresia and stenosis based on pathologic findings. J Pediatr Surg 14:370, 1969
30. Grosfeld JL, Cooney DR: Inguinal hernia after ventriculo peritoneal shunt for hydrocephalus. J Pediatr Surg 9:311, 1974
31. Grosfeld JL, Weinberger M, Clatworthy HW: Acute appendicitis in the first two years of life. J Pediatr Surg 8:285, 1973
32. Gross RE: Intestinal obstruction in the newborn resulting from meconium ileus. In The Surgery of Infancy and Childhood, pp 175-191. Philadelphia, WB Saunders, 1953
33. Hamilton JP et al: Subtotal pancreatectomy in the management of severe persistent idiopathic hypoglycemia in children. Pediatrics 39:49, 1967
34. Harken AH, Filler RM, Auruskin TW, Crigler JE; The role of "total" pancreatectomy in the treatment of unremitting hypoglycemia of infancy. J Pediatr Surg 6:284, 1971
35. Harrison MW, Connell RS, Campbell JR, Webb MC: Microcirculatory changes in the gastrointestinal tract of the hypoxic puppy: An electron microscope study. J Pediatr Surg 10:599, 1975
36. Haws EB, Sieber WK, Kiesewetter WB: Complications of tube gastrostomy in infants and children—15 years review of 240 cases. Ann Surg 164:284, 1966
37. Hays DM: Intestinal atresia and stenosis. Curr Probl Surg 31:22, 1969
38. Hendren WH et al: Traumatic hemobilia: Nonoperative management with healing documented by serial angiography. Ann Surg 174:991, 1971
39. Hey EN, Katz G: Evaporative water loss in the newborn baby. J Physiol (Lond) 200:605, 1969
40. Holgersen LO, Bishop HC: Nonoperative treatment of duodenal hematoma in childhood. J Pediatr Surg 12:11, 1977
41. Holliday MA, Segan NE: Parenteral Fluid Therapy, 2nd printing. Indianapolis, Indiana University Medical Center, 1956

42. Janik JS, Firor HV: Pediatric appendicitis, a 20-year study of 1,640 children at Cook County Hospital. Arch Surg 114:717, 1979
43. Jona JZ, Belin RP: Duodenal anomalies and the ampulla of Vater. Surg Gynecol Obstet 143:568, 1976
44. Kakos GS, Grosfeld JL, Morse TS: Small bowel injury in children after blunt abdominal trauma. Ann Surg 174:238, 1971
45. Kasai M, Kimura S, Asakura Y et al: Surgical treatment of biliary atresia. J Pediatr Surg 3:665, 1968
46. Kenney RA: Renal function. Pediatr Clin North Am 23:651, 1976
47. Kiesewetter WB: Imperforate anus. In Holder TM, Ashcraft KW (eds): Pediatric Surgery, p 415. Philadelphia, WB Saunders, 1980
48. Kirkpatrick JR: Injuries of the colon. Surg Clin North Am 57:67, 1977
49. Koop CE: Pyloromyotomy for pyloric stenosis. In Cooper P (ed): The Craft of Surgery, 2nd ed, p 1633. Boston, Little, Brown & Co, 1971
50. Koivista M, Blanco–Sequeiros M, Krause M: Neonatal symptomatic and asymptomatic hypoglycemia: A follow-up study of 151 children. Dev Med Child Neurol 14:603, 1972
51. Ladd WE, Gross RE: Malrotation of the intestine. In Abdominal Surgery of Infancy and Childhood. Philadelphia, WB Saunders, 1941
52. Lassaletta L, Fonkalsrud EW, Tovar JA et al: The management of umbilical hernias in infancy and childhood. J Pediatr Surg 10:405, 1975
53. Lilly JR: Total excision of choledochal cyt. Surg Gynecol Obstet 146:254, 1978
54. Lilly JR: In Terblanche J, Yakoob HI, Bornman PC et al (eds): Acute bleeding varices: A five-year prospective evaluation of tamponade and sclerotherapy. Ann Surg 194:530, 1981
55. Louw JH: Resection and end-to-end anastomosis in the management of atresia and stenosis of the small bowel. Surgery 62:940, 1967
56. Louw JH, Barnard CN: Congenital intestinal atresia: Observations on its origin. Lancet 2:1065, 1955
57. Lukash F, Zwiren GT, Andrews HG: Significance of absent vas deferens at hernia repair in infants and children. J Pediatr Surg 10:765, 1975
58. Lynn HB: Rectal myectomy for aganglionic megacolon. Mayo Clin Proc 41:5, 1966
59. Lynn HB: Intussusception. In Holder TM, Ashcroft KW (eds): Pediatric Surgery, p 438. Philadelphia, WB Saunders, 1980
60. McEntyre RL, Raffensperger JG: Surgical complications of Ehlers–Donlas syndrome in children. J Pediatr Surg 12:531, 1977
61. McParland FH, Kisewetter WB: Meckel's diverticulum in childhood. Surg Gynecol Obstet 106:11, 1958
62. Mahboudi S, Kaufman HJ: Intramural duodenal hematoma in children: The role of the radiologist in its conservative management. Gastrointest Radiol 1:167, 1976
63. Marks RM, Sieber WK, Girdany BR: Hydrostatic pressure in the treatment of the ileocolic intussusception in infants and children. J Pediatr Surg 1:566, 1966
64. Martin LW: Surgical management of total colonic aganglionosis. Ann Surg 176:343, 1972
65. Martin LW, Caudill DR: A method for elimination of the blind rectal pouch in the Duhamel operation for Hirschsprung's disease. Surgery 62:951, 1967
66. Mayer T, Black R, Matlak ME, Johnson DG: Gastroschesis and omphalocele: An eight-year review. Ann Surg 6:783, 1980
67. Nisson S, Bar–Moar J, Levy E: Anorectal myomectomy in the treatment of short segment Hirschsprung's disease. Ann Surg 170:969, 1969
68. Nixon HH, Tawes R: Etiology and treatment of small intestinal atresia: Analysis of a series of 127 jejunoileal atresias and comparison with 62 duodenal atresias. Surgery 69:41, 1971
69. Noblett HR: Treatment of uncomplicated meconium ileus by Gastroffin enema: A preliminary report. J Pediatr Surg 4:190, 1969
70. Noblett HR: Meconium ileus. In Ravitch MM, Welch KJ, Benson CD et al (eds): Pediatric Surgery, 3rd ed, pp 943-952. Chicago, Year Book Medical Publishers, 1979
71. O'Neill JA, Grosfeld JL, Boles ET Jr, Clathworthy HW Jr: Surgical treatment of meconium ileus. Am J Surg 119:99, 1970
72. O'Neill JA, Stahlman MT, Meng HC: Necrotizing enterocolitis in the newborn. Ann Surg 182:274, 1975
73. Ramstedt C: Zur operation der angelborenen pylorus—stenose. Med Klin 8:1702, 1912
74. Randolph JG, Lilly JR, Anderson KD: Surgical treatment of gastroesophageal reflux in infants. Ann Surg 180:479, 1974
75. Ravitch MM: Intussusception. In Ravitch MM et al (eds): Pediatric Surgery, 3rd ed, p 992. Chicago, Year Book Medical Publishers, 1979
76. Ravitch MM, Sabiston DC: Anal ileostomy with preservation of the sphincter. Surg Gynecol Obstet 93:87, 1951
77. Rickie SP, Fonkalsrud EW: Subcapsular hematoma of the liver—Nonoperative management. Arch Surg 104:781, 1972
78. Riechard SA, Helikson MA, Shorter N et al: Pelvic fractures in children—Review of 120 patients with a new look at general management. J Pediatr Surg 15:727, 1980
79. Root AW, Harrison HE: Recent advances in calcium metabolism. J Pediatr 88:177, 1976
80. Rosen FS: Neonatal immunity. In Smith CA, Nelson NM (eds): The Physiology of the Newborn Infant, 4th ed, p 740. Springfield, IL, Charles C Thomas, 1976
81. Rowe MI: Physiology of the pediatric surgical patient. In Holder TM, Ashcroft KW (eds): Pediatric Surgery pp 1-24. Philadelphia, WB Saunders, 1980
82. Rowe MI, Buckner D, Clatworthy HW Jr: Windsock web of the duodenum. Am J Surg 116:444, 1968
83. Santulli TV, Schullinger JN, Heird WC et al: Acute necrotizing enterocolitis in infancy: A review of 64 cases. Pediatrics 55:376, 1975
84. Scharli AF, Sieber WK: Surgical approach for the Ramstedt procedure in hypertrophic pyloric stenosis. Surg Gynecol Obstet 128:355, 1969
85. Shaw A: Safety of n-acetyl cysteine in the treatment of meconium obstruction of the newborn. J Pediatr Surg 4:119, 1969
86. Silverman WA, Sinclair JC, Scopes JW: Regulation of body temperature in pediatric surgery. J Pediatr Surg 1:321, 1966
87. Singer DB: Postsplenectomy sepsis. In Rosenbert HS, Bolander RP (eds): Perspectives in Pediatric Pathology, pp 285-305. Chicago, Year Book Medical Publishers, 1973
88. Soave F: Hirschsprung's disease: Clinical evaluation and details of a personal technique. Z Kinderchir (Suppl) 3:66, 1966
89. Solinas ED et al: Functioning islet cell adenoma in the newborn. Pediatrics 41:646, 1968

90. Soltero MJ, Bill AH: The natural history of Meckel's diverticulum and its relation to incidential removal. Am J Surg 132:168, 1976
91. Soper RT, Miller FE: Modification of Duhamel procedure: Elimination of rectal pouch and colorectal septum. J Pediatr Surg 3:376, 1968
92. Stanley–Brown EG, Frank JE: Mercury poisoning from application to omphalocele. JAMA 216:2144, 1971
93. Stewart DR, Colodny AL, Doggett WC: Malrotation of the bowel in infants and children: A fifteen-year review. Surgery 79:716, 1976
94. Stone HH: Preoperative and postoperative case (in hepatic surgery). Surg Clin North Am 57:409, 1977
95. Suruga K et al: A clinical and pathologic study of congenital biliary atresia. J Pediatr Surg 7:655, 1972
96. Swenson O, Sherman JO, Fisher JH, Cohen E: The treatment of postoperative complications of congenital megacolon: 25 year follow-up. Ann Surg 182:266, 1975
97. Thomas CG Jr: Jejunoplasty for correction of jejunal atresia. Surg Gynecol Obstet 129:545, 1969
98. Touloukian RJ: Neonatal necrotizing enterocolitis: An update on etiology, diagnosis, and treatment. Surg Clin North Am 56:281, 1976
99. Vinocur CD, Dinn WM, Dudgeon DL: Computed tomographic scanning in children. J Pediatr Surg 12:847, 1977
100. Wald MK: Problems in chemical adaptation. In Klaus MH, Fanaroff AA (eds): Care of the High-Risk Neonate. Philadelphia, WB Saunders, 1973
101. Wallace WM: Quantitative requirements of the infant and child for water and electrolytes under varying conditions. Am J Clin Pathol 23:1133, 1953
102. Wiedeman HR: E.M.G. syndrome. Lancet 2:626, 1973
103. Wilmore DW: Factors correlating with a successful outcome following extensive intestinal resection in the newborn infant. J Pediatr 80:80, 1972
104. Wolson AH: Ultrasound diagnosis of pelvic and wound abscess after appendectomy. Surg Gynecl Obstet 144:376, 1977
105. Yakovac WC, Baker L, Hummeler K: Beta cell neisidioblastosis in idiopathic hypoglycemia of infancy. J Pediatr 79:226, 1971

36
Complications of Biliary Tract Surgery and Trauma

David L. Nahrwold

OVERVIEW—PREVENTION AND MANAGEMENT OF INJURIES

Most of the complications of biliary tract surgery and of trauma to the biliary tract are related to leakage of bile, obstruction of the duct system, and infection. The surgeon can prevent some of the most serious and vexing postoperative problems by careful attention to detail during the operation. For example, the incision should be sufficiently large to ensure adequate exposure; this is essential to prevent injury to the hepatic artery, portal vein, and bile ducts. Of these, the bile ducts and hepatic artery are more commonly injured. Injury to the right hepatic and main hepatic arteries during dissection of the cystic artery can be avoided by ligating and dividing the cystic artery at its entrance into the gallbladder; this means that often the superficial (anterior) and deep (posterior) branches of the cystic artery will require ligation and division individually. Dissection of the presumptive cystic artery should proceed toward the gallbladder, not away from it. It is both an unnecessary and potentially dangerous routine to dissect out and identify routinely the right hepatic artery to facilitate identification of the cystic artery.

Mistaken identification of the cystic duct may result in injury to the extrahepatic bile ducts. This complication can be avoided by careful dissection of the junction of the cystic duct, common hepatic duct, and common bile duct. The anterior surfaces of the common hepatic duct and the common bile duct should be dissected free 1 cm superiorly and inferiorly to their junction with the cystic duct. Following this, the presumptive cystic duct should be dissected from its entrance into the common duct to its entrance into the gallbladder. Finally, an intraoperative cholangiogram should be done through a catheter placed in the most proximal portion of the cystic duct. It is as important to confirm the presumed anatomy through the use of intraoperative cholangiography as it is to identify calculi in the biliary duct system (Fig. 36-1).

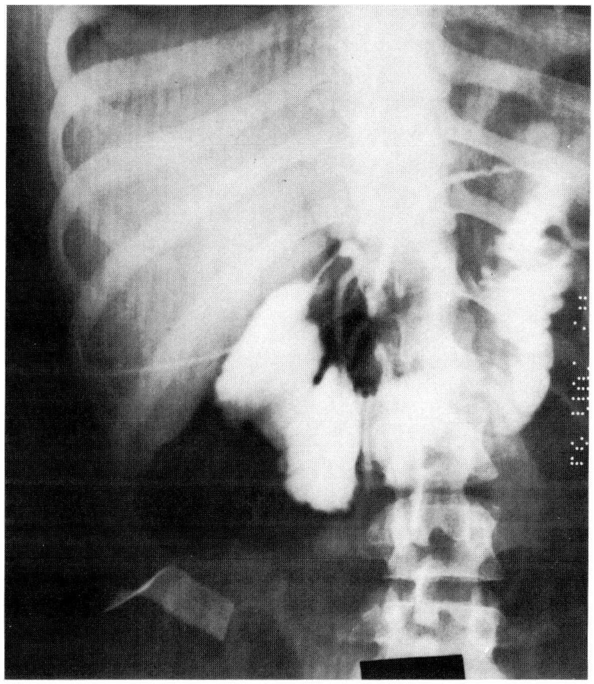

FIG. 36-1. Operative cholangiogram shows filling of the distal common duct, the pancreatic duct, and the duodenum, but not the duct system in the liver. Unknowingly, the surgeon placed the catheter in the common duct, which had been mistaken for the cystic duct.

IMMEDIATE REPAIR OF INJURIES

Any injury to the hepatic artery, portal vein, or bile ducts should be repaired immediately. Vascular clamps should be used to obtain control of hemorrhage, following which the artery or vein can be repaired with 6-0 monofilament suture. Magnification and microsurgical technique are usually necessary to repair an injured hepatic artery. Because, in some patients, ligation of the hepatic artery may result in hepatic necrosis and death, an attempt at repair should always be made.

Bile duct injuries that involve only a portion of the circumference of the duct can be repaired by interrupted 4-0 polyglycolic acid sutures. One limb of a large T tube should be placed through the repaired area. It is preferable to insert the tube proximal to the injury, but this cannot always be done.

When the common bile duct or common hepatic duct has been injured severely, primary repair may not be possible. In this case, the distal end of the duct should be sewn off, and the proximal end implanted into the intestine as a choledochoduodenostomy, or, if this requires too much tension, as a Roux-en-Y choledochojejunostomy. Either of these anastomoses should be splinted with a T tube placed into the duct proximal to the anastomosis. When the anastomosis is done to a large, obstructed duct, a splint is not needed; however, injury most often occurs during cholecystectomy in patients with ducts of normal caliber.

BILIARY TRACT TRAUMA

Iatrogenic injuries of the biliary tract are more common than are injuries sustained as the result of blunt or penetrating trauma. Organs adjacent to the biliary tract, such as the liver, duodenum, and pancreas, are frequently injured concomitantly, and therefore the complications of biliary tract trauma are not always due to injury of the biliary tract itself.

Blunt trauma to the upper abdomen may cause rupture, contusion, or avulsion of the gallbladder. Penetrating wounds result in lacerations. Injuries of the gallbladder should be treated by cholecystectomy. Unless it is very small, there is no reason to close a gallbladder laceration primarily. The complications of injury to the gallbladder are essentially the same as those of cholecystectomy done for disease of the gallbaldder, and they are discussed below.

Injuries to the extrahepatic duct system most commonly result from penetrating trauma and usually are associated with injuries to adjacent organs. The duct system may be lacerated, transected, or in the case of missile injuries, blown apart or avulsed. The injuries due to blunt trauma, which are very rare, usually result in transection of the common hepatic duct immediately distal to the confluence of the hepatic ducts or transection of the common bile duct near its entrance into the pancreas. Blunt extrahepatic bile duct injuries frequently are associated with a tear in the second portion of the duodenum. Surgical therapy for injuries of the extrahepatic duct system consists of primary closure of lacerations or, if this is not possible, restoration of bile flow from the liver to the intestine by primary ductal anastomosis, choledochoduodenostomy, or Roux-en-Y choledochojejunostomy. When these procedures are performed for trauma, the complications are similar to those that occur when they are undertaken for biliary tract disease.

Bile Leaks and Fistulas

ETIOLOGY AND PATHOGENESIS

Although most bile leaks from the liver or biliary duct system are the direct result of the surgical procedure, occasionally they are due to preexisting conditions. The most common site of leakage after cholecystectomy is the raw liver surface of the gallbladder bed. Leakage from the gallbladder bed occurs most often in patients who have severe chronic cholecystitis with extension of the inflammation and subsequent fibrosis into the hepatic parenchyma behind the gallbladder. This fibrosis and scar contraction pull one or more of the adjacent intrahepatic bile ducts toward the gallbladder where it is likely to be cut during the course of cholecystectomy.

Slippage of the ligature placed on the cystic duct at the time of cholecystectomy is a cause of postoperative bile leak, but it is rare. More often, there is leakage adjacent the cystic duct from inadvertent injury at the crotch formed by the junction of the cystic duct with the common hepatic duct. Since this injury is small and usually occurs on the posterolateral surface of the confluence of the ducts, it is not recognized easily at the time of surgery. The other common location of unrecognized injury is the distal common duct, where a perforation may occur during duct exploration. Usually, the perforation is made in the posterior aspect of the intrapancreatic portion of the common bile duct, an area not always surrounded by pancreatic tissue.

Other sites of possible leakage of bile after biliary tract surgery are at anastomoses between the gallbladder or a bile duct and intestine or at the site of insertion of a tube into the gallbladder or a bile duct.

The advent of percutaneous transhepatic cholangiography has introduced a new type of postoperative leak that, although rare, may be devastating to the patient. When this procedure is performed in the patient who has complete bile duct obstruction due to carcinoma of the pancreas or distal common duct, leakage from the hepatic puncture wound is not unusual. At laparotomy a few days after the cholangiogram there may be some bile stained peritoneal fluid, which may be mistaken for ascitic fluid in a jaundiced patient rather than seen as bilious ascites from the leaking puncture wound. If there is no hope for cure and a palliative cholecystojejunostomy is done, a small amount of pressure must be developed within the biliary duct system to enable bile to flow through the valves of Heister, through the gallbladder, and into the small intestine. This pressure may be sufficient to keep the hepatic puncture wound open, in which case the patient will develop bilious ascites and possibly bile peritonitis. Clearly, it is important to examine the lateral and superior aspects of the liver in patients who have had percutaneous transhepatic cholangiography for complete bile duct obstruction. If the puncture wound can be found, it should be closed with absorbable sutures.

CLINICAL MANIFESTATIONS

A drain, placed at operation, usually will control a bile leak and convert it to an external biliary fistula. Not all leaks will drain to the exterior, however; the drain may not be located immediately adjacent the leak, or it may become sealed off from the leaking duct by adjacent organs or adhesions. Depending on the amount of bile and the persistence of the leak, an accumulation of bile may be walled off in the upper abdomen, or the bile may spread throughout the peritoneal cavity.

Bile leaks have two general types of clinical presentations.[16] One is abrupt, with circulatory collapse early in the postoperative period, usually within 48 hours of surgery. Pain may be severe and generalized throughout the abdomen, or it may be absent. The physical findings usually include abdominal distention, but the presence and severity of tenderness to palpation vary. Because of the recent operation the abdominal findings may be difficult to interpret. The characteristic feature of this presentation is the presence of shock early in the postoperative period.

The second type of clinical presentation is insidious, with the development of symptoms as early as 4 or 5 days after the operation in some patients, or delayed for several weeks in others. Shock is not typical, and the symptoms are variable. Abdominal pain is often present; it may be episodic or constant, severe or mild. The location of pain is usually in the right upper quadrant or epigastrium, often with radiation to the right shoulder. A few patients have no pain. Nausea, vomiting, and a sensation of abdominal fullness may be present. In some patients the only clinical manifestation is that recovery from the surgical procedure does not progress at the anticipated rate. Physical examination may reveal mild jaundice, tachycardia, and abdominal distention. When there is bile duct obstruction or the leak is large, the stools will be acholic. The signs of ascites may be present. Elevation of the right diaphragm and rales in the right lung base may reflect upward pressure on the liver by a large collection of bile.

There is no relationship between the two types of clinical presentations and the presence or absence of localization of the leaking bile. Early and abrupt shock with severe abdominal pain and rigidity may occur in the patient with an accumulation of bile confined entirely to the subhepatic space or in another with bile spread throughout the abdominal cavity. By the same token, tense bile ascites may be present for several weeks with only mild symptoms and no circulatory collapse.[20] The causes of these paradoxes are unknown, but they could be related to the presence or absence of bacteria in the bile, the types and proportions of bile acids present, the rate of leakage into the peritoneal cavity, and other as yet undetermined factors. Circulatory collapse could be due to septicemia, loss of plasma volume by sequestration of several liters of bile in the abdominal cavity, absorption of large amounts of bile acids or other potentially toxic bile constituents from the peritoneum into the circulation, and several other processes. The mechanism probably is not the same in all patients.

The diagnosis requires a high degree of suspicion. The serum bilirubin may be elevated, but there is no characteristic pattern to the conjugated and unconjugated fractions. If the leak is due to biliary duct obstruction, the alkaline phosphatase will be elevated. Chest x-ray examination may show elevation of the right hemidiaphragm and atelectasis in the lower lobe of the right lung. Ultrasonography may be useful to delineate localized accumulations of bile (Fig. 36-2) and the presence of free bile in the abdominal cavity. The most direct and useful procedure in the diagnosis of bile ascites is abdominal paracentesis. Obviously, no fluid may be found when the bile is sequestered as a localized collection.

MANAGEMENT

Unless a bile leak is controlled by a drain, an operation should be planned as soon as the diagnosis is established or strongly suspected. The objectives of surgery are to evacuate the bile, to close the leak, and to remove its cause. In a large series of patients with postoperative bile leakage, the source was found in only about half.[16] In most cases, percutaneous transhepatic cholangiography will delineate the site of the leak. If this is not technically feasible, endoscopic retrograde cholangiography should be done. Every effort must be made to determine whether there is obstruction of the biliary duct system distal to the leak, because it is essential to relieve the obstruction when the leak is closed. Fur-

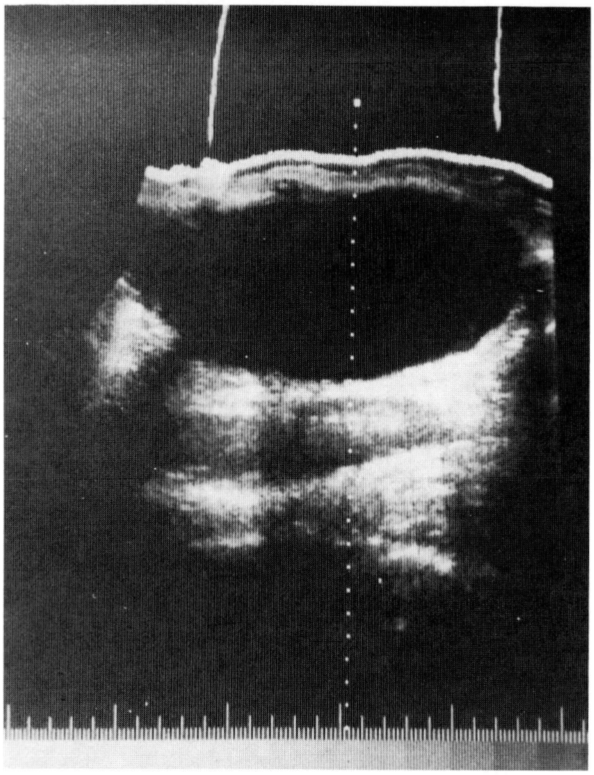

FIG. 36-2. Sonogram shows a large, localized collection of bile in the upper abdomen following cholecystectomy.

ther, if the leak is due to inadvertent transection of either a normal or anomalous bile duct, preoperative cholangiography will delineate the anatomy, and plans for reconstruction can be made preoperatively (Fig. 36-3). Preoperative antibiotic coverage should be instituted.

The bile should be cultured for aerobic and anaerobic organisms at operation and then completely evacuated. If the procedure was a cholecystectomy, the gallbladder bed, cystic duct stump, and all other areas of dissection should be examined carefully for the site of the leak. A leaking cystic duct or duct in the gallbladder bed should be ligated. If it was not done preoperatively, cholangiography will be necessary to check for distal duct obstruction, and choledocholithotomy or other appropriate procedure should be performed concomitantly. If the leak is due to severance of a major bile duct, it is important to dissect the entire extrahepatic duct system and possibly perform a cholangiogram to confirm the anatomy and choose the method of reconstruction. Usually, when a major normal or anomalous duct has been divided, it will be necessary to anastomose the proximal duct to a Roux-en-Y limb of jejunum, or, if it can be done without tension, directly to the duodenum (Fig. 36-4). We prefer to introduce a T

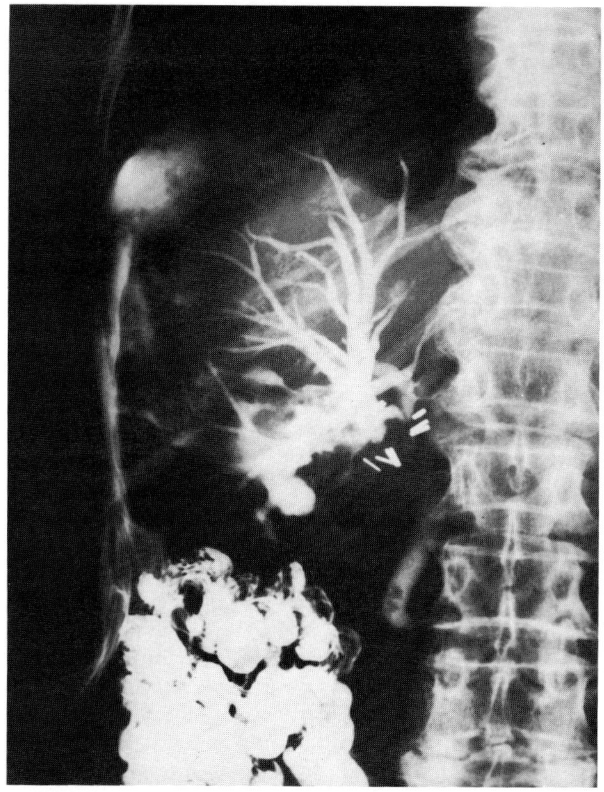

FIG. 36-3. Percutaneous transhepatic cholangiogram 7 days after cholecystectomy shows extravasation of contrast material from the partially transected common hepatic duct. Note the contrast material in the subphrenic space.

FIG. 36-4. Two methods of biliary tract reconstruction. (*A*) Choledochoduodenostomy. (*B*) Roux-en-Y choledochojejunostomy.

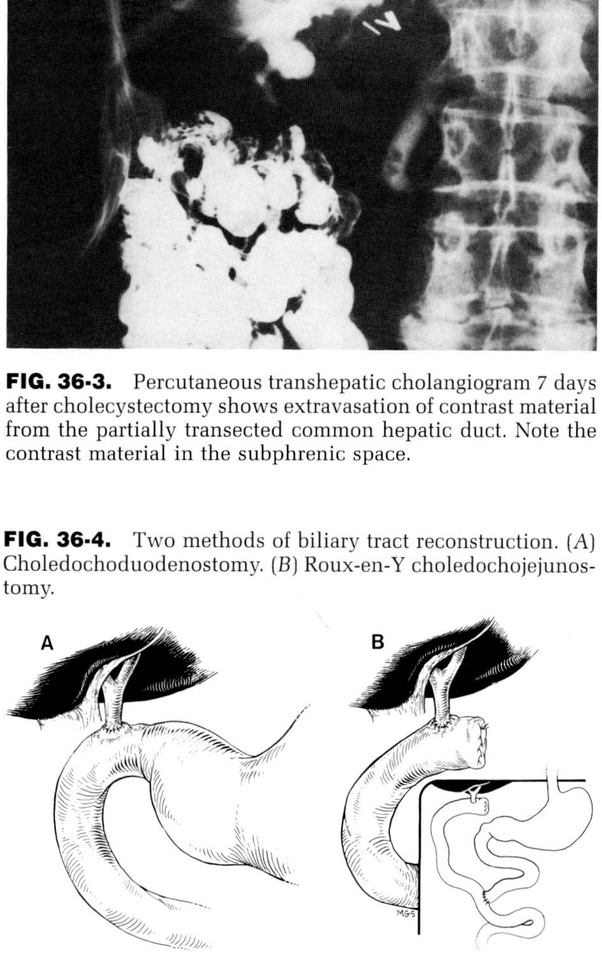

tube proximal to these anastomoses and insert one limb through the anastomosis. One or two U tubes may be used to splint a Roux-en-Y hepaticojejunostomy if the common hepatic duct or either hepatic duct was severed. One end is brought to the outside through the liver and the other through a Witzel enterostomy in the Roux-en-Y limb of jejunum. This technique is especially useful when there is insufficient room to insert a T tube proximal to the anastomosis. A two-layer anastomosis with careful apposition of mucosa to mucosa is preferable. Direct end-to-end or end-to-side anastomosis of bile ducts is almost never possible unless repair is undertaken at the time of injury.

When a bile leak is completely controlled by a drain, it is, by definition, an external biliary fistula. A fistula will close unless there is obstruction distal to the site of the leak. However, it is rarely possible to be certain that a leak is completely controlled by the drain. Thus, if drainage continues for more than 3 to 5 days, percutaneous transhepatic cholangiography or endoscopic retrograde cholangiography should be carried out, and whether to operate should be decided on the basis of the radiographic findings, as well as on the clinical course of the patient.

Postoperative Biliary Obstruction

ETIOLOGY AND PATHOGENESIS

Inadvertent, unrecognized ligation of a major bile duct is an uncommon, but serious cause of bile duct obstruction, which becomes manifest very early in the postoperative period. Excessive traction on the cystic duct during application of a clamp or ligation may result in tenting of the wall of the common duct and inclusion of a portion of its circumference in the ligature. This may be associated with failure to dissect and identify completely the junction of the cystic duct with the common hepatic duct and the common bile duct. Another cause of partial or complete ligation of a major duct is the imprecise application of a clamp in attempts to control major bleeding. Finally, the common hepatic or common bile duct may be ligated, divided, and partially excised when it has been mistaken for the cystic duct. Fortunately, with increasing frequency, this error is being recognized, and successful reconstruction is being done at the time of injury.

Most often, postoperative bile duct obstruction is due to a stone or stones. The obstruction may become manifest either in the immediate postoperative period or many years later. The incidence of "retained" or residual stones is reduced by routine use of operative cholangiography at the time of cholecystectomy, and by the performance of a completion cholangiogram through the T tube during choledocholithotomy.[19] The best evidence suggests that most common duct stones migrate from the gallbladder and grow to a larger size in the common duct. Fewer stones, about 5%, form *de novo* in the common duct after cholecystectomy. These tend to be soft, with an earthy appearance. They are amorphous and do not have the faceted appearance of the typical cholesterol stones found in the gallbladder.[22]

Very rarely, the development of a stricture after biliary tract surgery may be the result of an unrecognized injury to an extrahepatic duct. More frequently, stricture formation occurs at the site of an anastomosis in the duct system. The incidence of stricture can be minimized by the meticulous use of a two-layer technique when the duct is anastomosed to intestine and by splinting the anastomosis with a tube for about 8 weeks. In addition to stricture, the poorly constructed anastomosis leads to bile stasis, infection, and eventually stone formation.

In the absence of a previous suture line, extrahepatic bile duct strictures are nearly always located in the distal portion of the common duct. When the primary operation is done for obstruction due to stones impacted in the distal duct, mucosal damage and scarring from the presence of the stone, aggravated by instrumental trauma during choledocholithotomy, may lead to postoperative stricture. To circumvent the potential problems associated with stricture formation, some advocate concomitant choledochoduodenostomy or sphincteroplasty.[17] Pancreatitis, which may be associated with common duct stones or, much less common, result from operative trauma during biliary tract surgery, may cause a stricture in the intrapancreatic portion of the common duct (Fig. 36-5).

Finally, duct obstruction may result from complications associated with the use of tubes (Fig. 36-6). The proximal limb of the T tube inadvertently may be directed into the cystic duct stump, or, if it is too long, it may extend into one of the hepatic ducts. Either limb may be inserted so that it is kinked. Clearly, malposition of T tubes usually can be avoided by completion cholangiography, but if these technical errors are undetected, obstruction may result.

CLINICAL MANIFESTATIONS

Although the signs and symptoms of postoperative bile duct obstruction depend on the cause, jaundice is frequently the first clinical indication during the early postoperative period that all is not well. When a major bile duct has been ligated inadvertently, the patient becomes jaundiced within a day or two and remains so until the obstruction is relieved. Usually there are no other symptoms or signs save for the absence of bile in the nasogastric tube aspirate. Although the presence of bile in the aspirate rules out

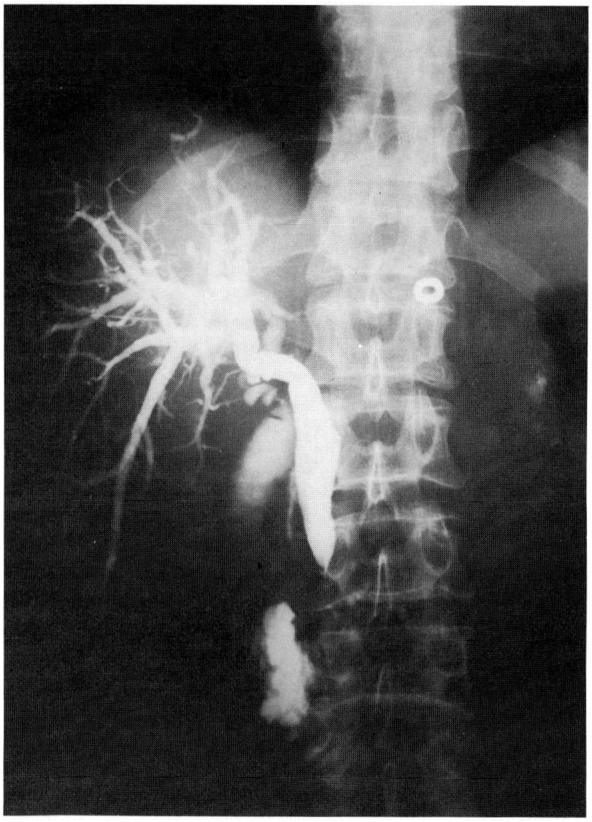

FIG. 36-5. Percutaneous transhepatic cholangiogram in a patient with chronic pancreatitis shows a stricture in the distal common bile duct.

FIG. 36-6. A malpositioned T tube may result in obstruction, inadequate drainage, or both. (*A*) Proximal limb directed into the cystic duct stump. (*B*) Proximal limb cut too long and directed into the right hepatic duct. (*C*) Proximal limb cut too long and kinked.

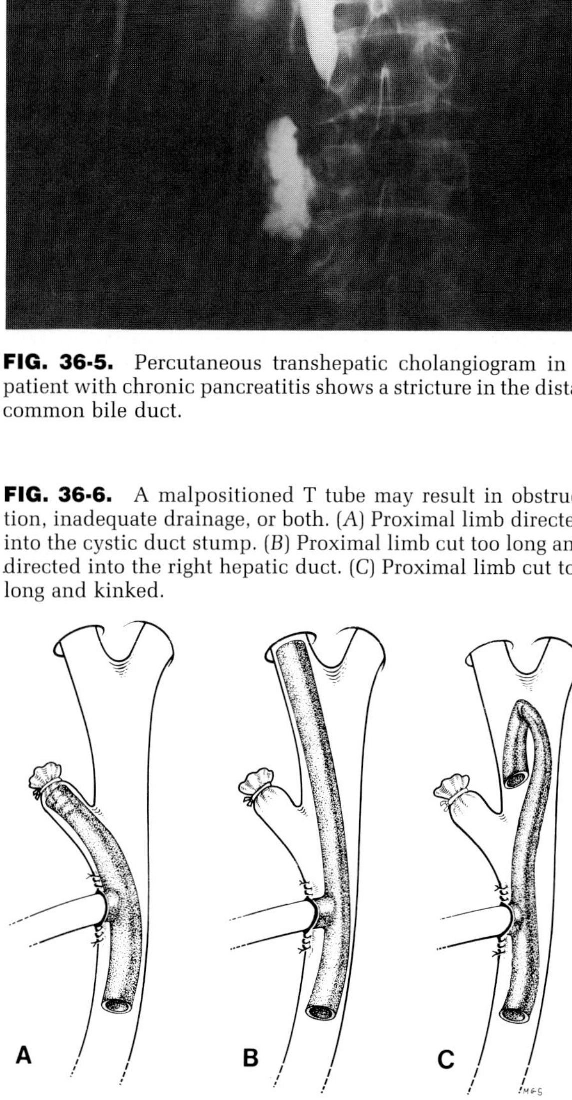

complete obstruction, the absence of bile is only supportive evidence for this diagnosis.

In the immediate postoperative period, obstruction due to stones almost always occurs in patients who have a T tube in place. When obstruction is complete, the first sign is an increase in the daily volume of bile drained by the tube, but this is not specific because resumption of a relatively normal diet also increases the volume of bile. Most stones overlooked at the time of choledochotomy will be found in the distal common duct, so that jaundice and a decrease in the volume of T-tube bile from a stone proximal to the T tube is rare. A stone proximal to the T tube usually does not cause complete obstruction.

Obstruction due to stones months or years after biliary tract surgery is rarely complete. The stone will be single in about half the cases, and when there is complete obstruction a stone will be impacted in the distal common duct. The signs and symptoms of retained stone do not differ from those of primary choledocholithiasis in patients who have had no previous biliary tract surgery. Jaundice, recurrent right upper quadrant colic, and chills and fever are the classic clinical findings. The chills and fever are manifestations of cholangitis, which may be so severe as to be associated with bacteremia. Sometimes the only symptom is vague dyspepsia; the discovery of retained stones does not necessarily mean that the symptoms were caused by the stones. Patients can harbor common duct stones for many years without symptoms. Any of these symptoms in the patient who has had a biliary tract operation is cause for further investigation.

The development of a stricture at an anastomosis between the common hepatic duct or the common duct and the small intestine is heralded by the same signs and symptoms caused by retained stone, namely, jaundice, chills and fever, upper abdominal pain, or dyspepsia. These symptoms also occur in strictures secondary to operative trauma or pancreatitis. Stasis in the biliary duct system predisposes patients to formation of sludge and stones proximal to the stricture; thus, minimal narrowing may culminate in complete obstruction from stones.

When postoperative biliary obstruction is due to malposition of a T tube, the clinical manifestations include jaundice and little or no output of bile from the T tube. The absence of T-tube drainage is evident immediately and can be discovered prior to completion of the operation.

DIAGNOSIS

Although the development of jaundice during the postoperative period is cause for serious concern, in most cases, emergency procedures are not needed.

The exceptions are when jaundice is accompanied by absent or scant T-tube drainage and when acute suppurative cholangitis has developed in the patient who does not have a T tube in place. It is essential to perform T-tube cholangiography immediately when the tube is not draining normal amounts of bile, because, if the tube is displaced from the duct, immediate operation to replace it is indicated. Malpositioned or kinked tubes also may require correction on an emergency basis. Acute suppurative cholangitis must be treated by emergency decompression and drainage of the biliary duct system.[7]

With these exceptions, the postoperative, jaundiced patient should have liver function tests to rule out nonobstructive causes such as transfusion hemolysis, jaundice associated with significant concomitant liver disease such as cirrhosis, and the jaundice that sometimes accompanies septicemia in patients who had sepsis preoperatively. Clearly, a T-tube cholangiogram should be done in all patients who have a tube in place. In those who do not, further investigation is necessary if serum conjugated bilirubin and alkaline phosphatase concentrations are elevated. Ultrasound examination is not likely to be helpful because the bile ducts do not dilate immediately. Either percutaneous transhepatic or endoscopic retrograde cholangiography is essential. The transhepatic route is preferred because visualization of the point of obstruction with the proximal duct system as a reference is more useful in planning a corrective procedure. Absence of dilatation of the intrahepatic ducts may preclude this route, however, and the endoscopic retrograde cholangiogram may be necessary, even though the nature of the obstruction is less easily discerned by this method.

As mentioned previously, an increase in the volume of T-tube drainage is a sign of overlooked stones. However, most overlooked stones do not give rise to signs or symptoms while the T tube is in place and draining. For this reason, a cholangiogram always should be done prior to removal of the tube, even though the intraoperative completion cholangiogram was normal. Also, discovery of an overlooked stone prior to removal of the tube preserves certain therapeutic options.

Progressive postoperative jaundice in the absence of ductal obstruction may be due to inadvertent ligation or division of the hepatic artery or one of its major branches. If the etiology of the jaundice is not clear, selective hepatic artery angiography is indicated and is especially urgent if technical difficulties or unexplained hemorrhage occurred at the time of surgery. While there is still controversy in the literature over whether the hepatic artery can be ligated in humans without sequelae, many experienced surgeons have observed necrosis of all or a portion of the liver after its arterial blood supply has been interrupted.

When symptoms of obstruction occur months or years after operation, the investigation should begin with liver function tests to determine whether serum conjugated bilirubin and alkaline phosphatase are elevated. Obviously, nonobstructive jaundice must be ruled out. Ultrasound examination of the liver and porta hepatis should be done to determine whether the ducts are dilated. Ductal dilatation is almost always present when there have been symptoms for 3 or more months. When the ducts are dilated, percutaneous transhepatic cholangiography should follow. Some have advised that the catheter should be left in place for decompression, particularly in patients who are completely obstructed.[10] To date there have been no controlled studies to show that this is advantageous to the patient. Endoscopic retrograde cholangiography is the less attractive alternative when percutaneous transhepatic cholangiography is unsuccessful or not possible. Thus, the key to diagnosis in late biliary tract obstruction is cholangiography. Once the nature of the problem—stones, neoplasm, or stricture—is discerned, the most efficacious procedure can then be planned.

THERAPY

Urgent reoperation is indicated in the immediate postoperative period if a major duct has been ligated or divided. Necrosis and perforation proximal to the ligature will occur in some patients, resulting in bile peritonitis and a proximal stump of questionable integrity for a reconstructive anastomosis. Thus, as soon as the patient is diagnosed and properly prepared, an operation should be undertaken. If the duct has been ligated but not transected, it may be possible to remove the ligature and place a T tube in the common duct with one limb through the ligated area. When there is too much damage from the ligature, the affected area may be excised and an end-to-end anastomosis done. Although it is desirable to do a two-layer anastomosis, generally this is not possible, and a single layer of simple, interrupted sutures of fine polyglycolic acid should be used. Magnification is very helpful in the performance of bile duct anastomoses.

Complete transections of the common duct or common hepatic duct rarely can be repaired by end-to-end anastomosis because so often a segment of duct has been excised. The distal end must be ligated with nonabsorbable material and the proximal end anastomosed either to the side of the duodenum or, if this cannot be done without tension, to a Roux-en-Y limb of jejunum. The cut end of the limb should be closed and the anastomosis done to the side of the jejunum an inch or two distal to the closure. Anastomosis of a bile duct to a loop of jejunum not fashioned into a Roux-en-Y limb is inadvisable because of the high incidence of cholangitis. The anastomosis of bile duct to duodenum or jejunum should be splinted with a T tube placed into the duct proximal to the suture line unless the duct and anastomosis are extremely large. The tube may be removed in about 6 weeks if a cholangiogram before removal is normal.

Attempts should be made to repair a transected or ligated hepatic artery. Magnification and microsurgical technique are essential. The distal segment may contain clots, which can be removed by passage of a small balloon catheter. Débridement of necrotic liver tissue and drainage are necessary.

Dislocation of a T tube within the first 5 postoperative days requires immediate reoperation and reinsertion of the tube. The likelihood of bile peritonitis and its potential mortality rate are too high to treat this complication nonoperatively during the early postoperative period, but if dislocation occurs after 5 days, the tube may be removed and the patient observed carefully for signs and symptoms of bile ascites or peritonitis. The same general guidelines apply to reoperation for the malpositioned T tube that is associated with complete bile duct obstruction.

The treatment of overlooked or retained stones varies with the circumstances under which they are discovered. The most common situation is the discovery of a retained stone or stones on the postoperative cholangiogram prior to the anticipated removal of the T tube. At present the definitive treatment of choice is extraction of the stones through the T-tube tract under fluoroscopic guidance.[5] This procedure requires that the T-tube tract be allowed to mature for 5 to 7 weeks, during which spontaneous passage is possible. Spontaneous passage of a stone is especially likely if its diameter is not larger than 7 mm, the duct lumen is less than 1.4 cm in diameter, and if there is no sharp angulation or stenosis in the intrapancreatic portion of the common bile duct.[23] Under these circumstances the T tube may be clamped. On the other hand, spontaneous passage is unlikely if the stone is more than 10 mm in diameter, especially if there are multiple stones, or if there is narrowing of the distal common duct. A choledochal sphincter yield pressure of over 13 cm of water, measured by simple manometry, also reduces the likelihood of spontaneous passage.[23] When these factors are present, caution should be exercised in clamping the T tube because cholangitis and obstructive jaundice may ensue. To facilitate the patient's return to normal activity, the open T tube may be attached to a plastic bile drainage bag worn at the waist. Care must be taken to encourage supplemental fluid and salt intake if the drainage is significant, particularly in the elderly.

After the tract has matured, the T tube is removed, and attempts are made to extract the stone or stones with the use of a basketing device. The procedure is facilitated by concomitant cholangiography. Stones may be crushed and the choledochal sphincter dilated to facilitate removal through the T-tube tract or passage into the duodenum, respectively. Successful removal of retained stones is possible in about 95% of patients.

Retained or recurrent stones also can be treated by endoscopic papillotomy, a procedure in which a wire-cutting device is inserted through the endoscope and used to cut the papilla of Vater by means of an electric current.[21] In experienced hands endoscopic papillotomy is successful in over 90% of patients. To date there have been serious complications, including death, duodenal perforation, pancreatitis, and hemorrhage. While the incidence of deaths and complications undoubtedly will decline with refinement of the technique and experience, the efficacy and precise indications for endoscopic papillotomy presently are not known. An obvious place for the procedure is in patients who have complete obstruction due to a stone impacted in the distal common duct and in whom the T-tube tract has not matured or is too small for extraction by this route.

Another alternative is the chemical dissolution of retained stones. Many agents have been tried, but in recent years the focus has been on perfusion of the duct with cholic acid or monooctanoin, both of which dissolve cholesterol.[25] Although cholate perfusion does dissolve stones in patients, monooctanoin dissolves gallstones more than twice as fast *in vitro* and appears to be effective and safe when perfused into the common duct through the T tube.[15] Recently, monooctanoin has been perfused into the common ducts of patients after T-tube removal by means of catheters inserted into the hepatic duct system percutaneously.[14]

The last resort is reoperation and choledocholithotomy. As the newer modalities are refined, the necessity for secondary operations probably will decrease.

Common duct stones that become manifest months or years after biliary tract surgery traditionally have been removed surgically. Primary common duct stones, which have an earthy appearance and are not faceted, are usually associated with marked common duct dilatation and are presumed to be due to stasis resulting from a faulty choledochal sphincter apparatus. Most experts advise that choledochoduodenostomy be performed at the time of stone removal to prevent recurrence, but this view is not universally held.

Although surgical therapy remains the standard

treatment for choledocholithiasis, endoscopic papillotomy is an attractive alternative. Prospective comparisons of the risks, efficacy, and long-term results will be necessary to determine which procedure is best.

Strictures are usually located in the distal common duct and are treated expeditiously and successfully by choledochoduodenostomy. Those more proximal usually require Roux-en-Y hepaticojejunostomy.

Infection

Sepsis and complications associated with infection are among the leading causes of death and morbidity after biliary tract operations. The reason that infectious complications are prevalent is that bacteria are present in the bile of many patients with diseases of the gallbladder and biliary ducts. In healthy persons, bacteria apparently enter the portal venous system from the bowel, are filtered by the liver, and are disposed of by its reticuloendothelial cell system. The precise mechanism by which bacteria enter bile in patients with extrahepatic biliary tract disease is unknown, but certain patients are more apt to harbor bacteria in their bile (bacterbilia) than others. Bacterbilia has been found in more than 50% of patients with certain types of biliary tract pathology, including acute cholecystitis, choleocholithiasis, and obstructive jaundice.[6] In patients who undergo elective cholecystectomy and do not have common duct stones or obstruction, the approximate incidence ranges from 15% to 25%.[12, 18] A definite relationship with age has been noted; the incidence of about 5% at age 20 progressively rises to about 90% at age 90.

A variety of organisms are found in the bile of patients with biliary tract disease. *Escherichia coli, Streptococcus viridans*, group D streptococci, *Klebsiella pneumoniae*, and *Enterobacter cloacae* comprise about 80% of the organisms cultured in several studies.[4, 8, 18]

ANTIBIOTIC PROPHYLAXIS

The incidence of septic complications following biliary tract surgery is reduced markedly by the prophylactic use of antibiotics. The demonstration of a relationship between bacterbilia and septic complications and the identification of groups of patients likely to have bacterbilia have led to two approaches to the use of antibiotics. One is to administer antibiotics to all patients who have acute cholecystitis, choledocholithiasis, or obstructive jaundice or who are over age 65. The rationale here is to use prophylaxis in patients who have more than a 50% chance of harboring bacteria in their bile. The other, more recent, approach is to perform a Gram stain on bile aspirated at the time of surgery and to institute antibiotic prophylaxis immediately if organisms are detected. Several studies have shown that organisms are seen on the Gram stain in almost 90% of patients who have bacterbilia.[4, 13] Both approaches are acceptable at present. The choice of antibiotic or combination of antibiotics varies among surgeons. We prefer a cephalosporin, currently cefazolin, in the dose of 1 g, intravenously, 30 minutes before operation or at the time of a positive Gram-stain report. No additional doses are given unless the operation is unduly long or attendant with a blood loss of more than 2000 ml.

Some antibiotics such as ampicillin and the cephalosporins are excreted by the liver and appear in high concentrations in bile. This characteristic is thought to be advantageous in biliary tract infections, but serum concentrations are also important, because antibiotics in bile cannot enter the obstructed, inflamed gallbladder, nor are they excreted into bile in patients with obstructive jaundice.

WOUND INFECTION

The simplest and most common septic complication is infection of the incision. The incidence is lower after simple cholecystectomy than after operations in which the biliary tract has been opened, such as choledocholithotomy. Drains and tubes should not be brought to the exterior through the incision because this practice increases the incidence of wound infection.

Wound infection is diagnosed by the usual findings of redness, swelling and tenderness. Fever and persistent elevation of the white blood cell count should prompt a careful examination of the wound. The treatment is to open the wound and irrigate it thoroughly free of purulent material. Many surgeons prefer to pack the open wound with gauze impregnated with povidone-iodine and to teach the patient to change the packing twice daily.

Clostridial wound infections are especially serious because they are associated with a very high mortality rate. *Clostridium perfringens*, an anaerobe that is found in a small percentage of patients who have bacterbilia, is the organism most frequently cultured from clostridial wound infections following biliary tract surgery. Other clostridial species may be found alone or in association with *Clostridium perfringens*. These uncommon infections develop during the first 2 postoperative days and are manifested by a high spiking fever and toxicity that may progress rapidly to delirium. The wound is tender and swollen and may exude a brownish discharge with a characteristic "sweet" odor. Crepitation is unusual. Gram-positive rods are seen on Gram stain.

The wound should be opened under anesthesia and débrided in a radical manner, excising all devitalized tissue. Intravenous penicillin, 20 million units per day, and intravenous tetracycline, 500 mg, every 6 hours, should be initiated as soon as the diagnosis is made. Erythromycin and clindamycin also have activity against clostridial organisms. Hyperbaric oxygen may be a useful adjunct, but gas gangrene antitoxin is not beneficial.

INTRA-ABDOMINAL COLLECTIONS AND ABSCESS

Leakage of small amounts of blood, lymph, bile, and peritoneal fluid in various combinations probably occurs after most biliary tract operations. Usually, these fluids migrate to the exterior by way of the drain placed in the area at the time of surgery. Localized collections of fluid occur when the drain does not function properly or is not located adjacent the source of leakage. When bacteria are present in the bile and contamination of the fluid has occurred, an intra-abdominal abscess may result, usually located in the subhepatic space. Continued leakage of infected fluid results in spreading peritonitis; this is especially likely in the case of a bile leak, as discussed previously. More often, the fluid collection or purulent material becomes localized and produces symptoms of right upper quadrant or epigastric pain and a sensation of upper abdominal fullness, which may be more pronounced after eating. Both a fluid collection and an abscess may cause jaundice as well as nausea and vomiting because of pressure on the extrahepatic duct system and on the stomach and duodenum. Fever is more likely associated with abscess.

On physical examination there is tenderness in the right upper quadrant and epigastrium, and a mass or sensation of fullness may be present.

The white blood cell count is usually elevated in patients with an abscess, or, when it is normal, there may be a shift to more immature forms. Plain abdominal and chest x-ray films may show elevation of the right hemidiaphragm, right pleural effusion, an upper abdominal mass, or gas bubbles in the right upper quadrant (Fig. 36-7). Upper gastrointestinal series with barium sometimes will show pressure on the stomach or duodenum by the mass. Computed tomography and ultrasound examination are especially helpful; they are the diagnostic procedures of choice when a fluid collection or abscess is suspected. The gallium scan has limited value in the early postoperative period.

The treatment of fluid collections and abscesses is drainage. Reoperation and thorough drainage should be carried out as soon as the diagnosis is made. Recently, abscesses and fluid collections have been drained by means of insertion of a catheter into the mass percutaneously with the aid of computed tomography or ultrasound. This approach, which obviates a surgical procedure, was successful in 89% of a group of 40 patients but must be considered an experimental approach at this time.[24] A full course of antibiotic therapy should be initiated at the time

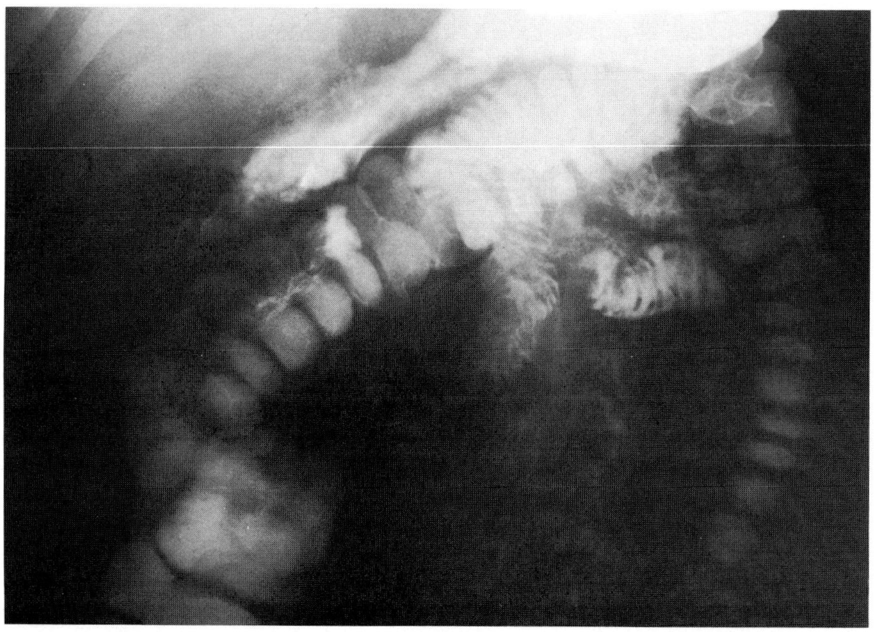

FIG. 36-7. Gas bubbles adjacent to the duodenum in a patient with a subhepatic abscess following cholecystectomy.

a postoperative intra-abdominal abscess is discovered. Our initial therapy is intravenously administered ampicillin, clindamycin, and tobramycin.

CHOLANGITIS

Clinically recognizable cholangitis occurs in the presence of bacterbilia and stasis within the biliary duct system, and it is usually the result of obstruction. Not all the clinical findings of fever, chills, upper abdominal pain, jaundice, and leukocytosis are manifested in every patient; but some indication of inflammation, such as chills, fever, or leukocytosis, is a requisite for the clinical diagnosis.

Cholangitis is frequently associated with postoperative cholangiography. The usual presentation is fever or a chill noted within a few hours after the performance of a T-tube cholangiogram. Experimental studies have shown that an increase in biliary tract pressure, such as might occur during rapid injection of contrast material, causes reflux from the bile ducts into the hepatic venous system, and that reflux of particles similar in size to bacteria is possible under these conditions.[11] Thus, cholangitis may be associated with bacteremia and may produce the clinical syndrome of gram-negative septicemia with hypotension, tachycardia, and delirium. Obviously, care should be exercised during postoperative cholangiography to maintain sterile technique and to avoid rapid injection and high pressures, especially when there is reason to suspect duct obstruction.

Other causes of postoperative cholangitis are retained or recurrent stones, stricture of a biliary-enteric anastomosis, and obstruction of an indwelling T tube or U tube by inspissated material. Tubes that are not removed within a few weeks of placement should be irrigated daily with sterile saline solution.

The treatment of cholangitis is to establish adequate drainage of the biliary tract and to administer antibiotics after blood and bile cultures are obtained. How adequate drainage is established depends on the circumstances. When a T tube or U tube is present, it should be opened. In the rare instance in which no tube is present and sepsis is not controlled by antibiotics within 12 to 24 hours, a T tube should be inserted. The goal is to prevent the most severe form of biliary tract inflammation, acute suppurative cholangitis, in which the ductal system becomes filled with pus under high pressure and septicemia continues until decompression is carried out.

HEPATIC ABSCESS

Acute suppurative cholangitis may lead to the development of one or more abscesses in the liver. Hepatic abscess is not often a postoperative complication of biliary tract surgery itself but usually results from an inflammatory condition for which an operation was done and becomes clinically manifest during the postoperative period. Most abscesses found in this manner are multiple. The symptoms include high, spiking fever, chills, right pleuritic or subcostal pain, nausea, vomiting, and jaundice. On physical examination, tenderness in the right upper quadrant or epigastrium and hepatomegaly are the most common findings. Occasionally, patients present in a state of shock, with bacteremia and sepsis. Laboratory studies reveal marked leukocytosis, hypoalbuminemia, elevated alkaline phosphatase, and hyperbilirubinemia. The chest x-ray film often shows pleural effusion, lower lobe atelectasis, and an elevated hemidiaphragm.

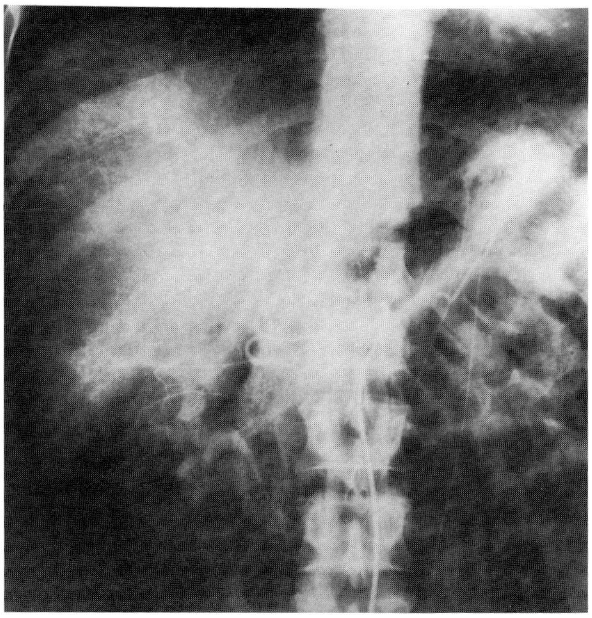

FIG. 36-8. Capillary phase of a celiac arteriogram shows a huge abscess in the right lobe of the liver.

The presence of an abscess or abscesses can be detected by hepatic scintigraphy, ultrasonography, computed tomography, and angiography (Fig. 36-8). Recently, percutaneous transhepatic cholangiography has been shown to be valuable in the diagnosis of multiple abscesses secondary to biliary tract obstruction.[9]

The treatment is surgical drainage combined with antibiotic therapy. Drainage of a large single abscess is simple, but multiple small abscesses may be difficult, if not impossible, to drain. The choice of antibiotic will be guided by culture of the blood or of the drainage from the abscess, but when these are not available, broad coverage should be instituted, such as ampicillin, clindamycin, and tobramycin. The organisms cultured from hepatic abscesses associated with biliary tract disease are those found in patients with bacterbilia. Mortality from hepatic abscess is very high; in one large series nearly a third of the patients died.[2]

Pancreatitis

Patients who have symptomatic cholelithiasis often have concomitant edematous pancreatitis, which is manifested by an elevated serum amylase concentration. There is swelling of the pancreas, but this tends to be a self-limiting process, and serum amylase returns to normal levels in a few days. The etiology of this condition is not entirely clear; strong evidence suggests that it occurs in association with passage of a stone through the common duct into the duodenum.[1] This type of pancreatitis, generally referred to as "gallstone-associated pancreatitis," may complicate the diagnosis of biliary tract disease, but it generally does not interfere with the appropriate surgical therapy or complicate the postoperative course.

Postoperative pancreatitis has been reported to occur after many types of surgical procedures, but it is especially frequent after gastric resection and biliary tract operations. The incidence after biliary tract procedures has been reported to be as high as 4%.[3] At least some, and perhaps all, cases of pancreatitis that complicate operations on the biliary tract are iatrogenic. Injury to the pancreas may result from retractors or from inadvertent perforation of the intrapancreatic segment of the common duct by a probe, stone forceps, or other instrument. Dilatation of the sphincter of Oddi by Bakes' dilators has been implicated also, but we have not observed this in the absence of bile duct perforation by the instrument. Long-arm T tubes, in which the distal limb resides in the duodenum and presumably obstructs the orifice of the pancreatic duct, may cause pancreatitis.

The diagnosis may be difficult in the postoperative period because of normal pain and abdominal tenderness. Otherwise unexplained fever, hemoconcentration, ileus, or prolonged abdominal pain and tenderness should lead to measurement of the serum amylase concentration. Values above about 300 international units are considered diagnostic.

Treatment of postoperative pancreatitis does not differ from treatment of other forms of the disease. Maintenance of fluid and electrolyte balance, nasogastric suction, and appropriate treatment of systemic and local complications such as pulmonary insufficiency, pancreatic abscess, and pseudocyst are all important.

References

1. Acosta JM, Ledesma CL: Gallstone migration as a cause of acute pancreatitis. N Engl J Med 290:484, 1974
2. Balasegaram M: Management of hepatic abscess. Curr Probl Surg 17:332, 1981
3. Bardenheier JA, Kaminski DL, Willman VL: Pancreatitis after biliary tract surgery. Am J Surg 116:773, 1968
4. Beinfield MS, Hayes RL: Use of intraoperative gram stain during cholecystectomy. Am J Surg 137:773, 1979
5. Burhenne HJ: Percutaneous extraction of retained biliary tract stones: 661 patients. AJR 134:889, 1980
6. Chetlin SH, Elliott DW: Biliary bacteremia. Arch Surg 102:303, 1971
7. Dow RW, Lindenauer SM: Acute obstructive suppurative cholangitis. Ann Surg 169:272, 1969
8. Farnell MB, van Heerden JA, Beart RW Jr: Elective cholecystectomy. The role of biliary bacteriology and administration of antibiotics. Arch Surg 116:537, 1981
9. Grossman RI, Ruig EJ, Oleaga JA, Perez MR: Diagnosis of pyogenic hepatic abscesses by percutaneous transhepatic cholangiography. AJR 132:919, 1979
10. Hansson JA, Hoevels J, Simert G et al: Clinical aspects of nonsurgical percutaneous transhepatic bile drainage in obstructive lesions of the extrahepatic bile ducts. Ann Surg 189:58, 1979
11. Huang T, Bass JA, Williams RD: The significance of biliary pressure in cholangitis. Arch Surg 98:629, 1969
12. Keighley MRB, Lister DM, Jacobs SI, Giles GR: Hazards of surgical treatment due to microorganisms in the bile. Surgery 75:578, 1974
13. Keighley MRB, McLeish AR, Bishop HM et al: Selecting patients requiring antibiotics in biliary surgery by immediate gram stains of bile at operation. Surgery 81:473, 1977
14. Mack E, Crummy AB, Babayan VK: Percutaneous transhepatic dissolution of common bile duct stones. Surgery 90:584, 1981
15. Mack E, Patzer EM, Crummy AB et al: Retained biliary tract stones. Nonsurgical treatment with Capmul 8210, a new cholesterol gallstone dissolution agent. Arch Surg 116:341, 1981
16. McKenzie G: Extravasation of bile after operations on the biliary tract. Aust NZ J Surg 24:181, 1955
17. Madden JL: Primary common bile duct stones. World J Surg 2:465, 1978
18. Metzger PP, Ecker HA Jr, Patterson LT: Biliary tract disease: Selection of patient and antibiotics. Pennsylvania Medicine 71:40, 1978
19. Nienhuis LI: Routine operative cholangiography: An evaluation. Ann Surg (Suppl) 154:192, 1961
20. Rosato EF, Berkowitz HD, Roberts B: Bile ascites. Surg Gynecol Obstet 130:494, 1970
21. Safrany L: Transduodenal endoscopic sphincterotomy and extraction of bile duct stones. World J Surg 2:457, 1978
22. Saharia PC, Zuidema GD, Cameron JC: Primary common duct stones. Ann Surg 185:598, 1977
23. Schein CJ: Postcholecystectomy Syndromes. A Clinical Approach to Etiology, Diagnosis, and Management, p 101. Hagerstown, Harper & Row, 1978
24. van Sonnenberg E, Ferrucci JT, Mueller PR et al: Percutaneous radiographically guided catheter drainage of abdominal abscesses. JAMA 247:190, 1982
25. Way LW, Admirand WH, Dunphy JE: Management of choledocholithiasis. Ann Surg 176:347, 1972

37 Complications of Pancreatic Surgery and Trauma

Robert E. Hermann

OVERVIEW

Operations on the pancreas are not performed as frequently as are operations on the biliary system or other intra-abdominal organs. For this reason, many surgeons have limited experience with the complications that may follow pancreatic surgery. In the past, the pancreas has been a difficult organ on which to obtain diagnostic studies. Recent improvements in diagnostic methods, along with an increasing incidence of biliary-related pancreatitis and of alcoholism and pancreatitis, an increasing incidence of pancreatic and periampullary malignancies, and an increasing awareness of endocrine problems of the pancreas have led to increased numbers of pancreatic operations in most medical centers.

Similarly, although injuries of the pancreas were occasional in the past, the increasing frequency of high-speed automobile accidents, blunt injuries of the upper abdomen, and gunshot and other penetrating injuries has increased the overall incidence of pancreatic injuries. It is important for all surgeons who operate within the abdomen on the pancreas to know how to avoid complications, how to manage these complications when they occur, and how to manage pancreatic injuries.

The pancreas lies in a relatively fixed position in the retroperitoneum of the upper abdomen, at about the level of the second lumbar vertebra, extending transversely across the abdomen. The neck and body of the pancreas cross the spine and are frequent sites of injury after blunt abdominal trauma. The pancreas lies in close association with the duodenum, common bile duct, aorta, portal and superior mesenteric veins, splenic vein, inferior vena cava, renal vessels, kidneys, and spleen (Fig. 37-1).[28, 57]

Pancreatic juice is formed by the pancreatic acinar cell, the basic cell unit of the exocrine pancreas. The amount of pancreatic juice produced daily varies from 700 ml to 1500 ml, depending on the state of hydration, health of the patient, and stimuli to secrete. A number of enzymes are secreted by the pancreas: amylase (hydrolizes starch and glycogen); trypsinogen, chymotrypsinogen, procarboxypeptidase A and B (all proteolytic enzymes); leucine aminopeptidase; trypsin inhibitor (inhibits the activation of trypsinogen to trypsin); lipase (hydrolizes fats); nucleases; elastase; collagenase; and lecithinase. Pancreatic juice contains a variety of potentially damaging proteolytic enzymes in an inactive (zymogen) form. When these enzymes become activated in the interstitial area of the pancreas, in the retroperitoneum, or in any area other than in the intestinal tract, cellular inflammation and necrosis occur. It is the effect of these enzymes, leaking outside the pancreatic duct system or gastrointestinal tract, that is the cause of many of the major complications after pancreatic operations or pancreatic injury. Both prevention of pancreatic juice leakage outside of the pancreatic duct system and appropriate external drainage of any leaks that occur are important in avoiding complications of pancreatic surgery or trauma.

General Complications of Pancreatic Surgery

ACUTE PANCREATITIS

Acute pancreatitis has a variety of causes, one of which is its occurrence as a complication of an operative procedure on the pancreas or an injury to the pancreas.[26, 48, 54, 67] Acute pancreatitis in this setting is usually a result of disruption of the pancreatic ducts, leakage of pancreatic juice into the retroperitoneal or peritoneal space, local hemorrhage, and

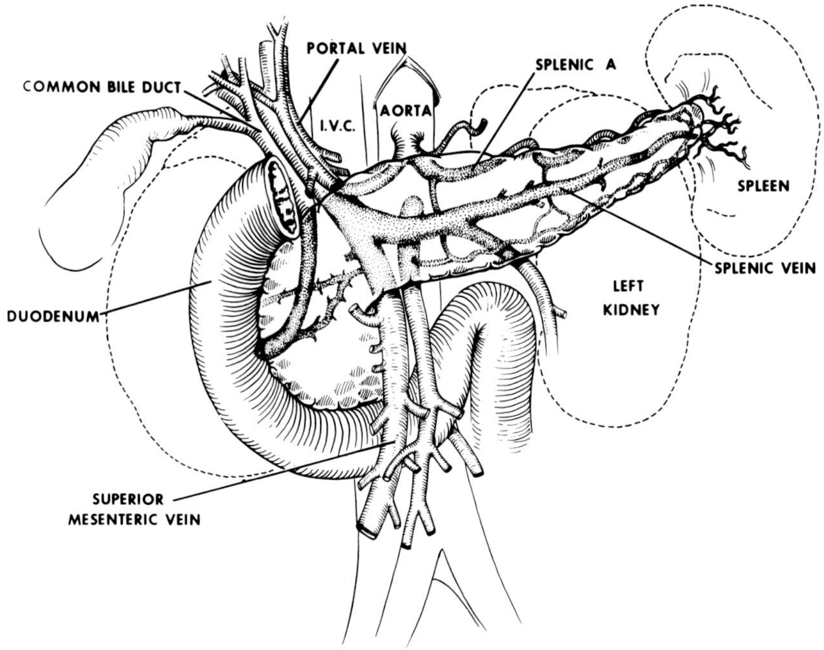

FIG. 37-1. The pancreas lies in close proximity to the duodenum, common bile duct, aorta, inferior vena cava, superior mesenteric artery and vein, splenic vein, portal vein, kidneys, and spleen.

activation of pancreatic proteolytic enzymes with resultant tissue destruction, necrosis, and infection. It has been the impression of many surgeons that acute pancreatitis is less likely to develop after a biopsy or other operative procedure in the fibrotic pancreas or pancreas previously involved with recurrent or chronic pancreatitis than in the normal pancreas. The fibrosis of previous pancreatitis appears to have a protective effect.

Clearly, an important preventive measure for acute pancreatitis is to avoid operations and injuries on the normal gland. When operating on the thickened or fibrotic pancreas, care should be taken that postoperative edema or bleeding does not obstruct the pancreatic duct and the flow of pancreatic juice. Most cases of postoperative acute pancreatitis occur because of leakage or obstruction to the flow of pancreatic juice from poorly performed anastomoses, from sutures inappropriately placed, or from postoperative edema or hemorrhage.[3, 12, 30] In such patients, acute pancreatitis occurs when postoperative oral feedings are begun with a stimulus to secrete pancreatic juice.

If postoperative acute pancreatitis is a concern, oral feedings should be delayed. Helpful diagnostic studies include serial serum amylase and calcium determinations and ultrasound or computed tomography (CT) scans of the pancreas to look for pancreatic or peripancreatic edema, fluid collections around the pancreas, or an acute pseudocyst or abscess.

Treatment should include prolonged nasogastric suction, fluid and electrolyte support, administration of calcium gluconate, and careful monitoring of central venous pressure and urinary output. Antibiotics should be prescribed if an elevated temperature or white blood cell count provides evidence of infection. Unfortunately, acute pancreatitis that develops postoperatively has one of the highest mortality rates of all acute pancreatitis, in the range of 30% to 40%.

PANCREATIC ABSCESS

A pancreatic (or peripancreatic) abscess may occur after an episode of acute pancreatitis in about 5% of patients.[33, 64] Its incidence after an operation on the pancreas or after pancreatic injury ranges from 2% to 4%. A spiking temperature, prolonged ileus, abdominal tenderness, and a persistent septic course from 10 days to 2 weeks after an operative procedure or pancreatic injury are suggestive of a pancreatic abscess. Ultrasound or a CT scan of the pancreas may be of great help in identifying a collection of pancreatic or peripancreatic fluid, pseudocyst, or abscess. A plain abdominal roentgenogram may show a "soap bubble" appearance of air fluid levels from gas-forming organisms in the abscess or retroperitoneum (Fig. 37-2).

When a pancreatic abscess is strongly suspected or diagnosed, operative exploration and drainage of the abscess are essential.[18] The entire retroperitoneal area should be opened and carefully inspected, areas of pancreatic necrosis débrided, and multiple drains and sump suction tubes placed into the area of the abscess. Multiple aerobic and anaerobic cultures should be obtained and the appropriate antibiotics instituted.

PSEUDOCYST

An area of pancreatic or peripancreatic necrosis that remains sterile may become acutely swollen and edematous with trapped fluid and pancreatic juice, forming a pseudocyst. A tender abdominal mass may be noted. Ultrasound or a CT scan should show a localized fluid collection in or around the pancreas. Serial serum amylase determinations will show hyperamylasemia persisting beyond that expected with resolving acute pancreatitis. In the absence of fever, an elevated white blood cell count, or other systemic signs of sepsis, this fluid collection will most likely be an acute pseudocyst rather than a pancreatic abscess. The correct initial treatment of this complication is observation.[7]

Over a period of 2 to 4 weeks, the pancreatic inflammation and acute pseudocyst will subside spontaneously in 50% to 60% of patients. In 10% to 20% of patients, increasing symptoms may force an urgent operation; in the remainder of patients (20%–30%) the pseudocyst will persist, maturing into a chronic pseudocyst that may require a later operation for drainage.

If an acute pseudocyst requires operation because of increasing size or severe pain, external drainage is the ideal treatment. The wall of this acute inflammatory collection is not sufficiently mature or fibrotic to hold sutures for an internal drainage procedure to the stomach or jejunum. A temporary pancreatic fistula may result but if given time will close spontaneously in 80% of patients.

PANCREATIC FISTULA

A pancreatic fistula may be either internal or external. An internal pancreatic fistula is usually the result of spontaneous perforation of a pancreatic pseudocyst or other area of pancreatic necrosis after an episode of acute pancreatitis or direct injury to the pancreas. Such an internal fistula permits leakage of pancreatic juice into the peritoneal cavity with resultant pancreatic ascites.[9, 58]

The diagnosis of pancreatic ascites should be considered whenever a patient develops ascites after an operation in which the pancreatic duct has been opened, after an episode of pancreatitis, or after pancreatic injury. The diagnosis is made by performing a paracentesis, obtaining an amylase determination of the ascitic fluid, and comparing it with a serum amylase level. Although the serum amylase may be moderately elevated, amylase levels in the ascitic fluid are usually very high, often ten times serum amylase levels. When this occurs, the diagnosis of

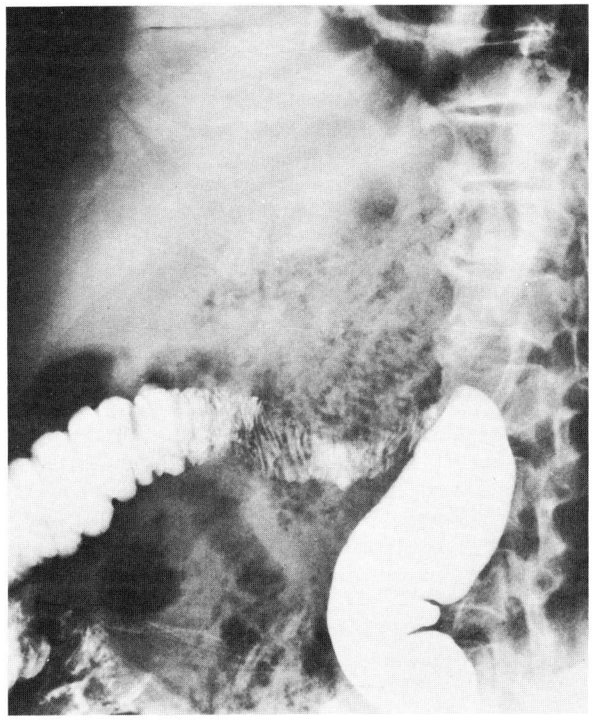

FIG. 37-2. A plain abdominal roentgenogram shows barium in the colon with an abscess cavity near the splenic flexure demonstrated by a "soap bubble" appearance in the retroperitoneum.

pancreatic ascites is secure. If the patient is otherwise stable, endoscopic retrograde cholangiopancreatography (ERCP) should be considered to identify the point of leakage of pancreatic juice from the pancreatic duct system. Identification of the point of leakage will be most helpful in planning an operation to close the fistula.

Medical treatment of pancreatic ascites should include putting the pancreas to rest by discontinuing oral alimentation and using total parenteral nutrition (TPN). If the ascites persists, operative closure of the fistula should be considered. At operation, the point of ductal rupture or pancreatic injury should be identified and a Roux-en-Y jejunal segment brought up to cover this point of injury, reentering pancreatic juice into this defunctionalized jejunal segment.

An external pancreatic fistula occurs most often after external drainage of pancreatic pseudocysts, after operations to explore or biopsy the pancreas, or after resective procedures on the pancreas.[37, 69] Pancreatic juice leaks from the point of ductal injury to the exterior, usually along an appropriately placed drain.

The diagnosis becomes obvious when clear, colorless fluid with a high amylase content is noted on the dressings or is collected in a postoperative stoma bag. An external pancreatic fistula, since it contains inactive pancreatic enzymes, causes little damage to the skin. Approximately 20% of pancreatic injuries are complicated by the development of a pancreatic fistula. The incidence of pancreatic fistula after operations on the pancreas ranges from 10% to 15%.

Most pancreatic fistulas discharge small to moderate amounts of pancreatic juice, from 100 ml to 300 ml per day. When a high-volume fistula occurs or persists, with discharge of 500 ml or more of pancreatic juice daily, partial or complete obstruction of the pancreatic duct system should be considered. High levels of amylase or lipase in the fluid confirm the diagnosis. With an established fistula, which persists for longer than 2 weeks, a fistulogram roentgenographic study should be obtained to assess fistula size and site of origin in the pancreas. The fistulogram may be repeated periodically while awaiting spontaneous closure of the fistula to assess changes in the size of the fistulous tract or any adjacent collections of pancreatic juice. In addition, ERCP may be useful in determining patency of the pancreatic duct and in helping to assess whether spontaneous closure of the fistula is likely.

Most pancreatic fistulas (80%) close spontaneously 3 weeks to 3 months after onset. Any pancreatic fistula contaminated by biliary drainage or intestinal contents is much less likely to close. Medical therapy consists of adequate replacement of fluid and electrolyte losses and limitation of oral intake with nutrition maintained by TPN, and appropriate skin care.

Any fistula that continues to put out pancreatic juice in amounts greater than 300 ml to 500 ml per day for longer than 4 to 6 weeks should be considered for operative closure. About 20% of external pancreatic fistulas require operative closure. The operative procedure is identical to that for internal fistulas; the site of the fistula should be identified and a Roux-en-Y jejunal segment brought up to cover the fistula tract so that pancreatic juice can reenter the intestine.

The overall mortality rate of patients with pancreatic fistulas is approximately 10%, depending on the cause of the fistula, the underlying complication or injury to the pancreas, and general condition of the patient.

HEMORRHAGE

Because of its retroperitoneal position and the fact that the pancreas overlies major blood vessels (vena cava, aorta, superior mesenteric artery and vein, portal vein, splenic artery and vein) and because of its rich vascular supply, operative injuries, acute postoperative pancreatitis, or external injuries carry a risk of hemorrhage. The combination of an injury to a major blood vessel from external trauma along with a pancreatic injury has an extremely high mortality rate. The mortality rate from pancreatic injury alone is from 3% to 6%, but associated vascular injuries increase the mortality rate dramatically. Hemorrhage is the cause of death after pancreatic injury in approximately 50% of patients.

Hemorrhage is also one of the major complications and most common causes of intraoperative death in patients undergoing major pancreatic resections. When pancreatitis develops postoperatively, hemorrhage is frequently delayed, occurring from 4 days to 3 weeks after the operative procedure. Hemorrhage at this time is usually due to pancreatic necrosis, infection, and erosion into a major blood vessel.

Hemorrhage as a complication of pancreatic surgery, pancreatitis, or pancreatic trauma is diagnosed on the basis of a sudden drop in hemoglobin and hematocrit, the rapid onset of shock, and an expanding tender abdomen.[14, 16, 31, 35, 50, 51] In the patient undergoing a pancreatic operation, hemorrhage, if it occurs, will be obvious. To control the hemorrhage, the entire pancreas must be mobilized, the major vessels that surround it inspected, and any bleeding vessels or bleeding areas carefully ligated or sutured. If a major vessel lying within the substance of the pancreas is bleeding, a partial pancreatic resection may be necessary to expose or ligate the bleeding vessel.

Hemorrhagic pancreatitis, occurring postoperatively, has a mortality rate of 30% to 50%. Intraoperative hemorrhage is the major cause of death during operative procedures on the pancreas, with a mortality rate of approximately 5% to 10%.

JAUNDICE

Jaundice is an uncommon complication of pancreatic surgery but may occur transiently in patients with postoperative acute pancreatitis or in patients who have had an injury to the head of the pancreas, distal bile ducts, or pancreatic duct. If the jaundice persists, as evidenced by continued elevated bilirubin levels, a percutaneous transhepatic cholangiogram should be performed to assess patency of the biliary system. If an obstruction of the distal bile duct is identified, biliary drainage transhepatically may be necessary. Alternatively, ultrasound or CT scan of the pancreas should be done to assess the pancreas itself for the cause of the jaundice, and operative exploration should be considered.[56]

At operation, an operative cholangiogram may be helpful. Edema, fibrosis, hemorrhage, gallstones, or pancreatic injury from a previous operative procedure may be the cause of the jaundice. Depending on the complication found, biliary–intestinal continuity should be restored.

GASTROINTESTINAL ULCERATION

Acute stress ulcerations of the stomach or duodenum may occasionally be a complication of operative procedures on the pancreas or of pancreatic injuries. Such stress ulcerations are diagnosed most often by the onset of gastrointestinal bleeding, rarely of gastrointestinal perforation.[24, 40] Similarly, late gastrointestinal ulceration occurs months or years after subtotal or total pancreatectomy.[21]

To confirm the diagnosis, upper gastrointestinal endoscopy is preferred to an upper gastrointestinal roentgenographic series utilizing barium. Intravenous cimetidine, intermittent nasogastric suction, and neutralization of gastric acidity to a *p*H of 5.0 or higher by the instillation of antacids into the stomach are most effective.

Occasionally a duodenal or gastric ulcer will perforate, with increased or generalized abdominal pain and tenderness. This diagnosis can be established by the evidence of free air in the peritoneal cavity, by paracentesis, or by the drainage of duodenal contents through previously placed drains or tubes.

If a gastrointestinal perforation is diagnosed, operative intervention, drainage of the right upper quadrant, and closure of the perforation are mandatory.

DIABETES MELLITUS

Diabetes may be a complication of patients operated upon for chronic pancreatitis if a major portion of the pancreas is resected. Ordinarily, as much as 80% of a normal pancreas can be resected without diabetes developing. However, when the pancreas is damaged or if the patient has chronic pancreatitis, resection of as little as 50% to 60% of the pancreas may cause mild diabetes. Diabetes occurs spontaneously in approximately 30% of patients with chronic pancreatitis.[27, 59]

If a total or radical subtotal pancreatectomy is performed, diabetes may result. This diabetes is often brittle, and only small amounts of insulin are required for control (10–20 units daily). Because of the loss of glucagon production from concomitant removal of the alpha cells, very small amounts of glucose ingestion or externally administered insulin may cause great swings in blood glucose levels from hyperglycemia to hypoglycemia.[17, 49, 66]

PANCREATIC INSUFFICIENCY

Pancreatic insufficiency, like diabetes, is predominantly a complication of chronic pancreatitis or radical subtotal or total pancreatectomy. Pancreatic insufficiency occurs in approximately 40% of patients with chronic pancreatitis. If the pancreas is totally or subtotally removed, pancreatic insufficiency will occur in most patients.

This is not a serious complication of pancreatic surgery or of injuries to the pancreas (an uncommon cause of pancreatic insufficiency). It can be treated by the oral ingestion of pancreatic enzymes utilizing Viokase, Cotazym, or Pancrease, 2 to 4 tablets with meals.

Complications of Operations for Acute Pancreatitis

CHOLECYSTECTOMY, BILE DUCT EXPLORATION, AND SPHINCTEROPLASTY

In the patient with acute pancreatitis related to gallstones, the surgeon may be tempted to perform an urgent cholecystectomy, bile duct exploration, or sphincteroplasty. At present, controversy has arisen in the surgical literature because of several reports by Acosta and colleagues, who have recommended early or urgent cholecystectomy and bile duct exploration for patients with gallstone pancreatitis.[1] They believe that this form of pancreatitis is caused by small stones migrating from the gallbladder into the bile duct, which impact at the sphincter of Oddi, obstructing the bile and pancreatic duct systems, with resultant pancreatitis. Their studies support the concept that patients wih acute pancreatitis should have urgent cholecystectomy and bile duct exploration.

A number of other studies, especially those of Kelly, support an opposite view.[39] It has been our experience that cholecystectomy, bile duct exploration, and sphincterotomy with attempts to remove impacted stones may cause an acute, mild pancreatitis to progress to an acute hemorrhagic pancreatitis.

I believe it is wisest to treat the patient with acute pancreatitis medically. In most patients, small stones in the bile duct will pass and the pancreatitis will resolve. In the few patients in whom the stones do not pass, urgent cholecystostomy or bile duct drainage should be performed, along with pancreatic exploration, débridement of necrotic pancreatic tissue, and drainage of the abdomen.

PANCREATIC EXPLORATION, DÉBRIDEMENT, DRAINAGE, AND CHOLECYSTOSTOMY

In the patient with acute pancreatitis, intensive medical therapy should be the initial form of treatment. Most patients (95%) will respond, and the pancreatitis will improve. However, in approximately 5% of patients, the acute episode may become increasingly severe with hypotension, hypocalcemia, massive fluid requirements, sepsis or the development of a pancreatic abscess, acute respiratory failure, and eventual hemorrhage. In this group of patients who initially respond to medical therapy but then worsen, operative exploration is indicated. At operation, as noted above, even though gallstones may be implicated in the cause of the pancreatitis, I believe that cholecystectomy and bile duct exploration should be avoided. I believe that exploration of the pancreas with débridement and resection of any necrotic pancreatic tissue, drainage of the peripancreatic area and lesser peritoneal cavity, and cholecystostomy with evacuation of gallstones and decompression of the biliary system are optimal (Fig. 37-3). I do not believe that gastrostomy and a feeding jejunostomy are advisable. In these situations, if the pancreatitis continues or progresses, it may be necessary to reexplore the abdomen, perform further débridement of the pancreas, and reinstitute drainage or drain additional areas of localized necrosis or sepsis.[41, 65]

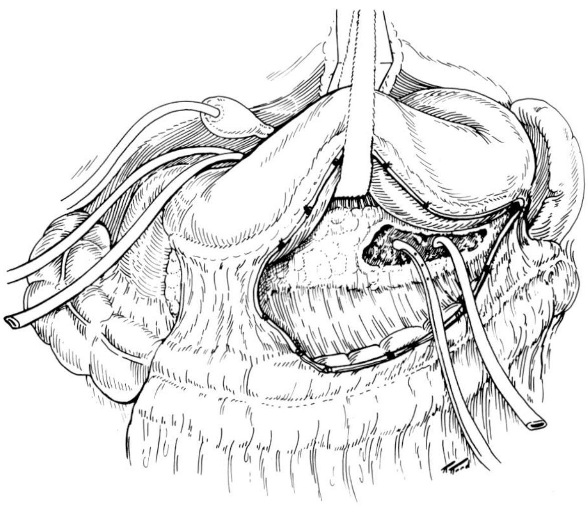

FIG. 37-3. The pancreas is explored through the gastrocolic omentum, opening the lesser peritoneal cavity. Necrotic pancreatic tissue is excised and multiple drains placed. Subhepatic drains are placed for inflammation in the head of the pancreas. A cholecystostomy has been performed.

In patients who require an urgent operation for acute pancreatitis, the postoperative mortality may range from 15% to 40%, depending on the severity of the disease, age of the patient, and other coexisting medical problems. Continuing complications of acute pancreatitis, despite operative exploration and drainage, may include the development of a pancreatic abscess or pseudocyst, progressive pancreatic necrosis with erosion into major blood vessels and hemorrhage, liver failure, renal failure, or respiratory failure.

DRAINAGE OF PANCREATIC ABSCESS

Pancreatic abscess occurs in approximately 5% of patients with acute pancreatitis. The diagnosis is made or suggested in a patient with spiking fever by the presence of an air-fluid cavity, as seen on ultrasound or CT scans or plain roentgenograms of the abdomen (Fig. 37-4). The mortality rate is approximately 35% for patients with a pancreatic abscess.[33, 64] When pancreatic abscess is diagnosed or strongly suspected, pancreatic exploration is indicated. The pancreas should be widely exposed by dividing the gastrocolic omentum and by opening the lesser peritoneal cavity. Any pancreatic or peri-

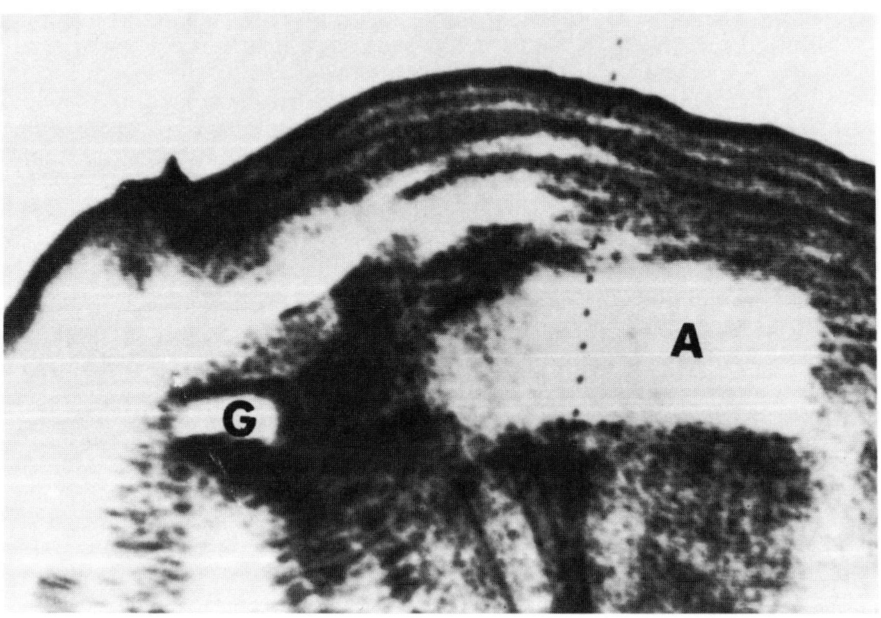

FIG. 37-4. An ultrasound study shows an abscess (*A*) in the area of the pancreas. The gallbladder (*G*) is also marked on this scan.

pancreatic abscess cavities should be drained widely with resection of necrotic pancreatic tissue.

The complications of pancreatic abscess that occur most frequently are erosion of the abscess into an adjacent major blood vessel or hollow viscus (colon, duodenum, stomach, or adjacent loop of small intestine). In my experience, colonic fistulas have been seen most frequently. The treatment of choice is a proximal diverting colostomy to permit the fistulous connection to close, with later resection of the colon and reanastomosis.

CONTROL OF HEMORRHAGE IN ACUTE PANCREATITIS

When an area of pancreatic necrosis or a pancreatic abscess erodes into a major blood vessel, acute and frequently massive retroperitoneal hemorrhage occurs. Hypotension rapidly develops with obvious blood loss confirmed by low hemoglobin or hematocrit levels. Abdominal distention, ecchymosis of the flank (Grey Turner sign), vomiting of blood, or the passage of a bloody stool by rectum is a sign of acute hemorrhage.

Rapid operative exploration through a long midline incision is necessary to stop the bleeding: by ligation or oversewing of the bleeding vessels in the pancreas, by splenectomy and ligation of the splenic vessels, or by vagotomy and pyloroplasty and oversewing of stress erosions in the stomach or duodenum. The mortality rate for patients with acute hemorrhage in pancreatitis is in the range of 40% to 45%.

Complications of Operations for Recurrent or Chronic Pancreatitis

BILIARY EXPLORATION AND SPHINCTEROPLASTY

In patients with recurrent episodes of pancreatitis or chronic pancreatitis with calcification seen on plain abdominal roentgenograms (Fig. 37-5), diabetes, or pancreatic insufficiency, bile duct exploration and sphincteroplasty may be indicated if gallstones are implicated in the etiology of the disease. Diagnostic procedures should include ultrasound or CT scans of the liver, bile ducts, and pancreas and ERCP. If bile duct stones, dilatation of the bile ducts, or stenosis of the sphincter of Oddi is found or if the pancreatic duct is obstructed at the termination of the duct where it empties into the ampulla of Vater, pancreatic duct sphincteroplasty may be indicated to improve drainage of the pancreatic duct system.[5, 29, 46]

Complications of these operations include acute pancreatitis, pancreatic abscess, jaundice and cholangitis, and hemorrhage.

In a series of 140 operations performed for recurrent and chronic pancreatitis (Table 37-1), Dr. Stanley Hoerr and I achieved satisfactory results in approximately 65% of patients, with an overall operative mortality rate of 5%.[29]

LONGITUDINAL PANCREATOJEJUNOSTOMY

The chronically inflamed, thickened, and fibrotic pancreas may be biopsied, transected, opened longitudinally to explore its duct system, or resected with less danger of complication than is likely with the normal pancreas or pancreas minimally affected by pancreatitis. In the operative procedure of longitudinal pancreatojejunostomy, the gland is mobi-

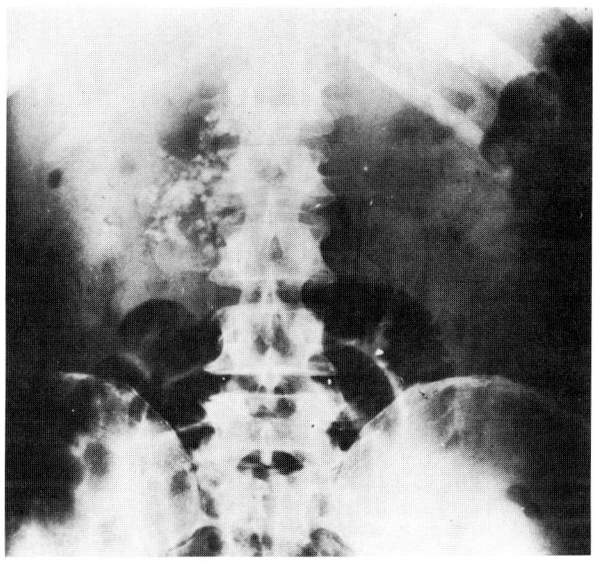

FIG. 37-5. A plain abdominal roentgenogram shows diffuse calcification in the head, body, and tail of the pancreas.

TABLE 37-1. OPERATIONS FOR RECURRENT AND CHRONIC PANCREATITIS (1961–1973)

Procedure	Number of Operations
Cholecystectomy, common bile duct exploration	37
Biliary bypass	23
Sphinctoroplacty and pancroatic duct exploration	21
Drainage of pseudocyst	19
Pancreatojejunostomy	9
Subtotal pancreatectomy, with or without pancreatojejunostomy	11
Others—exploration, biopsy, drainage of abscess, vagotomy, and pyloroplasty	20
Total	140

lized, the main duct identified by palpation along the ventral surface of the gland or by needling and aspirating in the region of the major duct, and the duct opened longitudinally throughout the major length of the pancreas. With the use of fine probes and scoops, stones and other calcareous material are cleansed from the pancreatic ducts, including secondary and tertiary ducts. A Roux-en-Y segment of jejunum is then brought up and joined to the opened pancreas, decompressing the obstructed pancreatic duct system into the jejunal loop.[38, 42, 53, 60] A two-layered anastomosis is created, with an inner row of interrupted Vicryl or Dexon sutures uniting pancreatic duct mucosa to jejunal mucosa and an outer row of interrupted 3-0 silk or other nonabsorbable suture material (Fig. 37-6).

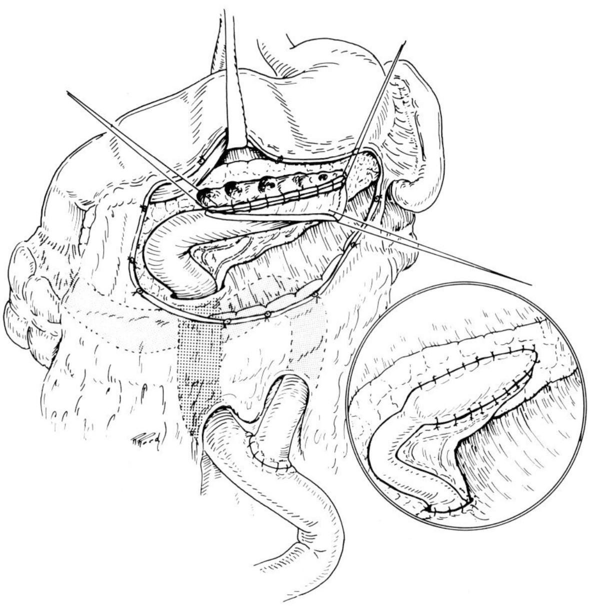

FIG. 37-6. The pancreatic duct has been opened widely and is being joined to a Roux-en-Y segment of jejunum.

Major hemorrhage, flare-up of pancreatitis, pancreatic abscess, and other complications of this operative procedure are rare. The major postoperative complication is leakage of the anastomosis with development of an external pancreatic fistula. Such a fistula will almost always close spontaneously within days or weeks. This operative procedure is a safe and effective treatment for chronic pancreatitis when pancreatic duct obstruction can be verified by ultrasound scans of the pancreas or by preoperative ERCP or intraoperative pancreatography.

DISTAL PANCREATECTOMY AND PANCREATOJEJUNOSTOMY

When chronic pancreatitis is so severe that the major duct system is converted from a single dilated duct into a multiple "chain of lakes" duct system with intermittent stenotic areas and areas of dilatation (Fig. 37-7), or when the pancreas is fibrotic and no pancreatic duct obstruction can be identified, then pancreatic resection and anastomosis of the residual proximal pancreas to a Roux-en-Y jejunal segment is indicated (Fig. 37-8).[42, 60, 63, 66] Again, the fibrotic or chronically inflamed pancreas tolerates operative resection and suturing well. Flare-ups of pancreatitis or hemorrhage are unusual. Intraoperative bleeding may be a problem during dissection of the pancreas while mobilizing it from the splenic vessels, celiac axis, or portal vein.

Postoperative drainage of the anastomosis

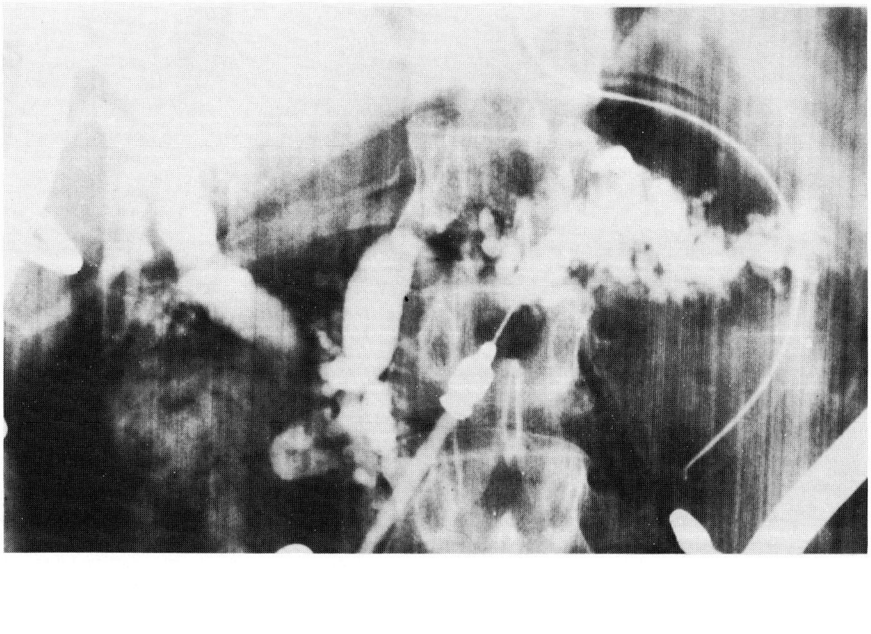

FIG. 37-7. An operative pancreatogram shows a dilated pancreatic duct in the head of the pancreas with multiple areas of stenosis and dilatation and a "chain of lakes" deformity in the distal pancreas.

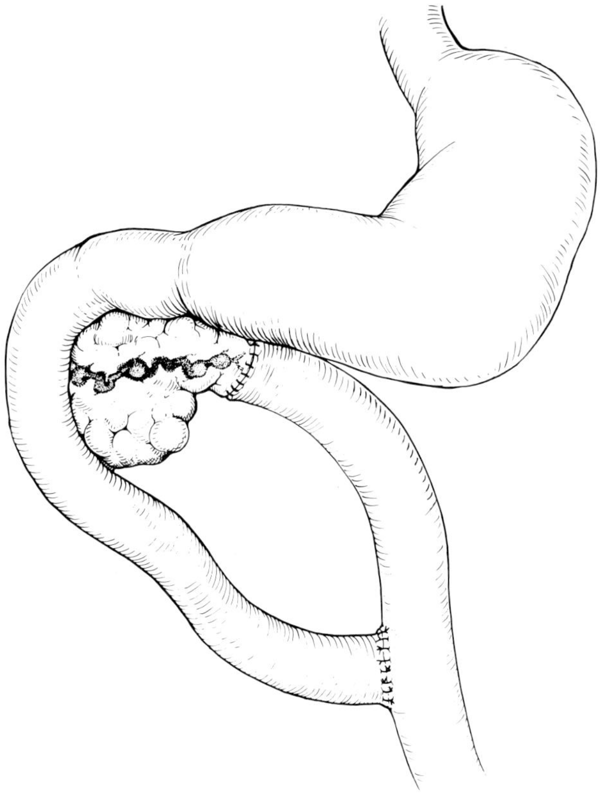

FIG. 37-8. The distal pancreas has been resected and the remaining proximal pancreas is joined to a Roux-en-Y segment of jejunum.

should be routinely employed; occasionally, pancreatic juice leakage with a temporary pancreatic fistula may result. This operative procedure, along with longitudinal pancreatojejunostomy, is relatively safe and has an overall operative mortality of approximately 5%.

SUBTOTAL PANCREATECTOMY

Subtotal pancreatectomy implies a larger pancreatic resection than does simple distal pancreatectomy.[17, 60, 66, 68] The procedure should be employed primarily for patients with fibrotic chronic pancreatitis when pancreatic duct obstruction is not seen. If subtotal pancreatectomy is performed, preserving 20% or less of the pancreas, it may not be necessary to join the residual pancreatic segment with a Roux-en-Y jejunal loop (Fig. 37-9). However, if there is any pancreatic duct obstruction at the ampulla of Vater, then distal decompression by pancreatojejunostomy should be performed.

The more radical the pancreatic resection, the greater the likelihood of postoperative complications and mortality. In resecting a greater amount of pancreas, care must be taken to identify the common bile duct so that it is not injured or divided during the resective procedure. Similarly, the gastroduodenal artery and superior and inferior pancreatoduodenal arteries provide blood supply to the duodenum and should be protected and preserved. The pancreas must be carefully resected from the superior mesenteric and portal veins. Complications of the procedure include common bile duct injury, injury to a major blood vessel with hemorrhage, duodenal necrosis, pancreatic juice leakage with postoperative infection, diabetes mellitus, and pancreatic insufficiency.

Because of the risks of the operative procedure and potential complications, we seldom employ subtotal pancreatectomy, reserving it for patients who do not respond to more conservative operations for treatment of the chronic pancreatitis.

PANCREATODUODENECTOMY

Resection of the head and body of the pancreas, preserving the distal gland, necessitates removing the duodenal segment and distal bile duct, a Whipple operation. This operative procedure is a major undertaking in patients with chronic pancreatitis. However, when chronic pancreatitis is confined to or involves predominantly the head of the pancreas, it is appropriate.[23, 60, 63] The pancreas must be carefully dissected from the superior mesenteric and

FIG. 37-9. A small remaining segment of the head of the pancreas in the C-loop of the duodenum is illustrated. A subtotal resection of the remainder of the pancreas has been performed.

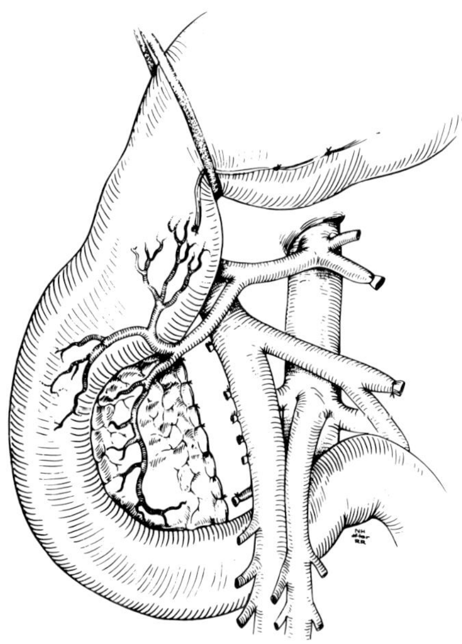

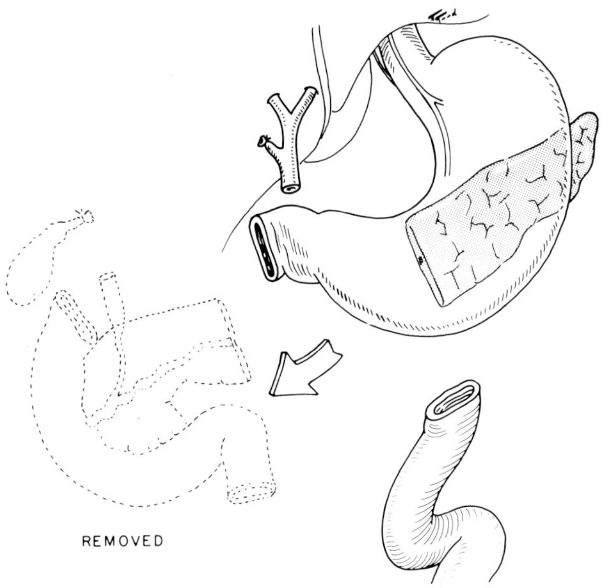

FIG. 37-10. The area of tissue removed during a Whipple resection is illustrated. The head of the pancreas, lower bile duct, duodenum, and gallbladder are resected. The stomach and pylorus are preserved.

FIG. 37-11. Reconstruction after a Whipple operation is depicted. The remaining pancreas is sewn into the open jejunum, and a choledochojejunostomy and a gastrojejunostomy are performed. The stomach and pylorus have been preserved.

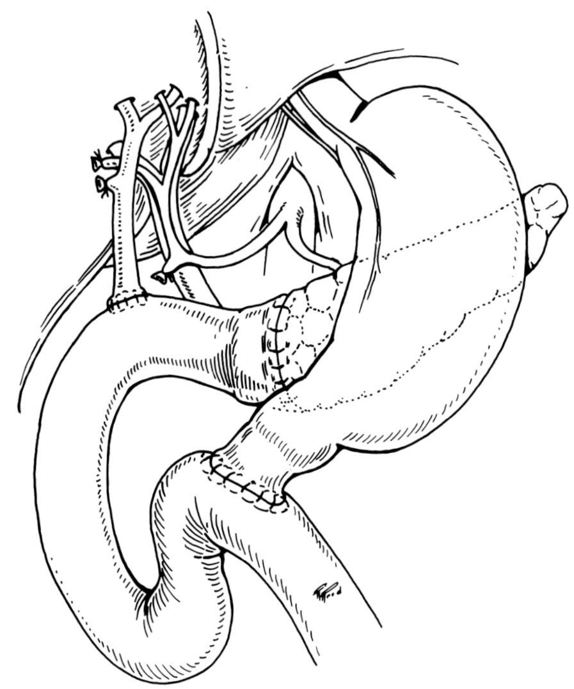

portal veins, the entire stomach and pylorus may be preserved; the gastroduodenal artery is ligated and divided; the common bile duct is divided; and the duodenum is removed. Reconstruction involves a proximal pancreatojejunostomy, a choledochojejunostomy, and gastrojejunostomy, in that order (Figs. 37-10 and 37-11).

Complications of the operative procedure include hemorrhage during the operative procedure, leakage of pancreatic juice from the pancreatojejunostomy postoperatively, leakage of bile from the choledochojejunostomy, and late gastrojejunal ulceration from inadequate neutralization of gastric juice at the gastrojejunostomy stoma.

These complications can be avoided by careful dissection and by a secure, two-layer anastomosis between pancreas and jejunum and bile duct and jejunum. Preserving the entire stomach and pylorus has improved gastric function after pancreatoduodenectomy and, surprisingly, has diminished the incidence of late gastrojejunal stomal ulceration.

Complications of Operations for Pseudocyst of the Pancreas

Pseudocysts of the pancreas are the result of pancreatitis in 75% of patients. In 20% of patients they result from trauma to the pancreas; in 5% they are caused by pancreatic duct obstruction from cancer of the pancreas or are idiopathic. In children, trauma to the pancreas is the major cause of pseudocysts.

The principal complications associated with pseudocysts are infection in the cyst with subsequent pancreatic abscess, jaundice as a result of bile duct obstruction from pressure of the cyst on the distal bile duct, perforation of the cyst into the peritoneal cavity with the development of an internal pancreatic fistula (pancreatic ascites), erosion of the pseudocyst into an adjacent organ such as the stomach or colon, and the development of aneurysms of the splenic or pancreatic arteries from the pancreatitis with erosion of the pseudocyst into these vessels or rupture, resulting in massive hemorrhage into the cyst.[11, 22]

Of these various complications, the most critical is massive hemorrhage into the cyst. Immediate operative exploration is required to control the bleeding. The mortality rate is approximately 50%. Occasionally a pseudocyst erodes into an adjacent organ and massive hemorrhage occurs, giving the picture of massive gastrointestinal bleeding with a pseudocyst as the underlying cause.

In managing pseudocysts of the pancreas, a selective celiac-superior mesenteric arteriogram should be obtained preoperatively to determine if aneurysms of any of the major vessels may be present.[15] If they are seen, it may be wise to ligate these vessels or resect the aneurysm at the time of operation for these pseudocysts.

The treatment of pseudocyst must be individualized. An acute pseudocyst or inflammatory mass of the pancreas will mature or resolve spontaneously in 50% to 60% of patients and should be treated medically. Ultrasound scans of the pancreas are most helpful in following the progress of an acute pseudocyst to resolution and disappearance, or to a persistent, chronic pseudocyst. If a pseudocyst of the pancreas enlarges progressively over a period of time, an operation should be performed. If the pseudocyst has not resolved in about 6 weeks, it is unlikely to do so and operation for drainage should be performed. Internal drainage is preferred to external drainage for a mature, chronic pseudocyst of the pancreas. The procedures most commonly performed are cystgastrostomy, cystjejunostomy using a Roux-en-Y jejunal segment, cystduodenostomy, or, occasionally, excision of a pseudocyst of the distal pancreas.[52, 55, 62] External drainage should be reserved for acute pseudocysts or for those without a mature, fibrotic cyst wall that can be safely joined to the gastrointestinal tract.

If operative exploration and drainage of a progressively enlarging pseudocyst are unduly delayed, infection of the cyst may develop or the cyst may rupture into the peritoneal cavity with the development of pancreatic ascites.

CYSTGASTROSTOMY

Cystgastrostomy should be performed only when a pseudocyst lies directly behind the stomach, and its anterior wall is firmly adherent to the posterior wall of the stomach. Attempts to anastomose a pseudocyst of the pancreas to the stomach when the cyst wall and the stomach are at some distance is hazardous; leakage of the anastomosis may occur, and peritonitis develop. When a pseudocyst is not closely applied to the posterior wall of the stomach, cystjejunostomy or cystduodenostomy is a preferable method of drainage.

The technique of cystgastrostomy is as follows: I usually perform a pseudocystogram prior to opening the stomach or the cyst. A large bore, 18-gauge needle is placed into the pseudocyst and approximately 30 ml to 50 ml of cyst fluid is withdrawn. Approximately 30 ml of contrast medium (Renografin-60) is instilled into the cyst cavity, and a roentgenogram is taken to define the outline of the cyst and its location in relationship to the stomach and other viscera and to identify multiple cysts (Fig. 37-12). When decompressing a pseudocyst, it is important to decompress all multiple pseudocysts or to excise a septum if the pseudocyst is bilocular. The stomach is opened through its anterior wall and the pseudocyst is approached through the posterior wall of the stomach. An incision is made through the posterior wall of the stomach and combined anterior wall of the pseudocyst, entering the cyst cavity. This opening is then enlarged, using a hemostat or Kelly clamp, and then incising it with a scalpel. A portion of the anterior wall of the cyst is excised for biopsy. An opening of approximately 4 cm to 5 cm is made, admitting two or three fingers. Any loose debris or pancreatic material lying freely within the cavity of the pseudocyst should be excised. The anastomosis is then sutured with interrupted 3-0 Vicryl sutures to unite firmly the anterior cyst wall and posterior stomach wall. These interrupted sutures also provide hemostasis for submucosal vessels in the wall of the stomach that may subsequently bleed. When the cystgastrostomy is completed, the anterior wall of the stomach is closed in the usual fashion.

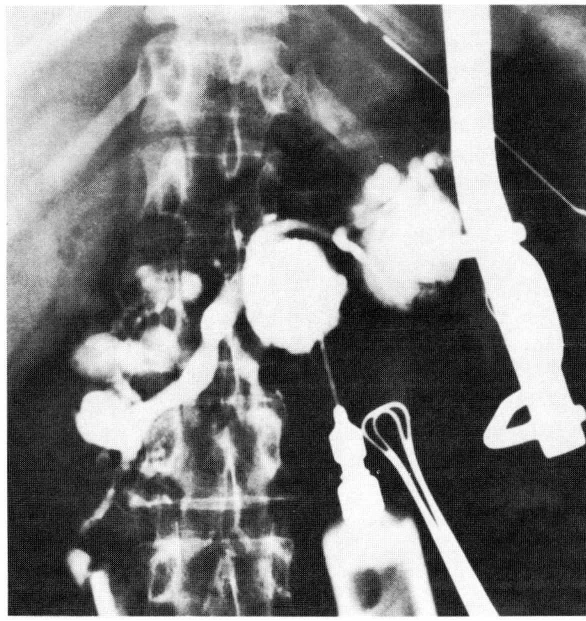

FIG. 37-12. This roentgenogram taken intraoperatively shows a pseudocyst in the body of the pancreas. The pancreatic duct is visualized. A second pseudocyst is identified in the distal (tail) pancreas.

The major complication of cystgastrostomy is bleeding. This may occur as a result of overly vigorous débridement of the pseudocyst itself, from delayed bleeding of submucosal vessels in the wall of the stomach or from gastritis that may occur 2 to 4 days after cystgastrostomy. Débridement of the pseudocyst cavity carries the risk of injuring the splenic artery or vein or other pancreatic vessels or aneurysms of these vessels, which can often be palpated in the posterior wall of the pseudocyst. Great care should be taken before any attached pancreatic tissue or other necrotic material lying within the cyst cavity is excised. If bleeding from the splenic or other vessels should occur, a wider opening into the cyst is required with suture ligation of the bleeding vessels. Occasionally this may require splenectomy and mobilization of the pancreas with control of the splenic artery and vein in their retroperitoneal, retropancreatic location.

Bleeding from one to several days after the operative procedure is caused by bleeding of the cystgastrostomy anastomosis from submucosal vessels in the stomach wall or from a hemorrhagic gastritis. Gastroscopic examination of the stomach and the pseudocyst anastomosis should be performed. Occasionally, a gastric or duodenal ulcer may be seen. If bleeding at the anastomosis is identified, it will usually stop spontaneously unless an arterial bleeding point is seen. In this situation, reoperation and ligation of the bleeding vessel may be necessary.

FIG. 37-13. An operative cholangiogram shows distortion of the distal common bile duct due to a large pseudocyst in the head of the pancreas.

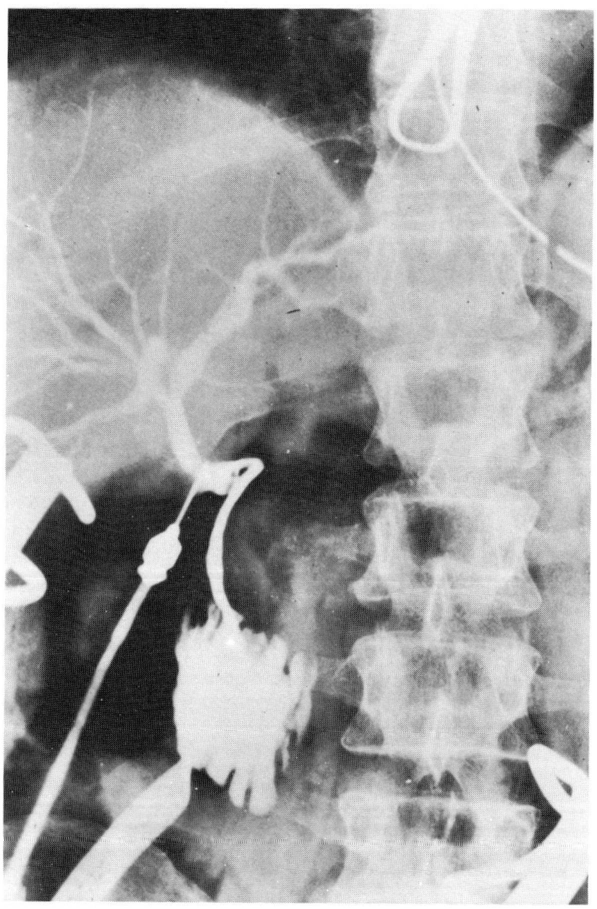

Hemorrhagic gastritis will usually resolve spontaneously and can be treated with cimetidine and antacids.

Postoperative gastrointestinal bleeding as a complication of internal or external drainage of a pseudocyst may occur after all methods of drainage but is slightly more common after cystgastrostomy. It occurs in less than 5% of patients.

CYSTJEJUNOSTOMY

The complications of cystjejunostomy are similar to those of cystgastrostomy. Whenever a pseudocyst of the pancreas is not firmly adherent to the posterior wall of the stomach but is located elsewhere, such as under the stomach or transverse mesocolon, a cystjejunostomy should be selected as the method of internal drainage. A pseudocystogram roentgenographic study is again obtained to identify the size and position of the pseudocyst and the presence of loculations or multiple cysts. A Roux-en-Y jejunal segment is constructed; the pseudocyst or multiple cysts are opened; and the defunctionalized jejunal segment is anastomosed to the cyst wall in two layers, using an outer row of interrupted 3-0 silk sutures and an inner row of interrupted 3-0 Vicryl sutures. Again, on opening the pseudocyst, great caution should be exercised in débriding its contents. A biopsy of the cyst wall should be obtained (to be certain the cyst is not a cystadenoma or cystadenocarcinoma of the pancreas). All significant pseudocysts seen on roentgenographic study should be individually joined to the Roux-en-Y loop for decompression.

Postoperative gastrointestinal bleeding may occur occasionally but is less common than after cystgastrostomy. Leakage of the cystjejunal anastomosis may occur, but can be prevented by good technique. Inadequate drainage of multiple pseudocysts may be a cause of recurrent pancreatic pain or recurrence (persistence) of an additional pseudocyst. The recurrence rate of pseudocysts (or of an undiagnosed, adjacent pseudocyst) has been reported to be from 10% to 15%.

CYSTDUODENOSTOMY

Cystduodenostomy should be performed only when a pseudocyst lies in the head of the pancreas, closely adjacent to the C loop of the duodenum and when dependent drainage may be undertaken without injuring the common bile duct as it passes through the head of the pancreas. A pseudocystogram should again be performed by needling the cyst cavity, withdrawing a portion of the fluid, and instilling contrast medium. Additionally, an intraoperative cholangiogram should be performed to identify the location and position of the common bile duct (Fig. 37-13).

If the pseudocyst appears closely adjacent to the duodenum, a duodenotomy is performed, and the cyst is entered through the medial or posterior wall of the duodenum. Injury to the common bile duct must be avoided even to the extent of opening the bile duct and passing a metal probe or sound into the bile duct to be assured of its location. The opening between cyst and duodenum is gradually enlarged; a segment of the cyst wall is excised or a biopsy obtained; and the internal wall of the anastomosis is sutured with interrupted Vicryl sutures for hemostasis.

Complications of cystduodenostomy include injury to the bile duct, gastrointestinal bleeding as after cystgastrostomy, and duodenal leakage as a result of technical failure in suturing the anastomosis.

EXCISION OF PSEUDOCYST

Excision of a pseudocyst of the pancreas should not be attempted unless it is small and localized in the tail of the gland. To attempt excision of a large pseudocyst or one in the center of the pancreas is hazardous.

A splenectomy is usually necessary to obtain exposure and to mobilize adequately the tail of the pancreas and the pseudocyst. After mobilizing and dissecting the pseudocyst free from its retroperitoneal location, the cyst may be excised and the distal pancreas ligated or oversewn. Special care must be taken to ligate the main pancreatic duct. If the duct is dilated or obstructed, a pancreatojejunostomy should be considered for distal drainage of the pancreas.

The major complication of excision of a pseudocyst is hemorrhage during the operative procedure. A second complication is development of a pancreatic fistula. Subdiaphragmatic or left upper quadrant abscess may occasionally result as a complication.

EXTERNAL DRAINAGE

External drainage should be reserved for acute pseudocysts or for those with an immature, thin wall. The pseudocyst is opened and any necrotic material or pancreatic debris is gently excised. Several Penrose drains or suction catheters are laid into the pseudocyst and brought out through lateral drainage stab wounds for external drainage.

Complications of this operative procedure include hemorrhage, which may occur intraoperatively from overly vigorous débridement of the cyst wall, or may be delayed from late erosion of the cyst into major vessels. Infection may develop as a late complication from progression of the necrotizing process or from infection caused by external drainage tubes or catheters. For this reason, postoperative closed suction drainage or drainage into a sealed stoma bag is advisable.

TABLE 37-2. OPERATIONS FOR PSEUDOCYST (1962–1973)

Procedure	Number of Operations
Internal drainage	
Cystgastrostomy	21
Cystjejunostomy (Roux-en-Y)	6
Cystduodenostomy	1
External drainage	11
Excision of cyst	3
Total	42

A late complication may be persistence of an external pancreatic fistula after all tubes and drains are removed. If this complication develops, a fistulogram should be obtained to determine whether there is communication with the main pancreatic duct system and whether there is proximal pancreatic duct obstruction. Additionally, ERCP may be helpful in identifying pancreatic duct obstruction. If there is no obstruction to proximal pancreatic juice flow, the external pancreatic fistula should close spontaneously within 6 weeks to 3 months. An operation is necessary for fistulas that fail to close spontaneously; they must be drained internally into a Roux-en-Y jejunal segment.

The operative mortality rate of cystgastrostomy, cystjejunostomy, cystduodenostomy, excision of the pseudocyst, or external drainage is approximately 5%. Our experience at the Cleveland Clinic, from 1962 through 1973, with the management of 42 patients with pseudocysts of the pancreas is given in Table 37-2.[29]

Complications of Operations for Pancreatic Injury

Injuries to the pancreas are increasingly being seen in most major medical centers during the past 10 to 20 years.[36, 47, 61] In the past, pancreatic injuries accounted for approximately 2% of all abdominal injuries. This incidence has increased so that pancreatic injuries are now being observed in 10% to 12% of all patients with abdominal injuries.[20] Although the incidence of blunt injuries of the pancreas is increasing, penetrating injuries are still seen more commonly in most centers.

Blunt trauma to the pancreas usually occurs as a result of a high-speed automobile steering-wheel injury, from bicycle or motorcycle handlebar injuries, or from forceful blows to the abdomen. Gunshot and stab wound injuries of the pancreas occur more frequently and are about twice as common as blunt injuries.

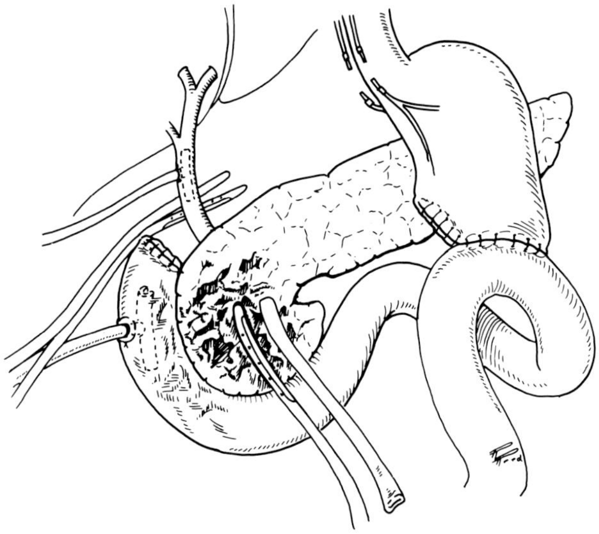

FIG. 37-14. A blunt, crush injury of the head of the pancreas with injury to the duodenum is illustrated. A diverticularization procedure has been performed, including vagotomy, resection of the antrum and gastrojejunostomy, T-tube drainage of the duodenum, and T-tube drainage of the bile duct. Multiple drains are placed in the subhepatic space and around the head of the pancreas.

Three areas of injury to the pancreas have been noted: injuries of the head of the gland, midpancreas, and distal pancreas.[2, 47, 61] Injuries to the head of the pancreas frequently include the common bile duct, duodenum, portal and superior mesenteric vein, liver, gastroduodenal artery, right kidney, and right colon. These injuries frequently crush the gland and are the most difficult to treat. They have the highest mortality rate (28%) of all pancreatic injuries.[25]

Injuries to the central pancreas are frequently transection injuries; the pancreas is compressed against the spine. Injuries to this area may also include the superior mesenteric vessels, splenic vein, liver, stomach, or transverse colon.[36, 47, 61]

Injuries of the distal pancreas are the least serious and least difficult to manage. These injuries are often associated with injuries to the spleen, splenic vessels, left diaphragm, left kidney, stomach, and splenic flexure of the colon. The mortality rate (16%) is about one half that of injuries to the head of the pancreas.

The mechanisms of injury to the pancreas are crush injury with destruction of pancreatic substance, penetrating injury of a localized segment of the pancreas, and complete transection of the pancreas. At operative exploration, it is important to assess the extent of injury, exposing the entire gland to operative view. Important in the assessment is whether or not the pancreatic duct has been injured or transected. In addition, the duodenum, major vessels, common bile duct, spleen, kidneys, and other adjacent organs must be carefully inspected.

The overall mortality rate from pancreatic injury is approximately 18% to 20%. A pancreatic injury alone has a mortality rate of only 3% to 6%. Associated injuries, especially vascular or duodenal injuries, sharply increase the mortality rate. The mortality rate from high-speed, blunt injuries is approximately 50%; from gunshot wounds approximately 25%; shotgun injuries, 60%; and knife wounds, approximately 8%. The overall mortality rate of pancreatic injuries is dependent to a large extent on associated injuries. The major causes of death after severe pancreatic injury are hemorrhage in 50% of patients, renal failure in 16%, and persistent sepsis in 12%.

Late complications of pancreatic injury include pancreatic fistulas, pseudocyst, and pancreatic abscesses. Pancreatic fistulas occur in approximately 20% of patients after treatment of the injury. Pseudocysts occur in approximately 10% of patients with pancreatic injuries and are more common in patients who have had blunt trauma than in those with a penetrating injury. Pancreatic abscess occurs in about 5% of patients.

INJURIES TO THE HEAD OF THE PANCREAS

Injuries to the head of the pancreas are the most severe, can be the most lethal, and are the most difficult to manage. If associated organs or structures are not injured, simple suture repair of the pancreas and drainage may be adequate. With more severe injuries, especially with coexisting injury to the duodenum, common bile duct, or superior mesenteric or portal vein, debridement and Roux-en-Y jejunal segment coverage of the area of injury; distal gastrectomy and Billroth II gastrojejunostomy with closure of the duodenal stump (diverticularization of the injury; Fig. 37-14); or pancreatoduodenectomy to remove the injured areas may be necessary.[2, 20] The magnitude and resulting mortality rate of these three operative procedures is, obviously, on an ascending scale. Pancreatoduodenectomy should be reserved for massive combined injuries of the head of the pancreas and duodenum; the mortality rate associated with the Whipple operation in this setting is from 20% to 30%.[45]

Complications of injuries to the head of the pancreas include massive hemorrhage encountered at operation or occurring postoperatively; persistent leakage of pancreatic juice, bile, or duodenal contents from inadequate repair or closure of the injury; and sepsis postoperatively from undrained collections resulting from the injury. These complications can be prevented by meticulous hemostasis and repair of all vascular structures at the time of operation; coverage, closure, or suturing of all injured structures; and appropriate wide drainage of the area including T-tube drainage of the bile duct and tube duodenostomy when these structures are involved in the injury.

INJURIES TO THE NECK AND BODY OF THE PANCREAS

Most injuries of the neck or body of the pancreas are transection injuries of the gland as it crosses the spine. The most appropriate method of management of these injuries is to resect the distal pancreas and repair the remaining proximal gland.[2, 20, 36] Minor injuries that have not involved the main pancreatic duct may be repaired by suturing the gland.

Complications include hemorrhage encountered at operation or during the postoperative period from inadequate repair of associated vascular injuries, pancreatitis with pseudocyst in the remaining head of the pancreas, persistent leakage of pancreatic juice with subsequent pancreatic fistula, and abscess formation and sepsis as a late consequence of inadequate repair or drainage. As with all such injuries, complications can be prevented by meticulous hemostasis, resection of all injured tissue, repair of the remaining proximal pancreas, and liberal postoperative drainage.

INJURIES TO THE DISTAL PANCREAS

Injuries to the distal pancreas should always be treated by resection of the distal gland and spleen, which is often injured as well. Rarely, minor injuries may be sutured and drained only. Careful closure of the remaining pancreas at the point of transection is important; an effort should be made to identify the pancreatic duct and ligate it separately. The left upper quadrant and subdiaphragmatic area should be drained postoperatively using closed suction drainage.[20, 36]

Complications of injuries to the distal pancreas alone are not usually serious. One should always look for concomitant injuries to the spleen, left hemidiaphragm, stomach, and left kidney. Associated injuries to these structures must also be repaired. With careful repair of the injury, the complications of hemorrhage, persistent leakage of pancreatic juice, pancreatitis with pseudocyst formation, and the development of a late abscess are not likely.

Complications of Operations for Cancer of the Pancreas

PANCREATIC BIOPSY

Biopsy of the pancreas in a patient with a mass lesion identified at operation should be performed cautiously. The site of the biopsy should be selected

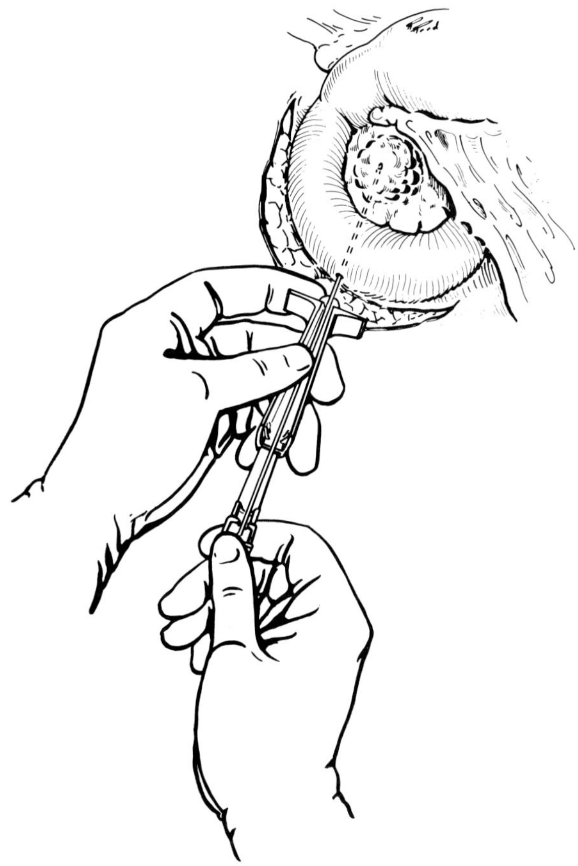

FIG. 37-15. The technique of transduodenal needle biopsy of a mass in the head of the pancreas, using a Tru-cut needle is depicted.

to avoid injury to any major vascular structures or to the common bile duct. The pancreas and duodenum should be mobilized adequately so that the lesion is elevated from its retroperitoneal position and grasped firmly. If the lesion is on the surface of the pancreas, a shave or wedge biopsy using a surgical scalpel may be safe. However, if the lesion is deep within the gland, a Tru-cut needle biopsy into the mass should be performed. preferably going through the duodenum if the lesion lies adjacent to the duodenum (Fig. 37-15). Needle aspiration cytology, using a 21-gauge needle, is safe and may provide adequate cytologic material to confirm the diagnosis of carcinoma.

The value of pancreatic biopsy, its accuracy, and the complications of the procedure are subjects of controversy. Evidence from many reports indicates that the accuracy of pancreatic biopsy is approximately 85%, with a 15% incidence of false negatives (inability to confirm the diagnosis of carcinoma).[34, 44] The morbidity rate of the procedure is approximately 5% and the mortality is less than 1%.

Complications of pancreatic biopsy include hemorrhage from injury to a vascular structure, persistent leakage of pancreatic juice with development of a pancreatic fistula, and acute pancreatitis from trauma to the gland or disruption of the pancreatic duct. Occasionally, bile duct leakage may result from an inappropriately placed biopsy.

These complications can be avoided by careful handling of the gland, careful biopsy technique avoiding vascular structures and the dilated pancreatic duct if it is obstructed, and entering through the duodenum for lesions in the head of the gland so that any pancreatic juice leakage will pass into the bowel and not into the peritoneal cavity.

Since introduction of the Tru-cut biopsy needle and with liberal use of 21-gauge needle aspiration cytology, our incidence of complications after pancreatic biopsy in the last 100 patients has been less than 2%.

PANCREATODUODENECTOMY

Pancreatoduodenectomy should be performed only for cancers of the head of the pancreas, ampulla of Vater, distal common bile duct, and periampullary duodenum that can be resected or cured. Additionally, the procedure may be performed for large or malignant islet cell tumors located in the head of the pancreas and for sarcomas or other rare tumors involving the head of the pancreas. Occasionally, the operative procedure is performed for massive injury of the head of the pancreas involving the duodenum, distal common bile duct, or portal vein.

The operative mortality rate for the procedure, when performed for a localized carcinoma, should be from 5% to 10%. Actual mortality rates reported in a number of series of patients studied range from 5%, in some major medical centers where the procedure is performed frequently by expert surgeons, to 32% in community hospitals where surgeons do the procedure infrequently.[4, 6, 19, 32, 43,*] When pancreatoduodenectomy is performed for major injuries of the head of the pancreas, the postoperative mortality is from 20% to 30%.[45]

Complications of pancreatoduodenectomy include hemorrhage and uncontrolled bleeding during and immediately after operation, leakage of pancreatic juice from the pancreatojejunal anastomosis, sepsis and intra-abdominal abscess from subhepatic or peripancreatic collections inadequately drained, and late anastomotic gastrojejunal ulceration that may occur several years after operation. Hemorrhage is the major complication and usually occurs during dissection of the pancreas from the superior mesenteric and portal veins, from injury to these large veins or to one of their branches. Injury to the hepatic artery or gastroduodenal artery may also be a cause of major hemorrhage. These complications are likely to be greater when attempts are made to dissect large tumor masses off the vessels than when dealing with small tumors.

Delayed leakage of pancreatic juice from the pancreatojejunal anastomosis is the most common postoperative complication. If drainage has been inadequate, a localized intra-abdominal abscess may result. To avoid this, careful construction of the anastomosis is critical. We have found that the entire end of the pancreas should be sutured into the jejunal segment, using a two-layer technique (Fig. 37-16). If the pancreatic duct cannot be sutured to the jejunal mucosa, it is wise to splint it with a small polyethylene catheter inserted as a free-lying splint. This anastomosis should always be drained by closed-suction drainage catheters left in place for 5 to 7 days postoperatively.

The most common late complication of pancreatoduodenectomy is anastomotic or stomal ulceration of the jejunum from the effect of gastric acid on the jejunum. Attempts to control or prevent this complication in the past have included the routine use of vagotomy when antral resection or hemigastrectomy was performed with pancreatoduodenectomy. Recently, the gastric or pylorus preserving modification of the Whipple operation has been introduced. The entire stomach, including the pyloric sphincter and vagal nerves are left, anastomosing the stomach and pylorus to the jejunum distal to the pancreatic and biliary anastomoses. Early experience with this operative procedure indicates that patients eat better and have less morbidity and that stomal ulceration does not develop as a late complication. Further experience with this modification of the Whipple operation is accumulating.

TOTAL PANCREATECTOMY

Total pancreatectomy is advocated by some surgeons for the treatment of cancer of the pancreas because it completely removes all pancreatic tissue and any multicentric foci of cancer, observed in approximately 10% to 30% of patients (usually as *in situ* or noninvasive areas of ductal atypia), and because total pancreatectomy avoids the necessity for pancreatojejunal anastomosis and the complication of leakage from this anastomosis.[8, 49]

Complications after total pancreatectomy are similar to those after pancreatoduodenectomy, with the exception of pancreatic leakage at the pancreatojejunal anastomosis. The overall operative mortality rate of the procedure and the incidence of post-

*Commission of Profession and Hospital Activities: Personal communication, 1972

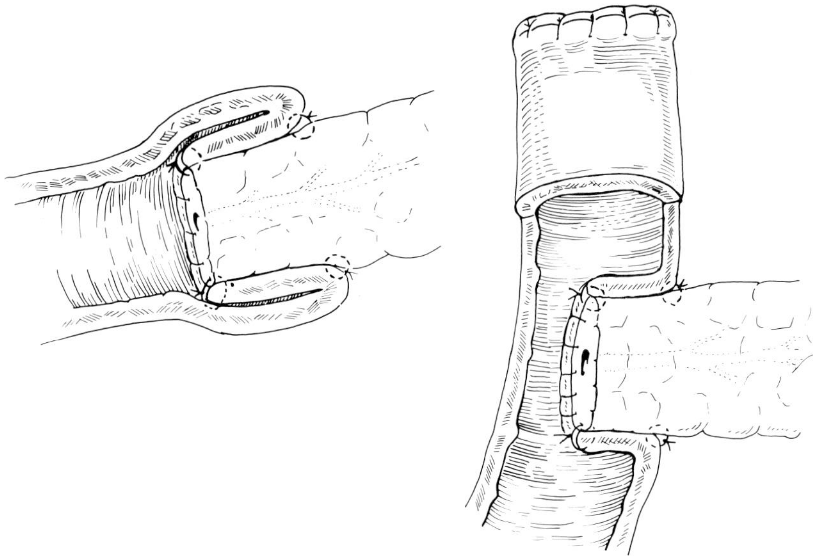

FIG. 37-16. The technique of pancreatojejunostomy is depicted. The pancreas may be invaginated into the end of the jejunum with a two-layer technique. It may also be invaginated through an opening in the side of the jejunum, again with a two-layer technique.

operative morbidity are almost identical to those of pancreatoduodenectomy.[13] However, the incidence of hemorrhage during the operative procedure and of postoperative subhepatic or left subdiaphragmatic abscess formation and sepsis is somewhat higher. The incidence of late complications and of gastrojejunal anastomotic ulceration is slightly higher after total pancreatectomy than after partial resection of the gland.

The major complication of total pancreatectomy is brittle diabetes caused by removal of all islet tissue, including the beta cells that produce insulin and the alpha cells that produce glycagon. The loss of alpha cells, in this instance, may be more critical. The diabetes that results is very brittle and difficult to control in about one fourth of the patients. The amount of insulin required daily is small, from 10 to 20 units. Daily food intake and exercise must be carefully regulated. Small overdosages of insulin or too little insulin may result in profound swings from hyperglycemia to hypoglycemia. Deaths from complications of the diabetes may occur as a late complication. The quality of life and the ability to eat a normal diet and pursue normal activities are clearly more diminished after total pancreatectomy than after pancreatoduodenectomy, with preservation of the distal pancreas.

CHOLEDOCHODUODENOSTOMY OR CHOLEDOCHOJEJUNOSTOMY

Biliary bypass should be performed when a cancer of the pancreas or periampullary region cannot be resected by virtue of its local size, invasion of other vital structures (especially the superior mesenteric or portal vein), or when metastases are identified outside the field of resection at operation.

Complications of these operative procedures include leakage of bile or intestinal contents from a poorly constructed anastomosis, postoperative infection as a result of abscess formation from inadequate drainage of the area of anastomosis, and, occasionally, hemorrhage from dilated vascular structures injured during the dissection or biopsy procedure. These complications can be avoided by careful technique. They occur in probably no more than 5% to 10% of patients. The operative mortality rate from these procedures is approximately 5% to 8% and is usually a result of the disease process and poor nutritional status of the patient rather than of the operative procedure itself.

GASTROJEJUNOSTOMY

Gastrojejunostomy is performed when a large, nonresectable carcinoma of the head of the pancreas or uncinate process appears to obstruct or may obstruct the duodenal segment. Complications of this procedure are few. Predominantly, they consist of inadequate emptying of the stomach through the gastrojejunostomy stoma or the development of postoperative nausea and vomiting from the reflux of duodenojejunal contents into the stomach when gastric emptying through the normal passageway continues. Why a gastrojejunostomy stoma malfunctions is not well understood. This problem occurs in probably 10% to 15% of patients and can be overcome by constructing a Roux-en-Y gastrojejunostomy, completely diverting the jejunum so jejunal contents cannot reflux into the stomach.

Late gastrojejunal ulceration is rarely a problem, and it is usually not necessary to perform a concomitant vagotomy when a gastrojejunostomy is performed for cancer of the pancreas.

When gastrojejunostomy is not performed routinely, gastric outlet obstructon from encroachment of the pancreas on the duodenum will develop in approximately 15% to 20% of patients. Many surgeons advocate routine gastrojejunostomy during all palliative bypass operations on patients with cancers that cannot be resected. Other surgeons, including us, perform gastrojejunostomy selectively only when obstruction or impending obstruction of the duodenal segment is identified at operation.

SPLANCHNIC RESECTION

When operations are performed upon patients with a cancer of the body or tail of the pancreas who also have upper abdominal and back pain preoperatively and a nonresectable lesion is found, consideration must be given to providing pain relief. This can be achieved by phenol or alcohol injection into the celiac ganglion or the periaortic splanchnic nerve trunks during operation. Identification of these structures, especially when the tumor has invaded retroperitoneally, can be difficult. For this reason, we most often utilize bilateral splanchnic resection, performed under the same anesthesia as that given for the exploratory laparotomy. After the abdomen has been explored and all biopsies or bypass procedures have been performed, the abdomen is closed; the patient is turned onto the abdomen; and separate paraspinal incisions are performed through the back. Splanchnicectomy relieves postoperative pain in about 80% of patients and is gratifying.

Complications of this procedure may include bleeding, injury to other nerve structures, and postoperative infection. Complications in the hands of an experienced neurosurgeon are rare.

Management of Pancreatic Ascites and Pancreatic Fistulas

As mentioned previously, pancreatic ascites from internal pancreatic fistulas and external pancreatic fistulas can occur as complications of pseudocysts that rupture into the peritoneal cavity, from external drainage of pseudocysts, from external drainage of areas of pancreatic necrosis, after pancreatic biopsy, or after pancreatojejunal anastomoses.

The point of leakage from the pancreatic duct system should be identified preoperatively by ERCP.[10] Additionally, ultrasound or CT scans of the pancreas may be helpful in identifying a residual pseudocyst. Pancreatic ascites can be disagnosed by finding amylase levels in the peritoneal fluid higher than are present in the serum.[9, 58]

Pancreatic ascites from an internal pancreatic fistula will rarely close spontaneously, but a trial of medical therapy should be instituted, by TPN with nothing given orally. The same treatment should be used for patients with external pancreatic fistulas.

External fistulas usually close in 3 weeks to 3 months after the onset of the fistula; approximately 80% will close spontaneously. Any internal fistula with persistent ascites or any external fistula that continues to secrete pancreatic juice in amounts greater than 300 ml to 500 ml per day for longer than 4 to 6 weeks should be closed by operative repair.

At operation, the site of pancreatic duct leakage should be exposed. Suturing or closing the fistula directly should not be attempted, but it should be diverted into a Roux-en-Y jejunal segment. This effectively reroutes the pancreatic juice back into the intestine and is the safest operative procedure for this problem.

Complications of pancreatic fistulas or of the underlying pancreatic problem (pancreatic injury, pseudocyst, or previous pancreatic resection and anastomosis) include postoperative sepsis, hemorrhage, and erosion into adjacent viscera. These complications occur in approximately 5% to 10% of patients. The mortality rate of patients with pancreatic fistulas is now less than 10%.

References

1. Acosta JM, Ross R, Galli OMR et al: Early surgery for acute gallstone pancreatitis. Evaluation of a systematic approach. Surgery 83:367, 1978.
2. Anane–Sefah J, Norton LW, Eisman B: Operative choice and technique following pancreatic surgery. Arch Surg 110:161, 1975
3. Anderson MC, Needleman SB, Gramatica L et al: Further inquiry into the pathogenesis of acute pancreatitis. Arch Surg 99:185, 1969
4. Aston SJ, Longmire WP: Pancreaticoduodenal resection. Twenty years' experience. Arch Surg 106:813, 1973
5. Bartlett MK, Nardi GL: Treatment of recurrent pancreatitis by transduodenal sphincterotomy and exploration of the pancreatic duct. N Engl J Med 262:643, 1960
6. Braasch JW, Gray BN: Considerations that lower pancreatoduodenectomy mortality. Am J Surg 133:480, 1977
7. Bradley EL III, Gonzalez AC, Clements JL: Acute pancreatic pseudocysts: Incidence and implications. Ann Surg 184:734, 1976
8. Brooks JR, Culebras JM: Cancer of the pancreas. Palliative operation, Whipple procedure, or total pancreatectomy? Am J Surg 131:516, 1976
9. Cameron JL, Kieffer RS, Anderson WJ, Zuidema GD: Internal pancreatic fistulas: Pancreatic ascites and pleural effusions. Ann Surg 184:587, 1976
10. Cooperman AM, Sivak MV, Sullivan BH et al: Endoscopic pancreatography. Its value in preoperative and postoper-

ative assessment of pancreatic disease. Am J Surg 129:38, 1975
11. Cordero OC, Khademi M, Lazaro E, Swaminathan AP: Intracystic hemorrhage: A complication of pseudocyst of the pancreas. Br J Radiol 48:602, 1975
12. Dumont AE, Martelli AB: Pathogenesis of pancreatic edema following exocrine duct obstruction. Ann Surg 168:302, 1968
13. Edis AJ, Kiernan PD, Taylor WF: Attempted curative resection of ductal carcinoma of the pancreas. Mayo Clin Proc 55:531, 1980
14. Facey FL, Weil MH, Rosoff L: Mechanism and treatment of shock associated with acute pancreatitis. Am J Surg 111:374, 1966
15. Frey CF: Pancreatic pseudocyst—Operative strategy. Ann Surg 188:652, 1978
16. Frey CF: Hemorrhagic pancreatitis. Am J Surg 137:616, 1979
17. Frey CF, Child CG, Fry W: Pancreatectomy for chronic pancreatitis. Ann Surg 184:403, 1976
18. Frey CF, Lindenauer SM, Miller TA: Pancreatic abscess. Surg Gynecol Obstet 149:722, 1979
19. Gilsdorf RB, Spanos P: Factors influencing morbidity and mortality in pancreaticoduodenectomy. Ann Surg 177:332, 1973
20. Graham JM, Mattox KL, Jordan GL: Traumatic injuries of the pancreas. Am J Surg 136:744, 1978
21. Grant CL, Van Heerden JA: Anastomotic ulceration following subtotal and total pancreatectomy. Ann Surg 190:1, 1979
22. Greenstein A, De Maio EF, Nabseth DC: Acute hemorrhage associated with pancreatic pseudocysts. Surgery 69:56, 1971
23. Guillemin G, Cuilleret J, Michel A et al: Chronic relapsing pancreatitis. Surgical management including sixty-three cases of pancreaticoduodenectomy. Am J Surg 122:802, 1971
24. Haller JD, Pena C, Dargen EL: Massive upper gastrointestinal hemorrhage due to pancreatitis. Arch Surg 93:567, 1966
25. Heitsch RC, Knutson CO, Fulton RL et al: Delineation of critical factors in the treatment of pancreatic trauma. Surgery 80:523, 1976
26. Hermann RE: Basic factors in the pathogenesis of pancreatitis. Cleve Clin Q 30:1, 1963
27. Hermann RE: Clinical aspects of pancreatitis. Postgrad Med 36:135, 1964
28. Hermann RE: Exocrine pancreas. In Manual of Surgery of the Gallbladder, Bile Ducts, and Exocrine Pancreas, Ch 7, pp 155–165. New York, Springer–Verlag, 1979
29. Hermann RE, Al–Jurf AS, Hoerr SO: Pancreatitis. Surgical management. Arch Surg 109:298, 1974
30. Hermann RE, Davis JH: The role of incomplete pancreatic duct obstruction in the etiology of pancreatitis. Surgery 48:318, 1960
31. Hermann RE, Knowles RC: Lethal factors and response to therapy in experimental bile-reflux pancreatitis. Ann Surg 161:456, 1965
32. Hoffman RE, Donegan WL: Experience with pancreatoduodenectomy in a cancer hospital. Am J Surg 129:292, 1975
33. Holden JL, Berne TV, Rosoff L: Pancreatic abscess following acute pancreatitis. Arch Surg 111:858, 1976
34. Isaacson R, Weiland LH, McIlrath DC: Biopsy of the pancreas. Arch Surg 109:227, 1974
35. Jacobs ML, Daggett WM, Civette JM et al: Acute pancreatitis: Analysis of factors influencing survival. Ann Surg 185:43, 1977
36. Jones RC: Management of pancreatic trauma. Ann Surg 187:535, 1978
37. Jordan GL Jr: Pancreatic fistula. Am J Surg 119:200, 1970
38. Jordan GL Jr, Strug BS, Crowder WE: Current status of pancreatojejunostomy in the management of chronic pancreatitis. Am J Surg 133:46, 1977
39. Kelly TR: Gallstone pancreatitis. The timing of surgery. Surgery 88:345, 1980
40. Kisken WA: Gastrointestinal bleeding secondary to pancreatitis. JAMA 202:287, 1967
41. Lawson DW, Daggett WM, Civetta JM et al: Surgical treatment of necrotizing pancreatitis. Ann Surg 172:605, 1970
42. Leger L, Lenriot JP, Lemaigre G: Five to twenty year follow-up after surgery for chronic pancreatitis in 148 patients. Ann Surg 180:185, 1974
43. Levin B, Re Mine WH, Hermann RE et al: Cancer of the pancreas. Am J Surg 135:185, 1978
44. Lightwood R, Reber HA, Way LW: The risk and accuracy of pancreatic biopsy. Am J Surg 132:189, 1976
45. Nance FC: Pancreatic injuries. Discussion at American College of Surgeons Program. New Orleans, April, 1981
46. Nardi GL: Remediable chronic pancreatitis. Surg Clin North Am 54:613, 1974
47. Northrup WF III, Simmons RL: Pancreatic trauma: A review. Surgery 71:27, 1972
48. Peterson LM, Collins JJ, Wilson RE: Acute pancreatitis occurring after operation. Surg Gynecol Obstet 127:23, 1968
49. Pliam MB, Re Mine WH: Further evaluation of total pancreatectomy. Arch Surg 110:506, 1975
50. Ranson JHC, Rifkind KM, Roses DF: Prognostic signs and the role of operative management in acute pancreatitis. Surg Gynecol Obstet 139:69, 1974
51. Ranson JHC, Rifkind KM, Turner JW: Prognostic signs and non-operative peritoneal lavage in acute pancreatitis. Surg Gynecol Obstet 143:209, 1976
52. Ravelo HR, Aldrete JS: Analysis of forty-five patients with pseudocysts of the pancreas treated surgically. Surg Gynecol Obstet 148:735, 1979
53. Sato T, Saitoh Y, Noto N et al: Appraisal of operative treatment of chronic pancreatitis. With special reference to side-to-side pancreaticojejunostomy. Am J Surg 129:621, 1975
54. Schiller WR, Suriyapa C, Anderson MC: A review of experimental pancreatitis. J Surg Res 16:69, 1974
55. Shatney CH, Lillehei RC: Surgical treatment of pancreatic pseudocysts; Analysis of 119 cases. Ann Surg 189:386, 1979
56. Sidel VW, Wilson RE, Shipp JC: Pseudocyst formation in chronic pancreatitis: A cause of obstructive jaundice. Arch Surg 77:933, 1958
57. Skandalakis JE, Gray SW, Rowe JS et al: Anatomical complications of pancreatic surgery—Part II. Contemp Surg 15:21, 1979
58. Smith RB III, Warren WD, Rivard AA et al: Pancreatic ascites: Diagnosis and management with particular reference to surgical technics. Ann Surg 177:538, 1973
59. Stobbe KC, Re Mine WH, Baggenstoss AH: Pancreatic lithiasis. Surg Gynecol Obstet 131:1090, 1970
60. Taylor RH, Bagley FH, Braasch JW, Warren KW: Ductal drainage or resection for chronic pancreatitis. Am J Surg 141:28, 1981
61. Thompson RJ, Hinshaw DB: Pancreatic trauma: Review of 87 cases. Ann Surg 163:1, 1966

62. Van Heerden JA, Re Mine WH: Pseudocysts of the pancreas. Arch Surg 110:500, 1975
63. Warren KW: Surgical management of chronic relapsing pancreatitis. Am J Surg 117:24, 1969
64. Warshaw AL: Pancreatic abscess. N Engl J Med 287:1234, 1972
65. Warshaw AL, Imbembo AL, Civetta JM et al: Surgical intervention in acute necrotizing pancreatitis. Am J Surg 127:484, 1974
66. Weiland DE, Kuntz DJ, Kimball HW: Subtotal pancreatectomy for chronic pancreatitis. Am J Surg 118:973, 1969
67. White TT, Morgan A, Hopton D: Postoperative pancreatitis. A study of seventy cases. Am J Surg 120:132, 1970
68. White TT, Slavotinek AH: Results of surgical treatment of chronic pancreatitis. Report of 142 cases. Ann Surg 189:217, 1979
69. Zinner MJ, Baker RR, Cameron JL: Pancreatic cutaneous fistulas. Surg Gynecol Obstet 138:710, 1974

38 Complications in Hepatic Surgery and Trauma

William R. Rout | George D. Zuidema

OVERVIEW—HEPATIC METABOLISM

Hepatic insufficiency as a consequence of major liver resection usually does not occur if the remaining liver is normal, represents at least 20% of the original functioning hepatic parenchyma, and its vessels and ducts are intact. As little as 10% functional hepatic tissue is enough to sustain life.

Major hepatic trauma or resection will cause marked catabolism and a negative nitrogen balance. Negative nitrogen balance (catabolism) in the severely injured patient is associated with a significant increase in rates of morbidity and mortality. A related and equally foreboding observation is the occurrence of immunologic anergy, which is associated with malnutrition, sepsis, shock, and trauma.[58] It is mandatory that patients suffering major hepatic insult or subjected to liver resection receive adequate nutrition. Those patients who cannot tolerate enteral alimentation must receive total parenteral nutrition (TPN) starting early in the postoperative period. The amount of nitrogen (protein) and calories required by the patient depends upon the degree of injury to the liver and the amount of remaining functional hepatic tissue. The patient is monitored for signs of liver failure. The nitrogen and caloric content of the diet are adjusted as necessary. Selected patients with an intact functional gastrointestinal tract can be frequently maintained on enteral alimentation through a nasogastric feeding tube, gastrostomy, or a jejunostomy. Metabolic monitoring is identical for patients supported by either parenteral or enteral nutrition. The major difference between total parenteral and enteral feeding is the absence of catheter-related sepsis in total enteral feeding. TPN should be continued until the patient demonstrates the ability to maintain adequate enteral alimentation.[3, 4, 55, 65, 72]

Maintenance of a sufficient blood sugar concentration and production of albumin are two of the metabolic functions that are affected by massive liver resection. One rarely observes hypoglycemia because of continuous intravenous infusions of glucose-containing solutions in the postoperative period. Nevertheless, the sugar concentration must be closely monitored. Hypoglycemia can be easily managed by an intravenous infusion of 10% or 20% dextrose solutions. Hypoproteinemia manifested by hypoalbuminemia can be temporarily managed by intravenous infusions of salt-poor albumin. The serum albumin concentration should be kept within the range of normal values.

Abnormalities in the biochemical parameters of liver function are similar whether hepatic dysfunction was produced by trauma or resection. The abnormality is dependent upon the amount of functional liver tissue lost, hepatic parenchymal anoxia and congestion, antecedent liver disease, and sepsis. A healthy liver undergoing resection will rapidly regenerate to normal metabolic function. Injured, resected cirrhotic liver tends not to regenerate, but there may be some improvement and partial restoration of preoperative liver function. However, the cirrhotic remnant will never completely regain preoperative levels of metabolic function.

The most common laboratory tests that are affected by traumatic loss or resection-induced hepatic dysfunction are elevations in lactic dehydrogenase (LDH), serum glutamic-oxaloacetic transaminase (SGOT), serum glutamic pyruvic transaminase (SGPT), alkaline phosphatase, and bilirubin. Cephalin flocculation, thymol turbidity, serum ornithine, and carbamoyl transferase are also elevated. Decreases occur in levels of serum cholesterol, triglycerides, nonesterified fatty acids, and cholesterol esters. Elevations of LDH and SGOT appear to be proportional to the extent of parenchymal injury. There are no patterns to the degree or dura-

tion of elevation. Unless there are major complications, the serum elevations of LDH, SGOT, and SGPT do not usually persist beyond 4 to 6 days. One value in following enzyme levels is to establish trends. The bilirubin elevations observed in sepsis are often preceded by enzyme elevations. Alkaline phosphatase tends to remain elevated for a longer period of time, ranging from several weeks to several months, depending upon the degree of injury and associated complications.

Jaundice is consistently observed in liver injury. Hyperbilirubinemia in the patient suffering liver trauma is usually caused by extravasation of blood into injured tissues and multiple blood transfusions. Hepatic parenchymal anoxia, regardless of its etiology, is a significant factor in producing jaundice. Hemorrhagic shock, heart failure, and the use of vasopressors cause hepatic anoxia by markedly decreasing total liver blood flow. General anesthesia, infection, and the administration of hepatotoxic drugs are additional causes of jaundice.

The majority of patients tend to develop jaundice early, within 48 to 72 hours, and then progressively clear it within several weeks. The serum bilirubin concentration is dependent upon three factors: pigment load, liver function, and the ability of the kidneys to excrete the bile pigment. With the visible jaundice caused by transfusions, most hepatic injuries, moderate-sized soft tissue hematomas, or hemorrhagic shock, the serum bilirubin will rise on the day of insult and peak in the range of 5 mg to 7 mg/dl. The elevation is usually transient, typically lasting only 3 days. Severe jaundice, with the bilirubin exceeding 20 mg/dl, may be observed in patients with large retroperitoneal hematomas. The severity and delayed onset of the jaundice can present a diagnostic problem to the physician since it is the pattern observed in septic liver failure. Fever with recurring or suddenly increasing hyperbilirubinemia is particularly ominous, since it connotes the presence of or impending sepsis.

Abnormalities in blood coagulation may be observed after liver resection. Prothrombin; factors V, VII, and X; and plasminogen can be decreased. Prothrombin and factor IX levels usually return to normal within 3 to 6 weeks. Factor V normally will rise to low normal to normal values at the end of 1 week. Platelet counts are frequently depressed for 1 to 2 weeks and then slowly return to normal concentrations. Within several weeks, without complications, all of these values will return to normal. Fibrinolytic activity and fibrin split products will be intermittently increased in the postoperative period. Hemorrhagic diathesis after hepatic resection is uncommon. It is usually caused by a consumptive coagulopathy or fibrinolysis.[16, 42, 60, 70]

Primary and Metastatic Hepatic Neoplasms

There is no difference in the diagnostic approach to primary or metastatic hepatic neoplasms. Unfortunately, most hepatic tumors are quite advanced at the time of diagnosis and cannot be resected. Smaller tumors, especially those in the hilus of the liver, may involve major blood vessels and cannot be resected. Although relatively uncommon, there is no question that isolated primary benign or malignant hepatic neoplasms should be considered for curative resection. Until recently, the concept of liver resection for commonly occurring metastatic liver carcinomas had gained little support. Extensive review of the literature and experiences at several large hospital centers reveal that under certain circumstances surgical intervention is indicated. Liver resection can play an integral part in multimodality therapy of children with Wilms' tumors. In the adult population, reports have indicated that to date only patients with resectable liver metastases from a colonic or rectal carcinoma have shown increased survival rates. The liver must be inspected at the time the patient is subjected to excision of a primary colorectal tumor. Synchronous liver metastases will be present 10% to 20% of the time. Approximately 25% of these patients will have resectable metastatic disease.

The natural history of patients with untreated liver metastases is grim, with postoperative survival ranging between 5 to 9 months.[6] Chemotherapy may prolong survival for a few additional months. A 5-year survival is rare in a patient with synchronous liver metastases at the time of excision of the colorectal primary. The mortality associated with liver resection for metastatic colorectal primary has been reduced in the past several years to about 5%, and recent studies have reported no mortality in carefully selected patients. Patients undergoing liver resection for a solitary metastatic nodule have the best prognosis. Five-year survival for liver resection in this group of patients is about 30%. Survival appears related to the amount of liver resected. Patients undergoing a lobectomy have a 5-year survival of 13%, while those undergoing a segmental or wedge resection have a 5-year survival of 21% and 24%, respectively. The amount of liver that must be resected allows for tumor-free margins.[2, 18, 19, 21]

DIAGNOSIS

The initial steps in the diagnostic workup for a hepatic neoplasm include an adequate history and physical examination supplemented by the appropriate laboratory studies. The history should include a search for suspected etiologic factors and for extrahepatic primary tumors. About 95% of the patients, especially those suspected of having metastatic liver disease, will present with nonspecific complaints such as weight loss, anorexia, fever, and gastrointestinal tract problems. About half of the patients will complain of pain, usually localized to the right upper quadrant. It may be sharp or intermittent and can radiate into the shoulder or right flank area. The pain may be exacerbated by deep inspiration, coughing, and changes in posture. On physical examination, tenderness on palpation will often be elicited in the area of the pain. Anywhere from 50% to 90% of the patients will present with hepatomegaly, ascites, or jaundice.[80]

There are no biochemical tests that will definitely establish the diagnosis of a liver tumor. The most reliable laboratory test aiding in the detection of carcinoma in the liver is an increased serum alkaline phosphatase. It is elevated in both primary and metastatic carcinoma in the liver. Liver function tests such as the transaminases, bilirubin, LDH, and sulfobromophthalein sodium retention have all had some value in the detection of liver tumors but add very little to the significance of an elevated serum alkaline phosphatase level.

Approximately 80% of patients with a primary hepatocellular carcinoma have an elevation of the alpha-fetoprotein. Serum concentrations of alpha-fetoprotein also are abnormal in other malignant conditions, such as malignancies arising from the stomach, bronchial, and reproductive systems. Any benign condition with rapid regeneration of hepatic parenchyma will cause an elevation. Examples include viral or alcoholic hepatitis.[83]

Serum carcinoembryonic antigen (CEA) assay can be an important adjunct in the detection of liver metastases. Marked elevations ($>$ 9 ng/ml) under certain conditions are accurate indications of metastatic disease in the liver even in the presence of a negative liver scan.[40] There are many diseases, as well as smoking, that can cause elevated CEA levels.

Following the initial clinical evaluation, additional noninvasive studies should be considered. Chest roentgenography reveals primary or metastatic disease in the lungs. Abdominal roentgenography is performed to evaluate the size of the liver, presence of calcifications, and organ displacement by the tumor. Upper GI series, barium enema, and intravenous urography are studies that are frequently indicated. Isotopic liver scanning with technetium-99m sulfur colloid aids in detecting a tumor mass. One of the most helpful noninvasive studies is ultrasonography of the liver. It can readily detect space-occupying lesions and is helpful in differentiating a cystic from a solid lesion. Sonography can also be used to differentiate nonobstructive from obstructive jaundice. Computed tomography (CT) under certain conditions is superior to sonography. The presence of gas-filled bowel makes sonography inferior to CT scanning. On the other hand, the presence of large amounts of fat will enhance the accuracy of ultrasonography, while decreasing the likelihood of obtaining a satisfactory CT scan. The resolution of both ultrasonography and CT is generally limited to the detection of lesions 2 cm or greater in diameter. Using ultrasonography in association with CT scans frequently makes it possible to detect smaller lesions.[8, 48]

Once the noninvasive evaluation has been completed, the workup needs to be completed by invasive diagnostic tests. A patient being evaluated for metastatic or primary liver carcinoma, if feasible, should have the lesion biopsied prior to major surgical exploration. A specimen for histologic evaluation may be obtained by percutaneous needle biopsy. The performance of blind biopsies usually will yield an adequate specimen about 55% of the time. Fine-needle-aspiration biopsy with the needle guided by ultrasonography or CT scans will markedly increase the diagnostic yield.[52] Laparoscopy can be considered in selected patients and 75% of the time will yield an adequate biopsy. Minilaparotomy may be considered and allows for gross inspection as well as adequate tissue sampling. Frequently CT scans can determine the etiology of obstructive jaundice, if the proper "cuts" are scanned. Percutaneous cholangiography is an excellent technique to evaluate patients presenting with obstructive jaundice. An additional advantage to percutaneous cholangiography is that the obstructed biliary tree can be provided with adequate drainage after the completion of the diagnostic study. One study vital to adequate preoperative evaluation of the patient with a liver tumor is selective hepatic arteriography. It differentiates a benign from a malignant process and accurately visualizes the blood supply of the tumor. A diagnostic accuracy of about 90% has been achieved through the use of selective hepatic angiography. The resectability of a liver tumor is usually determined by selective angiography.[32, 50, 74, 84]

Using the structured approach, moving from noninvasive to invasive examination, the surgeon will be able to determine the site, the extent, tumor histology, and resectability of the tumor prior to any determination of operative intervention. If the patient's lesion appears resectable, a celiotomy should be performed. If the extent of the tumor involvement is isolated to a resectable portion of the liver, it should be removed, taking adequate margins.

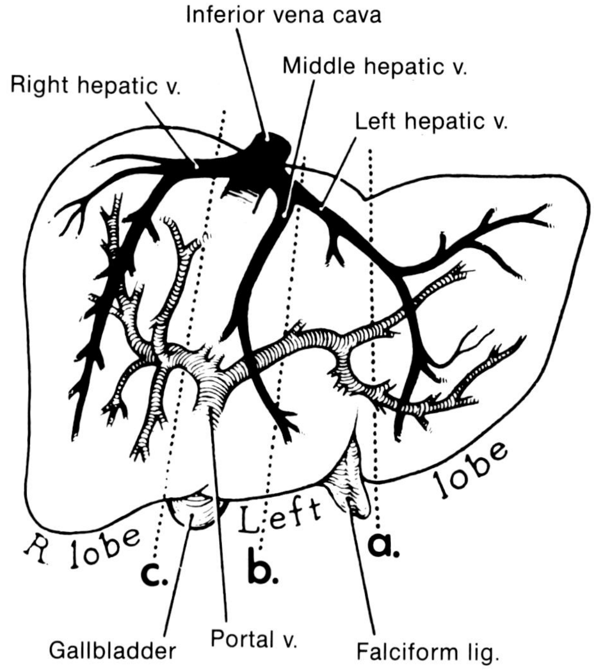

FIG. 38-1. The major lobar and sublobar vascular divisions within the liver. *a*, *b*, and *c* indicate the optimal planes for hepatic resection. (Zuidema GD, Rutherford RB, Ballinger WF [eds]: The Management of Trauma, 3rd ed, p 463. Philadelphia, WB Saunders, 1975)

LIVER RESECTION

An adequate comprehension of liver anatomy is necessary for the successful completion of a liver resection or controlling liver hemorrhage. There are several excellent articles that vividly illustrate modern concepts of normal liver anatomy.[26, 46, 73]

Hepatic resection can range from a wedge to a lobar or extended (trisegmentectomy) resection. Although the mortality rate of emergency liver resection is 50% or greater, an elective resection is different, with a mortality rate ranging from 0 to 15%. The techniques for performing an elective or an emergency hepatic resection are similar; circumstances differ. Liver parenchyma divided during an elective procedure is usually not friable or ischemic. Anatomical planes used for resection are easily identified in the uninjured liver. However, a large tumor can markedly distort liver anatomy. During an elective resection major vessels and ducts are isolated, ligated, and divided prior to removal of tissue. Extensive liver trauma often will cause the surgeon to pack, compress, mobilize, and débride in order to control hemorrhage so that he can search for major ducts and vessels that will need to be ligated and transected prior to performing a resection.

The anatomy of the liver is an important factor in determining the planes of resection. If the lateral segment of the left lobe is to be removed, the resection planes should be 1 cm to 2 cm to the left of the falciform ligament (*a* in Fig. 38-1; see also Fig. 38-2*A*). A left lobectomy is performed by dividing the liver in a plane extending from the left gallbladder margin to a plane just to the left of the vena cava (*b* in Fig. 38-1). A right lobectomy is performed when the plane of resection would traverse the liver from the right margin of the gallbladder to the right side of the vena cava (*c* in Fig. 38-1). An extended right lobectomy (trisegmentectomy) creates a plane of dissection running from the left margin of the gallbladder to the right side of the vena cava. These planes are used in the attempt to preserve as much as possible of the major intrahepatic ductal and vascular systems. The intralobar plane should be avoided in either a right or left hepatic lobectomy so as not to injure the middle hepatic vein (Fig. 38-2*A*). An anatomical plane produced by the falciform ligament should be avoided in order to avoid damage to the umbilical portion of the left portal vein (Fig. 38-2*B*). This plane also contains a number of small branches of the left hepatic artery, portal vein, and bile ducts.

Longmire and colleagues have outlined the steps for elective hepatic resection:[37]

1. Abdominal incision
2. Exploration and biopsy
3. Extension of incision into thorax (for right hepatic lobectomy)
4. Mobilization of lobe
5. Division and individual ligation of lobar branch of hepatic artery, portal vein, and hepatic duct; cholecystectomy
6. Division of segmental hepatic veins on dorsal surface of liver
7. Division of right or left hepatic vein
8. Division of parenchyma with ligation of biliary-vascular branches
9. Drainage
10. Closure of incision

A midline incision that can be extended in the chest is used for an emergency traumatic liver resection, while a right subcostal incision is used for an elective resection. In the latter, if after initial exploration the liver lesion can be resected, the incision can be extended into a chevron configuration by a left subcostal incision. Further exposure for a right lobectomy may require extending the incision into the eighth intercostal space. The diaphragm is opened about its periphery in a radial fashion in order to avoid injury to the phrenic nerve. Techniques of obtaining adequate hemostasis are described below and are used when indicated.

In general the outline for emergency hepatic re-

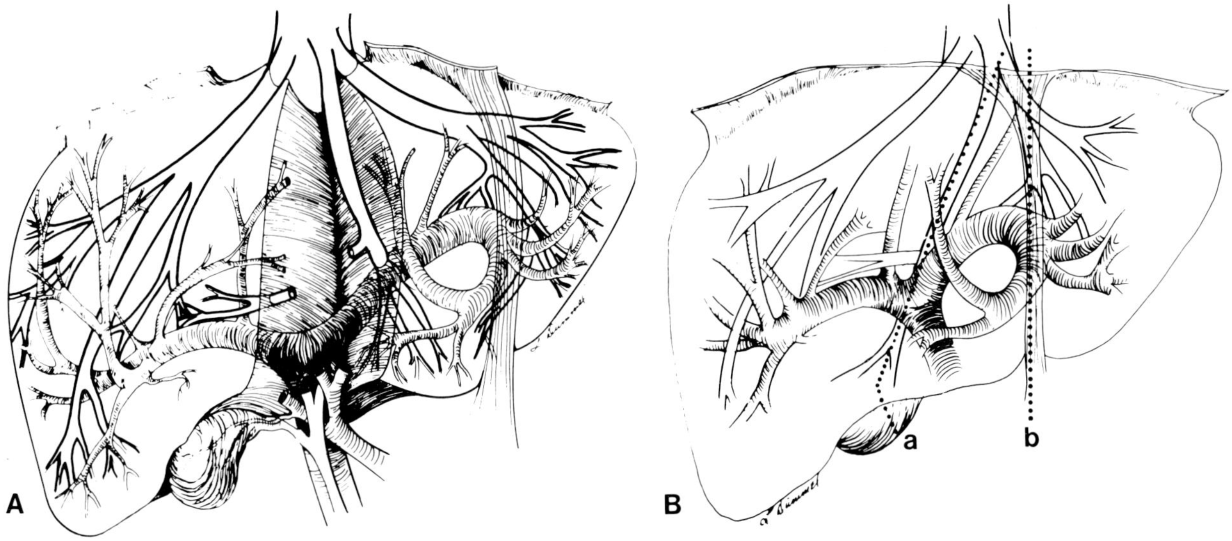

FIG. 38-2. (*A*) Intrahepatic anatomy. The liver is opened in the interlobar plane, and the intrahepatic anatomy of the portal and hepatic venous systems is depicted. The middle hepatic vein lies in the interlobar plane and joins with the left hepatic vein proximal to the vena cava, and the umbilical portion of the left portal vein may be seen in the plane of the falciform ligament. This latter plane divides the medial and lateral segments of the left lobe. (*B*) Planes to avoid in hepatic resection: *a*, the interlobar plane, is interdicted in either right or left hepatic lobectomy so as to avoid middle hepatic vein injury; *b*, the plane of the falciform ligament, is interdicted in extended right lobectomy or left lateral segmental resection so as to avoid injury to the umbilical portion of the left portal vein. (Donovan AJ, Turrill FL, Facey FL: Hepatic trauma. Surg Clin North Am 48:1313, 1968)

section would be patterned after elective resections. The main difference is that by necessity some of the steps would be performed in a different order during an emergency resection.

Numerous authors have described the techniques of liver resection. Quattelbaum and Quattelbaum, Byrd and McAfee, and McClelland and colleagues have given excellent descriptions of operative management of emergency hepatic resections.[10, 41, 62] Longmire and colleagues, Ong and Lee, Starzl and colleagues, Adson and Beart, and Foster and Lundy have adequately described the techniques for elective hepatic resections.[1, 20, 37, 53, 67, 68]

Small peripheral lesions can usually be excised by wedge resection. Hemostasis is obtained by interlocking mattress sutures or heavy chromic sutures placed prior to excision.

Liver Injury: Blunt and Penetrating Trauma

In patients suffering blunt abdominal trauma, the liver is second only to the spleen in frequency of injury. Five percent to 10% of patients sustaining blunt abdominal trauma will present with liver injury. The liver is second to the small bowel in incidence of injury resulting from penetrating abdominal trauma. Gunshot wounds account for an estimated 60% of all liver injuries. The remaining 40% is divided equally between hepatic injury from stab wounds and from blunt trauma.

The mortality rate associated with hepatic injury in the United States ranges from 8% to 20% with a mean of about 12% in most institutions. Many factors contribute to this mortality rate. Two elements that play a great part are the skill of the surgical team caring for the patient and the time elapsed between injury and operative intervention. Patients sustaining hepatic injury in a rural setting have a higher mortality rate than do those encountering similar injuries in the urban environment where paramedic services are available for resuscitation and transport to a trauma center.

Additional factors that determine survival after hepatic injury are as follows:

- Type of agent inflicting the injury
- Extent of damage to other organ systems—adjacent organs, thorax, lungs, brain, etc.
- Severity of hemorrhage
- Development of sepsis

Blunt injuries to the liver, frequently the consequence of an automobile accident, have a mortality rate approaching 20%. Stab wounds to the liver have an overall mortality rate of 1%. Mortality rates are higher in patients suffering from portal hypertension or a coagulopathy. Gunshot wounds approach an overall death rate of 15%. However, shotgun injuries to the liver have a mortality rate of 25%. The shot pattern is designed for scatter and produces not only liver but multiple-organ injuries.

Injuries to other organs frequently occur with liver trauma. Only 10% of gunshot or blunt injuries to the abdomen damage a single organ. Isolated liver injuries are associated with a mortality rate of about 5%, progressively increasing with the number of organs injured. Persons with six or more organs injured will risk dying in numbers greater than 60%.

Hemorrhage from either the liver or adjacent organs causes two thirds of the deaths associated with hepatic injury. Another one sixth of the deaths are brought about by sepsis. Accompanying head injuries will generate an additional one sixth of the mortality rate associated with hepatic injuries.[81, 82]

INITIAL EXAMINATION

The patient sustaining either penetrating or blunt injury to the liver will present with the general findings of significant intra-abdominal injuries. In haste, the obvious is unfortunately often disregarded. The importance of even a brief but accurate history and complete physical examination cannot be overemphasized.

Diagnosis of Liver Injury

- Right upper quadrant
  - Tenderness
  - Guarding
  - Rigidity
  - Mass
- Right shoulder pain
- Right side of chest—lower rib fracture
- Positive peritoneal lavage
  - Blood, red cells > 100,000/mm³
  - Amylase
  - Leukocytes > 500/mm³
  - Bilirubin
  - Bacteria
- Shock or hypotension—transient to refractory
- Peritonitis (in absence of blood loss, may be bile leak)

The most common initial finding with liver injury is abdominal tenderness. It is observed in 70% of patients with liver injuries. The patient will often complain of right shoulder pain, the result of blood and bile irritating the right diaphragm, producing the pattern of referred shoulder pain. Many patients exhibit abdominal guarding and rigidity, hypoactive or absent bowel sounds, and unexplained shock. Many victims of blunt trauma frequently have other injuries that obscure abdominal findings of significant liver trauma.[45, 82]

INITIAL THERAPY

Penetrating injuries to the lower chest and abdomen usually require prompt operative intervention. Blunt trauma to the area of the liver or suspected intra-abdominal injury is an indication to perform a diagnostic peritoneal lavage. Needle aspiration or "four quadrant tap" should not be attempted, since neither technique has been shown to be accurate.

Diagnostic peritoneal lavage is very accurate, the incidence of false-positive and false-negative lavages each being about 3%. The procedure is contraindicated in patients who have undergone multiple abdominal operations. Adhesions and loculations of the lavage fluid affect the safety and decrease the accuracy of the procedure. Diagnostic peritoneal lavage is usually contraindicated in the pregnant patient; however, if indicated, it can be performed in the first trimester before significant uterine enlargement. The reported incidence of complications in peritoneal lavage is about 5% in the patient with no contraindications. Lavage can be performed in the presence of penetrating trauma. Prior to performing a lavage, the bladder should be evacuated by Foley-catheter drainage. One of the best descriptions of the technique of peritoneal lavage has been offered by Thal and Shires.[76] A standard peritoneal dialysis catheter should be used, and the incision to insert the catheter should be extended through fascia of the linea alba and to, but not through, the peritoneum.[38]

During the initial resuscitation and evaluation of the patient suspected of having significant hepatic injury, gray scale ultrasonography, radionuclide and CT scans, and angiography are of little diagnostic value. Most of these patients are unstable and require aggressive support, but if the patient is easily resuscitated and remains stable, some of these procedures, if indicated, may be worthwhile.

RESUSCITATION

The initial therapy given to the patient with suspected liver injury is identical to that rendered to someone who has experienced severe abdominal or multisystem traumatic injuries. An adequate airway must be established and maintained. Vigorous attempts must be made to control hemorrhage and shock before attempting diagnostic or therapeutic endeavors.

Resuscitation in Liver Injury

1. Maintain airway, insert endotracheal tube if indicated or if patient unconscious
2. Complete physical examination
3. Cross match for blood
4. Insert two large-bore IV catheters
5. Insert one CVP or Swan–Ganz catheter
6. Infuse Ringer's lactate and colloid until blood is available
7. Attempt to "stay ahead" of fluid loss
8. Use military antishock trousers (MAST), if indicated
9. Insert nasogastric tube
10. Insert Foley catheter and maintain urinary output at 30–60 ml/hour

Any procedure performed by the staff during the initial resuscitation must not further compromise the condition of the patient. At least two large-bore intravenous catheters should be inserted in the upper extremities. Placement of central venous catheters or a Swan–Ganz catheter into the subclavian vein should be attempted only after the patient has been stabilized or conditions are well enough under control to permit the correct technique of insertion. An iatrogenically induced pneumothorax in a hemodynamically unstable patient or subsequent sepsis from a contaminated subclavian catheter is a likely complication that is best avoided. If additional venous access is initially required, attempts should be made to introduce a large-bore catheter in the external jugular or common femoral vein or to perform a cutdown into the greater saphenous or other accessible lower extremity veins.

Rapid infusion of 2000 ml of crystalloid (Ringer's lactate) will usually restore and maintain the patient's normal blood pressure if the blood loss has been limited to only 15% of total blood volume without continued significant bleeding. If the blood loss has been greater than 15% of blood volume or if hemorrhage persists, the blood pressure will often rise to near normal levels and then begin to fall. The patient will then need to receive not only additional crystalloid but also blood and albumin. At present, other available oncotically active compounds (dextrans and hydroxyethyl starch) should have very limited, if any, use during the resuscitation of someone with suspected liver injury. Dextran can cause a severe allergic reaction. Even though hydroxyethyl starch may be the superior colloid plasma expander, neither it nor dextran should be administered to a patient susceptible to hemorrhagic diathesis.[64] Refractory hypotension due to intra-abdominal hemorrhage frequently can be temporarily reversed by the use of MAST while rapidly infusing fluids.[29, 56]

Fortunately, in 50% to 70% of the patients suffering hepatic injury, hemorrhage will have ceased by the time the abdomen is explored. Only about 15% of liver injuries require complicated surgical procedures for control of bleeding.[81]

The patient remaining unresponsive to crystalloid, colloid, and blood infusions requires immediate operative intervention. This patient or one presenting with a tense hemoperitoneum and refractory hypotension will suffer profound cardiovascular collapse when the abdomen is opened. Accordingly, a thoracotomy and temporary thoracic aortic occlusion should be performed prior to celiotomy. Another approach to this problem is to take the patient to the operating room and infuse 2 units of blood (crossed or uncrossed type specific or type O Rh negative) while preparing and draping the chest and abdomen. If the systolic pressure rises to above 100 torr, the abdomen is opened and the abdominal aorta is compressed. There are several instruments designed for aortic compression. One simple and effective method is take a large or medium Richardson retractor and wrap the blades with a pack to prevent slippage. The padded flat surface of the retractor is pushed against the abdominal aorta between the retractor blade and vertebral column. The clenched fist of an assistant can accomplish the same goal.

If the systolic pressure remains less than 80 torr despite the blood infusion, a left anterior thoracotomy or median sternotomy is performed and the descending thoracic aorta cross clamped. The abdomen is then entered, and compression is applied below the diaphragm. The thoracic clamp is slowly released as additional blood is infused, attempting to maintain the systolic pressure above 120 torr.

While an assistant maintains pressure upon the abdominal aorta, the surgeon attempts to control the hemorrhage temporarily and assess the extent of intra-abdominal damage.[34]

The majority of complications due to traumatic injury to the liver are the result of bleeding. This bleeding may range from massive hemorrhage to a slow continuous ooze. Bleeding may be delayed, present intrahepatically, or manifest as hematobilia. Infection is another common complication of liver trauma. It occurs later and may present as a solitary or multiple intrahepatic abscesses, or it may exhibit the characteristics of walled off or generalized extrahepatic infection.

A number of problems will arise from interruption of biliary drainage or from retained devitalized liver tissue. Cardiopulmonary and renal problems are very common after hepatic trauma. The physician must be aware and prepared to treat multiple organ-system disease.

MANAGEMENT

The fundamental principles necessary for management of liver injuries are as follows:

1. Midline incision
2. Adequate control of bleeding
3. Removal of all devitalized liver
4. Examination for biliary duct damage; then repair and adequate drainage if necessary
5. Adequate drainage of operative field
6. Early reexploration for persistent bleeding[49]

When a patient with the diagnosis of liver injury is explored, the abdomen is entered through a midline incision. Then the surgeon has the ability adequately to examine the liver and the remainder of the abdomen for concomitant injuries. A midline incision, if necessary, can be rapidly extended into the chest by median sternotomy. The combined incision allows for better visualization of the superior surface of the liver with its attachments and peritoneal reflection, as well as allowing quick access to the intrapericardial and suprarenal vena cava if internal caval shunting is required. The thoracoabdominal incision enables the surgeon to displace the liver partially into the mediastinum, providing better exposure when performing subhepatic dissection or obtaining control of the smaller hepatic veins that enter the inferior vena cava. A median sternotomy is a well-tolerated chest incision, usually causing less pain to the patient and producing less respiratory impairment than is observed with an anterior lateral thoracotomy.[47]

HEMOSTASIS

Frequently no one method of hemostasis will adequately control liver hemorrhage; and the surgeon must utilize several modes of hemostasis. First attempts are to attain satisfactory temporary hemostasis.

Packing

Upon entering the abdomen, large packs are immediately placed to produce compression upon the bleeding liver wound to obtain adequate interim control. The surgeon is then given time to explore the remainder of the abdomen. Obvious bleeding sites are clamped. Leakage from intestinal wounds is closed with Babcock or linen-shod clamps or is oversewn.[81, 82]

Gauze rolls or sponges may be used to pack and maintain compression upon a bleeding liver injury for 24 to 72 hours. Initial resuscitation of the patient can then be completed in a hospital that is not equipped to care adequately for the patient's injury. Under these circumstances, after the wound is packed and the patient has stabilized, he is transported to a better equipped facility. Mortality and morbidity rates are markedly reduced by this method of triage.[11]

The escalation to major liver resection (lobectomy) in the patient suffering from massive liver injury with shock and tissue anoxia has a mortality rate approaching 50%. Packing to stop bleeding, utilizing additional hemostatic techniques, and then closing the incision with the intention of performing a reexploration within 24 to 72 hours will allow the physician to stabilize and study the patient and to prepare for more extensive surgery under more optimal conditions. Intravenous broad-spectrum antibiotic therapy must be instituted and the patient monitored for recurrent hemorrhage and sepsis.

A general rule to follow when the injury is severe and hemostasis appears impossible, even after the most vigorous attempts, is to use large packs, attempting to obtain sufficient pressure upon the liver to maintain hemostasis. The abdomen is closed, and the packs can be removed by celiotomy as long as 5 to 6 days postoperatively. This is not recommended, but it should be considered when one has employed all other alternatives.[11, 38, 81]

Bleeding capsular tears and small lacerations of the liver will readily respond to compression. Frequently, this bleeding will have ceased by the time the abdomen is entered.

Small hepatic vessels in the range of 1 mm to 1.5 mm in diameter can be electrocoagulated. Vessels greater than 2 mm in diameter must be ligated. Chromic or synthetic absorbable sutures should be used for ligation. Considerable time can be saved by using stainless steel hemostatic clips for vessel ligation. Large hepatic vessels should be meticulously tied or suture ligated.[1, 62]

A careful examination of liver laceration after initial control of bleeding will usually allow for cauterization or ligation of individual bleeding vessels. Some of the deeper or more complex injuries require opening more of the liver parenchyma to visualize the source of bleeding.[78]

Microcrystalline collagen, absorbable gelatin, or oxidized-regenerated cellulose can be applied with a pressure pack to minor venous oozing from the surface of the liver parenchyma. The collagen compound is probably the best of the three materials. Used judiciously, it causes no tissue reaction and is completely absorbed. It does not work well in the presence of thrombocytopenia. Use of these materials should be minimized since they are foreign bodies and can predispose the patient to infection and tissue necrosis. None of these compounds should be used to control large vessel bleeding or as a substitute for meticulous surgical techniques.[38, 45]

Pringle Maneuver

In conjunction with packing, the Pringle maneuver should be attempted.[61] The portal vein and hepatic artery are temporarily occluded by compressing the hepatoduodenal ligament (portal triad). This is accomplished either by digital or atraumatic vascular clamp compression.[61] Hemorrhage from the intrahepatic branches of the hepatic artery and the portal vein are usually controlled by this action. The one disadvantage to the Pringle maneuver is that it usually occludes most of the blood supply to the liver. This can further compromise marginally viable anoxic liver tissue. In the shocked patient, the use of the Pringle maneuver should not exceed 10 to 15 minutes. Bleeding persisting after the Pringle maneuver is usually hepatic venous in origin. An uncommon source of further bleeding after the Pringle maneuver may be an anomalous branch of the left gastric artery supplying the left lobe of the liver.[82]

Hepatic Artery Ligation

Considerable controversy over the indications, the effect, and the complications of hepatic artery ligation has arisen. The most recent consensus is that less than 5% of patients with hepatic injury are candidates for selective hepatic artery ligation. Hepatic arterial but not hepatic venous hemorrhage can be controlled by selective ligation, although if a venous branch of the portal or hepatic vein to a bleeding area is identified, it can be ligated. Selective hepatic artery ligation should be performed only after persistent attempts to gain local control of bleeding have failed. Ligation should be as selective as feasible, ligating the artery as far distally as possible. Devitalized tissue distal to the point of ligation should be débrided if the patient is stable. A cholecystectomy should be performed if the right hepatic artery is ligated. Rebleeding after hepatic artery ligation is not uncommon and may require reexploration.

Hepatic necrosis and sepsis are complications of selective hepatic artery ligation. Further tissue hypoxia may be caused by ligation. Some collateral flow to the liver can be maintained by not incising the coronary ligaments. The patient should be placed upon adequate antibiotic coverage. During the postoperative period the staff must carefully monitor the metabolic and oxygen requirements of the patient in order to prevent further anoxic insult.[17, 38, 45, 81, 86]

Finger Fracture

Finger fracturing is used bluntly to dissect in liver tissue. Glisson's capsule is incised by either sharp dissection or electrocautery. The forefinger and thumb are used to crush hepatic tissue. Resistant ducts and blood vessels are clamped, divided, and ligated or hemostatically clipped and divided.

Modifications are required with cirrhotic or fibrotic liver parenchyma. Finger fracturing is then combined with scissor dissection. This has been described as a "nibbling, spreading, and nudging of tissue." Finger fracturing may be expedited by assistance from a small blunt-suction tip or flat (scalpel) handle.[1, 35, 62]

Other Methods of Compression of Liver Tissue

The surgeon may control bleeding by mobilizing the right lobe of the liver by dividing the coronary and triangular ligaments. The right lobe is then rotated to the left. Care must be taken not to tear or injure further the hepatic venous system. Rotation of the right lobe of the liver to the left places tension on the inferior vena cava and hepatic veins and will often slow the bleeding to a manageable degree.[54]

Compression of liver tissue and control of hemostasis can be assisted by specially designed liver clamps. Most of these instruments were designed for use in elective hepatic resection. One usually has to mobilize the liver before they can be used. Application of these instruments can be tedious and time consuming; they are most useful to the surgeon who frequently resects liver. Flexible linen-shod clamps used during an open intestinal anastomosis can also be used as liver clamps.[13, 31, 35, 71]

Another method of controlling bleeding is the placement of mattress sutures immediately adjacent to the bleeding edge of the liver parenchyma. This is best used when liver tissue is to be resected. Large chromic sutures swedged onto blunt tip "liver" needles are the materials of choice. Even though synthetic suture has some advantages, it tends to saw through liver parenchyma. One can also get better control of tension when tying down the chromic suture. Large vessels within the suture-compressed tissue still must be individually ligated. Care must be taken not to damage the remaining viable tissue and blood vessels, or to interrupt major ducts.[38, 54, 66]

The Penrose drain can be used as a tourniquet to control liver hemorrhage. A 2.5-cm wide Penrose drain is placed around the liver proximal to the damaged parenchyma and is tied down until bleeding has ceased. The ends are brought out through the abdominal wall if it is to be left in place. If the patient is not to be reexplored, all devitalized hepatic tissue must be excised prior to closing the abdomen. Several days later in the intensive-care unit or operating room the tied Penrose can be removed by pulling the knot up through the abdominal wound and cutting below it. Advocates of this technique report that the Penrose tourniquet can be left in place as long as 1 week, and when it is removed bleeding usually does not recur.[49]

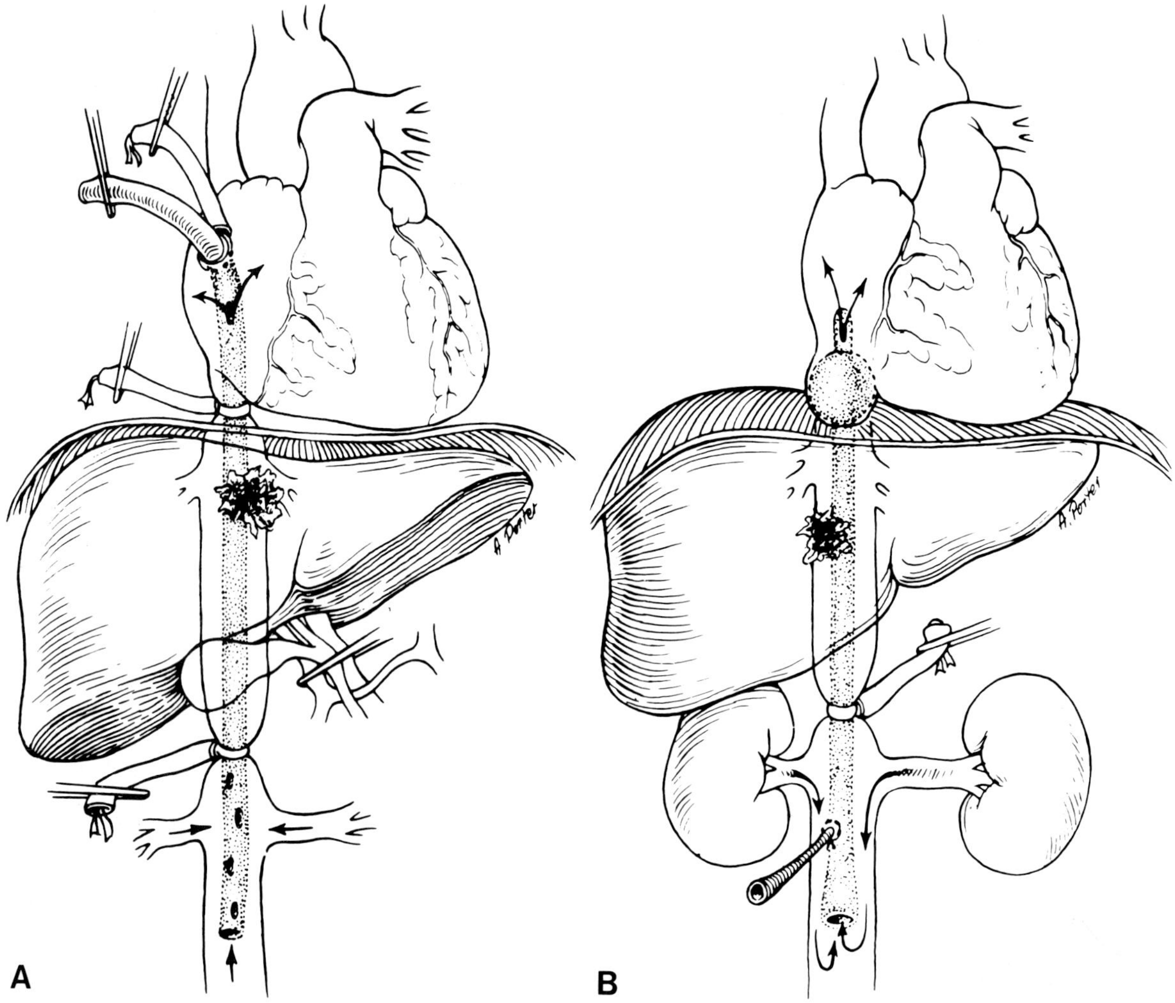

FIG. 38-3. (*A*) Inserting a shunt by way of the right atrial appendage to bypass the retrohepatic inferior vena cava. (*B*) Inserting a Foley catheter in the infrarenal inferior vena cava to bypass the retrohepatic vena cava. (Zuidema GD, Rutherford RB, Ballinger WF [eds]: The Management of Trauma, 3rd ed, p 466. Philadelphia, WB Saunders, 1979)

Hepatic Vein and Inferior Vena Caval Injuries

Fortunately, injuries to the retrohepatic inferior vena cava and adjacent hepatic veins are uncommon. The mortality rate from this injury exceeds 80%. Mobilization of the right lobe of the liver over to the left will frequently, as previously mentioned, reduce hemorrhage. Only rarely can one appose the margins of the lacerated vena cava with clamps and then suture the defect.

The most direct approach to obtain vascular control of hepatic venous and caval injuries is to use an intracaval shunt. Hemorrhage is initially controlled by tamponade with gauze packs. Many shunting devices have been described in the literature. Shunts can be made from a 36-French plastic chest tube, endotracheal tube, or a large Foley catheter (Fig. 38-3).

The shunt can be inserted downward through the right atrial appendage. Side holes are cut in the tube so blood flowing up through the tube will exit into the right atrium. The tube is inserted through a purse string placed in the atrial appendage. The shunt is pushed in to the level where the tip is just above the renal veins. Umbilical-tape tourniquets must be placed around the inferior vena cava just above the diaphragm and just above the renal veins. The supradiaphragmatic inferior vena cava is quickly isolated through a pericardiotomy incision. Placement of the suprarenal vein tourniquet will require the mobilization of duodenal loop and head of the pancreas (Kocher maneuver). With the shunt in place and the performance of the Pringle maneuver, the surgeon should have effectively isolated the vascular supply to the liver. If an endotracheal tube is used, the cuff is inflated just above the renal veins.

As an alternative, a Foley catheter can be inserted upward from an incision made in the vena cava above the renal veins. The balloon is inflated above the diaphragm to where it is larger than the vena caval hiatus. The surgeon then pulls the catheter back so the balloon will impact on the diaphragm, isolating the intrahepatic vena cava. Some specially designed tubes eliminate the need for the umbilical tourniquets and have a balloon that is inflated to occlude the lumen of the intrahepatic vena cava.[59, 66, 75, 78, 85]

Sometimes a hepatic vein will have torn and complicate control of bleeding. Small Fogarty embolectomy catheters can be inserted proximally and distally and inflated to obtain hemostasis.

Warm Ischemia Time

Inflow occlusion by the Pringle maneuver, intracaval shunting, and compression of the liver by a variety of techniques can produce ischemia of varying degrees. The limit for warm ischemia has been generally accepted to be a maximum of 20 minutes during emergency hepatic surgery. Warm ischemia of greater than 20 minutes with no significant hepatocyte injury has occurred during elective liver surgery. Steroids (methylprednisolone, 30–40 mg/kg of body weight, as an intravenous bolus) and hypothermia have been used to extend warm ischemia time. Topical hypothermia may be attempted by the use of iced Ringer's lactate poured over the surface of the liver.[54]

Drains

If permanent hemostasis has been attained without evidence of a bile leak, the liver wound is not drained. Until recently drains have always been used, but they can be harmful and should not be used if they are not needed. An unnecessary drain can predispose the patient to intra-abdominal infection and sepsis by retrograde entrance of bacteria along the drain tract into the abdomen. Drains should be used when bleeding continues or a bile leak is present or anticipated. After hepatic resection, large areas of dead space will require drainage. The ideal drain is a closed-system suction sump drain. Usually Penrose and open-suction sump drains are used, but they increase the risk of bacterial contamination of the peritoneum. Drains are removed as soon as there is no longer appreciable drainage.[15]

Omental Packing

Hepatic venous hemorrhage originating in large fractures of the liver can be temporarily controlled by having the assistant grasp the liver and compress the edges of the wound together, pushing the liver posteriorly to impede flow through the retrohepatic vena cava. A wound of this magnitude often requires major resection or packing. The mortality and morbidity rates associated with resection are substantial. Packing with a foreign body predisposes the patient to sepsis. Its removal usually requires reexploration. Large mattress sutures may be used, but injured viable liver tissue is often friable. If sutures are not placed deep enough into the liver, the tension placed on the suture while tying will tear through liver parenchyma.

Hepatic venous hemorrhage is from a low-pressure system, requiring less compression for hemostasis. If the wound is adequately débrided, the defect can often be filled with an omental pack. The pedicle of omentum utilizes the gastroepiploic vessels for its blood supply and is wedged into the depths of the wound cavity. A running absorbable synthetic or chromic suture is used to carefully oppose the edges of fractured liver under "mild tension." These wounds tend to ooze into the subhepatic space and require drainage. This technique has been quite successful in selected patients with liver fractures and hepatic venous hemorrhage.[69]

PORTAL VEIN INJURY

Portal venous blood is a nutrient source for the liver and provides venous drainage to the intestine. Fortunately, portal vein injury is uncommon, but its occurrence is frequently associated with severe liver injury. The injury is difficult to repair and usually is associated with other vascular injuries. Rapid and adequate exposure of the damaged portal vein is difficult. Initial management of portal vein hemorrhage is to achieve control, if possible, by packing. Temporary compression of the porta hepatis is attempted, followed by occlusion of the portal vein by using a vascular clamp. The optimal exposure of the portal vein requires mobilization of the cecum, ascending colon, and the mesentery of the small intestine. The duodenum and pancreas must also be mobilized. All of these structures are then retracted to the left, exposing the portal vein. The vein injury is isolated, and the packing and clamps, which provided temporary hemostasis, are removed. If vessels adjacent to the portal vein have been injured, they will have to be isolated and controlled.

The preferred method of portal vein repair is a lateral venorrhaphy. Alternative approaches have been an end-to-end anastomosis, interposition of a vein graft, insertion of a prosthetic graft, ligation, and portacaval or mesocaval shunt. A major disadvantage of using a portacaval shunt for reconstruction after portal vein injury is that it takes a long time to create the shunt in a compromised patient with multiple injuries. The preferable alternative when repair cannot be easily performed is portal vein ligation, in which the patient must be closely monitored for the risk of small bowel infarction secondary to venous hypertension. After portal vein ligation, it may be necessary to reexplore the patient in 24 to 48 hours to evaluate the condition of the intestine. If the intestine is very edematous or cyanotic and approaching the stage of venous infarction, a mesocaval shunt should be performed to provide adequate venous drainage of the intestine. This seldom is needed, however.[57]

INTRAHEPATIC HEMATOMA

Most significant injuries to the liver produce capsular disruption and hemorrhage into the abdominal cavity. Unruptured intrahepatic hematomas represent a small group of liver injuries that are caused by blunt trauma disrupting the liver parenchyma with subsequent bleeding beneath an intact liver capsule.

Small intrahepatic hematomas are given the opportunity to resolve spontaneously. Recent studies have supported this approach and report successful nonoperative therapy of even larger intrahepatic hematomas. Surgical intervention encompasses a celiotomy, evacuation of the hematoma, and ligation of the bleeding vessels. Too often surgery is unsuccessful. Bleeding recurs, and the patient requires a more extensive resection with its accompanying high morbidity and mortality rates.

Since the injury is confined to the liver parenchyma, it is difficult to elicit specific symptoms or complaints. Bleeding may cause capsular distention and subsequent pain, usually in the right flank. Examination may reveal a right pleural effusion or elevated right hemidiaphragm. Associated injuries such as rib fracture or chest wall contusion over the liver should suggest possible liver injury.

The liver function tests, SGOT, SGPT, and LDH levels are frequently elevated. Alkaline phosphatase is usually normal. Bilirubin may exhibit a transient elevation.

A filling defect in a lever-spleen technetium-99m sulfur colloid scan is seen with an intrahepatic hematoma. CT scans with or without contrast enhancement will also demonstrate intrahepatic hematomas. CT scans usually are more expensive than the technetium scan and provide no added improvement in diagnostic accuracy.

Sonography can be used to aid in the diagnosis of intrahepatic hematomas and has great value in following their course.

The nonoperative management of intrahepatic hematomas demands frequent observation and examination. The patient must be closely observed for at least 4 weeks. It is uncommon to see this complication after 1 month. Initially, bed rest is mandatory with slow return to full activity. Activity should be restricted for at least 6 weeks.

Nasogastric tube decompression of the gastrointestinal tract should be part of the initial therapy. The patient is then placed upon a 10-day course of intravenous broad-spectrum antibiotics. For the first several days, the hemoglobin and hematocrit should be frequently examined. Even if the lesion is stable, the hematocrit should be checked at least once a day. If the patient is on anticoagulant therapy, it must be reversed.

Any sudden deterioration in the patient's condition is an indication for surgical intervention. Blood loss is an early complication of intrahepatic hematoma. The hematoma can continue to expand slowly and rupture into either the abdomen or into the intrahepatic ductal system, causing hematobilia. Selective hepatic arteriography can identify the source of bleeding. Hemorrhage or persistent bleeding may be controlled by selective embolization. If angiographic control is unsuccessful, immediate operative intervention is indicated.

The late complications of intrahepatic hematoma include recurrent or persistent bleeding, sepsis, and intrahepatic abscesses. Slowly resorbing blood or bile mixed with devitalized hepatic parenchyma is an excellent culture medium.

Sepsis is managed by organism-specific antibiotic therapy and removal of the infected intrahepatic material. If an abscess can be easily located, percutaneous catheter drainage may be considered. Open drainage and débridement–resection are most frequently indicated.[12, 24, 25, 33]

Complications

HEMATOBILIA

One of the complications of liver trauma or liver surgery is hematobilia. It is easily detected in the postoperative period if the patient has had a catheter placed in the common bile duct. Hematobilia can occur any time from several days to weeks after the injury or surgical insult. The diagnosis of hematobilia is easily made in the patient with the classical presentation: colicky right upper quadrant pain, jaundice, and gastrointestinal tract hemorrhage. Unfortunately most patients have a much more subtle, even obscure presentation. Usually the patient will present with a history of intermittent gastrointestinal tract hemorrhage. Infrequently the patient may present with exsanguinating hemorrhage. Jaundice may be present. Any patient with a history of abdominal trauma, right upper quadrant pain, and upper gastrointestinal bleeding should be examined for the presence of hematobilia.

Hematobilia is secondary to injury of a hepatic arterial vessel. The artery bleeds into the low-pressure liver parenchyma and forms a false aneurysm. The aneurysm eventually erodes and ruptures into the low-pressure biliary tract. Laboratory studies in patients with hematobilia often reflect some liver damage. The SGOT, SGPT, and LDH levels are (even though transiently) usually elevated. Alkaline phosphatase level is elevated. The definitive diagnosis of hematobilia can be made by selective angiography. If angiography is not available, the lesion can be localized by gray scale ultrasonography, CT scan, and technetium-99m sulfur colloid scanning.

Treatment

The standard treatment of hematobilia has been surgical resection. The technique that is now recommended for control of hematobilia is selective angiography and therapeutic hepatic dearterialization by embolization. Gelfoam fragments have frequently been injected to clot bleeding vessels. The material is not ideal since it does dissolve. The patient then may rebleed, requiring reembolization. Therefore some angiographers have used Silastic or nonabsorbable beads for selective embolization. One of the risks of selective embolization is hepatic infarction.[77] Pyogenic abscesses can develop in the necrotic tissue. Liver necrosis will cause low-grade fevers, leukocytosis, and elevation of liver enzymes. After embolization, the patient can be noninvasively monitored by isotopic scanning, gray scale ultrasonography, or CT scan. Prior to discharge from the physician's care, the patient must undergo another selective arteriogram in order to ascertain that therapy has been successful.

Surgical intervention may be necessary in selective patients. Failure to stop hematobilia by selective arterial embolization will require operative intervention. Angiographic control may be successful, but the patient may present with a large, necrotic, infected intrahepatic cavity that requires débridement and drainage. A celiotomy and unroofing a small anterior lesion and direct ligation of bleeding vessels can be performed without much risk of morbidity and mortality. The deep lesions are much more difficult to treat. They have to be unroofed and drained, and the cavity is packed with omentum after direct ligation of the bleeding vessels. The deep lesions have a rate of rebleeding of about 40% and a mortality rate approaching 30%. In selected cases a major hepatic resection may have to be performed. Ligation of the hepatic artery has been tried and has met with some degree of success. Extrahepatic arterial ligation has a mortality rate of about 10%, and approximately 20% of these patients will rebleed. Ligation of either the right or the left hepatic artery will often control hematobilia. Within 24 to 48 hours collaterals within the liver will reestablish the blood supply and the patient may rebleed.[14, 22, 27, 51]

PYOGENIC LIVER ABSCESSES

One of the most feared complications of liver trauma or resection is the development of pyogenic liver abscesses. The reported mortality rate for undrained liver abscesses approaches 100%. Even with appropriate therapy the mortality rate is still at least 50%.

The hepatic reticuloendothelial system has a remarkable capacity to clear bacteria. Cultures obtained from healthy human liver tissue are sterile despite portal vein blood continuously exposing hepatic tissue to gastrointestinal tract bacteria. Hepatic tissue that has been contused, producing parenchymal hemorrhage, bile extravasation, ischemia, or devitalized tissue, can become secondarily infected.

Decreased host resistance, the consequence of a multiplicity of factors such as multiorgan system injury, burns, immunosuppression, and malnutrition predispose patients with marginally viable hepatic tissue to develop pyogenic liver abscesses. The bacteria that colonize the injured liver are from the portal vein or injured bowel, sepsis or bacteremia in the recovery/postoperative period, or "dirty," penetrating injuries.

Diagnosis

There is no "classic" presentation of a pyogenic liver abscess; the clue to diagnosing this problem is the knowledge that it may occur. Pyogenic liver abscesses present as a systemic febrile illness (Table 38-1). Patient histories are variable. The physician should be suspicious if the patient has suffered traumatic liver injury or liver surgery. The most common symptoms of a liver abscess are fever and pain. There is no pattern to the fever, which may be intermittent or continuous. A third of the patients complain of shaking chills. Pain usually presents in the right upper quadrant over the liver and is described as dull and constant. Patients with a liver abscess rarely complain of referred pain to the right shoulder but do complain of pleuritic pain. Many other complaints such as weight loss, malaise, nausea, and vomiting are nonspecific. Postoperative multitrauma patients may have their symptoms masked by injuries in other organ systems.

Physical findings are not specific. The examiner will observe hepatomegaly and tenderness on pal-

TABLE 38-1. PRESENTING SIGNS AND SYMPTOMS OF 490 PATIENTS WITH PYOGENIC HEPATIC ABSCESSES

	Number	Percentage
Symptoms		
Fever	398	81
Pain	252	51
Rigors	174	36
Nausea and vomiting	164	33
Weight loss	155	31
Anorexia	132	27
Malaise	96	20
Signs		
Hepatomegaly	246	50
Tenderness	246	50
Jaundice	131	27
Abnormal chest x-ray film	87	18

(McDonald AP, Howard RJ: Pyogenic liver abscesses. World J Surg 4:369, 1980)

TABLE 38-2. LABORATORY AND RADIOGRAPHIC FINDINGS IN 445 PATIENTS WITH PYOGENIC HEPATIC ABSCESSES

Finding	Number	Percentage
Leukocytosis (WBC $> 10^4/mm^3$)	316/445	71
Anemia (high < 12 g/dl)	165/349	47
Elevated serum bilirubin (> 2 mg/dl)	117/299	39
Hypoalbuminemia (< 2 g/dl)	130/238	55
Elevated serum alkaline phosphatase	139/300	46
Abnormal chest x-ray film	181/344	53
Abnormal liver–spleen scintiscan	85/106	80

(McDonald AP, Howard RJ: Pyogenic liver abscesses. World J Surg 4:369, 1980)

pation of the right upper quadrant. Jaundice in association with a pyogenic liver abscess is ominous. If a patient has been progressing satisfactorily and has cleared jaundice, the reappearance of jaundice with fever should be considered a manifestation of a pyogenic hepatic abscess until disproven.

Auscultation of the chest in many patients afflicted with an hepatic abscess reveals diminished breath sounds, rales, and ronchi at the right lung base. Percussion of the right chest frequently exhibits dullness at the right lung base and possibly an elevated right hemidiaphragm. Laboratory studies tend to be nonspecific (Table 38-2). Patients with hepatic abscesses usually exhibit a leukocytosis greater than 10,000 with a shift to the left. Two of the most frequent findings observed in the presence of hepatic abscesses are anemia and an elevation of the serum alkaline phosphatase. Elevation of liver enzymes (SGOT, SGPT, LDH) is unpredictable and follows no particular pattern. Serum bilirubin elevations greater than 2 mg/dl and hypoalbuminemia are commonly observed.

Abnormalities are seen in the chest x-ray film and are usually confined to the right lung base. They include atelectasis, an infiltrate, elevation of the right hemidiaphragm, or a right-sided pleural effusion. Subphrenic air fluid levels may also be present. Large abscesses in the left lobe of the liver will frequently displace the bowel downward and laterally. A barium meal upper GI study will demonstrate this shift and reveal indentation of the stomach by an enlarged left lobe.[48, 55, 56]

If one suspects a pyogenic liver abscess, one of the initial diagnostic studies should be gray scale ultrasonography. Ultrasonic scanning differentiates solid from fluid-filled lesions. It also assists in determining the location, number, and size of the hepatic abscesses. Radioisotope scanning of the liver with gallium-67 citrate is another method of discriminating abscesses from other space-occupying lesions. The gallium isotope has an affinity for inflammatory tissue and will concentrate in the hepatic abscesses. Indium-labeled leukocytes are similar to gallium-67 in their affinity for inflammatory tissue and have the additional advantage of no isotopic concentration in the colon. Both isotopes not only have the ability to detect liver abscesses but also reveal other intra-abdominal abscesses. Selective hepatic angiography has been utilized to detect isolated or multiple abscesses in the liver. The abscesses will appear as avascular lesions. Arteriography has very limited use as an aid to diagnosis of hepatic abscesses and offers no advantages over CT, ultrasonic, or radioisotope scanning. Hepatic scans in one collective study have been found to be abnormal 89% of the time when ultrasonography was noted to be abnormal 96% of the time.

CT scan is probably the most valuable adjunct in detecting and localizing intrahepatic abscesses. Even though CT scanning has been reported to detect lesions as small as 0.5 cm, the general consensus is that all scanning techniques can accurately detect intrahepatic lesions 2 cm to 2.5 cm in diameter. If the diagnostic workup is nonconclusive and an abscess is still suspected, operative exploration is indicated.[5, 9, 43, 63, 79]

Treatment

The only acceptable treatment for a pyogenic liver abscess is drainage. The success of therapy is dependent not only upon adequate drainage but also upon the general support provided to the patient. The patient must be provided with adequate nutrition, using TPN if indicated. Anemia, hypoalbuminemia, and electrolyte imbalances must be corrected. Adequate antimicrobial coverage is essential, and the patient should receive intravenous broad-spectrum antibiotics with coverage for both anaerobes and aerobes. Initial coverage would include the administration of a penicillin, with an aminoglycoside and clindamycin. Broad-spectrum coverage should be continued until specific pathogens are isolated by culture. Many of the isolates will be enteric organisms. Approximately two thirds of pyogenic abscesses are due to gram-negative enteric organisms of lower gastrointestinal tract origin. Antibiotic coverage is continued for at least 1 month when treating an isolated pyogenic liver abscess and up to 6 weeks if the patient has multiple liver abscesses.

SURGICAL EXPOSURE. Prior to the availability of broad-spectrum antibiotic therapy, drainage of a liver abscess was usually accomplished by the extraperitoneal approach or through an area of adhesions. It was hoped that this technique would keep the purulent drainage from the remainder of the peritoneal cavity. Mortality rates when the pleural or peritoneal cavity was contaminated were high. Many liver abscesses in the posterior portion of the right lobe of the liver were drained by a posterior retroperitoneal approach through the bed of the 12th rib.

Most surgeons now drain liver abscesses by transperitoneal exploration, made possible by adequate antibiotic coverage. Compared to the extraperitoneal approach, there appears to be no increase in rates of morbidity and mortality. One of the genuine advantages to transperitoneal approach is that it enables the surgeon to examine the entire abdomen adequately for the presence of extrahepatic abscesses, examine the liver for the presence of multiple abscesses, and have the ability to explore and decompress, if indicated, the biliary tree.

When the transperitoneal approach is used, the abdomen is entered through either a subcostal or midline incision. A meticulous search is made throughout the abdomen for the presence of infection or the primary source of seeding to the liver. Bimanual palpation of the liver is performed. Abscesses that have not been diagnosed prior to exploration can be detected since they will present as a change in consistency of the liver parenchyma. The area of the liver suspected to be harboring an abscess can be aspirated. Once the known or suspected areas have been determined, these portions of the liver are then packed off from the rest of the abdominal cavity. If the abscess is tense, it is first partially decompressed by needle aspiration. The abscess cavity is then opened and drained. Loculations are broken up.

A liver abscess may be associated with a large amount of necrotic tissue. All of the devitalized tissue must be excised even if it means performing a major liver resection. All abscesses must be drained. The effect of leaving one undrained abscess is as serious as not draining any abscess at all. The cavity is unroofed as much as possible and is drained. Dead space can be reduced by loosely filling wih a pedicle of omentum.[5, 23, 43, 63, 79] Soft drains should be used, since hard rubber drains may erode into the liver parenchyma and may cause hemorrhage. The ideal drain is a Silastic sump drain or a closed-system Silastic drain that can be converted into a sump. Although some prefer Silastic drains, any soft drain will suffice. Penrose drains can be used to provide some additional dependent drainage. It is important to have at least one good sump drain in each abscess cavity to provide irrigation when necessary. Postoperatively many physicians choose to irrigate the cavity through a drain with an antibiotic-containing solution. If the abscess is adequately drained, irrigation is not necessary. A drain may be used to inject radiopaque material in order to follow the closure of the abscess cavity. At least one large drain is left in place until the cavity has closed down and around it. The drain is gradually removed, allowing the tract to close.

Percutaneous drainage has been demonstrated to be a safe, effective method to drain selected pyogenic liver abscesses.[28] CT and ultrasound are used to detect and localize the abscess. Diagnostic needle aspiration is performed, and a guidewire is inserted through the needle. Using a modified Seldinger angiographic technique, a large pigtail catheter is inserted into the abscess cavity. A trocar catheter may also be used to drain the abscess after diagnostic aspiration. The cavity is then aspirated and irrigated. The catheter is connected to a catheter bag. Reduction in size of the abscess can be monitored by injecting radiopaque irrigant by way of the catheter into the cavity.

The success of percutaneous drainage is dependent upon several factors. The abscess must be completely drained. Loculated or multiple abscesses are best managed by open drainage. However, the high-risk patient with several large unloculated abscesses could be successfully managed by multiple percutaneous catheters. Thick fluid may not be easily drained through the small-bore catheter; this problem can be remedied by progressively increasing the size of the catheter and its side holes. If the material still does not adequately drain through the catheter, operative intervention is necessary. Many hepatic abscesses contain considerable debris and are surrounded by necrotic tissue. These abscesses require open drainage and débridement.

Although the diagnostic percutaneous aspiration of a liver abscess for culturing, followed by intravenous antibiotic therapy, is successful in selected cases, it should still be regarded as a mode of therapy with unacceptable risk to the patient. Patients being treated by percutaneous drainage should be carefully monitored. If there are signs of therapeutic failure, surgical drainage is mandatory.[25, 30, 44, 63]

EXTRAHEPATIC BILIARY TRACT DRAINS

Routine "controlled extrahepatic biliary drainage" as a component of the treatment of liver injuries is to be discouraged. It offers few advantages and increases rates of morbidity and mortality. Increases in the incidence of upper gastrointestinal bleeding, intra-abdominal abscesses, massive wound infection, jaundice, and cholangitis occur with routine T-tube choledochostomy in the treatment of penetrating liver injury.

One reason commonly given for T-tube drainage of the common bile duct is the ability to lower the intrahepatic biliary pressure. This would theoretically decrease the chances of bile extravasation from the edge of débrided or resected liver, but this has never been supported by any laboratory evidence. Bile leakage is best prevented by meticulous ligation of all transected bile ducts and adequate débridement of devitalized tissue.

The common duct has been opened and cannulated with a T tube in order to identify severed biliary ducts. One can accomplish the same goal by compressing the common bile duct with a noncrushing clamp and using a small-gauge pediatric scalp vein needle to inject fluid proximal to the clamp into the common duct (or into the gallbladder), observing back flow through the severed ducts.

T tubes have been used in the postoperative period to demonstrate ductal obstruction and aid in the early diagnosis of hematobilia. The possible complication of hematobilia is not an indication to use a T tube. Ultrasonography, percutaneous transhepatic cholangiography, and ERCP make it possible to visualize accurately the area of obstruction that may occur after major liver surgery. Routine extrahepatic biliary drainage would require cannulation of a normal-sized common bile duct, a task that can be difficult and time consuming. Furthermore one risks injury to the cystic and common bile ducts.

Extrahepatic biliary ductal disruption is not common. If it is not recognized, it can cause death. Patients suffering from a transection or rupture of the extrahepatic bile duct may experience a very prolonged hospital course, if there is a delay before the injury is recognized. Bile peritonitis as a consequence of a leaking bile duct can cause ascites, jaundice, acholic stools, prerenal azotemia, and a deteriorating clinical state. Bile staining of tissue without any apparent source is an indication for intraoperative cholangiography.

T-tube drainage of the common bile duct should be performed when injury to the extrahepatic biliary duct requires suturing and stenting or when major damage to the intrahepatic biliary ducts may require drainage to control bile leaks. An alternative to the T tube for decompression would be direct cannulation of the injured duct, bringing the catheter out through a stab wound in a dependent position, or using a Roux-en-Y intestinal loop to provide drainage after stenting an extensively damaged biliary ductal system. Another alternative would be transhepatic percutaneous stenting by inserting a Rodney–Smith tube through the liver parenchyma to stent an anastomosis and provide bile drainage.[7, 36, 39]

References

1. Adson MA, Beart RW Jr: Elective hepatic resections. Surg Clin North Am 57:339, 1977
2. Adson MA, Van Heerden JA: Major hepatic resection for metastatic colorectal cancer. Ann Surg 191:576, 1980
3. Almersjo O, Bengmark S, Hafstrom LO, Olsson R: Enzyme and function changes after extensive liver resection in man. Ann Surg 169:111, 1969
4. Aronsen KF, Ericsson B, Pihl B: Metabolic changes following major hepatic resection. Ann Surg 169:102, 1969
5. Balasegaram M: Management of hepatic abscess. Curr Probl Surg 18:285, 1981
6. Bengtsson G, Carlsson G, Hafstrom L, Jonsson P: Natural history of patients with untreated liver metastases from colorectal cancer. Am J Surg 141:586, 1981
7. Bowen JL, Fleming WH: Upper gastrointestinal bleeding associated with biliary diversion after hepatic injury. Ann Surg 177:402, 1973
8. Bryan PJ, Dinn WM, Grossman ZD et al: Correlation of computed tomography, gray scale ultrasonography, and radionuclide imaging of the liver in detecting space-occupying processes. Radiology 124:387, 1977
9. Buchman TG, Zuidema GD: The role of computerized tomography scanning in the surgical management of pyogenic hepatic abscesses. Surg Gynecol Obstet 153:1, 1981
10. Byrd WM, McAfee DK: Emergency hepatic lobectomy in massive injury of the liver. Surg Gynecol Obstet 113:103, 1961
11. Caine RY, McMaster P, Pentlow BD: The treatment of major liver trauma by primary packing with transfer of the patient for definitive therapy. Br J Surg 66:338, 1979
12. Cheatham JE, Smith EI, Tunell WP, Elkins RC: Nonoperative management of subcapsular hematomas of the liver. Am J Surg 140:852, 1980
13. Doty DB, Kugler HW, Moseley EV: Control of hepatic parenchyma by direct compression. A new instrument. Surgery 67:720, 1970
14. Fagan EA, Allison DJ, Chadwick VS, Hodgson HJF: Treatment of haemobilia by selective arterial embolization. Gut 21:541, 1980
15. Fischer RP, O'Farrell KA, Perry JD Jr: The value of peritoneal drains in the treatment of liver injuries. J Trauma 18:393, 1978
16. Flint LM. Liver failure. Surg Clin North Am 62:157, 1982

17. Flint LM Jr, Polk HC Jr: Selective hepatic artery ligation: Limitations and failures. J Trauma 19:319, 1979
18. Fortner JG et al: Major hepatic resection for neoplasia: Personal experiences in 108 patients. Ann Surg 188:363, 1978
19. Foster JH: Survival after liver resection for secondary tumor. Am J Surg 135:389, 1978
20. Foster JH, Lundy J: Liver metastasis. Curr Probl Surg 18:157, 1981
21. Foster JH, Lundy J: Liver metastases. Surg Clin North Am 28:161, 1981
22. Franklin RH, Bloom WF, Shoffstall RO: Angiographic embolization as the definitive treatment of posttraumatic hemobilia. J Trauma 20:702, 1980
23. Gaisford WG, Mark JBD: Surgical management of hepatic abscess. Am J Surg 118:317, 1969
24. Geis WP, Schultz KA, Giacchino JL, Freeark RJ: The fate of unruptured intrahepatic hematomas. Surgery 90:690, 1981
25. Gerzof SE, Robbins AH, Johnson WC, Birkett DH, Nabseth DC: Percutaneous catheter drainage of abdominal abscesses: A five-year experience. N Engl J Med 305:653, 1981
26. Healey JE Jr: Clinical anatomic aspects of radical hepatic surgery. J Internat Coll Surgeons 22:542, 1954
27. Heimbach DM, Ferguson GS, Hanley JD: Treatment of traumatic hemobilia with angiographic embolization. J Trauma 18:229, 1978
28. Herbert DA, Rotman J, Simmons F et al: Pyogenic liver abscesses: Successful non-surgical therapy. Lancet 1:134, 1982
29. Hibbard LT: Spontaneous rupture of the liver in pregnancy: A report of eight cases. Am J Obstet Gynecol 126:334, 1976
30. Johnson WC, Gerzof SG, Robbins AH, Nabseth DC: Treatment of abdominal abscesses. Ann Surg 194:510, 1981
31. Joishy SK, Balasegaram M: Hepatic resection for malignant tumor of the liver: Essentials for a unified surgical approach. Am J Surg 139:360, 1980
32. Kim DK, McSweeney J, Yeh SDJ, Fortner JG: Tumors of the liver as demonstrated by angiography, scan and laparotomy. Surg Gynecol Obstet 141:409, 1975
33. Lambeth W, Rubin BE: Nonoperative management of intrahepatic hemorrhage and hematoma following blunt trauma. Surg Gynecol Obstet 148:507, 1979
34. Lederwood AM, Kazmers M, Lucas CA: The role of thoracic aortic occlusion for massive hemoperitoneum. J Trauma 16:610 1976
35. Lin T: Results in 107 hepatic lobectomies with a preliminary report on the use of a clamp to reduce blood loss. Ann Surg 177:413, 1973
36. Lin T, Chen C: Metabolic function and regeneration of cirrhotic and non-cirrhotic liver after hepatic lobectomy in man. Ann Surg 162:959, 1965
37. Longmire WP, Trout HH, Greenfield J, Tompkins RK: Elective hepatic surgery. Ann Surg 179:712, 1974
38. Lucas CE, Ledgerwood AM: Prospective evaluation of hemostatic techniques for liver injuries. J Trauma 16:422, 1976
39. Lucas CE, Walt AJ: Analysis of randomized biliary drainage for liver trauma in 189 patients. J Trauma 12:925, 1972
40. McCartney WH, Hoffer PB: Carcinoembryonic antigen essay in hepatic metastases detection: An adjunct to liver scanning. JAMA 236:1023, 1976
41. McClelland R, Shires T, Poulos E: Hepatic resection massive trauma. J Trauma 4:282, 1964
42. McDermott WV Jr, Greenberger NJ, Isselbacher KJ, Weber AL: Major hepatic resection: Diagnostic techniques and metabolic problems. Surgery 54:56, 1963
43. McDonald AP, Howard RJ: Pyogenic liver abscesses. World J Surg 4:369, 1980
44. Martin EC, Karlson KB, Fankuchen EI et al: Percutaneous drainage of postoperative intraabdominal abscesses. AJR 138:13, 1982
45. Mays ET: Hepatic trauma. Curr Probl Surg 13:1, 1976
46. Michels NA: New anatomy of the liver and its variant blood supply and collateral circulation. Am J Surg 112:337, 1966
47. Miller DR: Median sternotomy extension of abdominal incision for hepatic lobectomy. Ann Surg 175:193, 1972
48. Moss AA, Schrumpf J, Schnyder P et al: Computed tomography of focal hepatic lesions: A blind clinical evaluation of the effect of contrast enhancement. Radiology 131:427, 1979
49. Murray DH Jr, Borge JD, Pouteau GD: Tourniquet control of liver bleeding. J Trauma 18:771, 1978
50. Nagasue N, Inokuchi K, Kobayashi M et al: Angiographic evaluation of hepatoma for surgical treatment. Surg Gynecol Obstet 143:184, 1976
51. Nielsen ML, Mygind T: Selective arterial embolization in traumatic hemobilia. World J Surg 4:357, 1980
52. Nosher JL, Plafker J: Fine needle aspiration of the liver with ultrasound guidance. Radiology 136:177, 1980
53. Ong GB, Lee NW: Hepatic resection. Br J Surg 62:421, 1975
54. Pachter HL, Spencer FC: Concepts in the treatment of hepatic trauma. Ann Surg 190:423, 1979
55. Pack GT, Molander DW: Metabolism before and after hepatic lobectomy for cancer. Arch Surg 80:685, 1960
56. Pelligra R, Sandberg EC: Control of intractable abdominal bleeding by external counterpressure. JAMA 241:708, 1979
57. Petersen SR, Sheldon GF, Lin RC Jr: Management of portal vein injuries. J Trauma 19:616, 1979
58. Pietsch JB, Meakins JL, MacLean LD: The delayed hypersensitivity response: Application in clinical surgery. Surgery 82:349, 1977
59. Pilcher DB, Harman PK, Moore EE Jr: Retrohepatic vena cava balloon shunt introduced via the sapheno-femoral junction. J Trauma 17:837, 1978
60. Pinkerton JA, Sawyers JL, Foster JH: A study of the postoperative course after hepatic lobectomy. Ann Surg 173:800, 1971
61. Pringle JH: Notes on the arrest of hepatic hemorrhage due to trauma. Ann Surg 48:541, 1908
62. Quattlebaum JK, Quattlebaum JK Jr: Technic of hepatic lobectomy. Ann Surg 149:648, 1959
63. Rubin RH, Swartz MN, Malt R: Hepatic abscess: Changes in clinical, bacteriologic and therapeutic aspects. Am J Med 57:601, 1974
64. Rudowski WJ: Evaluation of modern plasma expanders and blood substitutes. Br J Hosp Med 23:389, 1980
65. Sarfeh IJ, Balint JA: The clinical significance of hyperbilirubinemia following trauma. J Trauma 18:58, 1978
66. Schrock T, Blaisdell FW, Mathewson C Jr: Management of blunt trauma to the liver and hepatic veins. Arch Surg 96:698, 1968
67. Starzl TE, Bell RH, Beart RW, Putnam CW: Hepatic trisegmentectomy and other liver resections. Surg Gynecol Obstet 141:429, 1975
68. Starzl TE, Loep LJ, Weil R III et al: Right trisegmentectomy for hepatic neoplasms. Surg Gynecol Obstet 150:208, 1980

69. Stone HH: Use of pedicled omentum as an autogenous pack for control of hemorrhage in major injuries of the liver. Surg Gynecol Obstet 141:92, 1975
70. Stone HH, Long WD, Smith RB, Haynes CD: Physiologic considerations in major hepatic resections. Am J Surg 117:78, 1969
71. Storm FK, Lonmire WR Jr: A simplified clamp for hepatic resection. Surg Gynecol Obstet 133:103, 1971
72. Strawn TS, Williams HC, Flint LM Jr: Prognostic significance of serum biochemical changes following liver trauma. Am Surg 46:111, 1980
73. Suzuki T, Nakayasu A, Kawabe K et al: Surgical significance of anatomic variations of the hepatic artery. Am J Surg 122:505, 1971
74. Takashima T, Matsui O: Infusion hepatic angiography in the detection of small hepatocellular carcinomas. Diagnostic Radiology 136:321, 1980
75. Testas P, Benichou J, Benhamou M, Chanzy M: Vascular exclusion in surgery of the liver: Experimental basis, technic and clinical results. Am J Surg 133:692, 1977
76. Thal ER, Shires GT: Peritoneal lavage in blunt abdominal trauma. Am J Surg 125:64, 1973
77. Trojanowski JQ, Harrist TJ, Athanasoulis CA, Greenfield AJ: Hepatic and splenic infarction: Complications of therapeutic transcatheter embolization. Am J Surg 139:272, 1980
78. Trunkey DD, Shires GT, McClelland R: Management of liver trauma in 811 consecutive patients. Ann Surg 179:722, 1974
79. Verlenden WL III, Frey CF: The management of liver abscess. Am J Surg 140:53, 1980
80. Viamonte M, Schiff E: Diagnostic approach to heptic malignant neoplasms. JAMA 238:2191, 1977
81. Walt AJ: The mythology of hepatic trauma—Or Babel revisited. Am J Surg 135:12, 1978
82. Walt AJ: Hepatic injuries. S Afr Med J 16:658, 1980
83. Wepsic HT, Kirkpatrick A: Alpha-fetoprotein and its relevance to human disease. Gastroenterology 77:787, 1979
84. Williamson BWA, Blumgart LH, McKellar NJ: Management of tumors of the liver: Combined use of arteriography and venography in the assessment of resectability especially in hilar tumors. Am J Surg 139:210, 1980
85. Yellin AE, Chaffee CB, Donovan AJ: Vascular isolation in treatment of juxtahepatic venous injuries. Arch Surg 102:566, 1971
86. Zuidema GD, Rutherford RB, Ballinger WF (eds): The Management of Trauma, 3rd ed, p 465. Philadelphia, WB Saunders, 1979

39 Complications of Portal Decompressive Surgery

Seymour I. Schwartz

OVERVIEW

Operative procedures directed at reducing the extent of portal hypertension have, as their prime indication, esophagogastric varices that are bleeding or have bled significantly in the past. In unusual circumstances the decompressive procedure is carried out for intractable or rapidly evolving ascites. The other manifestation of portal hypertension, hypersplenism, does not constitute a specific indication for a decompressive procedure.

ETIOLOGY OF PORTAL HYPERTENSION

The etiologic factors indicated as causes of portal hypertension include increased hepatopetal flow, extrahepatic venous outflow obstruction, obstruction of the extrahepatic portal venous system, and intrahepatic obstruction. Increased hepatopetal flow without either presinusoidal or postsinusoidal venous obstruction is a rare circumstance caused by either a splenic arteriovenous fistula or a marked increase in splenic circulation; this is characteristic of massive tropical splenomegaly and occasional cases of splenomegaly associated with a myeloproliferative disorder. In these circumstances splenectomy alone effectively reduces portal pressure, and a portal decompressive procedure is not mandated.

Obstruction of the hepatic veins caused by an idiopathic endophlebitis is an unusual but dramatic indication for a decompressive procedure directed at reversing the rapid evolution of hepatic failure and massive ascites. By contrast, portal hypertension secondary to impaired flow in the extrahepatic portal venous system usually is not complicated by hepatocellular dysfunction or ascites. This is commonly caused by a cavernomatous transformation of the portal vein, which probably represents organization and recanalization of thrombi within the vessel. The lesion may be caused by infection that involves the umbilical vein, but in most cases the cause cannot be defined. The sinusoidal and hepatic vein wedge pressures in these patients are normal.

The overwhelming majority of patients with portal hypertension have intrahepatic obstruction due to a variety of hepatic diseases. The most common of these is cirrhosis of a nutritional or postnecrotic variety. Biliary cirrhosis, hemochromatosis, and Wilson's disease may also cause postsinusoidal obstruction. Congenital hepatic fibrosis and the early pathologic lesions of schistosomiasis are causes of presinusoidal obstruction.

Hemodynamic Effects of Major Portalsystemic Shunts

Portalsystemic shunts include end-to-side portacaval shunts (Fig. 39-1), side-to-side portacaval shunts; inferior venacaval–superior mesenteric venous anastomoses; end-to-side splenorenal shunts, usually with splenectomy; end-to-side portacaval shunts with arterialization of the hepatic stub; and selective distal splenorenal shunts. Each of these procedures effects decompression of the venous hypertension within the esophagogastric varices. Functionally, the shunts may be categorized either as totally or as partially diverting portal venous flow away from the liver, and also as decompressing or failing to decompress hepatic sinusoidal hypertension.

The end-to-side portacaval shunt prevents blood from reaching the liver since the portal vein is totally disconnected. This disconnection also prevents the portal vein from serving as an efferent conduit draining sinusoidal blood from the liver. Following an end-to-side portacaval shunt the hepatic vein wedge pressure, reflecting sinusoidal pressure, declines in the majority of patients. The hemodynamically func-

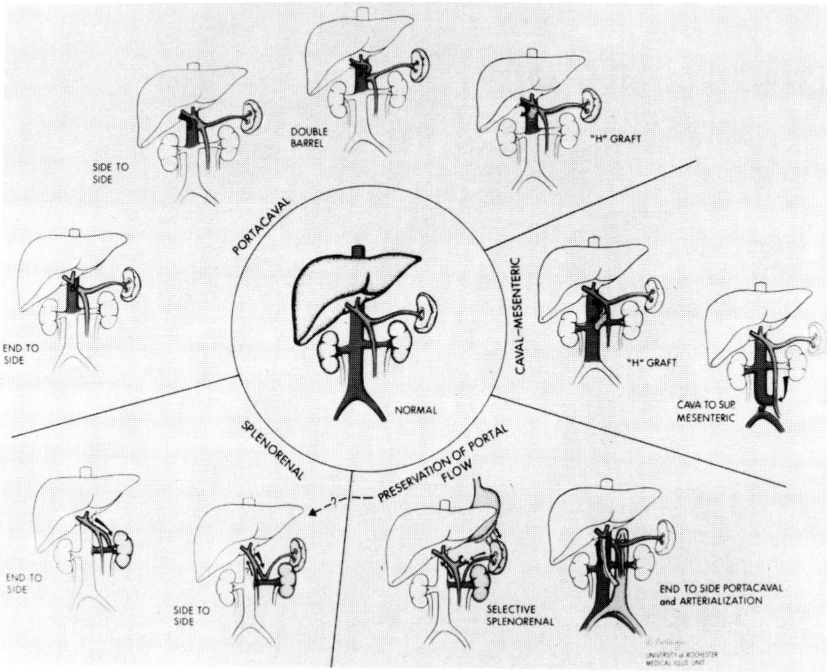

FIG. 39-1. Variety of portal decompressive procedures.

tional, side-to-side shunts include side-to-side portacaval shunts, central splenorenal shunts, and the mesocaval anastomoses; each of these procedures rarely provides adhepatic flow of splanchnic venous blood. However, each allows for potential decompression of sinusoidal hypertension. Therefore, a functional side-to-side anastomosis is mandated in patients with Budd–Chiari syndrome and rapidly evolving ascites since therapy is directed at reducing sinusoidal hypertension.

Patients with cirrhosis show no consistent difference in the extent of reduction of sinusoidal hypertension between a side-to-side shunt and an end-to-side portacaval shunt. Following a side-to-side shunt, the portal vein may effectively decompress the liver. This may be disadvantageous because it may siphon arterial blood and reduce the amount available for hepatic parenchymal cells. Under most circumstances the classic end-to-side splenorenal shunt and the H-graft interposition mesocaval shunt do not permit significant portal venous flow to enter the liver.

The only two procedures that assure a continuance of adhepatic flow along the course of the portal vein are the hepatic arterialization, as introduced by Maillard and associates, and the selective distal splenorenal shunt.[3] In the arterialization procedure, which has had little acceptance in the United States, the maintenance of inflow is related to arterial blood under arterial pressure. The distal splenorenal shunt proposed by Warren and associates is truly selective because it decompresses the esophagogastric varices while it maintains portal hypertension within the portal veins and sinusoids.[10] Portal perfusion persists initially, but accumulating literature indicates that in the course of time there is a stealing from the adhepatic portal flow into the newly established collateral veins, and portal perfusion eventually may be lost.[5]

Complications

Complications of portal decompressive procedures include intraoperative complications such as bleeding and shunt thrombosis and an "unshuntable" situation. Postoperative complications include continued bleeding, increasing ascites, renal failure, hepatic failure, encephalopathy, peptic ulcer, and other disorders that occur only sporadically.

INTRAOPERATIVE COMPLICATIONS

Bleeding

Intraoperative bleeding is related to several factors. Portal hypertension and consequent dilatation and increased pressure in collateral veins in the operative field lead to increased bleeding. Coagulopathy related to hepatic disease plays an additive role. The amount of intraoperative and early postoperative bleeding can be minimized by the conduct of the operation; this should be carried out expeditiously, and the shunt should be accomplished as rapidly as possible. Since the majority of collaterals are located in the retroperitoneum, the dissection of the portal vein, mesenteric vein, or splenic vein precedes the dissection of the recipient systemic vein, that is, the inferior vena cava or left renal vein. Intraoperatively the portal pressure may be reduced by intravenous infusion of vasopressin, 0.2 μ/ml/min. This infusion should be continued until the shunt is completed.

It is generally felt that a platelet count below the level of 70,000/mm^3 is critically low and should be corrected by administering 10 to 20 fresh frozen platelet packs and repeating the platelet count to determine the effect. Splenectomy may be required in rare circumstances of massive enlargement of the spleen, which acts as a platelet-sequestering or destructive organ. Any deficiency of specific coagulation factors, including factors II, V, and VII, should be corrected by administering fresh frozen plasma. Occasionally patients with cirrhosis also have a factor VIII deficiency that can be corrected by administration of a cryoprecipitate.

A small percentage of patients with cirrhosis undergoing shunt procedures have increased bleeding, related to augmented fibrinolysis, and a diffuse ooze associated with increased activation of plasminogen. This is particularly pertinent in patients who have received more than 10 units of blood. This bleeding has been corrected by the judicious administration of epsilon aminocaproic acid with a loading dose of 5 g, followed by 1 g/hour for 8 hours, and then 1 g every 8 hours.[2]

Shunt Thrombosis

Another complication of portal decompressive surgery is shunt thrombosis. With the use of natural tissues such as those employed in the portacaval shunt or splenorenal shunt, thrombosis usually develops intraoperatively and is related to technical factors. The incidence of shunt thrombosis can be minimized by measuring pressures after the construction of the shunt and by demonstrating a lack of gradient across the anastomosis. Pressure determinations are less informative in the selective splenorenal shunt. Patency of the shunt can be demonstrated in the early postoperative phase by ultrasonography or by computed tomography (CT) scan. Late thrombosis rarely follows these procedures. This is not true, however, of H-graft interposition mesocaval shunts. Here a significant percentage, sometimes as high as 25% in reported series, thrombose late and are responsible for recurrent bleeding. There is no therapy that can prevent this complication.

Situations in Which Shunts Are Precluded

In order for a portal decompressive procedure to be effective, low pressure in the systemic venous circulation is required. In rare cases, most of which have been reported in Japan, a web obstructs the suprahepatic vena cava, causing hypertension in the infrahepatic cava and precluding a shunt. This situation is readily addressed by fracturing the web transatrially. The more common circumstance resulting in inferior vena caval hypertension and precluding a shunt is caused by encroachment and compression of the inferior cava by a nodular caudate lobe (Fig. 39-2).[12] In some patients, resection of the caudate lobe can reduce pressure and still permit a shunt, but if this is not feasible, an intra-abdominal shunting procedure is precluded. The portal venous system in this circumstance has been decompressed by anastomosing the splenic vein to an isolated pulmonary artery by means of an interposed graft, but long-term patency has not been maintained. If a differential between the portal venous pressure and the inferior vena caval pressure exists despite the latter's elevation, a portal systemic decompressive procedure should be carried out.

EARLY POSTOPERATIVE COMPLICATIONS

Bleeding

In the patient who bleeds in the early postoperative period a differential diagnosis must be established to discriminate between thrombosis of the shunt with consequent bleeding from varices and acute gastric erosion or peptic ulceration. The great majority of cases of rebleeding are due to thrombosis of the shunt. The site of bleeding may be established rapidly by esophagoscopic evaluation. Shunt thrombosis can be defined by ultrasound, a CT scan, or most precisely, a splenoportogram. If the shunt is occluded, a decision regarding early reoperation and establishment of the functional shunt must be made. Most bleeding related to ulceration is caused by stress, and cimetidine may be employed postoperatively prior to reinstitution of oral intake.

Ascites

Ascites may develop rapidly or slowly during the postoperative period. There is a higher incidence of ascites associated with an end-to-side portacaval shunt than with a side-to-side shunt; perhaps this is related to the capabilities of the portal vein in the side-to-side shunt to act as an effluent from the hepatic sinusoids. Also, it has been stressed that patients with significant ascites should not undergo a selective distal splenorenal shunt since rapidly evolving ascites frequently has followed this procedure. Ascites that evolves in patients with hepatic

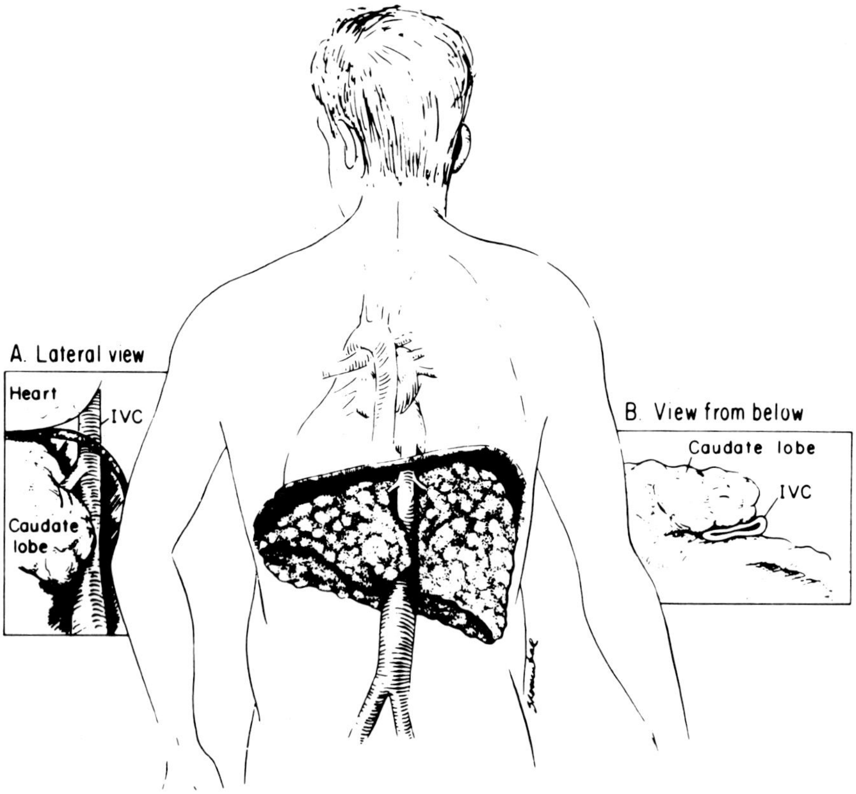

FIG. 39-2. Anatomic location of the retrohepatic inferior vena cava compression in a lateral, inferior, and posterior projection.

cirrhosis is caused by intrahepatic vascular obstruction and increased portal hypertension, resulting in increased intraperitoneal sequestration of hepatic lymph. Also contributing to the production of ascitic fluid is defective albumin synthesis, causing a low plasma osmotic pressure and an increased serum aldosterone level with consequent sodium retention.

Ascites that follows, or that is accentuated by, a portal decompressive procedure should be managed initially by a medical regimen that includes bed rest and daily measurement of weight and urine output to assess response to treatment. The 24-hour urinary sodium output should be monitored. The patient with hepatocellular failure who has accumulated ascites generally excretes less than 10 mEq of sodium daily in the urine, and a sodium intake in an excess of 0.75 g will result in ascites, every gram of sodium retaining 200 ml of fluid. The basis of therapy, therefore, is a very strictly restricted sodium intake of less than 22 mEq, or 0.5 g daily; the preferred intake is actually less than 10 mEq daily.

Furosemide generally is the first diuretic employed. The drug inhibits the reabsorption of sodium and chloride in the proximal and distal tubules and also in the loop of Henle. The action in the distal tubule is independent of any inhibitory effect on aldosterone. The usual daily dose is 20 mg to 80 mg, but the dose can be titrated up to 600 mg daily for short periods in severe cases. Periodic assessment of serum electrolytes, particularly potassium, should be performed. Spironolactone, an aldosterone antagonist, may be used in doses of 200 mg daily in combination with furosemide. In addition, a water diuretic such as mannitol may be considered in some patients. Ethacrynic acid, usually in doses of 100 mg daily, is a potent diuretic that has been effective when other medications have failed, but its administration requires close supervision of serum electrolytes.

Blood products, such as plasma, and saline solutions are contraindicated in patients with ascites despite their low serum sodium levels. Human albumin, if required, should be given in a salt-free preparation in doses of 25 mg to 50 mg daily. Abdominal paracentesis may be useful in ruling out postoperative peritonitis, but repeated paracenteses are contraindicated since they may result in withdrawal of large amounts of protein and may accentuate the hypoproteinemia already present.

If tense ascites develops after a decompressive procedure and fails to respond to a medical regimen, a peritoneovenous shunt may effectively reverse the process. Antibiotics are administered preoperatively and 72 hours postoperatively. A transverse abdominal incision, a supraclavicular incision, and a subcutaneous tunnel are made. The shunt is placed into the peritoneal cavity, and the valve is secured below the anterior rectus fascia. The tunnel may be medial or lateral to the nipple. The venous tubing is passed by way of the internal jugular vein, and the tip is positioned in the caudad segment of the superior vena cava.

Patency of the shunt should be established during the procedure. Flow is demonstrated before inserting the venous limb. After securing the venous tubing, a No. 23 needle is inserted and 10 ml of contrast medium injected to demonstrate patency radiographically. A colored solution of indigo carmine can be used to demonstrate flow in the venous tubing prior to closure of the cervical incision.

Postoperatively a large diuresis is anticipated, and a Foley catheter is mandatory to monitor intake and output. Forty milligrams of furosemide are administered every 6 hours for 24 hours with 40 mEq potassium for replacement. Total fluid intake is restricted to 1 L daily during this period. An abdominal binder is applied, and breathing exercises are begun on the third day. In the case of ascites that evolves rapidly in the postoperative period, the shunt may be removed in 2 to 3 weeks. In cases of chronic ascites, the device is maintained permanently.

The renal and hemodynamic effects of the peritoneovenous shunt are complex, and they include an increase in cardiac output, an increase in creatinine clearance by nearly 50%, and a decrease in plasma renin activity and aldosterone.[1] Subsequently, there is a steady rise in the level of serum aldosterone, but the plasma renin level remains below the preoperative mean. The procedure is associated with a significant complication rate, including spontaneous closure of the shunt, infection, and coagulopathy. Bleeding from esophagogastric varices has also been noted in patients with alcoholic cirrhosis after placement of the peritoneovenous shunt.

Renal Failure

Renal failure, considered as part of the hepatorenal syndrome, may occur in cirrhotic patients following shunting procedures. It usually is accompanied by a significant increase in ascites. The syndrome is characterized by progressive azotemia, a rising serum creatinine level, hyponatremia, and oliguria.

The genesis of functional renal failure accompanying ascites is characterized by a reduction of the effective circulation volume and peripheral perfusion of the kidney. Insertion of peritoneovenous shunt increases both renal flow and urinary output without further depleting effective intravascular fluid volume.[9] The peritoneovenous shunt is contraindicated in patients who have severe encephalopathy or marked derangement of the coagulation process.

LONG-TERM COMPLICATIONS

Postshunt Encephalopathy

Although the clinical manifestations of postshunt encephalopathy have often paralleled those of hyperammonemia, the etiology has not been defined. The complication cannot be related solely to shunting of blood directly into the systemic circulation since it does not follow shunts for hyperlipidemia and cavernomatous transformation of the portal vein; in these situations the liver function is normal. Encephalopathy is thus best related to hepatic dysfunction.

The clinical manifestations should be specific and include disturbed consciousness, personality changes, intellectual deterioration, slowed and slurred speech, liver "flap," and difficulty in writing. These are accompanied by changes in the electroencephalogram (EEG). Ill-defined neuropsychiatric features may be caused by multiple hospitalizations and should not be used to establish the diagnosis.

Postshunt encephalopathy is the one complication that has led to the introduction of new procedures, particularly arterialization of the portal vein and the selective distal splenorenal shunt. The consensus is that any decompressive procedure can be used for bleeding varices in a patient with cavernomatous transformation of the portal vein and normal liver function, since encephalopathy is not a problem. In patients with schistosomiasis, postshunt encephalopathy occurs with almost prohibitive frequency following a standard portacaval, splenorenal, or mesocaval shunt, and the incidence is reduced by selective distal splenorenal shunt, making this the procedure of choice in that disease. The major controversy relates to the shunt of choice in the alcoholic cirrhotic. Champions of the selective distal splenorenal shunt report a significantly lower incidence of encephalopathy although no difference was noted by others in prospective randomized series.

Treatment incorporates control of bleeding, infection, constipation, acid–base balance, and electrolyte abnormalities and the judicious use of analgesics and sedatives.[11] Intestinal cleansing either with enemas or with cathartics constitutes the first line of defense. Dietary protein restriction is effective as a short-term measure. Maintaining an intake of below 0.5 mg/kg of body weight for a long period is to be avoided. Specific therapy most often incorporates neomycin, which decreases ureolytic and proteolytic colonic bacteria, but this may be complicated by ototoxicity, nephrotoxicity, and staphylococcal enterocolitis. Lactulose, the effect of which is probably related to the metabolism of the drug by enteric bacteria, can also reverse the encephalopathy. Sorbitol has been shown to be as effective as lactulose. Additional drugs have been used, but with less uniform results. Intravenous amino acids to normalize the plasma profile have not had consistent effects. Ornithine salts of branched-chain amino acids have had some effect in patients with portal systemic encephalopathy. Most controlled studies fail to show a benefit for L-dopamine and bromocriptine.

Miscellaneous Complications

Although it had been thought that cirrhosis was accompanied by an increase in peptic ulceration, such is not the case; most cirrhotics are gastric hyposecreters. However, following a portacaval anastomosis there is an increase in gastric hypersecretion thought to be due to histamine bypassing the action of hepatic histaminase. This process may lead to the increased incidence of peptic ulceration that has been noted to develop in approximately 15% of patients after successful decompressive procedures. A case can be made for the use of antacids, bicarbonates, or cimetidine in the early postoperative phase, but long-term therapy is not indicated.

Following successful decompression of their portal systems, alterations of the liver function tests are the same as those expected in cirrhotic patients without surgical intervention. Jaundice is likely to increase immediately following the procedure, but hyperbilirubinemia generally returns to the preoperative level. In rare cases a more specific hyperbilirubinemia of unknown etiology develops; this is due to unconjugated pigment but not hemolysis.

Edema of the ankles may develop following a shunting procedure. This is not related to increased pressure in the vena cava since little change occurs and the edema is presumably part of fluid retention of cirrhosis. Permanent myelopathy with paraplegia has evolved very rarely after portacaval anastomosis. A few patients with cirrhosis have developed classic hemochromatosis following portacaval anastomosis, and an intensification of previously present hemochromatosis has occurred.

Mortality Rates and Survival

The figures for mortality are variable. Those selected here represent either a consensus or are found in particularly critical reports. Between 48% and 58% of patients who undergo an emergency portal systemic shunt and die are considered operative mortalities.[4, 7] Lower rates occurred in series of patients operated on without a medical trial, while the higher rates occurred in patients actively bleeding at the time of the operation. Increases in operative mortality rates have been correlated with ascites, Bromsulphalein (BSP) retention, serum glutamic oxalacetic transaminase (SGOT) elevation, and an increased "liver index" that considers BSP, prothrombin time, and bilirubin cumulatively. Elective shunts are accompanied by a 4% to 10% 30-day hospital mortality rate that best correlates with Child's classification of hepatic function.[6, 8] Five-year survival rates range between 42% and 88%, but most would place the figure at 50%. No specific type of shunt has been shown to offer a genuine advantage in this regard, for survival is based on adequacy of hepatic function.

References

1. Blendis LM, Greig PD, Langer B et al: The renal and hemodynamic effects of the peritoneovenous shunt for intractable hepatic ascites. Gastroenterology 77:250, 1979
2. Grossi CE, Rousselot LM, Panke WF: Coagulation defects in patients with cirrhosis of the liver undergoing portasystemic shunts. Am J Surg 104:512, 1962
3. Maillard JN, Rueff B, Prandi D, Sicot C: Hepatic arterialization and portacaval shunt in hepatic cirrhosis: Assessment. Arch Surg 108:315, 1974
4. Malt RB, Malt RA: Tests and management affecting survival after portacaval and splenorenal shunts. Surg Gynecol Obstet 149:220, 1979
5. Nabseth DC, Johnson WC, Widrich WC et al: Splenorenal shunts in portal hypertension. J Cardiovasc Surg 20:201, 1979
6. Newman MM: Portal hypertension. In Eiseman B (ed): Prognosis of Surgical Disease, p 262. Philadelphia, WB Saunders, 1980
7. Orloff MJ, Bell RH Jr, Hyde PV, Skivolocki WP: Long-term results of emergency portacaval shunt for bleeding esophageal varices in unselected patients with alcoholic cirrhosis. Ann Surg 192:325, 1980
8. Resnicoff SA, Schwartz SI: Portal decompressive surgery: Comparative evaluation of patients with Laennec's cirrhosis and other causes. Arch Surg 97:371, 1968
9. Wapnick S, Grosberg S, Kinney M et al: Renal failure in ascites secondary to hepatic, renal, and pancreatic disease. Treatment with a LeVeen peritoneovenous shunt. Arch Surg 113:581, 1978
10. Warren WD, Zeppa R, Fomon JJ: Selective transsplenic decompression of gastroesophageal varices by distal splenorenal shunt. Ann Surg 166:437, 1967
11. Weber FL: Therapy of portal-systemic encephalopathy: The practical and the promising. Gastroenterology 81:174, 1981
12. Welling RE, McDermott WV Jr: Combined caval and portal hypertension with cirrhosis of the liver. Ann Surg 177:164, 1973

40 Complications of Gastrointestinal Trauma

Alexander J. Walt

OVERVIEW

Many complications of trauma of the gastrointestinal tract can be avoided and are in essence iatrogenic. Nevertheless, an appreciable number of complications are inevitable and derive from the spillage of intestinal content, damage to adjacent organs, or the associated changes caused by hemorrhage and shock. Faced with anticipated morbidity, the surgeon should from the start seek to attenuate these predetermined complications. Gastrointestinal injuries cannot be viewed in isolation and are very frequently overshadowed both clinically and in terms of survival by head, thoracic, and nongastrointestinal intra-abdominal injuries. No consideration is given to injuries outside the gastrointestinal tract in this chapter and only the complications immediately pertinent to the gastrointestinal tract are discussed.

In penetrating wounds of the abdominal wall, the need for laparotomy is usually obvious; in blunt injury, however, the decision may be much more difficult. At laparotomy, injuries to the gastrointestinal tract are frequently obscured by concomitant injuries to the solid viscera or adjacent blood vessels. In practice, damage to these latter structures may initially overshadow the injury of the gut. The surgeon should therefore always consciously resolve to examine the entire gastrointestinal tract meticulously after any life-threatening or major lesions have been attended, even without obvious evidence of free intestinal content.

If isolated lesions of the gastrointestinal tract are recognized early, they are easily managed. Some lesions present few clinical signs initially and only become apparent after hours or days when sepsis and ileus are well established, by that time sometimes irreversibly.

Clinical efforts must obviously be directed toward early recognition of loss of intestinal integrity. This may not always be easy because clinical signs are somewhat unreliable; about 20% of patients with subsequently proven significant injuries in the abdominal cavity initially present with no clinical signs. The routine acceptance of negative results from a laparotomy as a small price for definitive information has been largely abandoned, since occasional complications result; negative results from laparotomy constitute a considerable expense to society.

Very few perforations of the gastrointestinal tract are self sealing. Unsuspected, neglected, or improperly treated injuries will inevitably result in considerable morbidity and often avoidable mortality. The clinical picture may be deceptively benign in the early stages or may be masked by the more florid manifestations of concomitant injuries. Sepsis is the most immediate threat to the patient.

Clinical pitfalls, adjuvant aids to diagnosis, and the general principles of management of injuries of the gastrointestinal tract are outlined.

PRINCIPLES IN THE AVOIDANCE OF COMPLICATIONS

A number of likely clinical pitfalls need always to be kept in mind in order to avoid complications.

1. The assumption that the absence of abdominal pain excludes the possibility of a perforated viscus is dangerous. It should always be remembered that tenderness may be delayed for hours, especially in the intoxicated patient or the patient who is under the influence of drugs. Even more obviously, patients who are paraplegic or in whom consciousness is obtunded owing to head injury may have a severe intestinal injury with no obvious clinical signs on abdominal examination.

2. Failure to recognize that any penetrating wound between the nipples and the costal margin may have passed through the diaphragm into any part of the intestinal tract is not uncommon. Less frequent, a gunshot wound entering the neck or subclavicular area may track downward into the peritoneal cavity. En route, the missile may damage the heart, causing a pericardial tamponade, or the lungs, resulting in a hemothorax, and these lesions may distract attention away from the abdomen. Consequently, peritoneal lavage may be invaluable in excluding visceral damage when the entrance wound is in the thoracic region.
3. The presence of peristalsis is perfectly compatible with the presence of a ruptured intestine for many hours after injury; ileus may be slow in appearing. Reliance on radiologic studies is dangerous because free air may not be detected for hours or even days, especially in patients in whom the distal small intestine is injured or in whom the ischemia of the intestinal wall occurs so gradually that perforation is delayed for several days.
4. One should be cautious about guessing the direction the missile may have taken because the position of the patient at the time of injury is not known, and missiles can follow capricious pathways, especially when deflected or shattered by bony structures.
5. Even in the presence of an intact peritoneum, gunshot wounds of the abdominal wall may cause visceral disruption from the effect of the blast. Selective laparotomy may be advisable on such occasions even though the peritoneum has not been transgressed.
6. Penetrating stab wounds of the peritoneal cavity may be followed by careful observation in the absence of overt clinical signs. Nevertheless, a negative peritoneal lavage, while reassuring, does not exclude significant intestinal injury. Although a few surgeons favor observation of patients with penetrating gunshot wounds, most prefer routine laparotomy for this group because almost all of these patients will have some degree of visceral or structural damage.
7. Injuries to the back should not be overlooked, especially in the flanks. Both penetrating wounds and blunt injuries may be confined to the retroperitoneal aspect of the ascending or descending colon or duodenum, in which case abdominal signs may be absent initially and the patient only recognized as having a serious lesion when sepsis supervenes or when a fistula appears.
8. Careful attention must be given to wounds of the perineum and gluteal region. It is not possible to predict the depth of penetration in such cases, and the size of the entry wound may not reflect the severity of the internal injury, especially the amount of bacterial leakage and proliferation.
9. Constellations of injury are often significant, for example, the association of a fractured pelvis and femur with rupture of the diaphragm and possibly rupture of the arch of the aorta in patients who have fallen from heights. Whenever ecchymosis of the anterior wall following trauma is noted—however small—the distinct possibility of visceral disruption must be entertained. This is especially likely with seatbelt injuries associated with damage to any part of the vertebral column or pelvis, in which case the likelihood of concomitant disruption of intestine pinned between the seatbelt and bone is almost certain. No part of the gastrointestinal tract is immune. Whereas the distal ileum has most often been regarded as being at greatest risk, the duodenum, midgut, colon, or indeed any part of the gastrointestinal tract is vulnerable. Furthermore, abdominal symptoms may be grossly delayed. Associated ileus is sometimes incorrectly attributed to the spinal injury or concomitant retroperitoneal hematoma.
10. Hyperamylasemia is a common finding in the injured patient. It has long been an accepted axiom that this abnormality alone does not justify laparotomy to exclude a pancreatic or intestinal injury. Recent studies of isoamylase fractions show that the hyperamylasemia is due to an elevation of amylase of nonpancreatic origin in many cases.[19] Hyperamylasemia is also not an uncommon feature of head and thoracic injuries. In blunt abdominal injuries, the finding of hyperamylasemia is used as a guide to treatment but is not an absolute indication for exploration because, in most cases, the hyperamylasemia will return to normal. Persistence of hyperamylasemia or a continuing rise in the level when the amylase is of pancreatic origin raises immediate suspicion of a significant intra-abdominal injury, which may be a perforation of the bowel or the development of a pseudocyst of the pancreas.
11. In penetrating wounds, the surgeon should always be reluctant to accept an odd number of holes in the bowel. Although from

time to time a tangential wound to the bowel is encountered, more often the second hole is hidden in the fat of the mesenteric border. The presence of ecchymosis or hematoma in the region of the stomach suggests the need to open the lesser sac for thorough visualization of both surfaces. Hematomas around the duodenum mandate a Kocher maneuver for inspection of the entire circumference. When the mesenteries of any part of the intestine contain hematoma, careful dissection of the borders of the gut must be undertaken to exclude a hidden laceration.

12. Pelvic fractures constitute a special problem.[12] Approximately 25% of patients with pelvic fractures have associated intestinal injuries. The likelihood of intestinal injury in the individual case is proportional to the severity of the pelvic fracture—over 30% in Malgaigne and bilateral pelvic fractures but less than 10% in unilateral fractures of the pelvic rami. Intestinal damage in association with pelvic fractures may be particularly difficult to diagnose because of the degree of local tenderness, abdominal distention, and frequent bloodstaining of the peritoneal fluid, which often results from seepage of a large retroperitoneal hematoma into the peritoneal cavity. This is the same feature that makes peritoneal lavage less reliable as a measure of significant intraperitoneal trauma. A negative laparotomy may need to be accepted in these cases as the lesser of two evils to ensure that a ruptured viscus is not overlooked.

AIDS IN THE RECOGNITION OF GASTROINTESTINAL INJURIES

A suspicious clinical attitude should be cultivated toward all injuries of the torso. Clinical observations may be deceptive but are often helped by radiologic data and information derived from peritoneal lavage.

Peritoneal Lavage

Peritoneal lavage (PL) is a valuable but fallible tool for determining whether a patient with a penetrating or, even more so, a blunt abdominal injury requires laparotomy.[14, 16] Certain caveats are pertinent. PL has its greatest value in helping to exclude the grounds for laparotomy especially in the unresponsive patient who is drunk, drugged, paralyzed, or unconscious or exhibits an ambiguous clinical picture. It is much less reliable in duodenal, small intestinal, diaphragmatic, and retroperitoneal injuries in that false-negative and false-positive results are more likely to be found in this group than from patients with other intra-abdominal injuries.

Different techniques for PL have been proposed, of which open subumbilical introduction of the dialysis catheter has been the safest and most effective. Careful technique is important if perforation of major vessels, the mesentery, or the bowel is to be avoided. The bladder should always be emptied first by Foley catheter and, in most cases, the stomach by a nasogastric tube. The procedure is carried out under sterile conditions with surgeon and patient properly prepared. The site of the small skin incision, made after local infiltration with 1% Xylocaine with 1/100,000 epinephrine, is made close to the umbilicus or in the infraumbilical ring, except in patients with a pelvic fracture in whom the catheter is inserted above the umbilicus to avoid the possibility of a false-positive lavage from passage of the catheter through any anterior extraperitoneal hematoma that may be present. Hemostasis is meticulously obtained before the linea alba is elevated under direct vision, and the trocar of a dialysis catheter is inserted into the peritoneal cavity. The trocar is withdrawn, and the catheter is gently advanced toward the pelvis. If free blood is obtained, the test is obviously positive. If no blood is obtained, 700 ml to 1000 ml of Ringer's lactate is allowed to flow into the peritoneal cavity by gravity. The patient is then moved from side to side as much as his injuries permit to ensure satisfactory circulation of the lavage fluid. The lavage fluid is then recaptured by lowering the bottle. The contents are analyzed for RBC and WBC counts and for the presence of bile, fibers, and sometimes feces. Measurement of amylase content has been abandoned by many because the elevation of the amylase level in the absence of other positive findings is too low to justify the expense of the test.

A crude way to assess blood in the lavage is to try, and fail, to read a newspaper through a tube containing the returned lavage fluid. Actual measurement is obviously much more reliable, but many questions have been raised about the most valuable indices for the interpretation of the data. Approximately 9 ml of blood in 1 L of fluid produces a concentration of 100,000 RBCs per mm^3. Traditionally, this level was accepted as the watershed, indicating the need for laparotomy. Over the past few years this figure has been challenged in the continuing attempts to reduce further the incidence of negative results from laparotomy. As perfection is pursued, some have worried that the zeal of surgeons in avoiding laparotomy may cause some patients to develop complications from injuries not reflected in the peritoneal lavage.

Varying criteria for a positive determination have been advanced, the most recent being those of Alyon and Perry, who suggested on the basis of 105 patients with penetrating trauma and 1812 with blunt abdominal trauma that the highest accuracy is obtained in penetrating trauma when the positive lavage criteria are fixed at greater than 50,000 RBCs per mm^3 or WBCs greater than 500 per mm^3 (it requires 3 or more hours for the WBC count to rise).[1, 6] The level of 100,000 RBCs per mm^3 must be retained in patients with blunt trauma. These criteria provided 95.2% and 99.1% accuracy with excellent specificity. The blood in these and similar series originates mostly from nonintestinal sources. It is well recognized, for example, that isolated injuries of the small bowel and colon may sometimes give false-negative results unless evidence of bile, feces, or fiber is seen on examination of the lavage return. Similarly, excessive reliance should not be placed on PL in reaching clinical decisions when the possibility of diaphragmatic injury is present. In patients with a thoracostomy tube in place, performance of PL has occasionally proven the presence of a hole in the diaphragm when the lavage fluid has appeared through the tube. In contrast, PL may be helpful in disclosing subdiaphragmatic injury in penetrating wounds of the chest, but a negative result should not be given total credence.[16]

Specific Injuries

DIAPHRAGM

About 4% of major blunt thoracoabdominal injuries have an associated diaphragmatic rupture.[17] The tear is on the left side in about 80% of patients, but lesions on the right side are increasing in incidence, either because of enhanced recognition or possibly because of the greater use of the shoulder harness in automobiles. Most lesions are greater than 10 cm in length with the posterolateral attachment of the diaphragm most often involved. Rarely, both sides of the diaphragm may have tears; this possibility should always be sought.

Blunt injury sufficient to rupture a diaphragm is almost invariably severe. Most of these patients are occupants of automobiles, but about 20% are pedestrians or have fallen from heights. The important feature is that the diaphragmatic rupture, although hazardous in its own right by permitting the herniation of organs into the chest, may be asymptomatic or completely overshadowed by the concomitant head injury, thoracic injury, assorted fractures, or abdominal visceral damage that occurs in over 95% of these patients.

Rupture of the diaphragm should always be sought but may be difficult to diagnose.[2] In 80% of patients with subsequently proven diaphragmatic hernias, radiologic studies show no lesion or only a slight fuzziness often attributed to atelectasis or a small effusion. A definitive diagnosis may be made by use of one of a number of techniques, such as a plain film after insertion of a nasogastric tube, fluoroscopy, a barium enema, pneumoperitoneum (but a resulting tension pneumothorax should be guarded against), liver–spleen scan, angiography, or a CT scan.

The salient fact, however, is that most ruptures are first diagnosed at a laparotomy undertaken to deal with some other suspected intra-abdominal injury. The herniation of specific organs is related largely to the site of injury. Since most tears are posterior, the spleen is the most common viscus to be discovered in the chest, and because of the intensity of the impact, the spleen is frequently injured. Splenectomy may be unavoidable. Similarly, the splenic flexure of the colon, sometimes lacerated, may have passed through the same tear. When intestinal content has spilled, the pleural cavity must be thoroughly irrigated and a thoracostomy tube inserted with full therapeutic antibiotic coverage. The development of an empyema may be anticipated in a significant number of patients. More anteriorly placed tears and tears in the central tendon allow passage of the stomach and small intestine.

In patients in whom the rupture has not been noted early—and this is more common in penetrating injuries such as stab wounds—development and presentation of complications may be delayed for weeks to years. The complications most commonly encountered in these circumstances are

1. Incarceration of intestine, with associated dyspepsia, pain, and vomiting and a mortality rate of about 20%
2. Strangulation of intestine with signs of septic shock when diagnosis is unduly delayed and a mortality rate of about 40%
3. Shortness of breath and hypoxemia due to atelectasis of the left lung following compression by the herniated viscera, which may dominate the clinical picture (Rarely, an intense ileus occurs, acutely displacing the heart to the right, and unless the herniated organs are reduced as an emergency, death may result rapidly.)
4. At operation, dense adhesions between the lung and herniated viscera, necessitating thoracotomy as the operative approach in long-standing cases

Ruptures on the right side constitute a special group that is less readily recognized, partly because right side ruptures are less common and partly because the liver blocks the area so that other viscera seldom pass into the right chest cavity. In addition, the contour of the herniated liver is often mistaken for the normal leaf of the diaphragm. The main complication associated with these injuries is concomitant damage to the liver.

The diaphragm should be repaired with two layers of nonabsorbable suture. Since the tension of this muscle in movement may be considerable, the rupture may occur if closure is carelessly performed.

STOMACH

The stomach is usually easy to manage in trauma except in a septic patient. Then the stomach often reacts by developing acute erosive gastritis and upper gastrointestinal hemorrhage. Wounds of the stomach are sutured in two layers, care being taken to ensure hemostasis. It is vital that an exit wound be meticulously sought because one is almost invariable present. This search sometimes requires the greater omentum to be taken down so that the posterior wall of the stomach and the area of the lesser curvature may be thoroughly inspected.

The gastric lesion most difficult to treat is a penetrating wound situated close to the gastroesophageal junction. In these cases, an approach is adopted similar to that for the repair of a large hiatal hernia. Satisfactory exposure is obtained, and with the proximal portion of the stomach adequately mobilized, the gastric wounds are repaired in two layers. If the repair appears to be tenuous by virtue of its anatomical location, a Nissen wrap may be added for insurance. If the vagus nerve is thought to have been damaged, a pyloroplasty is added. From the location of these lesions, concomitant injury to the diaphragm, liver, possibly the pericardium, the spleen, and the transverse colon often is present and must be sought carefully. Subsequent subphrenic abscess is the most common complication of this wound.

DUODENUM

Complications of duodenal injuries result from being overlooked early or from the initial sheer destructive nature of the injury.

Blunt injuries may result in intramural hematoma or laceration. Intramural hematomas are more frequent in children but occur in adults, too. Clinically, the patient develops gradual obstruction, complete or incomplete, with gastric distention, nausea, and vomiting. Diagnosis is easily made by a Gastrografin swallow, which reveals a characteristic "bird's beak" appearance. The clinical problem is whether operation—evacuation of the hematoma and possible bypassing of the area by gastrojejunostomy—should be undertaken. Nasogastric suction and total parenteral hyperalimentation will usually permit the hematoma to resorb spontaneously, and the duodenal lumen will open in about 10 to 14 days. In a few patients, however, the hematoma will rupture, and this observation has led some surgeons to advocate early operation. Most surgeons, however, adopt a middle ground of careful observation with the expectation that the hematoma will resorb. Operation is necessary only if obstruction persists beyond 10 days, if pain increases, or if any evidence of bleeding into the lumen of the bowel or into the peritoneal cavity appears.

Rupture of the duodenum is much more serious; all these patients need operation.[10] The second part of the duodenum is most often injured but in about one third of cases the injury is found in the first, third, or fourth parts of the duodenum. If the operation is performed within 24 hours of injury, virtually all patients with an isolated duodenal injury should survive. Although many of these lesions are retroperitoneal, some extend to the anterior wall of the duodenum with consequent spillage into the free peritoneal cavity. Early diagnosis depends upon clinical suspicion and radiologic proof provided by free or retroperitoneal air or by leakage of contrast material. Repair is obtained by a two-layer closure. Drainage usually is added but is probably unnecessary without concomitant pancreatic injury. If the quality of the closure of the duodenum is in question, a loop jejunum may be brought up to the repair and sewn around it as an onlay graft.

Complications in the more severe duodenal and duodenopancreatic lesions often directly relate to technical decisions. Large lesions involving only the duodenum, such as may result from a gunshot wound, are very difficult to repair with the assurance of primary healing. The penalty of failure is a duodenal fistula, possibly with generalized peritonitis. The area of repair is bathed by chyme, bile, pancreatic juice, and sometimes a variety of microorganisms. The principles of intestinal wound care must prevail, however, and the duodenum is débrided until satisfactory blood supply is obtained. When closure of the duodenal wound is not feasible without tension, a Roux-en-Y loop may be brought up to the area, and the end of the distal jejunum sewn over the defect. To reduce the secretions in the area of healing, a type of diverticulization has been successfully used in which stapling of the pylorus and the addition of a gastroenterostomy to bypass the repair are performed.[5] This technique is not often necessary unless pancreatic injury is associated, but it has been very effective. In many respects, this sequence has tended to replace the earlier diverticulization in which a duodenostomy, antrectomy, and gastrojejunostomy were done. Vagotomy is not usually added unless there is a history of peptic ulceration, and the pylorus can be expected to open spontaneously in about 3 to 4 weeks. Drainage by a very carefully placed sump drain and a collection of

Penrose drains brought through separate incisions and left for 4 to 8 days are usually added. Some surgeons also elect to place a small duodenostomy tube through an area of healthy duodenum for decompression, leaving the tube under gentle suction for about 14 days as a controlled fistula.

The incidence of complications is much higher with concomitant damage to the head of the pancreas (see Chap. 37).[10] Duodenual fistula occurs in about 10% of patients and should be managed nonoperatively at first by thorough drainage of the region, total intravenous parenteral nutrition, and the evacuation of any septic pockets. Most fistulae will close spontaneously, but if the fistula has not closed in about 6 to 10 weeks, operation is necessary. Distal obstruction should be excluded and adherence of the margins of the opening to the area of the liver or surrounding tissues is likely to be present. This indurated area needs to be freed until pliable tissue is defined, at which point repair is best achieved by the use of a Roux-en-Y loop of jejunum brought to the defect without tension.

The only indications for a pancreatoduodenectomy in duodenal injuries are associated extensive destruction of the pancreatic head and distal common bile duct or uncontrollable bleeding and shattering of the duodenum itself.

SMALL INTESTINE

Blunt injury to the intestine is most often associated with automobile accidents, especially when seat belts have trapped a loop of bowel against the vertebral column or after direct blows to a relaxed anterior abdominal wall. Although the fixed portions close to the ligament of Treitz and the ileocecal valve are more liable to this injury, the small intestine may be damaged anywhere along its length. Complications relate mostly to the clinician's failure to recognize the intestinal leak. Repair of lacerations is usually easy and effective unless a technical error is made, such as failure to débride the bowel adequately or to ensure a vascularized mesentery. Unlike the colon, the upper half of the small intestine is relatively sterile, and the microorganisms of the lower half are limited in number and invasiveness.

Although not common, failure to recognize a transection occurs more frequently than is generally appreciated. Symptoms may be few and may be grossly delayed. Free air may not be visible radiographically, and ileus may appear very slowly. Patients may even continue to eat initially, since adjacent bowel and omentum occlude the laceration in the wall. Eventually, ileus supervenes; the abdomen becomes tender; and evidence of localized peritonitis becomes apparent.

Treatment consists of nasogastric suction and operation under cover of appropriate broad-spectrum antibiotics. The area of injury is excised and an end-to-end anastomosis performed. Although it is customary to wash out the peritoneal cavity with about 2 L to 4 L of saline, a prospective randomized study has failed to show the benefit of this procedure.[8] The peritoneum can be closed without drainage, but it is probably advisable to close the subcutaneous tissues of the operative wound by secondary suture.

The complications of penetrating wounds are similar to those of blunt injuries although penetrating wounds as a rule tend to declare themselves earlier. Precautions to obviate subsequent complications such as leakage or obstruction include adequate resection of the injured area, identification of all holes (especially on the mesenteric border in the presence of adjacent hematoma), and extra careful examination of the bowel in the presence of multiple shotgun pellets.

COLON

The colon is thin walled, fixed in half its course, the reservoir of 10^{12} invasive microorganisms, and relatively poor in vascularity, and it faces directly into the peritoneal cavity; it is the least forgiving of the intra-abdominal intestinal organs.[18] The median mortality rate from colonic injuries is about 12%. Only about half of the deaths are due to the colonic injury itself; the other half are attributable to concomitant injury to other abdominal organs or to extra-abdominal systems (e.g., cardiopulmonary or neurologic). Infection is the most feared complication because colonic injuries seldom bleed excessively.

In the colon, above all other organs, complications should be assiduously avoided by the performance of the appropriate initial operation. Paradoxically, because of its well-deserved respect from surgeons, the colon has been treated with what is probably excessive conservatism. Over the past decade, much more flexible judgment has been exercised, and over 50% of colonic injuries are now being repaired primarily.[11, 15, 20]

The principles underlying surgical decisions may be outlined as follows:

1. A primary repair should be done whenever the surgeon's experience, judgment, and technical ability suggest that this is safe for the patient.
2. Patients with suspected colonic wounds are operated upon with a minimum of delay in order to reduce any further leakage and proliferation of bacteria.

3. Antibiotic coverage is given immediately when the possibility of colonic injury is suspected and should consist of an aminoglycoside and clindamycin intravenously. It is customary to add penicillin or ampicillin, but the enterococcus is so rarely the cause of subsequent infection that this is probably unnecessary. Some surgeons prefer intravenous cefazolin alone, but if anaerobic contamination is considerable, this single drug is likely to be inadequate. The advocacy of tobramycin rather than gentamicin as the aminoglycoside of choice rests on the purportedly reduced renal toxicity of tobramycin. Gentamicin is significantly cheaper, and since the appropriate dosage is monitored by regular measurements of blood levels and adjusted to match the degree of contamination or infection, the strong trend toward abandoning gentamicin needs to be questioned.
4. Patients in whom a primary repair should *not* be performed fall into the following categories:
    a. An elapsed time of more than about 6 hours between the injury and surgical repair
    b. Hypovolemic shock, pre- or postoperatively as defined by blood pressure below 80/50 torr for longer than 30 minutes
    c. Two or more concomitant visceral injuries, although a single severe visceral injury, particularly of the liver, pancreas, or kidney, often suffices to preclude primary repair
    d. Extensive fecal contamination of the peritoneal cavity
    e. The presence of 1 L of blood in the peritoneal cavity; this reflects severity of injury and the possibility of future infection
    f. Damage to the muscles of the posterior abdominal wall, necessitating wide débridement and assuring that there will probably be a fair amount of drainage postoperatively
    g. Destruction of a substantial segment of the anterior abdominal wall, which may render repair of this area difficult
    h. Age of the patient above 60 years, especially if he is in poor physiologic condition, as evidenced by marked emphysema, poor renal function, cirrhosis, or reduced cardiac performance

In penetrating wounds and in patients who have undergone operations for colonic injury, infection may declare itself overtly or subtly. The relatively occult manifestations of colonic leaks or pericolonic infection include an unexplained oliguria, fall in blood pressure, tachycardia, arrhythmia, or restlessness. Above all, tachypnea and hypoxemia as a reflection of an early adult respiratory distress syndrome originating from the intra-abdominal sepsis are the urgent warning signs most often clinically neglected. The overt signs include discomfort, pain, localized or generalized tenderness or guarding, ileus, or a palpable mass.

In questionable cases, an attempt may be made to localize the infection radiographically by a flat plate of the abdomen or by ultrasonography or CT scan. The use of ^{67}Ga scans or isotopically labeled leukocytes has not been effective in these acute circumstances. Whenever doubt persists about the presence of infection, an operation should be undertaken. At laparotomy, extensive exploration may be necessary because abscesses frequently become multiple once sepsis supervenes and may be found anywhere between the diaphragm and the levators, often between loops of bowel. In addition, the possibility of intrahepatic abscess formation must be remembered for patients who do not improve following apparently thorough evacuation of pus and adequate drainage.

The other relatively common complications in colonic injuries are associated with the colostomy that is performed in about 40% to 55% of patients. The performance of colostomy depends largely upon the type of wounding agents employed, being highest with shotgun wounds and lowest with stab wounds. The complications that relate to the establishment of the colostomy or to the subsequent colostomy closure are basically the same as those encountered in elective surgery. A difference in trauma, however, is to be found in patients in whom colostomy is established in the face of sustained shock, fecal spillage, and widespread organ damage; allowance must be made for slower healing and postoperative nutritional depletion. Similarly, closure of any colostomy after trauma should wait until other wounds are healed; catabolism has ceased; and all sepsis has been eradicated. This may necessitate waiting many months. In a series of 167 colostomy closures (103 were done for trauma), a 29.9% morbidity rate ensued, wound infection being the most common complication. There were no deaths, but 3.5% patients developed a fecal fistula.[13] The absence of distal obstruction must be established before the colostomy is closed. The added cost of the colostomy closure in 1982 dollars is about $10,000 in patients who developed complications and $7,500 in those who did not.

In about 15% of colonic injuries, the bowel may be repaired, but the surgeon is reluctant to return the anastomosis to the peritoneal cavity because he believes that the patient's general condition may militate against certain healing. Exteriorization of the repaired colon with "interiorization" 7 to 10 days postoperatively is successful in about 60% of such patients. This compromise entails careful attention to a number of points:[9]

1. The repaired bowel selected for exteriorization must lend itself to adequate mobilization.
2. The fascial bridge under the loop should be at least 5 cm in length. If any other bridge is placed under the loop, it must be adjusted so that the bowel describes a relatively gentle curve and is not kinked, with consequent proximal obstruction. If this detail is not followed, the repair will probably break down.
3. The skin of the colostomy wound must not be tightly closed.
4. The bowel must be carefully tended postoperatively to avoid dessication. This is best done by saline soaks, vaseline gauze dressings, and, possibly, the humidity provided by a covering colostomy bag.

If at any time the viability of the repair is questionable or if the patient's general condition is unsatisfactory, the repair should be opened and a colostomy established. This final decision should not be prolonged beyond 10 days at the most.

Blunt injuries of the colon constitute only about 5% of all colonic injuries, but they present a special set of complications.[7] By their nature, blunt colonic injuries, most often caused by direct blows or seat belts, may present few symptoms initially, especially in the 10% of patients in whom the colon alone is injured. In those in whom the colonic wall is badly contused or whose subtended mesentery is torn, gradual ischemia may result in gangrene and perforation over a period of a week, at which time typical sepsis and peritonitis appear. In most patients, however, the colonic injury is discovered at a laparotomy performed because of symptoms and signs produced by some other organ in the abdominal cavity, and the colonic injury comes as something of a surprise. The treatment of blunt colonic injury is much the same as for penetrating wounds, with particular care being taken to ensure that the margins of the bowel used for repair have a satisfactory blood supply because the blunt trauma may have been diffusely distributed.

The subcutaneous tissues of the laparotomy incision should not be closed when colonic content has spilled. Wound sepsis is thereby avoided, and these wounds heal well by secondary intention or on delayed closure. Similarly, infection is reduced if bullet wounds of the abdominal wall are débrided and drained but not closed primarily.

ANORECTUM

Rectal injuries have in the past carried a higher mortality rate than have colonic injuries, partly because they were poorly managed. Even today, the mortality rate is still appreciable and morbidity very high, although it is widely recognized that these lesions should be treated by the establishment of a proximal defunctioning colostomy (with or without a temporary Hartmann procedure), repair of the rectal lesion to the extent possible, washing out of the rectal contents, and provision of extensive perirectal presacral drainage. The complications of rectal injury may be due to failure to follow the principles outlined above, but they may also result from failure to pay proper attention to the frequently associated genitourinary injuries and the less frequent but even more debilitating neurologic injuries found in these patients. In addition, extensive and sometimes fatal sepsis may result from neglect or ignorance of the extent of the intrapelvic injury. This failure to explore and thoroughly débride damaged rectal and perirectal tissues is most often seen in three circumstances:

1. The extent of apparently minor penetrating wounds of the buttocks that in fact produce widespread internal damage that becomes rapidly infected may not be appreciated. Such wounds must be noted, explored throughout their length, and débrided thoroughly. A temporary colostomy is often needed.
2. In patients with pelvic fractures, a sliver of bone may penetrate the rectum, or they may have an adjacent rectal tear, and patients with compound fractures of the pelvis (e.g., with penetrating wounds from without) may also have a rectal component to the injury.
3. The impact of falls on the buttocks from a height may cause extensive but overlooked damage to gluteal muscles, the subcutaneous fatty tissues, and the perineal skin. Ecchymoses and hematomas may dominate the picture initially, but infection is liable to supervene, and the establishment of a colostomy after débridement of the perineal–gluteal area is essential. In addition, injury to the genitourinary system must be excluded.

PERFORATIONS FROM WITHIN

The colon and rectum may be injured from within by perforations caused by enema tips; endoscopic procedures; biopsy and polypectomy; excessive pressure in the course of the barium enema; insufflation or high jet compressed air; insertion of a foreign body, often for autoerotic purposes; swallowing of a bone or other sharp object; impalement; and laceration by bone from adjacent fractures.

The clinical picture varies widely. The incidence of perforation after colonoscopy is estimated at approximately 0.4%, but this figure varies considerably with the experience of the endoscopist and the condition of the diseased bowel for which the endoscopy is done. The incidence of perforation following biopsy is about 1%.[3] Perforation is most often due to pressure from the tip of the instrument, in which case the lesion is small, or a long laceration on the antimesenteric side of the rectosigmoid due to buckling and stretching of the segment, in which case the tear may be large. In some patients, the only evidence of this complication is the presence of air under the diaphragm on a postendoscopic roentgenogram. If the bowel has been well prepared and the perforation is small, the patient may be given antibiotics after all oral intake is discontinued and then very carefully observed. Most surgeons, however, prefer to perform a laparotomy to effect a simple repair of the injured bowel to avoid the risk of a slowly developing peritonitis. If the patient experiences immediate pain as the bowel is perforated, the diagnosis is obvious, and operation is usually advised without delay.

Perforation associated with a barium enema is a far more serious matter and occurs in about one in 2250 barium enemas.[4] Barium sulfate, when mixed with feces, causes a severe chemical peritonitis and is accompanied by a mortality rate of almost 50%. The mixture of barium, microorganisms, and intestinal content is a severe peritoneal irritant, which results in a great outpouring of exudate and subsequent dense adhesions in patients who survive. The treatment is rapid laparotomy and removal of as much of the barium and contaminating material as possible. Intravascular volume is replaced by Ringer's lactate to compensate for the third-space effect of the outpouring of fluid into the peritoneal cavity, and penicillin, an aminoglycoside, and clindamycin are administered (a larger than usual dose of aminoglycoside may be needed as a loading dose to obtain effective serum levels in these adverse circumstances). The peritoneal cavity is irrigated, and a proximal colostomy is established to divert the fecal stream. The damaged bowel should be exteriorized or resected.

Foreign bodies may produce perforation, although this is not common. When a foreign body has been removed per anum, the bowel must always be examined endoscopically to make certain that no tear of the wall is present.

Finally, attention must be given to the anal sphincter when this critical apparatus has been lacerated. To the extent possible, an accurate repair employing semisynthetic absorbable sutures should be performed and a defunctioning colostomy established. In rare cases in which the rectum pulls free from the sphincteric area and retracts proximally as an intact tube, the retracted end must be identified, brought down to the anal canal, and anchored firmly to the anal musculature. A temporary proximal colostomy is added for defunctioning purposes.

References

1. Alyono D, Perry JF Jr: Reappraisal of diagnostic peritoneal lavage criteria for operation in penetrating and blunt trauma. Surgery (in press)
2. Arendrup HC, Jensen BS: Traumatic rupture of the diaphragm. Surg Gynecol Obstet 154:526-530, 1982
3. Ecker MD, Goldstein M, Hoexter B et al: Benign pneumoperitoneum after fiberoptic colonoscopy: A prospective study of 100 patients. Gastroenterology 72:226-230, 1977
4. Gardiner H, Miller RE: Barium peritonitis: A therapeutic approach. Am J Surg 125:350-351, 1973
5. Graham JM, Mattox KL, Vaughan GD, Jordan GL Jr: Combined pancreatoduodenal injuries. J Trauma 19:340-346, 1979
6. Hornyak SW, Shaftan GW: Value of "inconclusive lavage" in abdominal trauma management. J Trauma 19:329-333, 1979
7. Howell HS, Bartizal JF, Freeark RJ: Blunt trauma involving the colon and rectum. J Trauma 16:624-632, 1976
8. Hunt JL: Generalized peritonitis: To irrigate or not to irrigate the abdominal cavity. Arch Surg 117:209-212, 1982
9. Kirkpatrick JR: The exteriorized anastomosis: Its role in surgery of the colon. Surgery 82:362-365, 1977
10. Lucas CE: Diagnosis and treatment of pancreatic duodenal injury. Surg Clin North Am 57:49-65, 1977
11. Matolo NM, Wolfman EF: Primary repair of colonic injuries: A clinical evaluation. J Trauma 17:554-564, 1977
12. Murr PC, Moore EE, Lipscomb R, Johnston RM: Abdominal trauma associated with pelvic fracture. J Trauma 20:919-923, 1980
13. Smit R, Walt AJ: The morbidity and cost of the temporary colostomy. Dis Colon Rectum 21:558-561, 1978
14. Soderstrom CA, DuPriest RW Jr, Cowley RA: Pitfalls of peritoneal lavage in blunt abdominal trauma. Surg Gynecol Obstet 151:513-518, 1980
15. Stone HH, Fabian TC: Management of perforating colon trauma: Randomization between primary closure and exteriorization. Ann Surg 190:430-435, 1979
16. Thal ER: Evaluation of peritoneal lavage and local exploration in lower chest and abdominal stab wounds. J Trauma 17:642-648, 1977
17. Waldschmidt ML, Laws HL: Injuries of the diaphragm. J Trauma 20:587-592, 1980
18. Walt AJ: Management of injuries of the colon and rectum. In MacLean LD (ed): Advances in Surgery, vol 16, pp 277–297. Chicago, Year Book Medical Publishers, 1983
19. Weaver DW, Bouwman DL, Walt AJ et al: A correlation between clinical pancreatitis and isoenzyme patterns of amylase. Surgery 92:576–580, 1982
20. Wiener I, Rojas P, Wolman FJ: Traumatic colonic perforation: Review of 16 years' experience. Am J Surg 181:705-715, 1975

Part Six

Complications of Endocrine System Surgery

41 Complications of Adrenal Gland Surgery

H. H. Newsome, Jr.

Metabolic and Pharmacologic Aspects

THE ADRENAL CORTEX

Cushing's Syndrome (Hypercortisolism)

PREOPERATIVE CONSIDERATIONS. OVERVIEW. The entire spectrum of metabolic derangements that we collectively term *Cushing's syndrome* results from excessive cortisol secretion by the adrenal cortex.[19] The persistent exposure of various tissues of the body to increased concentrations of cortisol eventually produces a wide range of changes in such diverse functions as fibroblastic proliferation, leukocyte migration, distribution of fat, lipogenesis, carbohydrate metabolism, and blood coagulability. Almost all of these changes have important implications for the clinician and the patient. Details of the effect of excess cortisol, or carbohydrate-active steroids, are listed in Chapter 18 as complications of immunosuppressive therapy. An understanding of these details will alert the clinician to the various postoperative complications that may be experienced with Cushing's syndrome.

Familiarity with the genesis of the hypercortisolemia is important from both the diagnostic and therapeutic standpoints.[12, 24] The causes of Cushing's syndrome can be divided into two general categories. An excessive production of ACTH initiates and sustains an overproduction of cortisol. Less commonly, the adrenal cortex may be the primary site of pathology, and autonomous production of cortisol results.

Causes of Cushing's Syndrome

- ACTH
  - Pituitary microadenomata
  - Ectopic tumor source
- Adrenal
  - Adenoma
  - Carcinoma
  - Nodular hyperplasia

It is obvious that results from diagnostic tests and therapy may differ according to the various causes of Cushing's syndrome. Since the treatment of choice for the pituitary origin of Cushing's syndrome is hypophysectomy, this cause of Cushing's disease is covered in Chapter 45. Ectopic (nonpituitary) production of ACTH requires treatment, which varies according to the accessibility of the tissue responsible for ACTH production. Finally, when Cushing's syndrome is produced by a primary adrenal process, direct surgical attention to the adrenal gland is indicated.

DIAGNOSIS. Documentation of an increased secretion of cortisol is the first diagnostic step in a suspected case of Cushing's syndrome.[3, 12, 13, 17] Increased cortisol secretion can be demonstrated by an increased basal plasma cortisol concentration, a loss of the diurnal variation in plasma cortisol concentrations, and an increased urinary excretion of 17-OHCS, or free cortisol. Since many otherwise normal obese persons will have a slightly increased excretion of cortisol or 17-OHCS in the urine, the low-dose dexamethasone suppression test is used to demonstrate a persistent increase in cortisol production in patients having Cushing's syndrome. With intact negative-feedback mechanisms, dexamethasone will suppress pituitary ACTH secretion and result in a decrease in cortisol secretion in simple exogenous obesity. The high-dose dexamethasone test will suppress ACTH-cortisol secretion in patients with the pituitary form of the disease, whereas in patients having an adrenal cause or ectopic production of ACTH, cortisol secretion remains unaffected by even high doses of dexamethasone. As the ACTH radioimmunoassay becomes more widely available, a combined cortisol and ACTH determination in a single plasma sample will become the standard means to differentiate the various types of Cushing's syndrome. For example, both ACTH and cortisol will

TABLE 41-1. DISTINGUISHING THE CAUSES OF HYPERCORTISOLISM

	Obesity	Pituitary	Adrenal	Ectopic
Low-dose dexamethasone	+	–	–	–
High-dose dexamethasone	+	+	–	–
Hypercortisolism	±	+	+	++
Plasma ACTH	Normal	Moderately high	Absent	Very high

be elevated with the pituitary source of the syndrome. Marked elevation of plasma ACTH is characteristic of an ectopic ACTH production. The adrenal tumor will result in an elevated plasma cortisol, but plasma ACTH will be undetectable because of the negative-feedback effect of the hypercortisolemia on pituitary ACTH secretion. These diagnostic considerations are summarized in Table 41-1.

In recent years, noninvasive localizing techniques have been quite helpful in confirming the results of laboratory testing and in directing surgical therapy to the appropriate area of the body. The tomogram of the sella turcica is abnormal in a certain percentage of patients with the pituitary cause of the syndrome. Currently available computed tomography (CT) is highly accurate in localizing the adrenal tumor, provided the lesion is greater than 1.0 cm to 1.5 cm in diameter. This scan is probably as accurate as, and considerably safer than, arteriography in localizing adrenal tumors. Once an adrenal tumor is diagnosed, the lateralization of the tumor allows the surgeon to confine the operation to a unilateral approach and eliminates the 50-50 chance inherent in empirical, sequential bilateral incisions.

PREPARATION FOR SURGERY. There are no specialized preparations required for this syndrome. The patient should be carefully instructed in the use of ventilatory aids during the postoperative period. Because of the increased risk of infection, we customarily wash the skin with antiseptic soap twice daily for a couple of days prior to surgery. There is a tendency to overtreat the patient preoperatively with excessive amounts of exogenous steroids. But with the excessive amount of endogenous cortisol already present, this is really unnecessary, and we have customarily waited until the intraoperative period to give steroids.

INTRAOPERATIVE CONSIDERATIONS. The intraoperative period for this surgery is devoid of metabolic or pharmacologic problems related to the disease. During the operation, we generally give the patient 100 mg of hydrocortisone intravenously. Should the surgery become protracted, the steroid is given again in 4 hours. The remainder of the steroid regimen is started in the recovery room.

POSTOPERATIVE CONSIDERATIONS. The steroid requirements during the perioperative period can be met by several schedules. We prefer a regimen that alternates intramuscular and intravenous routes. Fifty milligrams of cortisone acetate is given intramuscularly every 12 hours. On an alternate 12-hour schedule, 100 mg of hydrocortisone is given intravenously. This results in 200 mg of cortisol-equivalents per 24 hours. We have shown that this amount of steroid produces plasma concentrations that are probably more than adequate to cover the stress of the surgery in the ordinary patient.[36] In a patient with Cushing's syndrome, however, clinical impressions suggest that these patients require more steroids than usual. At the end of the first 48 hours postoperatively, the daily steroid dosage is reduced to 100 mg. Usually by the end of the third or fourth postoperative day, the patient begins oral nourishment, and the intravenous cortisol is eliminated. It is important to continue to give the steroid parenterally until intestinal absorption of oral steroid is assured.

Long-term steroid administration may initially be required at a dose as high as 75 mg to 100 mg per day. When the dose is lowered below this level, patients may develop malaise, joint aches, diarrhea, and even a low-grade fever. In cases of total adrenalectomy, the dosage should be gradually tapered to a permanent maintenance dose of 50 mg per day of cortisone acetate. In most patients, cortisone acetate alone is sufficient, but serum sodium and potassium levels should be monitored to detect a need for mineralocorticoids. Administration of 0.1 mg of fluorohydrocortisone per day will usually suffice to correct hyperkalemia, hyponatremia, and hypotension. Most patients can eventually be tapered from the steroid as the contralateral adrenal cortex becomes functional following unilateral adrenalectomy. At about 3 months postoperatively, pituitary secretion of ACTH resumes, but another 3 months is usually required before the adrenal cortex responds to ACTH. Exogenous ACTH administration (40 Units per day, for 5 days) will induce adrenocortical responsiveness and can be tried at 3 to 4 months postoperatively. ACTH infusion affords a means to hasten adrenal recovery once endogenous ACTH secretion returns. Obviously, the entire process of pituitary–adrenal recovery can be prevented by injudicious continued overdosage with exogenous steroids.

Conn's Syndrome (Primary Hyperaldosteronism)

PREOPERATIVE CONSIDERATIONS. OVERVIEW. Both major forms of primary aldosteronism manifest an autonomous, persistently excessive production of aldosterone from the zona glomerulosa of the adrenal cortex.[27] Approximately 80% of the cases of primary aldosteronism are due to a cortical adenoma. The other 20% of cases are due to hyperplasia of the zona glomerulosa. With either cause, the production of aldosterone is considered to be the initiating event in the pathogenesis of the syndrome. Several features of the hyperplasia variety bring into question the primacy of aldosterone in producing the hypertension.[38] Since aldosterone acts to stimulate the sodium–potassium exchange in the distal renal tubule, renal sodium retention and potassium excretion occur. These events lead to the onset of hypertension, muscle weakness, and hypokalemic nephropathy.

DIAGNOSIS. In addition to the hypertension, sodium retention leads to a suppression of plasma renin activity.[47, 50] Plasma renin remains suppressed in this syndrome even in the face of measures that would ordinarily stimulate renin secretion, such as those of an upright posture or of diuretic administration. The demonstration of a suppressed plasma renin activity during these stimulatory measures represents one of the essential laboratory diagnostic features. In contrast to measurement of plasma renin activity during conditions stimulatory to release of this enzyme, measurement of plasma or urinary aldosterone should be done during maneuvers (for example, infusion of sodium) that ordinarily suppress secretion of the steroid. Evidence of persistent hypersecretion of aldosterone during suppressive maneuvers must be obtained to confirm the diagnosis of primary hyperaldosteronism. These features are summarized as follows:

- Hypertension
- Hypokalemia, alkalosis
- Hyperaldosteronism (in spite of suppressive maneuvers)
- Suppressed plasma renin (in spite of stimulatory maneuvers)

It should be noted that during measurements of plasma or urinary aldosterone and plasma renin activity, sodium intake must be controlled and monitored. A low sodium intake or negative sodium balance will produce a physiologic hyperaldosteronism in normal subjects while a high sodium intake or positive sodium balance will normally suppress plasma renin activity. Control of dietary sodium intake is best achieved on an in-patient basis in a metabolic unit, but a low-sodium regular hospital diet, with carefully measured sodium chloride added to it, will suffice. Measurement of 24-hour urinary sodium excretion is the best device for confirming intake. Potassium intake is more difficult to control but can likewise be monitored by measurement of urinary excretion of potassium.

Once primary aldosteronism has been diagnosed by demonstrating increased aldosterone secretion and suppressed plasma renin under different conditions of posture and sodium balance, the surgeon then faces the problem of diagnosing tumor versus hyperplasia.[15] Localization of a tumor by noninvasive means will establish the etiology and facilitate surgery.[2, 51, 52] The occasional small size of these tumors may preclude the reliable use of either arteriography or CT scans for localization. A radioactive scan based on the uptake of iodinated cholesterol by the steroidogenic pathway has been used to localize the tumors (unilateral uptake) or to demonstrate hyperplasia (bilateral uptake).[11] Adrenal vein catheterization is another maneuver to distinguish hyperplasia from tumor.[18] The adrenal venous blood is assayed for aldosterone and cortisol. An elevation of the aldosterone:cortisol ratio on one side compared to that on the other is indicative of a tumor. Bilaterally equal ratios would indicate hyperplasia in a patient in whom autonomous secretion of aldosterone and a suppressed plasma renin have been demonstrated.[4] Other observations that may serve to differentiate hyperplasia from adenoma have been made. There is an anomalous fall in plasma concentrations of aldosterone with upright posture in patients with aldosteronomas.[23, 32] This response to posture may be related to the different response seen with angiotensin infusion.[53] Evidence for etiologic factors of hyperplasia different from those for adenoma include suppression of aldosterone secretion by cyproheptadine.[25] The rare dexamethasone-suppressible aldosteronism may be confused with adenomas because of similar plasma aldosterone responses to posture.[21]

PREPARATION FOR SURGERY. Correction of hypokalemia should be carried out in the preoperative period. Use of the aldosterone antagonist spironolactone, which promotes renal retention of potassium, and use of oral potassium chloride supplements facilitate the normalization of the serum potassium within 1 to 2 weeks.[6] Sodium restriction also aids in potassium repletion. Since sodium serves as a substrate for the sodium–potassium exchange, a diminution in sodium concentration in the renal tubular lumen results in a decreased urinary potassium excretion.

INTRAOPERATIVE CONSIDERATIONS. Once the hypokalemia has been corrected, the intraoperative course of the patient is usually benign. In the occasional patient who may have borderline hypokalemia and probably inadequately replaced potassium losses, an intraoperative blood sample should be checked for potassium concentration. As a rule, the problems seen with the other adrenal syndromes, such as obesity, fluctuations in blood pressure, or arrhythmias, are not present in primary aldosteronism.

POSTOPERATIVE CONSIDERATIONS. Analogous to postoperative functional recovery in Cushing's syndrome, the zona glomerulosa of the remaining adrenal gland remains hypofunctioning. A relative deficiency in aldosterone will be manifested by a tendency toward hypotension and hyperkalemia.[5] Administration of a mineralocorticoid such as fluohydrocortisone (Florinef) is the treatment of choice. Apparently, the renal production of renin and consequently the tropic hormone to the zona glomerulosa, angiotensin, remain suppressed postoperatively.[34] The renin–angiotensin system becomes activated, after 1- to 2-week trials of intermittent Florinef therapy, and stimulates the zona glomerulosa to full production of aldosterone.

The opposite—residual hyperaldosteronism—arises postoperatively when the diagnosis is hyperplasia, confirmed only by the indicated adrenal biopsy. Spironolactone therapy is the best available treatment for this subset of patients. A dose of 25 mg, twice daily, may suffice in some patients, but an increase in dose to 300 mg to 400 mg per day may be required in others to control the hypertension and correct the hypokalemia. As mentioned above, dietary sodium restriction will aid in decreasing urinary potassium loss.

ADRENAL MEDULLA

Pheochromocytoma

PREOPERATIVE CONSIDERATIONS. OVERVIEW. Since a pheochromocytoma is a tumor arising from the adrenal medulla or from an extra-adrenal sympathetic ganglion, it is not surprising that a functioning tumor becomes clinically evident through excessive catecholamine production.[14] Alpha- or beta-adrenergic receptors are stimulated by the circulating catecholamines. The relative degree of stimulation of these two types of receptors determines the particular constellation of signs and symptoms manifested by any given patient. Classically, norepinephrine stimulates alpha-adrenergic receptors to result in peripheral vasoconstriction and an elevation in blood pressure. Epinephrine stimulates the beta receptors, which produces a tachycardia and a dilatation of blood vessels in some vascular beds. In actuality, the alpha and beta functions overlap so that norepinephrine, when present in large amounts, can become chronotropic, although high concentrations of epinephrine can raise the blood pressure just as effectively. Pharmacologic use of alpha- and beta-blocking agents likewise may have hybrid effects. We have recently observed a patient with a pure norepinephrine-secreting tumor whose hypertension and symptoms completely disappeared with treatment by the beta blocker propranolol.[37] Although rare cases of pure epinephrine-secreting tumors have been reported, norepinephrine is secreted by almost all functioning pheochromocytomas. Most tumors also produce some epinephrine, and a wide range of norepinephrine:epinephrine ratios is seen.

Regardless of the secretory characteristics, the clinical features may not be distinctive. The diagnostic emphasis should be placed on considering the possibility of pheochromocytoma in any hypertensive patient, which the large number of clinically unsuspected pheochromocytomas reported in one series shows to be difficult.[48]

DIAGNOSIS. These tumors can now be diagnosed simply by demonstrating by radioenzymatic assay an elevated concentration of the catecholamines in the plasma and detecting a tumor by use of the CT scan.[8, 22, 29, 46] The radioenzymatic assay of plasma epinephrine and norepinephrine has brought a new dimension of sensitivity and accuracy to the measurement of these substances. Further diagnostic accuracy has been added using clonidine or pentolinium to suppress plasma catecholamines in patients with only essential hypertension.[7, 10] Where this method is not available, the old fluorometric determination of urinary catecholamines or measurement of the urinary excretion products of catecholamine metabolism, namely, vanillylmandelic acid or metanephrines, can be employed. The preoperative localization of these tumors can be more helpful than simply proving the presence of a pheochromocytoma. Not only can the adrenal tumors be lateralized, but the 10% of tumors that occur outside of the adrenal gland can be found. Because it is accurate and safer than arteriography, the CT scan is probably the localizing procedure of choice, for both the adrenal tumors and those in other areas. Oblique views of the thorax by ordinary x-ray film can demonstrate the mediastinal pheochromocytoma arising from the sympathetic chain. In the patient whose pheochromocytoma cannot be located by any of the above means, determination of catecholamines in blood sampled from various points in the superior and inferior vena cava can point to the tumor location.

PREPARATION FOR SURGERY. Pharmacologic blockade of alpha- or beta adrenergic receptors should be carried out with the appropriate agents.[41, 48, 49] Although no randomized, prospective study of patients with this uncommon tumor exists, use of these adrenergic blocking agents has apparently considerably reduced the incidence of cardiovascular mishaps during surgery for pheochromocytomas. Indications for the preoperative use of alpha-adrenergic blockade include sustained diastolic hypertension above 90 torr or paroxysms of hypertension in an otherwise normotensive patient. Phenoxybenzamine has been the agent of choice. Because of possible sensitivity to small amounts of this drug, patients should be started on 10 mg daily. In consideration of the slow onset of action, dosage should not be increased more frequently than every 48 hours. The dose is best titrated in each patient to a precise therapeutic point by routinely measuring blood pressure after 6 minutes in the upright position. A drop in diastolic pressure of over 40 torr indicates the approach of effective adrenergic blockade. Should any further blockade be desired, the patient is more appropriately maintained supine in bed as dosage is increased. Selection of patients for beta blockade is perhaps more arbitrary, but a useful guideline is that of a resting pulse rate of above 100 per minute, or the presence of more than three premature ventricular contractions per minute. Since beta blockade may decrease myocardial contractility, it is recommended that alpha blockade be instituted to lower ventricular afterload prior to the use of beta blockade with propranolol. Propranolol should be used with care owing to the existence of myocardopathy in some cases of pheochromocytoma. Proponents of preoperative blood transfusions for patients with pheochromocytomas cite the demonstration of a blood volume deficit, presumably due to sustained hypertension. This finding is not universal in patients with pheochromocytoma, and we prefer to start transfusion intraoperatively only if hypotension occurs after removal of the pheochromocytoma.

INTRAOPERATIVE CONSIDERATIONS. Anesthesia is selected to minimize the release and consequent effects of the catecholamines.[9, 40] By the time the patient arrives in the operating suite, the patient should have been well premedicated with morphine and diazepam. The second precaution is to establish a reliable radial artery line for intra-arterial monitoring. The EKG is also attached as soon as the patient enters the room. Anesthesia is induced by thiopental sodium (Pentothal) and the endotracheal tube inserted after succinylcholine takes effect. The patient is maintained with nitrous oxide-oxygen, fentanyl, curare, and pancuronium. Some anesthesiologists prefer supplementation with properidol, while others would add ethrane to the nitrous oxide-oxygen mixture. This anesthetic regimen results in little, if any, increase in the concentrations of plasma catecholamines.

Large quantities of catecholamines may be released during manipulation of the tumor and produce adrenergic effects in spite of full preoperative beta or alpha blockade.[20] In order to counteract sudden rises in blood pressure, phentolamine may be given as a bolus from a syringe or, more appropriately, as an intravenous infusion made to a concentration of 40 mg to 80 mg per 100 ml of fluid. Nitroprusside, another hypotensive agent, may be preferred because of its short half-life, which facilitates close titration of the blood pressure. Arrhythmias may be controlled by either lidocaine or propranolol. Propranolol must be used with caution because of its depressive effect on the myocardium. The congestive failure seen in the occasional patients with myocardopathy is particularly difficult to treat because it is refractory to digitalis or glucagon. Both the arrhythmias and the congestive failure may be improved by lowering the systemic blood pressure, thus reducing ventricular afterload and work.

In successfully treated cases, the blood pressure usually comes down to normal immediately upon removal of the tumor. Occasionally, the blood pressure will drop below normal. One mechanism for the hypotension is probably tachyphylaxis, and supranormal amounts of catecholamines are needed to maintain the blood pressure at a normal level. Toward this end, norepinephrine (Levophed) infusion is required. An additive mechanism for the hypotension is probably a low blood volume. A transfusion of 500 ml to 1000 ml of whole blood usually is associated with a return of the blood pressure to normal and of the ability to discontinue the norepinephrine drip. If, however, upon removal of a pheochromocytoma the blood pressure remains significantly elevated, the patient may harbor a second pheochromocytoma. Therefore, the surgeon must search, usually in the contralateral adrenal gland. Except in children, the coexistence of adrenal and extra-adrenal pheochromocytomas is distinctly unusual. Undetected metastases from a malignant pheochromocytoma would be likely in the adult with sustained hypertension and normal contralateral adrenal.

POSTOPERATIVE CONSIDERATIONS. With pheochromocytomas, postoperative complications of a metabolic or pharmacologic nature are distinctly uncommon, beyond the hypotension of tachyphylaxis or low blood volume. In the long view, it is extremely important to monitor the patient for a possible return of hypertension.[26] Perhaps the most likely cause of recurrent hypertension is the asynchronous growth of a pheochromocytoma in the contralateral adrenal gland, which was missed at the initial surgery. In sporadic cases, the incidence of bilaterality is approximately 10%, while that in children or in patients with the familial syndrome is as high as 50%. An infrequent cause of recurrent hypertension is the incomplete removal of a benign pheochromocytoma and the regrowth of residual tumor. A third cause of recurrent hypertension is the local recurrence or distant metastases of a previously removed malignant pheochromocytoma.[33] Unfortunately, there are no certain histologic criteria for diagnosis of malignancy in the primary pheochromocytoma, and the first indication of the tumor's malignancy may well be its subsequent reappearance.

SIPPLE'S SYNDROME. The familial occurrence of pheochromocytoma, medullary carcinoma of the thyroid, and primary hyperparathyroidism was described by Sipple in 1961.[45] The clinical presentation of the pheochromocytomas is indistinguishable from that of sporadic cases.[30] An important difference is the 50% incidence of bilateral pheochromocytomas in the familial form as compared to 10% in sporadic cases.[31] Although medullary thyroid carcinoma and primary hyperparathyroidism as separate entities can exist in the familial form, whenever familial forms of either entity are found, family members should be carefully questioned for history of pheochromocytomas or of symptoms suggesting the tumor. Even in seemingly sporadic cases, when the patient has suggestive symptoms or the family history is unclear, care should be taken to rule out pheochromocytoma by plasma or urine catecholamine determinations. Anesthesia and surgery in a patient with a pheochromocytoma, without adrenergic blockade or proper choice of anesthetic agents, may precipitate a disaster.

Operative Aspects

SURGICAL APPROACHES

Particular surgical approaches to adrenalectomy all involve several general considerations and review of potential complications.[39] Whether the operative approach is anterior, lateral, or posterior, the close proximity of the right adrenal gland to the vena cava and the consequent short adrenal vein should elicit extra care from the surgeon. The complication of a torn adrenal vein or an avulsion of a tumor attached to the vena cava is better avoided than dealt with *post facto*. If the adrenal vein is torn at an early stage of dissection, temporizing tamponade of the bleeding area should be done until extirpation of the tumor is complete. This tamponade can usually be accomplished by a judiciously placed sponge stick. Blind clamping with a right-angle or Satinsky clamp risks further tearing the vena cava. The vena cava should be visualized under adequate suction and light so that an accurate, gentle placement of a Satinsky clamp will stop, not exacerbate, the bleeding. In the posterior approach, the thoracic cavity must be entered, in extreme situations with bleeding, even at the expense of cutting the higher ribs. Blood loss of a more leisurely nature from the adrenal bed may also be problematic. Although opinions on details of technique vary, either ligation or hemoclip application is indicated before incising the generally vascular periadrenal tissue. It is usually customary to use a soft rubber drain brought from the adrenal bed out through the incision. The drain can be removed within the first 24 to 48 hours postoperatively.

Abdominal Approach

The abdominal approach may at times be preferred. When an adrenocortical tumor is large (greater than 300–400 g), the chance of carcinoma increases, and the prospect of possible removal of the surrounding structures makes the posterior approach unattractive. An abdominal approach is a reasonable alternative to bilateral posterior incisions when the tumor cannot be localized preoperatively or when known bilateral processes exist. The standard transabdominal incision is that of a "rooftop" or bilateral subcostal orientation. Because the anterior approach to the left adrenal gland entails the dissection around and retraction of the pancreas, the incidence of pancreatitis may be greater with this approach.[35] Similarly, an inadvertent splenectomy is seen almost exclusively with the abdominal approach. On the right side, a tear in the vena cava is perhaps somewhat more easily controlled through the large abdominal incision. Also, there is no problem transabdominally with pneumothorax, in contrast to that occasionally seen with the posterior approach.

Posterior Approach

The posterior approach entails placement of the patient in either the face-down or the half-lateral position. The paravertebral incision is used in the face-down position while the half-lateral position allows a flank incision, which can be carried somewhat more anteriorly. With the posterior approach, the adrenal area is entered through the bed of the 11th or 12th rib. In most instances of the 12th rib approach, it is obvious when the pleura is entered, and the surgeon may simply close the pleural hole with absorbable suture. The ventilator is held in positive pressure insufflation during the last closure step. Because a hole in the pleura may be unrecognized, the patient should always have a routine postoperative chest x-ray film. Only if for some reason the lung itself has been severed is there any significant difficulty. The pleural space is usually deliberately entered from the 11th rib bed. The posterior approach easily places the surgeon into the area of the adrenal gland on either side. Again, it should be mentioned that this approach is problematic for removal of a large tumor. The disadvantages of each surgical approach to the adrenal gland are listed below.

Transabdominal Approach
Pancreatitis
Splenic injury
Wound dehiscence

Posterior Approach
Pneumothorax
Large tumor
Vena caval control

APPROACH FOR SPECIFIC SYNDROMES

Cushing's Syndrome

Except for a large tumor thought to be carcinoma, the posterior approach is preferred for an adrenal tumor that produces hypercortisolism.[16, 44] The patients almost always have obese trunks, and the abdominal approach is unpleasant. The most common postoperative complication in Cushing's syndrome is that of wound infection. It is obvious that an infected posterior wound does not carry the same potential for dehiscence and evisceration that an abdominal wound does. In addition, the patient may have a greater propensity for pancreatitis under sustained cortisol excess than do patients with other syndromes not involving hypercortisolism. Obviously, the posterior approach does not necessitate handling of the pancreas. Other postoperative complications in Cushing's syndrome, such as the increased risk of thrombosis or of cardiovascular events, appear to be independent of the surgical approach.

Conn's Syndrome

If the tumor can be localized preoperatively by any of the means mentioned above, a unilateral posterior approach to Conn's syndrome is the most simple.[1, 3, 28] Because these patients are within the normal range of body habitus, the abdominal approach may be preferred when the tumor cannot be localized preoperatively. A considerable number of the aldosteronomas are quite small and not easily detected by casual palpation of the adrenal gland. If a tumor is not obvious, the lateral edge of each gland should be completely mobilized to allow careful palpation of the entire gland between the thumb and forefinger. If no tumor is palpable, the tip of each adrenal gland should be removed and immediately examined histologically by the pathologist for the presence of hyperplasia of the zona glomerulosa. Should the zona glomerulosa appear normal, the adrenal gland should be segmentally resected from the tip inward with the removed tissue sliced in 1-mm sections and searched for tiny tumors. When 60% to 70% of the adrenal gland has been removed thus, and the tumor is still undetected, a choice between possible residual tumor and certain adrenal insufficiency must be made. We believe that with the availability of postoperative spironolactone therapy, the surgeon should exercise the wiser option of stopping at this point rather than rendering the patient adrenally insufficient. Further postoperative studies, as mentioned above, can be performed to assess residual adrenal function. Should the initial histologic examination reveal hyperplasia of the zona glomerulosa (and no tumor palpable), the adrenals are left intact. Total adrenalectomy for hyperplasia does not affect the hypertension, and spironolactone is the treatment of choice.

Pheochromocytoma

Because of the possibility of multiple pheochromocytomas and in view of the normal body habitus of most of these patients, the transabdominal approach is preferred.[43] This philosophy may change as more confidence and improvements come with the newer noninvasive techniques of CT scan or venous arteriography. Other than the possible metabolic–pharmacologic complications or the general complications related to adrenalectomy covered above, there are no specific risks in removal of a pheochromocytoma. Because most of the release of the catecholamines from the tumor is caused simply by mechanical compression of the gland, it is obvious that gentle handling of the tumor will moderate the cardiovascular risks during surgery. Since some handling of the gland is necessary, an effort should be made to ligate the adrenal vein as early in the dissection as possible in order to inhibit escape of catechols from the tumor. Although some fall in blood pressure will occur soon after adrenal vein ligation, residual auxiliary venous channels still exist, and the remainder of the dissection must also be done carefully and gently. It is important to note, as mentioned previously, that a second tumor should be sought if the blood pressure does not fall significantly following removal of a pheochromocytoma.

References

1. Ackerman NB, Johnson–Giannopoulos N, Winer N: Pitfalls in the surgery of aldosterone-producing tumors. Am J Surg 124:774, 1972
2. Adamson U, Effendié S, Granberg PO et al: Preoperative localization of aldosterone-producing adenomas. Acta Med Scand 208:101, 1980

3. Aron DC, Tyrrell JB, Fitzgerald PA et al: Cushing's syndrome: Problems in diagnosis. Medicine 60:25, 1981
4. Auda SP, Brennan MF, Gill JR: Evolution of the surgical management of primary aldosteronism. Ann Surg 191:1, 1980
5. Biglieri EG, Slaton PE, Silen WS et al: Postoperative studies of adrenal function in primary aldosteronism. J Clin Endocrinol Metab 26:553, 1966
6. Bravo EL, Dustan HP, Tarazi RC: Spironolactone as a nonspecific treatment for primary aldosteronism. Circulation 48:491, 1973
7. Bravo EL, Tarazi RC, Fouad FM et al: Clonidine-suppression test: A useful aid in the diagnosis of pheochromocytoma. N Engl J Med 305:623, 1981
8. Bravo EL, Tarazi RC, Gifford RW, Steward BH: Circulating and urinary catecholamines in pheochromocytoma. N Engl J Med 301:682, 1979
9. Brown BR: Anesthesia for pheochromocytoma. In Brown BR (ed): Anesthesia and the Patient with Endocrine Disease. Philadelphia, FA Davis, 1980
10. Brown MJ, Allison DJ, Jenner DA et al: Increased sensitivity and accuracy of phaeochromocytoma diagnosis achieved by use of plasma-adrenaline estimations and a pentolinium-suppression test. Lancet 1:174, 1981
11. Conn JW, Cohen EL, Herwig KR: The dexamethasone-modified adrenal scintiscan in hyporeninemic aldosteronism (tumor versus hyperplasia). A comparison with adrenal venography and adrenal venous aldosterone. J Lab Clin Med 88:841, 1976
12. Cook DM, Kendall JW, Jordan R: Cushing syndrome: Current concepts of diagnosis and therapy. West J Med 132:111, 1980
13. Crapo L: Cushing's syndrome: A review of diagnostic tests. Metabolism 28:955, 1979
14. Cryer PE: Physiology and pathophysiology of the human sympathoadrenal neuroendocrine system. N Engl J Med 303:436, 1980
15. Davis WW, Newsome HH, Wright LD et al: Bilateral adrenal hyperplasia as a cause of primary aldosteronism with hypertension, hypokalemia and suppressed renin activity. Am J Med 42:642, 1967
16. Delaney JP, Solomkin JS, Jacobson ME, Doe RP: Surgical management of Cushing's syndrome. Surgery 84:465, 1978
17. Eddy RL, Jones AL, Gilliland PF et al: Cushing's syndrome: A prospective study of diagnostic methods. Am J Med 55:621, 1973
18. Egdahl RH, Kahn PC, Melby JC: Unilateral adrenalectomy for aldosteronomas localized preoperatively by differential adrenal vein catheterization. Surgery 64:117, 1968
19. Fehm HL, Voight KH: Pathophysiology of Cushing's disease. Pathobiol Annu 9:225, 1979
20. Feldman JM, Blalock JA, Fagraeus L et al: Alterations in plasma norepinephrine concentration during surgical resection of pheochromocytoma. Ann Surg 188:758, 1978
21. Ganguly A, Grim CE, Weinberger MH: Anomalous postural aldosterone response in glucocorticoid-suppressible hyperaldosteronism. N Engl J Med 305:991, 1981
22. Ganguly A, Henry DP, Yune HY et al: Diagnosis and localization of pheochromocytoma. Am J Med 67:21, 1979
23. Ganguly A, Melada GA, Luetscher JA, Dowdy AJ: Control of plasma aldosterone in primary aldosteronism: Distinction between adenoma and hyperplasia. J Clin Endocrinol Metab 37:765, 1973
24. Gold EM: The Cushing syndromes: Changing view of diagnosis and treatment. Ann Intern Med 90:829, 1979
25. Gross MD, Grekin RJ, Gniadek TC, Villareal JZ: Suppression of aldosterone by cyproheptadine in idiopathic aldosteronism. N Engl J Med 305:181, 1981
26. Harrison TS, Freier DT, Cohen EL: Recurrent pheochromocytoma. Arch Surg 108:450, 1974
27. Horton R: Aldosterone: Review of its physiology and diagnostic aspects of primary aldosteronism. Metabolism 22:1525, 1973
28. Hunt TK, Schambelan M, Biglieri EG: Selection of patients and operative approach in primary aldosteronism. Ann Surg 182:353, 1975
29. Jones DH, Reid JL, Hamilton CA et al: The biochemical diagnosis: Localization and follow-up of phaeochromocytoma: The role of plasma and urinary catecholamine measurements. Q J Med 49:341, 1980
30. Keiser HR, Beaven MA, Doppman J et al: Sipple's syndrome: Medullary thyroid carcinoma, pheochromocytoma, and parathyroid disease. Ann Intern Med 78:561, 1973
31. Lips KJM, van der Sluys Veer J, Struyvenberg A et al: Bilateral occurrence of pheochromocytoma in patients with the multiple endocrine neoplasia syndrome type 2A (Sipple's syndrome). Am J Med 70:1051, 1981
32. Luetscher JA, Ganguly A, Melada GA, Dowdy AJ: Preoperative differentiation of adrenal adenoma from idiopathic adrenal hyperplasia in primary aldosteronism. Circ Res (Suppl) 34,35:1, 1974
33. Mahoney EM, Harrison JH: Malignant pheochromocytoma: Clinical course and treatment. J Urol 118:225, 1977
34. Morimoto S, Takeda R, Murakami M: Does prolonged pretreatment with large doses of spironolactone hasten a recovery from juxtaglomerularadrenal suppression in primary aldosteronism? J Clin Endocrinol Metab 31:659, 1970
35. Nash AG, Robbins GF: The operative approach to the left adrenal gland. Surg Gynecol Obstet 137:670, 1973
36. Newsome HH, Manalan SA: Plasma cortisol and cortisone concentrations following postoperative adrenal steroid replacement. Surgery 73:429, 1973
37. Newsome HH, Weir GC, Daniel TM: Norepinephrine-secreting tumor of the organ of Zuckerkandl: Response to propranolol alone. JAMA 242:540, 1979
38. Padfield PL, Brown JJ, Davies D et al: The myth of idiopathic hyperaldosteronism. Lancet 2:83, 1981
39. Pezzulich RA, Mannix H: Immediate complications of adrenal surgery. Ann Surg 172:125, 1970
40. Pratilas V, Pratila MG: Anaesthetic management of phaeochromocytoma. Can Anaesth Soc J 26:253, 1979
41. Ross EJ, Prichard BNC, Kaufman L et al: Preoperative and operative management of patients with phaeochromocytoma. Br Med J 1:191, 1967
42. Schmidt FE, Lewis ML, Kahle HR: Chemodectomas of the carotid body and glumus tympanicum. JAMA 240:1266, 1978
43. Scott HW, Dean RH, Oates JA et al: Surgical management of pheochromocytoma. Am Surg 47:8, 1981
44. Scott HW, Foster JH, Rhamy RK et al: Surgical management of adrenocortical tumors with Cushing's syndrome. Ann Surg 173:892, 1971
45. Sipple JH: The association of pheochromocytoma with carcinoma of the thyroid gland. Am J Med 31:163, 1961
46. Stewart BH, Bravo EL, Meaney TF: A new simplified approach to the diagnosis of pheochromocytoma. J Urol 122:579, 1979
47. Streeten DHP, Tomycz N, Anderson GH: Reliability of screening methods for the diagnosis of primary aldosteronism. Am J Med 67:403, 1979

48. Sutton MGS, Sheps SG, Lie JT: Prevalence of clinically unsuspected pheochromocytoma. Mayo Clin Proc 56:354, 1981
49. Temple WJ, Voitk AJ, Thomson AE, Downs AR: Phenoxybenzamine blockade in surgery of pheochromocytoma. J Surg Res 22:59, 1977
50. Vaughan NJA, Jowett TP, Slater JDH et al: The diagnosis of primary hyperaldosteronism. Lancet 1:120, 1981
51. Vetter H, Brecht G, Fischer M et al: Lateralization procedures in primary aldosteronism. Klin Wochenschr 58:1135, 1980
52. White EA, Schambelan M, Rost CR et al: Use of computed tomography in diagnosing the cause of primary aldosteronism. N Engl J Med 303:1503, 1980
53. Wisgerhof M, Brown RD, Hogan MJ et al: The plasma aldosterone response to angiotensin II infusion in aldosterone-producing adenoma and idiopathic hyperaldosteronism. J Clin Endocrinol Metab 52:195, 1981

Suggested Reading

General

Block MB, Roberts JP, Kadair RG et al: Multiple endocrine adenomatosis type IIB. JAMA 234:710, 1975
Dunnick NR, Schaner EG, Doppman JL et al: Computed tomography in adrenal tumors. AJR 132:43, 1979
Egdahl RH: Surgery of the adrenal gland. N Engl J Med 278:939, 1968
Harrison TS, Gann DS, Edis AJ, Egdahl RH: Surgical Disorders of the Adrenal Gland: Physiologic Background and Treatment. New York, Grune & Stratton, 1975
Javadpour N, Woltering EA, Brennan MF: Adrenal neoplasms. Curr Probl Surg 17:1, 1980
Maddi R, Gabel RA: Anesthetic considerations for adrenalectomy. In Brown BR Jr (ed): Anesthesia and the Patient with Endocrine Disease. Philadelphia, F A Davis, 1980
Raker JW: Surgery of the adrenal glands. Adv Surg 5:129, 1971
Symington T: Functional Pathology of the Adrenal Gland. Baltimore, Williams & Wilkins, 1969
Tank ES, Bartlett JD, Herwig KR, Lapides J: Surgery of the adrenal glands in infancy and childhood. J Urol 106:280, 1971
Wells SA: Multiple endocrine neoplasia type II[1]. Annu Rev Med 27:263, 1976

Cushing's Syndrome

Lipsett MB, Hertz R, Ross GT: Clinical and pathophysiologic aspects of adrenocortical carcinoma. Am J Med 35:374, 1963
Macfarlane DA: Cancer of the adrenal cortex. Ann R Coll Surg Engl 23:155, 1958
Montgomery DAD, Welbourn RB: Cushing's syndrome: 20 years after adrenalectomy. Br J Surg 65:221, 1978
Orth DN, Liddle GW: Results of treatment in 108 patients with Cushing's syndrome. N Engl J Med 285:243, 1971
Plotz CM, Knowlton AI, Ragan C: The natural history of Cushing's syndrome. Am J Med 13:597, 1952
Rapaport E, Goldberg MB, Gordan GS, Hinman F: Mortality in surgically treated adrenocortical tumors. Postgrad Med 11:325, 1952
Richie JP, Gittes RF: Carcinoma of the adrenal cortex. Cancer 45:1957, 1980
Urbanic RC, George JM: Cushing's disease—18 years' experience. Medicine 60:14, 1981
Welbourn RB: The natural history of treated Cushing's syndrome. Br J Surg 58:1, 1971

Conn's Syndrome

Bartter FC, Biglieri EG: Primary aldosteronism: Clinical staff conference at the National Institutes of Health. NIH Clin Staff 48:647, 1958
Herwig KR: Primary aldosteronism: Experience with thirty-eight patients. Surgery 86:470, 1979
Kahn PC, Kelleher MD, Egdahl RH, Melby JC: Adrenal arteriography and venography in primary aldosteronism. Diag Radiol 101:71, 1971
Menon M, Mersey JH: Primary aldosteronism—A review. Urol Surv 30:95, 1980
Neville AM, Symington T: Pathology of primary aldosteronism. Cancer 19:1854, 1966
Scoggins BA, Coghlan JP: Primary hyperaldosteronism. Pharmacol Ther 9:367, 1980
Silen W, Biglieri EG, Slaton P, Galante M: Management of primary aldosteronism: Evaluation of potassium and sodium balance, technic of adrenalectomy and operative results in 24 cases. Ann Surg 164:600, 1966
Weinberger MH, Grim CE, Hollifield JW et al: Primary aldosteronism: Diagnosis, localization and treatment. Ann Intern Med 90:386, 1979
Zimmerman B, Moran WH, Rosenberg JC et al: Physiologic and surgical problems in the management of primary aldosteronism. Ann Surg 150:653, 1959

Pheochromocytoma

Bloom DA, Fonkalsrud EW: Surgical management of pheochromocytoma in children. J Pediatr Surg 9:179, 1974
Deoreo GA, Stewart BH, Tarazi RC, Gifford RW: Preoperative blood transfusion in the safe surgical management of pheochromocytoma: A review of 46 cases. J Urol 111:715, 1974
Freier DT, Echhauser FE, Harrison TS: Pheochromocytoma: A persistently problematic and still potentially lethal disease. Arch Surg 115:388, 1980
Freier DT, Tank ES, Harrison TS: Pediatric and adult pheochromocytomas. Arch Surg 107:252, 1973
Gibbs MK, Carney JA, Hayles AB, Telander RL: Simultaneous adrenal and cervical pheochromocytomas in childhood. Ann Surg 185:273, 1977
Hume DM: Pheochromocytoma in the adult and in the child. Am J Surg 99:458, 1960
Manger WM, Gifford RW: Pheochromocytoma. New York, Springer-Verlag, 1978
Modlin IM, Farndon JR, Shepherd A et al: Phaeochromocytomas in 72 patients: Clinical and diagnostic features, treatment and long-term results. Br J Surg 66:456, 1979
Ram CVS, Engelman K: Pheochromocytoma—Recognition and management. Curr Probl Cardiol 4:1, 1979
Remine WH, Chong GC, Van Heerden JA et al: Current management of pheochromocytoma. Ann Surg 179:740, 1974
Scott HW, Oates JA, Nies AS et al: Pheochromocytoma: Present diagnosis and management. Ann Surg 181:587, 1976
Stackpole RH, Melicow MM, Uson AC: Pheochromocytoma in children. J Pediatr 63:315, 1963
Van Way CW, Scott HW, Page DL, Rhamy RK: Pheochromocytoma. Curr Probl Surg 1:59, June 1974

42
Complications of Endocrine Pancreas Surgery

H. H. Newsome, Jr.

Metabolic and Pharmacologic Aspects

GASTRINOMAS (ZOLLINGER–ELLISON SYNDROME)

Preoperative Considerations

OVERVIEW. Gastrin is produced not only in the gastric antrum but in nonbeta cells of the pancreatic islets and in cells scattered throughout the duodenum and early small bowel.[27, 42] Neoplasms of the pancreatic islet cells and of the intestinal cells (10%) are the cause of the hypergastrinemia in the Zollinger–Ellison syndrome. The acid-secreting cells of the stomach are stimulated by gastrin to produce excessive hydrochloric acid. The syndrome becomes manifest clinically when the continued hypersecretion of gastric acid produces an ulcer diathesis. The resulting ulceration can be particularly virulent with combined gastric, duodenal, or jejunal ulcers seen. Bleeding, perforations, or obstructions are complications seen in this syndrome at a higher frequency than in ordinary cases of ulcer disease. Approximately one third of the cases of Zollinger–Ellison syndrome will be associated with diarrhea. The diarrhea is a result of the stimulation of intestinal motility by the high-volume acid output of the stomach and a consequent flooding of the distal small bowel and colon with more liquid than can be absorbed. Chronic dehydration may further complicate the undernourished state of these patients, who experience chronic abdominal pain, vomiting, or both.

DIAGNOSIS. The basic diagnostic considerations are listed below.[10, 33]

Peptic Ulcer Disease
Recurrent, multiple ulcers, jejunal ulcers, large gastric folds, widened duodenum

Gastric Secretion
Volume greater than 100 ml/hour or 3 L/day
Basal acid: > 15 mEq/hour and > 60% of maximum

Hypergastrinemia
Fasting basal: > 200 pg/ml; when basal < 500 pg/ml, stimulate with calcium or secretin

The patient initially presents with a problem in management of ordinary peptic ulceration. Diarrhea usually seems secondary in importance to the ulcer symptoms. Findings on endoscopy and the upper GI series usually performed on these patients are not necessarily specific for the Zollinger–Ellison syndrome. In contrast, an ulcer seen beyond the ligament of Treitz in approximately 20% of the patients is virtually pathognomonic of the disease. Large gastric folds, a widened duodenum, and excessive intraluminal fluid should also raise suspicions.

Prior to availability of a radioimmunoassay for serum gastrin, gastric analyses yielded the most specific information. Gastric outputs of greater than 100 ml per hour or more than 3 L per 24 hours, produced by an unobstructed stomach, are suggestive of the syndrome. The basal acid output usually is greater than 15 mEq per hour and more than at least 60% of the maximum acid output under histamine stimulation. Since the advent of the gastrin assay, serum gastrin should be measured in paired fasting samples.[36] In most laboratories, the upper limit of normal is 200 pg per ml. In borderline cases (less than 500 pg/ml), gastrin can be stimulated by calcium infusion (15 mg/kg of body weight over several hours, with multiple samplings during that period) or by secretin (1–3 units/kg of body weight for 1 hour).[16] The differential diagnosis for basal hypergastrinemia must include an antrum retained after a previous gastrectomy as well as the presence of antral G-cell hyperplasia. In these conditions, secretin does not produce a rise in serum gastrin; in fact, in the presence of retained antrum, secretin infusion may decrease the serum gastrin levels. Other entities producing a high serum gastrin, such as renal failure, pernicious anemia, and atrophic gastritis are not ordinarily associated with hypersecretion of gastric acid. The finding of hypercalcemia in some patients is significant because of the possibility of hyperparathyroidism due either to a coincidental parathyroid tumor or to the patient's belonging to a family with multiple endocrine adenomatosis, as is mentioned below.[2]

PREPARATION FOR SURGERY. Many patients with this syndrome are inadequately nourished and may have problems with electrolyte and fluid balance. Although the diarrhea can usually be controlled by nasogastric suction, the consequent nutritional and fluid problems remain. Poor intake caused by the severe ulcer symptoms accentuates the protein–calorie malnutrition from the intestinal loss of nutrients. The use of the H_2 receptor antagonist, cimetidine, has considerably improved the preoperative metabolic condition of patients.[3, 20, 25, 29] This drug effectively blocks gastrin stimulation of the acid-producing cells, diminishes the diarrhea, and allows the ulceration to heal. Although the medication is only palliative, without arresting growth of the islet-cell tumor or its metastases, use of cimetidine is well worth the few weeks required preoperatively to restore the patient to a normal state of nutrition and fluid and electrolyte balance. It is important to increase the cimetidine dose as much as two to three times above that recommended for ordinary ulcer disease in order to achieve effective diminution in gastric hypersecretion. In addition to protein–caloric rehabilitation prior to surgery, adequate replenishment of calcium, magnesium, zinc, and potassium should be assured.

Intraoperative Considerations

There are no specific pharmacologic considerations during the procedure itself. The same attention should be given to details of metabolic management as for ordinary peptic ulcer surgery. Because of the possibility of lingering, covert electrolyte abnormalities, the electrocardiographic leads should be placed to generate standard, easily interpreted EKG complexes. Because a total gastrectomy may have to be performed, intravenous lines should be ample and blood and blood products available.

Postoperative Considerations

Especially in patients who undergo total gastrectomy with an esophagojejunostomy, continued nutritional support should be provided in the postoperative period. Where intravenous hyperalimentation is not possible, consideration should be given to placing a feeding tube directly into the jejunum at the time of surgery.

INSULINOMA

Preoperative Considerations

OVERVIEW. Insulin is produced by the beta cells of the pancreatic islet. Approximately 90% of adult patients with hyperinsulinism will have a solitary neoplasm of the beta islet cells. Roughly 5% to 10% of these are islet-cell carcinomas. The other beta-cell lesion appearing in adults is diffuse adenomatosis, which can usually be seen on gross inspection and, most certainly, microscopically. The most common lesion in the infant and child is nesidioblastosis. It may rarely be seen in the adult.[12] The beta cells are arranged in ribbons or sheets throughout the pancreas, rather than in discrete islets. The other islet lesion seen in children is hyperplasia in which every islet is affected. In each of these lesions, hyperinsulinism produces the clinical syndrome. Insulin promotes glycogenesis in the liver and glucose uptake and utilization by almost all cells in the body.[4] A profound hypoglycemia is thus produced by hyperinsulinism. The symptoms of confusion, mental obtundation, and even coma are due to glucose deprivation in the brain. Other symptoms, such as pallor, sweating, and nausea, are likely due to the increased sympathoadrenal activity seen as a consequence of the hypoglycemia. The initial differential diagnosis must include both the causes of mental confusion and coma and the conditions that produce sympathoadrenal hyperactivity. Once hypoglycemia has been documented as a cause of the symptoms, the differential diagnosis then becomes a problem of ruling out the many causes of hypoglycemia:[22, 23]

Hyperinsulinism
Pancreatic islet adenoma, adenomatosis, carcinoma, hyperplasia, and nesidioblastosis
Iatrogenic or factitious (insulin and oral agents)
Relative, anterior pituitary or adrenocortical hypofunctioning, glucagon deficiency

Decreased Glycogen Stores
Acquired liver disease
Alcoholism and food deprivation
Hepatic enzyme defects such as the glycogen storage diseases, galactosemia, or aglycogenesis

Miscellaneous and Idiopathic
Reactive functional hypoglycemia
Nonpancreatic tumors with hypoglycemia
Low-birth-weight newborn
Infant of diabetic mother
Ketogenic hypoglycemia, leucine-sensitive and leucine-insensitive hypoglycemia

DIAGNOSIS. The first positive step in the diagnosis of endogenous hyperinsulinism is the demonstration of an elevated serum insulin concentration in the face of a low blood sugar.[9, 14, 31] The patient fasts under observation, and at 12 to 24 hours or when symptoms supervene, serum samples for glucose and insulin are obtained. Ordinarily, serum insulin is quite low when blood sugar levels are low, with the normal insulin:glucose ratio being below 0.20. However, in the patient with autonomous hyperinsulinism, the lowering of blood sugar levels does not suppress serum insulin concentrations. Patients with endogenous hyperinsulinemia will almost always have a fasting insulin:glucose ratio of 0.30 or greater. Pharmacologic tests that stimulate insulin release have been employed to assist in the diagnosis. These tests are usually no more accurate than is the fasting insulin:glucose ratios. In borderline or unclear cases, however, the tolbutamide test may be used. The amino acid, leucine, can also be used to stimulate insulin. Both the decrease in blood glucose concentrations and the rise in immunoreactive insulin following tolbutamide or leucine stimulation can be used as test indices. One of the most difficult situations in which to evaluate hypoglycemia is that produced by surreptitious exogenous administration of insulin. A helpful maneuver is the measurement of the C-peptide fragment, which is cleaved from pro-insulin to form insulin and can distinguish the insulin derived from endogenous pro-insulin from that derived from exogenous administration of insulin.[13, 30] Also, the percentage of circulating insulin as pro-insulin is higher with insulinoma than with other causes. The list below summarizes these diagnostic features.

- Hypoglycemia demonstrated during symptoms
- Symptoms relieved by glucose administration
- Fasting insulin:glucose ratio above 0.30
- Positive tolbutamide or leucine test
- Presence of C-peptide in serum
- $>$ 20% circulating insulin as pro-insulin

PREPARATION FOR SURGERY. The main risk to the preoperative patient is hypoglycemia. Dietary management should aim to minimize the frequency of hypoglycemic attacks. Small, frequent meals and late-evening snacks that shorten the overnight fast are efficacious. Diazoxide in doses between 500 mg to 800 mg per day is effective in inhibiting insulin release in most patients. Diazoxide acts both indirectly by stimulating epinephrine release, which promotes glycogenolysis, and directly through an inhibitory action on the beta cells of the pancreas.

Localization procedures commonly available prior to surgery are arteriogram, CT scan, and sonography.[7, 15, 35, 37] Although the success rate with angiography has been reported as high as 60%, this has not uniformly been the experience in most series. The CT scan and sonogram are particularly useful when the lesion is greater than 2 cm or located on the surface of the gland, but these conditions also render tumor location upon abdominal exploration easy. An experienced surgeon can probably locate an insulinoma better himself than can preoperative tests, including transhepatic portal vein sampling for insulin.[5] In the presence of sound laboratory proof of an insulinoma, failure to detect the tumor preoperatively by localization procedures should not deter surgery.

Intraoperative Considerations

The most worrisome intraoperative complication is hypoglycemia. Fortunately, because of the effects of the counter-regulatory hormones (catecholamines, glucagon, growth hormones), blood glucose tends to rise during any surgical procedure, and hypoglycemia from insulinoma is not as frequent a problem during surgery as it is during the basal state. Some attention has been given the fact that ordinarily when insulin secretion is suddenly interrupted, blood glucose concentrations rise. Such a rise is not specific because the counter-regulatory mechanisms during surgery may make the blood glucose rise anyway. Unfortunately, the tendency toward a rising glucose level compromises the usefulness of monitoring blood glucose to indicate successful insulinoma removal and may lead to a false assurance that hyperinsulinism has been cured when, in fact, residual tumor or hyperplasia remains.[38] However, if the blood glucose remains low after removal of what is thought to be a solitary adenoma or after a blind distal pancreatectomy, the chances are good that hyperinsulinism will persist unless other hyperplasia or neoplasia is removed.

Postoperative Considerations

In the patient having undergone successful removal of an insulinoma, the recovery is remarkable. The effects of hypoglycemia are no longer present, and the patient soon returns to a normal existence. In patients with persistent postoperative hypoglycemia, causes such as nonresectable diffuse islet-cell disease, nonresectable residual malignancy, or unappreciated multiple islet disease can usually be surmised from the findings at operation. Should these possibilities not exist, a consideration must then be given to the noninsulin causes of hypoglycemia listed previously, and a repeat diagnostic workup must then be done. When a residual tumor mistakenly left behind could have been easily resected, reoperation is clearly indicated. Still, some patients, such as those with nonresectable metastatic disease, high-risk medical diseases, and tumors requiring pancreatoduodenectomy, may best be managed nonsurgically. Mention has already been made of diet and diazoxide in controlling hypoglycemia. Long-term diazoxide therapy is successful in most instances in controlling hypoglycemia, but it may be associated with several side-effects, such as gastrointestinal upset, edema, agranulocytosis, and hypertrichosis. Cortisone acetate, up to 200 mg per day, can be used to potentiate the effect of diazoxide. Diphenylhydantoin may raise blood glucose in some patients. Somatostatin is an endogenous peptide that suppresses the release of several other peptide hormones. It has been reported to suppress insulin from these tumors, but its action is short lived, which necessitates frequent administration. Finally, streptozotocin has been used to inhibit insulin secretion from islet-cell carcinoma. The drug is toxic to the liver and kidneys and should be used only in palliation of islet-cell carcinoma.

Wermer's Syndrome

The familial occurrence of pancreatic islet-cell tumors, pituitary adenomas, and primary hyperparathyroidism was described by Wermer in 1954.[44] The islet-cell tumors are apparently transmitted as an autosomal dominant trait and are evenly distributed as either insulinomas or gastrinomas. The clinical presentation in familial cases is identical to that seen with sporadic cases. Obviously a satisfactory family history for the known presence of these tumors or their symptoms should be obtained.

GLUCAGONOMA

Preoperative Considerations

OVERVIEW. Glucagon originates in the alpha cells of the pancreatic islets.[32, 40] Although the anti-insulin nature of glucagon's effects are well documented, many of the features of the glucagonoma syndrome cannot be explained solely on the basis of such of glucagon's known actions as stimulation of gluconeogenesis.[18] Most glucagonomas produce a cutaneous lesion (migratory necrolytic erythema), glossitis, anemia, hypoaminoacidemia, weight loss, diabetes mellitus, severe depression, and venous thrombosis.[21, 24, 34]

Patients with the cutaneous syndrome are usually first seen by dermatologists who, noting the characteristic skin lesions and the elevated blood glucose, should consider glucagonoma as a diagnostic possibility. Patients with glucagonomas who do not have the cutaneous syndrome are difficult to distinguish from the many patients with the diabetes mellitus of insulin deficiency.

DIAGNOSIS. The demonstration of markedly elevated plasma glucagon concentrations is sufficient to clinch the diagnosis. However, since the syndrome is so rare, this diagnosis is seldom entertained in patients with these clinical characteristics. The characteristic rash is an important clinical clue. It usually appears first as a raised, reddened patch in the perioral area and on the feet. The patches spread and leave an older central portion that may be healed. Before healing, the central areas are quite susceptible to loss of epidermis, and raw, exposed areas may appear. The overall appearance of the rash is a geographic outline of reddened, active edges with either denuded or healed central portions. A complication from the skin lesions may arise in that secondary infection may occur in the raw, central areas. Some typical laboratory findings are an elevated blood glucose, low hemoglobin and hematocrit, and low plasma amino acid levels.

PREPARATION FOR SURGERY. At the moment, diphenylhydantoin appears to be the only medication that may suppress glucagon secretion from these tumors. The mild inhibition of glucagon secretion by this drug is not enough to reverse the syndrome, and the patient cannot be metabolically stabilized effectively prior to surgery. Efficacy of treatment for the necrolytic migratory rash has been difficult to evaluate because of the spontaneous fluctuation in the severity of the lesions. Topical antiseptic and antifungal agents, as well as systemic antibiotics and steroids, have all been used with varying results.

Localization of the tumors can be done either by CT scan or by arteriography. Since most of the tumors are large, the CT scan can detect the majority of them. The tumors have a characteristic "blush" on arteriography and are usually readily detectable by this means also. Over half of the tumors are malignant, and liver metastases may be demonstrated by arteriography.

Intraoperative Considerations

There are usually no significant metabolic aberrations noted during the surgery. Although the plasma glucose level tends to be elevated during surgery, it has no reported complications.

Postoperative Considerations

Since many of these tumors cannot be completely resected, the same preoperative problems of anemia, hypoglycemia, and cutaneous lesions will be present postoperatively. Even when malignancies are resected, careful follow-up with monitoring of the plasma glucagon concentrations is required.

SOMATOSTATINOMA

Preoperative Considerations

OVERVIEW. Somatostatinoma is an extremely rare tumor of the delta cells of the pancreatic islets, which secretes somatostatin.[1, 11, 17, 39] Somatostatin is a peptide hormone that suppresses the release of both insulin and glucagon.[8] The net effect on the patient, however, is a tendency toward hyperglycemia. The weight loss, anemia, and diarrhea reported in some of the cases currently cannot be explained on the basis of the known actions of somatostatin, and it is likely that other humoral substances are involved.

DIAGNOSIS. Demonstration of suppression of both insulin and glucagon in a patient with diabetes mellitus should raise suspicion of this diagnosis. Unfortunately, only a few laboratories are capable of measuring somatostatin, but demonstration of an elevated concentration of this hormone in the plasma is the definitive method for diagnosis.

PREPARATION FOR SURGERY. There are no special pharmacologic or metabolic preparations for this type of tumor. The tumor can be located preoperatively with arteriography.

Intraoperative Considerations

As with glucagonomas, these tumors may be malignant with metastases to liver. Depending upon the tumor burden and degree of hypersecretion of somatostatin, insulin replacement may be required for hypoinsulinemia and consequent glucose intolerance.

Postoperative Considerations

No special metabolic situations have been reported postoperatively.

WATERY DIARRHEA, HYPOKALEMIA, AND ACIDOSIS (WDHA OR VERNER–MORRISON SYNDROME)

Preoperative Considerations

OVERVIEW. Neither the exact islet-cell of origin of the tumors, nor the causative agents of the WDHA syndrome have yet been definitely established.[41] The tumors clearly belong to the group of hormone-producing neoplasms arising from the cells that originate in the neural crest.[26] These cells, which have the ability to process amino acids and produce hormones, have been designated as amine processing uptake and decarboxylation (APUD), and tumors that arise from this group of cells are sometimes known as APUDomas. Approximately 10% of tumors producing the WDHA syndrome are found in the adrenal glands, retroperitoneal area, or lungs. Of the other 90% arising in the pancreatic islets, over half are carcinoma. Several substances, such as serotonin, prostaglandin E_2, pancreatic peptide, and vasoinhibitory peptide have all been incriminated as agents producing a hyposecretion of gastric acid and hypersecretion from the intestinal glands. About a third of these patients will demonstrate achlorhydria in spite of histamine administration. Marked hypersecretion by the small intestine appears to be the basis of the diarrhea. Huge quantities of fluid, potassium, and bicarbonate enter the colon. Colonic function is essentially normal, but the sheer volume of fluid and electrolytes exceeds the absorptive capacity of the large bowel. The large volume of fluid produces the watery diarrhea, and the loss of bicarbonate results in acidosis. The contracted fluid compartment stimulates aldosterone secretion, which augments the potassium loss, both through the colon and the kidney, to produce hypokalemia.

DIAGNOSIS. Without availability of measurements of the several agents mentioned above, the diagnosis rests on exclusion of other causes of marked diarrhea. The diarrhea seen in this syndrome is quite characteristic in that it resembles weak tea. There is no mucous as frequently seen in the diarrhea from a villus adenoma, for example. There is absence of hypermotility seen in diarrhea associated with the Zollinger–Ellison syndrome or medullary carcinoma of the thyroid. There is no steatorrhea such as usually accompanies the intestinal malabsorption syndromes. Since many of these tumors are fairly large, pancreatic scan, sonogram, or arteriography may be useful in diagnosis. Attention should also be given to such areas as the adrenals, retroperitoneum, and lungs.

PREPARATION FOR SURGERY. There are characteristic electrolyte imbalances of a marked degree in these patients. Approximately 10% of patients die from fluid and electrolyte imbalance prior to surgery. Potassium loss is perhaps the most critical of the features, and more than 100 mEq of replacement per day may be required simply to replace daily losses. Hypomagnesemia may be serious and can produce tetany, which is worsened by potassium administration. Fortunately, the administration of prednisone, 30 mg to 60 mg per day, partially inhibits the secretory activity of these tumors in many patients. With successful prednisone therapy, the replenishment of the electrolytes and correction of the acidosis can be achieved more readily. The response of indomethacin presumably reflects the role of prostaglandin E_2 in the clinical presentation of some patients.

Intraoperative Considerations

Once the fluid and electrolyte problems have been corrected, there are no special metabolic or pharmacologic considerations during surgery. If the patient has been placed on preoperative prednisone, attention should be given to the increased need for steroids during the surgery.

Postoperative Considerations

When tumors cannot be resected or even found, streptozotocin may be added to the steroid-indomethacin regimen.

Operative Aspects

GASTRINOMA (ZOLLINGER–ELLISON SYNDROME)

Throughout the past two decades, the standard surgical approach for gastrinoma had been total gastrectomy. Morbidity and mortality rates for any other surgical approach were significantly higher than those for total gastrectomy.[45] Because the tumors are frequently multiple or malignant with metastases, the gastrin source may not always be totally eradicated. Continued excessive production of gastrin following inadequate tumor resection will stimulate any acid-producing tissue left in the stomach, and ulcer recurrence is inevitable. The preoperative complications of bleeding, perforation, diarrhea, and obstruction from the ulcerations continue. Therefore, total removal of the stomach assured that no gastrin-responsive gastric tissue remained. Total gastrectomy represented the only means to prevent acid secretion in the face of continuing hypergastrinemia.

Prior to the introduction of cimetidine, the H_2 receptor antagonist, it was obvious that the penalty for incomplete removal of the gastrin-producing neoplasms was a recurrence of the ulcer diathesis. Currently, the postoperative availability of cimetidine has allowed some margin for error in the attempt to select patients with pancreatic lesions amenable to resection. Although perhaps only 20% of the tumors are confined to the distal half of the pancreas, unless the pancreatic tumors are obviously outside of the limits of pancreatic resection, it may well be worth attempting removal of an apparent single, distal pancreatic lesion and testing the patient postoperatively for persistent hypergastrinemia, rather than initially performing a total gastrectomy.[6, 19] In the absence of postoperative continued ulcer disease, the morbidity and mortality rates for distal pancreatic resection are, of course, much lower than those for total gastrectomy. The addition of a parietal cell vagotomy may lower the sensitivity to gastrin of the acid-producing cells.[28] Should the serum gastrin still be elevated postoperatively, cimetidine treatment can be continued. The patient and surgeon should be forewarned that a total gastrectomy may become necessary. The therapeutic possibilities are depicted in Figure 42-1. The complications of total gastrectomy are covered in Chapter 31, but unless the patient with a gastrinoma is nutritionally repleted prior to surgery, the complication rate of wound breakdown, anastomotic leak, peritoneal sepsis, and so on is increased above that associated with gastric resection for nongastrinoma lesions.

INSULINOMAS

Approximately 80% of insulinomas are single and easily palpable and can be enucleated. In obvious multiple adenomatosis, there is some debate whether a total pancreaticoduodenectomy is justified when a 90% to 95% distal pancreatectomy can be done with lowered morbidity and mortality rates than accompanying the addition of duodenectomy. The effective use of diazoxide in patients has some-

FIG. 42-1. Possible therapeutic pathways for the Zollinger–Ellison syndrome.

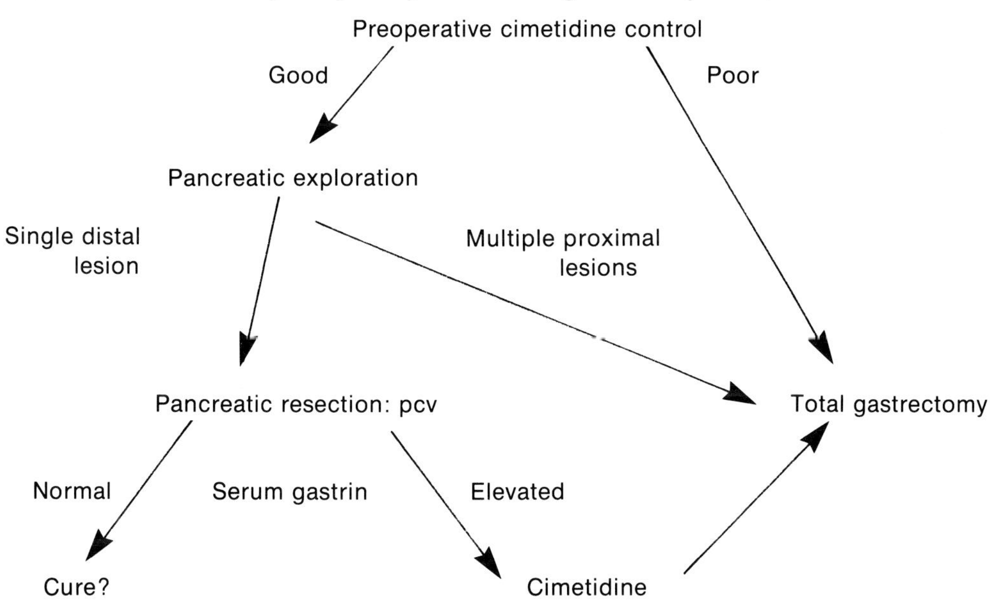

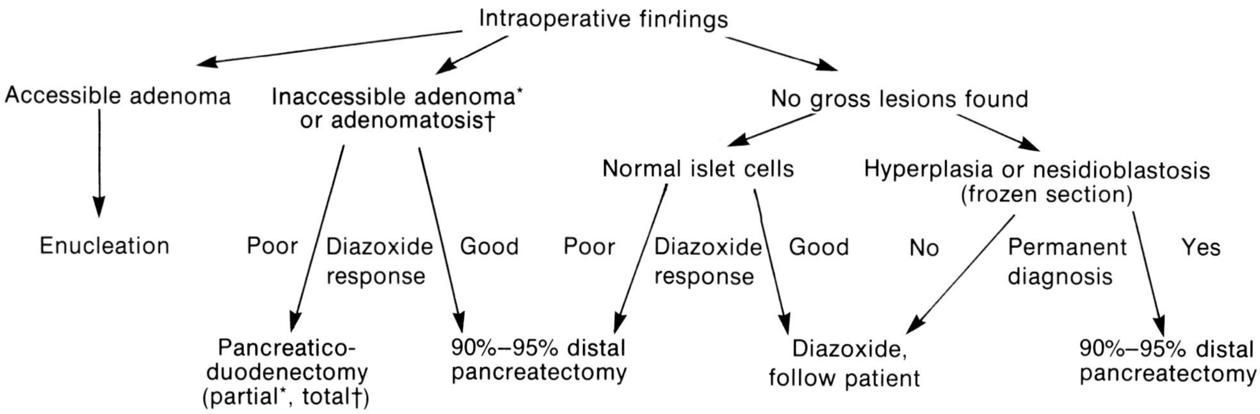

FIG. 42-2. Possible therapeutic pathways for B-cell hyperinsulinemia.

what swung the argument in favor of the less radical approach.[43] Failure to find the insulinoma is a difficult situation for the surgeon. One of the key steps in such an impasse is to perform a distal pancreatectomy with careful sectioning of the gland and checking the microscopic appearance of the islets by frozen section. If no islet-cell hyperplasia or microscopic adenomatosis is present, the surgeon can then choose whether to continue with blind pancreatic resection or to stop, place the patient postoperatively on long-term diazoxide therapy, and, at a later date, examine the patient again when the lesion becomes larger and more readily detected. The preoperative response to diazoxide is information invaluable to such a choice. Confirmation of islet-cell hyperplasia or nesidioblastosis by permanent pathology sections should delay embarking upon more radical pancreatic resection. A 95% pancreatectomy is probably the treatment of choice for these two entities in children. Figure 42-2 summarizes the diagnostic and therapeutic possibilities.

WDHA SYNDROME

As is true for the gastrinoma and the insulinoma, the islet-cell tumor producing WDHA syndrome may be located in ectopic positions. However, in contrast to the other ectopic tumors that are characteristically located somewhere within the duodenum, small intestine, or its mesentery, the WDHA tumor may also be found in the adrenal glands, retroperitoneal area, or lungs. Since these tumors are significantly larger than the average gastrinoma or insulinoma, locating the tumor within the pancreas is usually not a problem. The large carcinomas have usually invaded surrounding structures or metastasized to local lymph nodes or to the liver. Because of the virulence of this syndrome and of the mortality and morbidity from fluid and electrolyte imbalances, an attempt at resection should be made regardless of the tumor location. Even the debulking of carcinomas, limited by the risks of operative mortality, is recommended.

GLUCAGONOMA AND SOMATOSTATINOMA

Unfortunately, only a few of the patients reported with glucagonomas had tumors that could be resected. The majority of the tumors are malignant with a high incidence of metastases. If a single, resectable lesion is found, the results can be quite dramatic and prompt. If the primary malignancy can easily be resected, this should be done even for palliation, provided only a small tumor burden is left behind.

In the few reported cases of somatostatinomas, the lesions appeared to be resectable. This is especially the case when they are located in the tail of the pancreas.

References

1. Axelrod L, Bush MA, Hirsch HJ, Loo SWH: Malignant somatostatinoma: Clinical features and metabolic studies. J Clin Endocrinol Metab 52:886, 1981
2. Betts JB, O'Malley BP, Rosenthal FD: Hyperparathyroidism: A prerequisite for Zollinger–Ellison syndrome in multiple endocrine adenomatosis type I—Report of a further family and a review of the literature. Q J Med 49:69, 1980
3. Bonfils S, Mignon M, Gratton J: Cimetidine treatment of acute and chronic Zollinger–Ellison syndrome. World J Surg 3:597, 1979
4. Cahill GF: Physiology of insulin in man. Diabetes 20:785, 1971
5. Daggett PR, Kurtz AB, Morris DV et al: Is preoperative localization of insulinomas necessary? Lancet 1:483, 1981
6. Deveney CW, Deveney KS, Way LW: The Zollinger–Ellison syndrome—23 years later. Ann Surg 188:384, 1978

7. Dunnick NR, Long JA, Krudy A et al: Localizing insulin omas with combined radiographic methods. AJR 135: 747, 1980
8. Efendic S, Hokfelt T, Luft R: Somatostatin. Adv Metab Disord 9:367, 1978
9. Fajans SS, Floyd JC: Fasting hypoglycemia in adults. N Engl J Med 294:766, 1976
10. Friesen S: The Zollinger–Ellison syndrome. Curr Probl Surg, April 1972, pp 1–52
11. Ganda OP, Weir GC, Soeldner JS et al: Somatostatinoma: A somatostatin-containing tumor of the endocrine pancreas. N Engl J Med 296:963, 1977
12. Harness JK, Geelhoed GW, Thompson NW et al: Nesidioblastosis in adults. Arch Surg 116:575, 1981
13. Horwitz DL, Kuzuya H, Rubenstein AH: Circulating serum C-peptide: A brief review of diagnostic implications. N Engl J Med 295:207, 1976
14. Johansen K: Insulinoma: Clinical manifestations, diagnosis and treatment. The significance of the prolonged fasting test and of the fasting blood glucose-insulin relationship. J Endocrinol Invest 2:285, 1979
15. Kallio H, Suoranta H: Localization of occult insulin secreting tumors of the pancreas. Ann Surg 189:49, 1979
16. Kolts BE, Herbst CA, McGuigan JE: Calcium and secreting-stimulated gastrin release in the Zollinger–Ellison syndrome. Ann Intern Med 81:758, 1974
17. Krejs GJ et al: Somatostatinoma syndrome: Biochemical, morphologic and clinical features. N Engl J Med 301:285, 1979
18. Leichter SB: Clinical and metabolic aspects of glucagonoma. Medicine 59:100, 1980
19. McCarthy DM: The place of surgery in the Zollinger–Ellison syndrome. N Engl J Med 302:1344, 1980
20. McCarthy DM: Report on the United States experience with cimetidine in Zollinger–Ellison syndrome and other hypersecretory states. Gastroenterology 74:453, 1978
21. Mallinson CN, Bloom SR, Warin AP et al: A glucogonoma syndrome. Lancet 1:1, 1974
22. Marks V: Hypoglycaemia. 2. Other causes. Clin Endocrinol Metab 5:769, 1976
23. Merimee TJ: Spontaneous hypoglycemia in man. Adv Intern Med 22:301, 1977
24. Norton JA, Kahn CR, Schiebinger R et al: Amino acid deficiency and the skin rash associated with glucagonoma. Ann Intern Med 91:213, 1979
25. Orchard JJ: Cimetidine therapy in Zollinger–Ellison syndrome. JAMA 237:2221, 1977
26. Pearse AGE: The APUD concept: Embryology, cytochemistry and ultrastructure of the diffuse neuroendocrine system. In Friesen SR (ed): Surgical Endocrinology: Clinical Syndrome. Philadelphia, JB Lippincott, 1978
27. Rayford PL et al: Gastrin. Surg Gynceol Obstet 145:257, 1977
28. Richardson CT, Feldman M, McClelland RN et al: Effect of vagotomy in Zollinger–Ellison syndrome. Gastroenterology 77:682, 1979
29. Richardson CT, Walsh JH: The value of a histamine H_2-receptor antagonist in the management of patients with the Zollinger–Ellison syndrome. N Engl J Med 294:133, 1976
30. Scarlett JA, Mako ME, Rubenstein AH et al: Factitious hypoglycemia: Diagnosis by measurement of serum C-peptide immunoreactivity and insulin-binding antibodies. N Engl J Med 297:1029, 1977
31. Seyer–Hansen K, Lundbaek K: The clinical diagnosis of insulinoma. Scand J Gastroenterol 53:39, 1979
32. Sperling MA: Glucagon: Secretion and actions. Adv Exp Med Biol 124:29, 1979
33. Stadil F, Stage JG: The Zollinger–Ellison syndrome. Clin Endocrinol Metab 8:433, 1979
34. Stacpoole PW: The glucagonoma syndrome: Clinical features, diagnosis, and treatment. Endocr Rev 2:347, 1981
35. Stefanini P, Carboni M, Patrassi N et al: The value of arteriography in the diagnosis and treatment of insulinomas. Am J Surg 131:352, 1975
36. Thompson JC, Reeder DD, Bunchman HH: Clinical role of serum gastrin measurements in the Zollinger–Ellison syndrome. Am J Surg 124:251, 1972
37. Turner RC, Morris PJ, Lee ECG, Harris EA: Localisation of insulinomas. Lancet 1:515, 1978
38. Tutt GO, Edis AJ, Service FJ, van Heerden JA: Plasma glucose monitoring during operation for insulinoma: A critical reappraisal. Surgery 88:351, 1980
39. Unger RH: Somatostatinoma. N Engl J Med 296:998, 1977
40. Unger RH, Orci L: Glucagon and the A cell: Physiology and pathophysiology. N Engl J Med 304:1518, 1981
41. Verner JV, Morrison AB: Endocrine pancreatic islet disease with diarrhea. Arch Intern Med 133:492, 1974
42. Walsh JH, Grossman MI: Gastrin. N Engl J Med 292:1324, 1975
43. Wegienka LC, Simpson RG, Karam JH, Forsham PH: Clinical experience with diazoxide. Ann NY Acad Sci 314:383, 1968
44. Wermer P: Genetic aspects of adenomatosis of endocrine glands. Am J Med 16:363, 1954
45. Wilson SD, Ellison EH: Survival in patients with the Zollinger–Ellison syndrome treated by total gastrectomy. Am J Surg 111:787, 1966

Suggested Reading

Bloom SR, Polak JM: Glucagonomas, VIPomas and somatostatinomas. Clin Endocrinol Metab 9:285, 1980

dePeyster FA: Planning the appropriate operations for islet cell tumors of the pancreas. Surg Clin North Am 50:133, 1970

Frerichs H, Creutzfeldt W: Hypoglycaemia. I. Insulin secreting tumours. Clin Endocrinol Metab 5:747, 1976

Friesen SR, Tomita T: Pseudo-Zollinger–Ellison syndrome: Hypergastrinemia, hyperchlorhydria without tumor. Ann Surg 194:481, 1981

Galbut DL, Markowitz AM: Insulinoma: Diagnosis, surgical management and long-term follow-up. Am J Surg 139:682, 1980

Gauderer M, Stanley CA, Baker L, Bishop HC: Pancreatic adenomas in infants and children: Current surgical management. J Pediatr Surg 13:591, 1978

Harrison TS: The hypoglycemic syndrome: Endogenous hyperinsulinism. In Friesen SR (ed): Surgical Endocrinology: Clinical Syndromes. Philadelphia, JB Lippincott, 1978

Holst JJ: Gut endocrine tumour syndromes. Clin Endocrinol Metab 8:413, 1979

Jaffe BM: The diarrheogenic syndrome: Verner–Morrison, WDHA syndrome. In Friesen SR (ed): Surgical Endocrinology: Clinical Syndromes. Philadelphia, JB Lippincott, 1978

Kaplan EL, Lee CH: Recent advances in the diagnosis and treatment of insulinomas. Surg Clin North Am 59:119, 1979

Kavlie H, White TT: Pancreatic islet beta cell tumors and hyperplasia: Experience in 14 Seattle hospitals. Ann Surg 175:326, 1972

Kent RB, van Heerden JA, Weiland LH: Nonfunctioning islet cell tumors. Ann Surg 193:185, 1981

Lewis AE: The blucagonoma syndrome. Int J Dermatol 18:17, 1979

Mallinson C, Bloom SR: The hyperglycemia, cutaneous syndrome: Pancreatic glucagonoma. In Friesen SR (ed): Surgical Endocrinology: Clinical Syndromes. Philadelphia, JB Lippincott, 1978

Modlin IM: Endocrine tumors of the pancreas. Surg Gynecol Obstet 149:751, 1979

Newsome HH: Multiple endocrine adenomatosis. Surg Clin North Am 54:387, 1974

Rich RH, Dehner LP, Okinaga K et al: Surgical management of islet-cell adenoma in infancy. Surgery 84:519, 1978

Scholtz DA, ReMind WH, Priestly JT: Hyperinsulinism: Review of 95 cases of functioning pancreatic islet cell tumors. Proc Mayo Clin 35:19, 1960

Service FJ, Dale AJD, Elveback LR, Jiang N–S: Insulinoma: Clinical and diagnostic features of 60 consecutive cases. Mayo Clin Proc 51:417, 1976

Shatney CH, Grage TB: Diagnostic and surgical aspects of insulinoma: A review of twenty-seven cases. Am J Surg 127:174, 1974

Stefanini S, Carboni M, Patrassi N: Beta-islet cell tumors of the pancreas: Results of a study on 1,067 cases. Surgery 25:597, 1974

Suffecool SL: Anesthetic management for insulinoma resection. In Brown BR (ed): Anesthesia and the Patient with Endocrine Disease. Philadelphia, FA Davis, 1980

Wilson SD: Wermer's syndrome: Multiple endocrine adenopathy, type I. In Friesen SR (ed): Surgical Endocrinology: Clinical Syndromes. Philadelphia, JB Lippincott, 1978

Zollinger RM: Islet cell tumors of the pancreas and the alimentary tract. Am J Surg 129:102, 1975

Zollinger RM: The ulcerogenic (Zollinger–Ellison) syndrome. In Friesen SR (ed): Surgical Endocrinology: Clinical Syndromes. Philadelphia, JB Lippincott, 1978

43 Complications of Thyroid Surgery

H. H. Newsome, Jr.

Metabolic and Pharmacologic Aspects

HYPERTHYROIDISM

Hyperthyroidism is caused by a number of pathologic entities and has several therapeutic approaches.[42] The solitary toxic nodule is usually treated with radioactive iodine. The toxic multinodular goiter, unusual in the United States, can be treated with radioactive iodine, but surgery is preferred. Surgery for hyperthyroidism in this country is most commonly used for Graves' disease or diffuse enlargement of the thyroid gland. Standard initial therapy for these patients is usually antithyroid medications. Radioactive iodine and surgery are competing therapeutic modalities for patients with recurrence of disease after medical therapy. Since surgery is virtually restricted to Graves' disease, the following discussion dwells on the metabolic and pharmacologic aspects of the hyperthyroidism from diffuse thyroid hyperplasia.

Preoperative Considerations

OVERVIEW. Hyperthyroidism due to diffuse enlargement of the thyroid gland may be properly considered an autoimmune disease.[5] Ciculating immunoglobulins directed against a thyroid antigen have been demonstrated in the sera of almost all patients with Graves' disease. Several of these immunoglobulins are capable of stimulating thyroidal tissue to produce thyroxine (T_4) and triiodothyronine (T_3). Although T_4 is the major secretory product of the thyroid gland, T_3 is also produced by the thyroid gland.[17, 37] The primary sites of T_3 production are peripheral tissues through the conversion of T_4.[37] Thyroxine is also converted into reverse T_3 (rT_3), which is biologically inactive. The conversion of T_4 into active or inactive forms of T_3 can be modulated to serve as a further mechanism for control of peripheral thyroid hormonal effects on target tissues.[6] The multiple interactions of these hormones with the cell, such as binding with nuclear chromatin for anabolic effects or with the inner mitochondral membranes for activation of energy metabolism, and through the substitution for tyrosine in a variety of contexts, account for the myriad of biologic effects and clinical findings of Graves' disease.[30, 39]

Effects of the thyroid hormones may be differentiated on a temporal basis. An increase in oxygen consumption is an early biologic effect following thyroid hormone administration, but phenomena such as the increased heart rate and the increased sensitivity of lipolysis to epinephrine precede even the increase in oxygen consumption. Calorigenesis accompanies the increased oxygen consumption. Physiologic amounts of thyroid hormone potentiate both the glycogenolytic effect of epinephrine and the glycogen synthetic effect of insulin. With excessive amounts of thyroxine, there is a marked increase in the vitamin requirements. Some physiologic effects of T_3 and T_4 have an interesting biphasic dose dependency to the extent that physiologic effects may be reversed in thyrotoxic patients with a rise in circulating hormonal concentrations. The thyroid hormones have a biphasic effect on protein synthesis and somatic growth; normal concentrations promote protein synthesis and growth, whereas increased concentrations inhibit these activities. The same is seen in fat metabolism in that lipogenesis is stimulated at low levels of thyroxine concentrations, whereas lipolysis is promoted by superabundant concentrations. These effects are seen clinically in thyrotoxic patients as muscle weakness, growth retardation, and lowered body fat stores.

DIAGNOSIS. The clinical characteristics of thyrotoxicosis relate to three areas: the hormonal effects, the thyroid gland itself, and the eye signs. The hormonal features are similar to those produced by a pheochromocytoma; these features reflect, in part, the increased sensitivity of the patient to endogenous catecholamines. The features include sweating, heat intolerance, irritability, nervousness, increased appetite but persistent weight loss, fine tremor, tachycardia, arrhythmias, and cardiac failure. The thyroid gland is diffusely and usually symmetrically enlarged. A thyroid bruit is a useful diagnostic finding. In about half the patients, the eye signs seen most often are exophthalmos, lid retraction, widened palpebral fissure, and lid lag.

The diagnosis of hyperthyroidism is established through laboratory testing.[47] Total T_3 and T_4 are elevated in the serum. The T_3 resin uptake is increased. An elevated free thyroxine index, which is obtained by multiplying the total T_4 times the T_3 resin uptake, is probably the most reliable diagnostic laboratory finding. An exception to the accuracy of the free thyroxine index is the unusual situation in which only the T_3 is increased. Except in the rare pituitary cause, thyroid-stimulating hormone (TSH) is characteristically low in hyperthyroidism because of feedback suppression by T_4. Serum TSH does not respond with a normal rise following administration of thyrotropin-releasing hormone (TRH). The percentage uptake by the thyroid gland of radioactive iodine (RAI) is characteristically increased, although the enrichment of the diet in the United States by iodine sometimes results in a false lowering of the RAI uptake. In the hyperthyroid phase of silent thyroiditis, the RAI uptake is usually less than 5%. Radioiodine scan will show diffuse uptake in Graves' disease and unifocal uptake with a toxic nodule and faint, patchy uptake in thyroiditis.

PREPARATION FOR SURGERY. The increased vascularity of the thyroid gland in Graves' disease and the threat of perioperative thyroid storm have directed attention to adequate preoperative preparation. Plummer's introduction of iodine administration significantly lowered the surgical mortality rates from this disease.[32] Since the temporary suppressive effect of iodine administration may be followed by an accentuation of hyperthyroidism, the antithyroid drugs, such as the thionamides, were a welcome addition to the armamentarium.[2] A beta-adrenergic antagonist, propranolol, was subsequently introduced to ameliorate the peripheral effects of the thyroid hormone.[46] Most recent, reports of the combined use of potassium iodide and propranolol have documented both control of the effects of the thyroid hormones and a decrease in hormonal secretion.[10] Because of variable drug concentrations achieved in the blood of different patients on a fixed dose, oral dosage of propranolol should be adjusted in order to achieve a resting pulse rate of 60 to 80 beats per minute.[35] Apparently, hypervascularity of the thyroid gland under this regimen is also controlled. Thus, a decrease in the size of the gland and a disappearance of the cervical bruit are reassuring preoperative findings. Although the shortest time required for effective preoperative pharmacologic preparation has not been determined, 10 to 14 days is considered adequate for the standard regimen. Use of propranolol alone may allow a shortening of preparation time to 1 to 2 days.

Intraoperative Considerations

In the adequately prepared patient, the intraoperative period does not present any special problems. Although thyroid storm may occur at any time, the usual thyroid operation is of relatively short duration; thyroid storm most often makes its appearance during the immediate postoperative period. Attention should be paid during surgery to the pulse rate and the tachycardia treated with propranolol. An esophageal or rectal temperature probe should also be placed, and an ice mattress should be readily available.

Postoperative Considerations

Thyroid storm is a dreaded complication in the immediate postoperative period. The detection of the initial stages of thyroid storm may be difficult. Most of the clinical features are exactly those of ordinary thyrotoxicosis. In elderly patients, many of the clinical findings may be blunted or absent. Values for the thyroid function tests during thyroid storm may be in the same range as those in patients with uncomplicated thyrotoxicosis. Since the immediate need for treatment of thyroid storm precludes awaiting test results, the overlap of test values is not critical for therapy. The onset of fever is perhaps the earliest distinguishing feature of thyroid storm. Apparently, heat from excessive production can no longer be dissipated, and the core body temperature rises. Thyroid storm characteristically involves other organ systems. Cardiovascular decompensation can run the gamut from extreme tachycardia, dysrhythmias, high-output congestive heart failure to shock and death. Central nervous system effects, such as extreme irritability, agitation, marked tremors, and even frank psychoses, may be seen. Coma may ensue. Miscellaneous gastrointestinal features include nausea and vomiting, diarrhea, and jaundice.

Treatment of thyroid storm is directed toward blocking the peripheral effects of the hormone, decreasing the hormonal output from the thyroid gland, and providing systems support.[23, 24] Propranolol is the drug of choice for blocking the peripheral effects. Oral doses of 20 mg to 100 mg, every 4 hours, may be required to decrease the pulse rate. If necessary, propranolol can be administered intravenously at an infusion rate under 1 mg per minute.

Frequent monitoring of blood pressures and electrocardiographic patterns may be maintained during infusion. The effect of a milligram should be seen within a few minutes, and, if no slowing of the pulse rate occurs, this dose can be repeated. The total dose should be limited to 4 mg to 8 mg per 6 hours. Reserpine or guanethidine are also drugs that have been used effectively.

Propylthiouracil (PTU) or methimazole can be given to block thyroidal hormone synthesis. PTU has the added effect of blocking the conversion of thyroxine to triiodothyronine. The loading dose of PTU should be 600 mg to 1000 mg, with a maintenance of 300 mg to 600 mg, every 8 hours. It can be given by nasogastric tube, if necessary. It should be noted that since PTU blocks the synthesis of the hormone, PTU may take several days or weeks to decrease serum T_4 concentrations because previously synthesized hormone is being released from glandular storage during this period. In contrast, serum T_3 concentrations may begin to fall within 24 hours, probably owing to the inhibitory effect of PTU on the conversion of T_4 to T_3. The release of previously synthesized thyroid hormones can be blocked by sodium iodine, 1 g, intravenously, every 8 hours, or by supersaturated potassium iodide solution, orally 30 drops daily. Iodine should be given at least 1 hour after administration of the PTU in order to prevent iodine stimulation of hormonal synthesis. Finally, support must be given to the cardiovascular system by administration of a digitalis derivative, diuretics, and oxygen. Hypothermia should be maintained by icepacks or ice mattress. Steroids are also usually administered, and their beneficial effect may be due to enhanced conversion of T_4 to rT_3 (inactive) rather than to T_3 (active). The list below summarizes the treatment of thyroid storm.

Blocking Peripheral Thyroidal Effects
Propranolol, 20–100 mg, every 4 hours, orally, or 1-mg doses, IV; no more than 4–8 mg/8 hour

Decreasing Hormonal Output
Propylthiouracil, 600–1000 mg, followed by 300–600 mg, every 8 hours

Support of Other Systems
Digitalis, diuretics, and oxygen
Hypothermia
Corticosteroids

HYPOTHYROIDISM

Hypothyroidism in surgical patients may occur across a spectrum. Complete hypothyroidism is an expected outcome of total thyroidectomy usually performed for malignancies of the thyroid. However, it may not be appreciated that when surgery of the thyroid is limited to a lobectomy, euthyroidism is maintained only because of a compensatory increase in TSH secretion and a consequent stimulation of the remaining thyroid lobe to produce adequate quantities of T_4 and T_3. In surgery for Graves' disease, the most common operation is a subtotal thyroidectomy, which is designed to leave enough residual thyroid tissue to prevent hypothyroidism but not so much tissue that hyperthyroidism persists. In contrast to total thyroidectomy, which produces hypothyroidism at a time determined only by the biologic disappearance rate of the thyroid hormones, hypothyroidism following subtotal thyroidectomy in Graves' disease may appear later at variable times postoperatively because of continuing deterioration in the function of the remnant gland.

Overview

At one time, the hypothyroidism following subtotal thyroidectomy for Graves' disease was thought to be caused mainly by an extension of the autoimmune process originally producing the disease. Remnant size is now a more appreciated variable in that, when at least 6 g to 10 g of carefully measured remnant thyroid tissue is left behind, the incidence of hypothyroidism is acceptably low.[4, 21] Most hypothyroidism seen postoperatively in Graves' disease occurs within the first year, and only a slowly increasing incidence is seen thereafter.[9] Following the sudden withdrawal of thyroid hormone, such as after total thyroidectomy, clinically detectable hypothyroidism begins to appear only 3 to 4 weeks postoperatively. Because thyroxine is bound rather tightly to circulating proteins, its plasma half-life is about 1 week. The half-life of T_3 is only a few days, but T_4 is a prohormone for T_3 and serves as a precursor pool readily converted to T_3. The deficit of thyroid hormone produces physiologic changes, such as decreased oxygen consumption, low body temperature, and slow heart rate, which are obviously the opposite effects of those seen with excessive amounts of hormone.

Diagnosis

The full-blown picture of hypothyroidism can be recognized from symptoms such as lethargy, increased sleep requirements, weakness, easy fatigability, and cold intolerance.[13] The signs include coarse, thickened, dry skin and nonpitting edema, seen especially in areas of loose skin and around the eyes. There may be decreased mental acuity, poor memory, slow speech with the low voice of vocal cord myxedema, and a delayed relaxation phase of deep tendon reflexes. Unfortunately, almost all of these signs and symptoms are seen in the late stages of hypothyroidism and indicate neglect. The laboratory diagnostic tests must be used for early detection of hypothyroidism and prevention of its clinical sequelae. Characteristically, T_3 and T_4 concentrations in the serum are low; the TSH concentrations are high and can be markedly accentuated by administration of TRH. The T_3 resin uptake is low. Radioiodine uptake by the thyroid gland is characteristically below 15% at 4 hours and less than 35% at 24 hours. The RAI uptake may be unreliable in diagnosing hypothyroidism because of several factors, such as the sensitivity of the test to changes in iodine uptake, congenital thyroid conditions of failure to oxidize or place iodine on thyroxine, and the effects of diuretics.

Treatment

Once recognized, treatment of ordinary hypothyroidism is simply that of hormonal replacement.[7, 25] The symptoms of hypothyroidism are usually reversed within several days after the onset of treatment, but some of the findings, such as the skin changes, may take weeks or months to disappear. Levo-thyroxine is widely available commercially and is the drug of choice. The usual dose is 0.10 mg to 0.15 mg per day or, more precisely, 2.2 μg per kg per day. Triiodothyronine can also be used for replacement therapy; but because of its short half-life, multiple daily doses are required. Thyroid extract is a defatted preparation of bovine thyroid tissue and contains both T_3 and T_4. However, the biologic standardization of batches of this compound is not always homogenous. In the treatment of hypothyroidism in patients with cardiac disease, a gradual replacement should be attempted owing to the possibility of overdosing and inappropriately stimulating cardiac output.[19] The increased cardiac workload may result in angina pectoris or cardiac failure.

Operative Aspects

HOARSENESS

Edema affecting the intrinsic larynx is the most common cause of postthyroidectomy hoarseness. Direct effects of manipulation of the cricopharyngeal muscle and the cricoid and thyroid cartilages and, perhaps, of interruption of the lymphatics in the area account for most of the edema seen. Also, dissection around the larynx may repeatedly press and rub the vocal cords onto the relatively hard, immobile endotracheal tube. A mild degreee of edema produces a roughened, somewhat harsh, voice, but as edema progresses and the cords become more involved, voice volume may diminish. In the first few hours after surgery, the voice can be almost normal, but, later, as the edema progresses, a change in voice will become apparent. Such a progression is different from the immediate whispery voice seen with recurrent laryngeal nerve injury. Treatment for the laryngeal edema should include voice rest and vaporization of the inspired air. With progressive edema, dexamethasone, in 2-mg doses every 6 hours, may be indicated. When edema progresses to such a severity, the physician should anticipate airway obstruction, as discussed below.

RECURRENT LARYNGEAL NERVE DAMAGE

Damage to the recurrent laryngeal nerve can range from frank severance, immediate but temporary paresis, to delayed appearance of paralysis due to surrounding infection or scarring. The reported incidence of recurrent laryngeal nerve damage varies from 0% to 8%, with the higher figures seen in bilateral exposures, such as in total thyroidectomy, and in unilateral thyroid lobectomies combined with neck dissection. The incidences of recurrent laryngeal nerve injury reported in most series are probably underestimates because of the lack of routine indirect laryngoscopy.[34] Laryngoscopy is necessary in patients with recurrent laryngeal nerve damage whose voices are normal because of the compensatory movement of the contralateral cord across the midline.

Avoidance of Injury

Although no randomized, prospective studies are available to test the hypothesis, most surgeons seem to agree that identifying the recurrent laryngeal nerve and carefully tracing it to its entrance into the cricothyroid muscle is the best way to preserve it.[8, 15, 20, 22] The alternative method is simply staying out of the area of the nerve, perhaps only palpating without visualizing it.[14]

The nerve is best identified initially in the tracheoesophageal groove at approximately the level of the lower thyroid pole. The nerve can be recognized by its whitish, flattened appearance. The red, wavy filaments of vasa nervorum can be seen coursing longitudinally along the white wavy strands of the nerve. Our preferred technique for following the course of the nerve is to place the convex side of a small, curved hemostat down toward the nerve and successively spread the hemostat above and parallel to the nerve along its course. The nerve is easily visualized down below (dorsally) through the spread prongs of the hemostat, and care is taken not to disturb the nerve by any further dissection along its sides. All structures that are then dissected up from the ventral side of the nerve (between the hemostat and the ceiling) can be divided safely. Such structures that are divided must be clearly seen to be separate from the nerve. The course of the nerve should not be surmised but clearly visualized whenever structures are to be divided.

As experience is gained tracing the nerve past

the inferior thyroid artery, the almost endless variations of the relationship of the nerve to the artery become apparent. These variations almost preclude use of the thyroid artery as a reliable landmark in finding the nerve.[43] As the nerve is superiorly traced farther behind the thyroid lobe and closer to its entrance into the cricothyroid muscle, exposure is limited by the relative immobility of the thyroid upper pole fixed by its vascular pedicle. At this point, division of the superior thyroid vessels allows the thyroid lobe to be pulled more fully medially and ventrally, and excellent exposure of the nerve is once again possible.

A critical point is reached as the nerve approaches the vicinity of the so-called ligament of Berry. This tough, fibrous attachment of the posterior portion of the upper thyroid pole to the cricoid cartilage is usually medial to the recurrent laryngeal nerve, although the latter structure may sometimes course through the ligament. The course of the recurrent laryngeal nerve must be traced into the fibers of the cricothyroid muscle, because deviations are possible during the last few millimeters before the nerve disappears. An erroneous assumption about the course of the nerve may result in its damage during division of the ligament of Berry. Occasionally the nerve bifurcates prior to its entering the cricothyroid muscle. Since the branches innervate the intrinsic laryngeal muscles randomly, branch injury has an unpredictable effect, and care should be taken to preserve them. In approximately 1% of the cases, the inferior laryngeal nerve does not recur around the aorta or innominate artery.[16] Instead, a short branch of the vagus nerve crosses medially, at approximately the level of the inferior horn of the thyroid cartilage, to enter the cricothyroid muscle. Failing to find the recurrent laryngeal nerve after careful search of the tracheoesophageal groove, the surgeon should be exremely cautious in the region of the upper thyroid pole. Such an anomaly represents another sound reason why the recurrent laryngeal nerve should be identified early in the operation.

Detection of Injury

The main clinical evidence of unilateral recurrent laryngeal nerve injury is that of a weak, whispery voice (Table 43-1). There may also be some difficulty with complete glottic closure, for example, during coughing or the Valsalva maneuver. Inability to close the glottis may be quite marked with associated injury to the external branch of the superior laryngeal nerve and the recurrent laryngeal nerve. In isolated recurrent laryngeal nerve damage, the intact external branch of the superior laryngeal nerve innervates the cricothyroid muscle to maintain full adduction of the cord. When the superior laryngeal nerve is also damaged, though adduction is not possible, the cord is paralyzed in the intermediate position away from the midline, and full glottic closure is virtually impossible (Fig. 43-1). In most instances of isolated recurrent laryngeal nerve injury, the contralateral

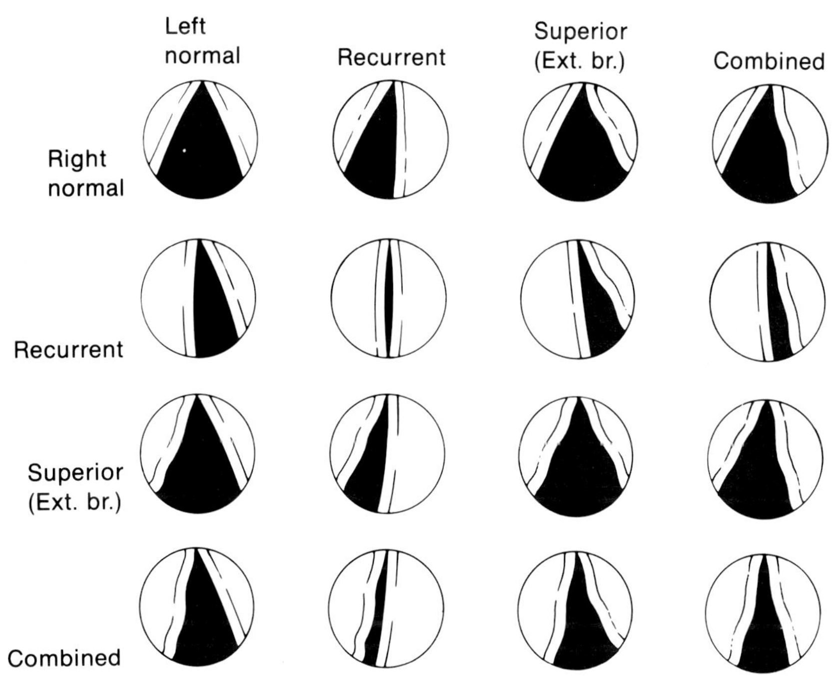

FIG. 43-1. The various types of laryngeal nerve injury as they appear on laryngoscopy.

TABLE 43-1. SIGNS AND SYMPTOMS OF LARYNGEAL NERVE INJURY*

	Voice	Glottic Close	Airway
Recurrent			
Unilateral	Weak	Weak	Good
Bilateral	Normal	Adequate	Poor
External branch, superior			
Unilateral	Lowered	Weakened	Good
Bilateral	Lowered	Loss of reflex	Good
Combined injury			
Unilateral	Weak	Poor	Good
Bilateral	Weak	Weak	Adequate

*Before compensatory cord changes occur

cord will move across the midline within a few weeks and abut the paralyzed cord to produce a normal voice. Therefore, unless indirect laryngoscopy is performed, it is not always possible to rule out recurrent laryngeal nerve damage. It is axiomatic that movement of the cord should be noted prior to a neck operation in any patient who has had previous neck surgery, regardless of the preoperative quality of the voice.

Management of the Injury

In isolated recurrent laryngeal nerve injury, the compensatory movement of the contralateral cord across the midline plus some fibrotic change in the paralyzed cord will produce a voice that may be acceptable to the patient. In some situations, the injection of Teflon into the paralyzed cord will stiffen it further and improve the quality of voice. With injury to the superior and inferior laryngeal nerve, arytenoidopexy will bring the partially abducted, paralyzed cord closer to the midline and improve the quality of voice.[18, 41]

Operations for Recurrent Laryngeal Nerve Damage

- Unilateral
  - Arytenoidopexy
  - Teflon injection
- Bilateral
  - Teflon injection
  - Arytenoidectomy
  - Innervated muscle transplant
  - Neurorrhaphy
  - Flap tracheostomy tube

SUPERIOR LARYNGEAL NERVE DAMAGE

The superior laryngeal nerve rises from the nodose ganglion of the vagus nerve. It divides into an internal and external branch at about the level of the hyoid bone. The internal branch enters the posterior aspect of the larynx through the thyrohyoid membrane to provide sensory fibers to the supraglottic larynx. The external branch continues downward in association with the superior thyroid vessels to innervate the cricothyroid muscle.

Avoidance of Injury

In considering that the external branch of the superior laryngeal nerve will be in close proximity to the superior thyroid vessels and that the nerve must diverge from this area to enter the cricothyroid muscle, it becomes evident that injury to the nerve is best avoided by dissecting in close apposition to the thyroid tissue of the upper pole and by separating this portion of the gland from the cricothyroid muscle.[26, 27] After encircling the upper pole of the thyroid in such a manner, blunt dissection can then be carried upward on the superior pole vessels to sweep the nerve away from the danger of ligation. The vessels can then be safely ligated. In contrast, if the superior thyroid vessels are initially encircled at a level above the tip of the upper pole, the external branch of the superior nerve may not be separated from the vessels, and the neural branch may well be ligated. If ligation of the thyroid pole is carried even higher, the internal branch of the superior laryngeal nerve may be injured, as well.

Detection of Injury

Since the external branch of the superior laryngeal nerve innervates the cricothyroid muscle, the signs and symptoms of damage to this branch naturally reflect loss of this muscle's function.[1, 27] (See Table 43-1 and Fig. 43-1). Contraction of the cricothyroid muscle brings the anterior portion of the cricoid and the anteroinferior portion of the thyroid cartilages closer together. Since these two cartilages are articulated upon each other at the midpoint of each side, movement of the anterior portions of these two cartilages toward each other results in a widening gap between their posterior portions. This widening gap pulls the arytenoid cartilages downward and backward and, thus, tenses and adducts the vocal cords. Therefore, loss of innervation to the cricothyroid muscle results in a loss of tension and full adduction of the ipsilateral vocal cord. Laxity of the cords produces several subtle changes in the voice, which may be of serious consequence to the frequent speaker, the singer, or anyone who talks a great deal.

The patient with superior laryngeal nerve damage typically feels that the voice is weak. Objectively, the voice is characteristically lowered in pitch, feeble and lacking in resonance and fails to project well. The maximum volume of voice is decreased. The flaccidity of the cord results in weak glottic closure, and a short phonation time occurs as the air is wasted during talking. Sensory loss from unilateral injury to the internal branch is usually not detected because sensation is still intact on the adjacent contralateral side. However, the fortunately rare bilateral internal branch damage may result in serious problems with aspiration because of the loss of reflex glottic closure when saliva or other material is in the hypopharynx. The changes seen on laryngoscopic examination with external branch damage may be subtle but are characteristic. Unilateral paralysis of the cricothyroid muscle will produce rotation of the cricoid cartilage in relation to the thyroid cartilage. The rotation results in an oblique glottis when viewed from above with the posterior commissure deviating to the side of the paralysis. Loss of external tension on the cord produces a flaccidity that may be evident as a difference in level of the paralyzed cord from that of the innervated cord. During inspiration, the paralyzed cord may be slightly aspirated to a level lower than that of the contralateral, innervated cord, or it may bulge outward to a level higher than that of the contralateral cord during expiration. Lack of external tension results in a slight shortening of the cord by the unopposed, intact vocalis muscle. The difference in length of the two cords may be more pronounced when the contralateral intact cord is tensed and lengthened during high-tone vocalization.

RESPIRATORY DISTRESS

Preoperative Respiratory Problems

An extreme difficulty may arise when a large colloid goiter impinges upon the tracheal lumen. It is the most common indication for removal of a goiter in the substernal position.[45] The symptoms are usually slowly progressive and begin as slight wheezing when the velocity of tracheal air flow is increased. Even minimal symptoms deserve attention, and a chest or soft-tissue cervical x-ray film should be obtained to assess the luminal diameter of the trachea. The airway obstruction may become slowly worse through growth of the goiter or rapidly worse, either by extrinsic causes, such as bleeding or swelling of the goiter, or intrinsic causes, such as obstruction by a mucous plug. Because of the pretracheal location of the huge goiter, tracheostomy is seldom possible, and reliance must be placed on deft intubation. Endotracheal intubation is so critical in these patients that we have adopted a method of trial breathing by facemask before proceeding. If after very light thiopental sodium (Pentothal) anesthesia, ventilation can be maintained adequately with a facemask, the patient is then paralyzed with a neuromuscular blocking agent and intubation done while the patient sleeps. However, if facemask ventilation is not possible, the patient is allowed to recover from the short-acting Pentothal, topical anesthetization is done, and the patient is intubated while awake. Occasionally, because of the marked distortion of the larynx by the goiter, a flexible fiberoptic bronchoscope is required for intubation. In the other preoperative circumstance of respiratory distress from a less bulky yet highly invasive, undifferentiated carcinoma, tracheostomy may be more vigorously pursued. The tumor is usually not as bulky as the huge goiter and tracheostomy may be inevitable so that there should be no hesitation in performing it.

Postoperative Respiratory Problems

Although respiratory problems in the postoperative period are relatively uncommon, they can be life threatening, and diagnosis and treatment must be prompt. Upper airway obstruction may be insidious at its onset. The clinical picture may be deceptive in that symptoms of hypoxia, such as restlessness, irritability, somnolence, and so on may erroneously suggest a primary cerebral rather than a respiratory problem. Of course, if stridor is present or dyspnea is appreciated by the patient or physician, appropriate attention can be given early. No matter how mild or trivial the degree of respiratory difficulty appears, the patient should be followed closely, and specific therapeutic maneuvers carried out promptly should the condition worsen.

EDEMA. Perhaps the most common cause of postoperative respiratory distress following surgery in the neck is edema of the larynx. As mentioned above, this results from the dissection and manipulation around the thyroid and cricoid cartilages and the hypopharyngeal muscles. Both inspiration and expiration may be difficult, but inspiration is typically more impeded and may be accompanied by stridor. In unusual instances in which the vocal cords are spared, stridor may not be present, and the physician is not alerted by this sign to the potential disaster of supra- or infraglottic closure. No matter how mild the edema appears, it is prudent to put the patient on voice rest and employ vaporization of inspired air. High doses of anti-inflammatory steroids have been suggested. The moderate degree of obstruction that forces extra respiratory effort is particularly pernicious as the patient tires, becomes exhausted, and can no longer maintain an adequate tidal volume. When a dangerous degree of respiratory obstruction has developed, as indicated by nasal flaring subcostal retraction and use of accessory respiratory muscles, the patient must be readied for possible tracheostomy. Deterioration of arterial gas concentrations is only confirmatory and may be a relatively late event. Intubation of the trachea may be extremely difficult through an edematous larynx. This method of airway restoration should be briefly attempted once, if at all, and immediate tracheostomy done.

HEMORRHAGE. Many small vessels are usually encountered during a neck operation. Any residual slight ooze can be handled by a drain left in place postoperatively for the first 24 hours. However, brisk bleeding may occur if there is inadvertent slippage of a ligature, usually from the superior or inferior thyroid artery. The bleeding may come out through the drain site and necessitate reexploration. Vigorous bleeding that does not drain externally may produce a large hematoma under considerable pressure, which may impinge upon the trachea to cause airway obstruction. Any sudden postoperative swelling in the neck is best handled by immediate reexploration, evacuation of the blood, and ligation of the bleeding point. The procedure can obviously be done in the patient's bed, if necessary, to prevent asphyxiation during transport to the operating room.

TRACHEOMALACIA. Softening of the cartilaginous tracheal rings may occur during chronic impingement by a goiter.[12] The softening is distinctly more common with large goiters, but it can occur in conjunction with small goiters or even the diffuse thyroid enlargement of Graves' disease. Appreciation of the condition at operation is the key to avoidance of difficulty. The quality and resilience of the tracheal rings should be noted during each thyroidectomy. If the rings feel soft, the patient should be extubated with full preparation for immediate reintubation. Since the thyroid gland and other surrounding tissues of the neck no longer support the softened rings, the negative pressure of inspiration collapses the trachea to produce an inadequate airway. Reintubation is usually accomplished with ease, and after several days, the surrounding tissues become supportive and usually allow extubation. If the second extubation attempt is unsuccessful, a nasotracheal tube can usually be safely left in place for several weeks to allow the tracheal rings to become more resilient. Tracheostomy is seldom necessary for this condition.

BILATERAL RECURRENT LARYNGEAL NERVE DAMAGE. In the unfortunate event that both recurrent laryngeal nerves are rendered functionless, the vocal cords are paralyzed in the fully adducted position, provided that the external branch of either superior laryngeal nerve is not damaged. On expiration the cords are blown open somewhat, but on inspiration, normal abduction is absent; the cords remain together at midline; and inspiratory stridor, or worse, may occur. Because the cords are apposed, the voice may be entirely normal. Thus, inspiratory difficulty and maintenance of voice may signal bilateral isolated recurrent laryngeal nerve paralysis. In the event of combined bilateral damage of the recurrent laryngeal nerves and of the external branches of the superior laryngeal nerves, the flaccid cricothyroid muscle prevents full adduction, and the cords are typically paralyzed in the intermediate position. With associated injury comes voice impairment, but the intermediate position of the cords also allows air to pass. Over a period of time, the cords may undergo fibrotic change, become more ridged, and meet at the midline. A gradual return of voice may signify the impending apposition of the cords and the onset of respiratory difficulty.

The immediate treatment of bilateral isolated paralysis of the recurrent laryngeal nerves with cords fixed in the midline can be either endotracheal intubation or tracheostomy. Intubation may be preferred in the immediate postoperative period because of the possible morbidity from a tracheostomy in a freshly dissected neck and also because either or both cords may be only temporarily paralyzed with a satisfactory return of function within a few weeks. If intubation has been done and the patient tolerates the intubation well, a trial extubation may be attempted after 1 to 2 weeks. Tracheostomy may then be inevitable if function has not returned by then. The patient is usually followed with the tracheostomy in place for 3 to 6 months. If nerve function has not returned at that time, other means of compensation for the disability should be considered. A flap tracheostomy tube that allows expired air to pass through the flap and over the cords to produce a voice has been advocated. As the flap closes during inspiration, the air comes in through the tracheostomy tube and bypasses the glottis. Arytenoidectomy is a permanent procedure that allows the cords to fall away from their bilateral midline position.[29, 38] Injection of the cords with Teflon and fixation in the intermediate position also permits the passage of air but destroys the quality of voice. If the cords have already stiffened naturally over time in the midline position, submucosal resection may be required.[38] The application of an innervated segment of omohyoid muscle has been described.[40] A successful operation results in the abduction of the reinnervated cord. Attempts have been made at immediate reexploration in the patient with nerve paralysis on the chance that the nerve has been cut and the ends reapproximated or a nerve graft placed by 6-0 or 7-0 monofilament sutures. The success of these maneuvers has not been high, perhaps because of the mismatch of nerve fibers going to abductor or adductor muscle groups.[28] In addition, neuroma formation at the anastomotic site may prevent the regenerated nerve fibers from reapproximating at all. In the chronic situation, before any of the reconstructive attempts in the larynx are performed, the patient must be checked for hypothyroidism, which can add materially to respiratory difficulties due to muscular weakness.

HYPOPARATHYROIDISM

Hypoparathyroidism seen after thyroid surgery almost always follows total thyroidectomy when all four glands are placed at risk. It occurs occasionally during subtotal thyroidectomy and rarely during simple lobectomy. Hypoparathyroidism of subtotal thyroidectomy was at one time thought related only to thyrotoxicosis and the osteodystrophy that resulted from that disease. However, mild hypocalcemia has since been reported after subtotal thyroidectomy in euthyroid patients. Perhaps the transient hypocalcemia is caused by release of calcitonin from the traumatized thyroid remnant, as well as from a mild degree of parathyroid insufficiency.[44] In contrast to the hypocalcemia seen following surgery for hyperparathyroidism, prolonged postthyroidectomy hypocalcemia is due solely to insufficient parathyroid hormone without accompanying bone disease, and hyperphosphatemia is the rule. The bone disease of preexisting hyperparathyroidism may produce hypocalcemia during postoperative bone remineralization, but the serum phosphate level is low or normal since this mineral is removed from the circulation along with calcium to form bone. The detection and treatment of the hypoparathyroidism following thyroid surgery is otherwise similar to that discussed for the hypoparathyroidism of parathyroid surgery.

Prevention of the hypoparathyroidism is of primary importance and is related to surgical technique.[3, 31, 33] In most instances, the parathyroid glands can be spared by staying adjacent to the thyroid capsule when dissecting the lobe free from surrounding tissues. This somewhat tedious method requires individual ligation of the branches of the inferior thyroid artery, as compared to the standard technique of simply ligating the artery as a single trunk well outside the area of the thyroid capsule. Parathyroids with a tenuous blood supply or those under the thyroid capsule may be saved by placing them in the substance of the sternocleidomastoid muscle.[11, 31, 36] The removed glands are immediately placed in cold saline, minced into 1-ml cubes, and imbedded among carefully separated muscle fibers.[48] Autotransplantation is recommended when the viability of the *in situ* parathyroid gland is in question. However, a parathyroid gland that, along with its blood supply, is easily separated from the thyroid and remains viable should probably be left *in situ*. In Stage II carcinoma of the thyroid, the neck dissection may require deliberate removal of the parathyroid gland. In this case, histologic identification of the glands must first be assured before it is autotransplanted.

DIFFICULTIES IN SWALLOWING

In most instances, difficulty in swallowing relates to soreness from the dissection or endotracheal tube. Extensive dissection in the retropharyngeal area may cause some genuine dysfunction of the hypopharyngeal muscles. These difficulties are usually temporary and disappear within several days. An occasional patient may undergo symptomatic fibrosis in this area, but the residual difficulty will gradually improve over a period of months. In the unusual instance of bilateral injury to the external branches of the superior laryngeal nerves, there is bilateral mucosal anesthesia of the hypopharynx and upper larynx. Liquids or other swallowed matter may not stimulate closure of the glottis, and aspiration can occur. This fortunately rare situation is a genuine problem in management, and a tracheostomy with a cuffed tube may be necessary. There is no satisfactory treatment for this condition.

CHYLOUS LEAKAGE

The major concern with lymphatics is injury to the left thoracic duct. The right thoracic duct may also be injured, but since its primary drainage is only the right lung, the volumes of lymphatic flow are relatively small, and spontaneous closure is the rule. Again, avoidance of injury is the most effective way of handling the problem, but almost equally important is prompt detection of the injury at the time of surgery and secure ligation of the duct. It is natural that some lymphatic loss occurs postoperatively through the drain site. However, if this drainage is so extensive that several dressing changes are necessary during the first 24 hours, injury to the thoracic duct should be suspected. If the drainage is copious, some advocate immediate reentry into the neck for an attempt at ligation. In many cases, with adequate fluid and electrolyte replacement, a high-protein, low-fat diet, and continuous local pressure, the chylous fistula may close spontaneously. Reoperation may be indicated if no progress is being made after weeks of conservative measures, but the cervical reoperation may be difficult and closure of the fistula not possible. The last available option is ligation of the thoracic duct through a left thoracotomy.

INFECTION

Because of the relatively clean nature of the cervical area and the rich vascular supply to the tissues in the neck, infection is distinctly uncommon. There is the occasional superficial infection involving the subcutaneous tissues down to the level of the platysma. This almost always responds to local measures of irrigation and sterile dressing. Use of chromic sutures to close the platysmal layer eliminates the phenomenon of chronic extrusion of nonabsorbable material from the infected wound. Occasional curettage of an old, granulating sinus may become necessary. A deep infection in the neck probably arises from a gross break in sterile technique or instrument sterilization. In the ordinary thyroid case, the cervical fascial planes have their superior boundary at the base of the skull and their inferior boundary around the anus. Therefore, a deep infection can be quite serious and demands prompt treatment with wide drainage and adequate antibiotic coverage. Infection may follow removal of the substernal goiter where adequate drainage is difficult. In these cases, a suction catheter may be preferred. Fortunately, the growth of the ordinary substernal goiter pushes tissue ahead of it so that, after extirpation, there is a fairly well delineated pseudocapsule that impedes generalized mediastinal infection.

References

1. Arnold GE: Physiology and pathology of the cricothyroid muscle. Laryngoscope 71:687, 1961
2. Astwood EB: Treatment of hyperthyroidism with thiourea and thiouracil. JAMA 122:78, 1943
3. Attie JN, Khafif RA: Preservation of parathyroid glands during total thyroidectomy. Am J Surg 130:399, 1975
4. Bradley EL, DiGirolamo M, Tarcan Y: Modified subtotal thyroidectomy in the management of Graves' disease. Surgery 87:623, 1980
5. Brown J, Solomon DH, Beall GN et al: Autoimmune thyroid diseases—Graves' and Hashimoto's. Ann Intern Med 88:379, 1978
6. Burman KD: Recent developments in thyroid hormone metabolism: Interpretation and significance of measurements of reverse T_3, 3, 3′T_2, and thyroglobulin. Metabolism 27:615, 1978
7. Capiferri R, Evered D: Investigation and treatment of hypothyroidism. Clin Endocrinol Metab 8:39, 1979
8. Elner A, Fex S, Ingelstedt S: Nerve injury in thyroid surgery. Acta Chir Scand 134:103, 1968
9. Farnell MB, van Heerden JA, McConahey WM et al: Hypothyroidism after thyroidectomy for Graves' disease. Am J Surg 142:535, 1981
10. Feek CM, Sawers JSA, Irvine WJ et al: Combination of potassium iodide and propranolol in preparation of patients with Graves' disease for thyroid surgery. N Engl J Surg 302:883, 1980
11. Gann DS, Paone JF: Delayed hypocalcemia after thyroidectomy for Graves' disease is prevented by parathyroid autotransplantation. Ann Surg 190:508, 1979
12. Green WER, Shepperd HWH, Stevenson HM, Wilson W: Tracheal collapse after thyroidectomy. Br J Surg 66:554, 1979
13. Hall R, Scanlon MF: Hypothyroidism: Clinical features and complications. Clin Endocrinol Metab 8:29, 1979
14. Holt GR, McMurry GT, Joseph DJ: Recurrent laryngeal nerve injury following thyroid operations. Surg Gynecol Obstet 144:567, 1977
15. Humphreys J: Exposure of the recurrent laryngeal nerves in thyroid operations. Surg Gynecol Obstet 98:239, 1944
16. Humphreys J: A hazard of thyroidectomy. Proc R Soc Med 65:169, 1972
17. Ingbar SH, Braverman LE: Active form of the thyroid hormone. Annu Rev Med 26:443, 1975
18. Isshiki N, Tanabe M, Sawade M: Arytenoid adduction for unilateral vocal cord paralysis. Arch Otolaryngol 104:555, 1978
19. Keating FR Jr, Parkin TW, Selby JB, Dickinson LS: Treatment of heart disease associated with myxedema. Prog Cardiovasc Dis 3:364, 1961
20. Kratz RC: The identification and protection of the laryngeal motor nerves during thyroid and laryngeal surgery: A new microsurgical technique. Laryngoscope 33:59, 1973
21. Liechty RD, Silverberg SG, Hernandez J: Limited subtotal thyroidectomy for Graves' disease. Arch Surg 116:561, 1981
22. Lore JM, Kim DJ, Elias S: Preservation of the laryngeal nerves during total thyroid lobectomy. Ann Otol Rhinol Laryngol 86:777, 1977
23. Mackin JF, Canary JJ, Pittman CS: Thyroid storm and its management. N Engl J Med 291:1396, 1974
24. Mecklenburg RS: Diagnosis and management of endocrine emergencies. Bull Mason Clin 31:101, 1977
25. Mecklenburg RS: Recognition and treatment of hypothyroidism. Bull Mason Clin 32:130, 1978
26. Moosman DA, DeWeese MS: The external laryngeal nerve as related to thyroidectomy. Surg Gynecol Obstet 127:1011, 1968
27. Moran RE, Castro AF: The superior laryngeal nerve in thyroid surgery. Ann Surg 134:1018, 1951
28. Murakami Y, Kirschner JA: Vocal cord abduction by regenerated recurrent laryngeal nerve. Arch Otolaryngol 94:64, 1971
29. Newman MH, Work WP: Arytenoidectomy revisited. Laryngoscope 86:840, 1976
30. Oppenheimer JH: Thyroid hormone action at the cellular level. Science 203:971, 1979
31. Paloyan E, Lawrence AM, Paloyan D: Successful autotransplantation of the parathyroid glands during total thyroidectomy for carcinoma. Surg Gynecol Obstet 145:364, 1977
32. Plummer HS: Results of administering iodine to patients having exophthalmic goiter. JAMA 80:1955, 1923
33. Reyes HM, Wright JK, Rosenfield RL: Prevention of hypocalcemia in children due to parathyroid infarction after thyroidectomy. Surg Gynecol Obstet 148:76, 1979
34. Roy AD, Gardiner RH, Niblock WM: Thyroidectomy and the recurrent laryngeal nerves. Lancet 270:988, 1953
35. Rubenfeld S, Silverman VE, Welch KMA et al: Variable plasma propranolol levels in thyrotoxicosis. N Engl J Med 300:353, 1979
36. Salander H, Tisell L–E: Incidence of hypoparathyroidism after radical surgery for thyroid carcinoma and autotransplantation of parathyroid glands. Am J Surg 134:358, 1977
37. Schimmel M, Utiger RD: Thyroidal and peripheral production of thyroid hormones. Ann Intern Med 87:760, 1977
38. Sessions DG, Ogura JH, Heeneman H: Surgical management of bilateral vocal cord paralysis. Laryngoscope 86:559, 1976

39. Sterling K: Thyroid hormone action at the cell level. N Engl J Med 300:117, 1979
40. Tucker HM: Human laryngeal reinnervation. Laryngoscope 86:769, 1976
41. Tucker HM: Management of the patient with an incompetent larynx. Am J Otolaryngol 1:47, 1979
42. Utiger RD: Treatment of Graves' disease. N Engl J Med 298:681, 1978
43. Wade JSH: Vulnerability of the recurrent laryngeal nerves at thyroidectomy. Br J Surg 43:164, 1955
44. Watson CG, Steed DL, Robinson AG, Deftos LJ: The role of calcitonin and parathyroid hormone in the pathogenesis of post-thyroidectomy hypocalcemia. Metabolism 30:588, 1981
45. Watt–Boolsen S, Blichert–Toft M, Folke K et al: Surgical treatment of benign nontoxic intrathoracic goiter. Am J Surg 141:721, 1981
46. Weiner L, Stout BD, Cox JW: Influence of beta sympathetic blockade with propranolol on the hemodynamics of hyperthyroidism. Am J Med 46:227, 1969
47. Wellby ML: The laboratory diagnosis of thyroid disorders. Adv Clin Chem 18:103, 1976
48. Wells SA, Gunnells JC, Shelburne JD et al: Transplantation of the parathyroid glands in man: Clinical indications and results. Surgery 78:34, 1975

Suggested Reading

Blum M: Easier understanding of the new thyroid tests. Res Staff Phys 27:72, 1981

Brennan MD: Clinical pharmacology: 5. Thyroid hormones. Mayo Clin Proc 55:33, 1980

Burrow GN: Hyperthyroidism during pregnancy. N Engl J Med 298:150, 1978

Caldarelli DD, Holinger LD: Complications and sequelae of thyroid surgery. Otolaryngol Clin North Am 13:85, 1980

Degroot LJ, Niepomniszcze H: Biosynthesis of thyroid hormone: Basic and clinical aspects. Metabolism 26:665, 1977

Edis AJ: Prevention and management of complications associated with thyroid and parathyroid surgery. Surg Clin North Am 59:83, 1979

Esmeraldo R, Paloyan E, Lawrence AM: Thyroidectomy, parathyroidectomy, and modified neck dissection. Surg Clin North Am 57:1365, 1977

Foster RS: Morbidity and mortality after thyroidectomy. Surg Gynecol Obstet 146:423, 1978

Freeman GC: Complications of thyroid surgery: Current concepts of prevention and treatment. Surg Clin North Am 70:409, 1970

Homburger HA, Hewan–Lowe K: Predictive values of thyroxine, thyrotropin, and triiodothyronine concentrations in serum. Clin Chem 25:669, 1979

Loré JM: Surgery of the thyroid gland. Otolaryngol Clin North Am 13:69, 1980

McClung MR, Greer MA: Treatment of hyperthyroidism. Am Rev Med 31:385, 1980

Scanlon EF, Kellogg JE, Winchester DP, Larson RH: The morbidity of total thyroidectomy. Arch Surg 116:568, 1981

Sedgwick CE, Cady B (eds): Surgery of the Thyroid and Parathyroid Glands, 2nd ed, vol 15

Stehling L: Anesthetic implications of hyperthyroidism. In Brown BR Jr (ed): Anesthesia and the Patient with Endocrine Disease. Philadelphia, FA Davis, 1980

Sterling K, Lazarus JH: The thyroid and its control. Annu Rev Physiol 39:349, 1977

Taylor S: The hypermetabolic syndrome: Hyperthyroidism, thyrotoxicosis, Graves' disease. In Friesen SR: Surgical Endocrinology: Clinical Syndromes. Philadelphia, JB Lippincott, 1978

Totten MA, Wool MS: Medical treatment of hyperthyroidism. Med Clin North Am 63:321, 1979

Werner SC, Ingbar SH (eds): The Thyroid, ed 4. Hagerstown, Harper & Row, 1978

Wesley JR, Buckingham BA, Gahr JA et al: Surgical treatment of hyperthyroidism in children. Surg Gynecol Obstet 145:343, 1977

Wool MS: Hyperthyroidism. Major Probl Clin Surg 15:102, 1980

44 Complications of Parathyroid Surgery

H. H. Newsome, Jr.

Metabolic and Pharmacologic Aspects

PRIMARY HYPERPARATHYROIDISM

Preoperative Considerations

OVERVIEW. Hypersecretion of parathyroid hormone (PTH) may arise from an adenoma, hyperplasia, or carcinoma of the parathyroid glands. Rarely, PTH is produced by tumors, principally of the lung, kidney, and pancreas. By definition, hypersecretion of PTH in primary hyperparathyroidism is autonomous, meaning continuous, in the face of hypercalcemia, ordinarily an inhibitor of PTH secretion. Therefore, hypercalcemia is characteristic of primary hyperparathyroidism. Tertiary hyperparathyroidism is also a hypercalcemic state, but it apparently evolves from a preexisting secondary hyperparathyroidism that is characterized by a normal serum calcium. Secondary hyperparathyroidism is discussed below.

Parathyroid hormone acts primarily on bone to stimulate osteoclastic activity, which results in bone demineralization and a consequent hypercalcemia. PTH also acts on the kidney to promote phosphate excretion and produce hypophosphatemia, which, in turn, inhibits the remineralization of bone. The deleterious renal changes of excessive PTH production are related primarily to the hypercalcemia and resulting hypercalciuria. An intracellular deposition of calcium in the kidney and a loss of urinary concentrating ability are the earliest renal effects. The deposition of intracellular calcium can progress to radiologically detectable nephrocalcinosis and to renal failure. High concentration of urinary calcium may promote formation of kidney stones. Nephrolithiasis may be seen in as many as 50% of cases of primary hyperparathyroidism.[14] Another target organ for hypercalcemia is the central nervous system. Neural activity becomes depressed and the mental state altered with marked elevation of serum calcium.

DIAGNOSIS. Through multichannel serum analyses, serum calcium determinations are easily performed—asymptomatic hypercalcemia is the most common mode of presentation for primary hyperparathyroidism. During the workup, the diagnosis becomes apparent as the many other causes for hypercalcemia are discarded.[8, 53] Before more recent developments, the diagnosis of hyperparathyroidism was limited to exclusion of such entities as carcinoma metastatic to bone, hyperthyroidism, sarcoidosis, multiple myeloma, thiazide therapy, vitamin D intoxication, milk-alkali syndrome, adrenal insufficiency, and so on. A more positive means of diagnosis became available through the measurement of urinary cyclic adenosine monophosphate (cAMP).[15] PTH stimulates cAMP production by the renal tubular cell and results in an increased urinary excretion of this moiety. Cyclic AMP excretion in the urine may be elevated in approximately 80% of proven cases of primary hyperparathyroidism.[49] A more convenient test is the radioimmunoassay of circulating PTH in the plasma.[9, 18, 55] Because problems of accuracy, sensitivity, and specificity may exist with any assay, the characteristics of the particular PTH assay in use should be known before clinical reliance is placed upon it. Although the early problem of production of antisera to PTH sufficiently sensitive to distinguish reliably between elevated and normal levels has largely been overcome, in most assays distinction between low normal and zero serum concentrations of PTH is still difficult. The detection of various fragments of the PTH molecule also presents some difficulties, especially in renal failure when such fragments may be differentially elevated. Some assays will measure predominantly the N-terminal portion of the PTH molecule while others measure the C-terminal part. The C-terminal portion, which is not biologically active, has a longer half-life than does the N-terminal fragment and, consequently, is more often elevated in primary hyperparathyroidism. Most commercial laboratories will provide data on the normal range of their PTH values (along with the relationship to serum calcium concentrations) and give some indication of the accuracy and specificity of the assay.

PREPARATION FOR SURGERY. Once primary hyperparathyroidism has been diagnosed by ruling out the other causes for hypercalcemia or by demonstrating an elevated serum PTH or urinary cAMP excretion, the patient is essentially ready for surgery. Preoperative localization of the hyperactive parathyroid glands may be of benefit to the surgeon. The selenomethionine scan has not proven sufficiently sensitive to be clinically useful.[83] An esophagram has been useful on several occasions, but the percentage yield is low because relatively few glands are located to indent the esophagus. Arteriography has been used for localization of the tumor, but a high percentage of false-negative results and the increased complications associated with this procedure in primary hyperparathyroidism have reduced its popularity.[46, 64, 80] A less dangerous, but highly time-consuming and expensive localization method is that of venous catheterization and sampling of the blood for PTH at various points in the neck and superior thoracic cavity.[5, 27, 61, 68] Both arteriography and venous catheterization have been proposed more frequently for persistent hypercalcemia after a previous neck exploration than for the initial workup. Ironically, in the neck operation in which localization is most needed, venous sampling is less reliable because of the distortion of venous drainage by the surgery. Of the several techniques available, sonography seems to have the best chance of developing adequate sensitivity, accuracy, and safety.[62, 77] Using the ordinary B-mode ultrasound, the enlarged parathyroid gland can be detected in over 50% of the cases. New technology may produce a sonographic system with sensitivity capable of detecting most of the cervical parathyroid glands.[29] Since sonography cannot penetrate into the mediastinum, the CT scan has been used for this purpose. Although successful localizations have been reported, the many vascular and other structures in this area may explain the rather low success rate of CT in detecting mediastinal glands.[39] It has not been shown that any of the above procedures are cost effective for the initial neck exploration.

Hypercalcemic crises may occur in primary hyperparathyroidism.[48, 57, 91] Hypercalcemia of greater than 13 mg/dl to 14 mg/dl should be lowered, if possible, in preparation for surgery. (Serum calcium concentrations in the range of 14 mg/dl or below can be simply monitored closely prior to surgery.) Certainly, above 15 mg/dl, hypercalcemia may cause dehydration, cardiac arrhythmias, and central nervous system depression, which add to the risk of anesthesia and surgery. Active steps should be taken to lower these concentrations.[37, 94] Rehydration with saline restores fluid balance and promotes the excretion of calcium, since sodium competes for reabsorption of calcium at the renal tubular level. Calcium excretion can be enhanced further by the diuretic, furosemide. During diuretic–saline therapy, serum magnesium and potassium levels should be carefully monitored because of the preexisting and continuing urinary losses of these electrolytes. The diuretic–saline therapy usually lowers the serum calcium and provides a period of time during which chest x-ray examinations, bone survey, and cervical sonography can be performed. Obviously, if the serum calcium is brought down within a safe range, more complete information such as serum PTH values can be obtained before neck exploration.

Other maneuvers to maintain the normal serum calcium, such as EDTA infusion (must be repeated often), mithramycin (slow in onset of action and with hepatorenal toxicity), or intravenous phosphate (risk of extraosseous calcification), are more problematic than the saline–diuretic regimen. Continuous infusion of thyrocalcitonin is currently being evaluated. The more complex modalities may be worth adding to extend the time if the diagnosis of primary hyperparathyroidism is still in question, especially if the patient is at high risk for surgery owing to other intercurrent diseases.[79]

Intraoperative Considerations

Optimal preparation for surgery, such as restoration of volume deficits, replacement of magnesium and potassium, and lowering of the serum calcium, is really the best intraoperative management of metabolic problems. For example, the premature ventricular contractions seen with hypercalcemia do not respond well to the antiarrhythmic agents until the serum calcium is lowered. Lowering of plasma PCO_2 by intraoperative ventilatory manipulations may temporarily lower the ionized portion of the serum calcium and ameliorate the arrhythmia. Intravenous EDTA or phosphate can also be used, but careful monitoring is mandatory. The complex intraoperative manipulations can be avoided by achieving lowered serum calcium levels prior to surgery. Hypophosphatemia below 1.5 mEq/dl may be associated with an increase in hemoglobin affinity for oxygen and a consequent decrease in release of oxygen to peripheral tissues. Inhalation anesthetics that lower the percentage of inspired oxygen should be avoided. Treatment during the short intraoperative period with intravenous phosphate is obviously more hazardous than is more leisurely preoperative correction of hypophosphatemia.

Postoperative Considerations

Intraoperative surgical goals should be mentioned as preface to a discussion of the postoperative period. The standard surgical treatment of an adenoma is its total removal. At least one of the remaining normal glands should be confirmed on frozen section before the operation is completed. Most experienced surgeons favor histologic identification of all the normal glands in order to rule out the possibility of a second adenoma or asymmetrical hyperplasia with near-normal small glands. Approximately 10% to 15% of primary hyperparathyroidism is caused by hyperplasia of all four glands. With known sporadic hyperplasia, it is customary to identify all four glands, remove three, and leave an approximately 100-mg viable portion of the fourth gland *in situ*.[6, 33] Total parathyroidectomy and autotransplantation of a remnant into the sternocleidomastoid muscle or into the muscle of the forearm have been most strongly recommended for the hyperplasia of secondary hyperparathyroidism when the activity of the gland remnants is likely to increase under the continued stimuli of renal insufficiency. The options of autotransplantation of fresh parathyroid tissue for easy removal with recurrent hypercalcemia or reimplantation of cryopreserved tissue for treatment for postoperative hypocalcemia should be strongly considered in the familial parathyroid syndromes. Because incomplete treatment of these syndromes with standard subtotal parathyroidectomy is common, total parathyroidectomy is advocated.[38, 50, 70] For the usual sporadic case of parathyroid hyperplasia, it is not clear that autotransplantation is less problematic than leaving the remnant *in situ*.[97]

PERSISTENT POSTOPERATIVE HYPERCALCEMIA. Etiologies of persistent postoperative hypercalcemia can be divided into those that are likely when four afflicted glands are found at surgery and those existing when three or fewer glands afflicted are found.

Four Glands Found at Operation
Nonparathyroid cause of hypercalcemia
Ectopic PTH production
Adenoma in fifth parathyroid
Apparently normal glands are really hyperplastic.
Inadequate resection of four obviously hyperplastic glands

Three or Fewer Glands Found at Operation
Missed adenoma
Residual hyperplastic gland

If four normal glands are found, perhaps the greatest likelihood is that of a nonparathyroid cause of the hypercalcemia.[54] A repeat serum PTH or cAMP test is indicated then and, if the subsequent results do not suggest hyperparathyroidism, a more diligent search for nonparathyroid causes for hypercalcemia must be undertaken. One of the most interesting and difficult causes is familial hypocalciuric hypercalcemia probably related to a defect in renal calcium excretion.[56] However, if the hypercalcemia still seems, on further testing, to be due to parathyroid hormone, the other three diagnostic possibilities are an adenoma in a supernumerary parathyroid gland that was missed at the time of surgery, PTH production from a nonparathyroid tumor, or small glands, actually hyperplastic, but erroneously diagnosed intraoperatively as normal.[16, 42, 43, 51, 59, 60, 66, 85, 92, 93] If four demonstrably hyperplastic glands were found, a persistent hypercalcemia might be due to an excessively large amount of parathyroid tissue left in the neck, either as part of the remnant fourth gland or as a hyperplastic supernumerary parathyroid gland. Where three or fewer normal glands are found, the most likely cause of persistent hypercalcemia is an overlooked adenoma. Of course, when three hyperplastic glands are found, the missing fourth gland is an adequate explanation for persistent hypercalcemia. The medical literature is replete with excellent reviews of causes and strategy for parathyroid reexploration.[4, 7, 12, 18, 19, 42, 51, 52, 54, 69, 73, 78, 86, 89] Considerations of localization and reoperation for missing glands are further discussed under operative aspects below.

RECURRENT HYPERCALCEMIA. The reappearance of hypercalcemia, months to years following neck exploration for hyperparathyroidism, commonly results from regrowth of a remnant hyperplastic gland.[42, 51, 73, 95] Occasionally, partial infarction of a missed adenoma will be followed by a return of hypercalcemia. A coincidental appearance of hypercalcemia due to nonparathyroid causes must also be considered. A less common cause is hypercalcemia from recurrence of a parathyroid carcinoma,[34] either previously recognized or erroneously diagnosed as an adenoma.

HYPOPARATHYROIDISM. The pathophysiology of hypoparathyroidism is the reverse of that described for hyperparathyroidism. Without the action of PTH on bone, calcium is deposited into bone at the expense of serum calcium concentrations. In the absence of PTH activity, renal tubular reabsorption of phosphate increases, and the resultant hyperphosphatemia further promotes calcium deposition into bone. The most obvious clinical effects of hypocalcemia are primarily those related to increased neuromuscular excitability. A magnesium deficit may develop during hyperparathyroidism, and hypomagnesemia can add to the hyperreflexia of postoperative hypocalcemia.[47, 84] Neuromuscular excitability may persist unless hypomagnesemia is also corrected.[81] Because the degree of PTH deficiency varies from case to case, the clinical syndrome may also vary in severity and duration.[67] For example, following removal of a large adenoma, hypocalcemia may arise from the avid remineralization of bone that occurs when the osteoclastic stimulation from PTH is removed. Although the function of the remaining normal glands is not completely suppressed, nevertheless, they respond to a fall in serum calcium with inadequate PTH secretion, and mild hypocalcemia results. In another situation, the three remaining glands may have been totally infarcted or removed, which results in absolute hypoparathyroidism and severe hypocalcemia. Serum phosphate concentrations may be useful in distinguishing relative from absolute hypoparathyroidism. With relative hypoparathyroidism and "hungry bones," the serum phosphate tends to be normal, whereas hyperphosphatemia is the rule with absolute PTH deficiency.

Postoperative hypoparathyroidism is suspected from the clinical features confirmed within this context by demonstration of a low serum calcium level.[13] Features such as perioral or acral paresthesias, increased neuromuscular irritability, such as demonstrated by the Chvostek's or Trousseau's sign, or carpopedal or laryngeal spasm exemplify a spectrum of severity. A low serum calcium level alone may not necessarily confirm hypoparathyroidism.[45] A decrease in ionized serum calcium and the clinical features of hypocalcemia can be produced by hyperventilation or severe systemic alkalosis. The total serum calcium level may be low because of low serum proteins that bind calcium, but the ionized calcium concentration may be normal. Therefore, with a finding of asymptomatic hypocalcemia, the serum protein concentration should be determined. Clinical symptoms disproportionately severe for the degree of hypocalcemia should suggest the presence of hypomagnesemia.[75] Confirmation of absolute hypoparathyroidism by demonstrating the absence of serum PTH is usually not possible because of the inability of most assays to distinguish reliably between normal and low or absent concentrations of the hormone. During the hypocalcemia of relative hypoparathyroidism coupled with active bone remineralization, serum PTH concentrations may be fixed at inadequate, but roliable, levels. Normal serum PTH and phosphate concentrations in the face of postoperative hypocalcemia usually indicate a state of relative hypoparathyroidism, from which recovery is probable.

The rate of development and the severity of the hypocalcemia determine therapy for postoperative hypoparathyroidism. These factors are dependent upon the degree of PTH deficiency and the rate of bone remineralization. The three main forms of medical mnagement are oral calcium, intravenous calcium, and vitamin D compounds. Details of these modalities are listed below.

Mild Hypocalcemia

Calcium lactate tablets; 325 or 650 mg, 2–6 tabs, qid (13% elemental calcium)

OR

Calcium glucinate liquid 20–60 ml/day in divided doses (5.75 mEq calcium/5 ml)

Moderate to Severe Hypocalcemia

Calcium chloride, 10% 10 ml slowly, IV (27% elemental calcium). Start oral calcium, also.

Persistent Hypocalcemia (in Spite of Oral Calcium Therapy)

Ergocalciferol (Calciferol), 200,000, IV, each day × 3 days, then 50,000, IV, each day (dose adjusted by serum calcium)

Dihydrotachysterol, 0.5 mg, initial dose, then 0.125 mg/day (dose adjusted by serum calcium)

For the patient with a gradual decrease in serum calcium concentration and resulting mild symptoms, oral calcium compounds may be all that are needed to treat the relative hypoparathyroidism. With a more precipitous fall in the serum calcium level and fairly severe symptoms, intravenous calcium should be administered after a blood sample for baseline calcium is obtained, and the patient should be placed immediately on oral calcium compounds. In many instances, the introduction of oral calcium at the onset of hypocalcemia will obviate the need for subsequent intravenous calcium. However, if, in spite of large amounts of oral calcium compounds, the patient continues to need intermittent intravenous calcium, vitamin D should be initiated in an effort to normalize the serum calcium and to allow discharge of the patient within a reasonable period of time. Although Calciferol is an inexpensive and widely available form of vitamin D, its action takes weeks to maximize and its withdrawal likewise requires weeks of monitoring the serum calcium in assessing vitamin D dependency. Another form of vitamin D, dihydrotachysterol, is fully active within 10 days of administration and has a short biologic half-life that permits abbreviated tapering of the compound at weekly intervals.[28]

Another modality for treatment of hypoparathyroidism is that of autotransplantation of cryopreserved parathyroid tissue.[11, 99] It is mainly useful in parathyroid hyperplasia. Should the gland left behind in the neck or transplanted into an ectopic site be inadequate to maintain normocalcemia, the implantation of cryopreserved tissue into the forearm or sternocleidomastoid muscles can alleviate the hypoparathyroidism. The cryopreserved tissue can remain viable *ex vivo* up to 1 year. Cryopreservation is also useful in reoperations for missed adenomas when search for an adenoma may lead to inadvertent removal or infarction of normal glands with consequent hypoparathyroidism. Permanent hypocalcemia following removal of a single adenoma at the initial operation is uncommon. Regrowth of transplanted hyperactive parathyroid tissue has been reported, but the excess tissue can easily be removed under local anesthesia.[10, 41, 98]

SECONDARY HYPERPARATHYROIDISM

Preoperative Considerations

OVERVIEW. The form of secondary hyperparathyroidism that sometimes commands the attention of the surgeon is associated with renal failure. A "nonsurgical" form of secondary hyperparathyroidism is that seen in some patients with a renal calcium leak, which results in hypercalciuria and stone formation. Because the hypercalciuria is related to a primary renal defect, parathyroidectomy is ineffective. This condition is sometimes known as *normocalcemic hyperparathyroidism.*

One of the earliest events in the course of renal failure is a tendency to retain phosphates. Hyperphosphatemia depresses the serum calcium concentration, which, in turn, stimulates the parathyroid glands to produce more PTH. A new steady state of normocalcemia is reached at the expense of increased parathyroid activity. As phosphate retention becomes more severe, the parathyroid glands become more hyperactive. A second mechanism in renal failure tending toward hypocalcemia and compensatory overactivity of the parathyroid glands is the decreased ability of the kidney to hydroxylate 25 OH_1D_3 to the active form of $1,25(OH)_2D_3$.[2, 24, 65] Hyperphosphatemia also accentuates the hypocalcemia indirectly by inhibiting the formation of this active form of vitamin D by the kidney. The vitamin D deficiency results in a decreased intestinal absorption of calcium and a consequent tendency toward hypocalcemia. Thus, both the hyperphosphatemia and the vitamin D deficiency of renal failure promote secondary hyperparathyroidism.[71]

Metabolic bone disease is the major consequence of the increase in parathyroid activity secondary to hypocalcemia.[20] The bone disease due specifically to excess parathyroid production is known as *osteitis fibrosa.* The bone disease may present as a generalized form or as localized cysts. In many patients, there may be a mixed pattern of osteitis fibrosa and osteomalacia on bone biopsy. Especially in the patients with pure osteitis fibrosa, the serum PTH and alkaline phosphatase levels are usually markedly elevated. Pure osteomalacia, in contrast, seems to be independent of excess parathyroid activity. Other nonosseous features of secondary hyperparathyroidism, such as pruritus, are poorly understood. Extraosseous calcifications are usually a result of vigorous treatment with vitamin D combined with failure to control the hyperphosphatemia by oral phosphate-binding gels.

Tertiary hyperparathyroidism is considered to be the form of parathyroid hyperactivity that arises after chronic stimulation of the parathyroid glands by conditions described above for secondary hyperparathyroidism. Apparently, the mass of parathyroid tissue becomes autonomous. The hormone secretory activity does not remain steady at the level just sufficient to maintain normocalcemia but continues to rise to produce a concentration of serum PTH that results in hypercalcemia. This condition can be seen both in patients currently on hemodialysis and in patients who had hemodialysis before having a renal transplant.[22, 36] Control of hyperphosphatemia is especially critical in the dialysis patient with tertiary hyperparathyroidism; failure to do so can result in extraosseous calcification prior to surgical correction.

DIAGNOSIS. Bone symptoms arising during chronic renal failure or prolonged hemodialysis usually suggest renal osteodystrophy. The symptoms include bone pain, with or without associated pathologic fractures, and joint pains. Muscle weakness may be a prominent part of the symptomatology. Many of these patients also suffer pruritis. The diagnosis can be established by demonstration of subperiosteal bone reabsorption on plain x-ray film or by using fine-grained x-ray film and magnification techniques to demonstrate cortical striations, especially in the shafts of the phalanges and metacarpals. The most definitive diagnosis is made from bone biopsies in which osteoid fibrosis is seen and in which increased bone turnover can be demonstrated by double labeling with tetracycline. Serum PTH is usually markedly elevated, especially if the radioimmunoassay employs an antibody directed to the carboxy terminal of the PTH molecule. Bone biopsy can exclude patients with osteomalacia characterized by unmineralized osteoid seams and slow rates of bone turnover. Serum PTH is usually not elevated in this subgroup of patients with osteomalacia.

PREPARATION FOR SURGERY. Other than the usual preparation of a patient on hemodialysis for surgery, there are no specific requirements for parathyroid surgery, and their normocalcemic state obviates calcium therapy. Patient selection is important. With the recent availability of the $1,25(OH)_2D_3$ form of vitamin D, many patients who were previously inadequately treated medically now can be helped with and even cured of their bone disease.[58] In the past, the serious risks of hypercalcemia and extraosseous calcification from the relatively large doses of vitamin D and even of dihydrotachysterol required in the treatment of renal osteodystrophy made many nephrologists understandably reluctant to increase the vitamin D preparations to their full therapeutic levels. Currently, the use of the dihydroxylated D_3, the phosphate-binding gels and high calcium concentrations in the dialysis fluid have largely prevented secondary hyperparathyroidism and renal osteodystrophy. Such a regimen results in increased serum calcium and decreased serum phosphorus levels. Parathyroid secretion is thereby suppressed by the normal serum calcium, and the bone lesions can heal. Only patients whose symptoms cannot be relieved by optimal adherence to this medical regimen are candidates for parathyroidectomy. Even within the subset of patients who do not respond to vitamin D are those with pure osteomalacia in whom parathyroidectomy is ineffective in healing the bone lesions.

Intraoperative Considerations

Typically, the parathyroid glands of secondary hyperparathyroidism are quite enlarged and easily found, when they are where they should be. For the successful operative treatment of this condition the surgeon must identify all four glands and remember that supernumerary glands, which, when left *in situ*, result in failure to treat adequately the osteodystrophy, have been reported. In considering gland remnant size, note should be taken that, unless renal transplantation is anticipated, the conditions originally stimulating the parathyroid glands will still be present postoperatively. Leaving behind too much residual glandular tissue will result in continuation of PTH hypersecretion and of the bone problems. However, excision of too much tissue will result in renal failure.

Parathyroid autotransplantation into a superficial muscle has been recommended to facilitate possible removal of excess residual glandular tissue at a later date.[98] Cryopreservation of removed glandular tissue and subsequent reimplantation have been suggested as treatment for the possible overzealous resection and the resultant hypocalcemia.[11, 99] Implantation of parathyroid tissue in the muscles of the forearm has the added advantage of allowing assay of the blood coming directly from the implanted gland and comparison of PTH concentrations to those found in blood from other sites. The ability to assess separately the implanted tissue in the forearm is especially useful for distinguishing between excessive implanted tissue in the arm and residual, missed tissue in the neck in patients with persistent bone problems. The location of the implanted gland in the muscles just under the volar skin of the forearm is also convenient in allowing excision of excessive glandular tissue on the one hand, or reimplantation of tissue for a deficit on the other. Either procedure can be done under local anesthesia.

Postoperative Considerations

Genuine proof of the adequacy of the operation is the healing of the bone lesions, demonstrated by x-ray film or bone biopsy. A decrease in serum alkaline phosphatase level is also a satisfactory indicator of effective treatment of secondary hyperparathyroidism. The carboxy terminal of the PTH molecule is the predominant peptide fragment that circulates during renal failure. Unfortunately, this fragment is biologically inactive, and although determining its concentration demonstrates the presence or absence of functioning parathyroid tissue, this does not necessarily reflect the actual amounts of biologically active hormone. Failure of bone lesions to heal may mean inadequate removal of parathyroid tissue from the neck or implantation of excessive amounts of parathyroid tissue in the forearm. Failure of lesions to heal may also indicate the presence of pure osteomalacia, rather than osteitis fibrosa.

Treatment of hypocalcemia in the face of renal failure may be particularly difficult because of the large doses of vitamin D that may be required. The calcium concentrations must be increased in the dialysate, and every effort should be made to decrease the intestinal absorption of phosphate by dietary means and by the use of phosphate-binding gel. The difficulty in this treatment emphasizes the importance of cryopreservation of removed parathyroid tissue. By implanting small slivers of the viable parathyroid tissue, the surgeon may effect a cure.

Operative Aspects

IDENTIFYING PARATHYROID GLANDS

Since persistent hypercalcemia most often arises from failure to locate pathologic parathyroid glands, some discussion of identification is warranted. In spite of recent emphasis on preoperative localization of the enlarged glands, identification of the gland by an experienced surgeon at the initial operation is essential to success. The normal parathyroid gland can vary in size from 4 mm to 10 mm and weigh up to 60 mg.[3, 10] The yellowish tan color, the homogenous appearance of the surface, and the soft consistency of these glands are most helpful characteristics in identification. Adenomas may be yellowish brown but more often are somewhat reddish brown, or, if their blood supply has been disturbed by dissection, they may become dark brown or almost black. They can vary in size from 1 cm to several centimeters. Hyperplastic glands are found in various colors, ranging from yellowish tan to dark brownish red.[17, 21] The configuration can be that of the round or oblong, unilocular tumor, similar to an adenoma, or they may be multinodular or lobulated.[88]

Toluidine blue has been given intravenously to patients during surgery in order to stain the parathyroid glands a darker blue than the surrounding tissue.[72] A critical dose of the dye must be used in order to avoid turning all tissues a dark blue. Many experienced parathyroid surgeons prefer to see the glands color coded in their natural hues, and this attitude, along with the cardiotoxicity of the dye, discredited this intraoperative method of identification. Other promising methods distinguish normal from hyperactive or adenomatous from hyperplastic glands on the basis of density, parenchymal cell mass, intracellular fat, or cell surface antigens.[1, 23, 93, 100] These methods may prove quite valuable after further clinical evaluation.

Locating the Gland at the Initial Operation

Although the parathyroid glands are capable of a notoriously wide anatomical distribution, they are most often located within a limited number of specific areas.[88] The upper parathyroid glands, which arise from the fourth branchial pouch, are usually located in close proximity to the posterior aspect of the upper pole of the thyroid. A second common location is along the cricopharyngeal muscle just posterior to the upper thyroid pole. The lower parathyroid glands originate in the third branchial pouch, along with the thymus, and usually descend to the level of the lower pole of the thyroid lobe. When adenomatous, either upper or lower gland tends to migrate downward, presumably under the pull of gravity. The upper gland can be found in the posterior mediastinum along the esophagus. The lower glands can migrate in a similar fashion into the mediastinum, but the lower glands are more commonly found within the thymic tissue. In fact, the lower glands can be found in the thymic tract anywhere from the level of the hyoid bone down into the mediastinum.[3, 31] Upper or lower glands have been found in such locations as the posterior surface of the sternohyoid muscle, within the carotid sheath, retrotracheal, retroesophageal, within the esophageal wall, above the hyoid, and intrathyroidal.

THYROIDECTOMY. The upper parathyroid glands, especially, may be found within the thyroid capsule.[44, 82, 87, 90] Careful subcapsular search should be made behind the upper thyroid pole for this gland. Parathyroid glands can actually be located within the substance of the thyroid gland; the incidence is as high as 5% in some series. Therefore, if after thorough neck exploration, only three normal glands have been found and an adenoma presumably missed or if only three hyperplastic glands have been found, a thyroid lobectomy should be done on the side of the missing gland. Thin slices are made of the removed thyroid lobe to allow identification of a parathyroid adenoma or hyperplastic gland. In theory, postoperative thyroid hormonal replacement may be indicated, at least to prevent chronic TSH stimulation of the contralateral thyroid lobe.

THYMECTOMY. As mentioned above, the lower parathyroid glands can be located in the thymus. The superior limits of the thymus can usually be detected on either side of the neck as a fibrous strand beginning near the anterolateral surface of the trachea, at the level of the lower thyroid pole, and expanding into a definite fleshy entity before entering the mediastinum behind each clavicle. By careful dissection, it is usually possible to free a large portion of the thymus from its mediastinal location.[35] Occasionally, small veins exiting from the lateral portions of the thymus need to be clipped or ligated. Approximately 20% of adenomas occurring in the lower glands will be located in the thymic tissue. Only a very small percentage of these cannot be retrieved from the mediastinum by the neck approach.

Reoperation

Reoperation is usually indicated for persistent parathyroid-related hypercalcemia. In postoperative hypercalcemia from an excessively large hyperplastic parathyroid remnant, the reoperative approach is simplified by knowing the details of the previous surgery, such as the histologic confirmation of glandular pathology and location. Cure is usually effected by further resection of the parathyroid remnant. Autotransplantation of parathyroid tissue into the forearm may prevent a second neck reoperation.[12, 30, 78] If on reexploration of the neck the remnant is only 50 mg to 100 mg, an effort should be made to find a supernumerary gland. In postoperative hypercalcemia following identification of only three normal glands, diagnosis is somewhat more complex because of the possibility of non-PTH causes of hypercalcemia. However, if the repeated diagnostic evidence still points to parathyroid-related hypercalcemia and no ectopic source can be found, a residual adenoma must be the presumed culprit. A similar presumption must be made if four normal glands were found at the time of surgery, but, here, the adenoma may be in a supernumerary gland. Finally, when only three hyperplastic glands were found, the persistent hypercalcemia is a certain indication that the missing gland is hyperplastic and the cause of the hypercalcemia. The decision whether to reexplore the neck first or to proceed directly with mediastinal exploration is influenced somewhat by what was found at the initial neck exploration; again, accurate information from the previous operation is most helpful. If the initial operation was properly done, including cervical thymectomy and thyroidectomy and a thorough search in all the ectopic cervical locations was performed, it may be justified to proceed with mediastinal exploration. Generally reasonable doubt about the absolute completeness of the cervical exploration remains so that a reexploration of the neck precedes the mediastinal exploration. Although preoperative localization procedures are not infallible, they may be useful in correctly leading the surgeon into a general area such as the left or right neck or the mediastinum.[32, 68, 96]

PREOPERATIVE LOCALIZATION PROCEDURES. Preoperative localization procedures were discussed in an earlier section so only points relevant to reoperation are mentioned here. Although barium swallow in the esophagus has a high false-negative rate, it is relatively innocuous and inexpensive and is justified prior to reoperation. Arteriography using the Seldinger technique has revealed the location of mediastinal parathyroid glands. Especially distinctive is the tracing of the small nutrient artery to the point of a tumor blush at the location of the hyperactive gland. Several centers have abandoned this technique because of the unusually high rate of cerebral complications. Arterial catheterization may infarct the tumor and should be considered as an alternative to surgery in the high-risk patient.[25, 26] Venous catheterization and assay of PTH in the blood sampled from various locations in the neck and the mediastinum depend upon the availability of a skilled radiologist, a reliable PTH assay, money, and time. Previous removal of the thyroid makes interpretation of the sonogram problematical in that one of the useful landmarks is gone. Because of the bone density, sonography cannot be used in the mediastinum. CT scan has been used in both the neck and the mediastinum, but the success rate is quite low in the neck. To date, several parathyroid adenomas have been detected in the mediastinum by this method, but not enough use has been made of the technique to assess it accurately. Refinements in CT scans and intravenous arteriography may make these procedures extremely useful in the future.

MEDIASTINAL EXPLORATION. With persistent hypercalcemia and a firm diagnosis of hyperparathyroidism, mediastinal exploration is indicated under several circumstances.[63,74,76] A mediastinal exploration should be done when significant hypercalcemia persists, a parathyroid source is again implicated, the preoperative localization tests have pointed toward the mediastinum as the location of the missing adenoma or hyperplastic gland, and, especially, when a thorough neck operation, including a cervical thymectomy and thyroid lobectomy, has been performed. In the absence of preoperative mediastinal localization, the operating surgeon probably cannot be absolutely certain that every possible cervical area was exhaustively searched at the initial exploration. Rather than proceeding directly to the mediastinum, the neck is usually reexplored in the second operation unless the gland is definitely not in that area. Unless the cervical reexploration was uncharacteristically easy, sternotomy should best follow the neck dissection, with time allowed to assess the serum calcium level and to stabilize any morbidity incurred from the difficult cervical procedure. An exception to the waiting approach might be marked hypercalcemia refractory to medical management. The sternum can be split from the suprasternal notch all the way to the xiphoid, although many surgeons take the sternotomy down to the level just below the third costochondral junction and the incision out into the third intercostal spaces. Hemostasis is as important for visualization in the mediastinum as it is in the neck. The pleura should be carefully stripped from the posterior edge of the sternum. The lower parathyroid glands are most often associated with the thymus, but a previously complete thymectomy through the cervical approach does not rule out a mediastinal adenoma. Adenomas have been found posterior to the aortic arch and even within the pericardial sac.

POSTOPERATIVE HOARSENESS

Postoperative hoarseness may arise either from edema of the vocal cords or from damage to the laryngeal nerve. Laryngeal nerve damage is more fully discussed in the chapter on thyroid surgery. Hoarsensss from edema is more apt to occur after a prolonged, thorough search for parathyroid glands than after a routine thyroidectomy. At particular risk is the patient in whom an extensive neck dissection is performed, particularly with exploration posterior to the esophagus and cricopharyngeous muscle. The voice may have a husky, rasping quality that is somewhat different from the quality of voice heard with pure laryngeal nerve damage. Of course, the edema is usually bilateral, and the development of such a voice during the postoperative period should alert the physician to the possibility of ensuing respiratory difficulty.

POSTOPERATIVE RESPIRATORY DIFFICULTY

Bilateral recurrent laryngeal nerve injury, though possible with parathyroid surgery, is more often encountered after total thyroidectomy and is discussed in the chapter on thyroid operations.

Vocal Cord Edema

Edema is probably the most common cause of respiratory difficulty in the patient who underwent parathyroid exploration. Inspiratory stridor may be the initial clue to impending respiratory embarrassment from edema of the cords. Both humidification of inspired air and high-dose dexamethasone administration have been advocated for laryngeal edema. It is imperative that a tracheostomy tray be maintained at bedside with the other necessary accompaniments, such as good lighting, gloves, and so on. Should there be any question of maintenance of a safe airway, performance of tracheostomy in the operating room is indicated. Attempts at endotracheal intubation through an edematous hypopharynx and larynx may result in critical delays.

Laryngospasm From Tetany

It is unusual for a hospitalized patient to reach such a severe stage of hypocalcemia as tetany. However, a fairly precipitous drop of serum calcium over several hours may follow a total parathyroidectomy in a patient with markedly dimineralized bones. The usual context for such severe tetany is the latent postoperative parathyroid insufficiency that may become clinically pronounced after the patient's discharge. The clue to diagnosis of laryngospasm as a cause of upper-airway obstruction is the concomitant peripheral signs of neuromuscular irritability, such as carpopedal spasm, tingling, and hyperreflexia. After a blood sample has been obtained for documentation of the hypocalcemia, intravenous calcium is given immediately (e.g., 1 g CaCl over 10 min) and an oral calcium regimen initiated. The serum magnesium concentration should also be determined from the same blood sample.

Pneumothorax

Pneumothorax should be within the differential diagnosis of postoperative dyspnea and hypoxia. This event might occur during a low neck dissection or a formal mediastinal exploration. From the cervical approach, searching the upper mediastinum for an adenoma brings the dissection near each dome of the pleura. A routine postoperative chest x-ray film is recommended following any cervical or mediastinal procedure for hyperparathyroidism. Should a pneumothorax greater than 10% occur, insertion of a chest tube connected to underwater seal is the safest treatment. A pneumothorax of lesser degree might be safely monitored with a second chest x-ray film soon after the initial one. Progression of the small pneumothorax warrants a chest tube insertion.

HORNER'S SYNDROME

The sympathetic ganglia and chain can be damaged in searching for parathyroid glands in the retroesophageal area or posterior to the carotid sheath. Especially vulnerable are the stellate ganglia, which lie on the anterolateral surface of the C7–T1 vertebral bodies. The patient will experience meiosis, narrowing of the palpebral fissure, and ipsilateral anhydrosis of the face and arm. Fortunately, the syndrome is usually temporary in this context.

References

1. Åkerström G, Grimelius L, Johansson H et al: Parenchymal cell mass determination in parathyroid glands and its application in a material of hyperparathyroidism. World J Surg 5:555, 1981
2. Avioli LV: Hormonal aspects of vitamin D metabolism and its clinical implications. Clin Endocrinol Metab 8:547, 1979
3. Beahrs OH, Edis AJ, Purnell DC: Unusual problems in parathyroid surgery. Am J Surg 134:502, 1977
4. Beazley RM, Costa J, Ketcham AS: Reoperative parathyroid surgery. Am J Surg 130:427, 1975
5. Bilezikian JP, Doppman JL, Shimkin PM et al: Preoperative localization of abnormal parathyroid tissue. Am J Med 55:505, 1973
6. Block MA, Frame B, Jackson CE: The efficacy of subtotal parathyroidectomy for primary hyperparathyroidism due to multiple gland involvement. Surg Gynecol Obstet 147:1, 1978
7. Block MA, Frame B, Kleerekoper M, Rao DS: Surgical management of persistence or recurrence after subtotal parathyroidectomy for primary hyperparathyroidism. Am J Surg 138:561, 1979
8. Bone HG, Snyder WH, Pak CYC: Diagnosis of hyperparathyroidism. Annu Rev Med 28:111, 1977
9. Bouillon R: Clinical applications and technical aspects of parathyroid hormone measurements. Ric Clin Lab 8:75, 1978
10. Brennan MF, Brown EM, Marx SJ et al: Recurrent hyperparathyroidism from an autotransplanted parathyroid adenoma. N Engl J Med 299:1057, 1978
11. Brennan MF, Brown EM, Spiegel AM et al: Autotransplantation of cryopreserved parathyroid tissue in man. Ann Surg 189:139, 1979
12. Brennan MF, Marx SJ, Doppman J et al: Results of reoperation for persistent and recurrent hyperparathyroidism. Ann Surg 194:671, 1981
13. Breslau NA, Pak CYC: Hypoparathyroidism. Metabolism 28:1261, 1979
14. Broadus AE, Horst RL, Lang R et al: The importance of circulating 1,25-dihydroxyvitamin D in the pathogenesis of hypercalciuria and renal-stone formation in primary hyperparathyroidism. N Engl J Med 302:421, 1980
15. Broadus AE, Rasmussen H: Clinical evaluation of parathyroid function. Am J Med 70:475, 1981

16. Carnevale N, Samson R, Bennett BP: Multiple parathyroid adenomas. JAMA 246:1332, 1981
17. Castleman B, Schantz A, Roth SI: Parathyroid hyperplasia in primary hyperparathyroidism. Cancer 38:1668, 1976
18. Christensen MS: Radioimmunoassay of human parathyroid hormone. Dan Med Bull 26:157, 1979
19. Clark OH, Way LW, Hunt TK: Recurrent hyperparathyroidism. Ann Surg 184:391, 1976
20. Coburn JW: Renal osteodystrophy. Kidney Int 17:677, 1980
21. Cope O, Keynes M, Roth SI, Castleman B: Primary chief-cell hyperplasia of the parathyroid glands: A new entity in the surgery of hyperparathyroidism. Ann Surg 148:375, 1958
22. David DS, Sakai S, Brennan BL et al: Hypercalcemia after renal transplantation. N Engl J Med 289:389, 1973
23. Dekker A, Watson CG, Barnes EL Jr: The pathologic assessment of primary hyperparathyroidism and its impact on therapy: A prospective evaluation of 50 cases with oil-red-0 stain. Ann Surg 190:671, 1979
24. DeLuca HF: The kidney as an endocrine organ for the production of 1,25-dihydroxyvitamin D_3, a calcium-mobilizing hormone. N Engl J Med 289:359, 1973
25. Doppman JL: The treatment of hyperparathyroidism by transcatheter techniques. Cardiovasc Intervent Radiol 3:268, 1980
26. Doppman JL, Brown EM, Brennan MF: Angiographic ablation of parathyroid adenomas. Diagn Radiol 130:577, 1979
27. Dunlop DAB, Papapoulous SE, Lodge RW et al: Parathyroid venous sampling: Anatomic considerations and results in 95 patients with primary hyperparathyroidism. Br J Radiol 53:183, 1980
28. Dymling J–F, Ryd H: Crystalline dihydrotachysterol (Dygratyl[R]) in the treatment of hypoparathyroidism. Acta Med Scand 184:333, 1968
29. Edis AJ, Evans TC: High-resolution, real-time ultrasonography in the preoperative location of parathyroid tumors. N Engl J Med 301:532, 1968
30. Edis AJ, Linos DA, Kao PC: Parathyroid autotransplantation at the time of operation for persistent hyperparathyroidism. Surgery 88:588, 1980
31. Edis AJ, Purnell DC, Van Heerden JA: The undescended "parathymus." An occasional cause of failed neck exploration for hyperparathyroidism. Ann Surg 190:64, 1979
32. Edis AJ, Sheedy PF, Beahrs OH, Van Heerden JA: Results of reoperation for hyperparathyroidism with evaluation of preoperative localization studies. Surgery 84:384, 1978
33. Edis AJ, van Heerden JA, Scholz DA: Results of subtotal parathyroidectomy for primary chief cell hyperplasia. Surgery 86:462, 1979
34. Flye MW, Brennan MF: Surgical resection of metastatic parathyroid carcinoma. Ann Surg 193:425, 1981
35. Freeman JB, Sherman BM, Mason EE: Transcervical thymectomy. Arch Surg 111:359, 1976
36. Geis WP, Popovtzer MM, Corman JL et al: The diagnosis and treatment of hyperparathyroidism after renal transplantation. Surg Gynecol Obstet 137:997, 1973
37. Goldsmith RS: Treatment of hypercalcemia. Med Clin North Am 56:951, 1972
38. Goldsmith RS, Sizemore GW, Chen I-W, Zalme E, Altemeier WE: Familial hyperparathyroidism: Description of a large kindred with physiologic observations and a review of the literature. Ann Intern Med 84:36, 1976
39. Goulliamos AD, Carter BL: Parathyroid adenomas: Identified by CT scan. Comput Tomog 5:59, 1981
40. Grimelius L, Åkerström G, Johansson H: The parathyroids: Location and histopathological diagnosis. Monograph, Institute of Pathology and Department of Surgery, University Hospital, Uppsala, 1981
41. Haase GM, Luce JM, Lock JP et al: Hyperparathyroidism following parathyroid autotransplantation. Surgery 86:694, 1979
42. Haff RC, Ballinger WF: Causes of recurrent hypercalcemia after parathyroidectomy for primary hyperparathyroidism. Ann Surg 173:884, 1971
43. Hardy JD, Snavely JR, Langford HG: Low intrathoracic parathyroid adenoma: Large functioning tumor representing fifth parathyroid, opposite eighth dorsal vertebra with independent arterial supply and opacified at operation with arteriogram. Ann Surg 159:310, 1964
44. Herbst JW, Neff WR, Freemant JB: Hyperparathyroidism: Ectopic parathyroid glands. Am J Surg 131:380, 1976
45. Juan D: Hypocalcemia: Differential diagnosis and mechanisms. Arch Intern Med 139:1166, 1979
46. Jelenko C, Teeslink CR, Herndon JR et al: Localization of parathyroid adenomata by selective arteriography. Am Surg 37:25, 1971
47. Jones CTA, Sellwood RA, Evanson JM: Symptomatic hypomagnesaemia after parathyroidectomy. Br Med J 3:391, 1973
48. Kelly TR, Zarconi J: Primary hyperparathyroidism: Hyperparathyroid crisis. Am J Surg 142:539, 1981
49. Lafferty FW: Primary hyperparathyroidism: Changing clinical spectrum, prevalence of hypertension, and discriminant analysis of laboratory tests. Arch Intern Med 141:1761, 1981
50. Lamers CBHW, Froeling PGAM: Clinical significance of hyperparathyroidism in familial multiple endocrine adenomatosis type I (MEA I). Am J Med 66:422, 1979
51. Livesay JJ, Mulder DG: Recurrent hyperparathyroidism. Arch Surg 111:688, 1976
52. McGarity WC, Goldman AL: Reoperation for primary hyperparathyroidism. Ann Surg 194:134, 1981
53. Mallette LE, Bilezikian JP, Heath DA, Aurbach GD: Primary hyperparathyroidism clinical and biochemical features. Medicine 53:127, 1974
54. Martin JK, van Heerden JA, Edis AJ, Dahlin DC: Persistent postoperative hyperparathyroidism. Surg Gynecol Obstet 151:764, 1980
55. Martin JK, Hruska K, Freitag J et al: Clinical utility of radioimmunoassays for parathyroid hormone. Mineral Electrolyte Metab 3:283, 1980
56. Marx SJ, Stock JL, Attie MF et al: Familial hypocalciuric hypercalcemia: Recognition among patients referred after unsuccessful parathyroid exploration. Ann Intern Med 92:351, 1980
57. Maselly MJ, Lawrence AM, Brooks M et al: Hyperparathyroid crisis: Successful treatment of ten comatose patients. Surgery 90:741, 1981
58. Massry SG, Goldstein DA, Malluche HH: Current status of the use of $1,25(OH)_2D_3$ in the management of renal osteodystrophy. Kidney Int 18:409, 1980
59. Max MH, Lawrence PH: Ectopic secretion of parathyroid hormone. Surg Gynecol Obstet 150:411, 1980
60. Monchik JM, Nelson TG, Powell DA: Adenoma in a fifth parathyroid gland: The role of selective venous catheterization. Surgery 73:782, 1973
61. Monchik JM, Pallotta JA, Sacks B, Shimkin PM: Role of selective venous catheterization of the small thyroid

veins as a diagnostic study in hypercalcemic states. Am J Surg 139:575, 1980
62. Moreau J–F, Dubost C, Buy J–N, Ferry J: Dépistage ultrasonographique pré-opératoire des adénomes parathyroidiens. La Nouvelle Presse Médicale 10:1923, 1981
63. Nathaniels EK, Nathaniels AM, Wang C-A: Mediastinal parathyroid tumors: A clinical and pathological study of 84 cases. Ann Surg 171:165, 1970
64. Newton TH, Eisenberg E: Angiography of parathyroid adenomas. Radiology 86:843, 1966
65. Norman AW: 1,25-Dihydroxyvitamin D_3 and 24,25-Dihydroxyvitamin D_3: Key components of the vitamin D endocrine system. Contrib Nephrol 18:1, 1980
66. Palmer JA, Sutton FR: Importance of a fifth parathyroid gland in the surgical treatment of hyperparathyroidism. Can J Surg 21:350, 1978
67. Parfitt AM: The spectrum of hypoparathyroidism. J Clin Endocrinol Metab 34:152, 1972
68. Powell D, Shimkin PM, Doppman JL et al: Primary hyperparathyroidism: Preoperative tumor localization and differentiation between adenoma and hyperplasia. N Engl J Med 286:1169, 1972
69. Prinz RA, Gamvros OI, Allison DJ et al: Reoperations for hyperparathyroidism. Surg Gynecol Obstet 152:760, 1981
70. Prinz RA, Gamvros OI, Sellu D, Lynn JA: Subtotal parathyroidectomy for primary chief cell hyperplasia of the multiple endocrine neoplasia type I syndrome. Ann Surg 193:26, 1981
71. Ritz E, Bommer J: Pathogenesis of renal secondary hyperparathyroidism. Dialy Transplant 10:479, 1981
72. Rosen IB, Bohnen DR, Walfish PG: The use of toluidine blue in locating abnormal parathyroid tissue at operation. Can Med Assoc J 110:393, 1974
73. Roslyn JJ, Mulder DG, Gordon HE: Persistent and recurrent hyperparathyroidism. Am J Surg 142:21, 1981
74. Rothmund M, Diethelm L, Brünner H, Kümmerle F: Diagnosis and surgical treatment of mediastinal parathyroid tumors. Ann Surg 183:139, 1976
75. Rude RK, Singer FR: Magnesium deficiency and excess. Annu Rev Med 32:245, 1981
76. Russell CF, Edis AJ, Scholz DA et al: Mediastinal parathyroid tumors: Experience with 38 tumors requiring mediastinotomy for removal. Ann Surg 193:805, 1981
77. Sample WF, Mitchell SP, Bledsoe RC: Parathyroid ultrasonography. Radiology 127:485, 1978
78. Saxe AW, Brennan MF: Strategy and technique of reoperative parathyroid surgery. Surgery 89:417, 1981
79. Schweitzer VG, Thompson NW, Harness JK, Nishiyama RH: Management of severe hypercalcemia caused by primary hyperparathyroidism. Arch Surg 113:373, 1978
80. Seldinger SI: Localization of parathyroid adenomata by arteriography. Acta Radiol [Diagn] (Stockh) 42:353, 1954
81. Slatopolsky E, Rosenbaum R, Mennes P, Klahr S: The hypocalcemia of magnesium depletion. Adv Exp Med Biol 103:263, 1977
82. Spiegel AM, Marx SJ, Doppman JL et al: Intrathyroidal parathyroid adenoma or hyperplasia: An occasionally overlooked cause of surgical failure in primary hyperparathyroidism. JAMA 234:1029, 1975
83. Stock JL, Krudy AG, Doppman JL et al: Parathyroid imaging after intra-arterial injections of [^{75}Se]Selenomethionine. J Clin Endocrinol Metab 52:835, 1981
84. Sutton RAL: Plasma magnesium concentration in primary hyperparathyroidism. Br Med J 1:529, 1970
85. Verdonk CA, Edis AJ: Parathyroid "double adenomas": Fact or fiction? Surgery 90:523, 1981
86. Vroonhoven TJ, Muller H: Causes of failure in the surgical treatment of primary hyperparathyroidism: Lessons from 51 successful reoperations. Br J Surg 65:297, 1978
87. Vellar ID, Shaw J, Brosnan G: Glandula in glandula: The intrathyroid parathyroid. Aust NZ J Surg 42:257, 1973
88. Wang C–A: The anatomic basis of parathyroid surgery. Ann Surg 183:271, 1976
89. Wang C–A: Parathyroid re-exploration: A clinical and pathological study of 112 cases. Ann Surg 186:140, 1977
90. Wang C–A: Hyperfunctioning intrathyroid parathyroid gland: A potential cause of failure in parathyroid surgery. J R Soc Med 74:49, 1981
91. Wang C–A, Guyton SW: Hyperparathyroid crisis: Clinical and pathological studies of 14 patients. Ann Surg 190:782, 1979
92. Wang C–A, Mahaffey JE, Axelrod L, Perlman JA: Hyperfunctioning supernumerary parathyroid glands. Surg Gynecol Obstet 148:711, 1979
93. Wang C–A, Rieder SV: A density test for the intraoperative differentiation of parathyroid hyperplasia from neoplasia. Ann Surg 187:63, 1978
94. Watson L: Diagnosis and treatment of hypercalcaemia. Br Med J 2:150, 1972
95. Wells SA: Hypercalcemia following parathyroid transplantation. Surgery 86:775, 1979
96. Wells SA, Doppman JL, Bilezikian JP et al: Repeated neck exploration in primary hyperparathyroidism: Localization of abnormal glands by selective thyroid arteriography, selective venous sampling, and radioimmunoassay. Surgery 74:678, 1973
97. Wells SA, Ellis G, Gunnells C et al: Parathyroid autotransplantation in primary parathyroid hyperplasia. N Engl J Med 295:57, 1976
98. Wells SA, Farndon JR, Dale JK et al: Long-term evaluation of patients with primary parathyroid hyperplasia managed by total parathyroidectomy and heterotopic autotransplantation. Ann Surg 192:451, 1980
99. Wells SA, Gunnels JC, Gurman RA et al: The successful transplantation of frozen parathyroid tissue in man. Surgery 81:86, 1977
100. Woltering EA, Emmot RC, Javadpour N et al: ABO(H) cell surface antigens in parathyroid adenoma and hyperplasia. Surgery 90:1, 1981

Suggested Reading

Anast CS: Parathyroid disorders in children. Pediatr Ann 9:28, 1980

Chan JCM, DeLuca HR: Calcium and parathyroid disorders in children. JAMA 241:1242, 1979

Clark OH: The hypercalcemic syndrome: Hyperparathyroidism. In Friesen SR (ed): Surgical Endocrinology: Clinical Syndromes. Philadelphia, JB Lippincott, 1978

Coe FL, Favus MJ: Does mild, asymptomatic hyperparathyroidism require surgery? N Engl J Med 302:224, 1980

Coffey RJ, Lee TC, Canary JJ: The surgical treatment of primary hyperparathyroidism: A 20 year experience. Ann Surg 185:518, 1977

Colacchio TA, LoGerfo P, Feind C: Surgical treatment of parathyroid disease: A review. Head Neck Surg 2:487, 1980

Dolgin C, Gerfo PL, Livolsi V, Feind C: Twenty-five year experience with primary hyperparathyroidism at Columbia Presbyterian Medical Center. Head Neck Surg 2:92, 1979

Egdahl RH: Surgery of the parathyroid glands. Surg Gynecol Obstet 130:901, 1970

Friedman EW, Schwartz AE, Spiro RH: Changing patterns in hyperparathyroidism. Surg Gynecol Obstet 137:941, 1973

Haff RC, Armstrong RG: Trends in the current management of primary hyperparathyroidism. Surgery 75:715, 1974

Harrison H, Duarte B, Reitz RE et al: Primary hyperparathyroidism: Four- to eight-year postoperative follow-up demonstrating persistent functional insignificance of microscopic parathyroid hyperplasia and decreased autonomy of parathyroid hormone release. Ann Surg 194(4):429-437, 1981

Heath H, Hodgson SF, Kennedy MA: Primary hyperparathyroidism: Incidence, morbidity, and potential economic impact in a community. N Engl J Med 302:189, 1980

Johansson H, Thorén L, Åkerström G: "Conservative" vs "liberal" approach to parathyroid neck exploration. Surgery 83:752, 1978

Kay S: The abnormal parathyroid. Hum Pathol 7:127, 1976

Kelly TR: Primary hyperparathyroidism: A personal experience with 242 cases. Am J Surg 140:632, 1980

McGarity WC, Mathews WH, Fulenwider JT et al: The surgical management of primary hyperparathyroidism. Ann Surg 193:794, 1981

Mannix H, Pyrtek LJ, Crombie HD, Canalis E: Hyperparathyroidism in the elderly. Am J Surg 139:581, 1980

Mansberger AR: Special article: Surgical diseases of the parathyroid glands. Am Surg 44:237, 1978

Schafer M, Economou SG: Ode to an indian rhinoceros: Or the evaluation and preparation of patients for parathyroid surgery. Surg Clin North Am 50:227, 1970

Schantz A, Castleman B: Parathyroid carcinoma: A study of 70 cases. Cancer 31:600, 1973

Scholz DA, Purnell DC: Asymptomatic primary hyperparathyroidism: 10-Year prospective study. Mayo Clin Proc 56:473, 1981

Scott HW, Richie RE, Crane JM et al: Surgical experience with hyperparathyroidism. Am Surg 47:54, 1981

Taylor GW: Surgery of hyperparathyroid disease. Br J Surg 67:731, 1980

Tsang RC, Noguchi A, Steichen JJ: Pediatric parathyroid disorders. Pediatr Clin North Am 26:223, 1979

Villar HV, Wangensteen SL: Surgery of the parathyroid glands. In Brown BR Jr (ed): Anesthesia and the Patient with Endocrine Disease. Philadelphia, FA Davis, 1980

Wang C–A: Surgery of the parathyroid glands. Adv Surg 5:109, 1971

Wells SA, Leight GS, Ross AJ: Primary hyperparathyroidism. Curr Probl Surg 17:398, 1980

45 Complications of Pituitary Gland Surgery

Richard L. Corales | Donald P. Becker

OVERVIEW

Since the first report of an attempted removal of a pituitary tumor by craniotomy in 1893, the operative approach to these tumors has varied according to the technical and scientific developments of each era.[1] *In 1905, Krause and, in 1906, Horsley advocated operative transcranial approaches through the anterior and middle fossas, respectively.*[17, 18] *Then, in 1907, Schloffer reported the first transsphenoidal approach to pituitary tumors.*[29] *Shortly later (1910), Halstead reported the first complication of the transsphenoidal approach, a patient who died shortly after surgery with symptoms suggestive of hypothalamic damage.*[11] *Between 1909 and 1928, Harvey Cushing adopted and popularized this approach, performing 242 transsphenoidal procedures, before the development of antibiotics and steroid replacement, with a mortality rate of 5.4%.*[4, 5, 15]

After 1928, Cushing abandoned the transsphenoidal approach for the midline transfrontal approach, which at that time allowed better direct visualization of suprasellar tumor and the optic chiasm, with a lowered incidence of cerebrospinal fluid (CSF) rhinorrhea and infection. Until the late 1950s, the transcranial approach to the sella remained the most widely used, despite the reports of several large series using the transsphenoidal procedure during this time.[6, 16] *The transsphenoidal procedure was revived in 1959, when Guiot reported the advantages of this approach using intraoperative image-intensified fluoroscopy and the routine use of antibiotics and replacement steroids.*[10] *Hardy later added the use of the operating microscope and microsurgical technique, which enabled the selective removal of both large and small tumors with less morbidity and mortality while preserving normal pituitary gland.*[12–14] *These and other recent refinements in the transsphenoidal procedure now allow neurosurgeons to remove pituitary adenomas efficiently and spare normal pituitary tissue, with a low incidence of morbidity and mortality.*[36]

Even though the microsurgical transsphenoidal approach has now gained widespread popularity, the transcranial approach has specific indications. Pituitary tumors with suprasellar extension and a normal sella turcica should be approached from above. Also, the transcranial approach may be more advantageous when the diagnosis of pituitary tumor is uncertain or in the presence of additional intracranial pathology. Tumors with loculated suprasellar extensions into the anterior and middle fossas may frequently require a transcranial approach, either primarily or staged with a previous transsphenoidal decompression. Generally, the operative approach employed depends upon the tumor's type, size, and extension and the goals of therapy for each individual patient. The surgical goals for each patient may vary according to the individual tumor type (hormonal secreting versus nonsecreting) and clinical presentation. Optimally, the surgeon should attempt complete removal of the pituitary adenoma while preserving normal pituitary tissue and function, with a negligible incidence of morbidity and mortality.

Intracranial Complications

Intracranial complications are the most severe, being the major cause of significant morbidity and mortality in most series. Injuries to intracranial structures adjacent to the sella such as optic nerves and chiasm, hypothalamus, carotid arteries, cavernous sinus, or cranial nerves usually occur with the removal of the suprasellar and parasellar extensions of the larger pituitary adenomas. Extensive knowledge of the microsurgical anatomy and anatomical variations of each of these structures is critical in avoiding devastating complications.[27] Because many of the complications related to craniotomy are discussed elsewhere in this text (Part 7), the emphasis here is upon the intracranial complications of the transsphenoidal approach.

When using the transcranial approach, the optic nerves and chiasm present a barrier to the exposure of the pituitary fossa. With this approach comes a 2% to 7.5% incidence of worsening of vision postoperatively.[7, 26] Preoperative knowledge of the anatomical position and variations of the chiasm in relation to the diaphragma sella and pituitary tumor may reflect the direction of suprasellar tumor growth as well as dictate the safest surgical approach needed for its removal. Injury to the optic nerves and chiasm is less likely when using the transsphenoidal approach and then only when the tumor "capsule" is disrupted during removal of suprasellar tumor.[21] However, from either approach, ischemic damage may result from injury to the small perforating vessels of the chiasm and optic nerves.

Postoperative visual impairment may result with compression of the chiasm from a postoperative hematoma, from overzealous packing of the evacuated tumor cavity, or secondary to prolapse of the chiasm and optic nerves into the evacuated sella cavity.[9] Optic nerve damage may also result from fractures through the optic foramen produced by the speculum retractors used in the transsphenoidal approach. Regardless of its etiology, a progressive postoperative visual loss generally warrants immediate reexploration for possible decompression of the optic nerves or chiasm. In selected cases, intraoperative monitoring of visual evoked potentials may aid the surgeon in recognizing and preventing injuries to the optic nerves and chiasm.

Postoperative meningitis may occur from introduction of organisms during surgery but is usually secondary to postoperative CSF leaks. Following transsphenoidal surgery, CSF leaks occur most commonly through the diaphragma sella, tumor capsule, and sella cavity, but they may result with any fracture of the base of the skull. The diagnosis of CSF rhinorrhea is best confirmed by the demonstration of glucose in the watery discharge dripping from the nostrils or from the development of pneumocephalus or intracranial air-fluid levels, as seen on routine brow-up lateral skull x-ray films (Fig. 45-1).

Initially, this condition should be managed with several days of spinal fluid drainage, by either multiple lumbar punctures or insertion of an indwelling lumbar subarachnoid catheter for continuous closed system drainage. The patient should be placed on appropriate prophylactic antibiotic coverage for pathogens common to the nasopharynx and should be positioned with the head elevated at least 45° at all times. If the CSF leak persists after 3 to 5 days of spinal drainage, the patient should be reexplored transsphenoidally for closure of the CSF leak by repacking of the sella or tumor cavity. Fortunately, postoperative rhinorrhea has become a relatively in-

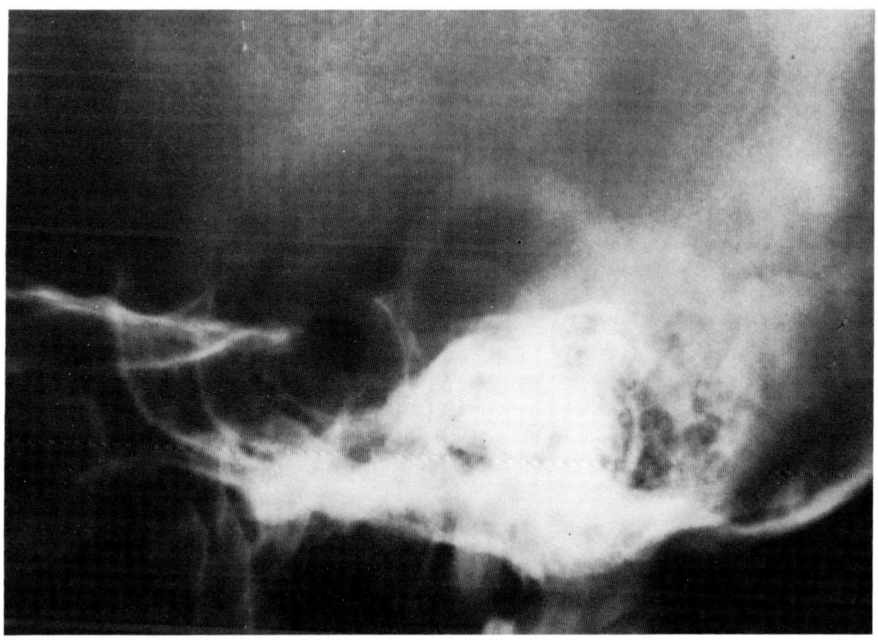

FIG. 45-1. Intracranial suprasellar air fluid level in a patient with postoperative CSF rhinorrhea.

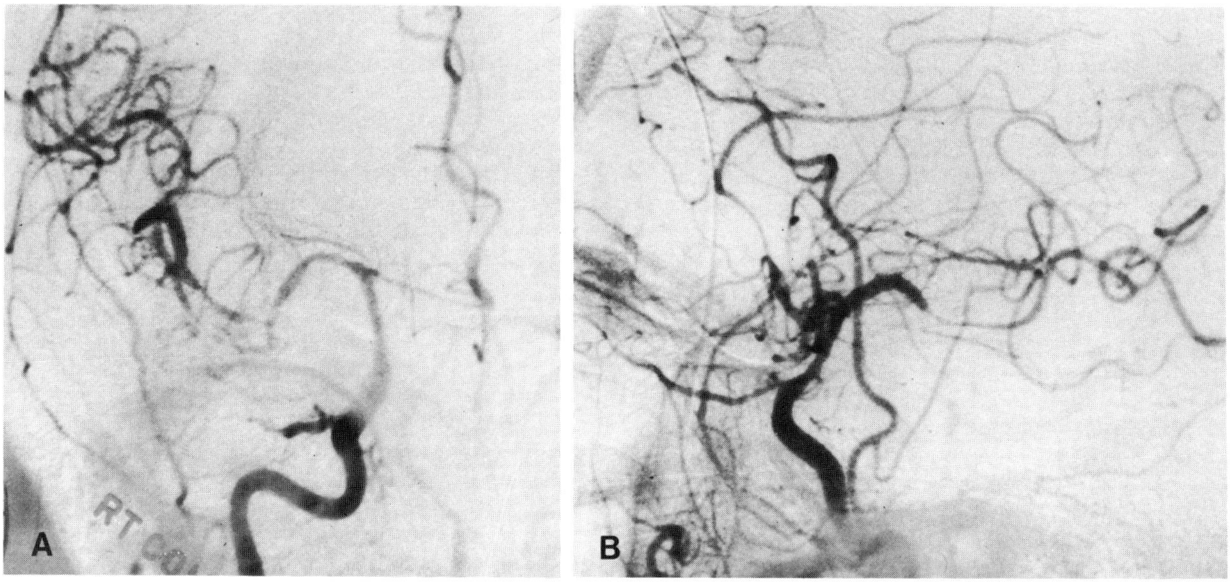

FIG. 45-2. (*A, B*) Postoperative AP and lateral right carotid angiogram in a patient having a significant subarachnoid hemorrhage resulting in severe vasospasm. All arterial vessels demonstrate the beaded appearance typical of arterial vasospasm.

frequent complication, occurring in less than 4% of cases, and with early recognition and prompt treatment, it usually resolves with a minimal threat of meningitis.[9, 20, 25]

Intracranial hemorrhage is an uncommon but devastating complication following transsphenoidal surgery. The hemorrhage may be primarily arterial (carotid artery and its branches) or primarily venous (cavernous sinuses and intradural connections). Postoperative intracranial hemorrhage usually presents as an expanding sellar and parasellar mass frequently associated with significant epistaxis and blood loss.

Carotid artery injury may result in death or serious morbidity, since it is difficult to control without compromising distal cerebral perfusion, resulting in significant cerebral ischemia or stroke. Carotid arterial hemorrhage may occur early in the postoperative period, or it may be delayed, as seen with the formation of a carotid-cavernous sinus fistula or false aneurysm. Associated subarachnoid hemorrhage or arterial wall injury may also provoke vascular occlusion or arterial vasospasm (Fig. 45-2). Preoperative carotid angiography often is helpful in recognizing and avoiding troublesome aberrant or tortuous carotid arteries or coexisting aneurysms coursing within the sella.[22, 34]

Other than hemorrhage, complications related to the cavernous sinuses include air embolism, sinus thrombosis, or damage to the cranial nerves (3rd, 4th, 5th, and 6th) coursing through the cavernous sinus.[24]

Hypothalamic damage may result from direct surgical trauma or by ischemia produced by vascular injury. Various hypothalamic syndromes characterized by disorders of thermal regulation, thirst and osmolality balance, endocrine function, level of consciousness, and changes in memory and behavior may occur and often are not reversible.

Extracranial Complications

Extracranial complications associated with the transsphenoidal approach to the pituitary gland are generally nonfatal but may cause a significant amount of morbidity. These usually involve the sphenoid sinus and nasofacial structures. Symptomatic sinusitis or the development of a mucocele may result with incomplete removal of the sphenoid sinus mucosa. Fractures of the hard palate and facial sinuses may occur from overaggressive dissection or retraction. Poor handling technique involving the nasal mucosa and cartilaginous septum may result in a postoperative nasoseptal perforation, nasal airway obstruction, persistent nasal discharge, and cosmetic nasal deformities. Nasal airway obstruction, symptomatic nasal septal perforations, and some of the cosmetic complications (saddle-nose deformity, broadened nose) may require surgical correction.

Endocrinologic Complications

The most common endocrinologic disorders following pituitary surgery are partial or complete hypopituitarism and diabetes insipidus. The detection and treatment of postoperative endocrine dysfunction, which require detailed pre- and postoperative endocrine evaluations, are two of the most important aspects in managing a patient undergoing pituitary surgery.

Diabetes insipidus (DI) is the most common endocrine abnormality resulting from pituitary surgery. Following transsphenoidal surgery, DI is usually transient, lasting several days, but it may persist for weeks to months, or it may be permanent in less than 5% of cases.[20, 30, 35] It usually results from damage to the anterior hypothalamus or median eminence, the pituitary stalk, or posterior pituitary gland. The diagnosis of DI is based on four factors, as listed below.

Polyuria, urine output > total intake by 250 ml/hour
Low urine osmolality, < 200 mOsmol/kg (1.001–1.005 specific gravity)
High serum osmolality, > 300 mOsmol/kg
Hypernatremia, serum Na > 150 mEq/L

After the diagnosis is confirmed by demonstrating an abnormally high serum osmolality with a low, dilute urine osmolality, the patient should be treated only after mild hyperosmolality of the serum is achieved. This avoids the erroneous treatment of a patient who is actually undergoing a water diuresis due to overhydration during surgery and postoperatively. Also, patients with acromegaly and Cushing's disease will frequently experience significant postoperative diuresis, which accompanies the sudden lowering of their postoperative growth hormone and adrenocorticotropin hormone levels, respectively. A high postoperative serum and urine osmolality level suggests an osmotic diuresis, often resulting from glucosuria as seen in the diabetic patient or following the administration of mannitol.

Frequent urine specific gravities, plasma osmolalities and electrolytes measurement, as well as accurate hourly intake and output records, are the basic requirements of the successful management of DI. Mild or partial DI may be managed simply by controlling fluid intake; however, more severe DI usually requires further treatment, initially with short-acting aqueous vasopressin (Pitressin) and chronically with Pitressin tannate in oil, clofibrate, or 1-desamino-8-D-arginine vasopressin (dDAVP).[3] Many excellent reviews on the management of postoperative DI have been published.[2, 3, 31, 38]

In the postoperative period, the syndrome of inappropriate secretion of antidiuretic hormone (SIADH) is uncommon and usually transient, but occasionally it persists for months or years. It usually results from damage to the hypothalamic neurohypophyseal unit and is characterized by a low serum sodium and osmolality, a high urine osmolality, and a urine sodium concentration of above 20 mEq/L.[2, 38] Untreated hypothyroidism, cirrhosis, and congestive heart failure may cause hyponatremia and decreased urine output and should be differentiated from SIADH in the early postoperative period. Management is primarily by fluid restriction, but SIADH may be effectively treated chronically with lithium carbonate and demeclocycline.[8, 35]

Acute symptomatic hypopituitarism usually occurs in patients not properly prepared for the stress of pituitary surgery. In the immediate postoperative period, the primary concern is adequate corticosteroid coverage for patients who may develop partial or complete adrenocortical insufficiency. Thus, pre- and postoperative steroids are routinely administered to all patients undergoing pituitary surgery, regardless of their preoperative endocrine status. Postoperatively, patients are either gradually tapered from steroids or are tapered to a maintenance physiologic dose over a period of 4 to 5 days. Then appropriate observation and endocrinologic testing can be used to assess the pituitary–adrenal axis and cortisol reserves. Generally, if patients have less than 15% to 20% of the anterior pituitary gland preserved or have significant preoperative hypocortisolism or if they undergo a total hypophysectomy, they will remain on replacement steroids for life.[28, 33] All patients with adrenal insufficiency, including those with normal baseline cortisol levels but impaired reserves, will require an increase in their maintenance steroid dose with stress. These patients should know about the symptoms of adrenal insufficiency and parenteral as well as oral administration of glucocorticoids.

If the patient is euthyroid preoperatively, hypothyroidism in the immediate postoperative period is of little consequence, because of the relatively long half-life (7 days) of circulating thyroxine. Preoperative hypothyroidism should always be recognized and corrected prior to surgery; however, thyroid replacement should never be given without complete assessment of adrenal reserve, because the institution of thyroid therapy increases the need for adrenal steroids and may precipitate an adrenal crisis.

Gonadotropin insufficiency is the most common impairment of anterior pituitary function following pituitary surgery. Long-term gonadotropin insufficiency not only results in decreased libido and infertility but may also be associated with accelerated osteoporosis and atherosclerosis.

TABLE 45-1. POSTOPERATIVE FATALITIES WITH TRANSSPHENOIDAL SURGERY: RICHMOND SERIES (1971–1980)

Cause of Death	Number of Patients (186 in all; 191 procedures)
Intracranial hematoma	1
Subarachnoid hemorrhage, vasospasm	1
Cardiomyopathy	1
Pulmonary embolism	1
Total	4

Systemic Complications

Patients undergoing pituitary surgery are prone to certain systemic complications, which are either inherent to the underlying hypersecretory syndrome (Cushing's disease, acromegaly) or directly related to the surgical procedure.

Patients with Cushing's disease may have increased risk of surgery because of their osteoporotic bones, vascular fragility, poor wound healing, and susceptibility to infection. Prolonged hypercortisolism in these patients may cause hypercoagulability with an increased incidence of deep vein thrombosis and pulmonary embolism.[32] Depression and other mental changes, which are common in Cushing's disease, may become dramatically exaggerated from a sudden decrease in postoperative cortisol levels following surgical removal of the adenoma. Gradually lowering the preoperative cortisol levels using aminoglutethimide or cyproheptadine may allow the patient to tolerate surgery better with a lessened incidence of postoperative depression and psychosis.[19, 23]

The natural history of untreated acromegaly, like that of Cushing's disease, is associated with increased morbidity and mortality.[37] The effects of excess growth hormone in stimulating tissue growth accounts for the majority of the clinical manifestations and complications of acromegaly. Hypertension, congestive heart failure, cardiomyopathies, hepatomegaly, and arrhythmias are all important contributors to the increased morbidity and mortality rates. For these patients, especially those with long-standing acromegaly, a cardiac evaluation should be obtained to bring the patient to the most optimal preoperative condition. Pituitary adenomas in acromegaly may be part of the multiple endocrine adenomatosis syndrome (MEA type I) and may be accompanied by adenomas of the parathyroid, pancreas (islet cells), and adrenal glands. Endocrinologic problems such as diabetes mellitus or hyperparathyroidism may occur and complicate the postoperative management of these patients.

Transsphenoidal Surgery for Pituitary Adenomas: Richmond Series (1971–1980)

In 1971, a prospective study was begun at the Medical College of Virginia on the utility of radical transsphenoidal surgery for pituitary adenomas. Between 1971 and 1980, 185 transsphenoidal procedures were performed on 180 patients with pituitary adenomas. An additional six patients underwent a transsphenoidal procedure for other pathology in the sella or for hypophysectomy as an ablative procedure for metastatic breast carcinoma.

Of the total series of 186 patients, four patients (2.1%) died within 1 month of their operation and are listed in Table 45-1. Two of these patients died as a result of an intracranial hemorrhage; in one, the hemorrhage resulted from an intracavernous carotid artery aneurysm that bled 3 weeks after surgery, the other from a subarachnoid hemorrhage that was followed by severe vasospasm 1 week after surgery (see Fig. 45-2). In both of these cases, the intracranial hemorrhage was probably attributable to arterial damage during surgery in attempting removal of lateral extensions of tumor. One patient with long-standing acromegaly died 3 weeks postoperatively from the severe cardiomyopathy that brought him to surgery. Another patient died from massive pulmonary embolism 1 week following apparently successful removal of her very large tumor. This patient weighed 375 pounds and had florid, long-standing Cushing's disease. All four of the postoperative fatalities had very large pituitary adenomas with significant suprasellar or parasellar extension.

Postoperative morbidity seen in these patients is summarized in Table 45-2. Seven of the total 186 patients (3.8%) experienced postoperative CSF rhinorrhea. Of these, four patients required reoperation for repacking of the sella and evacuated tumor cavity. Meningitis resulted in two of the four patients with postoperative rhinorrhea, one on the fourth postoperative day and the other 10 days after surgery. In both cases, meningitis resolved without sequelae with appropriate antibiotic therapy.

One patient who had severe osteoporosis associated with her Cushing's disease had permanent postoperative worsening of her vision. She had optic nerve damage from a fracture involving one optic foramen, resulting from excessive retraction during the procedure.

Four patients had postoperative cranial nerve (CN) palsies. Three had a transient sixth CN palsy, with one patient acquiring a permanent third CN palsy. The third CN palsy occurred during attempted removal of a very large thyroid-stimulating hormone (TSH) secreting adenoma that was invading the cavernous sinus. One patient had a transient cavernous sinus thrombosis that resolved after 2 to 3 months.

Although transient postoperative diabetes insipidus was relatively common, permanent DI occurred in only eight of the total 186 patients (4.3%). One of these patients had a total hypophysectomy as an ablative procedure for metastatic breast cancer, and another patient who presented with preoperative DI and an optic neuropathy had removal of a metastasis (oat cell carcinoma) to the sella. All of these patients have been well managed with appropriate vasopressin therapy (Pitressin, Pitressin tannate in oil, or dDAVP).

Four patients had postoperative complications related to the nasofacial structures. Two had a symptomatic nasal septal perforation, one of whom required subsequent corrective surgery. Another patient developed a significant saddle-nose deformity, which resulted from the erroneous removal of the superior one third of the nasal cartilaginous septum. A symptomatic diastasis of the hard palate occurred in another patient and was secondary to overzealous retraction (in an attempt to improve exposure to the sella floor) in a young woman having small, narrow nasal and facial structures. She required subsequent surgery for better reduction and fixation of her palatal diastasis.

A postoperative pulmonary embolism occurred in another patient with Cushing's disease who eventually recovered with appropriate medical management. Two patients wih significant pulmonary emphysema sustained a pneumothorax during the transsphenoidal surgical procedure. This undoubtedly resulted from the intraoperative use of multiple sustained Valsalva maneuvers with airway pressures up to 40 cm to 45 cm of water for 20 to 30 seconds in order to raise the intracranial pressure, thus facilitating delivery of suprasellar tumor into the sella and thus its removal.

Following surgery, anterior pituitary function (thyroid, adrenal, and gonadotropin axes) worsened in 13 of the 180 patients (7.2%) with a pituitary adenoma. The majority of these 13 patients became panhypopituitary postoperatively and are presently maintained on chronic hormonal replacement.

TABLE 45-2. POSTOPERATIVE MORBIDITY WITH TRANSSPHENOIDAL SURGERY: RICHMOND SERIES (1971–1980)

Complication	Number of Patients (186 in all; 191 procedures)	Incidence (%)
Mortality	4	2.1
Meningitis	2	1.0
CSF rhinorrhea	7	3.8
Requiring reoperation	4	2.1
Worsening of vision	1	0.5
Cranial nerve palsy		
Transient	3	1.6
Permanent	1	0.5
Cavernous sinus thrombosis (transient)	1	0.5
Diabetes insipidus (permanent) (One patient had total hypophysectomy as ablative procedure; one patient, preoperative DI)	8	4.3
Fractured hard palate	1	0.5
Nasal septal perforation	2	1.0
Saddle-nose deformity	1	0.5
Pulmonary embolism	1	0.5
Pneumothorax	2	1.0
Hypopituitarism	13/180	7.2

Surgical Considerations

Recent refinements of diagnostic radiologic and endocrine techniques have now increased the identification of smaller pituitary adenomas in younger patients. Also, recent advances in microsurgical techniques and procedures now allow neurosurgeons to remove pituitary microadenomas selectively with a negligible incidence of morbidity and mortality. However, as the tumor and its suprasellar and parasellar extensions increase, so does the risk of surgical complications. Other factors that increase risk are long-standing endocrinopathies, erosion of parasellar bony structures, previous craniotomy and radiation therapy, and poor general medical condition.

Extensive preoperative knowledge of the important anatomy and anatomical variations is essential to avoid complications. The anatomy of the sphenoid sinus, the sella and its surrounding neurovascular structures, and the nasal septum, as well as its role in nasal function, aids in avoiding postoperative dysfunction and cosmetic deformities.

A greater awareness of the systemic effects of long-standing endocrinopathies as well as a complete evaluation of a patient's endocrine status is necessary for the optimal intraoperative and postoperative management of patients with pituitary adenomas. Further technical developments such as the use of intraoperative evoked potential monitoring and image-intensified fluoroscopy will undoubtedly aid in preventing surgical complications.

Probably more than any other factor, the development and refinement of the microsurgical transsphenoidal procedure has enabled neurosurgeons to approach abnormalities of the pituitary gland safely.

References

1. Caton R, Paul FT: Notes of a cure of acromegaly treated by operation. Br Med J 2:1421, 1893
2. Cobb WE: Endocrine management after pituitary surgery. In Port K, Jackson I (eds): The Pituitary Adenoma. New York, Plenum Medical Books, 1980
3. Cobb WE et al: Neurogenic diabetes insipidus: Management with dDAVP (1-desamino-8-D-arginine vasopressin). Ann Intern Med 11:183, 1978
4. Cushing H: Surgical experiences with pituitary disorders. JAMA 63:1515, 1914
5. Cushing H: Intracranial Tumors, p 69. Springfield, IL, Charles C Thomas, 1932
6. Dott NM, Bailey AA: A consideration of the hypophyseal adenomata. Br J Surg 13:314, 1925
7. Fager GA, Poppen JL, Takaoka Y: Indications for and results of surgical treatment of pituitary tumors by the intracranial approach. In Kohler DO, Ross GT (eds): Diagnosis and Treatment of Pituitary Tumors. Amsterdam, Excerpta Medica, 1973
8. Graze K et al: Chronic demeclocycline therapy in the syndrome of inappropriate ADH secretion due to brain tumor. J Neurosurg 47:933, 1977
9. Guiot G: Transsphenoidal approach in surgical treatment of pituitary adenomas: General principles and indications in non-functioning adenomas. In Kohler PO, Ross GT (eds): Diagnosis and Treatment of Pituitary Tumors. Amsterdam, Excerpta Medica, 1973
10. Guiot G, Thibant B: L'extirpation des adenomes hypophysaires par roie transsphenoidale. Neurochirurgia (Stuttg) 1:133, 1959
11. Halstead AE: Remarks on the operative treatment of tumors of the hypophysis. Surg Gynecol Obstet 10:494, 1910
12. Hardy J: Transsphenoidal microsurgery of the normal and pathological pituitary. Clin Neurosurg 16:185, 1969
13. Hardy J: Microsurgery applied to neurosurgery. New York, Academic Press, 1969
14. Hardy J: Transsphenoidal surgery of hypersecreting pituitary tumors. Excerpta Medica International Congress Series 303:179, 1973
15. Henderson WR: Pituitary adenomata: A follow-up study of surgical results in 338 cases (Dr. H. Cushing's series). Br J Surg 26:811, 1939
16. Hirsch O: Life-long cures and improvements after transsphenoidal operation of pituitary tumors. Acta Ophthalmol 56:1, 1959
17. Horsley V: On the technique of operation on the central nervous system. Br Med J 2:411, 1906
18. Krause F: Hirnchirurgie Dtsch Klin 8:953, 1905
19. Krieger DT, Amorsa K, Linick F: Eypropheptadine-induced remission of Cushing's disease. N Engl J Med 293:893, 1975
20. Laws ER Jr, Kern EB: Complications of transsphenoidal surgery. Clin Neurosurg 23:401, 1976
21. Laws ER Jr, Trautman JC, Hollenhorst RW: Transsphenoidal decompression of the optic nerve and chiasm: Visual results in 62 patients. J Neurosurg 46:717, 1977
22. Lippman HH, Onaforio BM, Baker HL: Intrasellar aneurysm and pituitary adenoma: Report of a case. Mayo Clin Proc 46:532, 1971
23. Misbin RI, Canary J, Willard D: Aminoglutethamide in the treatment of Cushing's syndrome. J Clin Pharmacol 16:645, 1976
24. Newfield P, Ablin MS, Chestnut JS, Maroon J: Air embolus during transsphenoidal pituitary operations. Neurosurgery 2:39, 1978
25. Post K: Transsphenoidal surgery for pituitary tumors. In Post K, Jackson O (eds): The Pituitary Adenoma. New York, Plenum Medical Books, 1980
26. Ray BS, Patterson RH Jr: Surgical experience with chromophobe adenomas of the pituitary gland. J Neurosurg 34:726, 1971
27. Renn WH, Rhoton AL Jr: Microsurgical anatomy of the sellar region. J Neurosurg 43:288, 1975
28. Saglam S, Dragt CL, Wilson CB et al: Graded cryohypophysectomy in the rhesus monkey: Histopathology and endocrine function. J Neurosurg 36:169, 1972
29. Schloffer H, Erfolgreiche: Operation eines hypophysecentumors auf nasalem wege. Wien Klin Wochenschr 20:621, 1907
30. Schnall AM, Brodkey JS et al: Pituitary function after removal of pituitary microadenomas in Cushing's disease. J Clin Endocrinol Metab 47(2):410, 1978
31. Shucart WA, Jackson I: Management of diabetes insipidus in neurosurgical patients. J Neurosurg 44:65, 1976
32. Sjoberg HE, Blamback M, Grambert P: Thromboembolic complications, heparin treatment in increase in coagulation factors in Cushing's syndrome. Acta Med Scand 199(1–2):95, 1976
33. Van Buren JM, Bergenstal DM: An evaluation of graded hypophysectomy in man. Cancer 13:155, 1960
34. White JC, Ballatnine HT Jr: Intrasellar aneurysms simulating hypophyseal tumors. J Neurosurg 18:34, 1961
35. White MG, Fetner CD: Treatment of the syndrome of inappropriate secretion of antidiuretic hormone with lithium carbonate. N Engl J Med 292:390, 1975
36. Wilson CB, Dempsey LC: Transsphenoidal microsurgical removal of 250 pituitary adenomas. J Neurosurg 48:13, 1978
37. Wright AP, Hill DM, Lowy C, Frazier TR: Mortality in acromegaly. Q J Med 39:1, 1970
38. Zimmerman EA: Postoperative management following pituitary surgery. In Tindell GT, Collins WF (eds): Clinical Management of Pituitary Disorders. New York, Raven Press, 1979

Part Seven

Complications of Nervous System Surgery and Trauma

46
Complications of Craniotomy and Trauma

Michael J. Rosner | Donald P. Becker

OVERVIEW

The postcraniotomy or brain injury patient is often frightening to the general house staff or physician without extensive neurologic training. However, by applying basic principles for the physical examination, a few important anatomical considerations, combined with minimum physiologic principles, the general care of the postcraniotomy patient becomes much more straightforward. This chapter begins with a short review of the basic anatomy of consciousness, pupillary and oculocephalic reflexes, physiology, and a simplified but pertinent neurologic examination.

ANATOMICAL BASIS OF CONSCIOUSNESS

Consciousness may be disturbed when lesions involve either very large areas of the hemisphere or very small areas of the reticular activating system (RAS). Thus, a large ischemic infarct of the hemisphere or anoxic damage that has affected large areas of both hemispheres is often associated with decreases in the level of consciousness. The pathologic processes that affect large areas of brain (hypoxemia, hypoglycemia, ischemia, toxins, and mass lesions) will also affect areas of the RAS as well, and the distinction becomes difficult when made on the basis of level of consciousness alone. The presence of focal signs (e.g., hemiparesis, unilateral III nerve palsy) should suggest the possibility of a mass lesion.

However, the concept also applies to the relatively small hemispheric lesion, since this will rarely change the level of consciousness of a patient. An embolus to a distal branch of the middle cerebral artery may lead to complete paralysis of an arm but not to depression in the level of consciousness. A growing mass lesion, however, affects large areas of brain and typically alters the mentation and level of wakefulness of the patient *early* in its development, often before the development of limb paresis or cranial nerve deficit.

PUPILLARY RESPONSE AND DOLL'S EYES

Pupillary light reflexes are dependent upon an intact globe, retina, optic nerve, optic tract, the synapses of the optic radiation from the lateral geniculate body to the third nerve nuclei of the brain stem, and the third nerve itself. Any process affecting the integrity of this system may alter the light reflex, but our first concern is the mass lesion effect. Obviously, a mass lesion may affect this system at nearly any point, but the typical manner is by "uncal herniation." Here, the mass lesion causes shifting of the medial temporal lobe (uncus) and stretches or compresses the third nerve (Fig. 46-1). The pupil no longer reacts to light and is dilated. Pupillary dilatation always follows depression in the level of consciousness in the evolution of a mass lesion. Hemiparesis is variable and may occur at nearly any stage. The implication is that awake patients should be followed primarily in terms of their level of consciousness, since pupillary changes tend to occur late. A flashlight shined in the eye of an awake patient is much less helpful than is simply talking to the patient.

The oculocephalic reflex or "doll's eye" maneuver is also helpful. Anatomically, the afferent input is from the vestibular apparatus of the inner ear and proprioceptive receptors in the neck. This input is distributed in the brain stem to the vestibular nuclei and thence to the medial longitudinal fasciculus (MLF). The MLF coordinates the third nerve (medial rectus = medial eye movement) and the sixth nerve (lateral rectus = lateral eye movement). Thus, when the head is rotated from side to side in a supine,

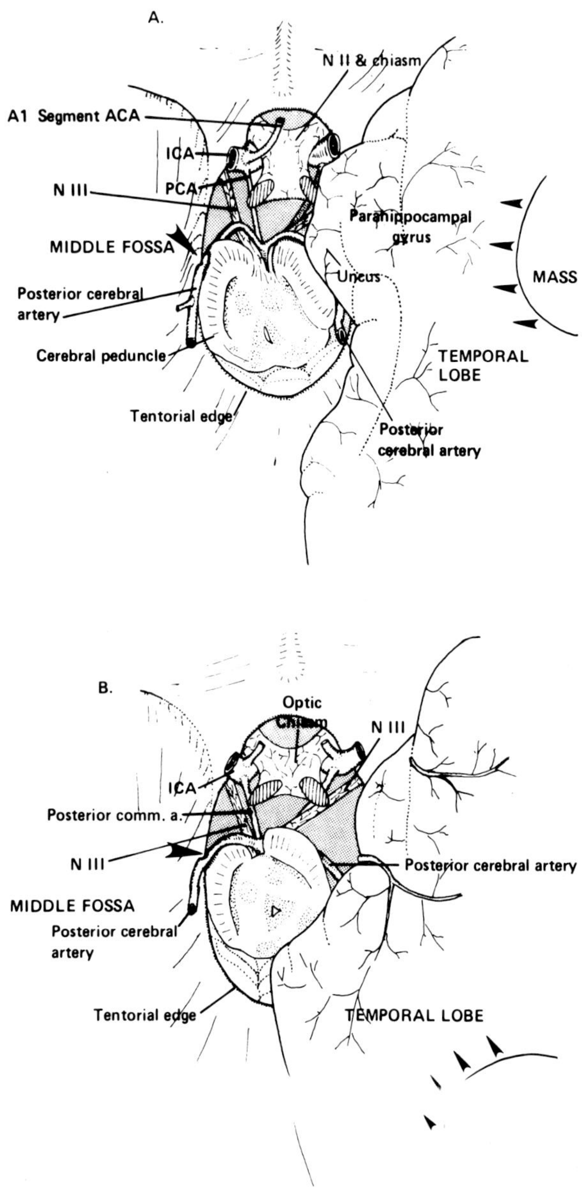

FIG. 46-1. (*A* and *B*) Uncal herniation is depicted to show how the mesial temporal lobe is "herniated" medially with distortion of the brain stem, stretching of the third (oculocephalic) nerve, and compression of the posterior cerebral artery. Distortion of the thalamus and brain stem causes a progressive decline in the level of consciousness, which may culminate in abnormal extension (decerebration) or flaccidity. Third nerve distortion may lead to pupillary dilatation; compression of the peduncle may produce contralateral hemiparesis. If the mass effect is great enough to cause the *opposite* cerebral peduncle to impinge on the tentorial edge (*large arrowhead*), a relative paresis on the *same* side as the mass may be observed; this phenomenon is known as "Kernohan's notch." This may lead the unwary examiner to assume incorrectly that the mass is contralateral to the hemiparesis when it is actually ipsilateral.

comatose patient, the eyes move together as if looking at a fixed point in space. If one eye does not move medially, a medial rectus paresis may be present; but, the movement of both eyes fully, medially and laterally, is normal. The implication is that both third nerves, both sixth nerves, and the brain stem (mesencephalon to pons) are anatomically intact. Fortunately, both the pupillary light reflex and the oculocephalic reflex are resistant to most metabolic and toxic insults and are essentially normal in the patient comatose due to nonstructural lesions. Lesions that disrupt the structural integrity of these systems (hematoma, tumor, infarct, etc.) usually affect the pupillary light and doll's eye reflexes by the time the patient passes into "coma" or no longer responds to voice or painful stimuli.[51] If, in the presence of decerebration or decortication, the pupils and oculocephalic reflexes are intact, then the coma is of metabolic origin.

PHYSIOLOGIC CONSIDERATIONS

Cerebral blood flow is normally in the range of 50 ml/min/100 g of brain, or about 700 ml/min for the whole brain. It is generally accepted that values of 20 ml to 25 ml/min/100 g of brain are associated with neurologic symptoms, but no permanent morphologic changes, if normal flows are restored. Below 15 ml to 20 ml/min/100 g of brain, permanent structural changes begin to appear. Therefore, under normal circumstances, the cerebral circulation delivers approximately twice the amount of blood necessary to sustain function and viability.[51, 76]

Cerebral autoregulation is the ability of the cerebral vasculature to change diameter in response to changes in pressure; this ability of the vasculature is able to maintain flow fairly constantly over the pressure range of 50 to 150 torr. Two important concepts modify the pressure actually "seen" by the cerebral vasculature: cerebral perfusion pressure (CPP) and hydrostatic pressure changes. Cerebral perfusion pressure is the difference between intracranial pressure (ICP) and the blood pressure (CPP = SABP − ICP) and is the pressure to which the vessels will respond by constriction or dilatation. The second point is that the SABP measured at head level is *less* than the pressure measured at the heart by the vertical distance of the head to the heart (usually about 30–40 cm when standing). Thus, when calculating the perfusion pressure, one must know the ICP, and the systemic pressure must be measured at the level of the *head*. With the patient supine, the SABPs at the heart level and the head are effectively the same, but if the patient is sitting or standing, the pressure at the head is 20 to 35 torr *less* than at the heart. Therefore, if the systemic pressure at the heart is 100 torr and the patient is sitting and has an ICP of 15 torr, his CPP will be about 55 torr (SABP at head level = 100 − 30 = 70; CPP = 70 − 15 = 55), a value near the lower limits of autoregulation.

Autoregulation is currently considered to occur primarily as the result of variation in the amount of oxygen delivered to the brain.[38] Oxygen delivery can be calculated by the following formula:

$$0_2\text{(ml/min)} = \text{Hgb (g/ml)} \times \%\ \text{saturation} \times 1.34\ \text{ml}\ 0_2\text{/g Hgb} \times \text{flow (ml/min)}$$

Clearly, if oxygen delivery is decreased and results in vasodilation, then this vasodilation can be brought about by anemia, hypoxemia, and decreasing pressure. Given a patient in whom oxygen delivery might already be at a critically low level, it is reasonable to raise oxygen carrying capacity (Hgb), saturation, or blood pressure to as near normal as possible. There is little rationale and less evidence to suggest that supranormal levels of these parameters are generally helpful.

Because the intracranial vasculature responds to pressure changes and other stimuli by changing diameter, it is immediately obvious that the vessels must also change their *volume* by a factor proportional to the *square* of the radius change. Thus, relatively small radius changes are consistent with relatively large changes in the cerebral blood volume.

When the intracranial pressure is low, these changes in cerebral blood volume are unimportant. But when the intracranial pressure is high and the compliance of the intracranial space is low, then relatively small volume changes become important. Therefore, if a patient is known to harbor a mass lesion or to have a diffuse increase in intracranial pressure with decreased compliance, further vasodilatation and increase in the cerebral blood volume could be expected to increase ICP even further. It should be noted that as the ICP increases, the CPP will decrease unless the arterial pressure increases. Therefore, increased ICP can be associated with decreases in cerebral blood flow, a conclusion supported by a great deal of experimental evidence.

Carbon dioxide is a powerful vasodilator when increased (hypercapnia); hypocapnia is an equally powerful vasoconstrictor. This relationship has been used to reduce the cerebral blood volume by vasoconstriction induced by hyperventilation. The treatment of increased ICP has utilized this concept and resulted in the placement of neurosurgical patients on mechanical ventilators, which allow rigid and reliable control of the arterial PCO_2. Secondary, but equally beneficial, effects are the avoidance of hypoxemia and hypercapnia. Muscle paralysis or sedation may be required in order to control respirations in this rigid manner.

To summarize, decreased oxygen delivery or hypercapnia is able to dilate the cerebral vasculature and increase cerebral blood volume. Clinically when the compliance of the intracranial space is low, increases in cerebral blood volume become important and result in higher levels of ICP. This can be damaging when it causes blood flow to drop to ischemic levels. Anemia, hypoxemia, hypercapnia, and hypotension are systemic factors capable of elevating ICP by increases in the cerebral blood volume and should be corrected when attempting to treat high ICP.

Additionally, since autoregulation is usually altered by intracranial pathology, a normally protective aspect of the cerebral physiology may be only partially functional in a particular patient. Recent evidence suggests that as autoregulation fails, the lower limits at which cerebral blood flow (CBF) begins to decline are 20 to 40 torr *higher* than normal. Thus, CBF may decline when the perfusion pressure is 70 to 80 torr, a value far higher than the normal 40 to 50 torr.[40]

ICP elevations associated with little or no brain shift tend to affect autoregulation less than does the elevation caused by focal mass lesions. One study noted a decline in CBF at 70 torr in the face of a mass lesion elevating ICP, as opposed to 40 to 50 torr when ICP was raised by cisternal perfusion and brain shift was not a factor. The reasons for this finding remain unclear, but the implication is that low CPP and hypotension are probably *less well* tolerated by the patient with a mass lesion than by the patient with a more diffuse process elevating his ICP.

NEUROLOGIC DETERIORATION

The most important concept necessary for the early detection of a postcraniotomy complication is *change*. Basically, the neurologic status of a patient who has undergone a craniotomy should be equal to, or better than, the preoperative level. This is most important with regard to the *level of consciousness*. Figure 46-2 lists the various aspects of the neurologic condition assessed by the Glasgow Coma Scale. The strength of this scale is the objectivity of its assessments and its format, which allows a changing neurologic status to be graphically displayed.

It is this change from one level to another that should alert the medical staff to the possibility of a postoperative or posttraumatic complication. The variables that constitute the grouping called "level of consciousness" are "eye opening," "verbal response," and "motor response." In essence, each scale is arranged to be sensitive to changing levels of stimulus necessary to obtain a particular behavior. For instance, the patient who, after surgery, has been a bit sleepy but opens his eyes briskly to a normal

GLASGOW COMA SCALE										
EYES	Spontaneous									
	Open to speech									
	Open to pain									
	Remain closed									
VERBAL	Oriented									
	Confused									
	Words									
	Sounds only									
	No response									
MOTOR	Obeys commands									
	Localizes pain									
	Withdraws									
	Abnormal flexor									
	Extension									
	No response									

FIG. 46-2. These three scales constitute the "Glasgow coma scale." Each is arranged such that the normal response will be recorded in the top portion of each scale, while progressively more abnormal responses are lower. If consciousness should deteriorate, the graph (usually assessed at least hourly) will show a gradually declining pattern. While eye opening tends to be the most sensitive indicator, important deterioration usually affects all three scales more or less in parallel.

NEUROLOGIC EXAM											
PUPILS	R.	Size									
		Reaction									
	L.	Size									
		Reaction									
OCR	R.	Medial									
		Lateral									
	L.	Medial									
		Lateral									
ARMS		Normal power									
		Mod. weakness									
		Severe weakness									
		Trace									
		None									
LEGS		Normal power									
		Mod. weakness									
		Severe weakness									
		Trace									
		None									

FIG. 46-3. This chart shows the important aspects of the neurologic examination that complement assessment of the level of consciousness. The pupils are judged as to size and reaction; the Doll's eyes (OCR = oculocephalic reflexes) are also assessed. Muscle strength in the upper and lower extremities is observed for change; this scale may also be used in the spinal surgery patient for the development or progression of paralysis.

voice command should be critically evaluated if he later begins to require louder voices, physical stimulation, or a painful stimulus in order to respond by "eye opening."

The Glasgow Coma Scale is simple, objective, and readily learned by nursing and ancillary staff. It is equally appropriate for the physician without extensive training in the neurologic sciences who finds himself responsible for the care of such patients. Regardless of the method of assessment, patients undergoing craniotomies and other neurosurgical procedures must be observed for deterioration, and the physician must be aware of the importance of even small changes.

The level of consciousness of the patient generally is the most sensitive indicator of a developing complication. However, examination of the cranial nerves and motor system should also be carried out at the same time as the assessment of the level of consciousness (Fig. 46-3). Very rarely, a pupil may begin to dilate, or react more slowly than it did previously, in the face of a developing mass lesion, while the level of wakefulness of the patient appears unchanged. The same may occasionally be true of motor signs, but these are exceptions rather than the rule. Both cranial nerve and motor signs have their greatest usefulness in patients in whom the preoperative level of consciousness was abnormal.

Table 46-1 (see under General Complications: Differential Diagnosis) lists the differential diagnoses that should be considered in any postcraniotomy patient who changes for the worse after sur-

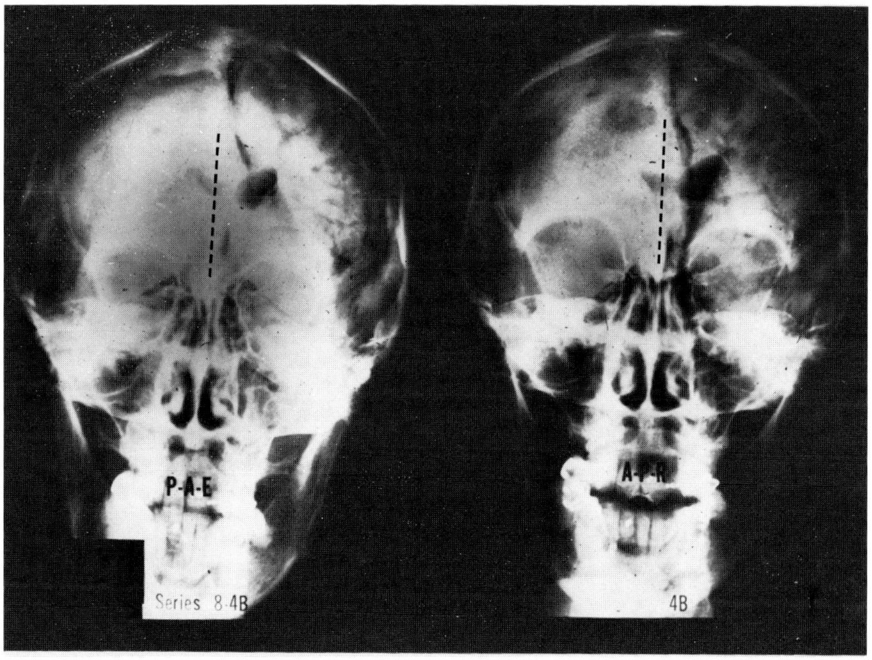

FIG. 46-4. An air ventriculogram allows estimation of the intracranial pressure at the time of air instillation into the ventricle. Further information is limited to the size, shape, and position of the ventricular system; note the shift of the ventricles across the midline (*dotted line*), compression of the right ventricle, and dilatation of the left. Brain edema, intracerebral hemorrhage, and extracerebral hematomas all may cause these findings. Because of the relative nonspecificity of the examination, ventriculography is used less and less; however, it remains relevant when the patient cannot be moved, or if the CT scanner is not available. If deterioration is due to acute hydrocephalus, the ventriculogram is diagnostic, and the ventricular tap initiates therapy. The patient without a ventricular drain who worsens after posterior fossa surgery is probably as well served by a ventriculogram and ventriculostomy as by CT scan, but this is one of the few such exceptions remaining.

gery. By far, the most serious class of problems occurring in the postoperative period is the hematomas, but hematomas are only a part of the larger classification of "mass lesion." By its nature, a mass lesion will, in the closed intracranial space, cause elevations in intracranial pressure and brain shift (Fig. 46-4).

Mass lesions that develop in the postoperative period may be hematomas (intracerebral, intraventricular, subdural, or epidural), contusions, brain edema, peritumoral edema, loculated ventricles, cysts, and even loculated collections of air. Often, combinations of these lesions will be present, such as the edema that may surround a contusion or area of hemorrhagic necrosis.

The general presentation of a mass lesion will be hallmarked by a decline in the level of consciousness followed or accompanied by third nerve paresis and progressive motor weakness. The rapidity with which these findings occur will depend upon the level of function existing before the decline and the speed with which the mass lesion develops and exerts its effects.

The awake patient developing a mass lesion will gradually require stronger stimuli to open his eyes and to establish contact with the observer. Initially, he will appear to be no more than sleepy after reacting from anesthesia, but as time passes, he will fall into a deeper and deeper "sleep" that will require first voice, then a loud voice, and then noise accompanied by a physical shaking, and eventually a painful stimulus will be necessary to arouse the patient to open his eyes. It should be established that after reacting from anesthesia, a painful stimulus should never be necessary to arouse the truly sleeping patient. Similarly, once awakened, the patient ought to be able to communicate to some reasonable degree with the physician. If he should immediately lapse again into a state requiring painful stimulation for arousal, then his level of consciousness is pathologic, and an explanation should be sought.[35, 51]

The decline in level of wakefulness in the face of a developing mass lesion is often accompanied by changes in the pupillary light responses. Often, the first response of the pupil on the side of a mass lesion will be miosis (constriction) rather than the more generally acknowledged mydriasis (dilatation). This is due to interference with the central origins of the sympathetic system and actually represents a "central" type of Horner's syndrome. This phase is transient and usually accompanied by restlessness, agitation, and combativeness. There will be no paralysis of ocular motility at this stage.

As the process continues, the third nerve itself will be affected, and the pupil will, as the next change to be noted, react more sluggishly to light than will the other side. There will be sluggish but often intact ocular motility responses; ultimately, the pupil no longer reacts to light and is dilated (but still round), and medial rectus function is lost. As the end stage is reached and the sympathetic system fails completely, there will be neither constrictor (parasympathetic, third nerve) nor dilator (sympathetic, cervical sympathetics) tone on the pupil, which will tend to become flaccid, midposition, nonreactive to light, and irregular in shape. Usually, both pupils are abnormal in this situation, and the patient is clearly in extremis.

The motor signs tend to follow a stereotyped course as well. After the patient has begun to demonstrate a decrease in his level of consciousness, his use of his arms will become asymmetrical, even if a painful stimulus is required to initiate a movement. A pinch on either side of the body should normally stimulate the patient to make a rapid grab at the pinched part with the arm on the pinched side. If a substantial difference develops between the two sides in the postoperative period, then the examiner should suspect that a mass may be developing. Eventually, the patient will simply not move the side where the lesion is when a painful stimulus is applied, and the term "hemiparesis" or "hemiplegia" becomes relevant. If the process continues, input from the hemisphere to the brain stem is gradually lost, and the patient first begins to show "abnormal flexor" or "decorticate" posturing, which evolves into "abnormal extensor" or "decerebrate posturing." If the mass lesion continues to exert its influence, the end-stage motor response is flaccidity.

By the time any one of these spheres (level of consciousness, pupillary response, and motor function) has progressed to even moderate levels, the patient will nearly always be demonstrating changes in complementary categories if a mass lesion is the etiology of the change. This is because mass lesions exert their effects by shifting the brain and *affecting large volumes* of tissue, including the diencephalon and brain stem, which contain the reticular activating system, or by leading to global reductions in CBF (by reducing CPP) so that the brain is diffusely affected by ischemia.

If the patient should develop a major deficit such as a hemiplegia, but remain perfectly awake, then a lesion capable of sparing the reticular activating system should be considered. An infarct involving the motor fibers from the hemisphere is one such lesion. The cortex, internal capsule, cerebral peduncle, or anywhere below these levels may be involved, but not the RAS. Therefore, the patient remains awake.

Similarly, if an infarct should involve the cerebral peduncle as the third nerve exits from the brain stem, then it is possible to have a hemiplegic patient with a contralateral third nerve palsy who is awake (Weber's syndrome). As a general rule, cerebral mass lesions have effects on level of consciousness, pupillary light responses, and motor function. One sphere alone is almost never significantly affected without concomitant and parallel changes in the other functions. If isolated changes in one group of responses should occur, then other classes of lesions should be considered (e.g., stroke, metabolic encephalopathy).

Before considering other entities, it should be pointed out that the side of pupillary involvement is ipsilateral to the mass lesion in about 95% of the cases. This makes the pupil a more accurate predictor of the side of the mass lesion than a hemiparesis, which is contralateral to the mass lesion only about 85% of the time (see Fig. 46-1). However, these figures represent the results of evaluation in patients with previously unknown lesions. They do not represent the probabilities in postoperative patients. Postoperative patients generally respond more in the expected manner with a third nerve palsy ipsilateral to the mass lesion, the hemiparesis contralateral to the mass, and the actual mass on the side of the surgery. Still, the examiner must remember that unusual lateralization of a mass is possible, and studies that confirm the impressions of a physical examination are desirable.

VITAL SIGN CHANGES

The classic combination of bradycardia and hypertension has been recognized as the "Cushing response" to an increasing ICP. Brain stem ischemia appears to be the essential stimulus to this hypertension. Although hypertension is a frequent concomitant of increasing ICP, bradycardia is extremely unreliable. Often, tachycardia is present, especially in the early phases of deterioration. Therefore, hypertension developing from a normotensive state should alert the physician to a possible rise in ICP; the pulse rate may change in either direction. But, bradycardia in the face of hypertension is ominous.

Respirations tend to increase as the ICP rises, and tachypnea should be considered evidence that something is not as it should be. Clearly, systemic etiologies for tachypnea such as atelectasis, pneumothorax, or improper endotracheal tube placement should also be considered and evaluated. The same applies to blood pressure and pulse changes. But if an immediate cause for such vital sign change is not apparent, then an intracranial lesion or complication should be considered. Cheyne–Stokes respirations and ataxic and apneustic breathing patterns occur in patients who are obviously deteriorating neurologically and require evaluation. But before patients reach this severe level of deterioration, their first respiratory change is often tachypnea.

Such hypertension, pulse changes, tachypnea, or abnormal respiratory patterns should be cause for alarm when accompanied by any changes in the level of consciousness of the patient. Intervention must begin early and is most effective at treating the patient before gross herniation occurs.

STUDIES

In summary, the cardinal symptom in the development of a postoperative mass lesion is a *changing mental status*. In the early phases, this change may be quite subtle. The patient may, over a period of hours, simply require a painful stimulus in order for the examiner to obtain an eye opening response. This degree of change is quite significant and should alert the physician that an intracranial mass may be developing. Vital sign changes may or may not be present.

The concomitant development of a motor paresis (facial paresis, arm or leg weakness) or pupillary changes in the face of a change in mental status should be considered presumptive evidence for a developing mass lesion and steps immediately instituted to define this problem. In general, an immediate CT scan should be performed in search of ventricular shift from extracerebral (subdural or epidural) hematoma or intracerebral mass (hemorrhage, contusion, or edema). Alternative diagnostic studies are ventriculography using air, measurement of the intracranial pressure, angiography, diagnostic tapping of the postcraniotomy site, or immediate reexploration in the operating room. However, the essential point is that suspicion that a lesion may be developing must precede the definitive steps needed to institute treatment.

General Complications: Differential Diagnosis

The preceding sections serve as the basis for evaluation of the patient who is worsening in the postoperative period. Table 46-1 lists a differential di-

TABLE 46-1. COMPLICATIONS THAT CAUSE NEUROLOGIC DEFICIT

	Diagnostic Examination				
Complication	*Air or Contrast Ventriculogram*	*Increased ICP*	*Angio-graphy*	*Plain X-ray Film*	*CT Scan*
Mass lesion					
Hematoma	+	+	+	−	+
Neoplasm + edema	+	+	+/−	−	+
Loculus	+/−	+	+/−	−	+
Edema	+/−	+/−	+/−	−	+
Pneumocephalus	+	+/−	+	+	+
Hydrocephalus	+	+	+	−	+
Infarct					
Swollen infarct	+	+	+	−	+
Nonswollen infarct	−	−	+/−	−	+/−
Infection					
Meningitis	−	+	+/−	−	+/−*
Ventriculitis	−	+	−	−	+/−*
Abscess	+/−	+/−	+/−	−	+
Empyema (subdural)	+/−	+	+	−	+/−
Metabolic					
Hypoxemia	−	+	−	−	−
Hypercarbia	−	+	−	−	−
Hyponatremia	−	+	−	−	−
Diabetes	−	−	−	−	−

* May show only hydrocephalus.

agnosis that includes common postoperative complications as well as several that are unusual. With a patient who deteriorates in the postoperative period, the greatest immediate concern is a mass lesion. The most common mass lesion historically has been the postoperative hematoma. This clot may be epidural, subdural, or intracerebral. Due to advances in surgical technique and hemostasis, postoperative hemorrhage is now fairly rare and often associated with coagulopathies, especially thrombocytopenia.

POSTOPERATIVE HEMATOMA

A postoperative hematoma may occur in the epidural or subdural space or within the parenchyma of the brain (Figs. 46-5 and 46-6). The clinical presentation of these lesions is not specific, and all are possible in the postoperative patient who is becoming more lethargic and developing focal signs such as hemiparesis, aphasia, and third nerve paresis with or without vital sign changes.

Since the treatment for these lesions is usually reexploration and evacuation of the mass lesion, it follows that the bedside evaluation need only be concerned that such a lesion may be developing. Little will be gained by worrying about whether it is an epidural or subdural hematoma.

Given such a suspicion, the examiner should attempt to define the problem by CT scan. However, if the patient is rapidly deteriorating, it may be more appropriate to return directly to the operating room for wound reexploration. Implicit in this is the fact that CT scans require time—time to arrange, to transport the patient, to obtain the scan and, when necessary, to return the patient to the operating room. No absolute criterion dictates which route to take, but decisions should be based upon good judgment considering the advantages of the greater amount of information offered by CT scans, possibly avoiding unnecessary reoperation, balanced against the inherent delay in obtaining this information.

FIG. 46-5. This cerebral angiogram of a patient after removal of a right acute subdural hematoma shows a partial reaccumulation of the hematoma. Note the avascular space between the inner table of the skull and the surface of the brain (*double-ended arrow*), and displacement across the midline (*dotted line*). Also, note that angiography demonstrates only the vessels; the presence of mass lesions is demonstrated indirectly by *displacement* of normal vasculature. Little information is conveyed about the density of the lesion as by CT scan.

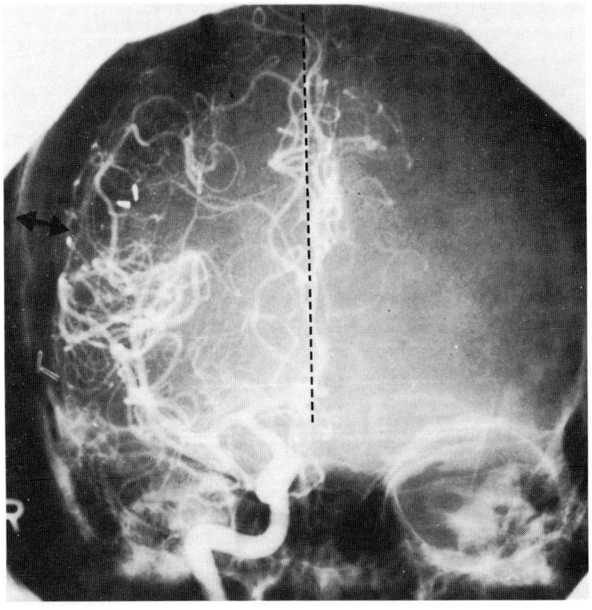

FIG. 46-6. Acute subdural hematoma. On the CT scan white areas represent high density such as bone and freshly clotted blood, while darker areas represent lesser degrees of density. Thus, the acute hematoma appears white on the scan; note the large left-to-right shift and ventricular collapse induced by the mass lesion.

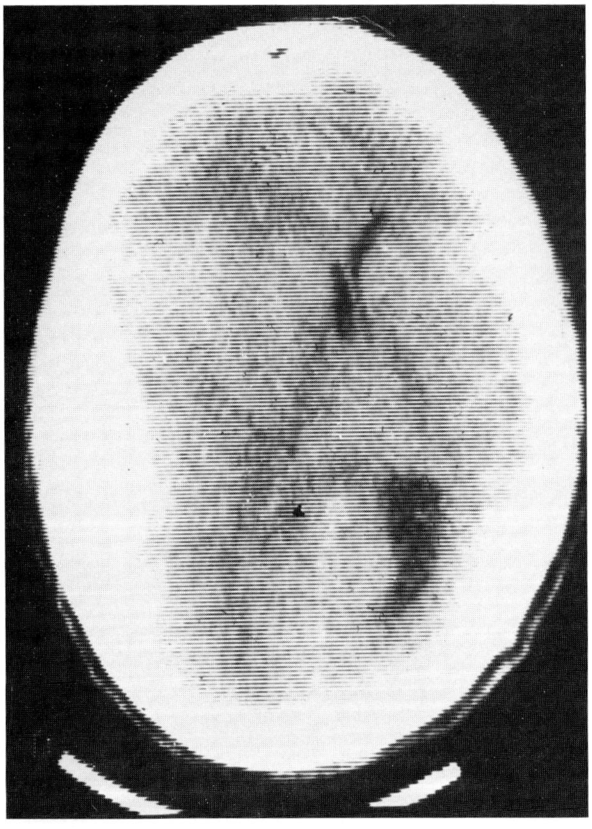

Regardless of whether the patient is to be returned directly to the operating room or evaluated first by CT scan (or any other radiologic techniques), procedures can be instituted immediately to increase the patient's tolerance to this potential mass lesion (Table 46-2).

1. *Mannitol.* This is an effective osmotic agent that will rapidly decrease intracranial pressure. It is given as a rapid intravenous infusion of 1 g to 1½ g/kg, or typically as a full bottle of 100 g (500 ml of 20%) for the average adult. It may be repeated as needed, but care must be taken to replace lost fluid lest hypovolemia and hypotension result. A urinary catheter is mandatory.
2. *Intubation.* If an endotracheal tube is not in place, it should be inserted immediately. Since arterial blood gas tests have probably not yet been undertaken, the patient should be begun on an F_IO_2 of 1.0. This is not dangerous in the short-term and may be lifesaving if the neurologic deterioration is due to hypoxemia. Ventilation should be adjusted to hyperventilation so that the PCO_2 is decreased to about 25 torr. A tidal volume of 10 ml to 15 ml/kg and rate of 12 to 15/min will usually accomplish this goal. A mild respiratory alkalosis with systemic *p*H values of 7.50 to 7.55 will result but is of no concern.
3. *Ventricular Drain.* If one is present, it may be opened and CSF drained for decompression. If a ventriculostomy is not in place, it is rarely worth delaying a CT scan for the additional 30 minutes required to insert it. An exception to this rule may be the patient who has undergone a posterior fossa craniotomy/craniectomy and who may deteriorate from acute hydrocephalus.
4. *Blood Work.* This should be limited to serum electrolytes, CBC, type and cross matching, and arterial blood gases. The serum sodium is important because hyponatremia may cause or aggravate brain edema with or without a mass lesion. Hypoglycemia may cause neurologic deterioration and seizures (especially in children) and is easily corrected. Hypoxemia and hypercapnia alone or together can lead to rapid neurologic deterioration and may be easily corrected. A current hemoglobin and sample for cross typing will be required if the patient is returned to the operating room; it makes little sense to draw and send these after a CT scan when they may be obtained at the same time as the electrolytes and blood gases.
5. *Central Venous Catheter.* If time permits, this catheter should be placed to aid in fluid replacement after administration of mannitol, which may rapidly lead to hypovolemia. It should be pointed out that the various forms of intravenous contrast used for CT scan and angiography are also osmotic diuretics and may potentiate hypovolemia. The diuresis occurring with mannitol is primarily a *water diuresis* with little Na^+ in the fluid; thus, replacement of this diuresis is generally best accomplished by fluids relatively low in sodium (D5/0.2% NS, D5/0.45% NS). If furosemide is added to enhance a mannitol diuresis, the urine will be very high in sodium, and replacement should be with normal saline.

TABLE 46-2. TRIAGE OF THE DETERIORATING PATIENT

Step	Basis
Recognition of possible complication	*CHANGE*
	1. Level of consciousness or
Begin treatment early* 1. Mannitol, 1 g/kg 2. Intubation TV 10–15 ml/kg, Rate 12 Aim at $PCO_2 \approx 25$	2. Hemiparesis, new or progressing, or 3. Pupillary changes 4. Progressive hypertension with or without bradycardia
R/O hypotension	Vital signs
R/O hypoxemia	Blood gases, physical examination
R/O hyponatremia	Serum electrolyte levels
R/O mass lesion and high ICP Hematoma Edema Hydrocephalus, etc.	CT scan or air ventriculogram or angiogram
R/O infection Meningitis Ventriculitis Abscess, etc.	Ventricular puncture or lumbar puncture

* Treatment must be instituted rapidly, often before a clear diagnosis is attained.

The theme for evaluating the patient who may be deteriorating from a mass lesion, either postoperatively or posttrauma, is speed. Rapid evaluation must be balanced against the increase in specificity of diagnosis and therapy that may be gained by a CT scan, angiogram, or ventriculogram. Although the postoperative patient may well deteriorate owing to a hematoma, he may also be the victim of brain edema, an infarct or some other lesion (vide infra) neither requiring nor responding to reoperation. The above steps have been outlined to extend the time

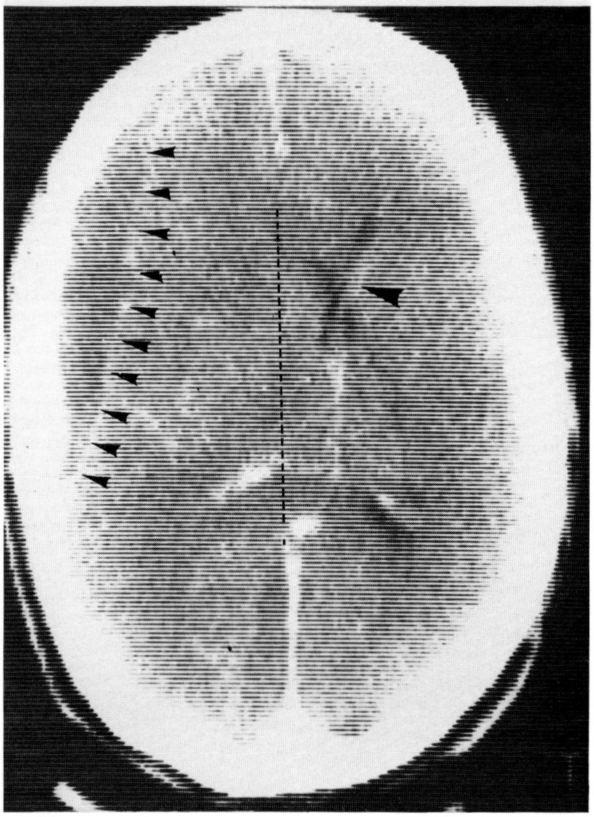

FIG. 46-7. Chronic subdural hematoma. Note the relatively lucent subdural collection, which represents liquefying hematoma. The CT scan is superior to most other diagnostic techniques because it gives information about the lesion density as well as precise location: it clearly labels this as a chronic subdural hematoma. Note the "enhancement" of the subdural membranes after contrast (*line of arrowheads*), and the shifted ventricles (*single arrowhead*). The treatment of this is twist drill or bur hole drainage and not usually craniotomy.

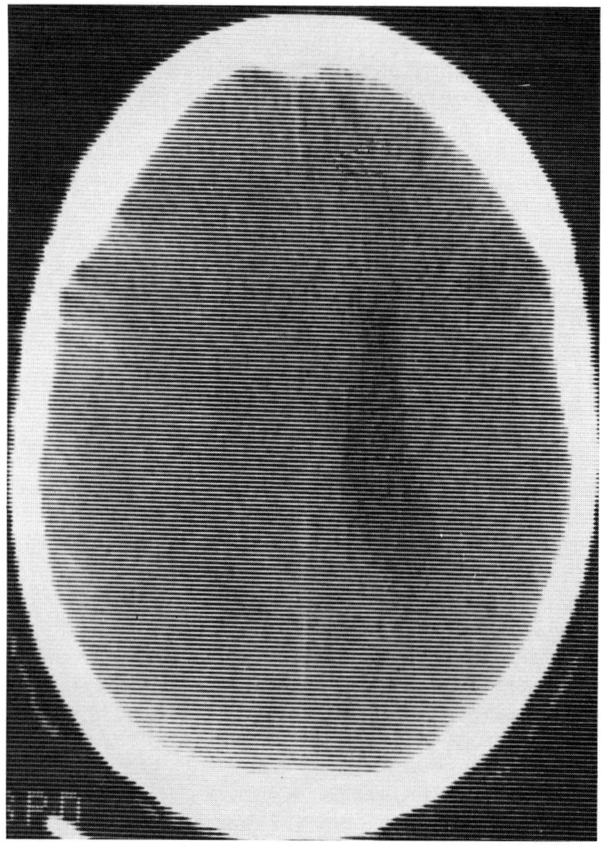

FIG. 46-8. The isodense subdural hematoma is difficult to diagnose by CT scan, especially if enhancing membranes cannot be demonstrated. Clues to its presence are the ventricular shift, collapse and compression of the ipsilateral ventricle, and the absence of sulcal markings. These findings could be duplicated by brain swelling, but an angiogram demonstrating an extracerebral collection (as in Fig. 46-5) or a diagnostic tap of the subdural space would confirm the presence of hematoma.

available to the physician to evaluate the changing patient more completely.

The patient who deteriorates many days or weeks following craniotomy may have a chronic subdural hematoma (Fig. 46-7). This lesion is a lucent, subdural mass lesion on CT scan and can be drained by burr holes or more easily by twist drill aspiration of the subdural space.[31] Of special concern is the "isodense" subdural hematoma (Fig. 46-8). This lesion represents an intermediate stage in the liquefaction of the dense, acute clot and the final lucent, liquid chronic subdural hematoma. Its presence is suggested by clinical change and a scan showing mass lesion effect (ventricular shift) with ipsilateral ventricular collapse and no sulcal markings.[68] It usually responds to twist drill aspiration.

BRAIN EDEMA

Brain edema occurring in the postoperative period may have its origin in excessive retraction or surgical trauma and appear as little more than decreased density on a CT scan associated with brain shift. However, brain edema is commonly associated with other etiologies and usually contributes to the total "mass" effect (Fig. 46-9). Edema often accompanies neoplastic lesions, especially metastatic tumors; it is common with intracerebral hemorrhage and contusion. Edema associated with cerebral infarction generally indicates a rather severe stroke and may cause the patient to herniate and die.[9, 32]

The treatment of brain edema is partially dependent upon the etiology of the lesion. The effectiveness of steroids is recognized for the brain edema associated with neoplastic and inflammatory (infectious) lesions; they are most effective when begun prior to surgery. Dexamethasone is the standard agent used in most centers and was initially chosen because of its low mineralocorticoid activity. The usual dosage range is 4 mg to 20 mg every 4 to 6 hours, and total doses of 100 mg or more per day are well tolerated. Other steroids are equally effective, but the dose should be adjusted for equivalent corticosteroid activity; the advantages of one steroid preparation over another are just theoretical; no solid evidence renders one more superior.

The use of steroid treatment of edema due to trauma, infarction, or anoxia is standard practice in some institutions, avoided in others, and irregularly used in some; the evidence for steroid effectiveness is minimal. However, steroids seem relatively safe and possess few adverse effects when used for short periods of time. Their doses are generally the same as for the edema of brain tumor. It is worth pointing out that a recent double-blind study of steroids in traumatic brain injury patients (placebo, low-dose, high-dose dexamethasone) demonstrated no beneficial effects of the steroid. But the rates of septic complications or gastrointestinal hemorrhage among any of the groups also did not differ.[12, 13]

Because brain edema represents increased tissue water, it exerts a mass effect and will usually be accompanied by an increase in intracranial pressure. Steroids may or may not be effective in all forms of edema and probably require hours to begin reducing edema at best. A more rapid reduction in ICP is required in the deteriorating patient and is best achieved with an intravenous infusion of mannitol. The dose is 1 g to 1½ g/kg, which is typically a 500-ml bottle of 20% mannitol. Some have advocated lower doses (0.25–0.50 g/kg), but these are generally not as effective nor will they lead to ICP reductions as long-lasting as the higher dose.

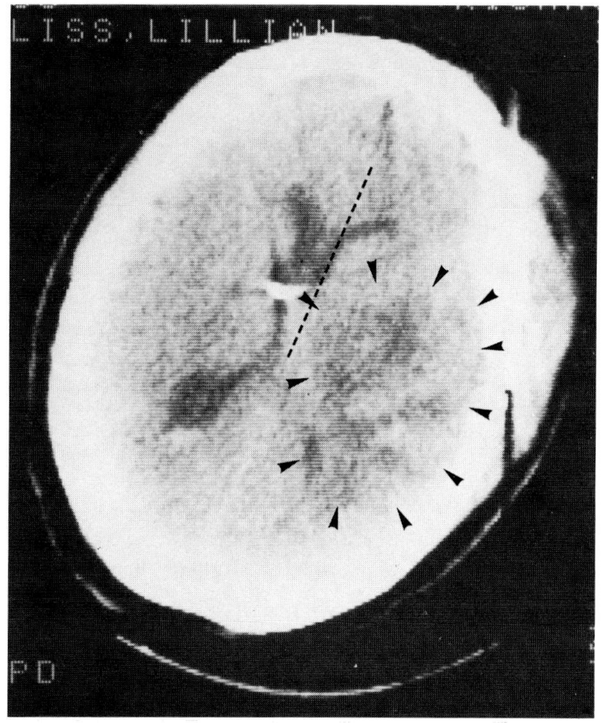

FIG. 46-9. This patient underwent right craniotomy and clipping of a posterior communicating aneurysm. She became progressively more lethargic with the development of a left homonymous hemianopia, and left hemiplegia. The ICP was elevated, and hydrocephalus was treated by ventriculostomy. Note the right-to-left shift of the ventricular system (*midline marked with dotted line*), compression of the right ventricular system and the areas of lucency (edema) in the right hemisphere (*outlined by arrowheads*). In essence, this represents the findings of an acute, severe right hemisphere infarct (swollen) with vasospasm as the etiology.

TRAUMA

The complications of trauma differ little from the complications to be expected after elective craniotomy.[67] However, in two essential points the trauma patient declares himself in need of special consideration: the frequency and severity of systemic complications and the frequency of intracranial hypertension and mass lesion.[66]

Systemic Complications

The systemic complications suffered by the patient with a traumatically injured brain are noteworthy for their frequency. Eighty percent of brain-injured patients who are unable to communicate with the examiner at the time of emergency-room evaluation have suffered multiple injuries. Hypotension, hypoxemia, and high blood ethanol levels all complicate the initial evaluation or potentiate the severity of the brain injury. Of those with significant systemic complications such as hypotension or hypoxemia, outcome is significantly worse than if such complication had not intervened.[46]

A substantial part of the physician's role in the care of the patient with a traumatically injured brain, indeed of any patient, is the prevention of systemic complications. Hypotension and hypoxemia are particularly devastating to the patient with brain injury, but are also the most avoidable complications. Carefully monitored hydration and pulmonary toilet are well worth the effort involved.

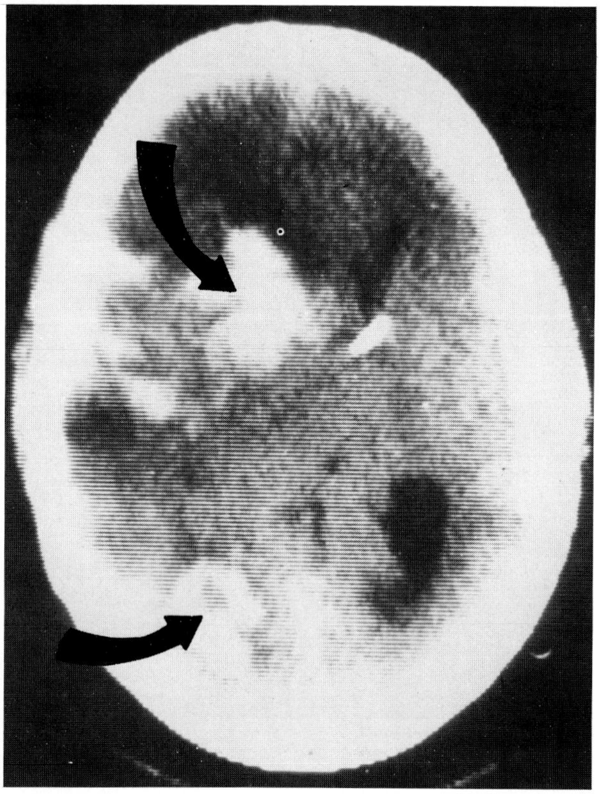

FIG. 46-10. The same patient as in Figure 46-6, but now 48 hours after removal of the subdural hematoma, the intracranial pressure again rose, and the patient's clinical condition worsened. A repeat CT scan demonstrated deep frontal and occipital intracerebral hemorrhage (*arrows*). These lesions have become known as "delayed traumatic intracerebral hematomas" and are most likely to occur in patients who have had significant hypotensive or hypoxic insults and who develop coagulopathies.

Intracranial Complications

Intracranial hypertension develops in approximately 50% to 80% of patients with severe injuries and is the direct cause of death in 50% of those dying after head injury. Generally, this intracranial hypertension is the result of traumatically induced *brain edema and swelling* and has been difficult or impossible to control using standard therapy such as hyperventilation, CSF drainage, hypothermia, barbiturate coma, and osmotic diuretics such as mannitol.[45]

This process often becomes apparent at the time of surgery when closing the dura is difficult because of brain swelling. It progresses in the postoperative phase and manifests itself by continuing neurologic deterioration in the face of an inexorably rising ICP. The end point is an ICP that plateaus at a level equal to the systemic arterial pressure. To date, we have been able only to slow the process and lack a definitive and effective therapy for this "malignant edema."

The patient with a traumatically injured brain also is subject to delayed intracerebral hemorrhage (Fig. 46-10).[28] About 10% of patients with severe brain injuries are subject to this lesion, and it is of interest to note that the incidence of shock, anoxia, acidosis, and anemia is about 90% in this group. This is twice the frequency of such insults in those not experiencing delayed hematoma.[25] The reasons for this are unclear but seem to relate to anoxic damage occurring at the time of injury. Thrombocytopenia occurring as the result of acute and chronic alcoholism, drug reactions, consumptive coagulopathy, disseminated intravascular coagulation, and sepsis all predispose the patient to this as well as to other hemorrhagic complications.[36] The presentation of the delayed intracerebral hemorrhage is not specific. The patient will usually be seen to deteriorate neurologically over a period of time, which will be paralleled by a rising ICP. CT scan is diagnostic and will demonstrate high-density intraparenchymal lesions with mass effect. However, not all patients will reveal these changes clinically, and only about two thirds will require evacuation of the mass.

The delayed intraparenchymal hemorrhage and high frequency of malignant brain swelling are unique to the patient with severe traumatic brain injury. It must be remembered that these patients are also subject to any of the other complications afflicting the postcraniotomy patient.

Infection (meningitis, ventriculitis) occurs in 10% to 15% of the severely brain injured; the risk of this increases arithmetically in the face of basal skull fracture with CSF leak (1–2%), craniotomy (5–10%), and ICP monitoring (5%). Prophylactic antibiotics appear not to prevent such infection in the face of trauma but remain in widespread use.[58]

Delayed hydrocephalus (3–5%) and chronic subdural (3–5%) hematomas occur with regularity in the severely brain injured and must be considered if a patient deteriorates or plateaus after a period of improvement.[14] Seizures also occur in the brain injured in about 10% to 15% of patients. They are about equally divided between focal and generalized epilepsy, are more likely if infection has occurred, and may reach a 40% incidence in those with missile injuries to the brain.

The care of the patient with a traumatically injured brain is complex. Most have additional injuries; they are prone to the same complications that any neurosurgical patient may experience and a few that are unique. They are especially susceptible to additional insults and may be further damaged by them. Thus, the overriding theme in the care of this group is vigilance and sensitivity to a change, however subtle, in their neurologic status. Complications must be anticipated, diagnosed, and treated early for maximal recovery to occur.

Dural Sinus Thrombosis

Fracture of the occiput predisposes the patient to thrombosis of one of the lateral sinuses, though it may also occur in the absence of fracture. Clinically, the patient demonstrates lethargy, occasionally seizures, headache, confusion, and papilledema. Intracranial pressure is high. Recovery tends to be spontaneous, possibly owing to recanalization of the sinus or development of collateral drainage. The entity should be suspected when ICP is high and no evidence of mass lesion or hemorrhage is found. Focal deficit is unusual, and the degree of trauma may have been minimal.[37]

VENTRICULAR LOCULATION AND PORENCEPHALIA

A loculated ventricle may act as a focal, expanding mass lesion under special circumstances.[1] In general, with neoplastic lesions in the region of the foramen of Monro, hemorrhage, or cysts, the drainage pathway from one lateral ventricle into the third ventricle may become blocked.[60] Since the choroid plexus in the lateral ventricle will continue to produce CSF, the blocked ventricle will expand, cause brain shift, and elevate the ICP.[62] The patient will generally become lethargic and demonstrate progressive signs of hemiparesis consistent with a hemispheric mass lesion. CT scan is diagnostic, and temporary or permanent drainage of the loculus is the treatment of choice. Following the triage flowsheet for the deteriorating patient will lead to the correct diagnosis, and treatment thereafter is drainage; a temporary ventriculostomy, needle aspiration of the loculus, and a permanent shunt are all effective therapies that may be employed according to the mechanism in a given patient.[1, 60, 62]

Porencephalia occurs if an area of brain infarcts or is damaged when in close proximity to the ventricles. The pulsations of the CSF dilate the area of "encephalomalacia" and produce the picture seen in Figure 46-14 (see under Pneumocephalus and CSF Leak). Porencephalia is important in the face of hydrocephalus because dilatation may occur in this region out of proportion to ventricular dilatation, thus causing further local tissue damage. In essence, the ventricles may decompress into the weakened cerebral parenchyma. These lesions require treatment if they are growing; therapy is usually ventricular shunting.

HYDROCEPHALUS

Hydrocephalus is a similar problem except that it is not usually associated with brain shift. The two major divisions of hydrocephalus are classically "communicating" (Fig. 46-11) and "noncommunicating" (Fig. 46-12); the former represents a ventricular system that is able to drain CSF into the subarachnoid space of the posterior fossa, while the latter does not allow this. Thus, dye placed into a lateral ventricle in the case of communicating hydrocephalus will emerge from the foramen of Luschka of the fourth ventricle and appear in CSF sampled from the lumbar canal. In noncommunicating hydrocephalus, the dye remains trapped within the ventricular system and lumbar CSF remains unstained.

Noncommunicating hydrocephalus may be the result of congenital lesions, but in the postoperative period it is usually due to residual tumor or edema blocking the ventricular system or even to a hematoma directly or indirectly causing a physical block to CSF reaching or exiting from the fourth ventricle (see Fig. 46-12). The diagnosis of noncommunicating hydrocephalus is generally made by CT scan demonstration of a mass or mass effect in a location capable of blocking these pathways in the face of an enlarged ventricular system, especially when the fourth ventricle is seen to be small in the face of lateral and third ventricular dilatation. When all ventricles are enlarged, the distinction becomes more difficult. Treatment is temporarily effected by ventriculostomy, and, if required, a permanent shunt is definitive.

Communicating hydrocephalus represents a functional block to the percolation of CSF from its exit at the foramen of Luschka to its point of absorption through the arachnoid villi into the major venous sinuses. The point of obstruction may be the tentorial incisure due to scarring from meningitis, the subarachnoid space itself, or damage to the arachnoid granulations. Any combination of these events is possible, but the most common cause of communicating hydrocephalus in the postoperative period is subarachnoid blood blocking absorption pathways. Deterioration from communicating hydrocephalus is generally slow, occurs over a period of days, generally lacks focal findings (though preexisting deficits may worsen), and occurs when a known etiology exists. CT scan demonstrates enlarged ventricles (as would angiography, ventriculography, or pneumoencephalography); lumbar puncture shows high pressure; and the fluid may or may not be abnormal. If the problem is thought to be transient, then temporizing measures such as ventriculostomy, lumbar punctures, a lumbar subarachnoid drain, or no treatment are possible. Particularly if the hydrocephalus is mild and due to a known

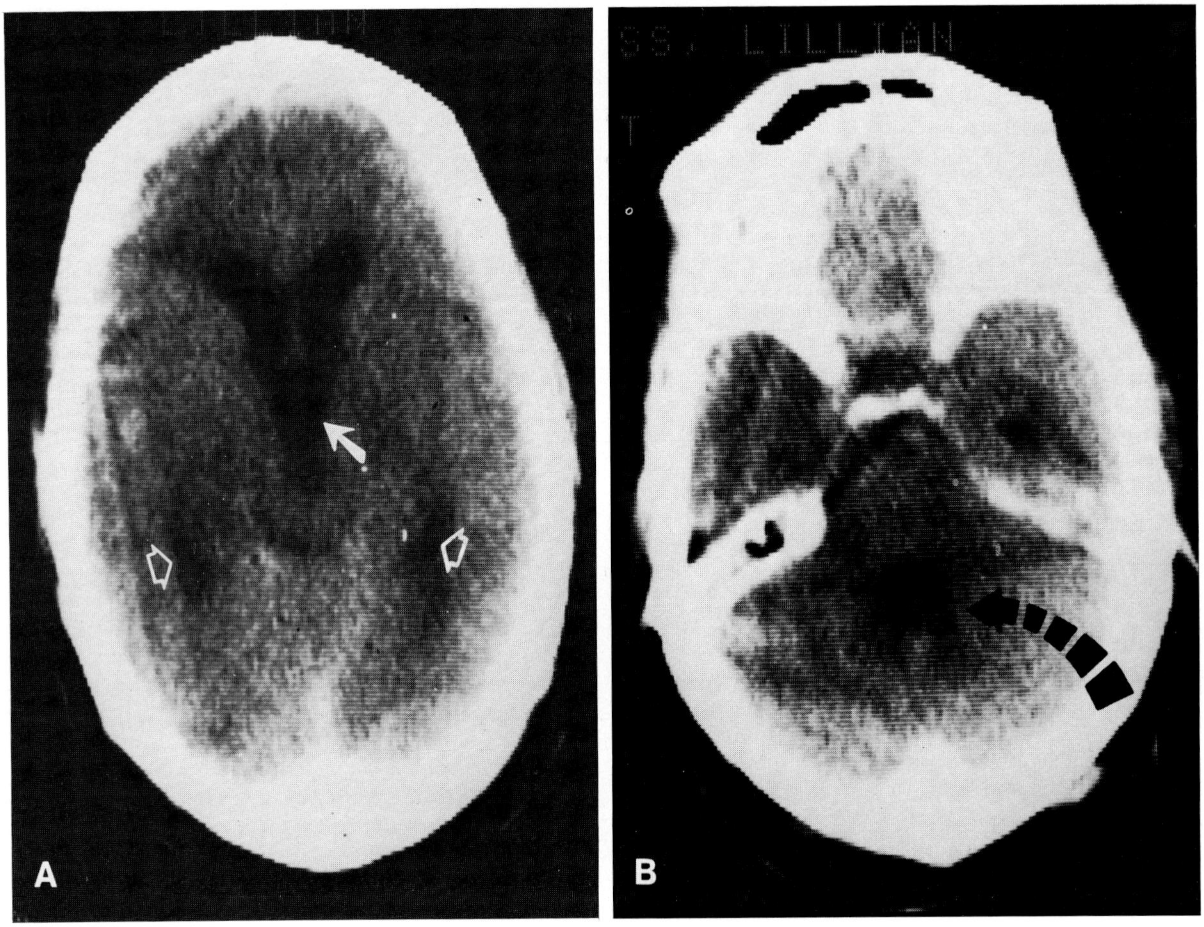

FIG. 46-11. (*A*) CT scan demonstrates enlarged ventricular system. The lateral ventricles are grossly enlarged as is the third ventricle (*solid white arrow*). This scan could represent either communicating or noncommunicating hydrocephalus; note dilatation of the temporal horns (*open white arrows*), which nearly always suggests hydrocephalus. (*B*) The lower cut of the scan of this patient clearly shows the enlarged fourth ventricle (*arrow*). The question of the size and location of the fourth ventricle must be specifically addressed when a scan is obtained for hydrocephalus. This set of scans is most consistent with communicating hydrocephalus.

etiology such as meningitis or subarachnoid hemorrhage that might improve with time, permanent shunting may be deferred; if required, it is the definitive treatment.

The concept of the two major divisions of hydrocephalus is helpful, but at times it is artificial. A cerebellar hemorrhage may well cause noncommunicating hydrocephalus by acting as a mass effect and blocking the fourth ventricular outflow pathways, but the same hemorrhage may also rupture into the subarachnoid space and cause an element of communicating hydrocephalus by an absorption block at the level of the arachnoid villi. In a given patient it may be impossible to decide which pathophysiological event might be occurring, but the difference is rarely important in treatment. Its importance derives from the fact that lesions capable of causing noncommunicating hydrocephalus are themselves generally more dangerous and lead to rapid deterioration of the patient. Noncommunicating hydrocephalus is itself more likely to lead to rapid deterioration of the patient, whereas communicating hydrocephalus rarely progresses rapidly. Thus, patients harboring lesions known to be capable of causing blockage of CSF flow from the ventricular system require more careful, anticipatory observation for deterioration due to acute hydrocephalus than does the patient in whom communicating hydrocephalus is likely to be the problem. In addition, *patients with noncommunicating hydro-*

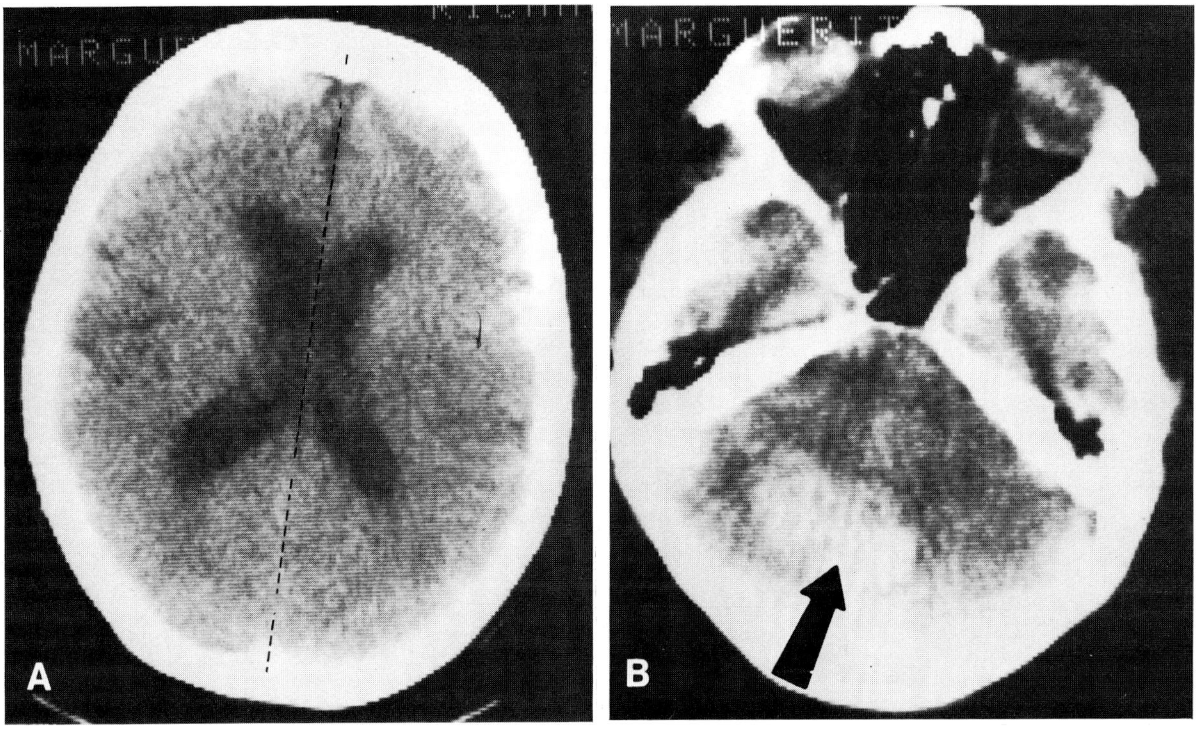

FIG. 46-12. (*A*) This scan is similar to Figure 46-11A. The lateral ventricles are enlarged (hydrocephalus) and in the midline (*dotted line*). (*B*) The lower scan demonstrates a high-density lesion in the left cerebellum (*arrow*). This was a cerebellar hematoma and led to noncommunicating hydrocephalus. Note the fourth ventricle is *not* seen. The mass lesion could equally have been a tumor, a postoperative hemorrhage, or even edema about an infarct. Patients with this form of hydrocephalus should *never* undergo lumbar puncture. Drainage should be by temporary or permanent shunt.

cephalus should never undergo lumbar puncture, since this procedure may lead to rapid deterioration from tonsillar herniation, respiratory arrest, and death. This is in contrast to communicating hydrocephalus, which may actually be safely treated by lumbar drainage.

Hydrocephalus, particularly noncommunicating, often is a prominent component of posterior fossa lesions and is a dreaded complication of posterior fossa surgery.[52] In patients undergoing posterior fossa surgery for any reason, this complication must be considered as dangerous as the development of a postoperative hematoma. Many surgeons always use a temporary ventriculostomy in such patients, while others may prefer to watch the patient clinically or even place a permanent shunt days or weeks before the more definitive procedure. If a permanent shunt has been placed and the patient deteriorates after posterior fossa exploration, shunt failure must be considered. Again, a CT scan usually suggests it, and shunt tapping and manometrics will confirm it.

A variation of noncommunicating hydrocephalus is found in the patient with "double compartment hydrocephalus." An aqueductal block may lead to hydrocephalus with a ventricular shunt providing drainage. But, if the fourth ventricular choroid plexus produces CSF at a rate in excess of the subarachnoid space's ability to absorb it, the fourth ventricle may dilate and cause symptoms. A second shunt in the posterior fossa may be required.[21]

PNEUMOCEPHALUS AND CSF LEAK

Pneumocephalus is simply the accumulation of intracranial air. Its common etiology is after a basal skull fracture that allows the subarachnoid space to communicate with the exterior, usually through the ethmoid, sphenoid, or frontal sinuses (Fig. 46-13). The air under these circumstances alerts the physician to observe for an active CSF leak, which may predispose the patient to meningitis, ventriculitis, or brain abscess. Although the most common cause of pneumocephalus is trauma, operative trauma that

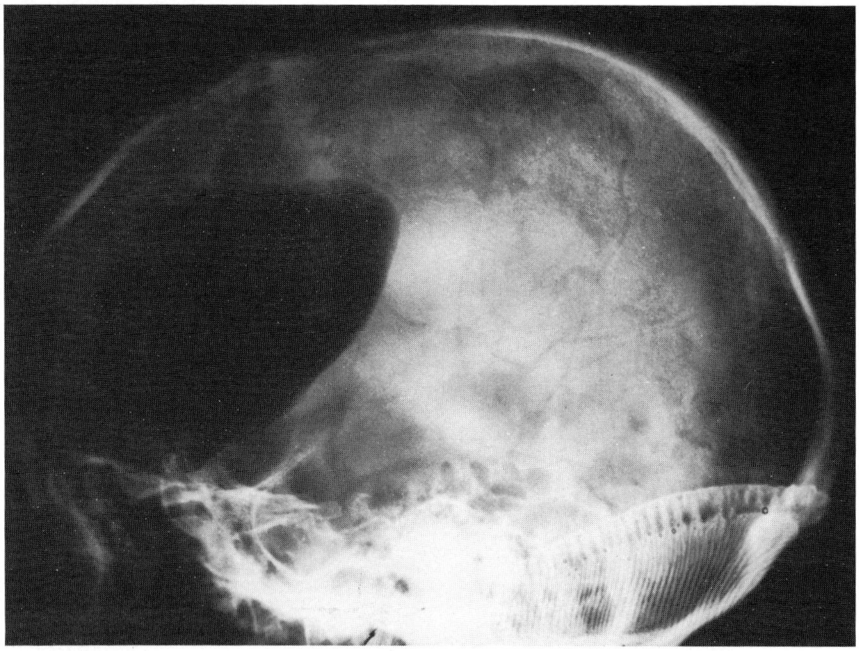

FIG. 46-13. Posttraumatic pneumocephalus. This is an extreme example of pneumocephalus occurring after trauma; there are multiple frontal fractures that extend into the air sinuses. Intracranial air may be located in the subdural space, in the subarachnoid space, or even within the ventricular system. Its importance is twofold: one, it implies CSF fistulas and suggests the possibility of infection; two, it may come under tension and act as a mass lesion and require aspiration.

violates the base of the skull, such as transsphenoidal surgery, or any of the other air sinuses must be considered capable of leading to CSF leak, which may be manifest not only by spinal fluid draining from the nose or into the pharynx but also by pneumocephalus. For this reason, a single brow-up lateral skull x-ray film should be obtained soon after any surgery or trauma capable of leading to this complication as a way to anticipate the problem before it manifests itself as meningitis or worse (Fig. 46-14).

Cerebrospinal fluid draining from the nose (rhinorrhea) or ear (otorrhea) after trauma is presumptive evidence of a fracture at the base of the skull. Occasionally, differentiation between CSF and other secretions is difficult. The definitive finding for CSF is a glucose level in the fluid greater than 25 mg to 30 mg/dl. Tears have a glucose of at most 5 mg/dl; nasal secretions, even when mixed with blood, usually are between 10 mg and 20 mg/dl glucose and are obviously mucoid in appearance. Dextrostix are generally too sensitive, and their accuracy at these low values is poor, so a milliliter of fluid should be obtained for laboratory analysis. However, if the Dextrostix examination is negative, the likelihood that the fluid is CSF is minimal.

The treatment of CSF rhinorrhea is generally conservative, though much argument has been directed at this point. Most rhinorrhea stops within 1 to 2 weeks of injury; nearly all will cease spontaneously by 4 weeks post-injury. If the rhinorrhea results from transsphenoid surgery, it is generally treated by diverting CSF through a lumbar subarachnoid drain. This should be effective within 5 to 10 days postoperatively, or reexploration and packing of the sella turcica should be carried out.[49]

The use of antibiotics is highly controversial. The fear of meningitis or other infection has prompted the routine use of prophylactic antibiotics in some centers. Others avoid their use in fear of selecting gram-negative or resistant strains of bacteria. Only a single randomized study found a very low incidence of infection ($\approx$2%) after basal fracture, and prophylactic antibiotics did not alter this. Indeed, the only infections occurred in the group of patients receiving antibiotics while none of the "nontreated" patients developed infection.[33] Regardless, it is wise to culture the nasopharynx or external auditory canal in the patient with a CSF leak before beginning treatment to provide a baseline culture. If infection should develop, antibiotics may be instituted on the basis of this culture. If they have previously been instituted, then a rational basis for a decision to change antibiotics has been provided. Similarly, given a patient with a CSF leak, once he has been shown not to harbor an intracranial mass lesion by CT scan, it is wise to obtain a CSF sample from lumbar puncture. This will aid the interpretation of future CSF analyses performed should meningism, fever, or other changes occur.

Although the vast majority of CSF fistulae cease draining without operative repair, some do not. A major concern before resorting to open craniotomy is the question of concomitant hydrocephalus. If hydrocephalus is present, a CSF fistula will rarely close

(Fig. 46-15). The patient will treat his own hydrocephalus by this abnormal drainage pathway. If the patient is treated by ventricular drainage or lumbar subarachnoid drain, then the fistula may heal. Care must be taken, however, lest the patient then become symptomatic from hydrocephalus. It should be noted that in the face of a CSF leak, the ventricular size may remain normal or small and the ICP low, so that possible hydrocephalus is not ruled out by these studies when CSF continues to leak.

A unique form of pneumocephalus may be seen after posterior fossa surgery performed on a sitting patient or when a lumbar subarachnoid drain is used to divert CSF for treatment of a basal fracture. In this situation, the arachnoid usually opens, and CSF is able to drain freely by gravity; most of the CSF is in the supratentorial space, and, as it drains, air may accumulate both in the intraventricular system and the subdural/subarachnoid spaces. Usually, this is of no consequence, but tension pneumocephalus may occur, act as a mass lesion, and lead to clinical deterioration in the postoperative period.[6, 17, 24] Diagnosis is based upon the clinical situation and a single lateral x-ray film is diagnostic. Treatment, if necessary, is by twist drill decompression of the air from the supratentorial space. A single aspiration should suffice, and the lesion should not recur.

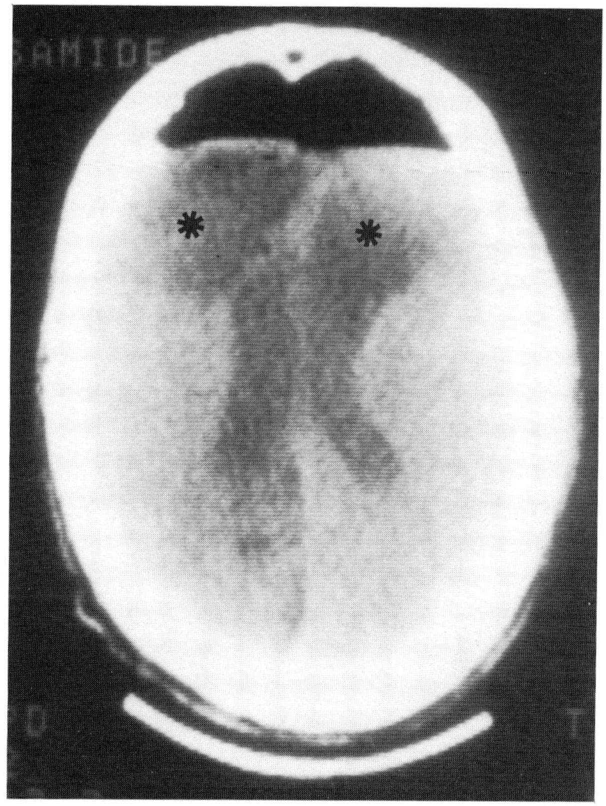

FIG. 46-14. CT scan of a patient after a transfrontal gunshot wound. The missile fractured the skull base with communication into the frontal *and* ethmoid sinuses. In the postoperative period, intracranial air was observed on plain x-ray film and CT scan. The patient had been observed to have CSF rhinorrhea. The CT scan also demonstrated hydrocephalus and bifrontal porencephalia (*asterisks*). Attempts to treat the CSF leak by temporary drainage were unsuccessful, and a permanent shunt for hydrocephalus was required. No further leak was experienced after the shunt was placed.

POSTCRANIOTOMY INFECTION

Between 2% and 5% of patients with clean craniotomies will experience infection in the postoperative period.[10] This rate may be decreased to less than 1% by prophylactic antibiotics.[43, 55] It is increased by reoperation by about 3% to 5% for each reexploration. It relates to length of surgery by about 0.5% to 1% for each hour of operation, so that patients who undergo very long operations are at substantially greater risk than those whose operations are short. Hypothermia has been associated with slightly greater risk of infection, but these operations also take longer so causality is difficult to determine.[75]

Interestingly, age, systemic disease, experience of the surgeon, and steroids have generally not been related to increased risk of infection. Wound drains add little or no risk of infection. Posterior fossa surgery was found by Wright to be less likely to result in infection in the face of long surgery or reexploration, which may relate to the more abundant vascular soft tissue exposed.[75]

The use of ventriculostomies and the subarachnoid screw for ICP monitoring carry about a 4% to 5% risk of infection, but their presence also increases the risk of wound sepsis in otherwise clean wounds, as do basal fracture and reexploration.[58] In our series of wound complications, we found that steroids were related to increased infection only if they were continuously used for periods of greater than 2½ to 3 weeks. In our ICP monitoring experience, prophylactic antibiotics have not altered the wound infection rate; however, in this situation we have an indwelling foreign body in more or less direct communication with the exterior, as opposed to a surgical wound that is opened for a short, finite period of time and then closed. The latter would seem to be more likely to respond to prophylactic antibiotics while the former less so; the data from our institution and those of Haines support this distinction.[27, 58]

The differential diagnosis of infection in the postoperative period is rather simple and includes meningitis, ventriculitis, subdural empyema, cerebritis-brain abscess as well as surgical wound sepsis

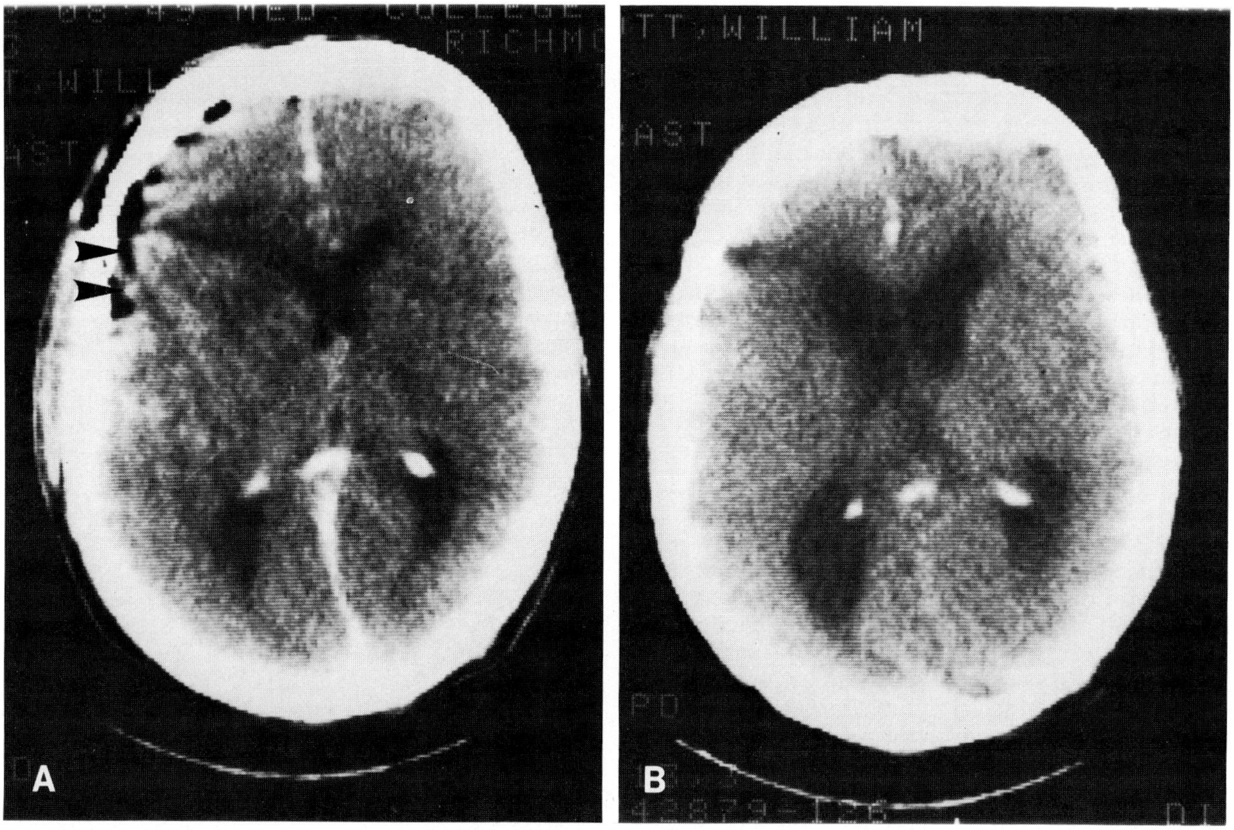

FIG. 46-15. (*A*) This patient underwent a left frontal craniotomy for a meningioma en plaque about the optic nerve. The sphenoid sinus was entered and the patient developed CSF rhinorrhea. During the period of CSF leakage, a CT scan revealed mild left frontal lobe edema and subdural air (*double arrowheads*), but *normal ventricular size*. (*B*) The same patient after successful treatment of the leak (reoperation and lumbar CSF drainage). His orientation deteriorated; he became lethargic and incontinent; and a CT scan revealed grossly enlarged ventricles. His earlier CSF fistula had effectively treated his hydrocephalus, which became symptomatic with ventricular enlargement when the leak was closed. It should be noted that CSF fistulas nearly never close spontaneously in the face of hydrocephalus.

itself. Because these different spaces are often brought into communication by surgical manipulation and other procedures, subsequent infection may well involve more than a single space, and use of a single term may be inaccurate and misleading. Because therapy may vary according to the precise locus and, occasionally, etiology of the infection, careful delineation of the infected spaces is desirable and, at times, crucial.

Meningitis and Ventriculitis

By definition, meningitis is infection that involves the leptomeninges (pia-arachnoid) and thus the subarachnoid space. This space is essentially in continuity from the hemispheric convexities to the lumbosacral subarachnoid space as well as the ventricular system. Thus, sampling fluid from the lumbar canal will generally reflect infection at higher levels. The same is true if fluid is obtained by cisternal puncture. However, since CSF is produced within the ventricles and exits from the small openings of the fourth, ventricular fluid may not reflect infection that is primarily subarachnoid; lumbar CSF would be the better fluid to examine.

Similarly, infection localized to the subdural space (subdural empyema) may leave the ventricular and lumbar fluids sterile with little more than a reactive pleocytosis. The same is true of cerebritis and brain abscess unless they erode into the ventricular system or subarachnoid space. In the postoperative patient, however, this communication often has been surgically created, and cerebritis may result in infected CSF early.

Meningitis typically presents as high fever, meningism, positive Kernig and Brudzinski signs, headache, depression in the level of consciousness, SIADH, and often seizures. To the extent that a given neurosurgical patient already has a depressed level of consciousness or is frankly comatose, he will not be able to complain of headache, confusion, and other subjective symptoms. Likewise, he is already subject to seizures. Even meningism and other signs of meningeal irritation may have their origin in subarachnoid hemorrhage induced by surgery or injury ("chemical" or "hematogenous" meningitis). In short, postcraniotomy patients may normally have all of the clinical signs of meningitis, including fever, so the diagnosis may depend entirely upon examination of the CSF and a high index of suspicion. The spinal fluid is often confusing since pleocytosis, hemorrhage and high protein and low glucose levels may be normal after surgery in the absence of infection.[70, 76]

Thus, if a patient changes for the worse, the first step is to rule out a mass lesion. Then, infection must be considered. It should be recognized that postoperative meningitis is often much more subtle in its manifestations than is the typical pneumococcal or meningococcal variety seen in the emergency room. Obviously, if signs of meningeal irritation should occur in isolation or associated with any other change, CSF examination is mandatory. Since the cell count and protein and pressure measurements are likely to be abnormal to some degree, absolute diagnosis must await culture results or the demonstration of bacteria on Gram stain of the CSF. It follows that *treatment must be begun before infection is clearly defined:* without culture and sensitivity reports. Simply, the risk of not treating actual meningitis is much greater than the dangers of a 5-day course of antibiotics given in the face of what might prove to be sterile, uncontaminated CSF.[30, 74, 76]

Treatment should be begun with the first suspicion of meningitis, but only after obtaining an adequate sample of CSF. The treatment requires that intravenous antibiotics be given in meningitic doses; because the organism will be unknown, antibiotics must be chosen on the basis of the most likely organisms, as listed below.

Common Postoperatively Encountered Organisms

- Gram-positive organisms
  - *Staphylococcus aureus*
  - *Streptococcus pneumoniae*
  - *Streptococcus pyogenes*
- Gram-negative organisms
  - *Escherichia coli*
  - *Proteus* species
  - *Enterobacter* species
  - *Pseudomonas aeruginosa*
- Anaerobic organisms*
  - Anaerobic streptococcus
  - *Bacteroides fragilis*
  - *Bacteroides melaninogenicus*

We prefer aqueous penicillin G, 2 million units, every 2 hours (24 million/day) and chloramphenicol (Chloromycetin), 1 g every 6 hours, intravenously. High doses of penicillinase-resistant penicillins are recommended for hospital-acquired infections combined with chloramphenicol. Regardless, therapy directed at gram-positive cocci and gram-negative organisms must be instituted. It may later be modified according to sensitivity test results, but if the clinical response is adequate then the antibiotic regimen may be left unchanged. Sensitivity results are helpful for two primary reasons: first, one can select an appropriate antibiotic if the clinical response has been poor with the initial agent(s); and second, one can discontinue an agent that is merely redundant.[15]

Ventriculitis

The clinical presentation of ventriculitis differs little from that of meningitis, though it is often much more subtle. Meningeal symptoms may be minimal and fever variable, while alteration in mental status and neurologic function predominate. Therefore, diagnosis requires a high degree of suspicion, and the only examination that is diagnostic is microscopic and bacteriologic examination of the ventricular fluid.

Both meningitis and ventriculitis tend to occur 3 to 5 or more days after violation and contamination of the subarachnoid or ventricular space in the postoperative period. This is usually when brain edema and the effects of operative trauma are clearly resolving, and a change or reversal in this pattern should alert the clinician to the possibility of infection in one of these spaces. While the triage diagram still applies to the deteriorating patient and a CT scan is advisable, the more delayed the complication, the more likely it is that one is dealing with infection or hydrocephalus. Both entities may be associated with elevated ICP, and infection should be considered in someone with a rising ICP, especially if this rise has no clear or reasonable explanation and occurs without mass lesion on the CT scan.

Meningitis may be delayed as much as 4 weeks or more after surgery, especially after violation of mastoid air cells or the air sinuses and in the face of CSF leak.[22, 23, 33, 41, 49]

Most patients remain on steroids in the postoperative period. It should be noted that steroids are particularly effective against inflammatory and neo-

*Usually limited to brain abscess.

plastic processes. Thus, if attempts to wean a patient from steroids meet with rising ICP or clinical deterioration, then masked infection or edema about a neoplastic process should be suspected. Because a brain tumor patient has no guarantee against infection, the possibility of both entities must be considered; that is, infection may supervene in the face of any underlying diagnosis and must always be considered in a deteriorating patient.

Brain Abscess and Cerebritis

Brain abscess, or its immediate precursor, cerebritis, is relatively rare in the postoperative period. The development of meningeal signs or infected CSF in the face of focal deficit suggests that this process should be ruled out. The absence of focal deficit does not rule out abscess. Abscess in the changing patient in the triage process that can be shown to have mass effect will be part of the differential diagnosis for such a mass.

If an abscess does not communicate with the ventricular or subarachnoid space, meningeal signs will usually be absent. Even *de novo* cerebral abscesses have completely normal CSF 5% of the time and the patient is usually afebrile. Steroids may suppress or delay neurologic change in the developing abscess, so this entity must also be specifically considered in the patient who worsens upon steroid withdrawal.

The treatment for brain abscess is bacteriologically the same as for meningitis or empyema, but drainage is mandatory. This process is also diagnostic, and one or two needle aspirations combined with high-dose antibiotics will clear about 80% to 85% of abscesses, The remainder require craniotomy for complete cure. If infection also involves the craniotomy flap, then reoperation, bone flap removal, and excision of the abscess should be carried out for definitive therapy.[2]

The use of intraventricular antibiotics has increased in the last decade and provides an effective means of treating certain forms of infection, especially meningitis and ventriculitis caused by highly resistant or gram-negative organisms.[15, 61]

Subdural Empyema

A specific form of abscess is the subdural empyema. This entity is also marked by neurologic worsening, the development of focal signs such as hemiparesis, and, in particular, seizures. The seizures associated with subdural empyema tend to begin focally, then become generalized, and quickly progress to status epilepticus. They are very difficult to control, and the patient often requires intubation, support from a mechanical ventilator, and sedation to the point of general anesthesia. The mass effect is often related to edema, since the actual amount of pus in the subdural space is usually minimal.

Subdural empyema is rare after craniotomy but may follow burr hole drainage of a chronic subdural hematoma. We have had one case occurring on the side of an ICP monitor. Most subdural empyemas occur in the face of chronic sinusitis in adults or after middle ear infections in young children and infants.

Diagnosis by CT scan may be difficult, and a high index of suspicion is required. More definitive diagnosis is offered by cerebral angiography and confirmed only by subdural tap or operation.[42]

Inflammatory effects are predominant and treatment characterized by drainage and high-dose antibiotics. The drugs and doses are the same as those recommended for meningitis, which may also be present. Drainage may be accomplished by reoperation or burr holes, and many surgeons recommend leaving subdural catheters for irrigation of this space with antibiotic solutions such as concentrated bacitracin (500 units/ml).[4]

Craniotomy Wound Sepsis

The principles of therapy for intracranial infection differ little from those for infection anywhere: drainage and antibiotics. The same apply to the treatment of craniotomy wound infections. These infections may arise and remain within the wound (but outside the dura) or be associated with intracranial infection. If the latter occurs, then early removal of an infected flap is nearly mandatory as well as identification of the offending organism. It follows that any evidence of a craniotomy wound infection should be accompanied by an immediate examination of the CSF. Most clinicians also begin antibiotics directed at preventing meningitis from developing, and these, once again, are usually in meningitic doses and directed at gram-positive and gram-negative organisms.

Various attempts to treat infection while preserving the bone flap have met with only partial success.[10] For this reason, we generally remove the bone flap, débride the inevitable infected granulations, and close the wound in a single layer with wire or Prolene suture over drains placed to allow irrigation of the subgaleal space. Usually 3 to 5 days of irrigation with concentrated bacitracin solution are adequate and the drains then removed. Antibiotics are continued for 10 to 14 days or longer, depending upon the clinical response, cultures, and CSF examinations.

CSF Shunt Infection

Shunt infection, which occurs with 5% to 15% of shunts, is handled according to similar principles. In addition to neurologic change, meningitis, ventriculitis, and seizures, shunt infections may also present as systemic sepsis-bacteremia and any of the subsequent complications of chronic seeding of the vasculature if the shunt drains into the venous system. "Shunt" nephritis is one of these entities. Peritonitis is also one of the presentations to remember in an infected ventriculoperitoneal shunt. The essential point is that a shunt is a foreign body and may serve as a nidus of infection; the type and presentation of the infection relate to the location of the shunt and its drainage. As in all such cases, treatment is removal of the foreign body, appropriate antibiotics in meningitic doses and usually a temporary CSF drain such as a ventriculostomy. Treatment is continued for 10 to 14 days or until the CSF is sterile. Generally, CSF is not considered sterile until cultures have remained negative for 5 days in the incubator. Occasional reports of successful management of infected shunts using antibiotics alone have been published, but this remains a technique with a high rate of recurrent infection (>70%) and is less definitive than shunt removal.[34] It should generally be reserved for situations in which shunt removal and replacement offer severe technical problems or when the patient is too ill to undergo surgery.

SUBGALEAL COLLECTIONS

In the postoperative period, blood in the subgaleal space may liquefy and CSF and other fluids collect in this very large dead space. Opinions vary widely as to the correct treatment. Some surgeons believe that these collections should never be drained, since violation of this space may lead to infection. Others drain such collections with impunity and regularity.[30]

There are three basic reasons to drain these collections. First, fluid can accumulate to the extent that tension is placed upon the suture line. Often one will enter a patient's room in the morning and find that the collection has drained from the incision sometime during the night. Second, the fluid may track along the loose areolar connective tissue that comprises the subgaleal plane and accumulate over the forehead, especially around the soft periorbital tissues. This is basically harmless, but uncomfortable and at least transiently disfiguring for the patient. Last, so much fluid in the subgaleal dead space may actually serve as a culture medium, and normally insignificant bacterial contamination from the time of surgery may flourish and lead to a craniotomy infection.

The only reason for not draining such a collection is fear that a sterile collection may become contaminated and infection result. There are no clear data to support either point of view. Because of this, our policy has been to avoid meddling with the subgaleal space unless the suture line or scalp flap is under tension or causing pain. It seems better to drain the fluid under controlled circumstances where the scalp can be prepared antiseptically and a sterile needle used to drain the collection than to trust to the cleanliness of the patient's pillow or to allow a portion of the wound to break down.

Since we have instituted the routine use of a subgaleal vacuum drain left at the time of craniotomy, the frequency of these collections has been reduced markedly. Additionally, we have observed that periorbital swelling has declined markedly, and, while patients are clearly more comfortable and less concerned about their eyes swelling closed, it has also been easier to examine the pupillary light reflexes and ocular motility in both awake and comatose patients.

A variation is the patient with occult or otherwise unrecognized hydrocephalus who decompresses his subarachnoid space into the subgaleal or subdural space by way of dural defects (Fig. 46-16). The bony closure is certainly never watertight, and it seems doubtful that even a perfectly closed dura

FIG. 46-16. This patient underwent transcortical resection of a left, lateral ventricular tumor. She developed a transient CSF absorption block, but instead of dilating her ventricular system, she decompressed the CSF into the subdural (*small arrowheads*) and subgaleal (*large arrowheads*) spaces. Note that there is a mild degree of left-to-right shift induced by the subdural CSF. She eventually absorbed CSF normally, and both collections resolved. In some patients the problem is severe and long lasting and requires a permanent shunt. It may also lead to hemiparesis and severe brain shift if the subdural collection (hygroma) becomes large; it may act in much the same way as a chronic subdural hematoma. It generally only occurs after transcortical entry into the ventricular system.

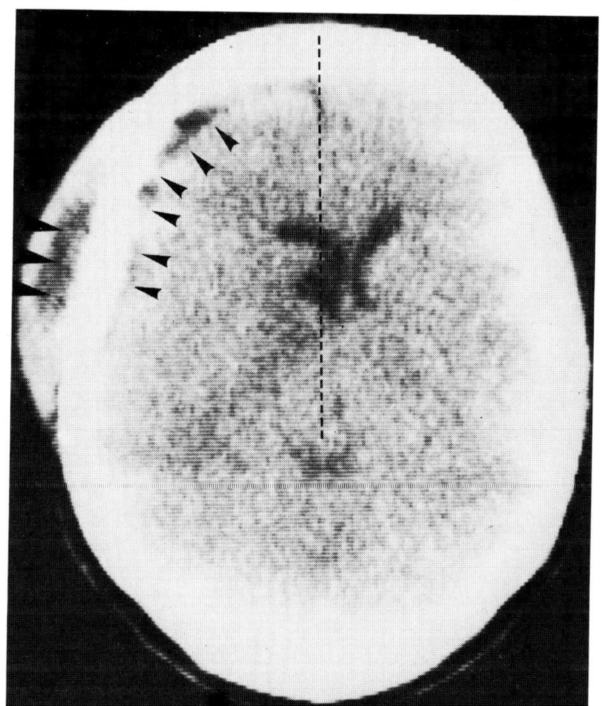

would be able to hold CSF under pressure and prevent its leaking into the subgaleal dead space. This collection is of concern for the previously mentioned reasons; however, treatment must be directed at the hydrocephalus. This etiology should be suspected when the fluid collection continues to reaccumulate after one or two aspirations of the wound and when it seems composed of almost pure CSF. Certainly, the danger is increased when multiple subgaleal taps are carried out, which may lead to fistulae or direct contamination of the space with subsequent meningitis.[30]

Diagnosis may be achieved in some patients by lumbar puncture; if the collection is decompressed by lumbar drainage, then this is presumptive evidence that the CSF pathways communicate with the subgaleal space. Failure to drain the collection with lumbar puncture does not rule out the possibility that it is accumulating owing to hydrocephalus; there may simply be a "one-way valve" effect prohibiting reentry of the CSF from the subgaleal space to the subarachnoid. Examination of the fluid and its prevention from recurring by CSF diversion provide presumptive evidence that CSF is leaking from the intracranial space to the subgaleal.

Since a proportion of hydrocephalus in the postoperative period is transient and will resolve on its own, serial lumbar punctures may be attempted, or a temporary lumbar or even a ventricular drain may be used to tide the patient over. A permanently installed shunt eventually may be required.

PERIORBITAL HEMATOMA

Periorbital hematoma is partially discussed under "Subgaleal Collections." There are a few circumstances under which marked edema and ecchymoses in the soft periorbital tissues may occur. Again, of itself, this edema is of little concern, but it can render an examination of the pupils nearly impossible, as well as frighten patients and families and be modestly uncomfortable. Because the periorbital tissues have no firm supporting matrix of connective tissue, edema and hematoma fluid do tend to collect about the eyes and cause them to swell closed. Usually, it is maximal on the side of operation, but may be bilateral, especially in trauma when it tends to be called "racoon eyes" or some similar name.

Usually little can be done about the problem, but if it becomes mandatory to examine the eyes, then 0.5 ml to 1.0 ml of hyaluronidase may be injected into the periorbital tissue to speed resolution of the swelling by allowing it to seep into the adjacent tissues more easily. The effect is often temporary and may need repetition; however, we have had only very few instances in which injection was required. Most patients who are alert would prefer to suffer a few days of edema than to have needles poked about their face.

As mentioned above, the use of a vacuum drain in the subgaleal space has reduced the incidence of periorbital swelling. In those in whom it still occurs, it is much less severe and of shorter duration than it used to be. Generally, this swelling is nearly resolved by the third or fourth postoperative day and rarely is a problem thereafter. A residual "black eye" may be apparent even weeks later but is of no concern.

The development of periorbital swelling where none has existed in the immediate 72 hours postcraniotomy suggests the possibility of CSF leaking into the tissues or even of early infection. Particularly if the periorbital tissues become erythematous and swollen several days after surgery, one should be alerted to the presence of infection. Sometimes this concern is unnecessary, and the swelling resolves spontaneously, but in others the craniotomy wound declares itself to be infected. Treatment at this stage is careful observation with the physician alerted to any signs suggesting meningitis, ventriculitis, or craniotomy flap suppuration.

POSTERIOR FOSSA EXPLORATION

The posterior fossa is an area with several specific and unique complications related to the sitting position and the potential for direct brain stem damage in the face of normal hemispheres.[20, 22, 23, 26, 29, 52]

Air Embolism

Air embolism is a complication caused by the negative venous pressure that occurs when a patient is sitting. Although a normal vein would simply collapse under negative pressure, the venous system of the skull is prevented from collapse either from the rigid walls of the dural sinuses or from the supporting bony structure of the diploic vessels. Thus air can be "sucked" into the venous system in amounts large enough to cause systemic hypotension due to cavitation within the heart. Usually this is manifest during surgery and not postoperatively, but it can cause prolonged unconsciousness after surgery, when anesthetic agents should have worn off.

A similar event occurs if air entering the venous system is able to cross a patent foramen ovale and enter the arterial circulation directly from the venous side (paradoxical air embolism). This air may embolize to the brain and lead to ischemic infarction. Its importance lies in the differential diagnosis of the patient who simply does not awaken from posterior fossa surgery or awakens with a neurologic deficit that does not relate to the posterior fossa exploration.

Hematoma

As mentioned in the discussion of pneumocephalus, the sitting position may result in CSF leaking from the ventricles, the hemispheres collapsing away from the inner table of the skull, and the space being filled with air. Usually, the air is under no tension and is absorbed over the next 48 to 72 hours; occasionally the air is under tension and requires aspiration. Similarly, as the hemispheres collapse from the inner table of the skull, a bridging vein from the cortex to the sinus may tear, with resultant hemorrhage. The result is that an acute hematoma will fill the dead space; it occurs in 1% to 2% of posterior fossa explorations in the face of hydrocephalus.[22, 30] This process would be exacerbated if the ventricular system were widely dilated from chronic hydrocephalus and the potential for the hemisphere to collapse further from the inner table correspondingly enhanced.[26] Bilateral subdural hemorrhage may also occur.[20] Probably by a similar mechanism, an epidural hematoma may form. About half of these have had their bleeding point localized to a burr hole made for ventricular decompression, but in the remainder the hemorrhage begins at a site distal to the burr hole.[71] Again, the importance lies in the differential diagnosis of the patient who remains comatose after anesthesia or who awakens with a deficit not existing preoperatively. A supratentorial lesion must be considered.

As previously mentioned, mass effect in the posterior fossa may lead to acute hydrocephalus and require ventricular drainage (see Fig. 46-12), or it may directly compress the brain stem. Brain stem compression is often manifest by acute coma and respiratory arrest, but lesser degrees of compression may manifest themselves by focal deficit, especially pupillary abnormality, sixth or seventh nerve paresis, gaze palsies, bradycardia, and hypertension. Although hematoma is the mass commonly thought of, contusion, edema, and swollen infarcts also can act as mass lesions and may require surgical débridement for relief of the compression and noncommunicating hydrocephalus.

Cranial Nerve Palsies

Although any of the cranial nerves may be damaged by surgical procedures, there are important ramifications when this damage involves the fifth, seventh, ninth, and tenth cranial nerves.

Damage to the fifth nerve may obliterate the corneal reflex. This leaves the eye prone to trauma, foreign bodies, abrasions, and infection. The diagnosis is easy, and usually warning the patient is adequate prevention. Obviously, direct section of the fifth nerve or its ophthalmic branch for the treatment of tic doloreaux may lead to this side-effect. Again, the patient requires a warning and should exercise increased awareness and care.

The seventh nerve functions in many ways, but the most important is closure of the eye. If the seventh nerve becomes paralyzed, eye closure is impossible. After resection of acoustic nerve tumors, paralysis of the seventh nerve may occur in up to 40% of the patients; only about half of this group regains function. Although function may still return as late as 2 to 3 years after damage to the nerve, the patient must be protected during the interim. The use of liquid tears may help prevent drying and exposure keratitis of the cornea, but if they should show signs of developing, then therapy is tarsorrhaphy. If function should return, the tarsorrhaphy can be revised. The presence of fifth and seventh nerve palsies can be disastrous, since abrasions, keratitis, and infection may develop to a more serious degree in patients with corneal anesthesia than in those in whom pain is prominent.

Acoustic nerve tumors are not the only lesions associated with these palsies; basal skull fracture, other cerebellopontine angle lesions, brain stem infarcts, and damage in the region of the parotid gland are all capable of causing this complication. The concern about the ophthalmic side-effects remains.

Paresis of the ninth and tenth nerves may also accompany posterior fossa exploration. Hypoactive gag reflex, depressed cough, and paralysis of the vocal cords may all result. These deficits leave the patient liable to pulmonary complications from acute and chronic aspiration. As with fifth and seventh nerve paresis, the diagnosis is not difficult. Examination of the gag reflex (9th and 10th nerves), listening to the voice for excessive hoarseness (vocal cord paralysis, 10th nerve), and having the patient swallow (9th and 10th nerves) are all easily performed. There is generally no specific therapy, but most of these problems are short lived and improve spontaneously.

When paresis is severe, feeding tubes, esophagostomy, gastrostomy, and tracheostomy may be required. For the marginal patient whose problem is resolving, it is important *not* to begin feeding with clear liquids such as broth, water, tea, and soups. Feeding should be begun with custards, gelatins, and other foods that can be manipulated easily, for they are less apt to lead to aspiration.[22, 23, 30, 35, 52, 76]

INTRACRANIAL HYPOTENSION

Intracranial hypotension is an unusual complication seen with very large craniectomies, overshunting (valve pressure too low), high-grade CSF leaks, and large free-floating bone flaps.[65] In any of these situations, the basic pathology seems related to shifting or compression of the brain in the face of no supporting CSF or bony structure.[6] The brain stem in particular is distorted and may lead to cranial nerve palsies (especially sixth nerve palsies), hemiparesis, lethargy, or other focal deficits. In general, placing the patient flat in bed alleviates most of the symptoms and suggests the diagnosis. The process is usually self limited in that CSF leaks usually stop on their own, and the soft tissues of the scalp provide more support.

If the problem originates in a valve that drains too quickly or too much, treatment must be directed at replacing the valve with one of higher pressure or higher resistance.[5] Subdural hemorrhage is the most serious complication resulting from not recognizing the "overshunted" patient. Usually this is a chronic subdural hematoma; it may be bilateral; and it responds to aspiration of the subdural space. Ligation of the shunt, or its removal, may be required to prevent recurrence. Again, the long-term treatment will require a higher pressure valve.

Fig. 46-17. Protocol for a diagnostic workup of postoperative seizures.

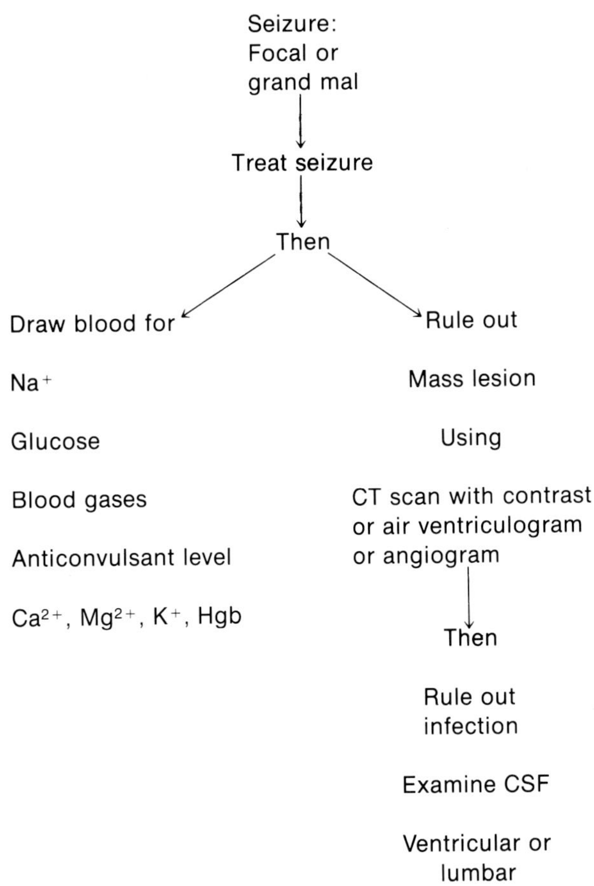

SEIZURES

Epilepsy in the postoperative period is a function of many variables, for example, preoperative seizures and type of pathology. It is difficult to estimate the risk of provoking a seizure just by craniotomy (*i.e.*, where the brain is normal and left untouched, and risks derive only from having the skull and dura opened and then closed). This figure is probably much less than 5%. It appears that most of the risk of epilepsy in the postoperative period originates in the cerebral pathology itself, which interacts with systemic events to reduce the seizure threshold.

An important concept to emphasize is that an epileptic event of any sort in a patient who was previously free of seizures (or under control) must be interpreted as a change in the neurologic status of the patient. If the patient awakens immediately and demonstrates little, if any, residual deficit, then following a protocol that emphasizes the systemic events that may precipitate seizures is reasonable (Fig. 46-17). In particular, low or less than therapeutic levels of anticonvulsants, hypoxemia, severe hyperglycemia, hypomagnesemia and hypocalcemia, hypoglycemia, and hyponatremia ought to be ruled out immediately.

An EEG obtained in the immediate postictal period is of little help because it often shows nothing more than diffuse or focal slowing. These findings may result from the postictal state or the underlying pathology, and both may be exacerbated by systemic abnormalities. Likewise, the question to be addressed is not "Does the patient have a seizure focus or a reason for epilepsy?" since the answers to both parts are clearly known. The primary question is "What has changed that caused the patient to have a seizure now?"

In addition to systemic metabolic events that may exacerbate an underlying seizure disorder, intracranial lesions must be considered. Postoperative hematomas, both extra-axial as well as intraparenchymal, are capable of epileptogenesis. Embolic stroke carries about a 7% risk of seizure and must be considered in the differential diagnosis. These lesions will tend to increase or produce focal neurologic deficit and may well be associated with lethargy or frank coma. Therefore, a mass lesion should be considered in the patient who does not return to his baseline status within a very short time after cessation of the fit. Infection is another intracranial process that significantly increases the risk of seizure and should be considered and actively ruled out. Infection is important, since the usual signs of meningitis, ventriculitis, and brain abscess often are already present or impossible to interpret in the postoperative period; the only way to be certain of their absence is by CSF examination. Again, this examination is usually grossly abnormal in the postcraniotomy patient, and steps may need to be taken on the basis of confusing information (more fully discussed under Infection).

TREATMENT. Most seizures are short lived and self limiting. With a patient in whom the seizure has stopped, the above workup should begin (see Fig. 46-17). In addition, treatment should be aimed at preventing recurrence, and after drawing an anticonvulsant level, additional parenteral doses of the patient's anticonvulsant should be administered. Practical points to be considered are the following:

Phenobarbital has a much faster onset of action than does phenytoin.

Diazepam has a period of action of only 10 to 20 minutes and should never be used as a maintenance anticonvulsant, but it is the drug of choice to halt a seizure immediately and is the first drug of choice in status epilepticus.

Both diazepam and phenytoin are extremely alkaline in their parenteral form (pH ≈ 11) and precipitate in the usually acidic (pH, 4.5–6) IV fluid, so they should not be mixed with such fluids and never given by "buretrol."

Phenytoin should never be given by IM injection since it precipitates, is poorly absorbed, and causes muscle necrosis.[48]

Paraldehyde dissolves the plastic of most syringes and IV lines and must be given in glass syringe directly into a vein, but with equal effectiveness may be given rectally or orally (in 30 ml of mineral oil per rectum). Paraldehyde in oil should never be given intravenously.

Seizures are indirectly dangerous, since they may signal a significant systemic or intracranial complication and lead to increased morbidity or mortality. Yet they represent a direct danger as well, since they nearly always interfere with respiration and may lead to systemic hypoxemia and acidosis and potentiate underlying cerebral pathology. With a damaged brain, such hypoxemia may produce more and greater insults than might otherwise be expected. Hypoxic injury is the significant complication of status epilepticus and may be fatal in the otherwise intact patient. Its effect on the postoperative patient is devastating. Table 46-3 outlines a treatment regime directed mostly at the patient in status epilepticus, though it is applicable to any patient. Of concern is the airway and systemic pressure of these patients, since all of the drugs that are effective anticonvulsants are respiratory depressants and may cause systemic hypotension at the required dosage. In particular, the patient being treated for status epilepticus should have continual monitoring of his blood pressure and will usually require intubation, additional oxygen, and probably mechanical respiratory support. This is particularly the case in the postcraniotomy patient.

TABLE 46-3. TREATMENT OF POSTOPERATIVE SEIZURES

Treatment	Precautions
1. Diazepam, 10–30 mg, IV push, until seizure stops; then	Watch blood pressure, airway, respirations
2. Phenobarbital, 1 mg/kg, IV, every 5–10 min until seizure stops, up to 10–15 mg/kg (about 700–1000 mg) over 30 min	Always support respirations, intubate, support blood pressure
3. Phenytoin, 500 mg, IV, over 10 min, then 100 mg, IV, every 1 hr × 5 to total loading dose of 15 mg/kg within 12–24 hr	Watch for asystole and other arrhythmias
4. If seizure continues, paraldehyde, 10 ml in 30 ml mineral oil per rectum, q 4–8 hr, or 10 ml, IV, q 4–8 hr (requires glass syringe and direct IV administration)	Patient on ventilator

ANEURYSM SURGERY

The direct operative treatment of cerebral aneurysms leaves the patient liable to the same complications as does any craniotomy: postoperative hematoma, infection, and hydrocephalus.[11] But, in addition to these complications, the patient suffering a subarachnoid hemorrhage due to aneurysm is subject to arterial vasospasm.[19] This condition is poorly understood, though a general consensus is that the vasospasm is somehow related to the breakdown products of blood in the subarachnoid space and has been shown more severe in patients with large amounts of subarachnoid blood defined on CT scan.[7, 18]

Clinically, vasospasm presents as a gradual deterioration in the level of consciousness of the patient with the concomitant development of neurologic signs related to the affected arterial supply. Basically, vasospasm causes a stroke with a subacute, gradual onset. If severe enough, the spasm and ischemia may cause brain swelling with edema, herniation syndromes, and death. A CT scan may show lucent areas related to infarction or tissue edema with shift; if the scan is done very early in the development of vasospasm, the study may appear normal, since time is required for infarction to become evident (see Fig. 46-9). Angiography will usually demonstrate a markedly narrowed and attenuated vasculature; these changes may be limited to the specific vascular bed of the operated aneurysm, or the changes may be generalized.

Treatment of vasospasm is difficult and controversial. However, certain principles are generally accepted. Since the basic pathology is analogous to that of ischemic infarction, steps should be taken to enhance the cerebral circulation. Increasing the systemic pressure by the use of pressor agents, reducing the ICP to enhance perfusion pressure, and expanding volume all seem at least partially effective.[16, 39, 44] Hypervolemia attained by overtransfusion and overhydration has recently been credited with nearly a 50% reduction in the incidence of vasospasm.[53] The use of a central venous pressure line or Swan–Ganz catheter to monitor the volume of these patients is mandatory. The use of direct vasodilators such as nitroprusside, dopamine, and nitroglycerine has been advocated, but their use remains controversial. Clearly, hypotension and hypoperfusion must be avoided. There is some rationale for the use of hemodilution as may be achieved with low-molecular-weight dextrans to reduce blood viscosity and enhance the capillary circulation, but, again, this remains controversial. Mannitol also causes a transient hemodilution and may be useful in the lowering of the ICP, but care should be taken to prevent the negative fluid balance that the diuretic may induce.[8]

In summary, vasospasm after the operative treatment of cerebral aneurysms is a difficult problem to treat. Its occurrence is unpredictable; its basic effect is the creation of ischemic infarction, which may be so severe as to lead to generalized cerebral edema and death. The most effective therapy has proven to be volume expansion with central venous pressure raised to 12 cm to 15 cm of water or more.[72, 73] Other manipulations designed to increase perfusion pressure (raising the systemic pressure, lowering the ICP) seem helpful. Direct vasodilators remain controversial.[3, 57]

Subarachnoid hemorrhage (SAH) results in hydrocephalus of some degree in about 10% to 15% of patients during their acute illness. Eventually, 5% to 10% of the patients afflicted by SAH will require a CSF shunt.[69]

EXTRACRANIAL–INTRACRANIAL BYPASS PROCEDURES

Extracranial–intracranial (EC–IC) bypass operations carry the same general risks as does any craniectomy, but a few complications are relatively limited to EC–IC.[56, 64]

Scalp Necrosis

Although careful technique and specific steps to avoid flap necrosis must be observed in the operating room, it should be noted that the blood supply to the scalp has been used for another purpose. Usually, with careful operative technique, flap necrosis is limited to a relatively small area of the surgical wound, often to the area in which the superficial temporal artery (STA) has been removed from the flap itself. Attention to the use of noncompressive dressings, not placing excessive pressure on the wound, and early suture removal all aid in avoiding problems with flap necrosis. Local wound care is usually sufficient to clear any minor eschar and areas of necrosis, and ultimate healing is satisfactory. Very rarely, reoperation and various plastic procedures may become necessary to effect healing.

Increased Deficit

There is about a 4% incidence of postoperative stroke after EC–IC; in our series, three patients worsened in the postoperative period. The worsening was minor, began 24 to 72 hours postoperatively, and resolved within an equally short time frame. All were shown to have patent anastomoses by angiography. One patient had been operated on with a high-grade stenosis in the high cervical, petrous, and cavernous carotid and was shown to have occluded this vessel completely. We believed that the occlusion was the result of a decreased pressure gradient across the stenotic region. Regardless, evaluation of a new deficit in the post EC–IC patient should be directed at demonstrating the absence of postoperative hematoma and then proving the patency of the anastomosis. A single case of aneurysm at the site of anastomosis has been described; undoubtedly, more such lesions will occur as time passes, and a postoperative angiogram will be required for detection.[50] Once these points have been confirmed, it has been our practice to hydrate patients according to the CVP (CVP≃ 12–15 cm H_2O) and to include low-molecular-weight dextran in normal saline (500 ml/day) in the hydration regimen. Because these patients are generally elderly, and also have cardiovascular disease, care must be taken to avoid overhydration and congestive failure.[64]

Late Complications

POSTRADIATION LEUKOENCEPHALOPATHY OR NECROSIS

The brain and spinal cord are generally considered to be radiation resistant, but when doses reach 5000 to 7000 rad, about 5% develop radiation necrosis. The pathologic lesion appears to be endothelial necrosis in the vasculature of the brain rather than a primary effect on neuronal or glial elements, though white matter seems preferentially affected.[63]

Clinically, this patient returns to the hospital

"not doing well." He may have new, or an exacerbation of old, neurologic deficit. The usual difficulty in diagnosis is resolving the problem of neoplastic recurrence *versus* radiation necrosis. Hydrocephalus and porencephalic cysts must also be considered. A CT scan will rule out the latter entities, but will often not clearly differentiate recurrent or residual tumor from radiation necrosis.

Treatment is symptomatic, and a trial or increase in the dosage of steroid medication is worthwhile. Differentiation between the tumor and radiation necrosis requires tissue examination, but there is usually little benefit to the patient in obtaining this antemortem.[60]

SHUNT FAILURE

Any patient with hydrocephalus treated by ventricular shunting is liable to malfunction of the shunt. Clinical presentation varies, but is often stereotyped to the individual patient. Either his symptoms will be similar to his initial presentation with hydrocephalus or he may have had a previous shunt failure. For this reason, a satisfactory history may be the best diagnostic examination.

Prominent symptoms are lethargy, headache, vomiting, confusion, incontinence, and gait ataxia. Diplopia, paralysis of upgaze (as in Parinaud's syndrome), and seizures all may occur. CT scan may demonstrate enlarged ventricles, which is best judged by comparison with a baseline study obtained when the patient was doing well.

The differential diagnosis will include chronic or subacute subdural hematoma (which may be bilateral), recurrent tumor if this was initially present, ventricular loculation, double compartment hydrocephalus, and anticonvulsant intoxication (especially with phenytoin) (Fig. 46-18).

Usually the progression of symptoms is relatively slow, but it may be rapid and life threatening. Treatment may be temporary ventriculostomy, tapping of the shunt if the obstruction is distal, or merely elective shunt revision. Care must be taken to rule out the presence of infection, which may have precipitated the shunt failure. If deterioration is extreme and life threatening, mannitol may be used in standard doses to allow time for a more thorough evaluation.[47, 54, 59]

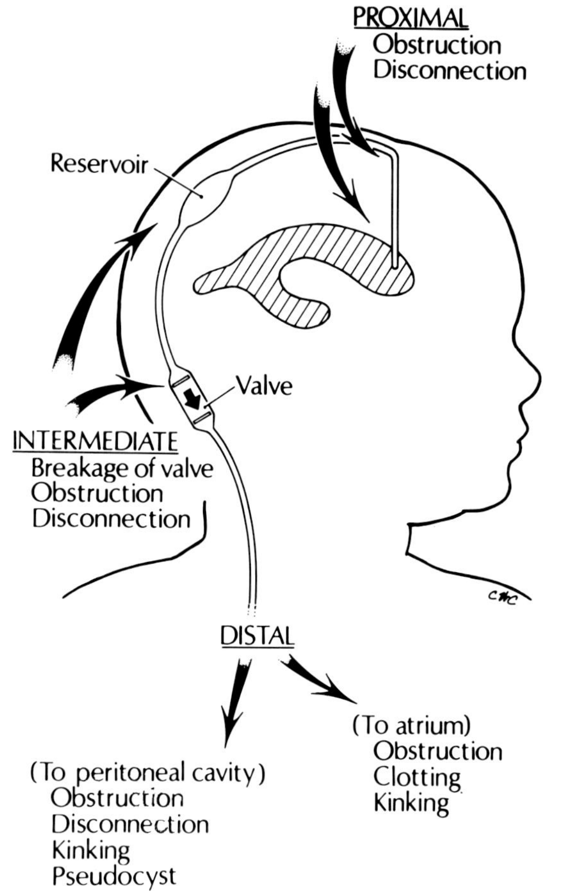

FIG. 46-18. A diagram of a typical shunt system and the various points at which obstruction may occur. Because detachment of the various components may be diagnosed by plain x-ray film (not CT!), a set of plain films is mandatory in the workup of suspected shunt failure. Note that infection may coexist with mechanical failure or *cause* obstruction, and an effort should be made to culture the CSF from such shunts even if mechanical failure seems most likely.

SPITTING SUTURES

Occasionally patients return to the outpatient clinic with suture material extruding from the line. This used to occur in about 5% of patients whose galea had been closed with silk; it is very rare since the advent of polyglycolic acid-based absorbable sutures. Generally the extruded sutures can be dealt with by grasping the thread in a hemostat and pulling gently until they are freed. Cleansing with saline or mild antiseptic is usually adequate, and a bandaid will suffice for a dressing.

DRAINING SINUS

The draining sinus without a visible suture at its base is ominous. Again, it is less frequent when absorbable suture is used in the galea. Often this problem occurs in patients with malignant disease who have received radiation and other immunosuppressive drugs such as steroids and chemotherapy. Culture usually yields staphylococcus or streptococcus species but often of low virulence; local wound care and antibiotics improve the gross appearance of the infection but inevitably fail. Treatment usually requires bone flap removal. The extent of epidural granulations and pus that typically occur is noteworthy and should be remembered whenever conservative therapy is tempting. However, there is little urgency, and suppression (not cure) of the infection with an appropriate antibiotic of low toxicity (sulfa compounds, tetracycline, penicillin) for a prolonged time may be appropriate.

Skull x-ray films should be obtained at intervals to observe bony changes suggesting osteomyelitis. Bone scans are usually positive because of craniotomy healing and are usually not helpful. Scalp tenderness may precede fluctuance and erythema, since many craniotomy infections are indolent. The sedimentation rate is usually elevated, but a significant leukocytosis is rare in the absence of fever.

HEADACHE AND SCALP PAIN

Headache following craniotomy is usually related to the basic disease process. However, for the first weeks postoperatively, headache may be present. It is usually mild to moderate, responds to mild analgesics, improves slowly, and is often localized to the side and site of the bone flap. It occasionally may have characteristics of common migraine but usually does not respond to antimigraine medications. It seems particularly common after surgery for arteriovenous malformations but is self-limited. The late occurrence of headache after a pain-free interval is ominous and should lead the examiner to consider new or recurrent pathology. Hydrocephalus, recurrent tumor, infection, or chronic subdural hematoma is a particular concern. Hyperesthesia and "funny" feelings not quite painful at the craniotomy (scalp) flap are common postoperatively and are probably due to damaged and regenerating nerves in the scalp. Time leads to resolution of these sensations, and simple salicylates suffice for control.

PAINFUL MASTICATION

Painful mastication is associated with temporal flaps and other exposures, which include incision of the temporalis muscle. This usually resolves in 6 to 12 weeks as scar forms, remodels, and softens. However, the occasional patient may alter his bite enough or splint during mastication to such an extent that secondary temporomandibular joint (TMJ) changes occur. Local pain or even muscle contracture headaches may occur; pain on palpation of the joint is presumptive evidence of the condition and tomography of the TMJ usually diagnostic. The condition may require oral surgery for correction, though initial management is salicylates, anti-inflammatory agents, moist heat, and time.

HYDROCEPHALUS AND CSF CIRCULATION

Disorders of CSF absorption and circulation (hydrocephalus) may well occur as the result either of the condition that leads to surgery, or of the surgery itself. This seems particularly likely when large amounts of subarachnoid hemorrhage or infection have supervened. Meningitis, hemorrhage, and scarring from surgery all may lead to increased resistance to CSF absorption and ventricular enlargement.

Occasionally, the CSF pathways may become blocked at one foramen of Monro and lead to unilateral ventricular dilatation, which will present as a mass lesion. Intraventricular tumors may cause loculation and dilatation of the portion of the ventricle unable to communicate with the foramen of Monro. Porencephalic cysts may form in an area of previous surgery, especially if hydrocephalus occurs. In these situations, headache, lethargy, and papilledema may be accompanied by hemiparesis and other focal findings. CT scan is diagnostic, angiography, usually suggestive; and positive or negative contrast ventriculography will confirm these findings. Lumbar puncture should not be done. Treatment is dependent upon etiology but will usually require shunting of the cyst, loculus, or the entire ventricular system. Operation (reoperation) is of little value since these are usually due to malignant gliomas, but it may be considered when the pathology is benign or under other specialized circumstances.

References

1. Albanese V, Tomasello F, Sampaolo S: Multiloculated hydrocephalus in infants. Neurosurgery 8:641, 1981
2. Alderson D, Strong AJ, Ingham MR, Selhon JB: Fifteen year review of the mortality of brain abscess. Neurosurgery 8:1, 1981
3. Allen GS: Cerebral arterial spasm: A discussion of present and future research. Neurosurgery 1:142, 1977
4. Bannister G, Williams B, Smith S: Treatment of subdural empyema. J Neurosurg 55:82, 1981
5. Black PM, Chapman PH: Transient abducens paresis after shunting for hydrocephalus. Report of two cases. J Neurosurg 55:467, 1981
6. Black PM, Davis JM, Kjellberg RN, Davis KR: Tension pneumocephalus of the cranial subdural space: A case report. Neurosurgery 5:368, 1979
7. Boullin DJ, Brandt L, Ljunqgren B, Tagari P: Vasoconstrictor activity in cerebrospinal fluid from patients subjected to early surgery for ruptured intracranial aneurysms. J Neurosurg 55:237, 1981
8. Burke AM, Quest DO, Chien S, Cerri C: The effects of mannitol on blood viscosity. J Neurosurg 55:550, 1981
9. Cervos–Navarro J, Ferszt R (eds): Advances in Neurology: Brain Edema, vol 28. New York, Raven Press, 1980
10. Chou SN, Erickson DL: Craniotomy infections. Clin Neurosurg 23:357, 1976

11. Clark K: Complications of aneurysm surgery. Clin Neurosurg 23:342, 1976
12. Conn HO, Blitzer BL: Non-association of adrenocorticosteroid therapy and peptic ulcer. N Engl J Med 294:473, 1976
13. Cooper PR, Moody S, Clark WK et al: Dexamethasone and severe head injury: A prospective double-blind study. J Neurosurg 51:307, 1979
14. Dongen KJ, Brookman R: Late computed tomography in survivors of severe head injury. Neurosurgery 7:14, 1980
15. Everett ED, Strausbaugh LJ: Antimicrobial agents and the central nervous system. Neurosurgery 6:691, 1980 ·
16. Fearnside MR, Adams CBT: The treatment of raised intracranial pressure following aneurysm surgery. J Neurol Neurosurg Psychiatry 43:957, 1980
17. Findler G, Hoffman HJ, Munro IR: Tension pneumocephalus complicating craniofacial surgery in a shunted hydrocephalic patient: Case report. Neurosurgery 7:525, 1980
18. Fisher CM, Kistler JP, Davis JM: Relation of cerebral vasospasm to subarachnoid hemorrhage visualized by computerized tomographic scanning. Neurosurgery 6:1, 1980
19. Fisher CM, Roberson GH, Ojemann RG: Cerebral vasospasm with ruptured saccular aneurysm—The clinical manifestation. Neurosurgery 1:245, 1977
20. Fishkin RD, Kurze T: Acute epidural hemorrhage complicating resection of acoustic neurinoma. J Neurosurg 21:58, 1964
21. Foltz EL, DeFeo DR: Double compartment hydrocephalus—A new clinical entity. Neurosurgery 7:551, 1980
22. Givre A, Olivecrona H: Surgical experiences with acoustic tumors. J Neurosurg 5:396, 1949
23. Gonzalez–Revilla A: Neurinomas of the cerebellopontine recess. A clinical study of one hundred and sixty cases including operative mortality and end results. Johns Hopkins Med J 80:254, 1947
24. Graf CJ, Gross CE, Beck DW: Complications of spinal drainage in the management of cerebrospinal fluid fistula: Report of three cases. J Neurosurg 54:392, 1981
25. Gudeman SK, Kishore PRS, Miller JD et al: The genesis and significance of delayed traumatic intracerebral hematoma. Neurosurgery 5:309, 1979
26. Haft H, Liss H, Mount LA: Massive epidural hemorrhage as a complication of ventricular drainage. J Neurosurg 17:48, 1960
27. Haines SJ: Systemic antibiotic prophylaxis in neurological surgery. Neurosurgery 6:355, 1980
28. Hirsh LF: Delayed traumatic intracerebral hematomas after surgical decompression. Neurosurgery 5:653, 1979
29. Horrax G, Poppen JL: Experiences with the total and intracapsular extirpation of acoustic neuromata. Ann Surg 110:513, 1939
30. Horwitz NH, Rizzoli HV: Postoperative Complications in Neurosurgical Practice. Huntington, New York, R Kreiger Publishing, 1973
31. Hubschmann OR: Twist drill craniostomy in the treatment of chronic and subacute subdural hematomas in the severely ill and elderly patients. Neurosurgery 6:233, 1980
32. Ignelzi RJ: Cerebral edema: Present perspectives. Neurosurgery 4:338, 1979
33. Ignelzi RJ, Vanderark GD: Analysis of the treatment of basilar skull fracture with and without antibiotics. J Neurosurg 43:721, 1975
34. James HE, Walsh JW, Wilson HD et al: Prospective randomized study of therapy in cerebrospinal fluid shunt infection. Neurosurgery 7:459, 1980
35. Jennett B: An Introduction to Neurosurgery, ed 3. Chicago, Year Book Medical Publishers, 1977
36. Kaufman NH, Moake JL, Olson JD et al: Delayed and recurrent intracranial hematomas related to disseminated intravascular clotting and fibrinolysis in head injury. Neurosurgery 7:445, 1980
37. Kinal ME: Traumatic thrombosis of dural venous sinuses in closed head injury. J Neurosurg 27:142, 1967
38. Kontos HA: Regulation of the cerebral circulation. Annu Rev Physiol 43:397, 1981
39. Kosnik EJ, Hunt WE: Postoperative hypertension in the management of patients with intracranial arterial aneurysm. J Neurosurg 45:148, 1976
40. Lewelt W, Jenkins LW, Miller JD: Autoregulation of cerebral blood flow after experimental fluid percussion injury of the brain. J Neurosurg 53:500, 1980
41. Love JG, Doge HW Jr, ReMine WH et al: Acoustic neuroma with meningitis and secondary communicating hydrocephalus: Successful treatment. Report of a case. J Neurosurg 13:400, 1956
42. Luken MG, Whelan MA: Recent diagnostic experience with subdural empyema. J Neurosurg 52:764, 1980
43. Malis LI: Prevention of neurosurgical infection by intraoperative antibiotics. Neurosurgery 5:339, 1979
44. Maroon JC, Nelson PB: Hypovolemia in patients with subarachnoid hemorrhage: Therapeutic implications. Neurosurgery 4:223, 1979
45. Miller JD, Becker DP, Ward JD et al: Significance of intracranial hypertension in severe head injury. J Neurosurg 47:503, 1977
46. Miller JD, Sweet RC, Narayan R, Becker DP: Early insults to the injured brain. JAMA 240:439, 1978
47. O'Brien MS (ed): Seminars in Neurological Surgery. New York, Raven Press, 1978
48. Olanow CW, Finn AL: Phenytoin: Pharmacokinetics and clinical therapeutics. Neurosurgery 8:112, 1981
49. Ommaya AK: Spinal fluid fistulae. Clin Neurosurg 23:363, 1976
50. Parent AD, Smith RR: Traumatic aneurysm complicating EC–IC bypass: Successful surgical clipping. Surg Neurol 15:229, 1981
51. Plum F, Posner JB: The Diagnosis of Stupor and Coma, ed 3. Philadelphia, FA Davis, 1980
52. Pool JK, Paya AA: The Early Diagnosis and Treatment of Acoustic Nerve Tumors. Springfield, IL, Charles C Thomas, 1957
53. Prity MB, Gianotta SL, Kindt GW et al: Treatment of patients with neurological deficits associated with cerebral vasospasm by intravascular volume expansion. Neurosurgery 3:364, 1978
54. Pudenz RH; The surgical treatment of hydrocephalus—An historical review. Surg Neurol 15:15, 1981
55. Quartley GRC, Polyzoidis K: Intraoperative antibiotic prophylaxis in neurosurgery: A clinical study. Neurosurgery 8:669, 1981
56. Reichman OH: Complications of cerebral revascularization. Clin Neurosurg 23:318, 1976
57. Ritchie WL, Weir B, Overton TR: Experimental subarachnoid hemorrhage in the Cynomolgus monkey: Evaluation of treatment with hypertension, volume expansion, and hyperventilation. Neurosurgery 6:57, 1980
58. Rosner MJ, Becker DP: Complications of ICP monitoring. Clin Neurosurg 23:494, 1976
59. Sayers MP: Shunt complications. Clin Neurosurg 23:393, 1976
60. Scanlon PW, Taylor WF: Radiotherapy of intracranial as-

trocytomas: Analysis of 417 cases treated from 1960 through 1969. Neurosurgery 5:301, 1979

61. Schiefer W, Klinger M, Brock M (eds): Brain abscess and meningitis. In Advances in Neurosurgery, vol 9. New York, Springer-Verlag, 1981
62. Smith HA, Moody D, Ball M et al: The trapped temporal horn: A trap in neuroradiological diagnosis. Neurosurgery 5:245, 1979
63. Sundaresan N, Galicich JH, Deck MDF, Tomita T: Radiation necrosis after treatment of solitary intracranial metastases. Neurosurgery 8:329, 1981
64. Sundt TM, Piepgras DG: Bypass surgery for vertebral artery occlusive disease: Technique and complications. Clin Neurosurg 26:346, 1979
65. Tabador K, LaMorgese J: Complication of a large cranial defect. J Neurosurg 44:506, 1976
66. Thompson RA, Green JR (eds): Complications of nervous system trauma. In Advances in Neurology, vol 22, Chap 65. New York, Raven Press, 1979
67. Tindall GT, Payne NS, O'Brien MS: Complications of surgery for subdural hematoma. Clin Neurosurg 23:465, 1976
68. Tsai FY, Huprich JE, Segall HD, Teal JS: The contrast-enhanced CT scan in the diagnosis of isodense subdural hematoma. J Neurosurg 50:64, 1979
69. Vassilouthis J, Richardson AE: Ventricular dilatation and communicating hydrocephalus following spontaneous subarachnoid hemorrhage. J Neurosurg 51:341, 1979
70. Vincent FM: Hypoglycorrhachia after subarachnoid hemorrhage. Neurosurgery 8:7, 1981
71. Weiss RM: Massive epidural hematoma complicating ventricular decompression. Report of case with survival. J Neurosurg 21:235, 1964
72. Wilkins RH: Attempted prevention or treatment of intracranial arterial spasm: A survey. Neurosurgery 6:198, 1980
73. Wilkins RH: Update—Subarachnoid hemorrhage and saccular intracranial aneurysms. Surg Neurol 15:92, 1981
74. Wise BL: Preoperative and Postoperative Care in Neurological Surgery. Springfield, IL, Charles C Thomas, 1978
75. Wright RL: Postoperative Craniotomy Infections. Springfield, IL, Charles C Thomas, 1966
76. Youmans JR (ed): Neurological Surgery, ed 2. Philadelphia, WB Saunders, 1982

47 Complications of Spine Surgery and Trauma

Harold F. Young | Donald P. Becker

Complications of Spine Surgery for Disc Disease

OVERVIEW

Spinal problems are the single most common cause of disability in persons under 45 years of age in the United States and the second most common cause of missed work days in North America.[61] Though most patients with back pain are treated nonoperatively and improve, approximately 165,000 patients per year are treated surgically for ruptured lumbar discs in the United States.[50] In the course of the evolution of surgery of the spine by neurosurgeons and orthopaedic surgeons, the indications for operation have broadened. Operations are now performed on the cervical, thoracic, and lumbar spine, not only for disc rupture or protrusion, but also for tumors, spinal stenosis, syringomyelia, and various nerve root entrapment syndromes, such as the articular facet syndrome.

LUMBAR SPINE SURGERY FOR DISC

In 1934, Mixter and Barr discovered that a protruded lumbar disc was a common cause of sciatica and that the pain could be relieved by removing the offending disc.[76] Total laminectomies were performed at several levels to discover a single protruded disc, which was removed through the dura. The mortality rate exceeded 20%. Today, lumbar laminectomy for lumbar disc herniation has become standardized to the point that operative complications are rare.[50] Dr R. E. Semmes, one of the pioneers of the procedure, reported a series of over 5000 cases without a single fatality.[103] Most contemporary series report a mortality rate of 0.2% to 0.4%, with deaths usually due to emboli and coronary disease rather than to the disc operation itself.

The peak age for incidence of disc disease is 30 to 50 years, with a slight predominance in men (63%). Lumbar disc protrusion in childhood and adolescence is relatively rare.[119] Only 1% to 3% of all lumbar disc protrusions occur in persons under 21 years, with trauma playing a distinct role in the etiology of about one half of these cases. Schöter and Entzian reported only 56 cases of lumbar disc protrusion in patients between 11 and 20 years of age from an overall series of 4695 patients with lumbar disc protrusion.[100] In a series of 43 cases of lumbar disc protrusion in childhood reported by Fisher and Saunders, only 10% of the patients required reoperation within 3 years.[45]

The majority of patients whose symptoms are from mechanical nerve root compression from a large protruded disc recover satisfactorily following the operation. However, failure of the operation to relieve symptoms is still common, and patients not infrequently have long-term increased pain and disability following surgery. This problem has colloquially been termed the "failed disc" syndrome. It is such a common cause of disability following an operation that it is appropriate to consider it a complication. Among 3238 patients whose operations for herniated disc were reported in a joint study, there were 757 complications, of which 206 (27%) represented reoperations.[101] About 75% of patients being evaluated and treated in pain clinics are patients with the failed disc syndrome who have had one or more operations for lumbar disc disease. The failed disc syndrome is defined as a recurrence of sciatica some time after an apparently successful lumbar diskectomy and is due to two factors, singly or in combination: improper selection of the patient and perineural fibrosis of the contents of the epidural spinal canal. In patient selection, the surgeon must be certain that the patient is psychologically stable without motivation of secondary gain from the operation. The surgeon should truly "get to know" the patient prior to the operation. Neurologically, the patient must have evidence of mechanical nerve root compression, which the operation can technically relieve. In every lumbar disc operation, the ligamentum flavum is removed from its protective barrier over the dura. If it is not replaced by an equally effective barrier, scar tissue may proliferate from torn muscle and bind dura and nerve roots to the walls of the canal.[43] When direct trauma to a nerve root is superimposed upon the indirect damage from hemorrhage and loss of epidural fat, the necessary ingredients for the development of failed disc syndrome are present. If reoperation for the failed disc syndrome is considered a complication, then reoperation may be considered the single most common complication in lumbar disc operations.

The most frequently occurring complications are listed below.

Anesthetic and Position Complications

Intra-abdominal Complications
Vascular injury including A–V fistula
Viscus injury (bowel and ureter)
Colonic ileus

Sepsis
Superficial sepsis
Meningitis
Interspace reaction

Injury to Neural Elements
Meninges
  CSF fistula
  Subcutaneous CSF
  Pseudomeningocele
Nerve root (battered nerve root)

Hemorrhage
Superficial bleeding
Epidural bleeding

Scarring
Epidural scarring
Arachnoiditis

Instability
Spondylolisthesis
Kyphosis
Angulation

Persistent Pain
Failed back syndrome

ANESTHETIC AND POSITION COMPLICATIONS

Anesthesia for lumbar disc surgery is generally routine and safe, yet there are a few potential pitfalls. The patient is usually intubated in the supine or face-up position, then rotated onto the abdomen, placing the body on rolls or a special frame. During the rotation and positioning of the patient, a poorly secured endotracheal tube may be easily dislodged or accidentally removed. Both the anesthesiologist and surgeon should be aware of this and carefully recheck pulmonary ventilation once the final position of the body is fixed. Blood pressure changes may occur during this change in position or when a special frame is elevated to produce flexion of the spine. Intra-abdominal venous compression may occur, distending the epidural venous plexus, thereby increasing epidural vascular problems during the operation. For this reason, some surgeons prefer the lateral position for lumbar disc operations. The position of the patient may lead to brachial plexus or peripheral nerve injury. The brachial plexus is especially prone to be compressed in the face-down position. The knee-chest position, favored by some surgeons, may lead to peroneal nerve palsy. The surgeon must carefully pad possible sites of nerve compression.

During the operation, muscle relaxants may be used for the large lumbar paraspinous muscles. The surgeon may, in fact, demand excessive use of muscle relaxants to gain exposure of the spine from a small incision and muscle retraction. If these drugs are not metabolized or reversed prior to the termination of the operation, respiratory problems may ensue.

Intra-abdominal Complications

VASCULAR INJURY. Since the initial report in 1945 by Linton and White, numerous reports have been published concerning injury to the great intra-abdominal vessels at the time of disc removal.[65] The frequently used pituitary rongeur is the instrument usually misused in retroperitoneal vascular injury. Any pathologic defect of the anterior longitudinal spinal ligament and anterior annulus will allow easy access to these structures (Fig. 47-1). Although the preponderance of injuries occurs at the L4–L5 level because of the proximity of the iliac vessels to the L4–L5 interspace, the aorta and vena cava have been injured as high as the L2–L3 level. In many cases the vessel wall is pathologically weakened after minor trauma by an instrument or anterior herniation of disc during the operation. In DeSaussaure's review of vascular injury occurring during lumbar disc operations, less than half of the instances of injury were associated with excessive bleeding during the course of the operation.[35]

There is both an acute injury and a more chronic injury, which is apparent weeks, months, or years after the operation. The acute injury is recognized during the operation or within the first 48 to 72 hours. Excessive bleeding into the operative field of the laminectomy usually is not noted but occurs into the intra-abdominal and retroperitoneal space and is announced by a sudden drop in blood pressure and signs of peripheral vascular collapse—obvious hemorrhagic shock. Immediate inspection of the depths

FIG. 47-1. Relationship of major abdominal vessels and viscera to the spine. Penetration of the anterior annulus easily results in injury to these structures.

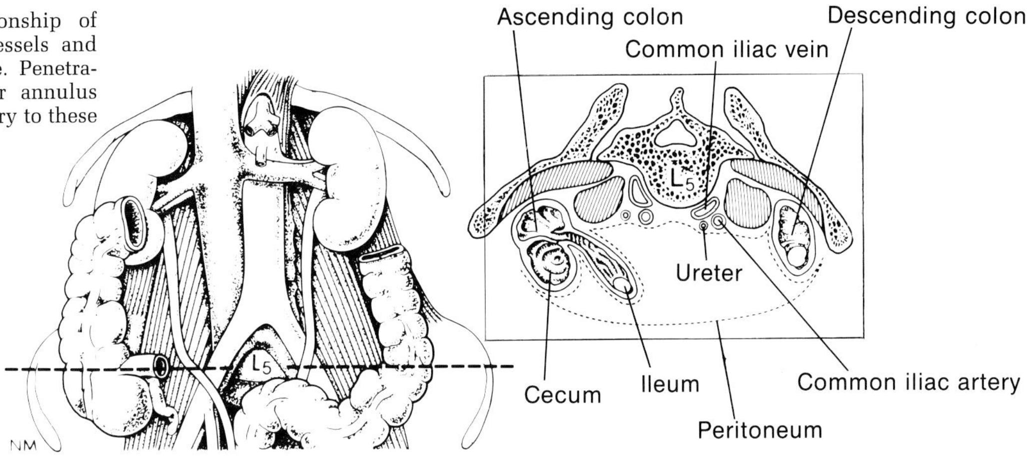

of the laminectomy site may reveal some signs of excessive bleeding. At least one report has suggested that upon wound irrigation with saline, rapid drainage of the saline pool should alert the surgeon to a perforation of the anterior annulus and the probability of intra-abdominal vascular injury.[106] If the bleeding is slow, then the injury may not be discovered until the postoperative period. Paralytic ileus and difficulty voiding may be associated symptoms. Examination of the patient may reveal deep lower abdominal tenderness, a palpable thrill, and a murmur if a fistula develops between the artery and vein. The murmur can be heard over the lower thoracic and lumbar vertebrae as well as the lower abdomen.

On occasion, the early stage of the injury may not be apparent, and the patient is discharged without recognition of the injury. Months or even years later, the patient presents with symptoms of high-output circulatory failure. The patient may exhibit breathlessness and varicosities of the groin, abdomen, and lower extremities. Compromise of the cardiovascular system is evident by increased pulse pressure, tachycardia, cardiac dilatation, arterialization of the venous system, and diminished arterial pulsation distal to the fistula. Anemia may be present and the chest x-ray film usually reveals cardiomegaly. Delays in diagnosis up to 7 or 8 years have been recorded before an acute hemorrhage occurs. This event often is associated with a very high mortality rate of about 50%.

TREATMENT. The acute stage of peripheral vascular collapse represents a surgical emergency. The laminectomy incision must be packed or rapidly closed and an immediate abdominal exploration undertaken. This will quickly reveal the location and extent of the injury. Sometimes the fistulous opening or vascular rent can be simply closed without wide vascular resection or grafting. In chronic cases, the technical problem of dissecting a false aneurysmal sac involving adjacent femoral nerve, ureter, and bladder may be formidable and may well involve excision of involved structures and replacement with grafts. Proximal and distal ligation of the artery and vein may lead to claudication or gangrene of the extremity, or vascular insufficiency of the spinal cord, especially if spinal branches from the aorta are involved.

VISCUS INJURY. Intra-abdominal viscus injury during the course of lumbar disc operations is exceedingly rare and certainly much less common than is great vessel damage. Only a few cases of small bowel injury have been reported, with one case recognized during the operation.[33, 35] If unrecognized at operation, the bowel injury is usually apparent soon because the patient develops a distended abdomen and complains of abdominal pain. Reports of ureteral injury are rare. Flank and abdominal pain, paralytic ileus, and low-grade fever may be present. Intravenous and retrograde pyelograms will usually define the injury.

TREATMENT. Treatment of either small bowel or ureteral injury is immediate operation and repair. Usually, repair of the lesion will have satisfactory results.

COLONIC ILEUS. Rarely, in uncomplicated lumbar laminectomy, without evidence of trauma to the contents of the abdominal cavity or retroperitoneal space, colonic ileus develops. Postoperatively, these patients develop constipation and severe abdominal distention associated with abdominal pain, fever, and leukocytosis. Radiologic studies reveal severe colonic enlargement, particularly of the cecum, with little or no distention of the small bowel. Barium enema rules out obstruction.

The clinical picture is different from that of paralytic ileus, which follows severe trauma and which probably results from cessation of all neural activity in the bowel. In paralytic ileus after trauma, peristalsis ceases and the entire bowel distends. The syndrome following laminectomy is characteristic of the illness known as Ogilvie's syndrome (acute colonic ileus).[83] The pathogenesis is unknown, but the ileus probably results from increased sympathetic activity that inhibits the bowel.

MANAGEMENT. Conservative management consisting of correction of any fluid or electrolyte abnormalities, continuous gastric suction with a nasogastric tube, and placement of a rectal tube may relieve the symptoms. Patients should be followed carefully and if distention of the cecum exceeds 12 cm, a decompressive operation is indicated.[51]

Sepsis

SUPERFICIAL WOUND INFECTION. The incidence of superficial wound infection in lumbar disc surgery varies from 0 to a maximum of 4%. The symptoms and signs and management of subcutaneous pus collections are similar to those appearing in other areas of the body. Buried nonabsorbable sutures may have to be removed because they may act as a foreign body. Removal of these sutures and adequate drainage usually result in prompt satisfactory healing. Persistent drainage, originating deep to the fascia, may be due to a foreign body such as a sponge, cottonoid, or spicule of bone. *Staphylococcus aureus* and streptococci are the two organisms most frequently involved. At times, a large collection of pus, up to 200 ml, may form beneath the fascia and be unrecognized for weeks.

INTERSPACE INFECTIONS. Postoperative interspace inflammation has been increasingly recognized since Giesiking's report appeared in 1951.[48] Many other reports have now appeared and since the septic origin of the condition is in question, the term *inflammation* is frequently used. Certainly, many cases are bacterial in origin. In the report of four cases by Brussatis, positive cultures were obtained in three of the four patients subjected to exploration, although pus was found in each case.[19] Other authors have noted that nonspecific abnormal tissue is frequently found on reexploration. The cause of "aseptic" diskitis remains obscure. In most cases, the evidence is against its being a bacterial infection. Both Teng and Williams suggested that trauma to the cartilagenous end plates of the vertebrae may be responsible for severe pain or aseptic diskitis.[115, 121] Many surgeons perform curettage of the end plates upon removal of the disc. Other authors even suggest that this maneuver may activate an occult infective process, such as the case of postdiskectomy tuberculous abscess reported by Kaplan.[60]

Clinically, there may be an acute or chronic disc space infection. Usually, the condition, regardless of whether it is acute or chronic, is heralded by the onset of severe back spasms, with the pain often referred to the groin, testis, flanks, or legs. These spasms are often extremely severe; the slightest body movement or movement of bed clothes may initiate a series of spasms. These are striking and will not be easily confused with the mild spasms that are often present during the first postoperative week when there is no evidence of superficial or deep infection. In interspace infection, signs of superficial wound infection are usually absent, but a genuinely septic process may appear with high fever, chills, leukocytosis, and an elevated sedimentation rate. Positive blood cultures can usually be obtained when this occurs. In some cases of inflammation with a nonspecific origin, the above responses may be absent or very mild.

These symptoms and signs may occur within 4 to 5 days of operation or may appear 2 to 4 months after operation. The symptoms may appear early and with partial or incomplete treatment reappear later. Symptoms that appear early after operation are more frequently bacterial in origin and are associated with high temperature and at some time during the course may show drainage through the skin. The usual organism is *Staphylococcus aureus*.[62] The delayed cases may indeed be a form of diskitis without a bacterial etiology. Though the pain may be less severe and temperature remain at normal levels, the presence of the inflammation is documented by x-ray changes of the spine. The x-ray findings are fuzziness and irregularity of the articular plates of the adjacent vertebrae with eventual dissolution of the cortical bony surface, sclerosis of the cancellous portion of the vertebral body, collapse of the involved interspace, and eventual fusion between the two involved vertebrae in 6 months to 2 years (Fig. 47-2).

TREATMENT. The initial treatment consists of antibiotics, analgesics, and immobilization. It is best to identify the responsible organism if possible by blood culture, incisional drainage, wound reexploration, or needle aspiration. Caution must be exercised in needle aspiration, which is done at the level of interspace inflammation and is best done under fluoroscopic control. If it is found necessary to obtain spinal fluid for culture, the needle should be introduced at a site distant from the operation and pain so as not to introduce infection through the dural barrier into the cerebrospinal fluid. All authors agree on the necessity of large doses of proper antibiotics over a 4- to 6-week course. Analgesics and muscle relaxants are important for relief from the spasms. Immobilization in a brace or bedrest is also helpful in relieving the pain and hastening recovery.

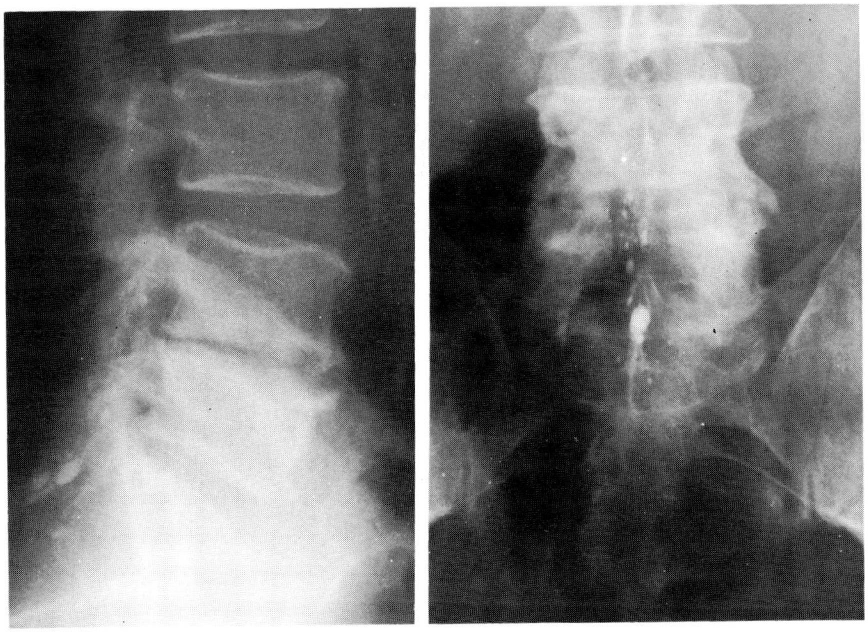

FIG. 47-2. Lumbar spine x-ray films shows fuzziness and irregularity of the articular plates of the adjacent vertebrae. The patient had severe back pain and spasms with an elevated sedimentation occurring 6 weeks after lumbar laminectomy and L4, L5 disc excision.

The need for reexploration is controversial. Some cases are best handled by early reexploration as soon as suppuration is suspected. Gallium isotope scanning and CT body scanning may be helpful in identifying a collection of pus requiring drainage. Reexploration is mandatory in the face of progression of symptoms or of neurologic defect. If an organism is cultured from the blood and is responsive to appropriate antibiotics, then reexploration may be avoided if the neurologic condition remains stable. Following reexploration, rather than leave the incision open, a closed irrigation–suction technique may be desirable.[47] The clinical course is usually satisfactory and correlates with the x-ray changes. Most often, stabilization and fusion of the spine occurs with resolution of the pain. However, meningitis and death may result. The diagnosis may be delayed and be finally evident only after a scrotal, groin, or psoas muscle abscess is identified.

In contrast with the ominous potential of interspace infections in the adult, children develop a more benign process. According to Onofrio, the treatment of childhood disc space infections consists solely of rigid spine immobilization for 6 to 12 weeks during the acute initial phase.[84] Disc space aspiration is seldom indicated or desirable unless recurrent clinical symptoms occur despite immobilization. Antibiotics are not generally recommended unless symptoms recur. The prognosis for most children is excellent and the duration of symptoms short. Any collection of pus such as in the psoas muscle should, of course, be drained. To explain this discrepancy for prognosis and treatment between children and adults, Boston and colleagues concluded that intervertebral disc space infections occur mainly by hematogenous spread of organisms in children, with the disease remaining localized within the interspace, whereas the adult disc involvement is by direct invasion from a contiguous paravertebral osteomyelitis.[14]

Injury to Neural Elements

Meninges, root sleeve, or caudal dural sac injury may occur during the course of lumbar hemilaminectomy for disc. This may occur at the initial operation, but it more often occurs at reexploration of a previously operated disc space. At the initial operation, the ligamentum flavum is easily identified between the lamina and at the hemilaminectomy site. The dura is protected until the ligamentum is opened. Improper use of sharp instruments or power drills has been implicated in injury to the meninges upon puncture or resection of the ligamentum flavum. The meninges may also be injured when attempts are made to remove the disc material itself. The disc material is usually beneath the nerve root and dura but if there are adhesions to the dura or nerve root sleeve, the dura tears as the disc material is being teased from the epidural space. When the dura is breached and arachnoidal continuity disturbed, CSF is visible at operation. Failure to repair the tear at that time leads to a subcutaneous fistula, subcutaneous CSF, or pseudomeningocele. The patient usually complains of headache when in the upright position, and a subcutaneous mass suggestive of fluid accumulation becomes evident.

MANAGEMENT. The treatment consists of closure by suture primarily, or if there is a significant dural defect, a graft of fascial lata will be necessary. This should be done at the initial operation as soon as the injury is recognized. When discovered postoperatively, reexploration and closure of the defect will be necessary.

ROOT INJURY. During lumbar spine operations, partial or complete cutting or stretching of a nerve root may occur. This occurs when a sharp instrument such as a rongeur, Kerrison punch, or drill injures the nerve in the course of lamina or ligamentum flavum removal. There may be no normal epidural fat tissue in the presence of a disc rupture and the nerve is in intimate contact with the ligamentum flavum, so the most careful and meticulous ligament opening is required. Sharp objects plunged through the ligament in these instances will often injure the nerve root.

The nerve root may also be injured during identification of the disc. The nerve root can be so stretched over the bulging disc that the compressed and splayed nerve root is mistaken for the annulus fibrosis or disc itself. Even upon recognition of the nerve root, undue retraction of the already stretched nerve by the surgeon or assistant may result in further stretching of the nerve and more or new neurologic deficit. Rarely, unrecognized nerve root anomalies may lead to inadvertent section of the nerve. Reexplorations of the lumbar spine are more frequently associated with nerve root injury than primary operations because scar formation obscures the normal anatomical appearances. With scar formation, the nerve root and dural sac are encased in epidural fibrosis (Fig. 47-3). Injury to the nerve root or contents of the dural sac in the course of scar dissection leads to increased neurologic deficit and sphincter problems. The patient will complain of increased numbness in the involved dermatome and weakness of the foot. In general, L4 root motor deficit produces quadriceps femoris weakness. L4 and L5 root injury produces footdrop, whereas S1 root injury produces weakness of plantar flexion.

MANAGEMENT. Nerve root injuries, especially sections of the root and cauda equina injuries, cannot be corrected by reoperation. If it is uncertain that such an injury occurred during an operation that is followed by serious new deficit in the immediate postoperative period, then a repeated myelogram is indicated to rule out an epidural hematoma. Clinically, the surgeon can offer little more than physical therapy and a leg brace if there is a footdrop. It is important to prevent such an injury, which is best accomplished by careful planning of the operation and in the case of a repeated operation, by finding normal anatomy and proceeding to abnormal areas.

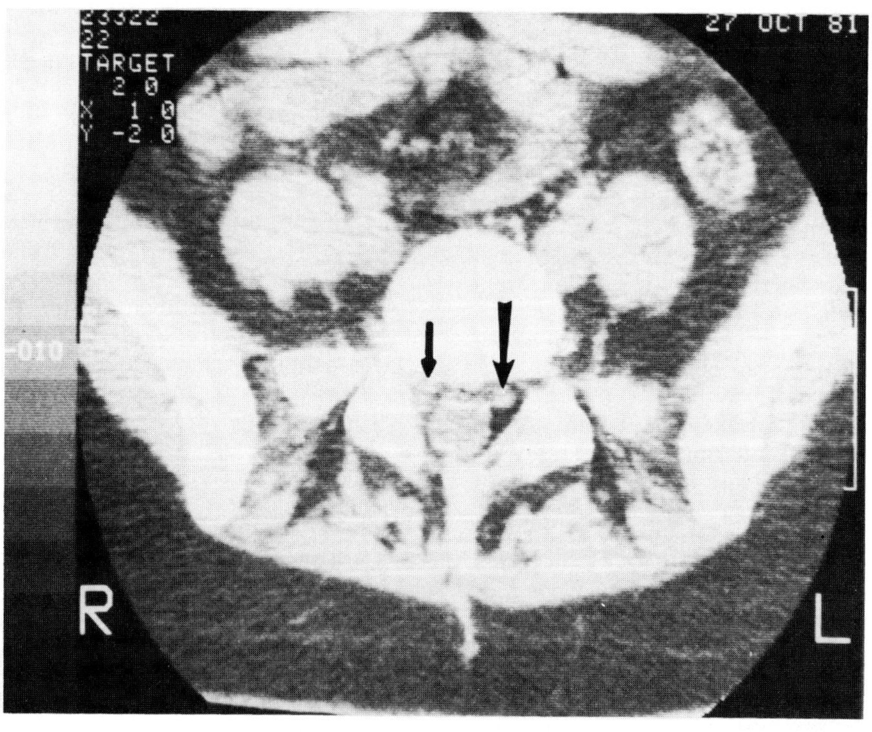

FIG. 47-3. CT scan of L5–S1 spine level in a patient experiencing recurrence of right leg pain 1 year after diskectomy at this level. The large arrow identifies the normal left L5 nerve root while the small arrow identifies the right L5 nerve root encased in epidural fibrosis, proven at reoperation.

Hemorrhage

Superficial hemorrhage is usually not a problem in lumbar surgery for disc protrusion, but deep or epidural hemorrhage, though rare, may be a cause or may contribute to arachnoiditis. Usually, during the operation, careful bipolar coagulation of any epidural veins in the operative field prevents serious epidural hemorrhage. Upon disc removal and relaxation of the dura, the pressure exerted by the dural sac, distended by CSF, will tamponade minimal venous bleeding. Unfortunately, many surgeons rely on this tamponade or use generous amounts of hemostatic agents such as Gelfoam in the epidural space for hemostasis. It is our firm conviction that any foreign body allowed to remain in the epidural space, coupled with blood and microscopic cotton filaments remaining from the use of cottonoids, is a major cause of epidural scarring or nerve root syndromes occurring after operation. Likewise, trauma or retraction causing intradural bleeding may contribute to arachnoiditis, especially if there is Pantopaque in the subarachnoid space from previous myelography.

MANAGEMENT. It is imperative that epidural hemostasis be complete without the use of hemostatic agents before closure of the incision. Acute epidural hematoma that is a cause of increasing or new neurologic defect in the immediate postoperative period requires prompt reopening of the incision and drainage. If possible, a myelogram should be done to reveal the cephalad and caudal extent of the hematoma, since full laminectomy will be needed for evacuation of the hematoma. If the blood is clotted, the existing hemilaminectomy used for disc removal will be insufficient for hematoma removal.

Cicatricial Processes

Intradural scarring (arachnoiditis) and extradural scarring are often the cause of the failed back syndrome (see Fig. 47-3 and Fig. 47-4). These processes are suggested when the patient complains of progressively severe burning leg pain unilaterally or bilaterally following initial relief of the back and leg pain after operation. Often the neurologic deficit is minimal in comparison with the magnitude of the pain syndrome. The pain is constant in nature, may not be aggravated by activity, and is severe and incapacitating.

MANAGEMENT. The best management is prevention. This is accomplished by performing the operation in a gentle manner without undue retraction of the nerve root or dura, which can excite hemorrhage intradurally. It has been proven experimentally that the combination of blood and Pantopaque will produce arachnoiditis.[58] Pantopaque remaining after a myelogram, coupled with hemorrhage associated with any trauma of the operation, initiates an inflammatory reaction, which results in arachnoiditis. Either poor hemostasis at the completion of the laminectomy or incomplete excision of pathologic disc material may be related to arachnoiditis. Prior to closure of the incision, placing a layer of fat over the dura and nerve root to replace the ligamentum may aid in preventing epidural scar formation.

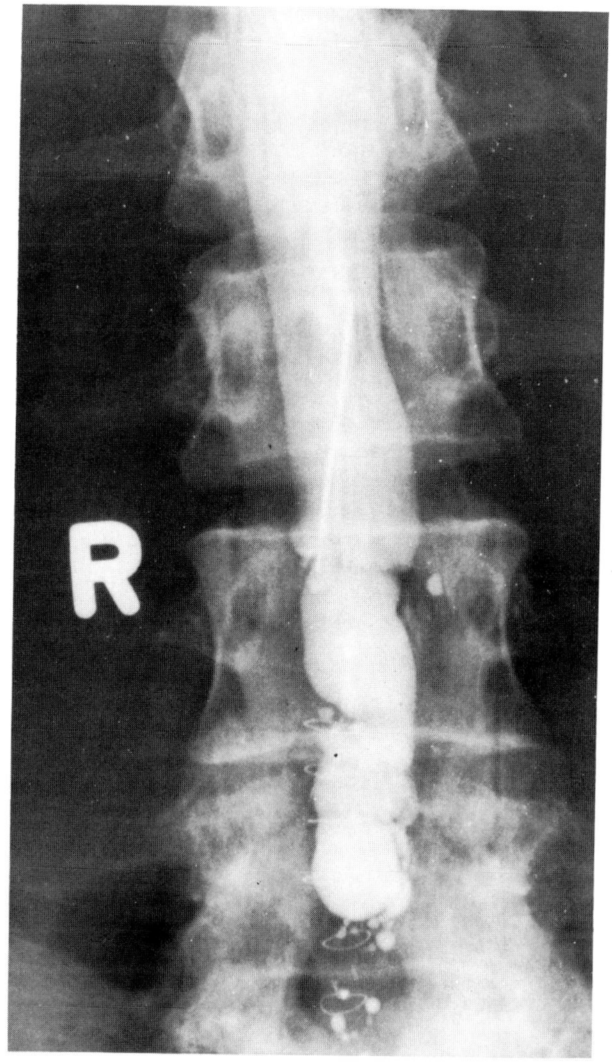

FIG. 47-4. The AP view of a lumbar myelogram of a patient experiencing bilateral burning leg pain following multiple lumbar laminectomies. The irregular lobulated column of pantopaque is diagnostic for arachnoiditis in this patient.

Once the diagnosis is established, the treatment is essentially conservative. Medications including analgesics and muscle relaxants must be used, but sparingly. Anti-inflammatory medication may be helpful and is at times dramatically beneficial, especially if the patient has a "rheumatoid tendency." Intrathecal injection of steroids has been advocated, though the complication of meningitis has been associated with this technique. Intradural or extradural rhizotomy or lysis of nerve roots have not been especially helpful. An exercise program and regular swimming may result in significant improvement. For the most part, the patient must learn to live with this disability and limit or modify his activities consistent with his symptomatic response. New therapies need to be initiated for the treatment of arachnoiditis, but at present, every effort must be made to prevent it.

Instability, Spondylolisthesis, and Bony Injury

Several structures provide for the stability of the spinal column: intravertebral joints, lamina, ligamenta flava, spinal processes, and intraspinous and paraspinous muscles. The vertebrae of the child are developing structures for which balanced mechanical stimulations are necessary to ensure normal growth. In the adult, stability depends mostly on the intervertebral joints and anterior and posterior longitudinal ligaments, while the role of the other structures is relatively less important. Spinal deformity or instability results from conditions in which there are bone and ligament deficiencies and neuromuscular imbalance occurs. Such conditions may be caused by multiple laminectomies that destroy growing bone structures (lamina and spinous processes), which separate interlaminar and interspinous muscle from adjoining vertebral arches, and allow substitution of scar tissue for insertion of paraspinous muscle masses into the lamina and spinous processes.

Instability is rare after unilateral or even bilateral hemilaminectomy for disc excision. The severe pain due to lumbar spondylosis is often treated by multiple-level, bilateral laminectomies, and facetectomies. Spondylolisthesis occurs after multiple bilateral laminectomies and facetectomies for lumbar spondylosis. Shenkin and Hash report that if only two levels (L4 and L5) are removed, the chance for slippage is only 6%, but if three or more levels are involved, the chance of slippage is markedly enhanced to 15%.[104] They also noted slippage only in patients under 70 years of age who were active. Specific bone and joint injury may occur during the operation and result in postoperative pain. Too wide a laminectomy carried into the facet joint may injure the joint or produce instability of the joint or intervertebral level. Even partial, bilateral facetectomy coincident with disc removal may result in instability and increased pain. In the course of decompression of the nerve root by resection of the superior articular facet and the inferior facet of the underlying vertebra, the posterior articular nerve of Luschka may be damaged, leading to persistent joint pain.

MANAGEMENT. If the operation involves wide bilateral laminectomies and facetectomies in an active patient under 70 years of age and the disc space is entered, posterolateral fusion should be considered at the initial operation. Instability or spondylolisthesis, which follows lumbar spine operations, and becomes symptomatic, will often require fusion as well.

Persistent Pain

There are many reasons for failure of lumbar disc surgery, as listed below.

- Error in judgment
  - Inadequate indication for operation
- Erroneous diagnosis
  - Missed tumors, benign and malignant
  - Intraspinal arteriovenous malformation (AVM)
  - Arthritis and rheumatoid disease
  - Hip and joint problems
  - Neuritis and neuropathies
- Improper operation
  - Missed fragment
  - Wrong level or side
  - Failure to deal with bilateral or complete lesion
  - Failure to deal with double level
  - Failure to recognize intradural fragment
  - Failure to deal with canal stenosis or lateral facet syndrome
  - Failure to treat instability
- Unforeseen root problems
  - Conjoined root
  - Extensive scarring and adhesions
  - Bilateral root syndrome
- Litigation, secondary gain
- Emotional instability
- Drug dependence

Some of these deserve discussion. Even when a pathological disc appears to have been successfully removed, there may still be coexisting pathology. This is rare in patients with symptoms and signs of disc rupture or disc protrusion. In a report from the Mayo Clinic by Love and Rivers of a series of patients who underwent operations for disc rupture, a few patients had malignant or benign tumors or intraspinal arteriovenous malformations which were initially not diagnosed.[67] This usually occurs only in patients who do not undergo preoperative myelography or who do not have an adequate myelogram. During myelography for suspected lumbar disc disease, the contrast material must be run into the lower thoracic spine to visualize the cauda equina. Only in this manner will another lumbar lesion be ruled out. Also, the level of spinal fluid protein is usually elevated in patients with intradural spinal cord tumor.

The disc material may be improperly handled at the time of the operation, or the lesion may not be located at the operation. When a small bulge of the annulus is identified and the bulge removed, a coexisting free fragment may be overlooked. One or more free fragments may be removed, but another or others may be missed, especially if these fragments have migrated from the interspace or down the nerve root into the neural foramina. At other times, the nerve root retractor may hide or move a disc fragment to the contralateral side.

The location of the fragment may be mistaken through improper study of x-ray films or by entering the incorrect level at operation, that is, performing a hemilaminectomy at L3–L4 instead of L4–L5 level. At times, a double disc lesion is missed because of disc protrusion at two levels or a lumbar stenosis associated with a one-level disc rupture. The lesion at times is bilateral or produces a complete block on the myelogram, and a hemilaminectomy is not sufficient for complete removal of a bilateral lesion. Rarely, the disc is intradural but should be so diagnosed on the myelogram.[70, 109] Last, failure to remove *all* pathologic degenerated disc material from the interspace may allow future extrusion of more disc material, and the symptoms will recur (Fig. 47-5).

MANAGEMENT. The management of missed or retained disc material is reoperation and removal upon discovery. At initial operation, the annulus should be carefully inspected for any hole, prior to further incision of the annulus. Such a hole will alert the surgeon that a fragment is free somewhere in the epidural space. All fragments must be meticulously sought and, at times, a foraminotomy done to expose any fragments along the nerve root if it is not free upon removal of interspace material. A blunt nerve hook or small right-angled instrument should be passed under the dura and nerve root to ensure complete removal of disc fragments. Bilateral lesions require a bilateral hemilaminectomy for removal of the disc fragments. If the lesion produces a complete block on the myelogram, then a bilateral laminectomy of adjacent levels is indicated for complete removal of the disc material.

Identification of the correct level of the operation is imperative. This is best done by careful study of preoperative x-ray films, noting the presence of anomalies such as six lumbar vertebrae or sacralization. Then at operation, the sacrum can be identified and used as a reference point to find the proper level. An intraoperative spine x-ray film should always be taken if the correct level or levels exposed during the operation are in doubt and particularly when the expected pathology is not found at exposure of the hemilaminectomy.

Summary of Lumbar Spine Surgery

The major complication of lumbar disc surgery today may well not be the acute complications of the operation itself but actually the so-called failed disc syndrome. The treatment for this syndrome is essentially one of prevention. If an operation is necessary, the best chance for success comes at the time of the initial operation and requires proper patient selection and the performance of the appropriate operation. This implies accurate diagnosis, proper preparation of the patient for the operation, and performance of the indicated surgical procedure with excellent technique. The decision to operate requires careful evaluation of the patient because the presence of the degenerative disc disease *per se* does not constitute an indication for surgery. Disc operation is usually helpful only when there is a significant degree of neural compression.

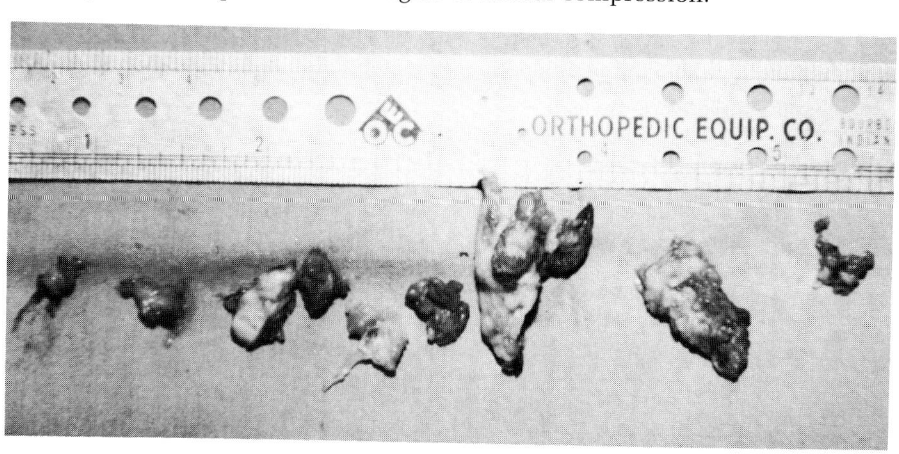

FIG. 47-5. Multiple degenerated disc fragments removed during course of lumbar diskectomy. Only two of these fragments were frankly ruptured into the epidural space. The remaining fragments were removed from the interspace. Failure to remove any single fragment could cause pain to recur.

THORACIC DISC SURGERY

Thoracic disc herniation is a rare spinal disorder. The incidence of protruded thoracic disc is about 2 to 5 per 1000 patients with herniated intervertebral disc. According to Patterson and Arbit, the incidence of operation for thoracic disc has been 0.15% to 0.8% of all disc operations.[86] Though symptomatic disc herniation has been described throughout the thoracic spine, most of the protruded thoracic discs are found in the lower levels, T11–T12 being the most common area. About 50% of herniated thoracic discs are associated with calcified material in the spinal canal, and Hochman and colleagues have confirmed that CT scanning will be an invaluable aid in the diagnosis of this disorder.[56]

The treatment of thoracic discs is extremely controversial and associated with at least one severe complication: the conversion of paraparesis to paraplegia. This is one of the most serious complications in neurosurgery and, when it occurs, almost invariably leads to a negligence claim. Thoracic discs and even tumors are so rare that one surgeon rarely gains experience in depth in treating this condition. The thoracic spinal cord has features that make it vulnerable to manipulation and trauma. The spinal canal in the thoracic region is small and mostly occupied by the spinal cord with a minimal subarachnoid space. The thoracic spinal cord has a tenuous blood supply, with the lower segments often dependent upon a single artery, the arteria radicularis magna, or artery of Adamkievicz. Thoracic discs tend to protrude not laterally but in the midline, and the protruded material is often hard and calcified and may be adherent to the dura mater. Sometimes a fragment can penetrate the dura and become embedded in the spinal cord, thereby simulating an intramedullary tumor. Finally, the diagnosis is often difficult to confirm. A thoracic disc rupture may produce the Brown-Séquard syndrome, exactly the syndrome produced by a benign extramedullary tumor.

Satisfactory myelography is difficult to achieve in the thoracic area and when not perfectly performed leaves the location of the pathologic mass in doubt. If a full-column technique is not performed or if lateral views are inadequate, the surgeon will not know if the mass is anterior, lateral, or posterior to the spinal cord. The surgeon then approaches the mass with a standard posterior laminectomy. Either this will allow the spinal cord to herniate posteriorly, or, in an attempt to remove the anteriorly located mass, undue traction and tension are placed on the cord. The cord must be moved laterally or rotated anterolaterally by a maneuver that is not tolerated by the thoracic spinal cord. In animals, a decompressive laminectomy alone, in the presence of an anterior epidural mass that obstructs the anterior spinal artery, always fails to restore normal spinal cord hemodynamics.[36] In addition to the effect on circulation, the anteriorly placed mass causes axial tension on the spinal cord, which increases with vertical distance and may reach a critical degree on the posterior surface of the cord, not relieved by decompressive laminectomy.

Management

The important concept with thoracic spinal cord lesions is to prevent further aggravation of the patient's neurologic condition. This is accomplished by meticulous attention to the details of the patient's symptoms, a scrupulous neurologic examination, and careful review of the plain x-ray films. Plain films may reveal evidence of calcification, which is characteristic of either a disc or a tumor. Myelography should include complete filling of the thoracic spine with contrast material with multiple lateral views to define the flow characteristics of the contrast material and relationship of the mass to the spinal cord. If the block is complete, contrast material must be introduced at the cervical spine level and allowed to flow down to the pathologic level. This will aid in defining a narrow disc space level defect (protruded or ruptured disc), as opposed to a larger defect usually with a meniscus in the dye column diagnostic of a tumor. In the future, CT scan of the thoracic spine will be increasingly helpful in revealing a spinal cord tumor. Although a small calcified meningioma or calcified disc may have a density similar to that of bone and again leave the diagnosis in doubt, the relationship of the lesion to the spinal cord should be clearly defined. When the exact location of the lesion is determined, the proper approach can be planned. If the lesion is a disc or anteriorly located tumor, then the lesion must be approached from anterior to the spinal cord. This can be done by the transpleural intrathoracic approach described by Perot and Munro and by Ransohoff and colleagues, by the lateral extrapleural approach, or by a lateral pedicle approach described by Patterson and Arbit.[86, 88, 92] It is almost impossible to remove a lesion located anteriorly to the thoracic cord from a standard posterior laminectomy approach without irreversible injury to the spinal cord or frank infarction. Postoperative paralysis requires skin and bladder care and long-term assistance in rehabilitation. Only if the patient awakens from anesthesia with leg function, then loses function rapidly in the postoperative period, are repeat myelogram and reexploration indicated. In this instance, worsening may be assumed to be due to hematoma formation.

CERVICAL DISC SURGERY

Posterior or Laminar Approach

The posterior cervical approach for lateral cervical discs has been standardized and increasingly employed since 1940.[41, 79, 102] In the past two decades, neurosurgeons have turned to the anterior approach for cervical disc disease, spondylosis, trauma, the removal of tumors located anteriorly in the cervical spine and foramen magnum, and in the performance of cordotomies, so that the posterior approach is being performed less often. The posterior laminectomy is still performed for cervical spondylosis with a narrow spinal canal for tumors, for lateral cervical discs, and for syringomyelia. The complications of anterior and posterior spinal operations are listed below.

Posterior or Laminar Approach
- Anesthesia and position complications
  - Hyperextension of the neck
  - Air embolus
  - Hypotension
  - Flexion over spondylitic bar
- Technical complications
  - Trauma to cord
  - Trauma to nerve roots

Anterior Cervical Approach
- Soft tissue injuries
  - Perforation of esophagus and trachea
  - Edema
  - Recurrent laryngeal palsy
  - Vertebral artery injury
  - Pneumothorax
  - CSF fistula
  - Horner's syndrome
  - Carotid artery or jugular vein injury
  - Hematoma
  - Wound infection

Neurologic Injuries
- Nerve root
- Spinal cord

Bone Graft and Donor Site Problems
- Failure of fusion
- Angulation deformity
- Aseptic necrosis and discitis
- Extrusion of bone graft
- Infection, seroma, hematoma
- Painful hip

PROBLEMS OF ANESTHESIA. Excessive manipulation of the neck during intubation for general anesthesia may produce myelopathy or quadriplegia. Though rare, the condition has been reported by Fender and others, who have estimated the incidence of myelopathy caused by manipulation of the neck during intubation and change of position during operation to be 2 per 1000.[44] In severe hyperextension of the head, the spinal cord may be compressed by anterior osteophytes (ridges) or actually pinched by the anterior osteophyte and posterior laminar processes. This can result in central hemorrhagic necrosis of the spinal cord.

MANAGEMENT. The potential problems encountered during induction of anesthesia are eliminated by awake intubation with the aid of a fiberoptic laryngoscope and topical anesthesia. With awake intubation, the patient can be reexamined prior to induction of general anesthesia. Actually, the position of the patient during surgery may be more important than intubation in producing myelopathy.

POSITION. Extreme positioning of the patient must be avoided at all costs. Formerly, most operations on the cervical spine and cerebellum were performed with the patient in the sitting position. This position is now recognized as potentially dangerous. Many authors have noted that the upright position, though supposedly making the operation easier for the surgeon, is hazardous for the patient. There are three well-recognized complications of the sitting position: venous air embolism; sudden hypotension resulting in cerebral thrombosis, ischemia, or anoxia; and quadriplegia or myelopathy from flexion of the spinal cord over an osteophytic bar. These three complications occur more often than has been reported.

VENOUS AIR EMBOLISM. The critical factor in entraining air is the development of a gravitational gradient between the open vessel and the dependent right atrium. Venous air embolism can develop no matter what position is used as long as this gravitational gradient exists. Venous air embolism during neurosurgical procedures on a patient in a sitting position has an incidence of 1.6% to 15%, and the mortality rate, generally from hypotension and cardiac arrest, approaches 93% in untreated cases and 0% to 28% in treated cases.[1, 25] The diagnostic signs of air embolism include millwheel cardiac murmur, sudden electrocardiographic changes, and alterations in respiratory patterns, but they may not be recognized until massive air embolism has occurred. Brechner and Bethune observed that during continuous monitoring of expired carbon dioxide (CO_2), air embolism consistently resulted in a reduction of end tidal CO_2 before physical signs appeared.[16] The Doppler tone can be overlooked by an anesthesiologist in a busy operating room, and the capnograph is a silent monitor.

MANAGEMENT. Preoperatively, if the sitting position is to be employed, the patient should have proper placement of a transvenous catheter into the right atrium for removal of air.[40, 75] Brechner and Brechner suggest the combination of the Doppler and end tidal CO_2 monitor with sound alarm for the detection of the occurrence of air embolism.[15] More recently, it has become recognized that the air accumulates in the entire pulmonary arterial tree and is best detected and treated by aspiration with a pulmonary artery catheter.[71]

During the operation all potential sources of air emboli should be promptly occluded. Bone wax should be generously applied to any bone bleeding, and all bleeding vessels should be occluded by bipolar coagulation. Generous use of saline to flood the incision is also helpful in preventing venous air embolism.

The successful treatment of air embolism is predicated upon early diagnosis and immediate institution of therapy, including aspiration of air from the right atrial catheter, use of an illuminator to facilitate demonstration of even small bubbles from the right atrial catheter, discontinuation of nitrous oxide and administration of 100% oxygen and injection of diazepam intravenously, performance of the Valsalva maneuver or institution of positive end-expiratory pressure (PEEP) with an in-line PEEP valve in the anesthesia circuit, return of the operating table to a horizontal position, and saline irrigation of the wound with compression and hemostasis of open vessels.[80]

HYPOTENSION. Blood pressure may fall significantly as the patient is placed into the sitting position, or during an operation in which the sitting position is used, especially if there is sudden hemorrhage. The hypotension may be profound and lead to cerebral ischemic thrombosis and infarction of the brain.

MANAGEMENT. An arterial line, preferably in the radial artery, should be established for accurate determination of mean arterial blood pressure during the operation. The patient's legs should be wrapped from the toes to the groin. The head should be elevated into the final position slowly, with serial blood pressure determinations. If blood pressure drops significantly, the patient should be returned to the supine position. Rarely, the patient cannot be placed in the sitting position because of hypotension. During the operation, intravascular volume must be meticulously maintained to prevent sudden hypotension. If fluid or blood replacement is not adequate, the onset of hypotension may be sudden and severe and require lowering the head of the patient. There must be excellent communication between the surgeon and the anesthesiologist because mere minor manipulation of the upper cervical spinal cord or brain stem may result in cardiac and blood pressure changes. The surgeon must warn the anesthesiologist when CNS tissue is being manipulated because vital signs may change, and the anesthesiologist, in turn, should alert the surgeon promptly if this occurs. Hypotension must not be allowed to persist when a patient is in the sitting position.

MYELOPATHY OR QUADRIPLEGIA RELATED TO POSITION OF THE NECK. Extreme positioning of the head, especially into the flexed position, may result in spinal cord injury, since 90% of men over 50 years of age and 90% of women over 60 years of age have cervical spondylosis of some degree. Since cervical spondylosis may actually be the indication for the operation, special care must be taken to avoid compression of the spinal cord.

MANAGEMENT. Usually, these patients will have had preoperative x-ray films, and the degree of spinal cord compression will be known. If the spinal canal is narrow or significant anterior ridges are present, then the spine must not be flexed whether the sitting or face-down position is used. A neutral or relatively straight position of the cervical spine will be necessary when the head is fixed to the headholder. Monitoring of spinal-cord-evoked potentials during positioning and intraoperatively should alert the surgeon to spinal cord compromise.[39]

MYELOPATHY OR QUADRIPLEGIA RELATED TO INTRAOPERATIVE TECHNICAL COMPLICATIONS. The surgical technique itself may well be the most important consideration in complications of the cervical spinal cord or nerve roots. Drilling the thickened bone at the junction of lamina and facet above and below the interspace can lead to injury of the nerve root. The slightest manual compression may permanently damage the spinal cord.

MANAGEMENT. If a lamina or hemilamina is removed, it should be done by the so-called *en face* technique. Drilling should be used only for trimming the bone rather than for complete bone removal. Ventral midline ridges should not be curetted by a posterior or posterolateral approach. Bony removal for lateral cervical disc must be adequate and not merely a "keyhole" exposure. Adequate removal of bone permits better exposure of hard spurs and allows more precise curettage of the spurs, without undue retraction of the nerve root, and better visualization of the spinal cord. The posterior approach to remove bone spurs at the oncovertebral joint or to decompress the root by foraminotomy is tedious. The most difficult and dangerous decompressions occur in the congenitally narrow canal, especially when the spine is straight. Even in the hands of the most skilled and careful surgeon, neurologic deficit may increase. The patient must be informed of these risks.

INSTABILITY. Wide cervical laminectomy in the treatment of cervical compressive root syndromes and in decompression of the spinal cord in cases of cervical spondylosis usually does not result in subluxation or angulation. In cervical spondylosis the burrlike facets have a wide girth, and the osteophytes beneath the anterior and posterior longitudinal ligaments almost always preclude the development of postoperative swan-neck deformities, even in the most extensive posterior decompressive procedures.

ANTERIOR CERVICAL APPROACH. The complications that follow surgery of the anterior cervical spine are varied because of the diversity of anatomical structures encountered during exposure of the spine, during the removal of disc or osteophyte, and during the interbody fusion. The two commonly used approaches—the Smith–Robinson technique and the technique advocated by Cloward—have been modified by a number of surgeons.[28, 107] More recently, following the suggestion of Hirsch, anterior single-level diskectomies are being done without fusion.[55]

The mortality rate from anterior cervical spine surgery is low, 1% or less in large series. Most deaths relate to unrecognized and untreated postoperative complications such as perforation of the esophagus and subsequent mediastinitis. The specific complications are divided into three types: exposure injuries, spinal cord or nerve root injuries, and complications of bone fusion.

Perforation of the pharynx, esophagus, or trachea may occur during exposure of the cervical spine (Fig. 47-6) by the use of misdirected sharp dissection or from sharp blade retractors. Sharp dissection can lead to carotid artery laceration and massive hemorrhage. The blade tips of fixed retractors must be placed beneath the longus colli muscles for safe protection of the trachea, esophagus, and neurovascular bundle, containing the carotid artery, jugular vein, and vagus nerve. Unrecognized esophageal perforation will lead to early postoperative chest pain, subcutaneous emphysema, and mediastinitis. Mediastinitis has a very high mortality rate if it is not recognized and immediately treated. Exposure of the cervical C7 level, especially in a patient who has a short neck, may result in penetration of the parietal pleura and a pneumothorax.

Vocal cord paralysis or paresis results from injury to the recurrent laryngeal or vagus nerve. Temporary hoarseness is noted by most patients, but voice changes are protracted in about 10% of patients and reported to be permanent in about 3% of patients.[116]

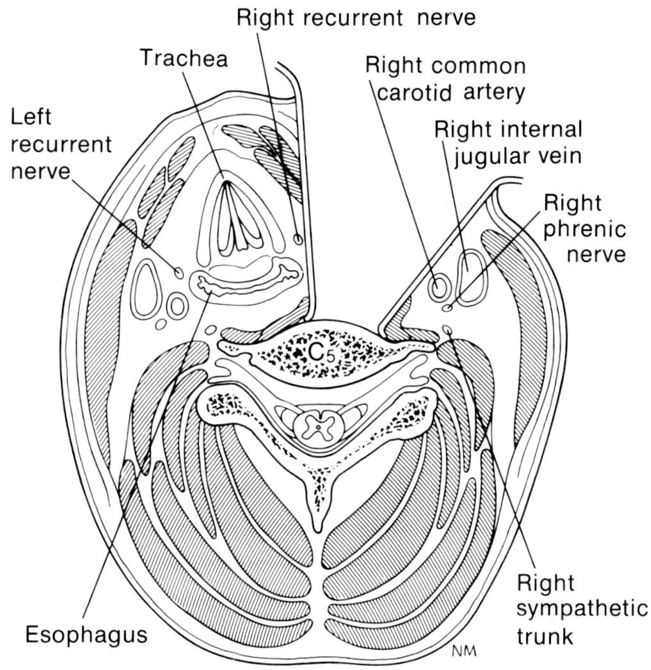

FIG. 47-6. Cross-sectional anatomy of the soft tissues that are encountered in anterior cervical spine operations.

Vertebral artery injury has been rarely reported. Vertebral thrombosis has resulted in infarction of the lateral medulla. This can produce a Wallenberg syndrome because of thrombosis of the posterior inferior cerebellar artery. The patient will have ipsilateral cerebellar ataxia, loss of pain and temperature sensation on the opposite side of the body and ipsilateral face. Bleeding rarely occurs from tears in the vertebral artery.

Cerebrospinal fluid fistula is usually caused by laceration of the dura over the spinal cord or nerve root by a power drill, sharp Kerrison punch, or curet.

Horner's syndrome results from injury to the sympathetic trunk when dissection extends lateral to the longus colli muscle. This is usually temporary and of no serious consequence.

Upon exposure of the anterior spine and visualization of the vertebral bodies and interspaces, x-ray film with a needle in one of the disc spaces must be obtained to identify the proper level for the operation. As a result of failure to obtain the x-ray film, the discectomy and fusion may be performed at the wrong level.

Postoperative wound hematoma is very rare. It is usually recognized easily in the recovery room and may be associated with stridor; unrecognized, it can lead to respiratory obstruction. The placement of a Philadelphia or other cervical collar around the neck at completion of the operation may conceal the early development of the hematoma. Superficial wound infections are also unusual and can be treated by drainage. They usually do not extend to the retropharyngeal space and, therefore, do not lead to bone graft infection or meningitis.

MANAGEMENT. It is easy to prevent most of the soft tissue injuries at the time of anterior cervical diskectomy. Sharp dissection should be limited to the skin and platysma muscle, then blunt dissection is primarily used for the remainder of the exposure. The surgeon must dissect between the sternocleidomastoid muscle laterally and the trachea and esophagus medially, avoiding sharp dissection in the paratracheal muscles. Overstretching of tissue and contusion of the recurrent laryngeal nerve must be avoided. It is important to place retractor blade tips beneath the longus colli muscle and not into the esophagus, trachea, or carotid artery. Careful fixation of the Cloward retractors before removing disc or drilling bone will aid in protecting the soft tissues from injury.

When the operation is followed by chest pain, subcutaneous emphysema, fever, and dyspnea, esophageal perforation should be suspected. Immediate cervical spine and chest x-ray examination will usually reveal air in the neck and mediastinum. Immediate thoracic surgery consultation is mandatory. Esophagoscopy or esophageal contrast study is indicated. Upon diagnosis, the wound will need immediate reexploration. The esophageal laceration should be repaired, drainage instituted, and proper antibiotics administered. Mediastinitis and respiratory distress usually will require tracheostomy.

Pneumothorax can easily be recognized at operation by filling the incision with saline, which will disappear into the chest. Aspiration of air at operation or closed chest tube drainage will be necessary if a significant pneumothorax exists postoperatively.

Carotid artery and jugular vein injury are avoided again by careful placement of the artery and vein lateral to the retractor blade. Firm fixation of the retractor blade under the longus colli muscle will prevent the vessels from slipping into the operative site where a sharp instrument, particularly the Cloward drill guide or drill, can lacerate the vessels. Primary vascular repair is immediately indicated if this injury occurs. In summary, soft tissue injuries are best prevented by gentle blunt dissection of deep structures of the neck. Careful inspection of the trachea, esophagus, carotid artery, jugular vein, and parietal pleura should be done prior to incisional closure.

INJURY OF THE SPINAL CORD AND NERVE ROOTS. Injury of the nervous system is decreasing in frequency from the level of incidence of anterior cervical disc surgery in early years. A paper on complications of anterior fusion presented by Flynn at the 1976 annual meeting of the American Association of Neurological Surgeons reported 129 cases of postoperative spinal cord deficit among 82,114 operations, an incidence of 0.15%.[46] It could be documented that in 53 cases, myelopathy was immediate, and in 17 cases it was delayed. In a report by Lunsford and colleagues of 295 operations for cervical disc disease done by the anterior approach when the symptoms were only radicular, there were no spinal cord injuries.[68] However, in 37 cases with preoperative myelopathy from cervical spondylosis, one patient had a permanent postoperative myelopathy, an incidence of 1 in 332 anterior cervical operations, or a 0.3% incidence.[69]

Myelopathy following anterior operations for removal of disc and fusion of the cervical spine may result when preexisting myelopathy or stenosis of the spinal canal predisposes the patient to this complication. Paralysis may be immediate or delayed for hours. The extent of neurodysfunction is variable and may fluctuate. Some cases are due to intraoperative trauma caused, for instance, by dowel impaction or by use of the osteotome or drill; some are surely due to clot. Others may be caused by edema or a vascular disorder. In some cases, rough instrumentation in the intravertebral foramen may be implicated. Initially, Smith and Robinson did not recommend total removal of the osteophyte so there was less opportunity to injure the cord or nerve root.[107] Subsequently, neurosurgeons who use the interbody technique, with or without magnification, often use a high-speed air drill or punch to remove the osteophyte. This can be exceedingly dangerous when the spinal canal is constricted and the patient has preexisting myelopathy. Care must be taken to penetrate the osteophyte at the most lateral margin of the interspace, but this may enhance the possibility of nerve root injury.

In addition to damage of the spinal cord by instruments, thrombosis of the anterior spinal or radicular arteries may occur, leading to spinal cord infarction. Excessive use of coagulation to control epidural bleeding or packing the epidural space has been suggested as an etiology for this rare event. Yet failure to control epidural bleeding upon penetration of the posterior longitudinal ligament can lead to compressive epidural hematoma formation, as reported by U and Wilson.[118] These patients awaken in the recovery room with paralysis or paresis, which proceeds rapidly to paralysis.

The spinal cord or nerve roots can be injured by an indriven bone graft. Excessive pounding can drive the bone graft into the spinal canal, resulting in irreversible spinal cord damage and paralysis or at least spastic paresis.

MANAGEMENT. Prevention, as always, is most important. Sharp instruments should be used in the posterior intervertebral space in conjunction with magnification techniques, employing the microscope or at least loops. Adequate operative illumination is critical. This will allow safe removal of the intraspinal osteophyte, thickened annulus, and longitudinal ligament. Excessive pressure or tamponade must not be applied against the spinal cord, but only against bone. Bipolar coagulation should be employed for minor epidural bleeding. The bone plug should be gently tapped in place while the anesthesiologist pulls lightly on the cervical traction. If the bone plug is driven too deeply, it must be removed at once. In every operation, a lateral cervical spine x-ray film should be taken before the patient leaves the operating room to check the level of the operation and placement of the bone graft. An unsatisfactory position of the bone graft should be corrected immediately.

Postoperative paralysis evident in the recovery room or that develops in the recovery room is an indication for immediate reexploration of the epidural space. A spinal epidural hematoma will be found unless direct spinal cord injury occurred during the operation. Reexploration is diagnostic and therapeutic. Only prompt evacuation of the rare epidural hematoma will restore neurologic function, and repeated cervical myelogram may delay the necessary reexploration. Hemostatic adjuncts such as Gelfoam or Avitene will invariably control the bleeding.

COMPLICATIONS RELATED TO BONE FUSION. Four methods of anterior cervical fusion have been described: the dowel technique of Cloward, the interbody methods of Smith–Robinson, the keystone technique of Bailey and Badgley, and finally the interbody approach without insertion of a graft as advocated by Hirsch.[8, 28, 55, 107]

Failure of fusion or nonunion appears to be highest with the dowel technique, with an incidence of from 2% to 20%.[28] With the interbody technique of Smith and Robinson, the incidence of pseudoarthrosis has been about 10% in most series. At least one series of 68 patients fused with the keystone technique had no cases of nonunion.[8] The technique of Hirsch nearly always results in bony fusion or fibrous union, but only long-term follow-up will reveal if fibrous union seen in simple disc resection is as satisfactory as is solid bony fusion seen in the other techniques. Anterior angulation deformity may follow anterior approaches of the spine, especially the dowel technique, and particularly when multiple level resections have been performed. Angulation deformity may develop in the technique of Hirsch, especially if the anterior margins of adjacent bone have been excessively removed.

Complications related to the iliac bone site are usually not serious but may cause significant problems in the postoperative period. Hematomas and infection are usually no problem. Persistent pain may be troublesome and is due to scar, fracture of the anterior superior iliac spine, or entrapment of the lateral femoral cutaneous nerve. Fracture of the iliac bone is caused by contraction of the sartorius muscle or direct injury to the region when the bone plugs have been removed without allowing 1.5 cm of bone between each dowel and also 1.5 cm to the edge of the ilium.[93, 94]

MANAGEMENT. Angulation deformity has been attributed to aseptic necrosis or resorption of the bone plug. Cloward claims that the incidence is reduced by use of cadaver bone grafts, while others prefer fresh autogenous graft or Kiel bone.[8] On multiple-level operations, it is imperative to perform the Smith–Robinson interbody procedure or use only the small Cloward drill so as not to remove too much of the vertebral body and its blood supply. If the angulation leads to myelopathy, cervical skeletal traction, reoperation, and bone replacement by an iliac graft or fibular graft will be necessary. In particular cases, posterior fusion may be indicated. Strict, prolonged postoperative immobilization of the spine by plaster jacket or halo vest will usually eliminate angulation of the spine.

Extrusion of the graft anteriorly or posteriorly occurs in about 2% of cases, but this rarely requires operation unless compression of the esophagus, trachea, or spinal cord is produced.[116] Fusion usually subsequently occurs, although in delayed fashion.

At the donor site, injury to the lateral femoral cutaneous nerve may cause persistent neuralgia paresthetica and require reexploration of the incision and possibly complete section of the nerve to obtain pain relief. The incision over the ilium and dissection to obtain the bone grafts should be lateral to the anterior superior iliac spine so as not to injure the lateral femoral cutaneous nerve.

In summary, the anterior approach is a low-risk operation with fewer overall complications than with the posterior approach to the cervical spine. In the series of 500 operations reported by Tew and Mayfield, there were no deaths related to the operation and only a 4.4% incidence of any complications, of which nearly all were minor.[116] It is a safe and effective operation when done properly for the correct indications.

Complications of Spine Surgery for Tumors

OVERVIEW

Primary spinal cord tumors are rare, but unfortunately compression of the spinal cord is a frequent and devastating consequence of systemic cancer. Skeletal metastasis occurs in about one quarter of patients with systemic cancer. The spine is most commonly involved, and one in 10 patients with skeletal metastasis develops pathologic fractures. Barron and colleagues estimated that spinal epidural metastasis develops in 5% of all patients with malignancy, and Black estimated that there are 18,000 new cases of spinal epidural metastasis in the United States each year.[10, 12]

Patients with spinal metastasis are often in poor general condition, but most series of patients undergoing operations for spinal metastasis indicate a relatively low incidence of death within the first month after surgical intervention. The operative mortality in reported series of patients with metastatic spine disease ranges from 3% to 9%.

Surgical morbidity must be evaluated in these patients, as well, when considering the complications of operation for patients with metastatic spinal disorder. The surgical series of Livingston and Perrin had a 10% morbidity rate from wound infection, wound dehiscence, epidural hematoma, cerebrospinal fluid fistula, meningitis, and instability.[66] The major complication is that seen when the patient with spinal metastasis who is ambulatory becomes paraplegic following surgical decompression. The risk of neurologic deterioration following operation ranges from 7% to 22% of patients, with an overall mean of 13% in respective studies (Table 47-1). Neurologic deterioration of these patients usually can be related to one of the following factors: errors in diagnostic evaluation and interpretation of x-ray films, excessive manipulation of the spinal cord during tumor removal, intraoperative and postoperative hemorrhage or edema, failure to perform adequate decompressive laminectomy, and postoperative angulation or instability of the spine because of wide destabilizing laminectomy or further destruction of stabilizing spinal elements by the tumor.

TABLE 47-1. MORTALITY, MORBIDITY, AND COMPLICATIONS OF SPINE SURGERY FOR METASTATIC TUMORS

Author(s)	Number of Patients	Patient Mortality		
		Number	*%*	*Mean*
Torma, 1957[117]	195	27	14	
Perese, 1958[87]	30	1	3	
Brice and McKissock, 1965[17]	139	8	6	
Smith, 1965[108]	52	2	4	
White *et al.*, 1971[120]	241	21	8.7	
Chade, 1976[24]	165	19	12	
Gilbert *et al.*, 1978[49]	31	1	3	
Livingstone and Perrin, 1978[66]	100	9	9	
Dunn *et al.*, 1980[38]	104	10	10	
Total	1057	98		9%
		Patients Worse After Operation		
Barron *et al.*, 1959[10]	38	7	18	
Brice and McKissock, 1965[17]	139	10	7	
Smith, 1965[108]	52	7	14	
Auld and Buerman, 1966[7]	41	9	22	
Chade, 1976[24]	149	25	17	
White *et al.*, 1971[120]	241	24	10	
Gilbert *et al.*, 1978[49]	65	8	12	
Dunn *et al.*, 1980[38]	104	23	22	
Total	829	113		13%
		Patients With Complications		
White *et al.*, 1971[120]	241	19	8	
Gilbert *et al.*, 1978[49]	31	13	42	
Livingston and Perrin, 1978[66]	100	10	10	
Total	372	42		11%

DIAGNOSTIC EVALUATION

Errors in diagnostic evaluation usually result from incomplete or inaccurate neurologic examination and inadequate contrast studies. The clinical examination should locate the level of the lesion but not its entire extent or the presence of multiple lesions. Plain x-ray films may show bony erosion or enlargement of a foramina by a benign tumor or destruction of a vertebra in metastatic carcinoma. Failure to visualize both the upper and lower extent of tumor with lumbar and cervical instillation of contrast material may lead to improper planning of the operation and subsequent inadequate bony decompression. Partial removal of tumor with inadequate decompression of the spinal cord will not reverse the neurologic condition. The other pitfall in diagnostic evaluation is failure to appreciate that the tumor is ventral to the spinal cord or that multiple sites are involved by tumor. In the former instance, the tumor invades and destroys the vertebral body and extends intraspinally against the spinal cord dura. The vertebral body, a major stabilizing element of the spine, is destroyed by the tumor. A posterior laminectomy not only removes the remaining normal stabilizing elements of the spine but also fails to decompress the spinal cord. The tumor mass cannot be removed by posterior laminectomy. Pressure on the spinal cord persists, and the spine is even more unstable than it was preoperatively. This leads to angulation and further compression of the spinal cord. Multiple sites of tumor invasion of the spine may be a contraindication for operation. Decompression at one site may be quickly followed by spinal cord compression and instability at another level.

Management

Complete myelography and tailored CT of the spine should be done on all patients with spinal cord tumor.[27, 73] When the flow of contrast material introduced by the lumbar route is obstructed, it should be introduced into the cervical spinal subarachnoid space as well. This will not only define the extent of the laminectomy necessary for tumor removal and spinal cord decompression but also define multiple sites of impending compression of the spinal cord. The myelogram should be carefully performed and studied to define the location of the mass in relation to the spinal cord. This permits the surgeon to approach the tumor directly, without sacrificing normal elements necessary for stabilization of the spine. In the future, CT scanning of the spine will most certainly replace myelography. CT will define the exact size of the tumor and its relationship to the spinal cord.

If the patient worsens or does not improve following operation, repeated myelography is indicated. If obstruction to the flow of contrast material remains from extradural mass, then reoperation is indicated because the original laminectomy may have been insufficient or epidural hematoma may have to be removed.

SPINAL CORD EDEMA OR INFARCTION

Another diagnostic uncertainty in a patient who fails to improve postoperatively is spinal cord edema, caused by trauma of the operation or from infarction of the spinal cord produced by compression and ischemia. Ischemia and hypoxia may result from occlusion or ligation of important radicular arteries, particularly the artery of Adamkiewicz, during the course of attempted radical tumor removal. Usually, preoperative, intraoperative, and postoperative steroid administration will diminish the incidence of spinal cord edema.

Excessive manipulation of the spinal cord during tumor removal may result in increased neurologic deficit or paralysis following operation. Retraction or rotation of the spinal cord in an attempt to remove a ventrally or a ventrolaterally located tumor may cause transient or permanent spinal cord damage through infarction of the spinal cord. Epidural hemorrhage may necessitate packing or compression of remaining tumor, but excessive pressure by injudicious packing against the spinal cord will almost certainly lead to spinal cord injury and further neurologic deficit.

Management

The postoperative myelogram will show an intradural intramedullary picture of a widened or splayed spinal cord from intramedullary swelling, unlike the preoperative myelogram, which demonstrated an extradural cord compression. A patient with spinal cord widening on myelography who is completely paraplegic usually will not be benefited from a repeated operation. At times, an extradural mass will produce so much compression and widening of the spinal cord that it is impossible to interpret the myelogram and reoperation is indicated.

HEMORRHAGE

Intraoperative and immediate postoperative hemorrhage is a serious problem in patients with metastatic tumors. Usually, the tumor cannot be completely removed. Some metastatic tumors such as the hypernephroma are very vascular, and piecemeal removal is associated with brisk bleeding. Residual tumor may bleed postoperatively. The potential for hemorrhagic complications may be enhanced by the fact that many of these patients are cachectic or have been on chemotherapy with resultant anemia and low platelet counts and other clotting deficiencies. In a small series of only 13 patients undergoing laminectomy for metastatic tumor causing spinal cord compression, Mayfield reported two deaths from hemorrhage.[72]

Management

Clotting deficiencies must be corrected before any operation is initiated. Usually, this will involve transfusion of platelets or the use of fresh frozen plasma. Meticulous hemostasis should be obtained at operation with the use of bipolar coagulation and hemostatic agents such as Gelfoam and Avitene. These hemostatic agents can be compressed laterally, against bone and the tumor mass, and not against the spinal cord.

When perfect hemostasis cannot be obtained at the operation, it is advisable to use a Hemovac drain for up to 24 hours. If the patient worsens in the postoperative period, then epidural wound hematoma must be suspected, and repeated myelography should be done. This is usually easily accomplished in patients with metastatic cancer because the contrast material is commonly not withdrawn from the subarachnoid space at the original myelogram. The finding of a complete block to the flow of contrast material is an indication for a repeated operation. If a patient worsens rapidly in the early postoperative period and myelography cannot be done promptly, then reoperation is indicated immediately upon recognition of neurologic deterioration.

INSTABILITY

Significant bone destruction with resulting spinal instability and deformity, usually anterior angulation and kyphosis, may be an important factor related to the effectiveness of various treatments of motor function disturbances in patients with spinal epidural metastasis. Deformities of the spinal cord caused by angulation with neurocompression cannot be treated effectively by radiation therapy alone.[85] Wide laminectomies with facetectomies in the cervical area performed in adults, without cervical spondylosis, cause a high incidence of mechanical instability and alterations in normal vertebral alignment.

In children, postoperative angulation may be a severe problem. Tachdjian and Matson reported a 31% incidence of postoperative scoliosis in 115 children treated for intraspinal tumors.[114] They stated that age at operation, type of tumor, level of tumor, irradiated muscle paralysis, and postoperative support were important in the pathogeneses of scoliosis. A recent report by Yasuoka and associates suggests that postlaminectomy deformity in children is due to a wedging change in the cartilaginous portion of the vertebral body and to the viscoelasticity of the ligaments in children.[124] The incidence of postoperative deformity is greater in the cervical and cervicothoracic region than in the lumbar spine; that is, the higher the level of laminectomy, the greater the likelihood of deformity.

Management

Management of spine angulation and instability involves operative procedures employing vertebral body excision or internal fixation with wire, rods, or bone fusion (Fig. 47-7). Traction for reduction and temporary stabilization of cervical spine dislocation or instability and external immobilization by means of halo apparatus may be useful here. Spinal stabilization is a key consideration in the management of patients with spinal epidural tumor associated with pathologic dislocation of the spine.

Frequent (at least every 3 months) postoperative x-ray films taken after wide laminectomy and facet removal must be obtained to identify early signs of angulation. If angulation is progressive or if pain or neurologic deficit occurs, immediate fusion is indicated to stabilize the spine.

In children, the lamina with the spinous process intact should be removed as a unit by bilateral section of the lamina (laminotomy) with a craniotome. Then the laminar element can be replaced postoperatively according to the method of Raimondi.[91] If serial, follow-up, spinal x-ray films reveal progressive angulation, early intervention by spinal fusion is indicated.

In summary, the complications of operation for metastatic cancer to the spine consist of an estimated 9% mortality rate, 13% rate of neurologic worsening, and 11% rate of other complications.

Spinal Trauma

OVERVIEW

Epidemiology

Spinal cord injury is a significant medical problem in the United States. Not only are serious spinal cord injuries devastating in themselves, but the long-term medical, social, and financial problems of paraplegia are staggering. There are 10,000 new cases of serious spinal cord injury per year in the United States. This is the number of people sustaining complete paralysis or severe paresis and not the much larger number who sustain bony spine fracture without neurologic deficit. This second group is of particular importance because medical mismanagement can result in serious neurologic deficit.

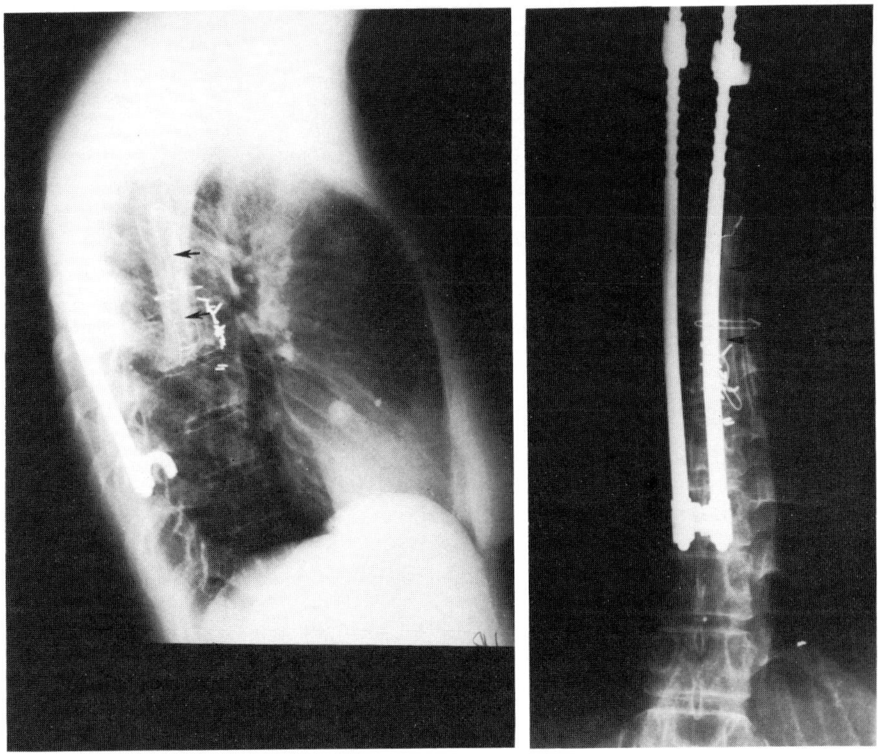

FIG. 47-7. X-ray films of patient who had removal of T3–T6 vertebral body for tumor. The vertebral bodies have been replaced by fibular and rib grafts (*arrows*), and Harrington rods have been used for posterior stabilization.

In the United States, Alker and colleagues found that 21% of 146 consecutive traffic accident autopsies showed radiographic evidence of cervical spine injuries.[3] When autopsy findings and cervical spine x-ray films were studied together, Bucholz and colleagues reported that of 100 fatally injured motor crash victims, 24% had fractures or fracture dislocations.[20] They indicated that neither gross inspection nor radiography alone will uncover all occult cervical lesions.

The mortality rate remains high and increases as the level of spinal cord injury ascends the cervical spinal canal. Although thoracic and lumbar spinal cord, as well as cauda equina injuries, are compatible with long life, the mortality rate increases with the level of the cervical spine involved. Most early deaths following acute traumatic quadriplegia and paraplegia are due to pulmonary complications. Autopsy findings reveal pulmonary edema, atelectasis, and pneumonia as common findings and that pulmonary emboli rarely occur the first month after injury. Wolman found severe pulmonary edema in 20 of 30 autopsies in quadriplegic patients who died in the first month following injury.[122] In a report by Bellamy and colleagues, autopsies were performed in 16 patients with cervical spinal cord injury, with the cause of death as pulmonary edema in most cases.[11] Meyer and colleagues noted massive pulmonary edema in four of nine acutely injured patients in Vietnam and suggested responsibility of a neurogenic factor for the pulmonary edema so frequently seen in these patients.[74] The lungs were edematous and congested; the average lung weight was 796 g, or more than twice normal.

Heiden and associates reported a 37% incidence of complications in nonsurgical patients with cervical spine injury with complete sensorimotor paralysis. These were mainly severe respiratory problems, thrombophlebitis or embolism, and upper gastrointestinal hemorrhage. They also reported that among patients undergoing anterior cervical fusion in the first week after injury, the incidence of severe respiratory problems was 46%.[54] This could be reduced to 27% when anterior fusion was delayed 1 to 4 weeks after injury. Late deaths in spinal cord injured patients are related to renal failure, but improving medical care has greatly reduced the late morbidity rate of spinal cord injury.

The outcome of spinal cord injury, in the minds of many authors, is largely predetermined by the extent of damage. Over the past decade, no less than 11 spinal cord trauma centers in the United States have been fully engaged in research on spinal cord injury; thus far no known therapy will reverse the severe spinal cord injury that results in paralysis. In fact, even as the 1980s begin, the treatment of spinal cord injury remains controversial.[113] Many advocate conservative care with immobilization of the spine, while others consider paralysis an indication for an operation, usually a laminectomy. No statistically significant reports of spinal cord function demonstrate that operation is superior to conservative therapy alone for severe spinal cord injury. Nevertheless, therapeutic modalities and the consequent postoperative complications vary with the nature and location of injury.

EARLY COMPLICATIONS OF SPINAL CORD INJURY

Hemodynamic and respiratory complications of spinal cord injury deserve special attention. The hemodynamic changes after high thoracic and cervical spinal cord injury are consistent with sympathetic denervation and failure of regulatory mechanisms mediated by both alpha- and beta-adrenergic peripheral vascular and myocardial receptors. Shown both experimentally and clinically, a very brief hypertensive response follows spinal cord injury immediately; it is quickly succeeded by hypotension. This hypotension may or may not be associated with multiple trauma. Blood pressure ranges of 80 torr, systolic, are usually encountered in high thoracic and cervical spinal cord injury. Improper early management leads to death of the patient.

"Spinal shock" causes profound inactivity of both the autonomic and somatic nervous systems in its early stages, but return of function is certainly much more rapid in the autonomic nervous system.[18] The early papers on spinal shock mechanisms stressed the dual etiologies of diaschisis of neurons and the effect of interruption of descending tracts *per se*. The fact that vasomotor tone is soon recovered in humans, making cardiovascular adjustments possible, indicates the initial arterial hypotension, bradycardia, and vasomotor relaxation are not solely the result of interruption of spinal tracts. Lesions in the spinal cord must be at or above the T6 level for spinal visceral reflexes to produce significant arterial hypotension.

Pulmonary edema secondary to overtransfusion is a major cause of death of patients with acute quadriplegia. It has been shown that the vascular space is expanded in acute quadriplegia patients, allowing accumulation of large volumes of infused fluid without an abnormal elevation of CVP. If the capacitance vessels retain the ability to constrict, then a sudden release of adrenal catecholamines or a sudden recovery and increase in autonomic neural activity could well trigger an acute overload of the vascular system.

Diagnosis is based on an awareness of the hazards of overtransfusion along with monitoring of the hourly urine volumes, Swan–Ganz catheterization, or blood volume studies. Presently, Swan–Ganz catheterization appears to be the only method that yields unambiguous information. Patients who are about to develop acute pulmonary edema have significantly higher heart rates, hematocrits, total blood volumes, and plasma volumes.

Management

Management of pulmonary edema from overtransfusion is based on the use of a volume-cycled respirator and diuretics. Along with reversal of significant hypotension, normal oxygenation must be maintained to prevent ischemia to the damaged spinal cord. Though no clinical proof of improved spinal cord recovery is shown by maintaining normal blood pressure and blood gases, experimental evidence suggests that this is true. Frequent blood gas determinations are a guide to proper respirator use.

CLOSED SPINE INJURIES

Injury to the cervical spinal cord may occur with or without concomitant fracture or subluxation of adjacent vertebrae. In subluxation or unstable fracture, the principles of therapy involve reduction of the deformity to relieve spinal cord pressure and immobilization of the spine to prevent further neural damage. Approximately 75% of all cervical spine injuries associated with neurologic deficits can be adequately aligned and decompressed without the need for immediate operative intervention. Of the remaining 25% of patients who continue to demonstrate some evidence of spinal cord compression after reduction, less than one half will have a lesion large enough to warrant emergency operation.[23] It is necessary to understand the mechanism of injury along with the accompanying ligamentous injuries for the proper management of unstable spinal injuries.

The four main complications in the management of cervical spine injuries are failure to obtain adequate cervical spine x-ray films or inadequate review of the films, complications of cervical traction or immobilization by halo brace, improper or unnecessary operation, and inadequate spine fusion.

Inadequate X-ray Films

It has been documented by Bohlman that 100 of 300 cases of spine injury were unrecognized in the emergency room at the Baltimore City Hospital.[13] One of the reasons is failure to show on x-ray film all the spinal vertebrae in the area of injury suggested by the clinical examination. Though many authors recommend complicated, costly, detailed series of cervical spine x-ray films, including pillar views and xeroradiography, the greatest pitfall involves inadequate plain x-ray films and their interpretation.

Management

In cervical spine injury, it is necessary to visualize the entire cervical spine, including the C7–T1 level. The films must be critically examined for fracture, dislocation, or locked facets as well as for a prevertebral mass from edema or hemorrhage. If plain x-ray suggests a fracture or if the cause of neurologic defect is not revealed, then thin film tomography must be done and will usually reveal or rule out the presence of a fracture. Absence of a cervical spine fracture on tomography should not be considered a normal result since the patient may still have significant ligamentous injury with cervical spine instability.[96] The muscles, ligaments, and discs play the major role in providing spinal stability, and injury to these tissues can be inferred only by the radiographic changes, since only the osseous structures are shown. In any cervical spine injury with or without spinal cord injury, stability of the spine must be determined. This is readily evident when there is subluxation on the initial x-ray film. In other instances such as fracture of the vertebral body or disruption of the posterior interspinous space, skilled flexion and extension x-ray films may be necessary to reveal the state of instability of the spine. Instability of the spine, a particular feature of injuries to the cervical spine, requires treatment by immobilization. In suspected unilateral cervical dislocation or jumped facet, tomograms are essential for accurate delineation of the bone involvement. Anteroposterior tomograms may show lateral displacement of the spinal process above the dislocation. Bilateral locked facets and the presence of a teardrop fracture are strongly suggestive of spinal instability.

Xeroradiography is a simple means of evaluating the C6–7 to T1 level of patients in whom conventional filming fails to penetrate the thick shoulder mass. The process, employing conventional x-ray generators and a patented selenium plate, has two unique properties. It exaggerates density differences between soft tissue and bone and exhibits the phenomenon of "edge enhancement," which sharpens the delineation of the interface between tissues of differing densities. The process allows excellent visualization of the cervical spine with a minimum of patient risk and manipulation.[89]

COMPLICATIONS OF TRACTION OR IMMOBILIZATION

Since Crutchfield perfected a technique for skeletal tong traction in 1933, it has become the standard technique to realign and immobilize the cervical spine.[32] In recent years, increasing numbers of neurosurgeons and orthopaedic surgeons employ early halo immobilization with four pins inserted into the outer table of the skull. There have been many modifications and advances in halo technique, but nearly all methods require insertion of metal pins into or through the outer table of the skull. Skull traction properly applied will tolerate up to 65 pounds of traction and usually realigns the spine very effectively. Because of continuous pressure exerted by traction, especially when spring-loaded points are used, the points tend to penetrate the outer table of the skull. After about 24 hours, they will have penetrated about 1 mm and will require retightening.

The following complications have been reported with the use of skeletal traction or immobilization:

WORSENING OF THE NEUROLOGIC DEFICIT. Several authors have documented onset of neurolic deficit or worsening of existing neurologic deficits and even death when traction is applied to the cervical spine.[97] Cloward reported a patient who extruded a disc against the spinal cord during reduction.[29] Others have suggested that worsening is due to excessive traction with application of weight over 70 to 80 pounds and stretching of the spinal cord or blood supply to the spinal cord. Hollin and associates reported a patient with a C5–C6 fracture dislocation who turned his head to cough while in Crutchfield traction, became paraplegic, and died 4 days later.[57]

MANAGEMENT. Worsening of the neurologic status during traction requires repeated x-ray films. Loss of reduction or excessive distraction may be visible on the film. The condition can sometimes be reversed by lessening the weight applied on the traction. Failure to improve warrants myelography, seeking an extruded disc, which must be removed immediately.

PRESSURE NECROSIS. It is possible with newer skeletal tongs such as the Gardner–Wells tongs and the halo to test the pressure of the contact points adequately. Though some scalp necrosis nearly always results from tong application, pressure necrosis of large areas of skin does not occur. If satisfactory tong hygiene does not prevent scalp necrosis and infection develops, the tong or pin sites will need to be changed.

PENETRATION OF THE INNER TABLE OF THE SKULL. Penetration may occur without serious sequelae. Yet brain abscess and extradural abscess, leading to the death of the patient, have been recorded following penetration of the skull by traction tongs. Osteomyelitis, meningitis, and even fatal ventriculitis may follow penetration of the skull by the pin of a halo brace.

MANAGEMENT. If penetration of the skull is proven by x-ray film or looseness of the tong, the tong should be inserted at a new site. Any evidence of osteomyelitis requires débridement of the infected bone.

INTRACRANIAL BLEEDING. Rare cases of intracerebral and extradural hematoma have been reported following tong penetration of the skull.[37] Extradural hematoma may occur from a tear of the middle meningeal artery by the pin as the artery courses in a deep groove in the skull.

Periodic x-ray films should be taken to diagnose skull penetration in patients who have long-term tong or halo placement before any complications occur.

LOSS OF REDUCTION. Loss of reduction occurs when tongs fall out, when they are improperly placed, or when the patient is turned. Tongs must not be neglected and must be periodically tightened. Use of excessive weight may pull out the tongs.

MANAGEMENT. Loss of reduction is treated by reinsertion of the tongs if they have fallen out. Reinsertion must be coupled with the proper weight. Excessive weight may so stretch the ligaments that removal of the tongs after a suitable period of time (6 weeks) leads to return of the deformity. This can be avoided by adhering to Crutchfield's view that the closer the dislocation is to the skull, the less weight is needed to attain reduction (5–10 pounds for the atlantoaxial region; 25–35 pounds for the C7–T1 level).

ATLANTOAXIAL DISLOCATION. Fracture of the dens (odontoid process) may occur during minor trauma and may easily be missed on initial clinical and radiologic evaluation. The treatment of cord involvement in this location represents a unique problem because of the atlantoaxial articulation. Most subluxations are anterior and are associated with a fracture of the dens because its attachment to the axis is weaker than to the ligament that anchors it to the atlas. This is fortunate because very few patients survive when forward displacement is unaccompanied by dens fracture. If the odontoid process is not fractured, the spinal cord is compressed between it and the posterior arch of the atlas. Neurologic deficit is noted about one half the time when dens displacement exists. Forward displacement of the fractured dens is often accompanied by delayed neurologic signs, and backward displacement of the fractured dens usually produces early symptoms. Excessive weight may pull the fragments of an odontoid fracture too far apart and lead to nonunion even after the weight has been diminished. Thus, a major complication of this fracture is failure of fusion and persistent instability.

The controversial issue in the handling of closed cervical spine injury, in general, is that of conservative treatment, cervical traction, and halo immobilization *versus* cervical traction plus operative fusion. This is no more of an issue than it is for atlantoaxial dislocations. Neurologic complications may be delayed for decades, and therefore accurately assessing the deaths of those treated conservatively is difficult. Amyes and Anderson suggest it is very low—only 8%.[4] Statistics on operative mortality are difficult to find because large surgically treated series are unavailable. Alexander and associates reported a 14% fatality rate in 16 operated cases while Apuzzo and associates reported no mortality or significant morbidity in 13 patients treated surgically.[2, 5] Operative fatalities are related to respiratory failure. In a careful clinicopathologic study of six patients with chronic medullospinal compression who died after upper cervical laminectomy, as presented by Dastur and colleagues, hematomyelia was revealed in five of the patients.[34] They attributed this to the sudden decompression of the anterior spinal artery and its branches at operation.

MANAGEMENT. All undisplaced odontoid fractures should be treated by external immobilization for at least 12 weeks. The mode of immobilization is not critical.[81] All fractures displaced more than 4 mm should be considered for primary operative management, especially if the patient is over 40 years of age. Most surgical approaches to the atlantoaxial dislocation involve either a laminectomy, especially of the arch of C1, or wiring of the arch of C1 to the lamina and spinous process of C2, and possibly C3, with the addition of a bone graft since wire alone may break. The addition of bone at C1–C3 level for fusion is considered essential, followed by 12 weeks of halo immobilization. In experienced hands, this usually results in solid fusion and stabilization of the atlantoaxial joint.

In children, fractures of the odontoid process are usually situated at the cartilaginous plate between the odontoid process and the body of C2, with the odontoid displaced anteriorly. Measurable distraction is rare, and upon reduction, excellent eventual healing occurs with long-term immobilization without operation.[105]

COMPLICATIONS OF HYPEREXTENSION INJURY OF THE CERVICAL SPINE

Hyperextension of the cervical spine has been found to be the mechanism of serious cervical spinal cord injury in approximately one half of all such injuries.[21] Burke classified hyperextension injuries as follows: (1) posterior vertebral body dislocation, (2) complete anteroposterior ligamentous rupture, (3) hyperextension injuries masquerading as flexion injuries, (4) extension disruption of the spine affected by ankylosing spondylitis, and (5) extension disruption without dislocation. More hyperextension injuries fit in the fifth category than in any of the other four. These patients are usually over 50 years of age and have some degree of degenerative change in the cervical spine and anterior longitudinal spinous ligament, kyphosis of the thoracic spine with compensatory cervical spine lordosis, and a spinal canal narrowed by hypertrophy of the ligamentum flavum and posteriorly protruding osteophytes and intervertebral discs. Most have a history of having fallen or sustained a blow to the forehead or upper part of the face.

Schneider and colleagues reported the sequelae of hyperextension cervical spine injuries to be the central cervical cord syndrome, anterior and posterior cord syndrome, central cervical hematomyelia, and complete transverse cord necrosis and transection.[99]

Soft tissue complications occur because of hyperextension of the cervical spine. In 1960, Morrison described a patient in whom hyperextension of the cervical spine had ruptured the esophagus.[77] The patient died from mediastinitis and bronchopneumonia 2 weeks after the injury. In 1980, Stringer and colleagues reported a patient with hyperextension cervical spine injury whose lateral cervical spine x-ray film showed a pocket of prevertebral air.[112] These authors suggested the mechanism by which the esophagus is ruptured to be either a trapping and pinching of the posterior wall of the esophagus as the anteroposterior ligament ruptures and the vertebral bodies separate, then snap back as flexion occurs, or an impingement on the sharp edge of one of the separated vertebral bodies.

Diagnosis and management are as described in the section on anterior cervical spine surgery. Early diagnosis will be made if prevertebral air is noted on cervical spine x-ray film. Immediate repair is mandatory to prevent mediastinitis, retropharyngeal abscess, aspiration pneumonia, or death.

LOWER CERVICAL INJURIES

As in high cervical trauma, controversy in management of lower cervical injuries perists. Advocates of the conservative approach *versus* the surgical approach with decompression and fusion confront advocates of the anterior approach *versus* the posterior approach as described for disc disease.[110]

The mortality rate is rapidly being reduced because of better early and late pulmonary care. In 1962, Drake reported an 18% mortality in 28 cervical spine patients undergoing operation.[37] In 1970, Norell and Wilson reported two operative deaths in 31 patients undergoing early anterior fusion while there were five deaths among 26 patients not undergoing surgery during the same period of time.[82]

The main complication of cervical spine injury with spinal cord involvement is failure to improve or worsening of the neurologic condition. Earlier reports reveal that 81% of the conservatively treated patients (by traction or other mode of immobilization) and 83% of those operated upon failed to improve neurologically.[26] If unnecessary major surgical intervention is to be avoided, the circumstances that constitute an indication for operation must be defined.

COMPLETE PHYSIOLOGIC SPINAL CORD TRANSECTION

Complete loss of spinal cord function, which persists more than 24 hours, most likely is permanent. Once the spine is realigned and immobilization is achieved, no evidence in the various series of patients reported indicates that any operation will improve the neurologic function in these patients. Surgical decompression may be justified for fracture of the facet, lamina, or pedicle of the vertebrae, which encroaches on a nerve root. Otherwise, operation is indicated only as a stabilization procedure to prevent painful angulation of the spine.

INCOMPLETE PHYSIOLOGIC SPINAL CORD TRANSECTION

The patient with a partial spinal cord injury who shows deterioration may well require operation. Disc herniation, bone fragments, or hematoma may be compromising the spinal cord.

Management

Myelography is indicated in a patient who worsens, and if a disc or hematoma is compressing the spinal cord, the lesion should be removed. The minimyelogram is safe and accurate and will reveal a complete block to the flow of Pantopaque if there is a large extruded disc fragment or epidural or subdural hematoma.[23] A disc lesion will usually be best removed from the anterior approach, and a hematoma will usually require a posterior laminectomy for removal. Both these conditions are rare in cervical spine injury.

More common, the myelogram shows a wide spinal cord consistent with edema or hematomyelia as found in the central cord syndrome. In general, patients with a widened spinal cord on myelogram will not benefit from operation. In fact, the patient with a partial injury may worsen neurologically following operation when only a "widened or edematous" spinal cord is observed at operation.

PERSISTENT PAIN FOLLOWING CERVICAL SPINE INJURY

Pain following cervical spine injury may of course be due to disc rupture, but more often it is due to angulation of the cervical spine or actual gibbus formation. Cone and Turner pioneered the treatment of cervical spine dislocations by posterior fusion.[30] Broken wires and absorption or sepsis of the bone graft have been the principal complications in this operation. Cloward as well as Smith and Robinson have advocated anterior interbody fusion as a superior method of stabilizing the spine and decompressing the spinal cord. The use of the anterior operation in "tear-drop" fractures for patients who have unstable spine fractures is frequently associated with failure to maintain the dowel or graft in proper position. The dowel easily displaces forward or even backward against the spinal cord (Fig. 47-8). This is especially likely if the posterior stabilizing elements of the spine are disrupted by the injury and if the operation on the anterior spine, involving a section of the anterior longitudinal ligament, increases spine instability.

Management

Cervical spine instability can lead to further spinal cord injury so that the treatment is critical. The spinal cord must not sustain a new or secondary injury because of instability or angulation. The x-ray films must be studied carefully and any operation planned so as not to increase instability of the spine. If the posterior spinal elements are disrupted, as is usually visualized by separation of the spinous processes, then posterior fusion will usuallly be indicated for stabilization. If the posterior elements are intact, an anterior fusion can be performed without aggravation of the instability. Usually, a trapezoid or kiel graft can be used in lieu of the round Cloward dowel so that displacement does not easily occur.

Either operation should be combined with rigid halo immobilization of the spine for at least 12 weeks. This will ensure fusion with proper alignment.[31]

Last, it should be stated that since an operation for cervical spine trauma rarely improves spinal cord function, a patient who is neurologically stable with a normal myelogram or a patient who is improving may be treated with halo immobilization for 12 weeks, at which time approximately 95% of patients will demonstrate spine stability.

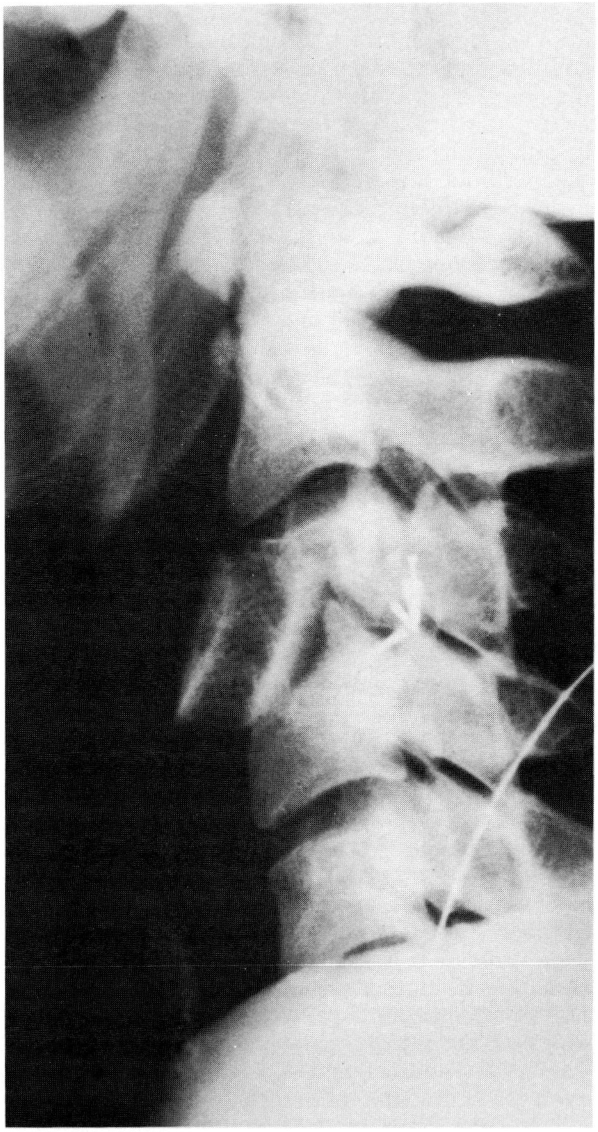

FIG. 47-8. Cervical spine x-ray film of bone-graft displacement in patient who had undergone a cervical spine fusion at C2–C3 level. This bone dowel was replaced at reoperation.

THORACIC SPINE INJURIES

The mortality rate for thoracic spine injuries ranges from 6% to 10% in most series. Most deaths are due to ruptured viscera and pulmonary embolism rather than to the spinal cord injury itself. Munro noted that 16.5% of 36 closed injuries of the thoracolumbar spine had associated hemothorax.[78] Most of the injuries to the lumbar and sacral cord segments occur in thoracic or thoracolumbar spine injuries. The thoracolumbar junction presents a special problem, since after the cervical region, the thoracolumbar junction is the most vulnerable region of the spinal column. Forty percent of all spinal cord injuries occur at this level. In 26 cases of T11 and L1 unstable fractures treated by a one-stage anterolateral decompression of the spine with Harrington rod alignment and posterior fusion, reported by Schmidek and colleagues, there were six complications.[98] The two judged to be procedure-related were a brachial plexus compression radiculopathy, probably secondary to intraoperative positioning on the table on a Stryker frame, and a dislodged Harrington rod.

Management

Complete thoracic spinal cord lesions are irremediable by a surgical procedure, and, therefore, since the ribs aid in stabilization, an operation should only be undertaken when definitely indicated for stabilization. The indications for operation are rare because spinal epidural hematoma requiring evacuation is rare. Stabilization of the thoracolumbar spine junction with Harrington rods and bony fusion is indicated to preserve cauda equina (root) function.

LUMBAR SPINE INJURIES

Injuries to the lumbar spine involve primarily roots, the capacity of which to recover exceeds that of the cord. The operative mortality rate is minimal, and the operation can be delayed while the patient's course is observed.[64]

Management

The spine must be realigned, if possible, and then the spine can be stabilized with Harrington rods and bony fusion. If the lumbar vertebral body is compressing the cauda equina anteriorly, then the anterior approach for partial vertebral body removal will be necessary for decompression.

COMPLICATIONS OF SACRUM FRACTURES

Isolated sacral fractures are rare and easily overlooked and, most often, occur in association with pelvic fractures. In almost 1000 cases of spine injury entered in the 1972 National Spinal Injury Registry, there were no isolated sacral fractures.[22] In the world literature, they appear only sporadically. The presence of a sacral fracture is easily missed. The neurologic abnormalities that accompany sacral fractures are presumably the result of damage to sacral nerve elements. Rarely, there are perianal sensory loss and bladder and anal sphincter disturbances. In 1938, Hallgrimsson reported three cases, the chief symptoms of which were dysuria and difficulty with defecation.[52]

Diagnosis

The diagnosis should be suspected in a patient who has signs of pelvic trauma such as perineal ecchymosis, lost sphincter control, or inability to micturate. It should also be suspected in patients with pelvic fracture, and persistent radiologic attempts, including an angled view 50° up from the horizontal, should be made. Examination will usually reveal anesthesia of the involved sacral dermatomes and a lax anal sphincter. A cystometrogram should support the diagnosis of cauda equina dysfunction.

Management

Byrnes and colleagues suggest that if the lesion is complete, treatment should be identical to that for peripheral nerve injury.[22] If the sacral fracture is displaced and the nerves are stretched, a sacral decompression can be done. However, if the lesion is incomplete, with retained sensation, then a conservative course can be followed, especially if bladder function begins to return.

COMPLICATIONS OF ANKYLOSING SPONDYLITIS

The cervical spine is the most common site for fractures of the ankylosed spine. The diagnosis of spinal fracture in patients who do not exhibit a neurologic deficit may be difficult because the pain may be ascribed to the condition of ankylosing spondylitis rather than to the fracture itself. X-ray demonstration of the fractures may be hindered by the presence of osteoporosis.

The fused vertebrae in ankylosing spondylitis behave as do long bones so that a fracture may be grossly unstable, increasing the chance of dislocation and spinal cord injury. Accompanying osteoporosis predisposes the patient to fracture even after minimal trauma.

The major problem with conservative therapy is instability of the spine because in an ankylosis of spine any movement of the trunk can cause movement of the fracture site by enhanced leverage, which may result in sudden paraplegia or death if the lesion is at the cervical level. Fazl and associates reported a patient with ankylosing spondylitis who sustained a T12–L1 fracture, resulting in paraparesis, anuria, and rupture of the aorta.[42] The laceration of the aorta resulted in formation of an aortic spinal subarachnoid fistula and the patient's death.

Management

Surgical therapy will help in obtaining rapid immobilization, and in thoracolumbar fracture, Harrington rod immobilization is of help. With vascular injury, the anterior approach is preferable to stabilize the spine and repair major vascular injuries.

COMPOUND SPINAL CORD INJURIES

The postoperative mortality rate for acute compound spinal cord injuries in World War II ranged from 5% to 12%. In war, many casualties result from fragmentation injuries, which are massive and must be considered contaminated. These differ from civilian bullet wounds inflicted by pistols ranging from 0.22 to 0.45 inches. In combat, higher-velocity bullets impart greater energy and may cause significant CNS injury as a result of a distant penetration with resultant shock waves. Thus, there may be a higher incidence of "concussion" in war wounds. Injuries restricted to the area of the bony vertebral column in civilian wounds without depression of fragments or with minimal soft tissue explosive effects probably do not cause transient spinal cord decompensation. A similar military high-velocity energy missile might have caused severe neurologic injury due to shock waves, in spite of noninvolvement of the CNS by the missile itself.

In Yashon's report on 65 civilian spinal cord, conus medullaris, or cauda equina bullet injuries, there were 15 deaths, but only two of these occurred from cauda equina wounds.[123] Laminectomy did not influence the course of the patients, and, of course, patients with cauda equina injuries fared better than those with spinal cord wounds. Most early deaths occur in patients who sustain high cervical missile wounds or severe cardiothoracic wounds.

Injuries to the spinal cord produced by missiles may be divided into three etiological groups as follows:

1. *Direct injuries due to missiles.* This group includes wounds produced by the passage of a bullet or shell fragment directly into or through the substance of the cord or cauda equina. The damage produced directly to the cord occurs in 2 ways, by destruction at the moment the metallic foreign body strikes or by subsequent compression of nervous tissue due to the presence of the foreign body in the spinal canal.
2. *Indirect injuries produced by bone.* The vertebrae are fractured by the missile, causing depressed or comminuted fragments of bone to lacerate the cord or protrude into the canal and compress the cord. The cord is injured either at the moment of injury or by subsequent pressure or movement of bony fragments within the spinal canal.
3. *Indirect injuries to the spinal cord due to concussion.* This group includes patients in whom a loss of neurologic function occurs after passage of a missile in the vicinity of the spinal column but not through the canal itself. Neural function is disturbed secondary to the velocity effects of the missile itself.

It is extremely rare to find extradural, subdural, or subarachnoid bleeding in any sufficient amount after a penetrating injury because space is adequate, both inside and outside the dura, for longitudinal infiltration of extravasated blood.

The main complications of penetrating muscle wounds of the spine are unusual neurologic deficit, spinal fluid fistula with subsequent development of meningitis, root pain, and compression of the spinal cord or cauda equina by retained intraspinal metal or bone.

UNUSUAL NEUROLOGIC DEFICIT

Gunshot injuries to the cervical spinal cord do not follow any particular clinical pattern. All degrees of symptoms occur, ranging from isolated radicular loss, to partial spinal cord injuries with mono-, para-, and hemiparesis, to tetraplegia. In addition to location of the fragment, other factors must be taken into account in a gunshot wound: in particular, the impact of the projectile, the deformation of the projectile in the tissue, and the related damage to the tissue itself. The gunshot injury to the cervical cord can lead to the syndrome of acute central cervical cord injury with more damage to the central portion of the spinal cord than to the periphery.[111] At times, retrospective analysis of the factors involved in the neurologic deficit for a missile wound is difficult. In many cases, the missile is lodged in the spinal canal and most of the energy dissipated before the missile reached the spinal canal.

Diagnosis

Plain x-ray films and tomography will usually reveal intraspinal bone or metal fragments. CT scan is proving extremely useful in detecting intraspinal bone or metal.

Treatment

If metal or bone is retained within the spinal canal, or bone is projecting into the spinal canal, and the patient has a partial lesion of the spinal cord, full laminectomy is indicated to remove all foreign and devitalized material from the spinal canal. This allows also for inspection of the neural elements and watertight closure of the dura to prevent CSF leakage and possible meningitis.

SPINAL FLUID FISTULA

When a spinal fluid leak persists following a gunshot wound to the spine, it usually means either a large laceration of dura or a spicule of bone or a foreign body is protruding through the dura, maintaining the opening. When wounds involve infected or contaminated paraspinal tissues as well as dura, closure of the dura is especially important to prevent meningitis. This is particularly the case when missiles initially pass through the bowel and then enter the spinal canal. Abdominal infection may penetrate the missile tract and spread to the spinal subarachnoid space, leading to meningitis.

Management

Proper management is based on establishing the diagnosis of a CSF fistula with certainty and then closing the dura. Diagnosis can be confirmed by the use of Pantopaque or metrizamide myelography, which should reveal the dural laceration by extravasation of contrast material or will reveal the filling defect of a persistent spicule of bone projecting into the subarachnoid space. In the latter instance, tomography of the spine and CT scanning will also be helpful in identifying the bone spicule.

In patients who have a sizable wound directly over or near the spinal column, the only way to débride adequately is to excise the wound to its depths and perform a formal laminectomy as widely as necessary to remove all comminuted and depressed bone fragments. The dura can be closed in watertight fashion primarily or with the use of a fascial graft if necessary. If the dura sac and spinal cord or cauda equina are completely severed with no possible return of neural function, then ligation of the open end of the dura may be carried out to accomplish closure. It is essential that spinal fluid leakage be sealed as soon as possible after the injury to prevent meningitis, but this operation should not take precedent over thoracic or abdominal operations to correct life-threatening situations. When necessary, the patient must be stabilized and placed on antibiotics until laminectomy and closure of the dura can be safely accomplished.

ROOT PAIN

Rarely, a compound wound of the lumbar spine or sacrum with involvement of the cauda equina in which the patient experiences severe radicular pain during the acute stage is seen. There is evidence of either incomplete transection or compression of nerve or nerve root by metal or bone. The pain may even grow more severe while the neurologic deficit recedes. This is characterized by recurring spasms of sharp, burning or stabbing pain, which radiates from a central to a peripheral location along the distribution of the nerve segments involved.

Management

Since this type of pain is very severe and usually untouched by ordinary medication, early operation is indicated. Nerve root compression usually can be confirmed by neural deficit found on examination and confirmatory electromyographic study, plus positive contrast studies. A cauda equina filling defect will be clearly visible on myelography. A laminectomy or at least a hemilaminectomy will be necessary for removal of the compression, whether it be metal or bone. Any dural laceration will need to be repaired after replacing herniated elements of the cauda equina inside the dura. The pain relief from removing compressive lesions of nerve roots is usually excellent. According to Pool, four out of five patients with root pain are aided by operation.[90]

COMPRESSION OF THE SPINAL CORD OR CAUDA EQUINA BY RETAINED INTRASPINAL METAL OR BONE

The importance of extrinsic cord pressure by bone fragments or metallic foreign bodies has always been a subject of great controversy. Early laminectomy for relief of cord compression is considered particularly desirable in the following types of cases:

1. Patients who exhibit a neurologic picture consistent with incomplete transection of the cord in whom the picture has definitely altered since the time of injury, especially if the neurologic deficit has increased. Even in patients showing improvement, however, recovery might well stop short of the maximum possible if the cord compression is allowed to persist; therefore, compression should always be relieved as soon as possible.
2. Patients with a neurologic picture of fixed but incomplete cord transection have x-ray films with clear-cut encroachment on the spinal canal by a metallic foreign body or definite fracture of a lamina or pedicle with or without depression of bone fragments. A Brown–Séquard type of incomplete lesion is seen occasionally and appears to indicate an especially favorable prognosis.
3. Patients with a neurologic picture of complete physiologic transection of the cord have x-ray films showing the presence of a metallic foreign body within or protruding in the spinal canal or have demonstrable fractures with depression of bone fragments into the canal. If a metallic foreign body lies on the same side of the spinal cord by x-ray film as the wound of entrance, this may be considered more favorable than if the foreign body has crossed the midline. What appears to be a complete physiologic transection may represent spinal shock, and removal of the localized pressure may hasten recovery of neural function.

Management

These patients should have early laminectomy, removal of the compressive metal or bone, and anatomical closure of the incision. Again, the dura should be closed in watertight fashion.

Lastly, from observation of patients with missile wounds of the spine, if examination of the patient and review of diagnostic studies leave any reasonable doubt in the surgeon's mind that the cord has been severed, there is little to lose and possibly much to gain by the earliest possible relief of localized cord compression.

DEEP VEIN THROMBOSIS

Deep vein thrombosis (DVT) is a particular problem in the patient with spinal cord injury, since early ambulation therapy is often not possible. In four series totaling over 1200 patients, the incidence of fatal pulmonary embolism in acute paraplegics was 2%. Joffe reported a 43% incidence of postoperative deep venous thromboses in neurosurgical patients. Of these, 90% were asymptomatic.[59]

Thus, this group of patients is especially vulnerable to the life-threatening complications of DVT. Furthermore, unless the patient is repeatedly reexamined for DVT by serial sophisticated methods for diagnosis of DVT, such as Doppler sonography, radioactive studies, or phlebography, fatal pulmonary embolism may occur. The patient with total motor and sensory paralysis will not have leg pain as one of the symptoms of DVT.

Management

The incidence of DVT can be reduced by the use of an intermittent, sequential pneumatic apparatus. In a report by Zelikovski and associates on neurosurgery patients, 50% of control patients developed DVT, whereas only 4.3% of the patients who were treated with the device were affected.[125]

The necessity of preventing DVT in neurosurgical patients must be seriously considered because of the high incidence of occult DVT. Following injury or surgery if the results of platelet count, prothrombin time, and partial thromboplastin time are normal, consideration must be given to the use of minidose heparin. If these determinations are within normal limits, 5000 units of aqueous heparin sodium are given subcutaneously every 12 hours after injury or postoperatively as long as the patient is confined to bed. Thus, it usually requires 3 days of minidose heparin therapy in postoperative spine patients, but much longer in the spinal cord injured patient. Early stabilization and halo application will allow these patients to arise earlier.

If pulmonary embolism or a mobile thrombus is detected by venography, a Greenfield filter should immediately be placed. This technique and the methods of removing life threatening pulmonary emboli are discussed in Chapter 30.

LATE COMPLICATIONS OF SPINAL CORD INJURY

Autonomic Hyperreflexia

Patients with paraplegia or quadriplegia often have subjective complaints and objective findings of autonomic hyperreflexia. Head and Riddoch first reported on the association of headaches with hypertension in patients with spinal cord injuries during World War I.[53] In 1962, Arieff and associates elaborated completely the clinical symptoms and signs of autonomic hyperreflexia or dysreflexia.[6] The most significant of these are acute hypertension, severe throbbing headache, sweating, and flushing of the skin above the level of the lesion, with pilomotor erection and peripheral vasoconstriction below the level of the lesion. At times, dilated pupils and occasional blurring of vision, bradycardia, and syncope are observed.

The precipitating factors of this significant rise in systolic blood pressure include distention of the bladder secondary to outlet or catheter obstruction, pelvic and rectal manipulations, bladder percussion, cold stimuli below the level of the lesion, pin prick and other noxious stimuli, and deep inspiration and distention of the hollow abdominal or pelvic viscera. This clinical picture occurs intermittently in spinal cord injured patients who have complete physiologic lesions from L2 to the cervical region, but most frequently above the T6 level. The mechanism of action is thought to be the release of uninhibited mass autonomic reflexes.[63] These etiologic factors activate and increase sympathetic activity on a peripheral or spinal cord basis below the level of the injury. Peripheral vasoconstriction produces decreasing blood flow to the musculature and skin of the extremities below the physiologic lesion. The bradycardia and syncope result from vagal inhibitory mechanisms that are activated to compensate for the sympathetic overactivity. A contributory physiologic factor is the interruption of descending cortical and parasympathetic inhibitory pathways.

MANAGEMENT. Various medical regimens and surgical procedures have been used to treat and abolish such sympathetic hyperreflexia. Ganglionic agents and vasodilators such as diazoxide, or nitroprusside, usually are ineffective at normal doses or produce unwanted side-effects. Anesthetic interruption of the sensory pathways from the stimulated areas is another method of therapy but often is only temporary. Bilateral carotid artery compression at the time of the acute episode and decompression of the distended bowel or bladder may be effective after the onset of acute hypertension.

Surgical procedures include deafferentiation of the T9 to T12 segments by bilateral rhizotomies, but these are destructive procedures. Others have reported modulation of the hyperreflexia by percutaneous epidural neurostimulation.[95] The implantation of a pulse-modulated epidural neurostimulation system below the level of a complete physiologic injury creates a synthetic central inhibitory mechanism between the initial "decerebrated" spinal cord and the peripheral elements.

Progressive Posttraumatic Syringomyelia

Syringomyelia is a late and probably progressive complication of spinal cord injury. Barnett and colleagues reported a 1.8% incidence, and in a review of the world literature, 143 cases of syrinx secondary to a fractured spine with spinal cord damage have been reported.[9] Syringomyelia has been diagnosed 5 to 23 years after spinal cord injury. In most patients, the initial neurologic deficit is sensory–motor. There is usually a long interval between the spinal cord injury and onset of symptoms, leading to the eventual diagnosis of the syrinx. The patient with spinal cord injury who experiences increased pain and numbness and the late appearance of new muscle weakness can be suspected of having a posttraumatic syrinx.

MANAGEMENT. The treatment is drainage of the cyst into the subarachnoid space or into the pleural or abdominal cavities.

SUMMARY OF COMPLICATIONS OF SPINAL CORD INJURY

A person with severe spinal cord injury is always subject to deterioration medically, psychologically, and socially. Many of these medical complications seen in the chronic phase are actually secondary to psychological and social problems. These, in turn, may be the residual of such developments as unnecessary or improperly treated medical complications accrued during the acute phase of treatment. The patient with spinal cord injury presents unique problems in diagnosis. Symptoms may be whimsical and are frequently marked or distorted by sensory impairment. Profound disturbances of reflex mechanisms controlling autonomic and endocrine functions require modification of standard surgical and medical protocols.

Complications of Cordotomy

Both open and closed (stereotaxic) cervical cordotomy are established procedures for relief of pain. The relief of pain in patients with cancer, as well as various benign pain syndromes, is achieved by interruption of the spinothalamic tract in the anterior quadrant of the spinal cord. If the lesion is enlarged beyond the limits of the anterolateral quadrant of the spinal cord, there are then associated, acknowledged complications, the most serious of which are respiratory and autonomic dysfunctions. This dysfunction includes respiratory arrest, apnea and vasomotor collapse, hypotension, hyponatremia, and urinary retention at varying intervals after cordotomy.

This syndrome of afferent respiratory dysfunction following cordotomy at the high cervical (C1–C4) levels is especially likely if the patient has preexisting pulmonary disease such as emphysema, has had a pneumonectomy, or has abnormal blood gas profiles. It almost invariably occurs if a bilateral lesion produced bilateral high analgesia. Following the procedure, the patient is usually confused, with associated hypotension, and will complain of inability to "get enough air." Sleep-induced apnea is especially likely to occur, and the patient, if unattended, may die quietly in his sleep.

No patient should have bilateral C1 level cordotomies. The patient who requires a bilateral cordotomy should have the second side done at a low cervical or thoracic level.

MANAGEMENT

Following cordotomy, the patient who has an impaired CO_2 response test and vital capacity will need intubation and support of respiration. Usually, these functions will improve with time and as CO_2 response approaches normal, the patient can be extubated. It must be remembered that the development of respiratory failure is usually insidious, and the surgeon should always be aware of this complication when performing a high cervical cordotomy.

References

1. Albin MS, Carroll RG, Moroon JC: Clinical considerations concerning detection of venous air embolism. Neurosurgery 3:380, 1978
2. Alexander E Jr, Forsyth HF, Davis CH Jr et al: Dislocation of the altas on the axis. The value of early fusion of C1, C2, and C3. J Neurosurg 15:353, 1958
3. Alker GJ Jr, Oh YS, Leslie EV: High cervical spine and craniocervical junction injuries in fatal traffic accidents: A radiological study. Orthop Clin North Am 9(4):1003, 1978
4. Amyes EW, Anderson FM: Fracture of the odontoid process. Report of sixty-three cases. Arch Surg 72:317, 1956
5. Apuzzo MLJ, Heiden JS, Weiss MH et al: Acute fracture of the odontoid process. An analysis of 45 cases. J Neurosurg 48:85, 1978
6. Arieff AJ, Tigay EL, Pyzik SW: Acute hypertension induced by urinary bladder distention: Headache and its correlates in quadriplegic patients. Arch Neurol 6:248, 1962
7. Auld AN, Buerman A: Metastatic spinal epidural tumors: An analysis of 50 cases. Arch Neurol 15:100, 1966

8. Bailey RW, Badgley CE: Stabilization of the cervical spine by anterior fusion. J Bone Joint Surg 42A:565, 1960
9. Barnett HJ, Jousse AT, Morley TP et al: Post-traumatic syringomyelia. Paraplegia 9:33, 1971
10. Barron KD, Hirano A, Araki S, Terry RD: Experiences with metastatic neoplasm involving the spinal cord. Neurology (Minneap) 9:91, 1959
11. Bellamy R, Pitts FW, Stauffer ES: Respiratory complications in traumatic quadriplegia. Analysis of 20 years experience. J Neurosurg 39:596, 1973
12. Black P: Spinal metastasis: Current status and recommended guidelines for management. Neurosurgery 5:726, 1979
13. Bohlman HH: Acute fractures and dislocations of the cervical spine. J Bone Joint Surg 61A:1119, 1979
14. Boston HC, Bianco AJ, Rhodes KH: Disk space infections in children. Orthop Clin North Am 6:953, 1975
15. Brechner TM, Brechner VL: An audible alarm for monitoring air embolism during neurosurgery. J Neurosurg 47:201, 1977
16. Brechner VL, Bethune RWM: Recent advances in monitoring air embolism. Anesth Analg (Cleve) 50:255, 1971
17. Brice J, McKissock W: Surgical treatment of malignant extradural spinal tumors. Br Med J 1:1341, 1965
18. Brisman R, Kouach RM, Johnson DO et al: Pulmonary edema in acute cervical spinal cord transection (Paper No 51). Presented at the Annual Meeting of the American Association of Neurological Surgeons, St Louis, April, 1974
19. Brussatis F: Osteomyelitis nach operation lumbalar diskushernien. Acta Neurochir (Wien) 3:209, 1953
20. Bucholz RW, Burkhead WZ, Graham W et al: Occult cervical spine injuries in fatal traffic accidents. J Trauma 19:768, 1979
21. Burke DC: Hyperextension injuries of the spine. J Bone Joint Surg 53(A):3, 1971
22. Byrnes DP, Russo GL, Ducker TB, Cowley RA: Sacrum fractures and neurological damage. Report of two cases. J Neurosurg 47:459, 1977
23. Carol M, Ducker TB, Byrnes DP: Minimyelogram in cervical spinal cord trauma. Neurosurgery 7:219, 1980
24. Chade HO: Metastatic tumours of the spine and spinal cord. In Vinken PJ and Bruyn GW (eds): Handbook of Clinical Neurology, vol 20, pp 415-433. Amsterdam, North-Holland Publishing, 1976
25. Chandler WF, Dinchiff DG, Taren JA: Acute pulmonary edema following venous air embolism during a neurosurgical procedure. Case Report. J Neurosurg 40:400, 1974
26. Cheshire DJ: The stability of the cervical spine following the conservative treatment of fractures and fracture dislocations. Paraplegia 7:193, 1969
27. Claveria L, Sutton D, Tress BM: The radiological diagnosis of meningiomas: The impact of EMI scanning. Br J Radiol 50:15, 1977
28. Cloward RB: The anterior approach for removal of ruptured cervical discs. J Neurosurg 15:602, 1958
29. Cloward RB: Treatment of acute fractures and fracture dislocations of the cervical spine by vertebral body fusion. A report of eleven cases. J Neurosurg 18:201, 1961
30. Cone W, Turner WG: The treatment of fracture—Dislocations of the cervical vertebrae by skeletal traction and fusion. J Bone Joint Surg 19(A):584, 1937
31. Cooper PR, Maravilla KP, Sklar FH et al: Halo immobilization of cervical spine fractures. Indications and results. J Neurosurg 50:603, 1979
32. Crutchfield WA: Skeletal traction for dislocation of the cervical spine. Report of a case. South Surg 2:156, 1933
33. Dandy WE: Serious complications of ruptured intervertebral discs. JAMA 119:474, 1942
34. Dastur DK, Wadia NH, Desai AD et al: Medullospinal compression due to atlanto-axial dislocation and sudden hematomyelia during decompression. Pathology, pathogenesis and clinical correlations. Brain 88:897, 1965
35. DeSaussure RL: Vascular injury coincident to disc surgery. J Neurosurg 16:222, 1959
36. Doppman JL, Girton M: Angiographic study of the laminectomy in the presence of acute anterior epidural masses. J Neurosurg 45:195, 1976
37. Drake C: Cervical spinal cord injury. Neurosurgery 19:487, 1962
38. Dunn RC Jr, Kelley WA, Wohns RNW, Howe JF: Spinal epidural neoplasia. A 15-year review of the result of surgical therapy. J Neurosurg 52:47, 1980
39. Engler GL, Spielholz NI, Bernhard WN et al: Somatosensory evoked potentials during Harrington instrumentation for scoliosis. J Bone Joint Surg 60A:528, 1978
40. Ericsson JA, Gottlieb JD, Sweet RB: Closed-chest cardiac massage in the treatment of venous air embolism. N Engl J Med 270:1353, 1964
41. Fager CA: Results of adequate posterior decompression in the relief of spondylotic cervical myelopathy. J Neurosurg 38:684, 1973
42. Fazl M, Bilbao JM, Hudson AR: Laceration of the aorta. Complicating spinal fracture in ankylosing spondylitis. Neurosurgery 8:732, 1981
43. Feild JR, McHenry H: The lumbar shield: A preliminary report. Neurosurgery 3:26, 1978
44. Fender FA: A new hazard in cervical laminectomy. JAMA 149:227, 1952
45. Fisher RG, Saunders RL: Lumbar disc protrusion in children. J Neurosurg 54:480, 1981
46. Flynn TB: Complications of anterior cervical fusion. Presented at the Annual Meeting of the American Association of Neurological Surgeons, San Francisco, California, April, 1976
47. Garrido E: Closed irrigation—suction technique in the treatment of lumbar laminectomy. Infection: Case report. Neurosurgery 5:354, 1979
48. Giesiking H: Lokalisierte spondylitis nach operiertem bandscheibenvorfall. Adl Chir 76:1470, 1951
49. Gilbert RW, Kim JH, Posner JB: Epidural spinal cord compression from metastatic tumor: Diagnosis and treatment. Ann Neurol 3:40, 1978
50. Goald HJ: Microlumbar disectomy: Follow-up of 147 patients. Spine 3:183, 1978
51. Haimovic IC, Arbit E, Posner JB: Colonic ileus complicating laminectomy. Neurosurgery 3:369, 1978
52. Hallgrimsson S: Three cases of fracture of the sacrum. Acta Orthop Scand 9:100, 1938
53. Head H, Riddoch G: The automatic bladder, excessive sweating and some other reflex conditions in gross injuries of spinal cord. Brain 40:188, 1917
54. Heiden JS, Weiss MH, Rosenberg AW et al: Management of cervical spine cord trauma in southern California. J Neurosurg 43:732, 1975
55. Hirsch D: Cervical disc rupture: diagnosis and therapy. Acta Orthop Scand 30:172, 1960
56. Hochman MS, Pena C, Ramirez R: Calcified herniated thoracic disc diagnosed by computerized tomography. Case report. J Neurosurg 52:722, 1980

57. Hollin SA, Gross SW, Levin P: Fracture of the cervical spine in patients with rheumatoid spondylitis. Am Surg 31:532, 1965
58. Howland WF, Curry JL: Pantopaque arachnoiditis. Experimental study of blood as a potentiating agent and corticosteroids as an ameliorating agent. Acta Radiol [Diag] (Stockh) 5:1032, 1966
59. Joffe SN: Incidence of postoperative deep vein thrombosis in neurosurgical patients. J Neurosurg 42:201, 1975
60. Kaplan ES: Post-disectomy tuberculous abscess. Case report. J Neurosurg 38:358, 1973
61. Kelsey JL, White AA, Pastides H, Bisbee GE: The impact of musculoskeletal disorders on the population of the United States. J Bone Joint Surg 61A:959, 1979
62. Kemp HBS, Jackson JW, Jeremiah JD, Hall AJ: Pyogenic infections occurring primarily in intervertebral discs. J Bone Joint Surg 55B:698, 1973
63. Kurnick NB: Autonomic hyperreflexia and its control in patients with spinal cord lesions. Ann Intern Med 44:678, 1956
64. Landau B, Ransohoff J: Late surgery for incomplete traumatic lesion of the conus medullaris and cauda equina. J Neurosurg 30:257, 1968
65. Linton RR, White PD: Arteriovenous fistula between the right common iliac artery and the inferior vena cava. Report of a case of its occurrence following an operation for a ruptured intervertebral disk with cure by operation. Arch Surg 50:6, 1945
66. Livingston KE, Perrin RG: The neurosurgical management of spinal metastasis causing cord and cauda equina compression. J Neurosurg 49:839, 1978
67. Love JG, Rivers MH: Intractable pain due to associated intervertebral disc and intraspinal neoplasm. Report of cases. Neurology 12:60, 1962
68. Lunsford LD, Bissonette DJ, Jannetta PJ et al: Anterior surgery for cervical disc disease. Part 1: Treatment of lateral cervical disc herniation in 253 cases. J Neurosurg 53:1, 1980
69. Lunsford LD, Bissonette DJ, Zorub DS: Anterior surgery for cervical disc disease. Part 2: Treatment of cervical spondylotic myelopathy in 32 cases. J Neurosurg 53:12, 1980
70. Lyons AE, Wise BL: Subarachnoid rupture of intervertebral disc fragments. J Neurosurg 18:242, 1961
71. Marshall WK, Bedford RF: Use of a pulmonary artery catheter for detection and treatment of venous air embolism: A prospective study in man. Anesthesiology 52:131, 1980
72. Mayfield FH: Complications of laminectomy. Clin Neurosurg 23:435, 1976
73. Memon MY, Scheck L: Ventral spinal tumor: The value of computed tomography in its localization. Neurosurgery 8:108, 1981
74. Meyer GA, Berman IR, Doty DB et al: Hemodynamic response to acute quadriplegia with or without chest trauma. J Neurosurg 34:168, 1971
75. Michenfelder JD, Martin JT, Altenburg BM et al: Air embolism during neurosurgery: An evaluation of right-atrial catheters for diagnosis and treatment. JAMA 208:1353, 1969
76. Mixter NI, Barr JS: Rupture of intervertebral disc with involvement of spinal canal. N Engl J Med 211:210, 1934
77. Morrison A: Hyperextension injury of the cervical spine with rupture of the esophagus. J Bone Joint Surg 42B:356, 1960
78. Munro D: Thoracic and lumbosacral cord injuries. A study of forty cases. JAMA 122:1055, 1943
79. Murphy F, Simmons JCH, Brunson B: Surgical treatment of laterally ruptured cervical disc. Review of 648 cases, 1939-1972. J Neurosurg 38:679, 1973
80. Newfield P, Albin MS, Chestnut JS, Maroon J: Air embolism during transsphenoidal pituitary operations. Neurosurgery 2:39, 1978
81. Norell H: The treatment of unstable spinal fractures and dislocation. Clin Neurosurg 25:193, 1978
82. Norell H, Wilson CB: Early anterior fusion for injuries of the cervical portion of the spine. JAMA 214:525, 1970
83. Ogilvie H: Large-intestine colic due to sympathetic deprivation: A new clinical syndrome. Br Med J 2:671, 1948
84. Onofrio BM: Intervertebral discitis: Incidence, diagnosis and management. In Clinical Neurosurgery, Chap 29, p 481. Baltimore, Williams & Wilkins, 1980
85. Patterson R: Metastatic disease of the spine: Surgical risk versus radiation therapy. Clin Neurosurg 27:641, 1980
86. Patterson RH, Arbit E: A surgical approach through the pedicle to protruded thoracic discs. J Neurosurg 49:768, 1978
87. Perese DM: Treatment of metastatic extradural spinal cord tumors. A series of 30 cases. Cancer 11:214, 1958
88. Perot PL Jr, Munro DD: Transthoracic removal of midline thoracic disc protrusions causing spinal cord compression. J Neurosurg 31:452, 1969
89. Peters ND, Ehni G: Xeroradiography in evaluation of cervical spine injuries. Technical note. J Neurosurg 49:620, 1978
90. Pool JL: Gunshot wounds of the spine: Observations from an evacuation hospital. Surg Gynecol Obstet 81:617, 1945
91. Raimondi AJ: Reflection of a laminar flap for exposure of the spinal canal in children. Clin Neurosurg 25:504, 1978
92. Ransohoff J, Spencer F, Siew F et al: Transthoracic removal of thoracic disc. Report of three cases. J Neurosurg 31:459, 1969
93. Reale F, Gambacorta R, Mencattini G: Iliac crest fracture after removal of two bone plugs for anterior cervical fusion. Case report. J Neurosurg 51:561, 1979
94. Reynolds AF Jr, Turner PA, Loeser JD: Fracture of the anterior superior iliac spine following anterior cervical fusion using iliac crest. Case report. J Neurosurg 48:809, 1978
95. Richardson RR, Cerullo LJ, Meyer PR: Autonomic hyperreflexia modulated by percutaneous epidural neurostimulation: A preliminary report. Neurosurgery 4:517, 1979
96. Ridderuold HO, Gandee RW: Diagnostic value of tomography for cervical spine injuries. Va Med 107:630, 1980
97. Rogers WA: Fractures and dislocations of the cervical spine. An end-result study. J Bone Joint Surg 39A:341, 1957
98. Schmidek HH, Gomes FB, Seligon D, McSherry JW: Management of acute unstable thoracolumbar (T 11 L1) fractures with and without neurological deficit. Neurosurgery 7:30, 1980
99. Schneider RC, Cherry G, Pantek H: The syndrome of acute central cervical cord injury with special reference to the mechanisms involved in hyperextension injuries of the cervical spine. J Neurosurg 11:546, 1954
100. Schöter L, Entzian W: Lumbar disc protrusion in childhood and adolescence. Adv Neurosurg 4:12, 1977

101. Schramm J, Oppel F, Umback W, Wüllenweber: Complications after lumbar operation on intervertebral discs: The results of a statistical survey. Nervenarzet (West Berlin) 49:26, 1978
102. Scoville WB, Dobrmann GJ, Corkill G: Late results of cervical disc surgery. J Neurosurg 45:203, 1976
103. Semmes RE: Ruptures of the Lumbar Intervertebral Disc, Their Mechanism, Diagnosis and Treatment. Springfield, IL, Charles C Thomas, 1964
104. Shenkin HA, Hash CJ: Spondylolisthesis after multiple bilateral laminectomies and facetectomies for lumbar spondylosis. Follow-up review. Neurosurgery 50:45, 1979
105. Sherk HH, Nicolson JT, Chung SMK: Fractures of the odontoid process in young children. J Bone Joint Surg 60A:921, 1978
106. Shevlin WA, Luessenhop, AJ, Fox JL, McCullough DC: Perforation of the anterior annulus during lumbar diskectomy. Case Report. J Neurosurg 38:514, 1973
107. Smith GW, Robinson RA: The treatment of certain cervical spine disorders by anterior removal of the intervertebral disc and interbody fusion. J Bone Joint Surg 40A:607, 1958
108. Smith R: An evaluation of surgical treatment for spinal cord compression due to metastatic carcinoma. J Neurol Neurosurg Psychiatry 28:152, 1965
109. Smith RV: Intradural disc rupture. Report of two cases. J Neurosurg 55:117, 1981
110. Stauffer EC, Kelley EG: Fracture dislocations of the cervical spine stability and recurrent deformity following treatment by anterior interbody fusion. J Bone Joint Surg 59A:45, 1977
111. Steudel WI, Inguinza W: The syndrome of acute central cervical spinal injury after a gunshot lesion. Case report. J Neurosurg 47:290, 1977
112. Stringer WL, Kelley DL, Johnson FR, Holliday RH: Hyperextension injury of the cervical spine with esophageal perforation. J Neurosurg 53:541, 1980
113. Sussman BJ: Fracture of the cervical spine: A critique of current management in the United States. Paraplegia 16:15, 1978
114. Tachdjian MD, Matson DB: Orthopedic aspects of intraspinal tumor of spinal cord and gliomas of the intradural portion of the filum terminale. Fate of patients who have these tumors. Arch Neurol 65:378, 1951
115. Teng P: Postoperative lumbar diskitis. Bull Los Angeles Neurol Soc 37:114, 1972
116. Tew JM, Mayfield FH: Complications of surgery of the anterior cervical spine. Clin Neurosurg 23:424, 1976
117. Torma T: Malignant tumors of the spine and the spinal extradural space: A study based on 250 histologically verified cases. Acta Chir Scand (Suppl) 225:1, 1957
118. U HS, Wilson CB: Postoperative epidural hematoma as a complication of anterior cervical disectomy. Report of three cases. J Neurosurg 49:288, 1978
119. Webb JH, Svien HJ, Kennedy RLJ: Protruded lumbar intervertebral disks in children. JAMA 154:1153, 1954
120. White WA, Patterson RH Jr, Bergland RM: Role of surgery in the treatment of spinal cord compression by metastatic neoplasm. Cancer 27:558, 1971
121. Williams RW: Microlumbar disectomy: A conservative surgical approach to the virgin herniated lumbar disc. Spine 3:175, 1978
122. Wolman L: The disturbance of circulation in traumatic paraplegia in an acute and late stage: A pathologic study. Paraplegia 2:213, 1965
123. Yashon D, Jane JA, White RJ: Prognosis and management of spinal cord and cauda equina bullet injuries in sixty-five civilians. J Neurosurg 22:163, 1970
124. Yasuoka S, Peterson HA, Laws ER, MacCarty CS: Pathogenesis and prophylaxis of postlaminectomy deformity of the spine after multiple level laminectomy: Difference between children and adults. Neurosurgery 9:145, 1981
125. Zelikovski A, Zucker G, Eliashiv A et al: A new sequential pneumatic device for the prevention of deep vein thrombosis. J Neurosurg 54:652, 1981

48 Complications of Nerve Injury and Nerve Repair

David G. Kline | Alan R. Hudson

OVERVIEW

The peripheral nervous system develops and is anatomically located in close proximity not only to muscles and their tendons but also to vessels, bones, and even lymphatics. Thus, injury to nerve is frequently complicated by injury to other important structures. In addition, attempts to repair injury to these non-neural structures can easily result in unintended nerve injury. Such occurrences are especially sad, for recovery is very genuinely limited even when these complications are readily diagnosed and repaired promptly and properly.

Errors in Diagnostic Judgment

Failure to recognize nerve injury, especially in a timely fashion, is usually the consequence of an inadequate initial neurologic examination. Such an oversight is more likely in the seriously injured patient in whom multiple and oftentimes life-threatening conditions compete for the physician's attention. Nonetheless, it is surprising how often this failure occurs when an associated nerve injury is overlooked during suturing of a simple, soft tissue wound (Fig. 48-1). A fracture or dislocation that requires immobilization or acute casting may make testing difficult but not impossible. Excessive delay in neurologic evaluation leads to late nerve repair. This may thwart successful regeneration, for with time distal end-inputs atrophy, and even if new axons reach them, functional regeneration will not occur. Students should be taught that evaluation of motor and sensory function distal even to the least complicated appearing soft tissue laceration is a must and should be done before any treatment is begun. Such examination is simple to accomplish. If there is serious nerve injury, the more distally innervated muscles will not contract, and sensory as well as autonomic loss will be present, especially in autonomous zones. With upper extremity injury, the examiner can check for function of not only the median and ulnar but also of the radial nerves by asking the patient to flex, extend, and even abduct and adduct fingers and thumb or to make a "cone" with fingers and thumb and then open up the cone. In lower extremity injury, the important distal components of the sciatic complex can be examined by asking the patient to flex and then extend his toes. Even in unconscious patients, presence or absence of beads of sweat in the autonomous zones of the fingers can be ascertained by the use of +20 lens of the ophthalmoscope. Absence implies a complete lesion, whereas sweating prevents exclusion of a partial lesion or, in the months after injury, one that is regenerating. O'Rian has also described immersing the finger or toe in warm water.[27] A normally innervated digit will wrinkle after a few minutes of immersion, while one without innervation will not.

Complications of Repair

LESIONS IN CONTINUITY

The majority of injuries to nerve—over 60% in our series—leave the nerve in gross continuity with a variable amount of internal damage. This is because most forces injuring nerves are blunt in nature with a variable amount of contusion and stretch that do not divide nerve. One of the largest sources of failure with surgical intervention is inaccurate assessment of the ability of some of these lesions to regenerate. Thus, incorrect resection of a lesion incontinuity that is predominantly axonotmetic and thus can regenerate at a rate with an efficiency greater than can be gained by resection and suture does the patient a great disservice. This is especially so with proximally located lesions in, for example, the lower trunk, medial cord and proximal ulnar nerve in the

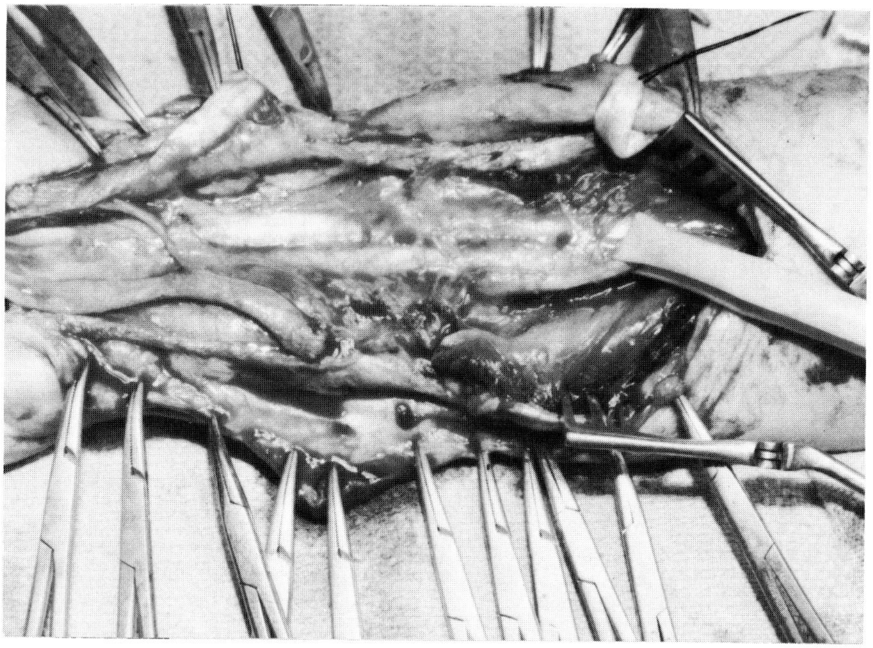

FIG. 48-1. Transected median nerve at the lower forearm level. This sharply cut nerve could have been repaired end-to-end with relative ease when the soft tissue wound was repaired primarily, had it been suspected. When explored some weeks after injury, stumps had retracted, making end-to-end suture difficult.

upper extremity, and the peroneal division of the sciatic in the lower extremity in which success with suture is small. In such lesions, proper preoperative evaluation of clinical and electromyographic completeness of the lesion as well as identification of any subsequent clinical or electrical evidence of recovery is most important. Of course, the reverse is also true, for leaving a lesion incontinuity behind in which there is little or no potential for functional regeneration is equally serious. Thus, for suspected lesions in continuity, several months' delay before exploration is advised.[13] If clinical or electrical loss does not reverse significantly, exploration is in order, and at the operating table, stimulation and recording studies can be used to prove or disprove the presence of significant regeneration.

Significant deficit persisting beyond several weeks necessitates referral to a surgeon experienced in nerve injuries. If function has not improved by several months, as shown by repetitive evaluation by clinical and electrical examinations, exploration is indicated since, if resection is necessary, results with repair will decrease dramatically after that period. Time is especially likely to play a role in nerve injuries resulting from surgical procedures. The attending surgeon may delay referral unduly, long hoping that the surgical accident will correct itself. Thus, if a motor or sensory loss is noted postoperatively, early referral should be sought and the exact details of the original procedure explained so that an early therapeutic program can be outlined.

Another common error results from evaluation of patients with multiple nerve injuries. Progressive return of function in the distribution of one nerve does not necessarily predict the fate of other nerves injured. Recovery of one nerve's function does not ensure recovery of another because the extent as well as the nature of the injuries affecting both may be greatly different.

SUTURE

Where a transected nerve or a lesion incontinuity is resected and sutured, lack of adequate regeneration is a serious complication (Fig. 48-1). This may be due to failure to resect the injury back to healthy proximal or to recognizable distal fascicular structure (Fig. 48-2).[31] This is especially so with attempted primary repair in which the longitudinal extent of the injury, except with sharp injuries, may be difficult to identify. When inadequate resection is done before suture, the damaged and scarred fascicles are reopposed. This results in a pattern of disorganized regeneration with penetrance of the distal stump by axons that stray into extrafascicular tissues. Even if they reach the intrafascicular environment, they do so with relatively poor axonal caliber and myelination secondary to more proximal repair-site branching or entrapment by scar. Of interest, the second leading cause of failure with suture is distraction at the repair site. This does not always produce frank loss of continuity but can

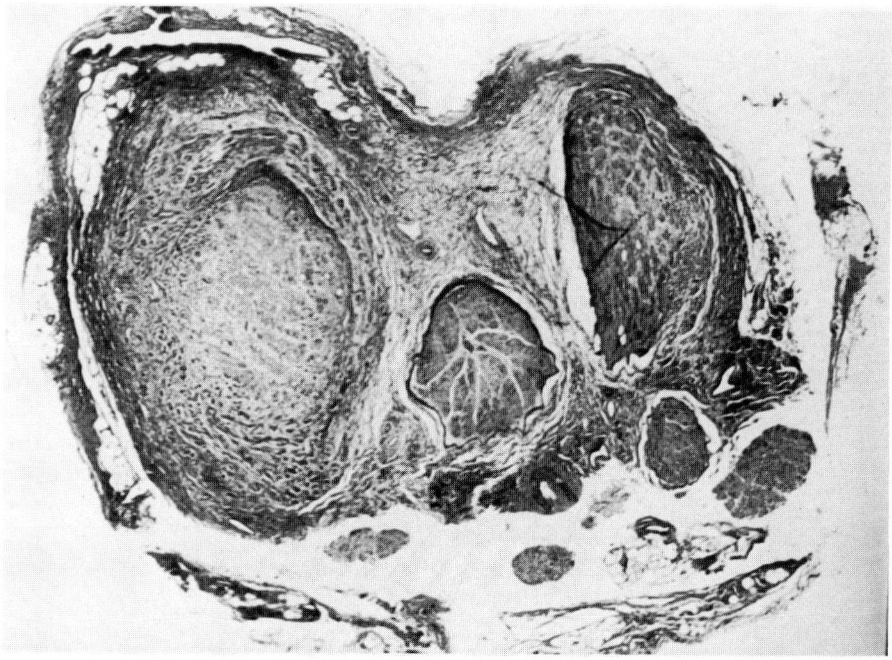

FIG. 48-2. Proximal section of a lesion in continuity. The amount of perifascicular and intrafascicular scar tissue and the lack of axonal maturity indicate the need for further proximal section. (Masson × 12).

cause separation of the proximal and distal stumps with an intervening connective tissue bridge that serves as a poor conduit for maturing axons.[34] Thus, if the surgeon trims each stump severely and persists with an end-to-end repair under undue tension, distraction may result. Fine metallic sutures as markers on the proximal and distal stump epineurium may avert this complication if radiographs of the limb are matched with the baseline or post-repair x-ray film as the limb is being extended. We do not believe that mobilization of the nerve to make up length is deleterious to successful regeneration, but this opinion is not shared by all. However, if the limb is flexed too acutely or immobilized too long, then serious secondary contractures at the joints can occur. In recent years, for this reason as well as because short interfascicular grafts do work under the proper circumstances, we mobilize the nerve ends, use mild flexion only, and apply no stretch to stumps to gain end-to-end repair under mild but not severe tension. If repair cannot be gained by these maneuvers, then transposition of the nerve can sometimes be used to make up length. If these maneuvers do not work, then we do not hesitate to use interfascicular grafts.

Despite what appears to be adequate resection of scarred nerve at the time of suture, the repair can fail. The sutured nerve then becomes a neuroma in continuity, which has to be resected and re-repaired. Availability of improved noninvasive and operative electrical methods of assessment supplements the classical inspection and palpation of the neuroma to aid in making this decision.[13] Results with re-repair, because of the lapse of additional time without distal end-organ innervation, are even more limited than with the original repair. Suture failure may be due to poor matching of fascicles or their misalignment due to unrecognized rotation of the stumps. It can also be due to the fact that fascicular topography or the position of the fascicles in relation to one another changes over the longitudinal course of the nerve.[34] Thus, even sacrifice of a few centimeters of neural tissue due to necessary resection of a neuroma in continuity or from overenthusiastic trimming of stumps of a transected nerve means that the fascicle that is at five o'clock on the proximal stump may have its distal fascicular component at seven or even nine o'clock on the distal stump, making matching difficult. This, by the way, provides a very genuine limitation to fascicular repair except for primary repair of sharp injuries to distal portions of nerve. Fascicular anatomy in distal nerve is well defined, with less of a mix of sensory and motor fibers, as well as motor fibers, to different muscle groups than occurs proximally.

MIS-SUTURE

Unfortunately, any surgeon treating a number of nerve injuries has seen nerves mistakenly sewn to tendons, since their gross appearance can be similar, especially when experience with them is limited and particularly if the procedure is done under tourniquet or with inadequate exposure and excessive bleeding. This occurs not infrequently at the forearm level where median or ulnar nerve is sewn to one of the flexor tendons (Fig. 48-3). We have also seen several examples in the lower leg where a slip of an extensor tendon has been sutured to a peroneal branch and one case where lower leg posterior tibial nerve was sutured to a flexor tendon slip. We have also found a bulbous intrapelvic femoral stump neuroma sutured to the femoral vein proximal to the inguinal ligament, while the distal stump had retracted and was adherent to external pelvic brim. Less frequent but equally devastating is misassortment of severed nerves at the level of the plexus or upper arm, where proximal stump of the median nerve has been found sewn to the distal stump of the ulnar nerve and the distal stump of the median nerve sewn to the proximal ulnar nerve.

At the plexus level, cord-to-nerve anastomoses may be readily confused, especially if heavy scarring or continuous bleeding complicates secondary operation. The likelihood of this problem is reduced with experience although with transection of the plexus, even experienced surgeons can be misled; suture of nerve ends to distal stumps of severed veins or arteries has even been seen. If the surgeon is uncertain about the macroscopic or microscopic anatomy or the extent of the pathology, skin closure is preferable to an inadequate or incomplete operation for the latter leads to confusion and uncertainty when the patient is evaluated later.

NEUROLYSIS

Failure of neurolysis, which as a procedure is usually an admission that resection of an area of injury is not necessary, is frequently due to a poor decision in favor of it.[25] This can be avoided if proper intraoperative electrical techniques are used to document the need, or lack thereof, for resection and repair. If nerve action potentials (NAPs) can be recorded through an area of injury in the early months or muscle function stimulated in the later months, then resection is not necessary, and some significant recovery will almost always occur. If the injured nerve with partial and yet significant distal sparing, or complete injury with the potential to recover because of a axonotmetic rather than a neurotmetic lesion, is handled too roughly, then the partial or axonotmetic lesion may be converted to a complete or neurotmetic lesion without any potential for significant sensory or motor recovery.

GRAFT REPAIR

There are many reasons for failure of graft repair, most of which relate to judgment over its use. Thus, a graft of the medial cord portion of the brachial plexus, or one of the lower roots or lower trunk of the plexus, seldom works, nor do those to the peroneal division of the sciatic nerve at the thigh, let alone buttock, level. Certainly, poor technique in harvesting grafts, improper preparation of the proximal and distal stumps, and poor apposition of the grafts to roots and fascicles can result in failure, as

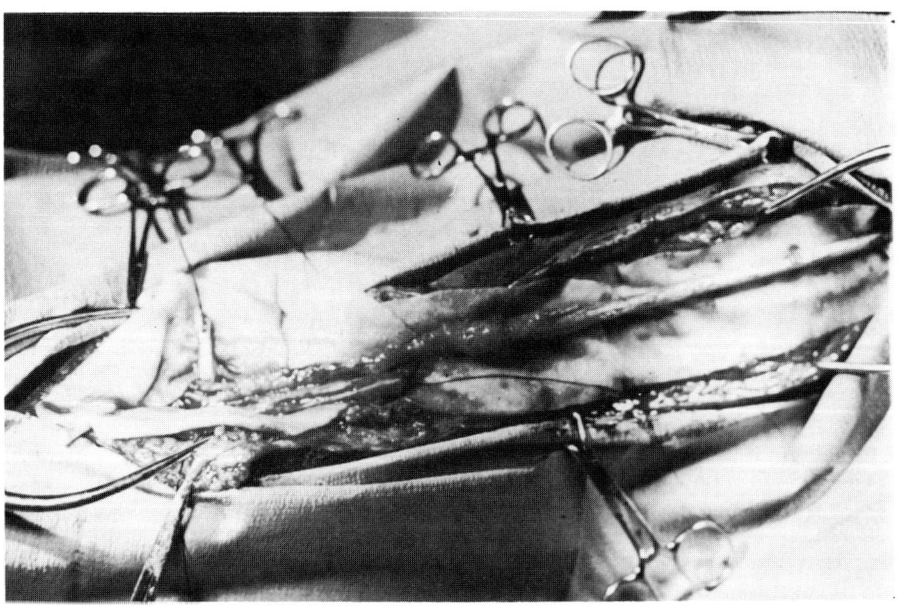

FIG. 48-3. Proximal median nerve found sutured to the distal palmaris longus at the midforearm level.

can undue expectations for regeneration through lengthy grafts, especially when used to replace proximal neural elements. Distraction should be infrequent since the primary reason that grafts are selected is for a lengthy gap that cannot be made up by careful mobilization, mild flexion of the extremity, and transposition where indicated. Nonetheless, distraction is a reported complication. To begin with, when grafts are used they should be 10% to 15% longer than the length to be covered since they tend to contract with time and thus can pull away from one or both stumps. Although the efficacy of lengthy grafts is controversial, our experience has shown that such grafts usually fail. Gaps of over 3 to 4 inches are difficult to repair successfully except for radial, musculocutaneous, and some distal tibial nerve lesions. With shorter grafts, failure can be due to excessive neuroma at either the proximal or distal stumps. This can be minimized by proper preparation of the fascicular groupings on either stump, careful placement of fine sutures under magnification, and use of a bed for the graft segment as clear of scar as possible.[19] There is some evidence that fine-caliber grafts, such as those provided by sural or antebrachial cutaneous nerves fare better than do large-caliber whole, even autologous, nerve grafts. Homologous grafts, whether irradiated or not, seem to fail; their use awaits further refinements in immunologic manipulation and tissue typing. Even autologous, fine interfascicular grafts may develop some areas of central necrosis, presumably owing to inadequate blood supply or perfusion by tissue fluids alone. Unfortunately, with some brachial plexus lesions, especially from stretch, placement of interfascicular grafts can be technically satisfactory but the procedure doomed to failure when proximal sections of root stumps show heavy scar or the presence of hundreds to thousands of ganglion cells (indicating more medial derangement, despite the apparent gross appearance of an acceptable root for anastomosis). Even when proximal input is healthy, if the surgeon overlooks a more distal or second and thus "skip" lesion, the results will be poor whether suture or graft is done.

INJURY TO ADJACENT STRUCTURES IN THE COURSE OF NERVE REPAIR

Vascular Injury

Owing to their close anatomical position to nerves, particularly in the upper extremity, vessels may not only be injured by the original lesion but inadvertently so by the surgeon. Chance of this increases greatly with a prior operation on the extremity, especially if it included a vascular repair, since the vessels as well as nerves will be encased in scar and adherent to one another. The wall of an arterial vein graft may be quite thin and readily come apart at a suture line. Needless to say, injury to major vessels such as subclavian and axillary arteries and veins should be repaired. This can usually be done by fine vascular sutures if temporary tamponade is employed. Vascular clamps may be necessary; which dictates exposure of the vessels proximal and distal to the lesion. Limb survival is more certain when flow has been lost in the brachial artery distal to the profundus branch than proximal to it, although the extremity will, in our experience, fare better with brachial artery input than without. On occasion, limbs with prior vascular damage in which extensive collateral circulation has developed may survive without ischemic symptoms despite loss of the brachial artery. Limbs with few collaterals, although surviving, will be symptomatic with use, and often these patients will have poor tolerance to cold. The decision whether or not to employ grafts and how extensive the vascular repair should be is best made by or with a surgeon with vascular experience. Nonetheless, at times an arterial injury may not need to be reconstructed. Ulnar artery is in close continuity with the ulnar nerve and can be readily injured during dissection. If direct suture does not effect repair and leakage is a significant problem, then ligation can be resorted to, providing there is a patent radial and the patient does not already suffer from arterial insufficiency in the hand.

Tendon Injury

Tendons can be inadvertently injured by the surgeon, especially in the forearm and in the distal lower extremity. With adequate exposure, this should be infrequent. On the spot repair is usually indicated just as with prior laceration or injury to large muscle bundles. Some exposures require that muscles be split or even transected. Thus, with a lateral subgluteal approach to the sciatic nerve, gluteus maximus and medius are sectioned close to their insertion on the ilium while adequate exposure of the brachial plexus may require not only transection of pectoralis minor but section of pectoralis major close to its insertion on humerus, as well as section of the clavicle. Adequate transposition and burial of the ulnar nerve includes section of pronator teres fascia and muscle as well as some of the flexor carpi ulnaris. These structures are then partially repaired after transfer of the nerve. Restoration of function to muscle or tendons either purposefully or inadvertently injured under these circumstances requires careful repair and some degree of approximation. Because of the extent of the original injury or the amount of mobilization needed to gain repair, some soft tissue wounds are lengthy and dissection of soft tissues extensive. Thus, with prior scar and much bleeding during a secondary dissection, infection of the wound is a threat. This complication can be minimized by the usual measures of thorough débridement of scar, careful hemostasis, and closure of soft tissue in multiple layers with opposition but without pressure on the underlying nerves. Careless handling of the limb while removing drapes or applying dressings also can undo the most skillfully performed neural anastomosis.

Injuries Associated With Nerve Injury

Nerve injury is frequently associated with concomitant injury to bones, tendons, and vessels or even injury to more central portions of the nervous system.[2,7] On occasion, such injuries can complicate those to the nerve itself and delay its recovery. Thus, a radial nerve injury associated with mid-humeral fracture may be complicated by envelopment of the nerve in callus, making spontaneous recovery and certainly intraoperative evaluation and repair more difficult. Peroneal nerve can also be involved with callus associated with fracture of the head of the fibula, as can the ulnar nerve in the olecranon notch. Occasionally, median and even ulnar nerve can be bound down in callus and secondary scar associated with a Monteggia fracture at mid-forearm level. An occasional consequence of fracture of the clavicle is formation of enough callus to compress the subclavicular portion of the brachial plexus, resulting in progressive and serious loss of function.[8]

It should also be remembered that soft tissue injuries can lead to swelling that will secondarily entrap nerves, especially where nerves are snugly situated. Injury to soft tissues close to the elbow can lead to cubital tunnel syndrome with ulnar entrapment. Median and ulnar nerves can be secondarily entrapped beneath the fibers of the transverse carpal ligament at the wrist and proximal level of the palmer when soft tissue swelling follows blunt trauma. Thus, dissection of and operation on the ulnar nerve close to the elbow should be accompanied by transposition of the ulnar nerve out of the cubital tunnel, while with distal ulnar or median nerve injuries, the transverse carpal ligament should be sectioned.[25]

Vascular injury can, of course, lead to clots, aneurysms, and arteriovenous fistulae, which may complicate the neural injury. The classical situation is that of an axillary artery aneurysm that compresses partially injured brachial plexus and is a cause of progressive deficit.[26] The patient often develops further deficit due to expansion of the aneurysm, which often is a pseudoaneurysm with clot (Fig. 48-4). Pain develops and usually but not always has a neuritic pattern with paresthesias, electric shocklike sensations, and sometimes a burning and even causalgiclike nature. This may be mistakenly treated by sympathetic block and even sympathectomy. Arteriography does not always resolve the issue, especially with pseudoaneurysms, for the vessel may fill smoothly past the lesion. Clots due to vas-

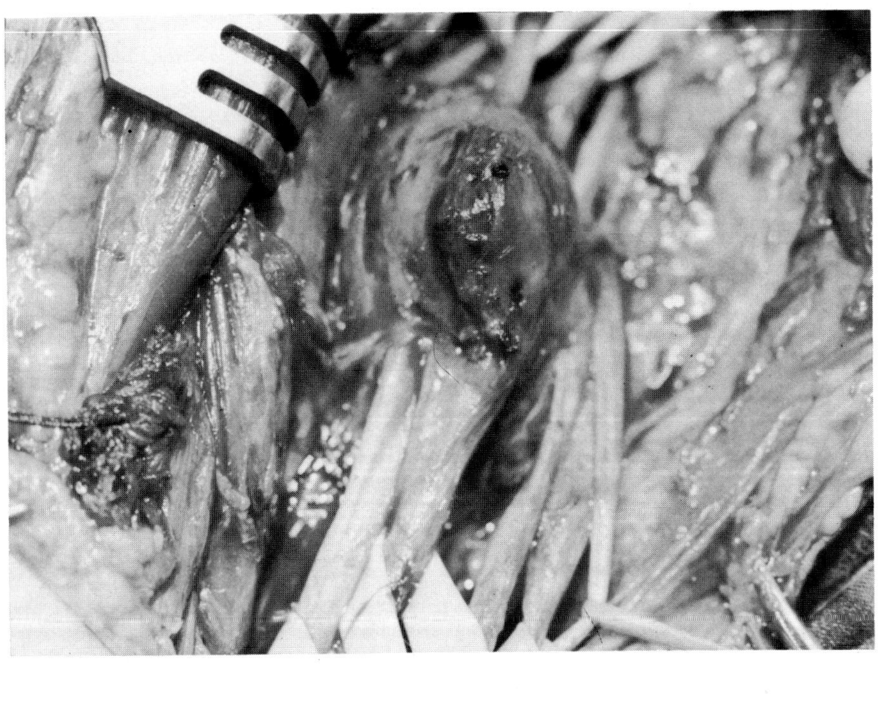

FIG. 48-4. Aneurysm of the axillary artery secondary to a gunshot wound compresses the lateral and medial cord contributions to the median nerve, as well as the posterior cord and radial nerve.

cular injury, particularly in the subgluteal, occasionally popliteal, and less frequently, subpectoral regions can acutely compress nerves and result in rapid and progressive loss of function. Expeditious surgical evacuation is indicated. This is not true of most retroperitoneal bleeding secondary to anticoagulation or trauma in which the pelvic plexus is involved. Here, expectant treatment usually but not always leads to reversal of lower extremity neural loss.[5] We have had experience with several arteriovenous fistulae associated with sharp injury to an extremity involving a nerve. These resulted in expansion of the size of the extremity as well as a thrill or bruit on auscultation, which was dampened by compressing the major feeding artery proximally (Fig. 48-5). Removal requires not only isolation of the feeding and draining vessels but a thorough exposure of the nerves involved. Occasionally, a venous aneurysm may complicate the injury and may invest or envelop the nerve. Although rare, we have had experience with venous aneurysms involving the posterior tibial and the median nerve in two patients who had been operated on unsuccessfully elsewhere. In both cases, neural symptoms became more evident with a dependent position of the extremity. Nerves had to be dissected over a length and epineurium opened in order to obliterate feeding vessels.

Unless proximal vascular injury is corrected, ischemia severe enough to result in loss of the limb is possible, as is death from hypovolemic shock. The latter can all too readily occur in conjunction with a brachial plexus injury in which major proximal vessels such as the subclavian artery or vein are avulsed or transected, as well as a femoral triangle injury in which the femoral artery or vein is involved.

Brachial plexus injury is not infrequently associated with bony injury involving ribs, clavicle, scapula, head of humerus, and cervical spine fractures, especially those of the transverse processes. Hemopneumothorax and, less frequently, lymphatic duct injury have been seen. We have seen patients who, along with their cervical spine fracture or dislocation, have had plexus injury as well as quadriplegia. In one nonquadriplegic patient with a severe plexus injury on the right, radicular pain developed on the left, and an acute cervical disc was found on myelography, as well as meningoceles, suggesting root avulsion on the right. Removal of the disc through an anterior approach helped the left-sided pain, but nothing substantial could be done for the right upper extremity paralysis. Plexus and head injury are obviously associated since the blow leading to unconsciousness and, in some cases, less reversible brain injury, may also distort the neck and shoulder enough to result in a stretch or avulsive injury to the plexus.

Two special categories of injury that can lead to neural loss, whether or not there was any to begin with, are *Volkmann's ischemic contracture* and the anterior *compartment syndrome.* Dislocation of the elbow with or without supracondylar fracture or even extensive soft tissue damage at the level of the elbow and volar forearm can result in direct injury or spasm to the brachial artery and secondary infarction of forearm musculature. Owing to swelling in this confined space, median and ulnar nerve and even the posterior interosseous branch of the radial nerve can be compressed and suffer ischemic damage. Immediate and extensive fasciotomy is necessary; we favor neurolysis of the nerves.[25] Delayed exploration exposes scarred and ischemic muscle and nerve but at a less reversible time, emphasizing the need for acute management.[6] We have seen several cases of forearm swelling, both with and without

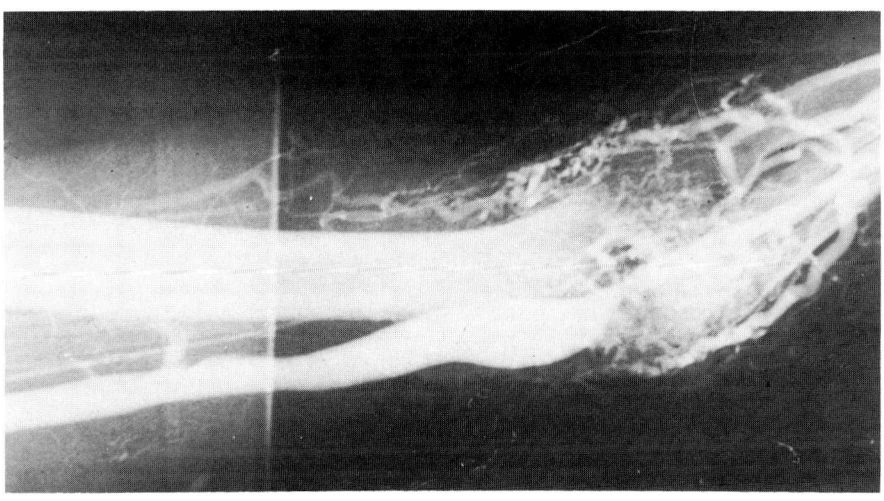

FIG. 48-5. Arteriovenous fistula at the level of the elbow involving brachial artery due to a stab wound. Both the median and ulnar nerves were secondarily involved by this lesion.

hematoma, from pool cue, baseball bat, and "billy club" injury to the forearm, requiring immediate fasciotomy and early neurolysis. These injuries were not associated with vascular or bony injury, but acute swelling in this relatively confined space threatened the nerves and necessitated the same treatment warranted by early Volkmann's contracture. Anterior compartment compression syndrome is secondary to contusive injury with or without fracture involving the lower extremity. Unless early fasciotomy is done, compression and vascular compromise can lead not only to irreversible infarction of soft tissues but also to severe damage to peroneal nerve branches, resulting in footdrop.[22, 39]

Complications to Nerves Resulting From Other Operative or Medical Procedures

NECK LEVEL

Laryngeal Nerve Injury

Close anatomical disposition of structures within the neck predisposes them to injury with surgery.[36] Palsy of the recurrent laryngeal nerve leading to hoarseness and loss of normal phonation can occur in conjunction with thyroidectomy, tracheostomy, anterior cervical decompression and fusion, and radical neck dissection as well as other less common procedures. As a branch of the 10th cranial nerve, the recurrent laryngeal leaves the carotid sheath in the lower neck and on the right courses around subclavian artery except when the latter arises directly from the aortic arch. On the left, the recurrent branch winds around the arch of the aorta. Nerves on both sides travel adjacent and somewhat between the trachea and esophagus to reach the criocoarytenoid muscles in the larynx. Owing to the nerve's position, close to the midline, it can be injured by traction or can actually be divided during the course of surgical dissection. Some hope for restoration of function through direct suture or graft has been provided by Miehlke and others.[18] Various muscle transplants have been tried experimentally for irreparable laryngeal palsy but have not been applied clinically to our knowledge.

Accessory Nerve Injury

Accessory nerve can be easily injured in conjunction with various neck dissections, especially since it takes a somewhat transverse course in the posterior triangle, whereas the other important structures to be spared take a more vertical or semioblique course.[40] Of the 16 accessory palsies we have seen, most required operation because there was no clinical or electromyographic evidence of trapezius reinnervation. Each case was secondary to operative injury due to biopsy or attempted removal of lymph nodes or some other relatively small mass located either in the anterior or posterior triangle of the neck. It is true that some of these lesions spare the more medial trapezius musculature, but most paralyze the entire muscle. It is rare, even with proximally located lesions, for the sternocleidomastoid to be paralyzed since in addition to its very proximal accessory input, it usually receives twigs from cervical roots, C2, C3, and even C4. In one case we operated on, the initial surgeon had taken a lymph node biopsy and had had it reported on frozen section examination as a malignant lesion. As a result, a modified radical neck dissection was done through the original, small neck incision used to biopsy the node. A severe lesion incontinuity to the accessory nerve resulted and required resection and repair since an NAP could not be evoked through it (Fig. 48-6). In another instance, lymph node biopsy resulted in a lesion incontinuity that had a small NAP when operated upon 3 months after the injury. This led to a split procedure in which a portion of the accessory nerve was replaced with an auricular nerve graft and the rest received a neurolysis. In the remaining cases, nerve had been either totally transected or severely enough contused that suture was necessary. One patient had also experienced pain and paresthesias in the forearm and hand, and at the time the accessory nerve was repaired, a substantial amount of scar was found enveloping the upper roots and truncal elements of the plexus. Node biopsy should be done through an adequate incision with good lighting and assistance. Linear structures suggestive of nerve should be identified by a stimulator.

Hypoglossal Nerve Injury

Hypoglossal nerve may be inadvertently injured in the course of neck dissection, particularly for carotid endarterectomy. This, of course, leads to paralysis and atrophy of the genioglossus muscle on the side of the lesion. Thus, with the tongue at rest, it will tend to deviate away from the side of the lesion and with protrusion toward the side of the lesion. Hypoglossal paralysis has serious consequences because speech can be affected as well as food handling. Suture repair can lead to recovery and is best done acutely if it is recognized that the nerve has been sharply divided. Contusive or stretch injury due to retraction may require a period of observation. Tongue musculature can be sampled by electromyography, although this is painful for some patients. If no clinical nor electrical recovery occurs in 3 months, then exploration, direct recordings, and either a neurolysis or resection and suture of the nerve is done.

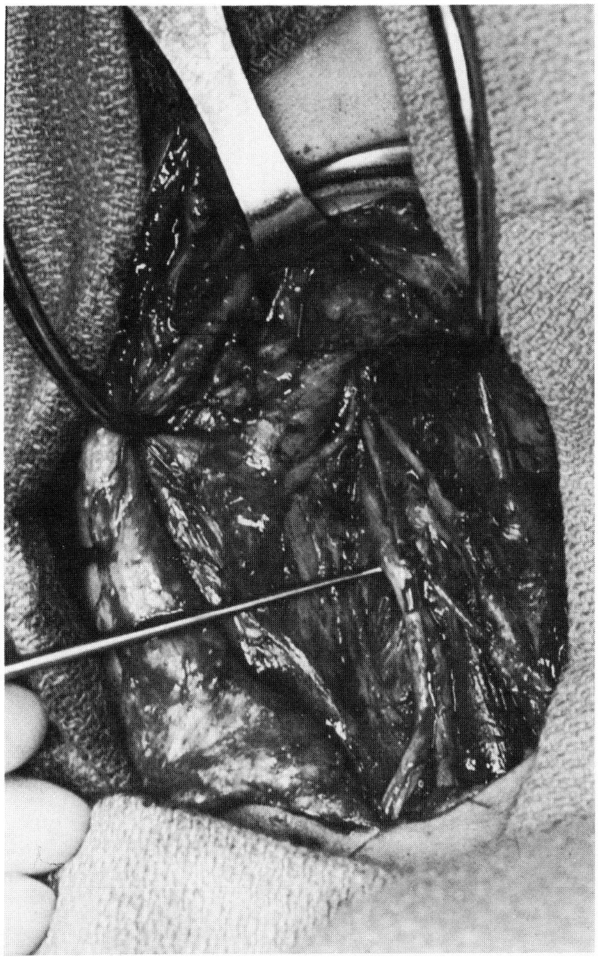

FIG. 48-6. Instrument points to a lesion in continuity involving the accessory nerve. The injury was sustained as a result of a lymph-node biopsy. An NAP could not be evoked through this lesion a number of months after injury, so resection and repair was necessary.

Other Cranial Nerve Injuries

Although injury to each cranial nerve is possible with many head and neck procedures, facial palsy as a result of parotid surgery and lingual palsy or lingual distribution paresthesias after dental blocks or extraction pose special problems in correction.[30] This makes avoidance of the complication all the more important.

Brachial Plexus Injury

Brachial plexus injury can result from a variety of surgical procedures on the neck, shoulder, and chest. A neuropraxic or even more severe injury can be secondary to axillary compression caused by an assistant wedged into the armpit area at chest or abdominal surgery. Either poor positioning of the shoulders or pulling them downward and backward by tape can lead to stretch injury of the plexus. Most, but unfortunately not all, of these positional or compressive palsies will reverse with time. Direct operative inspection, recordings, and even repair may be necessary. We follow these cases for at least 4 months before recommending exploration.

More direct injury to the plexus may result from a variety of operative procedures. Unfortunately, some of these procedures are done in an attempt to relieve pain thought to be of plexus origin. A not uncommon example is transaxillary resection of the first rib for presumed thoracic outlet syndrome. From a neurosurgeon's viewpoint, true thoracic outlet syndrome is a diagnosis of exclusion. Cervical disc disease, cervical spondylosis, or more peripheral entrapment of ulnar nerve at elbow or median or ulnar nerve at wrist can mimic some of the findings and most of the symptoms of this syndrome. There are no clinical findings in our experience that are specific for the diagnosis. Adson's sign can be present without the syndrome or supraclavicular and infraclavicular tenderness, or a Tinel's sign on tapping in the supraclavicular space or around the shoulder can occur due to other disorders. Lower root or trunk or ulnar distribution motor or sensory change can be difficult to localize to a specific level. Disappointing is the fact that conduction studies across the clavicle are not more diagnostic, but this is because of the need to stimulate supraclavicularly and to record from a more distal musculature or nerve. Since nerves are at a depth in the supraclavicular area and are covered by a variable amount of soft tissue, precise stimulation at an accountable locus is difficult to obtain, making calculation of distance and velocity measurements between stimulus and recording sites imprecise.

During first rib resection, particularly from the transaxillary approach, the plexus is not well visualized. Although it is usually protected by gentle retraction, it can nonetheless be injured. Some of the injuries due to retraction and milder degrees of stretch will recover with time but others (four in our series of plexus injuries) have partial division or contusion and stretch of the plexus and have required resection and repair. Since the damage was to lower roots and trunk, recovery has been poor. It would appear that the complication is most likely when an attempt is made to resect the posterior third of the rib by a transaxillary or infraclavicular approach. Unfortunately, in our experience, it is just this portion of the first rib and the attached scalene muscles that are responsible for the type of entrapment that constitutes true thoracic outlet syndrome. These structures are not well visualized by a transaxillary approach. As a result, one of us favors the posterior subscapular approach to the plexus for thoracic outlet syndrome. Here the posterior third of the rib as well as its middle third can be removed readily, as can the scalene muscles. Roots close to their exit from the intervertebral foramina can be traced down to trunks with ease and subclavian artery and vein readily protected since they lie inferior to the lower trunk of the plexus.

Median sternotomy can also injure the plexus by fracture of the first or second rib articulation with the thoracic transverse processes. If the rib retractors are placed too close to the manubrium and opened too widely, a posteriorly deflected rib fracture can impinge on the lower elements of the plexus. Thus, plexus palsy has been reported after cardiopulmonary bypass as well as other cardiac procedures. This needs to be considered in the postoperative differential diagnosis along with more straightforward compression of the plexus due to poor positioning of the patient or the surgeon and his assistants.[33]

Sympathectomy when done either by the transaxillary or supraclavicular route can lead to plexus injury. Other complications associated with this procedure include pneumothorax, Horner's syndrome (often the price for an effective and thus cephalad enough sympathectomy), and postsympathectomy neuralgia, an ill-defined but bothersome complication.[11] The surgeon must be careful to differentiate stellate ganglion from the first thoracic root and not mistake the latter for a ramus communicans and section it.

SHOULDER LEVEL

A variety of injuries to plexus can occur secondary not only to a shoulder injury but also to operations on the shoulder.[1, 15] Contusion and stretch due to inadvertent or excessive retraction during reconstruction of the shoulder capsule can occur as can entrapment or even division of a portion of plexus during a Putti Platt procedure to correct recurrent dislocation of the shoulder. In one case, the posterior cord of the plexus at the level of the profundus branch of the axillary artery had a suture through it. With removal of the suture 4 months later and neurolysis of the cord, recovery eventually occurred. NAP recording had shown early regeneration through the injury site. Vascular bypass or repair at the shoulder level can also lead to plexus injury. We have had patients with complicating plexus injuries following bypass from carotid to axillary artery as well as one complicating an axillary to axillary artery bypass from the right side to the left side.

Radical Mastectomy

Axillary dissection during radical mastectomy resulted in three completely paralyzed extremities we saw.[13] In one instance, the complication was not initially recognized by the surgeon and when first identified was mistakenly thought to be improving, resulting in late referral. All plexus elements had been transected, had with time retracted, and required grafts 3 or more inches in length to make up the deficit, with an anticipated poor outcome. In another instance, the complication was recognized, but a delay in referral for secondary repair led to a less than optimal result, once again because of the necessity of using grafts of some length. In the third case, the surgeon recognized that plexus had been transected when it happened, called for help, and a primary end-to-end repair was done with eventual excellent results for a plexus level lesion. Thus, when plexus or any nerve is transected surgically, acute repair is preferable unless the transecting injury is blunt. When the injury is blunt, stumps can be tacked down to adjacent fascial planes so that secondary exploration will provide nerve ends that can be brought together without undue tension or need for grafts. Injuries recognized as due to contusion or stretch are best left alone acutely, followed carefully, both clinically and electrically, and reexplored for intraoperative stimulation and recording studies at 3 to 4 months, if regeneration is not evident.

Radiation Plexitis

Another unfortunate iatrogenic cause of progressive plexus palsy is radiation damage. This is usually associated with x-ray therapy following radical mastectomy for breast carcinoma, but it has also been seen with irradiation for Hodgkin's disease and pulmonary tumors.[14] There is usually an interval of several years between the course of radiation and onset of symptoms. Skin changes, including hyperpigmentation, telangiectasia, and ruborous or thickened skin, may or may not be present. The extent of neural involvement may be from roots down to nerves of upper arm.[17] Painful paresthesias may be part of the problem. Pathologically, heavy scar envelops the nerve, but vascularization of the nerves themselves is often poor. After removal of the extraneural scar, the nerves have a yellowed and somewhat atrophic appearance consistent with direct intraneural irradiation damage. In addition to overdosage and failure to utilize multiple ports, idiosyncratic reaction may in some patients be causative.[29] Of great interest, most but not all of the patients seen by us who have had a radiation neuropathy due to treatment for breast cancer have been cured of their primary disease.[37] Plexus radiation neuropathy has also been seen as a consequence of treatment of hidradenitis of the axillary region and of soft tissue tumors and angiomas of the upper arm.

Unfortunately, operative decompression by first

rib resection and neurolysis of the plexus either with or without axillary dissection as a secondary procedure does not always help. The neurologic deficit was increased in several of our eight cases treated by operative decompression, even though pain and paresthesias were improved.

Neural Tumors

Another neural cause of plexus palsy or neural loss at any level is en bloc resection of a tumor arising from or involving nerve. This complication is especially devastating when the tumor has involved a proximal neural element, but we have seen this at almost every level. Many of these tumors were schwannomas and neurofibromas, most of which can be removed without destroying the total cross section of the nerve with proper microscopic and electrical monitoring techniques (Fig. 48-7). Repairs of the deficits following en bloc resection have almost invariably required the use of lengthy grafts with limited recovery of function. Biopsy without dissection of fascicles or fibers away from the bulk of the nerve can be equally deleterious.

ARM AND FOREARM LEVEL

Involvement of nerves secondary to fracture or callus formation has been mentioned previously, as has Volkmann's ischemic contracture. Either the radial nerve at the mid-humeral level or the posterior interosseous branch at the level of the volar supinator can be entrapped by manipulation of fractures, particularly in an operative fashion with the use of plates and screws. Nerve can also be compressed if the limb is casted before swelling has had a chance to resolve. Unfortunately, some operations for tennis elbow may also result in injury to the radial nerve. Posterior interosseous nerve palsy presents as a rather striking and diagnostic palsy restricted to the motor portion of the nerve; the superficial sensory branch leaves the radial nerve close to the level of the elbow itself. Wrist dorsiflexion is usually present but decreased in strength with a tendency for the wrist to deviate radially. This is because the branch to the extensor carpi radialis either leaves the radial nerve at a site proximal to the posterior interosseous nerve or more frequently the nerve travels a short distance with the superficial sensory nerve, then leaves it, and enters the extensor carpi radialis. However, the extensor carpi ulnaris fascicle leaves the posterior interosseous nerve more distally. Supination may or may not be decreased. Extensor communis and extensor pollicis longus function is absent so there is an inability to extend fingers or thumb. Decompression, not only dividing the volar head of the supinator but also tracing the posterior interosseous nerve through to the dorsum of the forearm, is necessary. With more severe injury associated with plating of the radius, a segment of the nerve has to be removed, and either direct suture or, more likely, graft repair done, using the superficial sensory branch that supplies sensation to a surprisingly small portion of the dorsum of the hand.

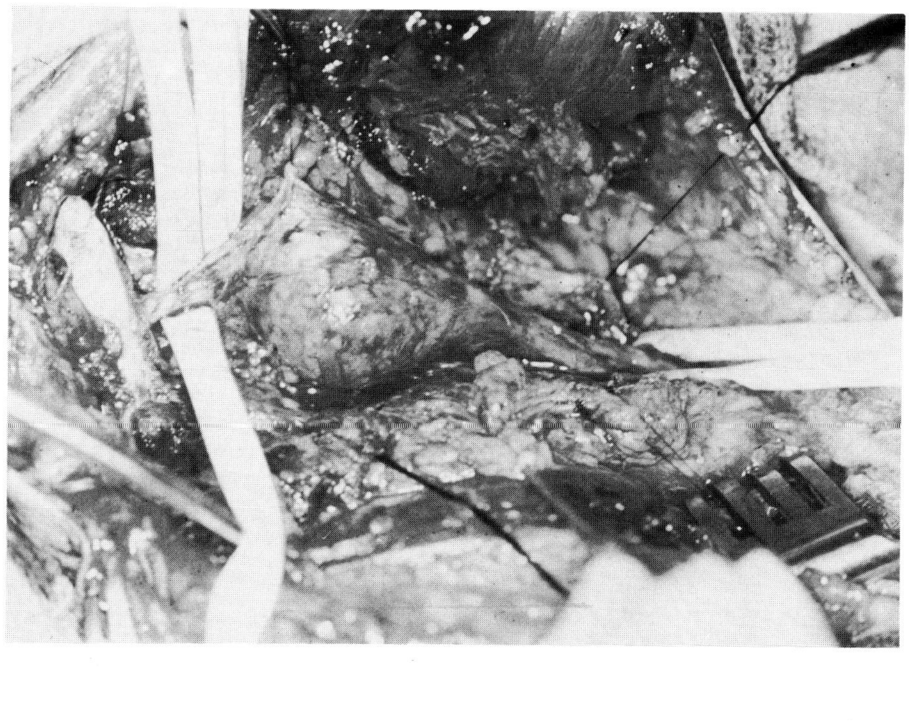

FIG. 48-7. Typical appearance of a neurofibroma involving an upper element of the plexus.

Repair of laceration of the superficial sensory nerve in the lower forearm or at wrist level due to excision of a ganglion can lead to a painful neuroma with especially bothersome paresthesias over the dorsum of the wrist and hand. Resection of the nerve is preferable, just as it is for sural nerve injuries. Resection is especially indicated when a soft tissue wound with an overlooked superficial sensory radial or sural nerve injury leads to a proximal stump neuroma. A variety of complications to median or ulnar nerve can occur as a result of ill-advised or improperly performed operations for carpal tunnel syndrome or tardy ulnar palsy. In addition to a deficit, extremely bothersome paresthesias may result. Poorly placed, short incisions leading to inadequate division of offending structures and an incomplete neurolysis are often causative.

LEG LEVEL

Lumbosacral Plexus Injury

Some of the most serious neural complications imaginable can be associated with retroperitoneal or pelvic operations. Thus, resection of retroperitoneal masses can be complicated by upper lumbosacral plexus loss with paralysis of psoas, iliopsoas, and quadriceps muscles. This complication occurs not infrequently when the retroperitoneal mass has been either a neurofibroma or a schwannoma with origin in upper lumbar roots with or without intraspinal involvement. These benign tumors are mistaken for a carcinoma or some other type of retroperitoneal mass, and en bloc resection is done by removing a portion of the lumbosacral plexus. Repair even by grafts is usually impossible because the injury extends to and often through the intervertebral level of the roots. The situation is analogous to that of a severe stretch injury to the brachial plexus in which technically grafts can be inserted but without enough healthy proximal root outflow to which to attach them. Lower pelvic plexus palsy includes loss in the distribution of the sciatic nerve and has resulted from pelvic tumor removal. This complication is occasionally seen with aortofemoral or iliofemoral bypass procedures as well. In one case, severe bleeding could only be controlled with difficulty, and the pelvis had to be packed leading to a nonoperable and largely irreversible pelvic plexus palsy.

Femoral Nerve Injury

Femoral triangle exposure, particularly for vascular repair, can be complicated by nerve injury. At this level, injury due to bypass or, on rare occasions, a high saphenous stripping and ligation can also occur.[3] Neural repair is difficult because an inch or so distal to the ilioinguinal ligament the nerve branches many times to form a pes of motor and sensory nerves going to various segments of the quadriceps and to sensory areas over the anterolateral thigh. Reconstruction requires grafts, making the outcome less certain.

Ilioinguinal and Genitofemoral Injury

One of the most vexing neural complications in surgery is injury to ilioinguinal or genitofemoral nerves associated with herniorrhaphy. Pain and paresthesias in the groin, scrotum, medial upper thigh, and even the penis result. Repair of these neural injuries is almost always impossible because normal anatomical planes are lost and scar is present. When the nerves are located, they are usually found to be injured over a length, making repair difficult. Neurolysis has been worthwhile in the few instances in which a suture went through or around a nerve or in which they were entrapped by tightly, restructured fascial planes. Unfortunately, the more usual case is that of injury and damage over a length of the nerve. The uncertainty surrounding the type of sensory regeneration gained through a suture or a graft to these nerves makes resection preferable to repair because imprecise sensory regeneration may lead to as much or more pain and paresthesias.

Sciatic Palsy due to Hip Surgery

Iatrogenic sciatic injury is not infrequently associated with management of dislocation of fractures of the hip and pelvis, even when not associated with the original injury.[28] Palsy is most likely to occur when open manipulation of the fracture or dislocation is required.[23, 38] The sciatic nerve is in close approximation to the posterior hip joint after it leaves the sciatic notch and thus can be adherent to injured capsule and muscles around the notch, as well as to bone fragments. This makes secondary injury difficult to avoid even for the surgeon with great experience with hip reconstruction. With the advent of hip replacement and especially the use of acrylates, the nerve may be found embedded in or even compressed by broken pieces of this material.[4] Since acrylate sets by an exothermic reaction, damage to the nerve can occur by heat, although more frequently the nerve is directly traumatized as well as encompassed by acrylate. Only a few of these injuries are reversible by reoperation.[10, 32] Sciatic repair at such a proximal level is difficult for a number of reasons. First and foremost, neural injury frequently extends proximal to the sciatic notch and involves the intrapelvic portion of the neural complex. Second, damage is usually extensive and over a length of the nerve, requiring replacement by grafts, a procedure of questionable value at this level, particularly for the peroneal portion of the nerve. In addition, the associated orthopaedic injury that led to the complication makes rehabilitation of the limb with neural damage difficult. Weight bearing is important, and this may be delayed by the hip or pelvic fractures and dislocation. It is sad to have to present this issue in such a negative light, but results with reconstruction of the sciatic nerve at this level for these complications are poor.

At the level of the knee, either tibial or peroneal nerves can be damaged by other operative procedures. Although rare, puncture of the posterior knee capsule by an arthroscope can injure popliteal artery and vein as well as nerves. This complication has been seen by one of us in a patient with total sciatic palsy. Some damage was due to the immediate complication of compression of the nerves by hematoma, but some was due to emergency surgery necessary to secure and repair vessels. Much more common is injury to the peroneal nerve in and around the head of the fibula—an area where the nerve is angulated, tethered, and naturally tight as it courses around the head of the fibula. Although a few months of conservative management is probably in order if gross continuity and not transection is suspected, exploration, electrical recordings, and repair, if so indicated, should not be delayed too long.[12] Unfortunately, results with repair are not satisfactory, making it very important to protect the nerve in any surgical procedure about the knee. Unfortunately, when peroneal palsy occurs and the surgeon explores the nerve, he often falsely selects neurolysis because some degree of continuity is found. Then he follows the patient for another period, hoping that the recovery not destined to come about will nonetheless occur. It is especially important, if a peroneal palsy following knee surgery is to be explored, to be able both to stimulate and to record from the nerve, to prove or deny the presence of meaningful regeneration. Neurolysis alone may not suffice even when this iatrogenic injury does not appear that serious upon inspection and palpation. An uncommon but devastating cause of sciatic or other peripheral nerve palsy is damage due to use of an implantable stimulator for pain. When a deficit is added to a painful disorder, the pain usually takes on even greater importance.[16, 21, 24, 35]

Injection Injury

Two common sites for injection injury are the buttock level for the sciatic nerve and the lower lateral arm or mid-humeral level for the radial nerve. Venipuncture or brachial or axillary artery catheterization may also be responsible for a painful palsy.[20]

Sciatic nerve palsy may occur even if the upper outer quadrant is selected as the site for injection, especially if the patient is thin or cachectic, if the needle is too long, or if it is inserted with sufficient force to depress or indent the soft tissues, reducing the distance between the tip of the needle to the nerve to less than that for puncture without compression. Whether or not placement adjacent to the nerve without puncture of the nerve can result in damage is uncertain. Certainly, the majority of cases appear to be due to direct puncture and deposition of the medication in the nerve, but a small percentage of patients develop injection palsy, especially to the sciatic nerve, with substantially delayed onset of symptoms, as well as sciatic loss. The usual pattern is that of pain and paresthesias, often radicular in nature, upon insertion of the needle and then recrudescence of these symptoms and rather abrupt onset of palsy upon deposition of the medication. If seen immediately and if the deficit is severe, then surgical exposure of the nerve and irrigation with saline can be tried, but this has not been documented because both diagnosis and referral are almost always delayed. Pain often requires management by more than just commonly used analgesics. Tegretol and Elavil are frequently required and less often sympathetic blocks or sympathectomy. Weight bearing with early use of a spring-loaded kick-up foot brace may be necessary because, unfortunately, the peroneal division is often preferentially injured. Both divisions may be initially involved, but fortunately the tibial division frequently recovers spontaneously. As with other diseases, the severity of injury ranges from very mild but very painful to very severe with total sciatic loss but little pain. If the loss is complete to one or both divisions and recovery is not evident in 4 months, then exploration and electrical recordings are indicated. If no NAPs to one or both divisions are found, resection and repair are indicated. Not all injection palsies recover spontaneously as was originally thought. Unfortunately, recovery with suture repair at such a proximal level does not always occur, especially with resection and repair of the peroneal division. Usually the tibial division receives the neurolysis, and the peroneal is repaired after recordings have sorted out the severity of the damage, but in the reverse case, results are more encouraging.[12] Fortunately, the majority of the injection injuries to sciatic nerve can be managed conservatively since loss in the distribution of both divisions is partial and some degree of recovery can be expected.

If a child jerks an arm away or upward at the right moment, injection in the deltoid region can be delivered too distally in the arm and strike the radial nerve as it runs between biceps, brachialis, and triceps or as it courses through the humerus. Radial palsy has even been seen with an automatic pressure injection deposition of a DPT shot. If the radial palsy is complete, which is most often the case, then exploration after a few months will be necessary. Most but not all radial nerve injection injuries leading to complete distal loss will require resection at the injection site and suture. Unlike the sciatic nerve, results with suture or graft repair even at a proximal level are satisfactory.

ANKLE LEVEL

Management of fractures or ligamentous tears about the ankle can be complicated by posterior tibial injury, particularly when collateral ligaments are too tightly approximated or reduction is done without proper protection of this nerve. Inadequate release of the tarsal tunnel or contusion during this procedure can lead to a serious and painful distal palsy. In these cases, exploration, recordings, and repair may be necessary.

References

1. Artz T, Huffer JM: A major complication of the modified Bristow procedure for recurrent dislocation of the shoulder. J Bone Joint Surg 54A:1293, 1972
2. Brynes D, Russo GL, Ducker TB, Cowley RA: Sacrum fractures and neurological damage. J Neurosurg 47:459, 1977
3. Cox SJ: Saphenous nerve injury caused by stripping of long saphenous vein. Br Med J 1:415, 1974
4. Edwards M, Barbaro N, Murray W: Delayed sciatic palsey after total hip replacement. Neurosurgery 9:61, 1981
5. Gilden DH, Eisner J: Lumbar plexopathy caused by disseminated intravascular coagulation. JAMA 237:2844, 1977
6. Goldner JL: Volkmann's ischemic contracture. In Flynn JE (ed): Hand Surgery, 2nd ed. Baltimore, Williams & Wilkins, 1975
7. Harris WR: Avulsion of lumbar roots complicating fracture of the pelvis. J Bone Joint Surg 55A:1436, 1973
8. Howard FM, Shafer SJ: Injuries to the clavicle with neurovascular complications. A study of 14 cases. J Bone Joint Surg 47A:1335, 1965
9. Hudson A, Kline D, Gentili F: Peripheral nerve injection injury. In Omer GE, Spinner M (eds): Management of Peripheral Nerve Problems. Philadelphia, WB Saunders, 1980
10. Johnson EW: Nerve injuries in fractures to the lower extremity. Minn Med 52:627, 1969
11. Kleinert H, Norberg H, McDonough J: Surgical sympathectomy—upper and lower extremity. In Omer GE, Spinner M (eds): Management of Peripheral Nerve Problems. Philadelphia, WB Saunders, 1980
12. Kline DG: Operative experience with major lower extremity lower lesions, including the lumbosacral plexus and the sciatic nerve. In Omer GE, Spinner M (eds): Management of Peripheral Nerve Problems. Philadelphia, WB Saunders, 1980
13. Kline DG, Hackett E: Reappraisal of timing for exploration of civilian peripheral nerve injuries. Surgery 78:54, 1975
14. Kori SH, Foley KM, Posner JB: Brachial plexus lesions in patients with cancer. Clinical findings in 100 cases (abstr). Neurology 29:583, 1970
15. Lohrhan PH: Isolated paralysis of the serratis magnus following surgical procedures. Report of a case. Ann Surg 54:656, 1947
16. Long DL: Electrical stimulation for relief of pain from chronic nerve injury. J Neurosurg 39:718, 1973
17. Match RM: Radiation induced brachial plexus paralysis. Arch Surg 110:384, 1975
18. Miehlke A: Functional rehabilitation of laryngoparalysis through vagus-recurrent nerve anastomosis. In Clinical Microneurosurgery, pp 253-272. Stuttgart, George Thieme Verlag, 1976
19. Millesi H, Meissl G, Berger A: Further experience with interfascicular grafting of the median, ulnar and radial nerves. J Bone Joint Surg 58A:209, 1976
20. Molnar W, Paul DJ: Complications of axillary arteriotomies. An analysis of 1,762 consecutive studies. Radiology 104:269, 1972
21. Nashold BS, Goldner BS, Bright DS: Electrical stimulation of peripheral nerves with micro-electrical implants for pain relief. In Omer GE, Spinner M (eds): Management of Peripheral Nerve Problems. Philadelphia, WB Saunders, 1980
22. Nghiem D, Boland J: Four-compartment fasciotomy of the lower extremity without fibulectomy: A new approach. Am Surg 46:414, 1980
23. Nicoll EA: The management of dislocations of the hip associated with fractures of the acetabulum. J Bone Joint Surg 35B:147, 1953
24. Nielson KD, Watts C, Clark WK: Peripheral nerve injury from implantation of chronic stimulating electrodes for pain control. Surg Neurol 5:51, 1976
25. Nulsen F, Kline DG: Acute injuries of peripheral nerves. In Youmans JR (ed): Neurological Surgery, vol 2, p 1089. Philadelphia, WB Saunders, 1973
26. Nulsen FE, Slade HW: Recovery following injury to the brachial plexus. In Woodhall B, Beebe G (eds): Peripheral Nerve Regeneration: A Follow-up Study of 3656 WW II Injuries. Washington, DC, US Government Printing Office, 1956
27. O'Rian S: New and simple test of nerve function in the hand. Br Med J 3:615, 1973
28. Patterson EP: Neurological complications of fractures and dislocations of the pelvis. J Trauma 12:1013, 1972
29. Salmer A, Botrickle A, Herzoq KG et al: Reversible brachial plexopathy secondary to irridation. Cancer Treat Rep 65:797, 1981
30. Samii M: Nerves of the head and neck. In Omer GE, Spinner M (eds): Management of Peripheral Nerve Problems. Philadelphia, WB Saunders, 1980
31. Seddon H: Surgical Disorders of the Peripheral Nerves, 2nd ed. New York, Churchill Livingstone, 1975
32. Spiegel PG: Complete sciatic nerve laceration in closed femoral shaft fracture. J Trauma 14:617, 1974
33. Stephens JW: Neurological sequelae of congenital heart surgery. Arch Neurol 7:450, 1962
34. Sunderland S: Nerves and Nerve Injuries. New York, Churchill Livingstone, 1978
35. Sweet WH, Wepsic JG: Stimulation of the posterior columns of the spinal cord for pain control. Indications, techniques and results. Clin Neurosurg 21:278, 1974
36. Swift TR: Involvement of peripheral nerves in radical neck dissection. Am J Surg 119:694, 1970
37. Thomas JE, Colby MY: Radiation induced or metastatic brachial plexopathy? A diagnostic dilemma. JAMA 222:1392, 1972
38. Weber ER, Daube JR, Coventry MB: Peripheral neuropathies associated with total hip arthoplasty. J Bone Joint Surg 58A:66, 1976
39. Whitesides TE, Haney JC, Harada H et al: A simple method for tissue pressure determination. Arch Surg 110:1311, 1975
40. Woodhall B: Operative injury to accessory nerve in the posterior cervical triangle. Arch Surg 74:122, 1957

49 Complications of Persistent Postoperative Pain

Richard P. Greenberg | Donald D. Price | Donald P. Becker

OVERVIEW

Postoperative pain arising from surgical incision, wound infection, or hematoma, and so on can usually be managed with analgesic medication, appropriate treatment, and good patient–surgeon rapport as long as the painful state resolves within weeks to a few months following surgery.[2, 4, 12] *However, if the painful process is not curable or self-limiting and persists for 6 months or more, a persistent postoperative pain syndrome can develop that may be refractory to treatment.*[5, 26] *Furthermore, an unfortunate complication can occur in such chronic pain patients, i.e., opiate addiction.*[4, 5, 26]

A chronic pain syndrome no longer dependent on an identifiable disease should itself be considered a pathologic process.[3] *It can be a complication of many surgical diseases and procedures and become a greater problem for the patient than was the original illness.*

Organic and psychological factors that influence persistent postoperative pain are incompletely understood.[5] *This chapter begins with a discussion of pain physiology, emphasizing central nervous system (CNS) mechanisms that may be responsible for chronic pain. The rationale, benefits, and drawbacks of medical or surgical treatment for chronic pain syndromes may be better understood by this review. The more common postoperative persistent pain syndromes and their possible treatments are also considered.*

Mechanisms of Nociception

Significant advances in our understanding of neurons, sensory pathways, and neural mechanisms important in signaling information about tissue injury have been made within the last 10 years. Moreover, data obtained recently have led to knowledge of brain mechanisms that inhibit pain. This information is undoubtedly of great potential value to physicians.

For a person to perceive an event as painful, a complex processing of sensory information must occur at all levels of the CNS—periphery, spinal cord, and brain. Furthermore, the ongoing natural pain-inhibiting mechanisms present in the CNS must be overcome in order for this perception to take place. Thus, the pain experience and nociceptive responses are not directly and simply related to activity in "pain" receptors but depend upon inhibitory and facilitatory factors within the CNS.[17, 19, 20] The gate control theory of pain proposed by Melzack and Wall attempted to summarize what was known about these factors and to integrate this knowledge with electrophysiologic data.[20] This theory, formulated in 1965, has inspired both innovations in pain treatment and extensive research on nociceptive and nociceptive suppression mechanisms. Therefore, a brief overview of the basic tenets of the gate theory introduces nociception and thereby provides a framework for discussing what is presently known about central nociceptive mechanisms.

The gate control theory proposed that pain phenomena are determined by interactions among three central systems: (1) the spinal cord dorsal horn sensory transmission neurons (called T cells), which receive input from both low- and high-threshold primary afferents; (2) substantia gelatinosa interneurons, which modulate the excitatory effects from these primary afferents; and (3) descending control systems, which originate within the brain and are at least partly triggered by somatosensory afferent input itself. The dorsal column pathway was proposed to be an important trigger of descending control systems.

This chapter was supported in part by NINCDS Teacher Investigator Award K07NS 346-03 (RPG), NIDR Contract 263-77-C-0623, and by Clinical Research Center Grant No. M01-RR0065.

These three central systems were proposed to converge in the spinal cord. The interactions of these components are shown in Figure 49-1 and are summarized as follows: Touch or other forms of gentle stimulation evoke impulses in large low-threshold mechanoreceptive afferents (A-beta), which are initially effective in activating the T cells. However, their subsequent effect is to evoke inhibition of the T cells either pre- or postsynaptically. In contrast, impulses in small high-threshold afferents (A-delta and C fibers) activate a positive facilitatory mechanism that augments the excitatory effects of subsequent afferent impulses. This effect could result from a disinhibition of ongoing effects from large afferents or to an active facilitatory mechanism that is independent of the influence from large afferents, as shown in Figure 49-1. Thus, the experience of pain is partly determined by the ongoing afferent activity that precedes the stimulus, the stimulus-evoked activity (*i.e.*, the relative number of impulses evoked in low- and high-threshold afferents), the relative balance of excitatory and inhibitory effects from low- and high-threshold afferents, and descending controls that can suppress or exaggerate synaptic transmission at the first central synapse. The details of these peripheral and central mechanisms are now presented in light of some of the modifications and additions that have altered the original gate control concept.[33]

Primary Cutaneous Afferents

Pain receptors that signal impending tissue damage are not uniformly sensitive. They fall into several categories depending on their responses to mechanical, thermal, and chemical stimulation and on the conduction velocities of the axons that supply them.[23] The primary afferents discussed below are among the best-known neurons that conduct painful information centrally (spinal cord, brain).

High-threshold mechanoreceptive afferents (HTM), A-delta fibers, respond only to intense mechanical stimuli and conduct between 4 m and 40 m/sec. Many respond only to stimulus intensities that produce overt tissue damage; others give threshold responses to nondamaging pressure applied to the skin (less than 1 g/cm^2). This group of mechanoreceptive afferents is particularly sensitive to excitation by sharp objects but relatively insensitive to heat. Therefore, they seem adapted for transmitting information related to localized pricking pain.

Heat nociceptive afferents, A-delta fibers, conduct between 3 m and 20 m/sec and also respond to intense mechanical stimulation. However, unlike the HTM afferents, heat-nociceptive afferents respond to increases in receptive field skin temperature. These responses accelerate positively, the steep portion of the curve occurring in the 45° to 51°C range. Threshold temperatures for these afferents are usually below noxious or painful levels (40°–44°C), but highly noxious skin temperatures (> 50°C) evoke maximum responses.

Polymodal nociceptive C afferents form an extremely important group of peripheral fibers since they constitute 80% to 90% or more of the C-fiber population of primates.[23] They innervate skin and are characterized by their responses to noxious mechanical, noxious heat, and chemical irritant stimuli. Some also respond to intense cold (< 10°C). There is little doubt that C-polymodal nociceptive afferents signal tissue damage and contribute directly to pain sensations in humans.

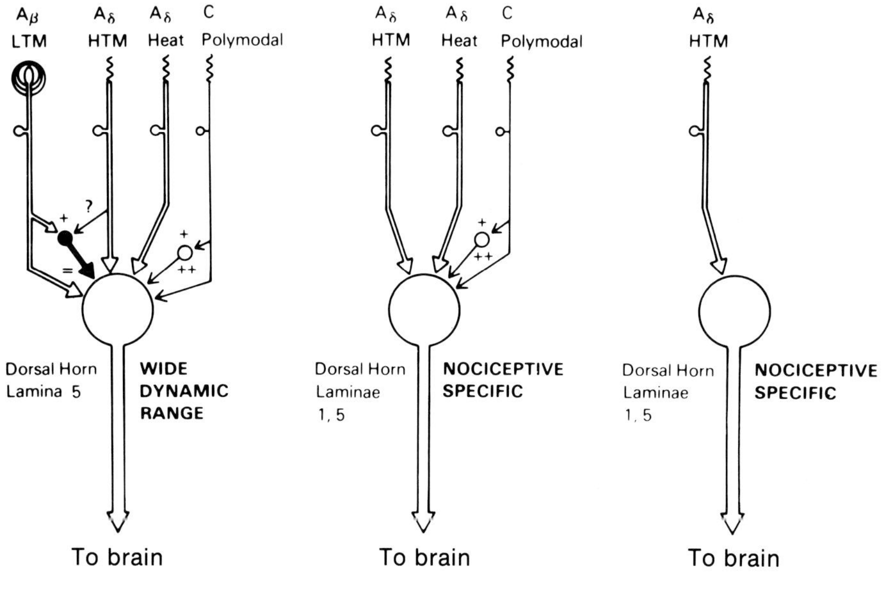

FIG. 49-1. Three types of spinothalamic tract neurons that could be involved in pain. Facilitory interneurons are indicated by small unfilled circles and plus signs. Inhibitory interneurons are indicated by small filled circles and minus signs. (*LTM*, low threshold mechanoreceptor; *HTM*, high threshold mechanoreceptor)

The above-mentioned fibers, among others, are interrupted when a peripheral nerve is sectioned (neurectomy) to relieve persistent postoperative pain.[3, 22, 29, 35]

Spinal Cord Neurons That Subserve Pain

DORSAL HORN SENSORY TRANSMISSION NEURONS

Primary afferents that signal tissue injury (discussed above) synapse on neurons in the dorsal grey matter of the spinal cord. Some of these neurons give rise to ascending sensory pathways to the brain, including spinothalamic and spinoreticular pathways (Fig. 49-2). The spinothalamic pathway is lesioned to relieve contralateral body pain during a spinal cordotomy.[27, 35]

There are three distinct types of dorsal horn neurons that convey information about tissue injury by way of the spinothalamic tract to the brain. Wide dynamic range neurons (see Fig. 49-1) exist within laminae I to VI of the dorsal horn but are most concentrated in laminae IV to VI.[9, 23–25] They receive synaptic excitatory effects from large, myelinated, (A-beta) low-threshold mechanoreceptive afferents, A-delta high-threshold mechanoreceptive afferents, and C-polymodal nociceptive afferents. As a result of this extensive convergence, these cells respond with increasingly higher frequencies of impulse discharge to gentle touch, firm pressure, and noxious pinching.

The second type of dorsal horn spinothalamic neuron (see Fig. 49-1) responds predominantly or exclusively to intense mechanical and thermal stimuli and is located primarily in the marginal layer. No responses can be evoked in this neuron by gentle tactile stimuli. It receives excitatory synaptic effects from A-delta high-threshold mechanoreceptive afferents, from A-delta heat nociceptive afferents, and from C-polymodal nociceptive afferents. As a result of these inputs, this type of neuron responds to firm pressure and pinch with an increasingly higher frequency of impulse discharge.

The third type of dorsal horn spinothalamic neuron (see Fig. 49-1), also found mainly in the marginal layer, is unequivocally specific for responses to noxious skin stimuli. It appears to receive input from only A-delta high-threshold mechanoreceptive afferents since it responds only to noxious mechanical stimulation of the skin. Therefore, like the A-delta primary afferent high-threshold mechanoreceptors, this type of spinal dorsal horn neuron is likely to be related to the first pain evoked by a sharp object. The identification of these *nociceptic-specific* neurons supports the theory that pain is subserved

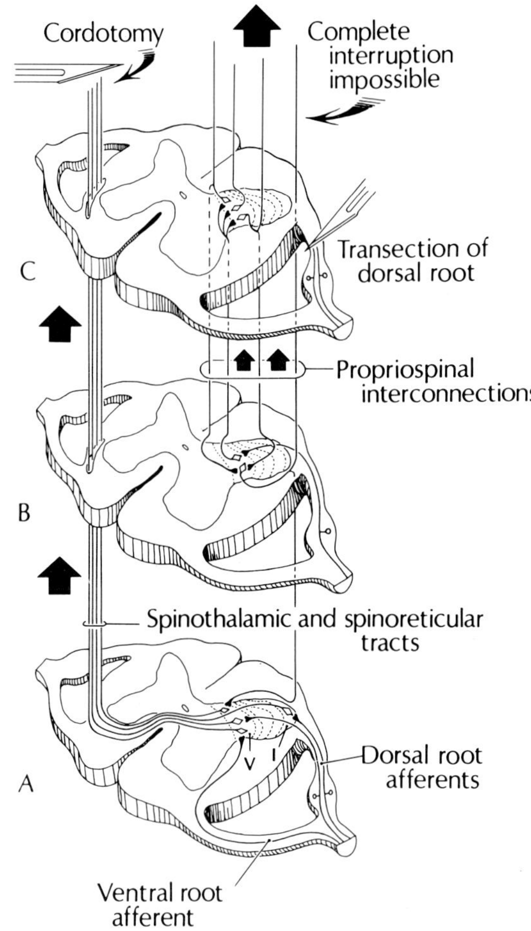

FIG. 49-2. Spinal cord and ascending pain pathways. Dorsal-root nociceptive afferents and some ventral-root afferents converge on spinal–dorsal-horn neurons in layers I and V. Axons from laminae I and V form the ascending spinothalamic and spinoreticular pathways. In addition to these pathways, propriospinal interconnections also subserve pain transmission. Propriospinal interconnections contribute to sensory projection neurons and can be an alternative means of channeling nociceptive input to the brain. Because of the widespread distribution of propriospinal interconnections, surgical lesions of the dorsal root (rhizotomy) or spinothalamic tract (chordotomy) often do not provide long-term pain relief. For example, a complete lesion of the spinothalamic tract between points *C* and *A* can be circumvented by the still intact propriospinal connections.

by neurons and pathways that are activated only by noxious stimuli and not other forms of somatosensory stimuli.[20, 23]

Both *wide dynamic range* and *nociceptive-specific* neurons give rise to ascending sensory pathways, and both are likely to be involved in pain. Marginal layer nociceptive-specific neurons have small receptive fields, somatotopic organization, and many respond only to one kind of stimulus energy. They seem well adapted to provide information about precise location and type of noxious stimulus. Wide dynamic range neurons also seem capable of providing this information but to a lesser degree. It has been shown that selective electrical activation of wide dynamic range neurons in humans is sufficient to evoke pain the location of which can be approximated and the intensity of which varies with the frequency and intensity of electrical stimulation of their axons in the anterolateral quadrant.[23]

PROPRIOSPINAL INTERCONNECTING NEURONS

Spinal cord processing of sensory information to signal tissue injury not only occurs in dorsal horn sensory transmission neurons but also in intersegmental spinal neurons by means of propriospinal interconnections (see Fig. 49-2). These spinal neurons undoubtedly play a major role in central summation and facilitation mechanisms of pain. Although the spinothalamic tract (spinal cordotomy), a relatively discrete neural pathway arising from dorsal horn transmission cells, can be surgically sectioned and pain thereby alleviated, it is very difficult to interrupt propriospinal interconnecting neurons surgically because of their widespread distribution in the cord (see Fig. 49-2).

The longest propriospinal connections, extending from cervical to lumbosacral levels, originate from layer IV to VI in spinal dorsal horn, a major site of origin for spinothalamic tract neurons.[36] Spinothalamic tract neurons are strongly influenced by propriospinal connections since such connections and sensory relay neurons originate from the same dorsal horn layers. This influence is reflected in the extensive receptive fields of some spinothalamic neurons, which often extend across several spinal dermatomes.[23, 24] Some of the input to these neurons, then, is likely to originate from interneurons many spinal cord segments away.

Centralization of Pain

The role of propriospinal interconnections in the dorsal horn input–output relationships is illustrated schematically in Figure 49-2. From this diagram it is evident that interruption of spinothalamic neurons at one level by spinal cordotomy would leave open the possibility that *somatosensory pain information could still pass by way of propriospinal connections* to sensory neurons at another level. Initially, the partial interruption of this pathway would result in a zone of analgesia related to the interruption of a critical pathway, as well as to a decrement in the total number of sensory neurons conveying nociceptive information. The gradual return of pain after 1 to 2 years following a cordotomy would depend on these preexisting interconnections and upon processes related to increased efficacy of synaptic transmission (e.g., denervation sensitivity).

Surgical interruption of any part of an afferent pain pathway in the peripheral or central nervous system, such as peripheral neurectomy, rhizotomy (section of dorsal root), or cordotomy (interruption of the spinothalamic tract), often fails to relieve pain for more than a few months to years because of the above-discussed mechanisms. Moreover, it has become increasingly apparent that the CNS is exquisitely sensitive to the peripheral neurologic damage that sometimes accompanies surgical procedures. Even very small peripheral lesions, such as tooth extraction, are followed by clear signs of degeneration within the medulla.[8] Drastic transneuronal changes occur in second-order neurons of pain pathways, such as retraction of dendrites and loss of dendritic spines.[8] Physiologic changes also take place in spinal cord somatosensory neurons as a consequence of deafferentation.[16] Two or more weeks after dorsal root rhizotomy, these neurons increase their spontaneous impulse activity and show intermittent high-frequency bursts of activity. These changes, which may reflect denervation hypersensitivity, are likely to account at least partly for central pain or the pain of deafferentation, for example anesthesia dolorosa or postcordotomy dysesthesia (see below), complications of surgical lesions of the nervous system. Similar physiologic changes resulting from interruption of afferent neurons have been observed at all levels of the CNS.

The effects of peripheral deafferentation on central nociceptive neurons may be so marked that removal of the original source of pain (e.g., a neuroma, or tumor) may fail to relieve the chronic pain. The pain has become centralized and no longer depends upon the original disease process. Centralized pain is more resistant to treatment by surgical deafferentation than is pain with a clear somatic origin.[5, 30, 35] This would explain the persistence of pain following surgery that successfully removes the diseased tissue yet fails to relieve the patient's primary presenting symptom—pain.

Descending Controls of Nociceptive Afferent Pathways

A major tenet of the gate control theory is that descending controls can augment or reduce transmission of nociceptive information at the level of the spinal cord dorsal horn. Considerable progress has been made in the last few years describing the anatomical, physiologic, and neurohumoral substrates of neural systems that modulate pain perception.

Indeed, the potency of these descending controls and their multiplicity are even more extensive than those envisioned by the gate control theory. Important therapeutic strategies for relief of chronic pain have been suggested by the descending pain inhibitory systems. For example, electrical stimulation of areas of the brain where descending pain pathways originate—periventricular grey deep brain stimulation—and of the spinal cord dorsal columns—dorsal column stimulation—has been successfully utilized in patients with persistent pain.[14, 15, 21, 31] Electrical stimulation for pain control has advantages over lesions of the peripheral and central nervous system. This mode of surgical therapy is reversible and does not have the unpleasant side-effects that can sometimes develop following lesion therapy such as anesthesia dolorosa (see below).

Particular progress has recently been made in elucidating the periventricular and periaqueductal grey neural systems that can be activated by electrical stimulation as well as by the narcotic analgesic drugs.[5, 14, 17] The pain inhibitory effects of both narcotic drugs and brain stimulation appear to be mediated by activity at brain sites surrounding the third ventricle, cerebral aqueduct, and fourth ventricle. Both narcotic-produced and brain-stimulation-produced analgesia are reduced by depletion of monoamines and by the narcotic antagonist naloxone.[10, 11] Much evidence now indicates that these two modes of pain suppression exert their effects by activation of a serotonergic pathway that originates in nucleus raphe alatus and descends by way of the dorsolateral funiculus of the spinal cord to the dorsal horn.[17, 18, 34] The ultimate site of inhibitory action involves the release of serotonin and its consequent inhibition of dorsal horn neurons that are the origin of nociceptive pathways. The discovery of an endogenous "pain suppressive" system that is activated by narcotic drugs and the identification of opiate receptors in the brain have led to the search for and discovery of endogenous "morphinelike" substances within the brain, termed *enkephalins*.[1] Moreover, the utilization of stereotactic implantation of stimulating electrodes in the periventricular grey region of the brain for relief of persistent pain was suggested by this discovery.[14] This procedure appears to have particularly successful applications for the control of chronic pain in the back and lower extremities.

Persistent Postoperative Clinical Pain Syndromes

Clinical pain may be divided into two broad etiologic categories: peripheral or neurogenic pain and central or deafferentation pain. Examples of pain syndromes in these groups are given in the following list:

Peripheral, Neurogenic Pain
Nerve compression syndromes
Cervical or lumbar rhizopathy
Peripheral nerve injury, neuroma
Cauda equina arachnoiditis
Peripheral neurectomy

Central, Deafferentation Pain
Causalgia
Anesthesia dolorosa, postneurectomy pain
Amputation, phantom limb pain
Postcordotomy dysesthesia
Spinal cord injury pain
Thalamic pain

Pain originating in a peripheral nerve can ultimately become centralized in the spinal cord or brain according to mechanisms described above. As the cause of a pain syndrome becomes more independent of peripheral stimulation, which is centralized, it often becomes more difficult to treat successfully.

PERIPHERAL PAIN SYNDROMES

Postoperative Peripheral Neuralgia

Pain caused by peripheral nerve injury, so-called peripheral neuroma pain, most commonly follows thoracotomy (intercostal nerves), flank incisions for urologic disorders (intercostal nerves usually T10–T12) and herniorrhaphy (ilioinguinal, iliohypogastric nerves).[23, 29, 35] However, persistent postsurgical pain may be present following incisions in many other areas of the body. Another cause of postoperative peripheral neuralgia is nerve compression due to surgical suture material, fibrous adhesions, organized hematomas, and so on.[35] Pain secondary to nerve compression often resolves following the removal of the offending mass.

It is difficult on occasion to separate the effect of nerve compression from that of nerve injury. For example, meralgia paresthetica caused by compression or injury of the lateral femoral cutaneous nerve manifests itself by paresthesias, hypesthesia, and persistent pain referred to the anterolateral thigh. This persistent pain syndrome may follow surgical procedures of the region of the anterior, superior iliac crest and pelvis that cause either *injury or compression* of the lateral femoral cutaneous nerve. Other examples of this phenomenon are in the cervical and lumbar regions where persistent root pain, rhizopathy, exists owing to nerve compression or injury in spite of appropriate laminectomy, diskectomy, or foraminotomy.

The mechanisms of altered neural activity responsible for neuroma or compression/injury pain are unknown. Among the possible causes of pain are peri- or intraneuronal scar formation, peripheral end organ damage, aberrant collateral sprouting of intact neighboring nerves or of the proximal end of the damaged axon, Schwann cell reaction, changes in spinal cord cells that have lost part of their normal input (central pain), and so forth.[3, 32] In light of all types of surgical approaches to diseased tissue, neuralgia with persistent pain develops in relatively few patients. Why some patients and not others with similar operations are afflicted with painful neuroma is unknown.

SIGNS AND SYMPTOMS. It is difficult for a patient with persistent pain in the site of an incision to pinpoint its onset. Initially, the stress of surgery and the presence of acute incisional pain, which resolves in a short period, mask the neuroma pain. However, whether detected early or late after surgery, the pain is described as having either a sharp knifelike quality that may be exacerbated by movement or as a toothache, throbbing, unremitting, and often not relieved with opiate medication.

The pain is most often present in the sensory distribution of the injured nerve. Thus, with intercostal nerve involvement pain may be present in all or part of the beltlike thoracic area that is innervated by that particular nerve. Palpation, especially of the incisional area, may cause a marked increase in pain. Skin sensation can be altered so that even innocuous stimuli produce pain (hyperpathia). Hyperpathia can sometimes be found to extend over a wider area of skin than is innervated by the injured nerves.

TREATMENT. Exploration of the wound to identify and resect the end bulb, the neuroma, which may have formed on the offending peripheral nerve, often provides short-term relief at best.[35] The painful neuroma can re-form for the same reasons that led to the original problem. However, if an incisional hernia, misplaced suture, or other secondary complication of the surgery is present, reoperation to correct the local problem is advised.[22]

Surgical or chemical interruption of the involved peripheral nerve proximal to the incision site or of the dorsal root (rhizotomy) may sometimes relieve the pain.[13] The surgeon must also section at least one nerve above and below the injured nerve because of overlapping sensory innervation. Although this procedure does provide pain relief in some patients, it may fail to provide long-term benefits to others. A neuroma can form on the proximally resected peripheral nerve, or the pain may have become centralized. Thus, nerve resection at any level may fail to help the pain. Furthermore, anesthesia dolorosa (described below) may result from nerve resection and manifest itself in the distribution of the original persistent pain.

There are nonsurgical treatments that may also be successful in relieving neuroma pain. Transcutaneous nerve stimulation of the involved dermatomes or acupuncture may be effective in some cases.[21, 31] These modalities have the benefit of not causing permanent changes in the peripheral or central nervous system.

Attempts have been made to potentiate the body's intrinsic pain suppression mechanisms by chemical manipulation. The amino acid L-tryptophan, when given in large doses (2 g daily, divided doses) is thought to increase the level of serotonin, one substance necessary for endogenous pain suppression. Amitryptaline also enhances central pain inhibition and in combination with L-tryptophan may have greater efficacy. This drug combination has also been effective in relieving unpleasant sensations felt by patients in areas surgically denervated.

Arachnoiditis

Cauda equina arachnoiditis, a condition encountered in patients who have had one or more myelograms or lumbar disc surgery, is also a peripheral neuralgia.[35] Fibrous bands and scar tissue form on and between the cauda equina axons, presumably because of bleeding in the subarachnoid space. Arachnoiditis is one of the causes of persistent pain following lumbar diskectomy or any procedure involving thecal sac manipulation.

SIGNS AND SYMPTOMS. Patients may initially have pain relief following surgical diskectomy only progressively to develop constant widespread pain in the back and legs several days to months later. The pain syndrome due to adhesive arachnoiditis often involves a wider distribution than the original radicular pain. Many patients complain of a knifelike, sharp pain that coexists with a background chronic aching pain. Both lower extremities may be involved even if the initial pain was confined to a nerve root on only one side. Progression of this condition can lead to paraplegia as well as bowel, bladder, and sex dysfunction.

TREATMENT. It is of little value to explore the cauda equina nerve roots in an effort to remove the scar tissue. Reoperation as well as injection of steroid medications may reduce pain levels initially but can also cause increased formation of adhesions.[3]

Operant conditioning, a psychological technique aimed at rehabilitating the patient by rewarding behavior consistent with tolerating and coping with persistent pain, should be tried in conjunction with acupuncture or transcutaneous nerve stimulation.[5, 18]

Surgical treatment of arachnoiditis should be judiciously utilized and limited to CNS stimulative procedures of dorsal column or periventricular grey stimulation, as opposed to CNS lesions like cordotomy.[14, 21]

CENTRAL, DEAFFERENTATION PAIN SYNDROMES

Causalgia and Reflex Sympathetic Dystrophy

On occasion causalgia and reflex sympathetic syndromes that most commonly follow peripheral nerve trauma, gunshot wounds, stab wounds, and so on may be caused by peripheral nerve injury in the course of various surgical procedures. The severity of nerve injury has not been correlated with the development of painful neuroma on the one hand or causalgia and reflex sympathetic dystrophy on the other. A completely interrupted nerve rarely produces these syndromes.

Because pain is associated with dystrophic and atrophic changes sometimes involving the entire limb, centralization of pain with abnormalities at the spinal cord or more rostral CNS levels probably plays a major role in this syndrome. A central mechanism may be postulated wherein loss of normal neural innervation produces aberrant central neural circuitry. The sympathetic nervous system is often thought to play a role in this syndrome because symptomatic relief can be obtained by sympathectomy. However, no evidence directly implicates the sympathetic nervous system.[35]

SIGNS AND SYMPTOMS. Although these pain syndromes are usually produced by peripheral nerve injury, causalgia and reflex sympathetic dystrophy differ from painful neuroma because of the symptom complex that accompanies pain. Causalgia manifests itself in days to weeks of surgery by the onset of intense, unremitting, burning pain initially limited to the distribution of the injured nerve. Eventually, the pain may involve the entire limb. The median, ulnar, and sciatic nerves are frequently involved, as well as is the brachial plexus. When causalgia persists for longer than 6 months, dystrophic changes occur. Initial edema, hyperthermia, and increased sweating give way to thin, cool, pale to cyanotic skin. Hair is lost, and trophic changes in the nails occur. Bone rarefaction is seen radiographically. Ultimately, limb atrophy and bone decalcifications develop.

Reflex sympathetic dystrophy is similar to but less intense than causalgia. The diffuse pain manifest in this syndrome can be increased by touch and pressure. Severe atrophy of muscles, joint fibrosis, and bone decalcification (Sudeck's atrophy) are also associated with reflex sympathetic dystrophy.

TREATMENT. Essential to the successful treatment of these syndromes is their early detection and vigorous management. Aggressive physical therapy, serial sympathetic Xylocaine blocks of the stellate ganglion, or lumbar sympathetic chain and surgical sympathectomy, when indicated, represent sound strategy.[3] Transcutaneous nerve stimulation can be very effective in reducing pain levels, especially when combined with the above regimen.[7]

Anesthesia Dolorosa

Persistent pain secondary to incomplete peripheral nerve lesions is described above. When a peripheral nerve is completely sectioned during a surgical procedure (e.g., ilioinguinal nerve resection during herniorrhaphy), an area of numbness that is moderately uncomfortable develops. Usually the numb area resolves within 3 to 6 months without sequelae. However, in a small number of cases an extremely painful area of numbness may be produced by neurectomy or rhizotomy (dorsal root section). Ten percent to 15% of patients who have trigeminal neurectomy (interruption of cranial nerve V) because of tic douloureaux develop anesthesia dolorosa (painful anesthesia) in the facial distribution of this cranial nerve.[35]

Centralization of pain most likely plays a rôle in the development of anesthesia dolorosa. As described above, denervated dorsal horn neurons develop new neural synaptic connections. These abnormal synapses may be responsible for the pain syndrome.

SIGNS AND SYMPTOMS. Shortly after neurectomy the patient will perceive paresthesias in the distribution of the nerves resected. In some cases the onset is delayed for several weeks. When the pain is completely developed, the patient describes unremitting paresthesias, drawing sensations, and burning and excruciating pain in the distribution of the sectioned nerve. A hallmark of anesthesia dolorosa is the unchanging intensity of the pain. If neurectomy or rhizotomy was performed to relieve pain, the 10% to 15% of patients who develop anesthesia dolorosa afterward state that this condition is far more difficult to tolerate than was the original pain.[22, 35]

Other complications that follow a neurectomy are trophic changes in the distribution of the interrupted nerve and herpes simplex of the skin, especially after trigeminal nerve resection.

TREATMENT. There is no satisfactory treatment for this condition. Surgery to resect the nerve further is unproductive. Other lesions of the peripheral or central nervous system aimed at relieving the pain cause additional problems. A course of carbamazepine or phenytoin should be tried.

Reports of the efficacy of transcutaneous nerve stimulation, dorsal column stimulation, or stimulation of the internal capsule and ventral posterior thalamic nuclei suggest that these surgical approaches should be judiciously used in selected cases.

Amputation, Phantom Limb Pain

Less than 10% to 15% of patients who require surgical amputation of a limb develop an intermittent severe pain syndrome the location of which is perceived to be in the missing extremity (see also Chap. 61).[28] Patients sense the presence of the entire limb after amputation, can feel it moving, and appreciate pressure when it is thought to be resting on another part of the body.

Loss of sensory input following amputation increases the likelihood of abnormal self-sustaining CNS neural activity. The perception of pain in a phantom limb attests to the validity of the mechanism of centralization of pain. Clearly the site of the pain is not in the amputated limb. Neither is it simply in sectioned nerve endings of the amputation stump because even rhizotomy fails to change the presumed location or intensity of the phantom pain.

SIGNS AND SYMPTOMS. The pain is described as having a stabbing, sharp, shooting quality. Severe paresthesias that can radiate into the phantom limb are present in the stump. Attacks are intermittent with pain relief between each episode. A number of events, such as movement, hot or cold temperature, defecation, and sexual intercourse, can precipitate an attack of pain. The episodes of pain may be most intense in the early postoperative period but generally persist unabated for the remainder of the patient's life. Trigger points may be present on the well-healed stump or even elsewhere on the body.

TREATMENT. The stump should initially be carefully evaluated so that small abscess formation can be corrected. Unfortunately, local stump care cannot be expected to reduce the pain of phantom limb in most cases. Other disease states that cause limb pain should also be investigated.

As in other persistent pain syndromes, CNS lesions either peripherally or centrally placed fail to alleviate phantom limb pain. Procedures such as transcutaneous electrical nerve stimulation, acupuncture, dorsal column stimulation, and internal capsule stimulation should be considered for pain relief in these patients. Local xylocaine nerve block may relieve the pain temporarily.[35]

Pain Following Lesions of the Central Nervous System

In addition to persistent postoperative pain syndromes initiated by peripheral nervous system injury, chronic pain may also follow postoperative lesions of the spinal cord or brain.[5, 6] Central nervous system lesions that develop during tumor removal or vascular surgery, as well as spinal cord and brain lesions made for the control of movement disorders or pain, can lead to chronic pain syndromes of severe intensity.

Postcordotomy Dysesthesia

Percutaneous or open surgical lesions in the anterolateral quadrant of the spinal cord (spinothalamic tract) for pain relief produce loss of pain and temperature sensation on the opposite side of the body. In 10% to 20% of cases, the patient develops painful dysesthesia in the neural distribution affected by the cordotomy.

SIGNS AND SYMPTOMS. Within days to several months following a cordotomy, patients feel a burning, constant pain that cannot be easily relieved by opiate medication and often represents pain greater than the original for which the cordotomy was done. The skin becomes hyperpathic, so that light touch or the feel of clothing augments the pain level. On occasion skin ulcerates. Infrequently, similar syndromes develop as a result of surgery of the spinal cord for tumors, vascular lesions, and so on.

Thalamic Pain

Vascular lesions of the thalamic sensory nuclei may produce a pain syndrome on the side opposite the lesion. This occurs very rarely postoperatively and is more commonly seen following a spontaneously occurring thalamic stroke (syndrome of Dejerine–Roussy).

SIGNS AND SYMPTOMS. Pain is often the only symptom, without other neurologic findings such as motor or sensory deficits. The pain is unremitting and burning, occasionally has a paresthetic component, and is not relieved by opiates. This problem may endure for the remainder of the patient's life. Following the causal event, the onset of pain is almost immediate.

TREATMENT. There is no satisfactory treatment for pain caused by lesions to the CNS. A trial of carbamazepine or phenytoin is advised. CNS lesions for pain relief are not usually successful.

Stimulative central procedures have the best chance of affording some relief of pain. Internal capsule or ventral posterolateral or ventral posteromedial thalamic nuclei stimulation with a stereotactically implanted depth electrode can produce moderate to satisfactory results.[15]

Summary

Early recognition and diagnosis of postoperative pain syndromes that can persist may allow the best treatment for patients with this surgical complication. It is difficult to cure postoperative pain once the condition becomes chronic. However, pain may be alleviated to some extent by reassurance and informative discussions with patients. Lesions of the peripheral and central nervous system for benign pain should be undertaken with circumspection. Electrical stimulation, acupuncture, operant conditioning, physical therapy, patient reassurance, the avoidance of narcotic medications, and so on would appear to be the measures of choice in dealing with persistent postoperative pain.

References

1. Basbaum AI, Clanton CH, Fields HL: Opiate and stimulus-produced analgesia: Functional anatomy of a medullospinal pathway. Proc Natl Acad Sci USA 73:4685, 1976
2. Collins WF, Venes JL, Wagner FC, Spencer DD: Pain. In Schwartz SI, Shires GT, Spencer FC, Storer EH (eds): Principles of Surgery. New York, McGraw-Hill, 1979
3. Cousins MJ, Bridenbaugh PO: Neural Blockade in Clinical Anesthesia and Management of Pain. Philadelphia, JB Lippincott, 1980
4. Eckenhoff JE: Management of pain. In Artz CP, Hardy JD (eds): Complications in Surgery and Their Management, pp 315-323. Philadelphia, WB Saunders, 1960
5. Fields HL: Pain II: New approaches to management. Ann Neurol 9:101, 1981
6. Fields HL, Adams JE: Pain after cortical injury relieved by electrical stimulation of the internal capsule. Brain 97:169, 1974
7. Foreman RD, Beall JE, Applebaum AE et al: Effects of dorsal column stimulation on primate spinothalamic tract neurons. J Neurophysiol 39:534, 1976
8. Gobel S: Neural circuitry in the substantia gelatinosa of Rolando: Anatomical insights. In Bonica JJ et al (eds): Advances in Pain Research and Therapy, vol 3, pp 175-195. New York, Raven Press, 1980
9. Handwerker HO, Iggo A, Zimmermann M: Segmental and supraspinal actions on dorsal horn neurons responding to noxious and non-noxious skin stimuli. Pain 1:147, 1975
10. Hayes RL, Bennett GJ, Newlon PG, Mayer DJ: Analgesic effects of certain noxious manipulations in the rat. Brain Res 155:69, 1978
11. Hayes RL, Price DD, Bennett GJ et al: Differential effects of spinal cord lesions on narcotic and non-narcotic suppression of nociceptive reflexes: Further evidence for the physiologic multiplicity of pain modulation. Brain Res 155:91, 1978
12. Hunt TK: Wound complications. In Artz CP, Hardy JD (eds): Management of Surgical Complications, pp 26-27. Philadelphia, WB Saunders, 1975
13. Hosobuchi Y: The majority of unmyelinated axons in human ventral roots probably conduct pain. Pain 8:167, 1980
14. Hosobuchi Y, Adams JE, Linchitz R: Pain relief by electrical stimulation of the central gray matter in humans and its reversal by naloxone. Science 197:183, 1977
15. Hosobuchi Y, Adams JE, Rutkin B: Chronic thalamic stimulation for the control of facial anesthesia dolorosa. Arch Neurol 29:158, 1973
16. Loeser JD, Ward AA: Some effects of deafferentation in neurons of the cat spinal cord. Arch Neurol 17:629, 1967
17. Mayer DJ, Price DD: Central nervous system mechanisms of analgesia. Pain 2:379, 1976
18. Mayer DJ, Price DP, Rafii A: Antagonism of acupuncture analgesia in man by the narcotic antagonist naloxone. Brain Res 121:368, 1977
19. Melzack R: The Puzzle of Pain, pp 1-232. New York, Basic Books, 1973
20. Melzack R, Wall PD: Pain mechanisms: A new theory. Science 150:971, 1965
21. Nashold BS: Electrical stimulation of the skin, peripheral nerves, or dorsal column for pain relief. In Morley TB (ed): Current Controversies in Neurosurgery, pp 502-509. Philadelphia, WB Saunders, 1976
22. Omer GE: Pain. In Epps CH (ed): Complications of Treatment of Peripheral Nerve Injuries, vol 2, pp 768-779. Philadelphia, JB Lippincott, 1978
23. Price DD, Dubner R: Neurons that subserve the sensory-discriminative aspects of pain. Pain 3:307, 1977
24. Price DD, Hayes RL, Ruda M, Dubner R: Spatial and temporal transformations of input to spinothalamic tract neurons and their relation to somatic sensations. J Neurophysiol 41:933, 1980
25. Price DD, Hu JW, Dubner R, Gracely R: Peripheral suppression of first pain and central summation of second pain evoked by noxious heat pulses. Pain 3:57, 1977
26. Reuter JB, Girard DE, Nardone DA: The chronic pain syndrome: Misconceptions and management. Ann Intern Med 93:588, 1980
27. Rosomoff HL, Carroll F, Brown J, Sheptak P: Percutaneous radiofrequency cervical cordotomy: Technique. J Neurosurg 23:639, 1965
28. Solonen KA: The phantom phenomenon in amputated Finnish war veterans. Acta Orthop Scand (Suppl) 54:7, 1962
29. Sunderland S: Nerves and Nerve Injuries, ed 2. Edinburgh, Churchill–Livingstone, 1978
30. Tasken RR: Clinical neurophysiology of deafferentation pain. Pain (Suppl) 1:96, 1981
31. VanderArk GD, McGrath KA: Transcutaneous electrical stimulation in treatment of postoperative pain. Am J Surg 130:338, 1975
32. Wall PD: Sensory physiology after various types of peripheral nerve injury (abstr). Pain 1:10, 1978
33. Wall PD: The gate control theory of pain mechanisms. A reexamination and restatement. Brain 101:1, 1978
34. Watkins LR, Mayer DJ: The neural organization of endogenous opiate and non-opiate pain control systems. Science 216:1185, 1982
35. White JC, Sweet WH: Pain and the Neurosurgeon. Springfield, IL, Charles C Thomas, 1969
36. Yezierski RP, Culberson JL, Brown PB: Cells of origin of propriospinal connections to cat lumbosacral grey as determined with horseradish peroxidase. Exp Neurol 69:493, 1980

50 Psychological Complications of Surgery

Michael R. Milano | Donald S. Kornfeld

OVERVIEW

Psychological complications occurring in the course of general surgery are at least as ubiquitous as physiologic complications. Even such physiologically grounded complications as postoperative delirium are, however, rarely given notice in surgical morbidity conferences. This reinforces the misconception that psychological complications are nebulous, difficult to evaluate and treat, and sometimes best ignored. It is our position that psychological complications can be assessed systematically and treated as part of a rational plan. It is also our position that such an approach will benefit the patient on a physiologic as well as a psychological basis.

It is useful to contrast psychological complications with the physiologic aftermaths of surgery. Some type of psychological response to general surgery is inevitable, for all people respond to major events impinging upon them. The range of psychological responses is broad and must be evaluated for each individual patient. The patient who successfully masters the stresses of surgery[19] may be psychologically better adapted after surgery or he may suffer varying degrees of lasting disability. The dividing line between normal responses and untoward psychological complications is not as clearly defined as it is for physiologic complications. Furthermore, the surgeon has virtually no useful laboratory procedures to guide him in his assessment of most psychological complications.

Imagine the treatment of postoperative paralytic ileus with only the aid of the physical examination. The management of this condition with its multiple causes could be determined only by following sequentially the unfolding symptom complex, which might range in significance from trivial to life-threatening.

The patient is the crucial participant in his psychological recovery, and the surgeon may be more of an enabler than a definitive source of cure. For example, the successful treatment of many psychological complications will often focus on issues of patient compliance; the "medicine" will not work without the patient's understanding and acceptance. Approaches that capitalize on the patient's active participation in recovery are most effective. Planning such an approach and eliciting the participation of ancillary medical staff and the patient's family receive specific attention later in this chapter.[2, 13, 29] It is, however, infinitely more complex than straightforward prescription of an antibiotic.

Many of the psychological complications of surgery arise in conjunction with a problematic surgical course or are, as in the case of delirium, largely manifestations of underlying physical disturbances. Optimal management involves dealing with all of the etiologic factors, which forces the surgeon to think across diagnostic categories. Blurring the boundary between physical and psychological is commonplace, and the surgeon should be prepared to abandon categorical thinking of mind versus body. Furthermore, psychological complications of surgery may involve not only the patient but also the surrounding social structure of the ward and the interpersonal network of work and family. Surgery is quintessentially dyadic and involves only the surgical team and the patient's body. The understanding of some psychological complications may, however, require assessing the patient's position in his family. The patient is alone in surgery, but not in his response to surgery.

Although this chapter focuses on the intraoperative and postoperative complications of surgery, some attention must be paid to the preoperative elements of surgical treatment. Certainly many of the psychological stresses of surgery are much in evidence before the patient reaches the operating room. For example, the first major peak of anxiety for mastectomy patients occurs at the time of initial diagnosis and in the several days before admission.[31] *Both patient and spouse may demonstrate the most intense emotional responses before surgery and may, in fact, be more relieved than distraught postoperatively.*[17, 18] *Furthermore, most of the psychological difficulties encountered postoperatively have their roots in the patient's fundamental character structure, which is fixed long before the surgeon's arrival on the scene. Frequently the surgeon, as a secondary physician, has no prolonged presurgical relationship with his patient upon which to build trust and no detailed knowledge of the patient's pattern of responding to illness. His first encounters with an emergency patient may be postoperative.*

The importance of preoperative assessment of the psychological coping mechanisms of the surgical patient, therefore, merits brief discussion before considering the complications of surgery. Frequently the nature of postoperative complications can be forecast by the patient's psychological expectations for surgery. Patients who anticipate severe psychological stress respond, in fact, to the anticipation rather than to the reality of the surgical experience. What the patient expects is often what he experiences. The surgeon should be alert to the probability of psychological complications in the patient with preexisting organic brain disease, severe anxiety about surgery, or markedly and unrealistically negative expectations of outcome. The surgeon should make careful note of the patient's response to his disease or diagnosis and should inquire about fears of anesthesia, hospitalization, and surgery. It is essential to watch the patient's facial and body reactions during the discussion of these issues. This requires only the use of simple questions such as, "Most patients are afraid of surgery, what are your fears? Can you describe them?" Patients may have distinct fears about their diagnosis, surgery, or anesthesia, and each should be noted separately.[6] *This is especially important for patients initially hesitant of or who reject a recommendation for surgery. Obviously all patients have some preoperative fears, but the capacity to respond with trust to explanation and reassurance is a good sign that the patient is coping well.*

There is a growing literature demonstrating that careful preoperative preparation of the surgical patient favorably alters the postoperative course, resulting in shortened hospital stay, decreased use of pain medication, increased patient satisfaction with the surgical experience, and decreased physiologic complications.[9] *A wide variety of preparation techniques have included structured information giving, relaxation techniques, and careful stepwise preparation for the postoperative sensations involved in recovery.*[11, 20] *In general, techniques that encourage the patient toward activity, either through use of relaxation to counter pain or encouragement toward ambulation and postoperative exercise, are more effective than educational techniques that leave the patient in an entirely passive state. Careful preoperative assessment and preparation for surgery are certainly the best preventive measures for forestalling postoperative psychological complications.*

Psychological Complications Occurring in the Operating Room, Recovery Room, and Surgical Intensive-Care Unit

Psychological factors can play a surprising role in events in the operating suite. The influence of psychotropic medications on anesthesia are primarily the responsibility of the anesthesiologist, but high levels of preoperative anxiety can substantially prolong thiopental induction and can be lowered by minor tranquilizers or supportive preoperative interviews.[34, 35] Furthermore, the patient's character structure may in fact affect his physiologic response to surgery. For example, patients with the type A coronary-prone-behavior pattern show a heightened blood pressure response during coronary artery bypass surgery.[21]

Of greatest interest to the general surgeon is the direct psychological effect of the operative experience upon the patient. Patients with spinal anesthesia and immediate recall of surgery show anxiety, irritability, demandingness, and tearfulness as evidence of recent psychic trauma.[38] Approximately 1% of general surgery patients will have accurate recall of important parts of the actual surgical experience.[36] Awareness of surgery is usually incomplete and is more common for surgery in which anesthesia is lighter (e.g., cardiac or obstetric). Hypnosis may enhance the patient's recall of the operative experience.[5] Although many patients seem undisturbed by the recall of surgical events, Blacher reports a syndrome of traumatic neurosis following awareness during cardiac surgery.[4] These patients experienced postoperative nightmares recounting specific details of the actual surgery and dreams about being attacked, had diffuse somatic manifestations of anxiety, and were preoccupied with fears of death. Guerra reported that his patients with postoperative awareness of surgery were less troubled by their recollection of pain or events than by their difficulties in communicating these events to the surgical team.[12] The opportunity to discuss operative awareness seems to be essential in successful treatment. Minor tranquilizers will also help with the daytime anxiety. No studies systematically report long-term psychological complications, but a number of the patients described above demonstrated a persistent refusal to utilize the hospitals, anesthesiologists, and surgeons associated with the undiscussed operative awareness.

The surgical recovery room is described anecdotally by many patients as traumatic.

What are the frightening aspects of the recovery room? Typically, a recovery room is a large, open area in which a group of patients lie at various levels of consciousness, an area in which one patient may be lying for 3 hours waiting for spinal anesthesia to wear off, while across the room, a patient who has suddenly begun to bleed is being frantically worked upon by a group of physicians and nurses. In the same room, a patient emerging from anesthesia is screaming loudly for pain relief while another patient, awaiting transfer to her floor, lies quietly, staring off into space apparently oblivious to what goes on about her. In another corner, a patient has been told that the analgesic she had been given an hour ago is all that was ordered and she must bear the pain until she returns to her floor where more medicine can be ordered. Across the room, a child who has just had a tonsillectomy lies terrified, watching this group of sick adults. The picture we have painted is perhaps not typical of all recovery rooms but demonstrates the psychological problems that are found there—the problems from unnecessarily exposing patients to frightening experiences by allowing them to observe all that goes on about them, from unnecessarily exposing them to frightening remarks by staff who believe that patients are oblivious to these comments, from inadequate analgesia that will be enhanced only upon the patients' return to their hospital floors. There is especially the problem of the impact of this generally horrifying scene upon the mind of a child.

What can be done to reduce the anxiety-provoking aspect of this room? One basic change can be made in the structure of the room itself. It should be feasible to construct a room with a central nursing station and individual cubicles for patients. In this way, patients would not be totally exposed to the sights and sounds of surrounding patients. Although it is true that with limited nursing staff, easy access to all patients must be provided, there is no reason why bed stalls cannot be separated by low-level partitions, so that the patient, lying in bed, is effectively screened from adjacent patients. Curtains can also be provided on an overhead track to provide complete privacy when needed and when someone remembers to close them.

There is a special danger that, with increasing reliance upon electronic monitoring equipment, the recovery room could too quickly become a place in which patients attached to machines are watched from afar by nurses and medical staff. This would be most unfortunate. Patients coming out of anesthesia are in particular need of human contact for reassurance that all is well. No machine can provide this. Although monitoring equipment can greatly increase our medical effectiveness, it cannot serve as a substitute for good nursing care and human contact.

The recovery room experience, however brief, can provide the surgeon with much information about the patient's ultimate psychological adaptation. Menzer noted the emergence of childlike, demanding, and uncooperative behavior in some posthysterectomy patients in the recovery room.[28] These were manifestations of preexisting psychological vulnerability and served as excellent indicators of subsequent difficulty in the psychological acceptance of hysterectomy.

Hay and Okun likened the effect of the surgical ICU on the medical observer to that of a tension-charged war bunker.[14] Studies of postcardiotomy delirium have noted the role of the open heart intensive-care unit environment in precipitating overt delirium.[22] The critically ill patient is less able to tolerate the sleep deprivation, the restriction of movement, and the atmosphere of recurrent emergencies. The rapid resolution of postcardiotomy delirium after transfer to a standard environment affirmed the suggestion that the setting contributed to the delirium.[15] Lazarus and Hagens were able to reduce the incidence of postcardiotomy delirium from 33% to 14% by having the OHRR nurses establish a relationship with the patient preoperatively, by maintaining frequent postoperative verbal contact, and by more prolonged sleep periods and more frequent orienting maneuvers.[23] Similar success has been reported by substituting family members as orienting, reality-guiding helpers postoperatively in the ICU. Although the ICU is admittingly stressful, it would appear that careful preoperative preparation and immediate postoperative maintenance of emotional contact; maneuvers orienting the patient to time, person, and place; and adequate sleep are important elements in the prevention of the dangerous postoperative psychiatric complication of delirium.

Psychological Complications of Surgery in the Immediate Postoperative Period

The surgical patient is most dependent upon his surgeon during the period of time from return to the surgical floor to hospital discharge. To a large extent the patient's response in this stage will depend upon the nature of the surgery. Patients with elective surgery will have had some time to prepare psychologically; however, patients who have had emergency surgery will be responding both to the surgery and the related antecedent trauma. The neurosurgical patient may have prolonged postoperative disturbances of consciousness. The cancer patient will be coping with the implications of his diagnosis as well as the surgery. Finally, many patients will be experiencing relief of pain or definitive cure, which are potent promoters of good psychological adaptation.

Prior to surgery, the surgeon must endeavor to prepare his patient for the immediate events of illness, hospitalization, and surgery itself. Postoperatively his role is to prepare the patient for pain, to educate the patient for active participation in convalescence, to explain complications when they occur, and to reassure the patient about the numerous novel and potentially frightening events occurring in that phase of treatment. In passing, he may observe a number of unpleasant feelings or affects in his patients. Differentiating these important but benign responses to surgery from incipient psychological illness should, in most cases, be within the skill of the surgeon.

THE POSTOPERATIVE PATIENT EXPRESSING DISCOURAGEMENT

The statement, "If I have to go on like this, I just don't want to live anymore," is relatively common but always necessitates further inquiry. The differentiation of the discouraged from the suicidal patient can be pursued with a number of questions:

Is the pessimism related to postoperative developments such as protracted pain or unexpected complications? If so, these patients state that their mood will improve as their physical state improves. Frequently the patient may need more pain medication or a more detailed and reassuring explanation of his postoperative symptoms.

A 45-year-old man, 1 month post-hemigastrectomy for duodenal ulcers, told a nurse, "I'd rather die than go on living like this." He had a postoperative anastomotic leak with pancreatitis, weight loss, and pain and had been on prolonged parenteral nutrition. On further discussion it was discovered that he was not well informed about the nature of the surgical complications and that he suspected a diagnosis of cancer. He stated that he did not wish to die, but he was discouraged and frightened by the unexpectedly difficult course of his surgery. With explanation his mood improved, and he expressed thanks for the encouragement when he eventually recovered.

Can the patient visualize being well and happy again? The suicidal patient is hopeless and cannot. The discouraged patient can, if only he recovers. *Does the patient feel guilty and deserving of his illness?* Most depressed and suicidal patients blame themselves, although statements such as, "Why is God punishing me?" need not necessarily mean that the postsurgical patient is suicidal. The suicidal patient relates his unhappiness to rejection, personal deficiency, or other evidence of worthlessness rather than to the immediate problems of the postoperative state. Somatic indices of depression or suicidal preoccupation such as insomnia, weight loss, constipation, or psychomotor retardation will be very hard to evaluate because these symptoms can commonly accompany the postoperative state. However, the depressed or suicidal patient will most often have a history of depression antedating surgery. Finally, the patient should be asked, "Do you feel so badly that you could take your own life if you had the means to do so?" Such a question will never initiate suicidal thoughts, it may only uncover them.

Depression usually has an insidious onset and is often present for weeks before it is evident to the patient or physician. Hence, an abrupt onset of negative feelings suggests the diagnosis of discouragement. Frequently the differentiation of discouragement from depression cannot be made definitively until the patient improves surgically. At that point, with sustained encouraging developments, the *discouraged* patient will improve. The *depressed* patient will not. It should be noted that classical depression is extremely rare in the immediate postoperative state. If uncertainty continues after the surgeon's investigation, then psychiatric consultation should be requested. Tricyclic antidepressants have a delayed therapeutic effect (1–3 wk), and their anticholinergic side-effects and effect on cardiac conduction can be troublesome. Therefore, these drugs are rarely indicated in the immediate postoperative period and should not be given without psychiatric consultation.

THE FRIGHTENED POSTOPERATIVE PATIENT

Most patients experience some degree of fear both pre- and postoperatively, and the surgeon needs a strategy to assess the extent to which fear is appropriate, pathologic, or even psychotic. The first indication of the patient's fears may appear in response to what, it is hoped, is a routine bedside question, "Do you have any questions for me?" Patients may thus describe their fearfulness directly. However, apprehension may be first noted on the patient's face during discussions or routine medical care, or it may present with somatic manifestations of tremulousness, diaphoresis, periodic tachycardia, nausea, chest pains or tightness, distractibility, agitation, or tearfulness. The surgeon's problem is to differentiate postoperative fearfulness from delirium or nonorganic psychoses.

Fearfulness is certainly a commonplace psychological sequel to surgery, and its management will be a day-to-day requirement of surgical care. A systematic follow-up of symptomatology is crucial. *Is the fearfulness relieved by discussion and reassurance or surgical improvement?* Or *does it intensify?* Minor tranquilizers (e.g., diazepam [Valium], 5 or 10 mg, tid or lorazepam [Ativan], 1–3 mg tid) may provide symptomatic relief but are not to be substituted for ongoing discussions with the patient about underlying concerns.

It is suggested that the surgeon state, *"You seem frightened, what is it that's frightening you?"*

It is expected that most fearful patients will relate their concerns to their health and will benefit from discussion with the surgeon. Many patients with a phobic or obsessive temperament are concerned that the fearfulness represents a break in self-control, which will lead to complications, "nervous breakdown," or death. They can be reassured that this is not true. Other patients will displace their concerns from important medical matters to worrying about relatives, their business, or minor hospital procedure details. Patients with a strong sense of identification with other persons may fear that abdominal surgery will reveal fatal cancer as it did for a parent, spouse, or friend. Some fearful patients may have a long preoperative history of hypochondriasis and expectation of bodily damage. Under these circumstances a sharp increment in fearfulness is of much greater significance than the mere presence of some measure of distress would be.

The classic psychoses of schizophrenia or manic–depressive disease are exceedingly rare in the immediate postoperative phase. There is no evidence that relapses of schizophrenia or manic–depressive diseases are likely to be triggered by surgery, unless a patient's prior psychopathology has focused on issues of body image or fears of physical damage. Psychiatric consultation is needed for the management of such patients. However, until such help arrives, the acutely agitated delusional psychotic patient can be treated with an antipsychotic agent such as haloperidol (Haldol) or chlorpromazine (Thorazine). Detailed advice regarding their use is outlined in the section on Delirium.

THE ANGRY POSTOPERATIVE PATIENT

Many patients are, of course, angry about their illness, and many are angry toward physicians long before treatment. One of the most distressing clinical problems for surgeons, however, is the apparently cheerful, jovial, unworried preoperative patient who in the days after surgery berates his physicians, nurses, or relatives and issues threats of legal actions. It is always possible that the patient has a legitimate cause for anger, but postoperative hostility, unaccompanied by psychosis, is unfortunately the psychological complication of surgery most likely to impel the surgeon to shorten his rounds with the patient.

A 54-year-old married truck driver responded with a carefree "macho" demeanor to discussion of his diagnosis of rectal cancer and to details of a projected abdominoperineal resection. Five days after surgery, his mood was angry, and his demands were incessant, but there was little evidence of fearfulness. Only after 20 minutes of discussion did he admit to shame about his colostomy and despair about impotence. He was enraged about his helplessness. And only after days passed and he had an opportunity to discuss these feelings was he able to visualize himself as a functioning person who in other respects would be able to deal with life as "aggressively" as before. At that point his anger abated.

Such patients are frequently ashamed to admit to feelings of helplessness or fear, and they assume a "strong" and frequently angry stance. They may be noncompliant with minor details of postoperative care and may be haughty or demeaning toward the surgeon or other caretakers. It is helpful to relate such behavior to prior character traits and to recognize that the patient is counterphobic, that is, denying fear or weakness by behavior he perceives as courageous or manly.

If clearly no elements of delirium are present, the surgeon will manage such angry responses best by recognizing the underlying source of the patient's distress. The patient can be reassured that his helplessness is temporary and that he can be allowed maximum activity. It is important to grant such patients every possible appearance of control. Engaging the patient in an argument usually exacerbates the patient's need for dominance and escalates his behavior. The surgeon may, therefore, have to allow the patient to "win" a minor argument. The surgeon must be sure to acknowledge the validity of the patient's legitimate criticism of hospital staff. He really does not want to take over the management of his own case, even though it might appear that way. The patient's hostility should recede as he becomes less helpless.

Although these responses to surgery are commonplace, several distinct psychiatric complications occur primarily in the early postoperative phase and are particularly worthy of attention.

POSTOPERATIVE DELIRIUM

The most common and most important psychological complication of surgery is postoperative delirium. Delirium in surgical patients was described in the 19th century as "interval psychosis," referring to the lucid postoperative interval of days that may precede the onset of delirium. The studies that assess patients preoperatively and follow them sequentially show a higher incidence of delirium than do purely retrospective studies. Titchener studied an aged, nonprivate-hospital surgical population and found 13.1% of patients exhibiting postoperative manifestations of organic brain disturbance.[32] Many of the determinants of postoperative delirium are physiologic. The higher incidences are found in patients who are aged; who have prior existing memory disturbance; who have compromised cardiovascular, renal, or hepatic functioning; who are alcoholic or drug dependent; or who have a history of delirium. Postcardiotomy delirium became a recognized syndrome because of its frequency after open heart surgery and has served as the model for understanding postoperative delirium. It demonstrates quite well how preoperative factors (e.g., personality, age, severity of illness), operative factors (e.g., bypass time, systolic blood pressure), and postoperative factors (e.g., cardiac output, sleep deprivation) can interact to produce delirium. Its incidence has dropped with refinements in surgical technique and more effective psychological intervention.

Delirium characteristically has a rapid onset, and symptoms may appear simultaneously in many areas of psychological functioning. Prototypically, the patient is disoriented to time, place, or person, but the severity of the disorientation may vary, and usually only orientation to person is preserved. The patient may show impaired perception, misidentifying shadows, sounds, and smells in a terrifying fashion. Hallucinations are characteristically visual. Cognitive capacity is severely impaired, and the patient is unable to appreciate correctly what is happening to him. Thoughts may be disorganized, concrete, or flighty and are dominated by the patient's panic. Recent memory is usually severely impaired.

Delirious patients are often agitated and pick at the bed clothes, hurl themselves out of bed to escape imaginary attackers, or strike out. At other times the delirious patient may be lethargic. Symptoms are characteristically exacerbated at night ("sundowning") or at times of stress (e.g., during postoperative care or in a noisy environment with ward confusion). The symptoms may fluctuate from hour to hour, creating diagnostic confusion. It is common to hear reports of delirious behavior from the night nursing staff and find a lucid patient on morning or afternoon rounds.

The major diagnostic problems arise from the disturbances of mood characteristic of delirious patients and patients with organic brain syndromes in general. Affective lability may lead to tears and abrupt outbursts of panic, which must be differentiated from more prosaic postoperative responses. The patient who persistently shouts is more likely panicked from derlirium than he is from pain. Irritability, anger, euphoria, apathy, or depression may be the presenting symptoms. When the diagnosis is in doubt, brief tests of orientation and immediate recall may help, as may the EEG.

Prompt diagnosis is crucial for several reasons. The delirious patient is difficult to manage and may, in a state of disorganized panic, pull out intravenous or central venous pressure lines, leap from bed, or attempt to flee from illusory demons. Delirium is primarily a manifestation of underlying physiologic disturbances of brain functioning, and the identification and removal of underlying causes is the basic goal of diagnosis. Delirium that presents immediately after surgery is most likely related to intraoperative factors perhaps interacting with a preoperative vulnerability. Delirium that develops after a 2- to 3-day lucid interval is usually related to postoperative factors. Drugs are a common cause, but virtually every metabolic or endocrine disorder; hypoxia; hyperthermia; cardiac, hepatic, renal, or pulmonary failure; and a long list of further causes may be present.[24] Alcohol and drug withdrawal are especially common causes of delirium in trauma patients. When hospitalization interrupts supplies, delirium may appear 24 to 72 hours later. Every effort must be made to determine the underlying physiologic cause of the delirium. Although the more acute symptoms can be managed with drugs, these potentially serious problems must be identified and treated. It should be noted that delirium is basically a transient (hours to days) phenomenon; if it persists beyond weeks, then the diagnosis of dementia, or chronic organic mental syndrome, must be entertained.

Psychological and environmental considerations play a role in the management of delirium. For example, early psychological preparation with careful preoperative discussion and support in the open heart recovery room lowered the incidence of postcardiotomy delirium from 33% to 14% in one series.[23] The delirious patient is highly vulnerable to his environment, and noise, confusion, day–night blurring, and unfamiliar faces all exacerbate symptomatology. The environment should, therefore, be made as simple and nonthreatening as possible. Gentle reassurance, especially if it is provided by familiar, trusted, and recognizable figures, may help more than restraints will. The patient needs to be reconnected with familiar routines and persons. Overly detailed explanations of procedures or problems to a patient with compromised cognitive functioning may deepen his confusion and exacerbate his delirium. A careful balance must be struck between helpfully informing the patient and detailed and confusing explanations.

The panic and psychotic thinking and perceptions of the delirious patient require immediate symptomatic management until the delirium clears. For most agitated patients phenothiazines are the treatment of choice. The highly agitated patient can initially be given chlorpromazine (Thorazine), 25 mg, intramuscularly. Larger doses should not be given. It is preferable to give smaller doses at shorter intervals. An elderly or debilitated patient should be given a test dose of 12.5 mg, intramuscularly. A regimen of repeated doses, such as 25 mg, intramuscularly, four times a day, while awake, should be established for each patient. This regular dosage schedule, based upon the patient's physical status and psychological response, is used until the panic and psychosis clear. This is preferable to the exclusive use of as needed doses, which often results in a more labile and extended course of the delirium. Vital signs must be monitored frequently; even though hypotension or oversedation result, lowering the dose is usually effective management. Additional 25-mg doses can be used when needed to supplement the basic regimen. The patient should be shifted to an oral dose of two to three times the intramuscular dose as soon as possible.

If fear of cardiovascular side-effects precludes the use of a phenothiazine, or if a less sedating agent is indicated, 0.5 mg to 2.0 mg of haloperidol (Haldol) can be given intramuscularly. Dose requirements will vary with the patient's age, weight, and general medical condition. If the drug is well tolerated, the dose can be gradually increased. A daily dose of more than 10 mg, intramuscularly, is not usually needed in patients with delirium. When the delirium has abated sufficiently to use oral medication, the patient can be switched to a three times daily schedule, with total daily dosage two to three times the amount needed intramuscularly. Benzodiazepines should not be used to treat the anxiety or agitation of delirium. Such medications will often overly sedate the patient without affecting the psychotic symptoms and may even aggravate the agitation and confusion.

TRAUMATIC NEUROSIS

Although delirium is a psychophysiologic condition, traumatic neurosis is the purest expression of psychological disturbance. It represents a response of the patient's ego or executive mental facilities to sudden and overwhelming traumatic events. The antecedent trauma may be surgery itself, as described in recovery room experiences of patients undergoing major surgical experiences while partially awake. Highly vulnerable patients may experience the entire surgical experience as traumatic. Frequently, the emergency surgical patient may be responding in the postoperative state to the traumatic experiences—automobile accidents, gunshot or knife wounds, or muggings—that were the cause of the surgical intervention. The incidence of traumatic neurosis has not been definitely established for surgery in general, but it is relatively high on services dealing with physical trauma.

The essential symptoms of traumatic neurosis are diffuse anxiety and repeated reliving of the traumatic event. The anxiety is felt to be the result of the frightening stimuli overwhelming the ego. It may present directly as diffuse fearfulness, with agitation, sensitivity to noise or startle reactions to minor stimuli, and a sense of impending doom. Autonomic manifestations such as tachycardia, palpitations, flushing and sweating, nausea, or diarrhea may predominate. The most pathognomonic features of traumatic neurosis involve repetitive recall of the traumatic event. The visual content of the trauma predominates, and patients can mentally reenact scenes during the day and have their sleep interrupted by vivid nightmares of the event. Typically the syndrome is self-limiting and diminishes with time. However, later stress may precipitate nightmares and memories of the original traumatic event. Diagnostic confusion may arise when the patient does not present with the immediate anxiety of a traumatic neurosis but rather shows a psychological pattern of defense against feelings of anxiety and helplessness.

A 23-year-old woman on the fourth postoperative day was in the midst of a protracted struggle with surgical and nursing staff over compliance with ward rules. She repeatedly removed intravenous lines, threatened to sign out of the hospital against medical advice, and threatened medical staff with "the kind of treatment" she had received (*i.e.*, multiple stab wounds). When interviewed, this patient was found to be overwhelmingly and overtly anxious and preoccupied with the traumatic event. Prior to hospitalization she had developed an aggressive, cocky facade and aggressive lifestyle to conceal feelings of helplessness. The abrupt onset of anxiety signified to her that she was in danger of losing control of her mind, becoming helpless and "going crazy." She dealt with this fear with defiant behavior. With the opportunity to ventilate her concerns and reassurance that she would soon be her old self again, her behavior became more appropriate.

The treatment of traumatic neurosis is as usually effective and gratifying as it was for the above patient. Patients need to be reassured that their symptoms are "normal and inevitable," that they will diminish with time, and that the repeated recollections and nightmares do not signify loss of mental control. Abreaction, or rediscussion of the traumatic event, is in itself therapeutic. The patient should be warned of the possibility of a return of the symptoms during times of similar stress. The autonomic manifestations of anxiety and the insomnia may be symptomatically ameliorated with minor tranquilizers (e.g., diazepam [Valium], 5–10 mg, or lorazepam [Ativan], 1–2 mg, orally, tid) or hypnotics (e.g., flurazepam [Dalmane], 30 mg, qhs).

POSTOPERATIVE PHANTOM PAIN

Phantom sensations and phantom pain following amputation represent a blend of physical and psychic factors. The ubiquity of phantom sensations has been underestimated. They have been described for limbs, breasts, rectum, penis, and face. Phantom representation of voiding or defecating sensations have been reported after total cystectomy and proctectomy. Approximately 54% of mastectomy patients in one series reported phantom sensations.[16] The nature of phantom sensation is protean, with virtually every type of feeling described. Phantoms of positioning of the absent limb are common. The surgeon must inquire about the presence of phantom sensations so that he can reassure his patient that they are normal and will gradually disappear.

Although phantom limb sensation is an almost universal phenomenon, phantom pain is less common but more important. A number of physical variables seem to enhance the prospect of postoperative phantom pain. Well-established preoperative pain patterns due to diabetic neuropathy or vascular claudication predispose the patient to pain, as does the presence of severe stump pain. Thus phantom limb pain has been reported in only 1% of young war amputees but in 56% of middle-aged amputees with preexisting vascular disease.[10, 30] The more intense and enduring the preoperative pain, the greater is the likelihood of persistent postoperative phantom pain.

In other cases the psychic contribution is predominant. Postmastectomy phantom pain, for example, is most frequent in younger patients, in patients with preexisting psychological problems, and in patients preoperatively expecting a traumatic psychological response to loss of the breast.[16] Indeed the phantom pain is associated with psychological trauma and is a useful indicator of a patient at risk for continuing difficulty. Patients with personalities based on rigid self-reliance and independence find the helplessness of the immediate postamputation state traumatic and experience a higher incidence of persistent phantom pain than do patients who accept disability more easily or are less inclined to perceive the amputation as a threat to their self-esteem.[30] The patient with persistent phantom pain will usually need referral for psychiatric help.

A 63-year-old widow experienced severe persistent phantom pain after a right, below-the-knee amputation for peripheral vascular disease. The claudication in her right leg had begun about 4 years after the death of an older sister who had lost both legs to peripheral vascular disease. Asked about her reaction to the loss of the person upon whom she had been psychologically dependent, the patient instead complained about intensive phantom pain. After continued questioning, she cried bitterly about her sister's death, but the pain diminished. As her grief was further explored, the pain disappeared, and she was able to begin a rehabilitation program. For this patient phantom pain allowed her to identify with the lost sister, and the process of grieving allowed her to relinquish the pain.

It is not to be expected that every surgeon will be able to deal with complex psychological contributions to postoperative phantom pain. It is, however, important to have a high index of suspicion for the contribution of depression, despair, helplessness, and grief to this syndrome. Only by considering all of the etiologic factors can the appropriate treatment be selected. The depression and despair must be treated psychodynamically and a dynamically oriented rehabilitation approach initiated. Tricyclic antidepressants (e.g., imipramine [Tofranil] or amitryptyline [Elavil]) also are useful both as analgesics and for treatment of underlying depression. A psychiatric consultant should be requested for help with the regimen.

POSTOPERATIVE PAIN

The surgeon is often faced with severe postoperative pain thought to be "out of proportion to the apparent physical causes." Unfortunately, a patient's failure to respond to an analgesic regimen too often reflects the surgeon's undermedication of the patient.[26] The physician's fear of addicting his patient leads to the use of inadequate doses of narcotics. For a patient preoperatively unaddicted to drugs, there need be little concern about "addicting" the patient. Although many patients will become temporarily physically dependent on narcotics, this will not lead to a genuine psychological craving unless a significant emotional problem is already present. The patient with underlying emotional problems is more likely to become addicted to a course of inadequate low doses than to effective levels of analgesia. For example, the usual adult dose of meperidine should be 75 mg, *every 3 hours*, since this is a short-acting drug. The dose will have to be adjusted for weight, age, and other factors.

Ascribing intense, puzzling postoperative pain to psychological factors is hazardous unless it can be demonstrated that the patient had preexisting difficulties in adaptation or unless the pain seems to serve a useful purpose in the patient's life. Thus pain "due to psychological factors" should not be merely a diagnosis of exclusion. Relief of pain by placebo injection is of no diagnostic value since approximately 40% of laparotomy patients experience significant relief from placebo injection.[3]

A 67-year-old widow employed as a governess complained of left upper quadrant pain after a fall bruised several ribs. The absence of clear-cut findings led to a presumptive diagnosis of "psychological overlay." However, the patient had a long history of good psychological functioning, had no recent life stresses or changes, and was happy, esteemed, and successful in her role as a governess. Her mood and prior adaptation ruled out psychological causes. After prolonged observation and extensive radiologic investigation, the diagnosis of splenic damage was confirmed.

On occasion, the surgeon needs to deal with a patient with postoperative pain whose prior life adaptation has been poor, who desires narcotics for both psychological and physical reasons, and for whom hospital dependency has become adaptive. Management issues frequently arise before weaning such patients from pain medication, and timing of withdrawal of pain medication becomes critical.

A 23-year-old single unemployed man had a 3-month hospitalization for partial surgical excision of an extensive hemangioma of deep structures of the right leg and pelvis. He had severe postoperative pain, extensive bleeding, an open wound slow to heal, and a doubtful postoperative prognosis for saving the leg. He had also been abandoned by his family, had a poor job record, and was known to use his pain medication freely. Attempts to wean him provoked angry interchanges with physicians and nurses.

A psychiatric consultant met with the patient and elicited his fears about the illness and concerns about the prolonged and only partially successful course of his surgery. This was coupled with provision for a rehabilitation program after discharge. Power struggles over pain medication were abandoned until the patient's concern for his future were dealt with. After the plan was worked out, a discharge date was established. A week before discharge he was told that he would be switched to oral analgesics over the remaining days. The patient coped well with his discharge and subsequent plans and left the hospital on minimal doses of oral analgesics.

It is important to be aware that such postoperative pain may be an expression of other dysphoric affects. The sedating effects of the narcotics are thus being used by the patient to deal with his anxiety, helplessness, or hostility. Once these underlying emotions are identified, the physician may be able to deal with them directly by discussing them with the patient. Tranquilizers can also be used to supplement the narcotics. The phenothiazines (e.g., chlorpromazine [Thorazine] provide both sedation and potentiation of the narcotic effects. The pain or the dependency on pain medication can be successfully managed when the surgeon or psychiatric consultant is able to provide the patient with an alternative mode of coping with the underlying issues.

The above list of immediate psychological complications describes only those most common and most typical of the immediate postoperative period. Even for the patient who has seemed to cope well with the hospital phase of surgery, specific attention should be given to the issues of discharge. The patient should be asked how he sees the surgery affecting his life. He needs to discuss return to work, to his family, to his sex life, and to his social life. Does he anticipate difficulties? Such information will be essential in helping to manage psychiatric complications occurring after surgery.

Delayed Complications of Surgery

It has been difficult to assess the long-term psychological complications of surgery. Surgery often occurs in the context of protracted illness, advancing age, and preexisting psychopathology. Each of these may dominate the patient's later postoperative years, and disentangling the effects specifically due to surgery may be impossible. Barker, for example, found that cholecystectomy patients had no increase in psychiatric referral in the 2 years after surgery.[1] Titchener, however, found 29 of 200 patients who improved surgically but declined psychologically in the first years after discharge.[33] Consequently, results must be considered in light of specific illnesses, age groups, and presurgery psychological groupings of patients. In addition, psychopathology arising 1 year after discharge may not be seen by the surgeon whose contact with the patient has been completed. The following guidelines are designed to help the surgeon in his postdischarge assessment and management of psychological complications of surgery. Later, the psychological effects of a specific surgical procedure, mastectomy, are considered.

The patient's psychological adaptation to surgery in the hospital is the most immediately available guide to his delayed adaptation. We have seen that even behavior recorded in the recovery room may be predictive of ultimate psychological adaptation. Patients whose primary concerns with anesthesia or the surgical procedure itself will, of course, be free of concern postoperatively. Patients with diagnostic fears may be reassured by cure. However, failure to respond psychologically in a fashion congruent with the surgical result bears particular concern.

A common feature of patients with prolonged psychiatric sequelae is a rise in guilty anxiety in the immediate postoperative period. Such anxiety is notable for its persistence despite reassurance. It is often associated with an emphasis on moral issues ("What did I do to deserve this? Why is God punishing me?") rather than medical issues and for its association with a sense of dread and ultimate doom. Such patients will shift their pattern of adaptation and relatedness from joking and mild denial to bitter pessimism, or from competence and activity to resigned dependency. When these new patterns persist on postoperative followups and when there is no obvious surgical reason for them, then a psychiatric referral should be made.

Sometimes the expected psychological complications bear little relationship to the nature of the surgical procedure. Ileostomy for ulcerative colitis presents significant adaptive problems, but most patients report that relief of prior symptoms leaves them feeling psychologically better.[7] Although permanent colostomy following abdominoperineal resection requires much less postoperative maintenance, it usually involves a diagnosis of cancer, occurs in a much older population, and usually produces impotence. Consequently, there is a high incidence of depression months after discharge, and the surgeon must maintain a high index of suspicion for psychological sequelae.[8]

The most helpful guideline to delayed psychological complications again may be the patient's expectations. Modified radical mastectomy may produce similar physical deficits in 10 patients, but two may have severe psychological responses to loss of the breast. For these patients, their breasts will have had a greater role in sexual self-esteem, as a source of either pride or shame. If the surgery affects organs critical to self-esteem, then a greater psychological response will occur. Loss of limb will have a deeper impact on an athlete than on a sedentary intellectual for a major source of gratification and self-esteem is impaired. The patient generally knows this before as well as after surgery but will usually see the impact most in the period of time after discharge.

The post discharge rehabilitation or recovery period requires some of the same evaluative skills already described. Anxiety, discouragement, depression, and defensive hostility have much the same meaning here as before. The process of rehabilitation proceeds best when such negative affects are effectively addressed and ameliorated. However, surgery often requires a passive acceptance that something will be lost or at least done to the patient. The patient in the post discharge rehabilitation phase is seeking actively to replace the lost limb with a prosthesis or to develop a new area of self-esteem to supplant lost sexuality after an abdominoperineal resection. The process may be either psychological or surgical (e.g., breast reconstruction or penile prosthetic implants). The active participation of family may be as important as the patient's participation. It is the surgeon's role to minimize the surgical impediments to recovery, but he must also orchestrate the early process of rehabilitation.

Assessing delayed psychiatric complications in the office after discharge will be most effective if the surgeon uses himself as a screening and referring agent rather than tries to be the treating physician for all of these problems. Certain general adaptational questions are best timed for the postdischarge follow-up. *How has the operation affected your life in general? Have you returned to work? Has it changed your family relationships? Have you resumed your social and sexual life? Are your spirits back to normal?* In answer to this brief sequence of questions, most delayed psychiatric complications will be reported to the surgeon. If reassurance and advice is offered, it is necessary to confirm at a later time that the intervention was effective and sufficient. Major or persistent psychological complications are best managed by referral to a psychiatrist.

DELAYED PSYCHOLOGICAL COMPLICATIONS IN THE MASTECTOMY PATIENT

Each disease has its own pattern of psychological complications. Mastectomy is a common operation the consequences of which cannot be hidden. It affects an organ granted sexual significance in our culture. Consequently, interest in the psychological consequences of mastectomy began 30 years ago and has led to a considerable literature.

What then are the delayed psychological consequences of mastectomy? Maguire studied 200 women and found that 1 year after mastectomy they reported a 20% incidence of depressed feelings, a 10% incidence of anxiety, and a 38% incidence of sexual difficulties.[23] A satisfactory surgical outcome was predictive of good psychological response, but 25% of the patients considered their psychological adaptation to be significantly poorer 1 year postoperatively. Jamison and colleagues found 10% incidence of poor psychological adaptation 1 year after mastectomy.[17] Silberfarb found that, apart from peaks of distress at the time of discovery of illness and at the time of first recurrence, patients who had had mastectomy did not differ psychologically from the population at large.[31] When Worden and Weisman compared such patients with other cancer patients, they found no evidence for a specific post-mastectomy syndrome of depression.[39] Perhaps phantom breast sensation is the only specifically operative complication of mastectomy.

As the treatment of breast cancer has changed, so have the delayed psychological consequences; for example, the advent of adjuvant chemotherapy has changed the symptom complex in the postoperative phase. Since the continued chemotherapy keeps the issue of cancer uppermost in the patient's mind, it may impede the repression common when the patient no longer needs to confront her illness through ongoing treatment.

Delayed postoperative complications of mastectomy are as prevalent in the patient's spouse as they are in the patient. This probably explains the preponderance of sexual difficulty, because adequate sexuality requires the participation of two persons relatively free of anxiety, inhibition, or despair. Sexual difficulties are best discussed briefly with patient and spouse, who may be referred as a couple for more extensive therapy.

The literature on the psychological complications of mastectomy offers some insight into the surgeon's evolving role in intervention. Retrospective and anecdotal studies have shown the highest incidence of complications. Older studies also show by far the highest incidence of psychiatric complications, and several explanations should be considered. In recent years, widespread publicity about mastectomy has diminished some of the sense of fear and shame associated with it. The surgeon can, therefore, deal with each patient more frankly and openly. Progress in the surgical approach to mastectomy, however, probably claims the greatest credit. Two-stage procedures minimize trauma and the feeling of not being prepared in sensitive patients. Modified radical, partial, and simple mastectomy, and lumpectomy, where surgically indicated, allow the patient some choice of procedure and have minimized postoperative morbidity. Finally, breast reconstruction has been of great psychological benefit for patients seeking to minimize physical residual effects.[27] Such options have offered mastectomy patients enhanced opportunity to find the surgical procedures most harmonious with their psychological needs.

Two interventive programs have also been demonstrated to be effective. Memorial Hospital's self-help group patterned after Reach to Recovery received favorable reports from 98% of participants, demonstrating that contact with other mastectomy patients facilitates psychological rehabilitation.[37] Maguire and colleagues provided routine counseling to mastectomy patients and lowered postoperative psychiatric morbidity from 38% to 12% of patients.[25] Note that the major effective agent was not the brief counseling but improved case finding. Patients developing postoperative psychiatric complications were referred for definitive and more extensive therapeutic intervention, and this accounted for a decreased morbidity rate. Such case finding and referral are well within the capacity of surgeons interested in minimizing postoperative psychological morbidity following mastectomy and other surgical procedures.

References

1. Barker MG: Psychiatric illness after hysterectomy. Br Med J 2:91, 1968
2. Baudry F, Wiener A: The family of the surgical patient. Surgery 63:416, 1968
3. Beecher HK: The powerful placebo. JAMA 159:1602, 1955
4. Blacher R: On awakening paralyzed during surgery: A syndrome of traumatic neurosis. JAMA 234:67, 1975
5. Cheek DS: Unconscious perception of meaningful sounds during surgical anesthesia as revealed under hypnosis. Am J Clin Hypn 1:101, 1959
6. Deutsch H: Some psychoanalytic observations in surgery. Psychosom Med 4:105, 1942
7. Druss RG, O'Connor JF, Prudden JF, Stern LO: Psychologic response to colectomy. Arch Gen Psychiatry 18:53, 1968
8. Druss RG, O'Connor JF, Prudden JF, Stern LO: Psychologic response to colectomy. 1. Adjustment to a permanent colostomy. Arch Gen Psychiatry 20:419, 1969
9. Egbert L, Battit G, Welch G: Reduction of postoperative pain by encouragement and instruction of patients. N Engl J Med 270:825, 1964
10. Ewalt JR, Randall GC, Morris H: The phantom limb. Psychosom Med 9:118, 1947
11. Flaherty GG, Fitzpatrick JJ: Relaxation technique to increase comfort level of postoperative patients: A preliminary study. Nurs Res 27:352, 1978
12. Guerra F: Letter: Awareness during anesthesia. Can Anaesth Soc J 27:178, 1980
13. Hackett TP, Weisman AD: Psychiatric management of operative syndromes. 1. The therapeutic consultation and effect of noninterpretive intervention. Psychosom Med 22:267, 1960
14. Hay D, Okun D: The psychological stresses of the intensive care unit. Psychosom Med 34:109, 1972
15. Heller SS, Frank KA, Malm JR et al: Psychiatric complications of open heart surgery: A re-examination. N Engl J Med 283:1017, 1970
16. Jamison K, Wellisch D, Katz RL, Pasnau RD: Phantom breast syndrome. Arch Surg 114:93, 1979
17. Jamison K, Wellisch D, Pasnau RD: Psychosocial aspects of mastectomy. 1. The woman's perspective. Am J Psychiatry 135:432, 1978
18. Jamison K, Wellisch D, Pasnau RD: Psychosocial aspects of mastectomy. 2. The man's perspective. Am J Psychiatry 135:534, 1978
19. Janis IL: Psychological Stress: Psychoanalytic and Behavioral Studies of Surgical Patients. New York, John Wiley & Sons, 1959
20. Johnson JE, Leventhal H, Daggs JW: Contribution of emotional and instrumental response processes in adaptation to surgery. J Pers Soc Psychol 20:55, 1971
21. Kahn JP, Kornfeld DS, Frank KA et al: Type A behavior and blood pressure during coronary artery bypass surgery. Psychosom Med 42:407, 1980

22. Kornfeld DS, Zimberg S, Malm JR: Psychiatric complications of open heart surgery. N Engl J Med 273:287, 1965
23. Lazarus HR, Hagens JH: Prevention of psychosis following open heart surgery. Am J Psychiatry 124:1190, 1968
24. Lipowski ZJ: Delirium: Acute Brain Failure in Man. Springfield, IL, Charles C Thomas, 1980
25. Maguire P, Tait A, Brooke M et al: The effect of counselling on the psychiatric morbidity associated with mastectomy. Br Med J 281:1454, 1980
26. Marks RW, Sachar EJ: Undertreatment of medical inpatients with narcotic analgesia. Ann Intern Med 78:173, 1973
27. Mendelson BC: The psychological basis for breast reconstruction following mastectomy. Med J Aust 11:517, 1980
28. Menzer D, Morris T, Gates P et al: Patterns of emotional recovery from hysterectomy. Psychosom Med 19:379, 1951
29. Miller WB: Psychiatric consultation. Part 1. A general systems approach. Int J Psychiatry Med 4:135, 1973
30. Parkes CM: Factors determining the persistence of phantom pain in the amputee. J Psychosom Res 17:97, 1973
31. Silberfarb PM, Maurer H, Crouthamel C: Psychosocial aspects of neoplastic disease: 1. Functional status of breast cancer patients during different treatment regimens. Am J Psychiatry 137:450, 1980
32. Titchener JL, Zwerling I, Gottschalk LA et al: Psychosis in surgical patients. Surg Gynecol Obstet 102:59, 1956
33. Titchener JL, Zwerling I, Gottschalk LA et al: Consequences of surgical illness and treatment. Arch Neurol Psychiatry 77:623, 1957
34. Williams J, Jones J, Williams B: The chemical control of preoperative anxiety. Psychophysiology 12:46, 1975
35. Williams J, Jones J, Workhaven M, Williams B: The psychological control of preoperative anxiety. Psychophysiology 12:50, 1975
36. Wilson SL, Vargin RW, Stephen CR: Awareness, dreams, and hallucinations associated with general anesthesia. Anesth Analg (Cleve) 54:609, 1975
37. Winick L, Robbins GF: Physical and psychologic readjustment after mastectomy: An evaluation of Memorial Hospital's PMRG program. Cancer 39:478, 1977
38. Winkelstein C, Blacker R, Weger B: Psychiatric observations on surgical patients in the recovery room. NY State J Med 65:865, 1965
39. Worden JW, Weisman AD: The fallacy in postmastectomy depression. Am J Med Sci 273:169, 1977

Part Eight

Complications of Genitourinary Surgery and Trauma

51
Complications of Ureteral Surgery and Trauma

Warren W. Koontz, Jr.

OVERVIEW

The ureters are muscular tubes that run from ureteropelvic junction of the kidney to the bladder.[13] The ureter, renal pelvis, and calyces are similar in composition, being made up of an inner transitional cell mucosa, longitudinal and circular muscular fibers, and an outer adventitial or fibrous layer. Peristaltic waves initiated by a bolus of urine move the urine from the ureteropelvic junction into the bladder. The average ureteral length is around 24 cm to 30 cm, depending upon the size of the patient and the distance from the kidney to the bladder. Proximally, the ureter courses immediately up and over (anterior) to the psoas muscle and lateral to the transverse processes. The middle third of the ureter passes posterior to the gonadal vessels (spermatic or ovarian). Distal to this area, the ureter crosses the iliac vessels and lies anterior to the sacroiliac joint. The ureter then courses posterior and laterally following the course of the hypogastric vessels and in close proximity to the walls of the pelvis. In the lower third, the ureter then courses medially toward the bladder, lying anterior to the hypogastric artery and medial to the obturator nerve and vessels. In the male, the ureter crosses the vas defferentia, penetrating the bladder wall posteriorly and above the prostate and seminal vesicles. In the female, the ureter crosses the uterine artery and vein and passes within 1 cm or 2 cm of the uterine cervix, coming in close proximity to the wall of the vagina, and from here enters the base of the bladder. The ureters enter the bladder obliquely by passing through a submucosal tunnel that, when the bladder is filling, prevents vesicoureteral reflux. There are three points of physiologic narrowing of the ureter. These include the ureteropelvic junction, where the ureter crosses the iliac artery, and the intramural portion of the ureterovesical junction.

The arterial blood supply of the ureter is multiple and depends upon the anatomical portion of the ureter. Branches of the renal artery supply the upper third of the ureter and the renal pelvis. Branches from the aorta, iliacs, gonadal, deep hypogastrics, and superior vesical arteries supply the middle third of the ureter. Branches of the uterine, vesical and middle hemorrhoidal arteries supply the lower third of the ureter. There is an apparent plexus of these vessels in the adventitia of the ureter and renal pelvis; hence, interruption of the arterial supply in one area does not ordinarily affect significantly the ureteral blood supply. This explains how one can perform a kidney transplant, remove 12 cm to 16 cm of ureter, and have the newly reimplanted ureter survive when the blood supply is dependent soley upon the renal artery. Venous drainage of the ureter arises from the submucosal and muscular layers and crosses the adventitia where it drains into veins parallel to the arterial supply. Lymphatics accompany the blood vessels and drain into three regional lymph nodes. These are the hypogastric, iliac, and lumbar or periaortic lymph node chain. The nerve supply of the ureter is derived from the autonomic nervous system and accompanies the blood vessels in distribution. An excised portion of the ureter will continue to contract even when deprived of its extrinsic nerve supply.

Anatomical variations of the ureter may occur. The most common variation is duplication. Duplication may be partial, with two ureters leaving the kidney and joining somewhere along the normal anatomical path. The duplication may be complete, with two ureters draining the kidney and emptying separately into the bladder. Duplicated ureters are unique in that the ureter draining the upper renal segment enters the bladder below the orifice of ureter draining the lower renal segment in virtually all instances. Duplicated ureters of the lower third may travel in the same ureteral adventitial sheath with a merging of the muscle bundle and blood supply as the ureter enters the bladder wall.

Ureteral Healing

For ureteral repair to occur, several factors affect epithelialization of the ureteral defect and final healing with no obstruction. These include no tension on the area to be repaired, no urinary leakage, and a mucosa-to-mucosa approximation of the defect, or a longitudinal strip of ureter with bridging of the defect, around which new epithelium can spread to develop a new ureteral lumen. Circumferential scar of the ureter may contract, causing a stricture, hydroureter and hydronephrosis, and possible renal damage.[2]

The ureter has a remarkable ability to close its own defects by regeneration of any or all of its components. In general, the defect is first bridged by transitional cell epithelium, then by fibrous tissue that will contract, pulling already present smooth muscle into the gap. This seemingly stimulates the growth of new smooth muscle in order to complete the repair. Following injury, active transitional cell epithelial proliferation occurs within 3 to 4 days of the creation of the defect. Regeneration of the epithelium is quite rapid since the entire defect may be bridged with a single layer of epithelium within a week to 10 days. Urinary flow across a repair may promote a lumen and stimulate transitional cell and muscle growth; however, newly formed epithelium may also be distracted, and urinary extravasation may lead to reactive fibrosis, stenosis, and obstruction. Adjacent tissue around a ureter in repair is also important. Rigid tissue such as fascia produces a disorderly repair, in which less rigid tissue such as fat allows the ureteral walls to renew with peristaltic activity.

Ureteral healing may be improved by the use of a stenting agent. The use or nonuse of a stenting tube has been argued for many years. The proponents of ureteral stenting believe that the stent will immobilize the ureter until healing has occurred; inhibit the growth of granulation tissue and allow the orderly regrowth of an intact epithelial layer, followed by its muscular covering; prevent the leakage of urine at the anastomotic site; help to maintain an adequate lumen of the ureter during the healing phase; and minimize any tendency to angulation of the ureter.[3,4,23] Other investigators believe that complications may follow the use of stenting catheters and that these outweigh the possible merits. One of the problems associated with stents is an inflammatory stricture and calcification at the site of repair. If the stent slips, angulation, distortion, and poor healing may result. The stent may develop deposits of amorphous phosphate material, causing obstruction with hydroureter and hydronephrosis, as above.

Healing of a ureteral defect may be watertight within 24 to 48 hours. Large defects may take 4 to 6 weeks to epithelialize completely and allow fibrotic tissue and smooth muscle to regenerate without functional obstruction. When a mucosal approximation is done, it should not have a suture through the mucosa, but sutures of small caliber should be used in the adventitia and muscularis to approximate the mucosa.

Methods of Injury

Injuries to the ureter may be surgical for ureteral disease such as stones or tumors. The surgical approach to the ureter must be planned carefully to allow complete healing without obstruction or leakage. Inadvertent injuries to the ureter may also occur at the time of another surgical procedure, characteristically during gynecologic surgery and involving the lower third of the ureter. Other surgery, such as repair of an aortic aneurysm, may also cause injury to the ureter, which may be affected in any portion. Urologists also are not immune to causing inadvertent injury of the ureter, which may be major or minor such as a partial clamping of the wall of the ureter or incisions into the ureter with no loss of tissue.

In addition to surgical injury, external penetrating injuries may affect the ureter. There may be involvement by stabbing or, more likely, a gunshot wound, which is important for the reestablishment of ureteral continuity. The blast effect from a high-velocity projectile may mean that more of the ureter will subsequently be lost than is apparent when first investigated.[9]

Irradiation therapy is being used for a number of abdominal and retroperitoneal tumors, such as those in the cervix, prostate, bladder, or bowel. The etiology of radiation-induced ureteral stricture or damage is poorly understood. Although frequently exposed to high doses of irradiation, the ureter is rarely injured. Ureteral injuries associated with irradiation therapy for carcinoma of the cervix are postulated to be caused by tumor necrosis with subsequent parametrial fibrosis. Localized ischemia has also been proposed as a possible cause of stricture formation.[1]

Blunt injuries of the ureter are rare, usually of the avulsion type, and tend to involve the upper ureter. Extreme hyperextension of the lumbar spine at the moment of impact, especially in children whose spines are extensible, combined with sudden deceleration of the kidney, may result in an avulsion.

The site is usually 1 cm to 2 cm below the ureteropelvic junction. The upper ureter is mobile and flexible and more easily avulsed than the lower end of the ureter, which is more or less immobilized along the pelvic wall.[20]

Injuries of the ureter should be recognized promptly and treated immediately. However, undiagnosed surgical or traumatic injuries may cause unexplained fever, inordinate postoperative pain, leakage of urine from a wound, or anuria, in the case of injury to both ureters or to one ureter in a patient with a solitary kidney. Any of the preceding developments should call for immediate radiographic study, especially excretory urography. Ureteral injury would be suggested by hydronephrosis, extravasation of contrast medium at the site of injury, or no visualization of the offended organ if the ureter has been completely obstructed. Fistula formation may occur both to the skin and, in the female patient who has undergone recent pelvic surgery, to the vagina, resulting in large amounts of urine drained vaginally. The late complication of such an injury is stricture formation, hydroureteronephrosis, and subsequent renal damage.

Signs, Symptoms, and Methods of Diagnosis of Ureteral Injury

The diagnosis of ureteral injury can be made intraoperatively in most cases of surgical damage. The surgeon should suspect ureteral injury if urine appears in the field. On occasion, hemostatic sutures must be placed to control bleeding deep in the pelvis, and ureteral injury may be difficult to discern. An ampule of indigo carmine may be administered intravenously, and the appearance of a blue discoloration as the contrast material is excreted through the laceration will confirm urinary leakage. Ureteral leakage may be ruled out by a catheter inserted preoperatively or by introducing a ureteral catheter cystoscopically or through a cystotomy intraoperatively. The best time to repair a ureteral injury is the time of the injury. The abdominal incision should not be closed until it has been confirmed that no ureteral injury has occurred. In the postoperative period an increase in abdominal pain, abdominal tenderness, a mass, or unexplained fever may occur. The leakage of urine through the vagina or through the surgical wound is an obvious indication of urinary tract injury. The absence of hematuria is not sufficient to exclude a surgical injury to the ureter. Excretory urography is extremely accurate, and the usual findings are extravasation, hydronephrosis, nonvisualization, delayed excretion, and evidence of ureteral narrowing. A retrograde pyelogram may be indicated and indeed may be the definitive diagnostic study to show urinary extravasation or obstruction.

Management

Certain general principles are paramount in the management of ureteral injuries. These include the following:

1. The injured segment should be stented to provide proper alignment of the lumen for healing. The stent may also provide urinary diversion.
2. Urinary diversion is an important aspect of ureteral healing since urine is very irritating. If allowed to remain in the area of a ureteral repair, it will usually cause an increased amount of fibrosis, scarring, and stricture formation. Drainage may be internal by stents or external to allow urine escaping from the repair to drain out and not form a urinoma.
3. There should be adequate débridement of any damaged ureter. This is especially the case in gunshot wounds of high velocity.
4. Any repair or anastomosis of the ureter should be as watertight as possible, but it should be without tension. A ureteral repair under tension will disrupt, extravasate, fibrose and scar and cause obstruction. The repair of the ureter must be tailored to the type and extent of injury, associated injuries, and location of the injury in the ureter.

NEPHRECTOMY

Management of ureteral injury by unilateral nephrectomy should be lowest on the list of options. The presence of a normal kidney and collecting system on the contralateral side may allow a nephrectomy to be performed on the injured side without risk to the patient. Although it solves the problem of the ureteral injury, preservation of renal function should be paramount. Nephrectomy is not appropriate in patients with a solitary kidney or a diseased or injured contralateral renal unit. The removal of a normal renal unit because of a ureteral injury should be limited to patients in whom extensive repair may be harmful because of associated injuries or disease.

Urinary Diversion

Urinary diversion is a temporary means of providing drainage of the kidney and preservation of renal function. It allows any reaction that has occurred at the site of injury to resolve prior to attempted reconstruction. It also may allow the surgeon to extricate a sick patient from a life-threatening situation.

Ureteral Stents

If the injury to the ureter has been minor, a temporary indwelling ureteral stent may be passed cystoscopically. If only a few days of drainage are necessary, then the standard ureteral catheter may be passed cystoscopically into the renal pelvis. This catheter would then be brought to the outside, through the urethra, and a closed-drainage system applied. The catheter is held in place by the passage of a urethral Foley catheter into the bladder to which the ureteral catheter can then be attached. This method of drainage is adequate for 5 to 7 days but may be used as long as 10 days. The problems with this technique are dislodgement of the ureteral catheter, due to the patient's movement, and the higher incidence of urinary infection associated with any external catheter.

This technique has been modified by the use of indwelling ureteral stents. There are two types available: First is the Gibbons stent, which is made of soft silicone and may be passed up the ureter. It is constructed so that it will not migrate up or down.[6] Second, the double pigtail stent is passed into the collecting system over a guidewire, and then, when the wire is removed, a coil results in the renal pelvis and in the bladder (Fig. 51-1).[7] The small coils stabilize the stent and allow it to be left in place from 4 to 6 weeks before either removal or replacement. Painful bladder spasms may occur because of the intravesical protrusion of these stents, and vesicoureteropelvic reflux may occur because the stents have no antireflux mechanism. This factor allows a check on the patency of the catheter by noticing whether or not reflux occurs as revealed on cystogram.

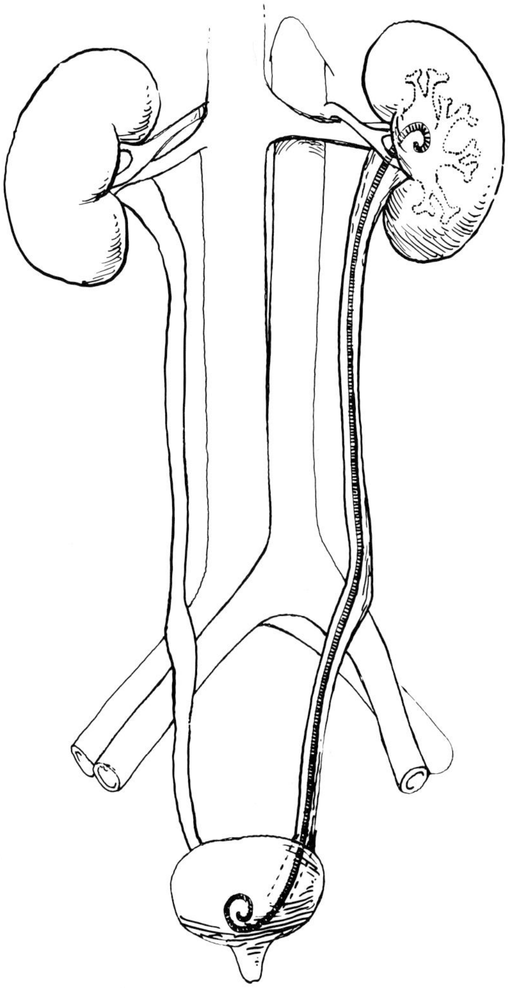

FIG. 51-1. A double pigtail ureteral stent has been placed in the left ureter with the coiled tips at each end to prevent migration.

Nephrostomy

Temporary or permanent urinary diversion may be accomplished by indwelling nephrostomy drainage. The technique is percutaneous radiographic or ultrasound methods of localizing the dilated renal pelvis in order to place a needle, followed by a guidewire, and then an indwelling catheter. The nephrostomy tract may then be dilated gently to an appropriate size of No. 16 to 18 French.[17]

Surgical exposure of the kidney through a flank incision, usually subcostal, may be utilized for the placement of a straight Foley or Malecot catheter (Fig. 51-2). An alternative is the use of the loop nephrostomy (Fig. 51-3), which is a continuous catheter that runs through the parenchyma of the kidney in two places with openings in the area of the renal pelvis. Since both ends of the loop nephrostomy come outside, it is much easier to change this type of catheter than the straight catheter.[22] If a satisfactory tract is formed, the straight catheter can be changed with ease. If the tract has not formed with a thick wall, then the replacement of a straight catheter may become difficult or impossible. The replacement loop nephrostomy catheter can be sewn onto the old one and the new one pulled through. It is easier to utilize a loop nephrostomy for semipermanent or permanent forms of urinary diversion. This form of diversion is utilized often in ureteral injury or trauma to allow healing of the area of injury so that a primary or secondary repair can be accomplished.

URETERAL REPAIR

Figures 51-4 through 51-8 reflect methods of primary repair of ureteral injuries. Figure 51-4 is a direct ureteral anastomosis. This is best accomplished in

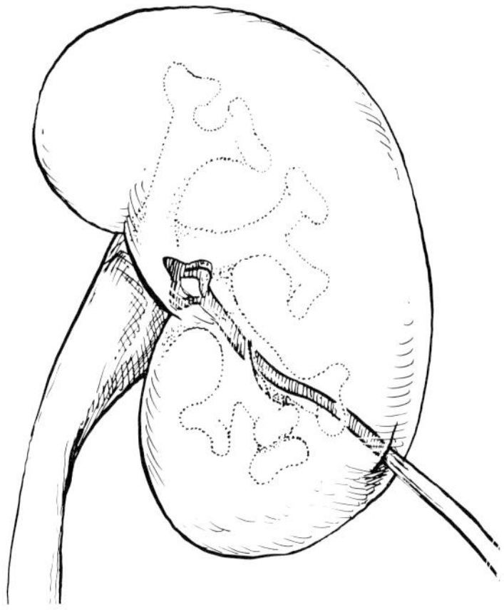

FIG. 51-2. A straight malecot nephrostomy tube has been placed through the renal parenchyma and into the renal pelvis for temporary urinary drainage.

FIG. 51-3. A loop nephrostomy (circle nephrostomy) is easier to change and maintain if nephrostomy drainage is required for a prolonged period of time.

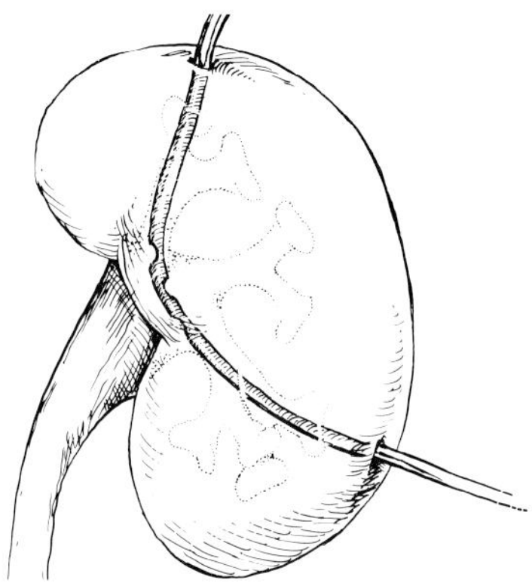

FIG. 51-4. A ureteroureterostomy is usually in the middle or upper third of the ureter.

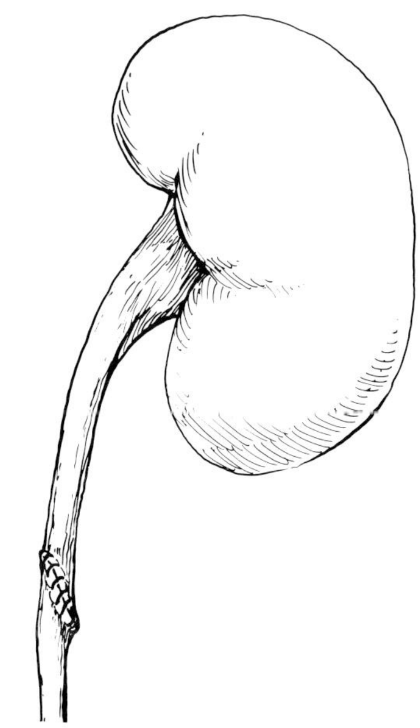

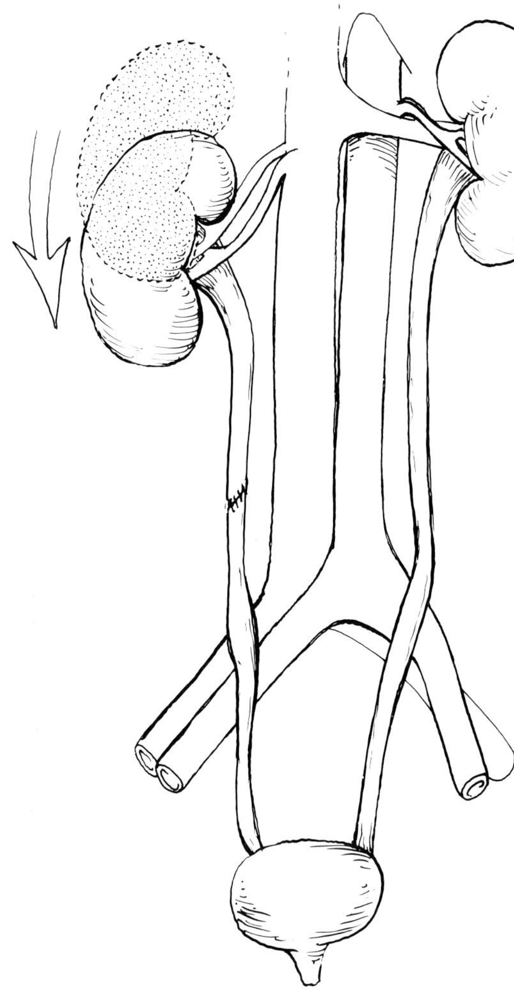

FIG. 51-5. To remove tension from a ureteral anastomosis, in selected cases, the kidney may be mobilized and moved downward.

lesions of the upper and middle ureter and may be used in the lower one third of the ureter if it is not too close to the ureterovesical junction. Both ends must have satisfactory blood supply; there must be débridement of any tissue that is not healthy, and the anastomosis should be done on an angle so that it will be as large as possible.[18] Repair should be done with interrupted sutures of absorbable material. A most important rule to follow in performing a ureteroureterostomy is that there must be no tension on the anastomotic site. Tension on the anastomosis will cause disruption, leakage, and failure of the repair. There are a number of ways in which tension on the anastomosis can be relieved. Figure 51-5 demonstrates that a kidney may be freed from all of its surrounding attachments and displaced downward on its blood vessels. This will allow the upper ureter to descend and in selected cases may be of benefit in a ureteroureterostomy.[15] When a ureteroureterostomy has been performed, I believe that it is important to utilize urinary diversion. This may

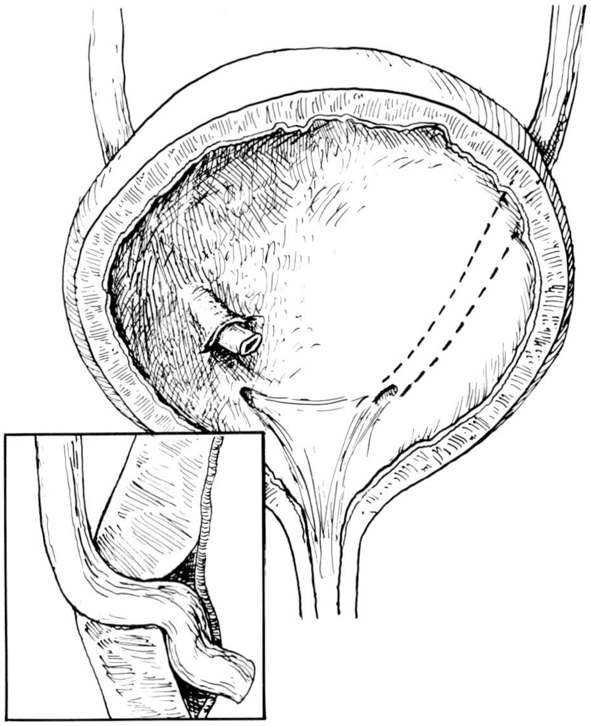

FIG. 51-6. The submucosal tunnel has been created for a ureteroneocystostomy.

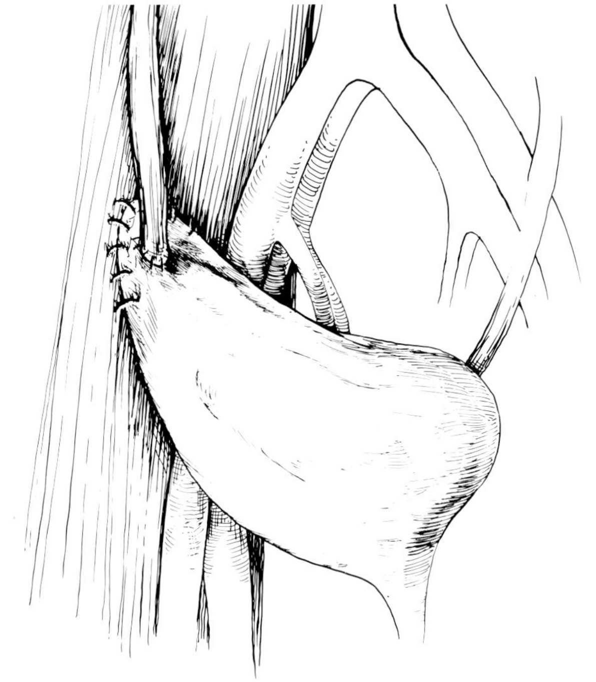

FIG. 51-7. In selected cases with absence of a portion of the lower ureter, the bladder may be mobilized and fixed to the psoas muscle.

be by means of an indwelling ureteral stent that can be removed through the bladder at 10 to 14 days or by using nephrostomy or ureterostomy drainage.

Figure 51-6 demonstrates a ureteroneocystostomy or ureteral reimplantation. If an injury has occurred to the lower ureter just above the bladder level, there may be enough ureter remaining so that the ureter can be reimplanted into the bladder. If the lower ureter has been injured and the anastomosis and reimplant cannot be performed without tension, Figures 51-7 and 51-8 demonstrate two methods in which a ureteral reimplant may be performed. In Figure 51-7, the bladder is mobilized partially and pulled over to the side of the injury. Here a portion of the ureter can be sewn to the psoas muscle belly lateral to the iliac vessels to stabilize the bladder in this area, allowing the ureter to be reimplanted without tension.[5,16] Figure 51-8 demonstrates a technique in which a flap of bladder is elevated, allowing the ureter to be reimplanted.[12]

Figures 51-9 through 51-11 demonstrate methods of restoring ureteral continuity when a large amount of ureteral length has been lost. Figure 51-9 demonstrates a transureteroureterostomy. Here, the upper portion of the ureter may be swung across anterior to the great vessels and an end-to-side transureteroureterostomy performed. The danger from this procedure is that the contralateral normal side may be damaged.[8]

Figure 51-10 demonstrates that a segment of small intestine may be utilized to substitute for a large loss of ureteral continuity.[11] Indeed this technique may be used to bridge a defect in the ureter all the way from the renal pelvis to the bladder. It may be used for bilateral defects as well. Small bowel, usually distal ileum with its mesentery intact, may be utilized as is or an incision made on the antimesenteric side, the same size as the normal caliber of the ureter. Such repairs are time consuming, and temporary urinary diversion with drainage of the anastomosis is mandatory.

Figure 51-11 demonstrates an autotransplant.[10] This technique may be utilized when the ureter is very short, and the kidney can be moved downward into the iliac fossa. Because of the vessel anatomy, it may be easier for the surgeon to take the right kidney and place it in the left iliac fossa or the left kidney into the right iliac fossa.

PERMANENT URINARY DIVERSION

Figures 51-12 and 51-13 reveal two common methods of permanent urinary diversion that may be utilized in patients who have a ureteral injury. Permanent urinary diversion should be avoided, if at all possible, owing to long-term sequelae such as pyelonephritis, stone formation, hydronephrosis, and renal failure. Figure 51-12 depicts a method of cu-

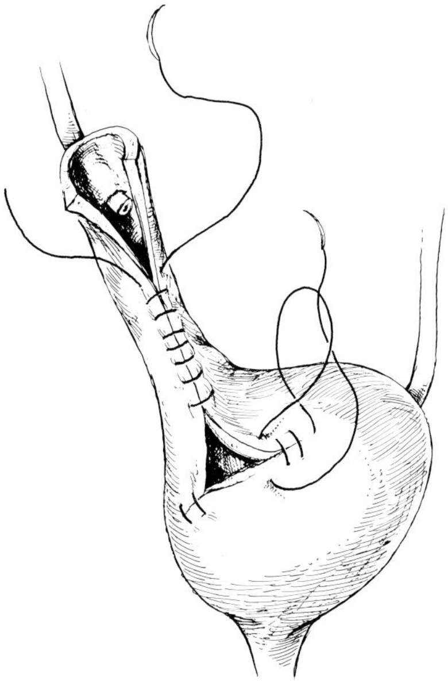

FIG. 51-8. With a large bladder and a defect in the lower ureter, a flap of bladder may be utilized to bridge a defect.

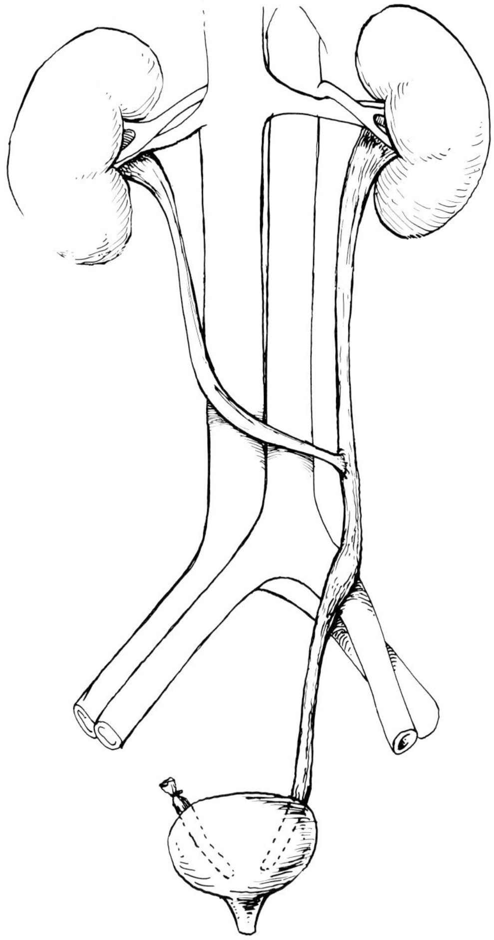

FIG. 51-9. For middle and some upper-third ureteral lesions, a transureteroureterostomy may be performed.

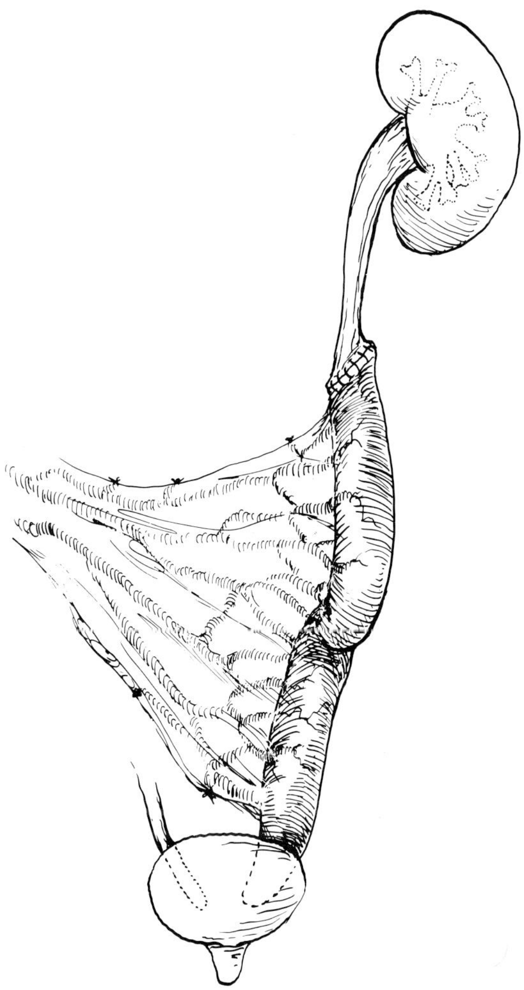

FIG. 51-10. Large defects in the ureter may be bridged by the utilization of an intestinal segment. This may be short or indeed may run from the renal pelvis to the bladder.

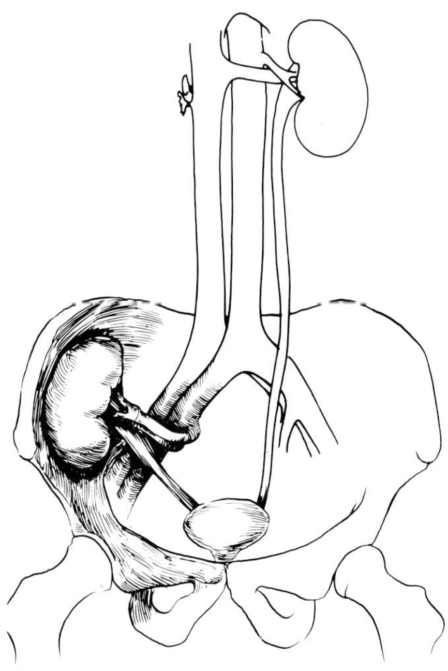

FIG. 51-11. If only a small portion of the upper ureter is remaining, the kidney may be autotransplanted into the ileac fossa.

taneous ureterostomy that is simple and easy to perform and with a low postoperative mortality.[14, 21] However, a major complication is stenosis of the cutaneous ureterostomy. It is difficult to free enough ureter to reach to the skin, form a stoma, and be in a location that is easily managed by an external appliance. The blood supply to the ureter must be excellent, and indeed the anastomosis to the skin must be as large an opening as possible. The method more widely used for permanant diversion is the use of intestine, usually small bowel (but possibly large bowel), to make a conduit to the lower abdominal wall (Fig. 51-13).[19] The ileal conduit or sigmoid conduit seems to be the best method of permanent urinary diversion. However, the technique of undiversion or utilizing the small intestine to bridge the gap into the bladder is preferable when the bladder is normal.

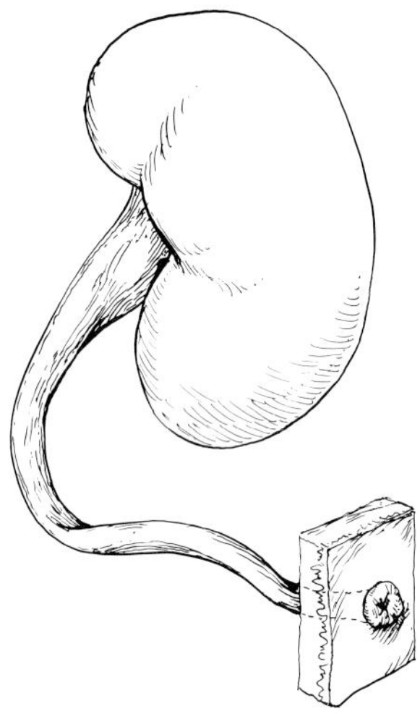

FIG. 51-12. Permanent urinary diversion may be by means of a cutaneous ureterostomy.

FIG. 51-13. The use of an intestinal segment, be it small bowel or large bowel, has fewer complications than the cutaneous ureterostomy, which should be utilized only in selected cases.

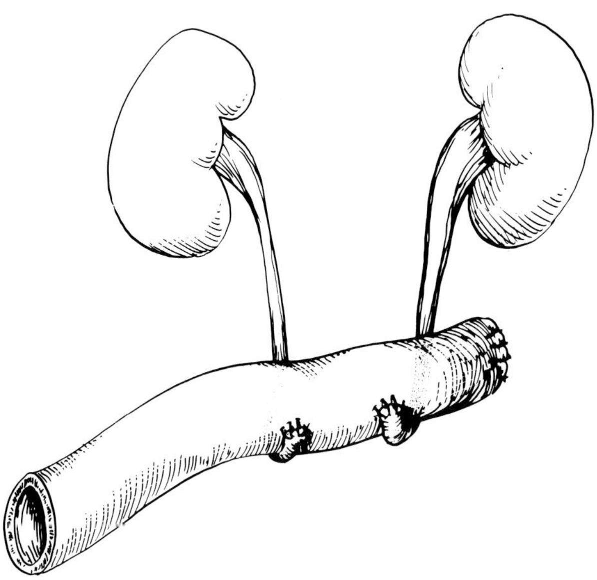

References

1. Alfert HJ, Gillenwater JY: The consequences of ureteral irradiation with special reference to subsequent ureteral injury. J Urol 107:369, 1972
2. Bergman H: The Ureter. New York, Hoeber Medical Division, Harper & Row, 1967
3. Boyarsky S: Ureteral surgery. In Glenn J (ed): Urologic Surgery. Hagerstown, Harper & Row, 1975
4. Carlton CE: Injuries to the kidney and ureter. In Campbell's Urology, 2nd ed, vol 1. Philadelphia, WB Saunders, 1978
5. Ehrlich RM, Melman A, Skinner DG: The use of vesicopsoas hitch in urologic surgery. J Urol 119:322, 1978
6. Gibbons RP, Correa RJ Jr, Cummings KB: Experience with indwelling ureteral stent catheter. J Urol 115:22, 1976
7. Hepperlen TW, Mardis HK, Kammandel H: The pigtail ureteral stent in the cancer patient. J Urol 121:17, 1979
8. Hodges CV, Moore RJ, Lehman TH, Behman AM: Clinical experience with transureteroureterostomy. J Urol 90:552, 1963
9. Lucy DT, Smith MJV, Koontz WW Jr: Modern trends in the management of urologic trauma. J Urol 107:641, 1972
10. Marshall VF, Whitsell J, McGovern JH, Miscall BG: The practicality of normal autotransplantation in humans. JAMA 196:1154, 1966
11. Morales DA, Askari S, Hotchkiss RS: Ileal replacement of the ureter. J Urol 82:304, 1959
12. Ockerblad MF: Reimplantation of the ureter into the bladder by a flap method. J Urol 57:845, 1947
13. Orkin L: Trauma to the Ureter. Philadelphia, FA Davis, 1964
14. Persky L, Hoch WH, Kursh ED: Surgical management of the ureter. In Campbell's Urology, 4th ed, vol 3. Philadelphia, WB Saunders, 1978
15. Popescu C: The surgical management of postoperative ureteral fistula. Surg Gynecol Obstet 119:1079, 1964
16. Prout GR Jr, Koontz WW Jr: Partial vesical immobilization: An important adjunct to ureteroneocystostomy. J Urol 103:147, 1970
17. Rutner AB, Fucilla IS: Percutaneous pigtail nephrostomy. Urology 14:337, 1979
18. Salvatierra O Jr, Bucklew WB, Morrow JW: Penetrating ureteral injuries. Surg Gyneol Obstet 119:1079, 1964
19. Skinner DG, Richie JP: Ureterointestinal diversion. In Campbell's Urology, 4th ed, vol 3. Philadelphia, WB Saunders, 1978
20. Stone HH, Jones HQ: Penetrating and non-penetrating injuries to the ureter. Surg Gynecol Obstet 114:52, 1962
21. Straffon RB, Kyle K, Corvalan J: Techniques of cutaneous ureterostomy and results in 51 patients. J Urol 103:138, 1970
22. Tressider GC: Nephrostomy. Br J Urol 29:130, 1957
23. Young JD Jr: Trauma to the kidney and ureter. In Karafin and Kendall (eds): Urology. Hagerstown, Harper & Row, 1978

52
Complications of Urethral and Penile Trauma

Robert H. Hackler

Urethral Injuries

OVERVIEW—ANATOMY

Sustaining a urethral injury, while not necessarily life threatening, often results in significant morbidity. Proper handling of the initial injury is vital to reducing long-term disability. This discussion is divided into injuries below the urogenital diaphragm (anterior urethra) and injuries at or above the diaphragm (prostatomembranous urethra).

The anterior urethra traverses the corpus spongiosum from the inferior fascia of the urogenital diaphragm proximally to the urethral meatus (Fig. 52-1). It is divided into the pendulous urethra distally and the bulbous urethra proximally, with the division being the attachment of the suspensory ligament. The posterior urethra extends from the urogenital diaphragm to the bladder neck. The membranous urethra is firmly fixed within the urogenital diaphragm, and the prostatic urethra extends from the superior fascia of the urogenital diaphragm to the vesical neck.

Fascial layers dictate the directional and limiting factors in the extravasation of blood and urine following extensive injury to the anterior urethra. Buck's fascia covers the erectile bodies (corpora cavernosum and corpora spongiosum) and ends distally at the inferior fascia of the urogenital diaphragm, where it fuses with Colles' fascia (see Fig. 52-1).

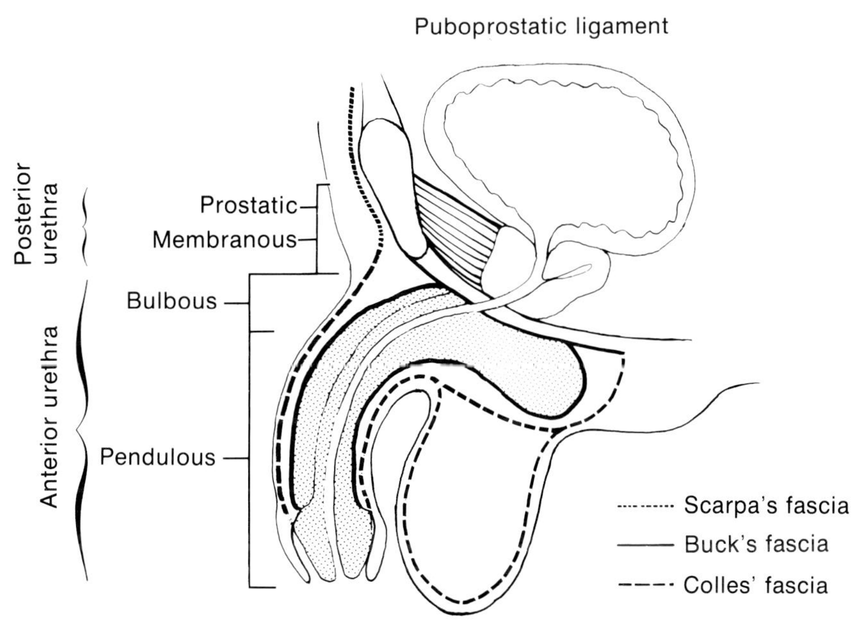

FIG. 52-1. Normal anatomy of the genitourinary tract.

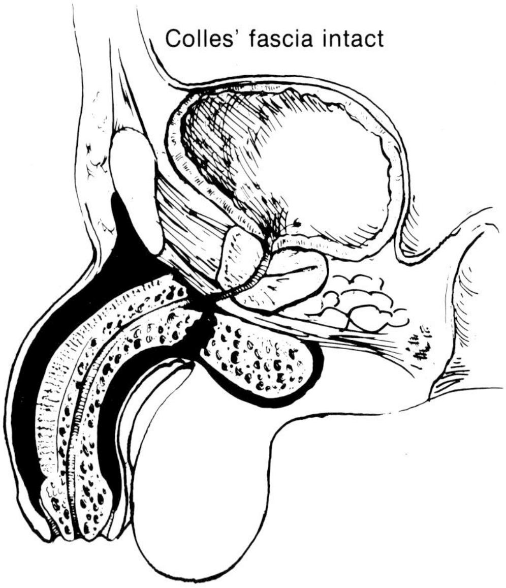

FIG. 52-2. In anterior urethral rupture, extravasation is limited to the penile shaft when Buck's fascia remains intact.

Rupture of the pendulous or bulbous urethra that fails to disrupt Buck's fascia limits the urine extravasation to the subcutaneous tissue of the penis (Figs. 52-2 and 52-3). Colles' fascia is the inferior extension of Scarpa's fascia and makes up part of the inferior fascia of the urogenital diaphragm. This fascia continues as dartos fascia of the scrotum and penis and attaches to the fascia lata of the thigh. Thus, injury to the anterior urethra that disrupts Buck's fascia is then confined within Colles' fascia, resulting in extravasation along the shaft of the penis, scrotum, and perineum (Fig. 52-4). It can gradually proceed anteriorly and superiorly to the axilla. Colles' fascia resists penetration of urine into the pelvis, thigh, and ischiorectal and perianal areas (anal triangle; Fig. 52-5).

INJURIES TO THE ANTERIOR URETHRA

Etiology

Most injuries to the anterior urethra are iatrogenic secondary to overzealous manipulation of endoscopic instruments or urethral catheters. This injury most commonly occurs in the bulbous urethra. Other causes of anterior urethral disruption are gunshot wounds, straddle injuries, and self-manipulation.

Diagnosis

Most minor injuries to the anterior urethra (contusion) are iatrogenic, resulting in disruption of the mucosa associated with minimal extravasation into

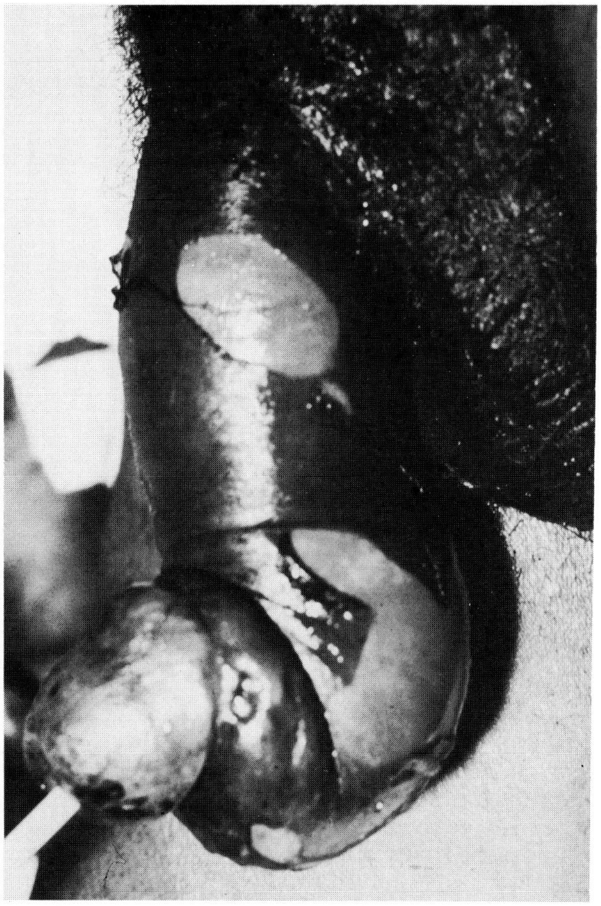

FIG. 52-3. Rupture of the anterior urethra with extravasation limited within Buck's fascia.

FIG. 52-4. Extravasation is limited within Colles' fascia in disruption of the anterior urethra and Buck's fascia.

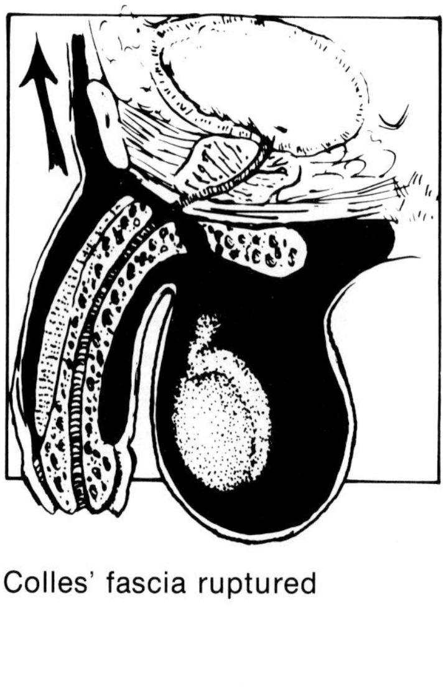

the corpus spongiosum (Fig. 52-6). This should be suspected by the physician for the catheter will not traverse the entire urethra or blood is noted in the urethral meatus. Retrograde urethrograms are contraindicated in this type of injury because of the risk of introducing bacteria into the vascular corpus spongiosum.

In more serious injuries to the urethra, the first diagnostic procedure should be a retrograde urethrogram performed in a sterile manner with the patient in the oblique position (Fig. 52-7). Since some contrast materials produce a sclerosing effect, the iodine solution should be diluted and in a water-soluble base. The urethrogram will differentiate between a partial and a complete disruption of the urethra, and this is extremely important for proper management. Passage of a urethral catheter should be condemned because entrance into the bladder does not exclude a partial urethral injury, further

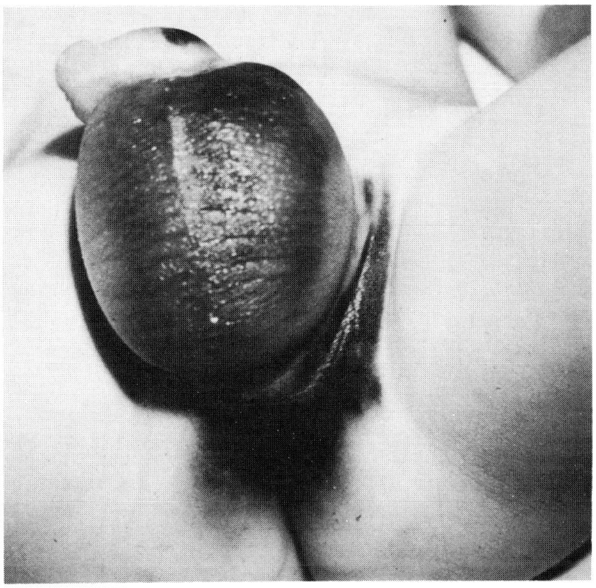

FIG. 52-5. Disruption of Colles' fascia allows extravasation along the penile shaft, scrotum, and perineum.

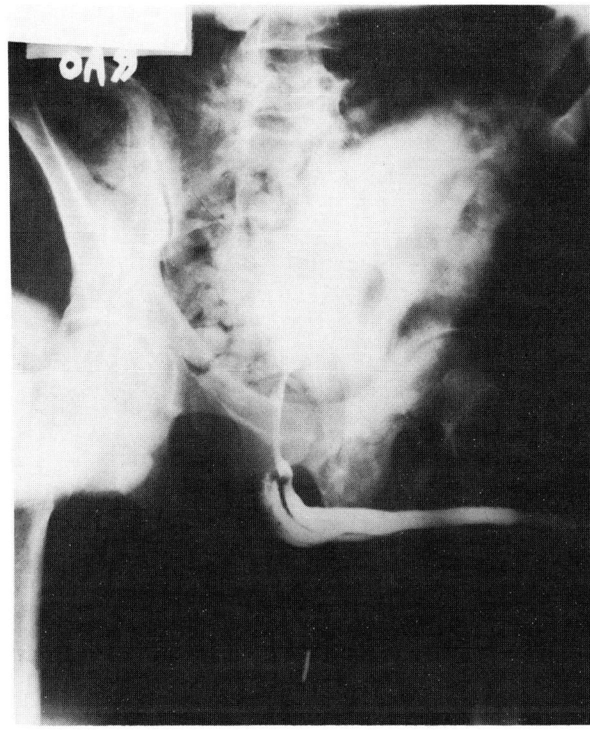

FIG. 52-6. Anterior urethral injury with extravasation into corpus spongiosum.

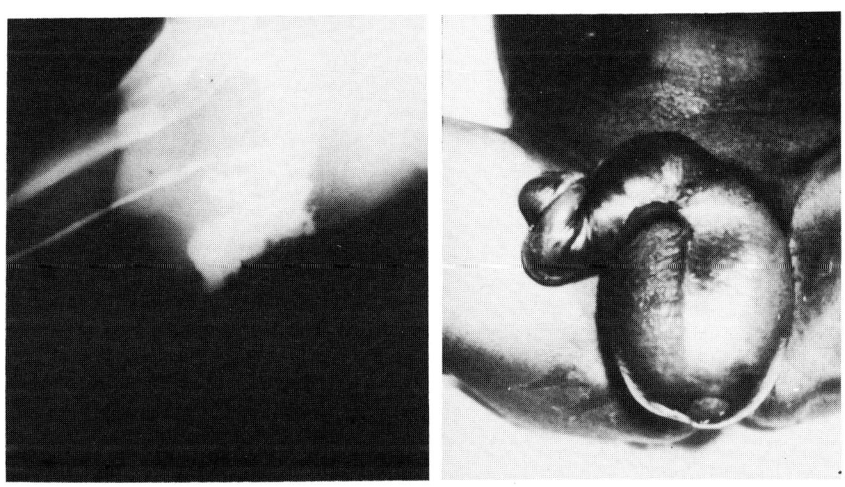

FIG. 52-7. Retrograde urethrogram (*left*) shows urethral disruption through Colles' fascia. (*Right*) Clinical appearance.

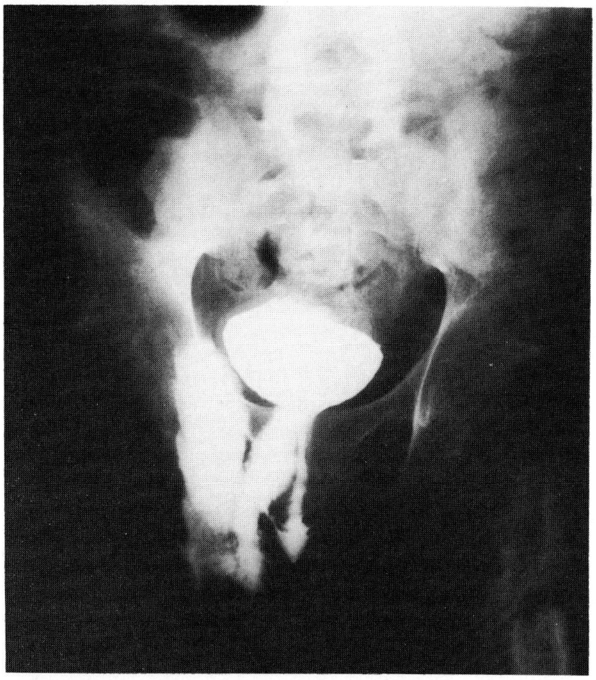

FIG. 52-8. Significant extravasation requires extensive drainage as well as suprapubic cystostomy.

damage to a partial injury is certain, and infection may be introduced. Unfortunately, many patients with urethral trauma are immediately catheterized after reaching the emergency room. In that situation, the catheter should not be removed if the cystogram shows proper placement within the bladder lumen. In order to determine the condition of the urethra, a small angiocath can be passed along the Foley catheter in order to perform a modified retrograde urethrogram.

Treatment

Minor injuries to the anterior urethra can usually be managed conservatively and without intraurethral catheterization. The patient needs close observation for sepsis, local signs of subsequent extravasation, and urinary retention. These minor injuries do not involve the entire circumference of the urethra and therefore rarely result in stricture formation. If a Foley catheter is in place, continued stenting should be maintained for several days.

Management of the more serious anterior urethral injury is predicated on the degree of urethral disruption and the amount of extravasation. If the retrograde urethrogram shows only partial disruption and physical examination reveals minimal extravasation still confined within Buck's fascia, then simple suprapubic cystostomy will suffice. Significant extravasation confined within Colles' fascia and associated with only partial disruption requires immediate drainage along with suprapubic cystostomy (Fig. 52-8). These partially disrupted urethras usually heal without stricture formation, especially if the urine extravasation is adequately evacuated.[18] If a urethral catheter is in place and draining clear urine, signifying only partial disruption, then no further therapy is necessary. The catheter should be of small diameter (less than No. 16 French) so as not to obstruct the free drainage of urethral secretions as well as tissue exudates from the damaged urethra.

Total disruption of the urethra requires immediate incision and drainage of the extensive perineal hematoma and urinary extravasation. The proper handling of the disrupted urethra is controversial. Several techniques are described according to personal experiences and philosophies. Some who believe that primary urethral repair at the time of injury could aggravate the problem recommend placing a suprapubic cystostomy and later correcting any urethral problems such as stricture.[14] This approach is certainly best for the surgeon inexperienced in perineal surgery. Another approach is marsupialization of both ends of the urethra to the skin. This is a safe approach, especially when tissue viability of the injured urethra cannot be determined.[11] Several months later, a second stage urethroplasty should successfully reconstitute the urethra. Direct end-to-end anastomosis is a third alternative. This procedure should be reserved for a urethral defect less than 1½ cm in length in order to effect an anastomosis without tension.[9] All devitalized urethra must be débrided and the urethra spatulated and then reapproximated over a No. 24-French catheter using 4-0 chromic catgut. After completion of the anastomosis, a No. 14- to 16-French Foley catheter is inserted for approximately 14 days. If there is any question of tension at the anastomotic site, then suprapubic cystostomy would be indicated.

In infants and small children with severe disruption of the anterior or posterior urethra, cutaneous vesicostomy is an acceptable method for bladder drainage.[3] It is easily accomplished in this age group owing to the intra-abdominal position of the bladder. All foreign materials (suprapubic cystostomy, intraurethral catheters) are eliminated, thus reducing infection, and the constant danger of the suprapubic cystostomy tube becoming malplaced is removed.

INJURIES TO THE PROSTATOMEMBRANOUS URETHRA

Etiology

Injury to the prostatomembranous urethra usually follows violent external force that separates the prostate from its attachments to the urogenital diaphragm and the puboprostatic ligaments (Fig. 52-9). Over

90% of these injuries are associated with a pelvic fracture; however, only about 10% of male patients with pelvic fractures have significant urethral injury. Approximately 13% will have accompanying bladder disruption.[11] In the female, pelvic fractures commonly result in bladder rupture but rarely cause urethral injury.[2]

Rarely gunshot wounds injure the posterior urethra, and perineal dissection associated with abdominoperineal surgery for colon cancer has resulted in urethral disruption.

Diagnosis

Patients with pelvic fractures need immediate evaluation of the urethra and bladder, especially if there is hematuria, blood dripping from the urethral meatus (urethral milking might be necessary to elucidate this sign), inability to urinate, and bladder distention. Often, urinary extravasation is minimal owing to a competent bladder neck, and a massive retroperitoneal hematoma is undetected behind the intact urogenital diaphragm. In complete ruptures, the prostate dislocates superiorly, but findings on rectal examination may be equivocal owing to the large retroperitoneal hematoma.

Following stabilization of the patient's vital signs, an immediate intravenous pyelogram is indicated. This will identify any upper urinary tract injury, and the delayed films may reveal the typical teardrop deformity of the bladder consistent with massive pelvic hematoma. Also, elevation of the bladder base is consistent with total disruption of the membranous urethra. A retrograde urethrogram is then indicated in order to determine the extent of the urethral injury (Fig. 52-10). As previously stated, urethral catheterization is inadvisable because inexpert continued manipulation often risks compounding the injury.

FIG. 52-9. Disruption of the prostatomembranous urethra allows extravasation into the retroperitoneal space.

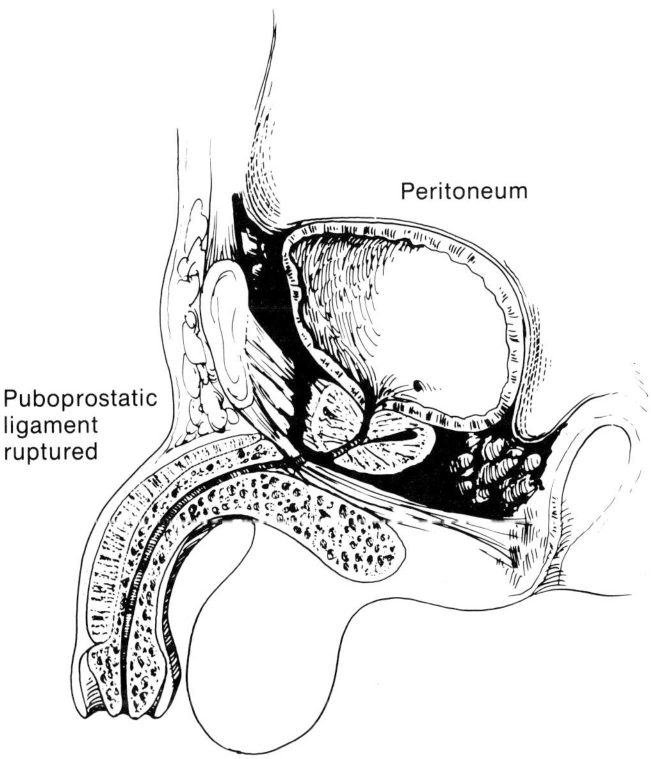

FIG. 52-10. Catheter in the retroperitoneal space. The initial diagnostic procedure for a patient with suspected urethral injury should have been a retrograde urethrogram.

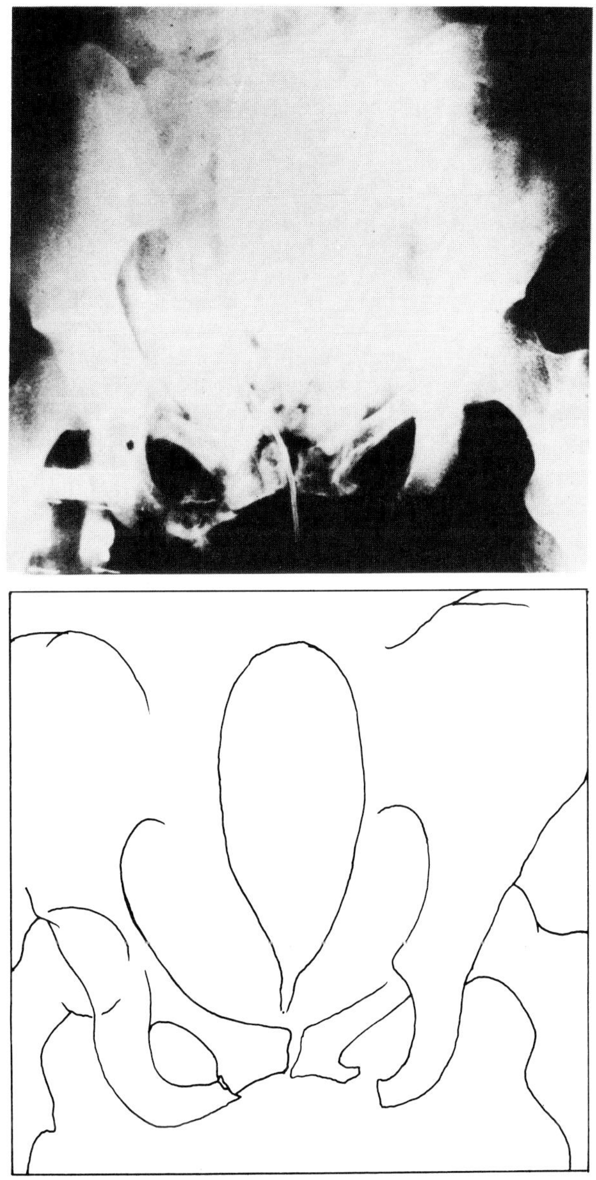

Complications

The development of urethral strictures following severe urethral trauma is serious and represents a major long-term disability. The incidence of impotency is also significant, especially if the injury is mishandled surgically. Incontinence is usually not a major problem, even though there may be significant damage to the external sphincter mechanism, because the bladder neck area remains competent and should preserve urinary control.

Treatment

The immediate concern following massive trauma is to preserve life. Many of these patients with pelvic trauma have associated life-threatening intracranial, intrathoracic, or intra-abdominal injuries. However, the urologic management is not a low priority because often the initial injuries are forgotten and the patient is left with a long-term urologic disability.

Incomplete injuries of the membranous urethra with no dislocation of the prostate should be treated by simple suprapubic cystostomy. Many of these patients do not develop strictures or impotency. If a stricture does develop, it is usually minimal and can often be treated with an occasional dilatation. The more severe stricture is usually short and easily repaired by a one-stage operation 3 to 6 months later.

Currently the proper management of the totally disrupted prostatomembranous urethra is highly controversial, confusing most urologists. The problem is whether to perform urethral realignment over a Foley catheter accompanied by suprapubic cystostomy drainage or a simple suprapubic cystostomy. It is difficult to determine the best method, because most reported series are small (the injury is uncommon) and many fail to differentiate adequately complete from incomplete lesions. This produces imprecise data on the incidence of postoperative stricture and especially impotence.

The time-honored and still the most commonly used procedure consists of suprapubic cystostomy and realignment of the urethra over an intraurethral catheter.[8, 10, 15, 19] Many urologic textbooks include excellent descriptions of the technique.[3, 14] There should be minimal pelvic dissection in order to prevent massive hemorrhage by release of the tamponaded pelvic hematoma. Some maintain the new position of the prostate apex to the membranous urethra by gentle traction on the Foley catheter balloon. They believe that the use of anchoring sutures from the lateral apex of the prostate to the perineal skin in order to anchor the urethra produces malalignment and subsequent obstruction.[10] Others maintain that constant traction on the bladder neck with a Foley catheter balloon may produce bladder neck incompetence, leading to incontinence.[19]

The long-term complication rate in many series from this realignment procedure has been significant, with approximately 80% developing strictures and greater than 35%, impotence.[1, 3, 5-7, 12, 16, 17, 20] However, the advocates of this procedure point that whereas simple suprapubic cystostomy always results in stricture formation requiring further surgery, the realignment procedure does not necessarily lead to strictures or may result in a stricture of such caliber that periodic dilatation suffices. To support this view, DeWeerd reported six strictures in 22 patients with only two requiring subsequent urethroplasty, and Crasswellar and colleagues encountered only approximately 35% of patients with strictures that necessitated further surgery.[8, 10] Some indirect evidence suggests that retropubic dissection in order to perform the realignment procedure significantly increases the impotency rate.[7, 16, 17] However, Crasweller and colleagues believe that the impotency is due to the extent of the injury rather than being secondary to surgical pelvic dissection.

Simple suprapubic cystostomy without any manipulation of the retropubic space was introduced by Johanson and popularized by Morehouse and associates.[16] The advocates of simple suprapubic cystostomy accept the inevitability of stricture formation but point to five major advantages: (1) the impotency rate is extremely low; (2) it is impossible to complete an undiagnosed incomplete rupture inadvertently; (3) it prevents infecting the hematoma, which would lead to extensive periureteral fibrosis and subsequent dense, complex strictures; (4) it prevents hemorrhage by manipulation within a previous tamponaded hematoma; and (5) it eliminates complications of a long-term urethral catheter such as urethritis, prostatitis, and epididymitis.[7, 13, 17] This procedure allows the prostate to descend to the urogenital diaphragm as the pelvic hematoma resolves and results in a simple, short stricture. This should result in a higher success rate some 3 to 6 months later when the stricture is corrected with urethroplasty.

Injuries to the Penis

OVERVIEW—ANATOMY

Penile injury is rare owing to its guarded anatomical position and mobility. Injury to the internal structures of the penis are usually caused by penetrating missiles, while avulsing power takeoff injuries result in loss of skin. Strangulation of the penis is due to constricting objects (rings, nuts, strings) and eventually leads to necrosis. Blunt trauma usually occurs in the penile erect state during intercourse and ruptures the tunica albuginea of the corpus cavernosum. Last, total amputation of the penis is rare and often self-inflicted.

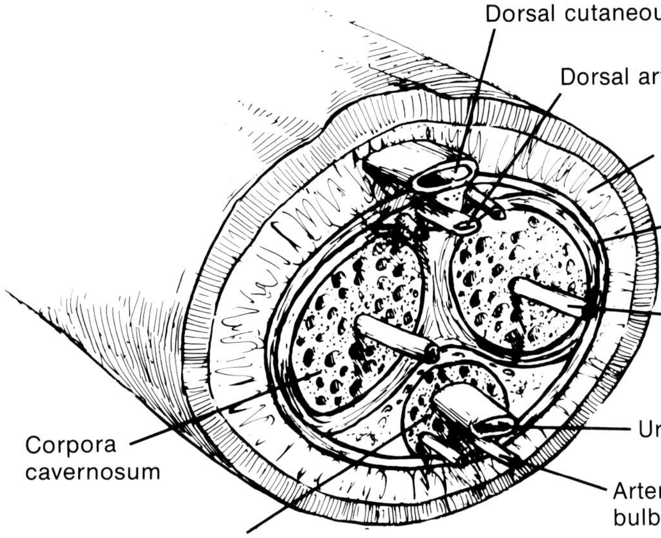

FIG. 52-11. Normal anatomy of the penis.

The paired corpora cavernosa and the corpora spongiosum (with the enclosed urethra) make up the main structures of the penis. The corpus cavernosum is enclosed within the sturdy tunica albuginea, and all three corpora bodies are covered by Buck's fascia (Fig. 52-11).

DIAGNOSIS

Physical examination usually reveals the extent of injury. Extravasation of blood localized to the penis signifies an intact Buck's fascia. Retrograde urethrography is needed if urethral injury is suspected. If Buck's fascia has been disrupted, then the extravasation of blood and urine will extend within the Colles' fascia attachments.

TREATMENT

Injuries that avulse the penile skin need total removal of all skin distally to 0.5 cm from the glans penis. This allows for split-thickness skin grafting from the defect to the coronal sulcus, thus preventing lymphedema.[4]

Injuries that rupture the corpus cavernosum need immediate exploration. Satisfactory exposure is afforded by incising the skin 360° at the coronal sulcus (circumcision incision), thereby allowing total retraction of the skin back to the penile base. The hematoma is evacuated, and any significant injury to the corpus cavernosum is repaired with 3-0 permanent suture. A urethral injury is easily detected and corrected.

Total amputation of the penis needs microvascular surgery if all vital structures are to survive.[9] Simple reanastomosis of the corpora bodies, urethra, and skin leads to necrosis of the glans penis and the skin, even though the corpus cavernosum usually survives. The amputated penis should be cleansed, kept in a sterile container, and chilled. Microscopic reanastomosis is performed to at least one of the dorsal arteries, the deep dorsal vein, and the superficial dorsal vein.

References

1. Allen TA: The transpubic approach for strictures of the posterior urethra superior to the urogenital diaphragm. Urol Clin North Am 4(1): 95, 1977
2. Bredael JJ, Kramer SA, Cleeve LK, Webster GA: Traumatic rupture of the female urethra. J Urol 122:560, 1979
3. Bright TC III, Peters PC: Injuries to the bladder and urethra. In Harrison JH, Gittes RF, Perlmutter AD, Stamey TA, Walsh PC (eds): Campbell's Urology, 4th ed, pp 906-930. Philadelphia, WB Saunders, 1978
4. Bright TC III, Peters PC: Injuries to the external genitalia. In Harrison JH, Gittes RF, Perlmutter AD, Stamey TA, Walsh PC (eds): Campbell's Urology, 4th ed, pp 931-945. Philadelphia, WB Saunders, 1978
5. Cass AS, Godec CJ: Urethral injury due to external trauma. Urology 11:607, 1978
6. Chambers HL, Balfour J: The incidence of impotency following pelvic fracture with associated urinary tract injury. J Urol 89:702, 1963
7. Coffield KS, Weems WL: Experience with management of posterior urethral injury associated with pelvic fracture. J Urol 117:722, 1977
8. Crassweller PO, Farrow GA, Robson CJ et al: Traumatic rupture of the supramembranous urethra. J Urol 118:770, 1977
9. Devine CJ, Devine PC, Horton CE: Anterior urethral injury: Etiology, diagnosis and initial management. Urol Clin North Am 4(1):125, 1977

10. DeWeerd JH: Immediate realignment of posterior urethral injury. Urol Clin North Am 4(1):75, 1977
11. Frick J, Schulman CL, Marberger H, Turner–Warwick R: Traumatic lesion of the urethra: Immediate and delayed treatment. Eur Urol 1:3, 1975
12. Gibson GS: Urological management and complications of fractured pelvis and ruptured urethra. J Urol 111:353, 1974
13. Grassberg KI, Kassner EG, Haller JO, Waterhouse K: The radiographic approach to injuries of the prostatomembranous urethra in children. J Urol 122:678, 1979
14. MacKinnon KJ: Lower urinary tract trauma. In Glenn JF, Boyce WH (eds): Urologic Surgery, 2nd ed, pp 688-696. Hagerstown, Harper & Row, 1975
15. Malek RS, O'Dea MJ, Kelalis PP: Management of ruptured posterior urethra in childhood. J Urol 117:105, 1977
16. Morehouse DD, Belitsky P, MacKinnon K: Rupture of the posterior urethra. J Urol 107:255, 1972
17. Morehouse DD, MacKinnon K: Posterior urethral injury: Etiology, diagnosis, initial management. Urol Clin North Am 4(1):69, 1977
18. Singh M, Blandy JP: The pathology of urethral stricture. J Urol 115:673, 1976
19. Turner–Warwick R: Complex traumatic posterior urethral strictures. J Urol 118:564, 1977
20. Waterhouse K, Gross M: Trauma to the genitourinary tract: A 5-year experience with 251 cases. J Urol 101:241, 1969

53
Complications of Scrotal Surgery and Trauma

Bruce Broecker

OVERVIEW

Scrotal surgery encompasses surgery performed for a wide variety of conditions. These conditions may be congenital (cryptorchidism) or acquired (varicocele), malignant (germ cell carcinoma of the testis) or benign (hydrocele), emergent (torsion of the spermatic cord) or elective (vasectomy), life threatening (Fornier's gangrene) or cosmetic (testicular prosthesis). The procedures may be therapeutic (vasovasostomy), prognostic (testicular biopsy), or diagnostic (seminal vesiculogram).

ANATOMY

Scrotum

The scrotum is composed of integument and underlying dartos tunic but virtually no underlying subcutaneous fat. The dartos tunic is a thin layer of smooth muscle directly beneath the scrotal skin and continuous with the superficial (Colles') fascia of the abdomen, groin, and perineum. This fascial continuity allows urinary extravasation within the scrotum to dissect into these areas and, more important, allows fascial infections to spread rapidly up the anterior abdominal wall.[24] In the midline the dartos tunic fuses to form a septum that divides the scrotum into two compartments at the median raphe.

The scrotal vascular supply is derived from branches of the perineal artery, which is a branch of the internal pudendal artery. The posterior scrotal branches provide a rich vascular network for the scrotum, and scrotal incisions will interrupt many of these small vessels. Hemostasis is generally easily accomplished with electrocautery, but it should not be left until the end of the procedure, when these small vessels are much more difficult to locate.

The venous and lymphatic drainage of the scrotum generally follows that of the arterial supply. The lymphatic drainage of the scrotum is to the superficial and deep inguinal lymph nodes.

The innervation of the scrotum is by the perineal nerve, which parallels the course of the perineal artery and vein and is a branch of the pudendal nerve. The nerve supply arises from branches of the second, third, and fourth sacral nerve roots.

Testis and Epididymis

Within the scrotum lie the testes, epididymis, and a portion of the spermatic cord. The testis and epididymis are covered by four fascial layers derived from the anterior abdominal wall during testicular descent. The first three fascial layers are single-layered structures that completely envelop the testes epididymis and distal spermatic cord. The tunica vaginalis is a double-layered membrane surrounding the same structures on all sides with fusion of the two layers posteriorly. The two layers of the tunica vaginalis correspond to the parietal and visceral layers of peritoneum picked up as the testicle descends from its retroperitoneal position of origin into the scrotum.

The testis is both an endocrine and exocrine gland. The endocrine function is androgen production, and the functioning cell is the Leydig cell. The exocrine function is spermatogenesis, and the primary cell is the spermatogonium in the seminiferous tubule. Also found in the seminiferous tubule is the Sertoli cell. The exact function of this cell is not clear, but evidence points toward a role in nourishment and protection of the spermatogonia and as part of the blood–testis barrier.[5]

The epididymis is divided into three portions: the head (globus major), located posteriorly at the superior pole of the testis and directly attached to the ductuli efferentes of the testis; a central portion, called the body (corpus); and a tail (globus minor), located at the inferior pole of the testis and leading directly into the ductus deferens. The epididymis is involved in sperm maturation, storage, and transport.[7]

The blood supply to the testis and epididymis is the same and is derived from three sources. The major arterial supply comes from the internal spermatic artery, which arises from the abdominal aorta. Collateral blood supply for the testis and epididymis comes from the deferential artery and the external spermatic artery (cremasteric artery) and branches of the internal and external iliac arteries, respectively. The venous drainage reflects the arterial supply, with the exception of the left internal spermatic vein, which drains into the left renal vein rather than into the vena cava.

The lymphatic drainage of the testis also reflects its retroperitoneal origin and is to the preaortic perirenal lymphatic chain. Previous inguinal or scrotal surgery or trauma, however, will alter this pattern to include the pelvic nodes, both superficial and deep.[13]

Spermatic Cord

The spermatic cord is located in the inguinal canal between the internal inguinal ring and the superior pole of the testicle, and it is made up of the internal spermatic artery, the pampiniform plexus, and the vas deferens. It is covered by the same four fascial layers that cover the testis and epididymis. However, the two layers of peritoneum in the spermatic cord fuse and obliterate the communication between the peritoneal cavity and the tunica vaginalis (processus vaginalis).

The pampiniform plexus is a convoluted network of veins draining the testes. At the level of the internal ring, these join to form one or two larger veins that become the internal spermatic vein and drain into the vena cava and left renal vein on the right and left side, respectively.

Inguinal Canal

The inguinal canal is a 4-cm long oblique tunnel created by descent of the testicle from its position of origin in the retroperitoneum to its final location in the scrotum. Structures of importance in proximity to the inguinal canal include the ilioinguinal nerve, the inferior epigastric vessels, and the iliofemoral junction. The ilioinguinal nerve lies deep to the external oblique fascia in the groin and provides sensory innervation to the root of the penis, medial thigh, and scrotum. Deep to the transversalis fascia in the medial aspect of the inguinal canal lie the inferior epigastric vessels and, in the lateral aspect, the junction between the iliac and femoral vein and artery.

Surgical Approach

There are two surgical approaches to the scrotum and its contents: transscrotal and inguinal. Either approach may be acceptable; the choice may be left to the preference of the surgeon. In the majority of the conditions, however, one approach holds a clear advantage over the other.

TRANSSCROTAL INCISION

The following conditions are preferentially approached through a scrotal incision:

Testicular Torsion

Detorsion of the testicle and spermatic cord is done through a scrotal incision so that the contralateral as well as the ipsilateral testicle may be fixed by pexis to the scrotal wall. Torsion of the spermatic cord results from improper attachment of the epididymis to the scrotal wall. This defect is congenital and bilateral. In order to prevent a future episode of torsion, both testes should be fixed by pexis.

Hydrocele Without Hernia

The elderly patient who develops a hydrocele following an episode of epididymitis or trauma, but does not have an inguinal hernia, may have the hydrocele drained through the scrotum. The advantages of this approach are better control of bleeding, easier exposure with less mobilization, better drainage, less postoperative pain, and shorter surgical time. If an underlying malignancy of the testicle cannot be excluded, however, the hydrocele should be repaired through an inguinal incision. In the elderly patient this is unlikely, but in the patient below the age of 40 years, its frequency is enough to demand that most, if not all, hydroceles be explored through the groin. Ultrasound is useful preoperatively to exclude tumor when the testicle cannot be palpated.[17]

Vasectomy and Vasovasostomy

Surgery on the vas deferens is best done through a scrotal incision. Exposure is better and operative time less, and, in the case of vasectomy, it can be done on an outpatient basis under local anesthesia.

Testicular Biopsy

Testicular biopsies for evaluation of infertility should be done through a scrotal incision. Both testes should be biopsied, and frequently a seminal vesiculogram will be part of the evaluation. Similarly, when a testicular biopsy is necessary to diagnose leukemic or lymphomatous infiltrates, both testes should be biopsied, and the transscrotal approach is indicated.

Epididymal Surgery

Epididymectomy and epididymovasostomy are both accomplished most easily through the scrotum.

Orchiectomy

A simple orchiectomy is generally done transscrotally.

Technique

Once the decision has been made to approach the condition through the scrotum, the incision may be either longitudinal or transverse and may be either in the midline or laterally. The choice rests largely with the preference of the operating surgeon; neither approach offers clear-cut advantages. Regardless of the approach chosen, if the principles of careful and meticulous hemostasis are applied, the outcome should be satisfactory.

The question of drainage elicits controversy in many surgical procedures, and certainly scrotal surgery is no exception. The general guidelines most universally accepted, however, are the use of drains with any infectious condition and the avoidance of drains with any malignant condition. With noninfectious, nonmalignant conditions, drainage is probably unnecessary when hemostasis has been meticulous, but once again the decision largely depends upon the surgeon's preference. When drains are used, they generally are needed no longer than 24 to 48 hours.

INGUINAL INCISION

An inguinal incision should be utilized whenever the spermatic cord as well as the intrascrotal contents must be exposed. The following procedures are preferentially done through an inguinal incision:

Hydrocele With Hernia

Congenital hydroceles are usually found to have a patent processus vaginalis. For this reason, all hydroceles in children should be repaired through an inguinal approach so that the processus vaginalis can be divided and ligated. Likewise, any adult patient with evidence of a patent processus vaginalis should also have his hydrocele repaired through the groin. As noted previously, if an underlying malignancy cannot be excluded as the etiology of the hydrocele, the approach should be through the groin so that a radical orchiectomy can be performed if a tumor is present.

Cryptorchidism

Eighty percent of undescended testes are located in the inguinal canal, and most of the remaining 20% are located just inside the internal inguinal ring.[10] The inguinal incision is the best approach for location and mobilization of the testicle and spermatic cord. Placement of the testicle into the scrotum is easily accomplished through the inguinal incision.

Testicular Cancer

Testicular malignancies *must* be removed through a groin incision. Not only does this allow removal of the spermatic cord up to the level of the internal inguinal ring, but, more important, the surgeon can clamp the spermatic cord prior to mobilization and examination of the testicle, which decreases the chance of hematogenous or lymphatic spread. It also prevents the contamination of the scrotal wall with tumor and potential spread of the tumor into the superficial and deep inguinal lymphatics.[13]

Varicocele

Ligation of the internal spermatic vein should be done at the level of the internal inguinal ring, where the multiple veins in the pampiniform plexus have converged into two or three larger veins. Attempts to ligate each of the varices in the scrotum usually result in significant hemorrhage and formation of a large postoperative hematoma as well as incomplete ligation of all varices.

Testicular Prosthesis

A testicular prosthesis can be inserted through either an inguinal or scrotal incision. The inguinal incision is less prone to contamination, however, and therefore is less likely to develop wound infection and extrusion of the prosthesis.[8]

Complications

In addition to the complications common to all scrotal surgery, which are discussed later, there are several complications unique to the inguinal approach. The ilioinguinal nerve passes through the inguinal canal on top of the internal oblique muscle and below the external oblique aponeurosis. Division of the nerve may occur inadvertently, resulting in temporary postoperative paresthesias. More important, the nerve may occasionally be entrapped during closure of the wound.[16] This results in persistent postoperative incisional pain, which may extend down into the scrotum. It must be differentiated from the normal postoperative incisional pain inherent in any operative incision and from pain caused by strangulation of the spermatic cord due to too tight a closure of the external inguinal ring. Differentiation of these conditions is on the basis of the persistence, long after incisional pain should have reasonably disappeared, of pain and the absence of the testicular swelling and tenderness seen with strangulation of the spermatic cord. It can be confirmed by infiltrating 1% Xylocaine along the course of the nerve in the groin. If this produces temporary relief, then nerve entrapment can be suspected and the wound reexplored.

Injury to the spermatic cord may occur with operations done by the inguinal approach. This may be either by direct damage to the spermatic artery, vein, or vas deferens, or by strangulation of the cord at the external ring. Injury to the vas, if recognized intraoperatively, should be repaired with 6-0 nonabsorbable suture. If unrecognized intraoperatively, it will probably remain so postoperatively, since it produces virtually no symptoms. Operative injury to the artery may produce hemorrhage, which is recognized immediately, but, more common, it results in late postoperative atrophy of the testicle. Unfortunately at that time it is too late for effective treatment. Too tight a closure of the external inguinal ring may strangulate the entire spermatic cord. This is recognized in the early postoperative period by enlargement and tenderness of the testicle due to venous obstruction. It is differentiated rather easily from postoperative scrotal hematoma, which also may produce scrotal swelling and tenderness on physical examination. The wound should be reexplored and several sutures removed from the external ring, or late postoperative atrophy will occur.

Common Complications

The complications common to all procedures involving the scrotum and its contents are hemorrhage and infection.

HEMORRHAGE

Postoperative bleeding and hematoma may be frequent sequelae of scrotal surgery and trauma. The scrotum is a richly vascularized structure, and the intrascrotal compartment readily expands to accommodate large postoperative hematomas. The loose scrotal skin does little in the way of compressing or tamponading capillary bleeders until quite sizable hematomas have formed. Recognition is easy. The scrotum in the early postoperative period will enlarge to three to four times its normal size. The testicle may be displaced by the hematoma and still be palpable, or it may be encased by the hematoma and no longer identifiable by palpation. The hematoma generally is moderately tender on manipulation. With a large hematoma, the diagnosis is obvious and unlikely to be confused with other conditions. Smaller hematomas may be confused with postoperative edema and thickening of the scrotal wall or strangulation of the spermatic cord.

Management depends upon the size and symptoms of the hematoma and whether or not it is continuing to expand. Small- to moderate-sized hematomas will resolve spontaneously with liquefaction and reabsorption of the blood and can be treated expectantly with compression dressings and elevation. However, if the hematoma is quite large and symptomatic or expanding, it should be drained surgically, bleeding vessels controlled, and compression dressings applied.

INFECTION

Because of the excellent vascular supply of scrotal skin, infections tend to be rather uncommon except when surgery is done for an abscess or other infectious condition and when a postoperative hematoma is present that becomes secondarily infected. Infection may also occur with scrotal trauma and devitalized, contaminated skin.

The local manifestations of infection in the scrotal wall or compartment are the universal signs of infection—erythema, warmth, and tenderness. Fever and other systemic manifestations of infection are generally present. Recognition is easy when local and systemic signs are present. It may be less obvious whether or not a smaller hematoma is infected when systemic signs are absent. Management of scrotal infections conforms to general surgical guidelines for dealing with surgical infections. Adequate drainage and débridement are the cornerstone of therapy and should be supplemented with appropriate antibiotics.

Specific Conditions and Their Complications

HYDROCELE

A hydrocele is an increase in the amount of fluid within the tunica vaginalis, and it results from an imbalance between the rate of fluid production and the rate of reabsorption.[14] Most commonly located in the tunica vaginalis surrounding the testicle, a hydrocele may also be found along the spermatic cord in the processus vaginalis. It may or may not communicate with the intraperitoneal cavity. Numerous repairs have been described for the treatment of hydroceles, the most successful of which are based on removal of most or all of the parietal layer of the tunica vaginalis, thus reducing the secretory surface. Complications specifically associated with repair of a hydrocele are failure to recognize an underlying malignancy and recurrence of the hydrocele. Hydroceles may be secondary to neoplasm, trauma, or infection, or they may be congenital, owing to a patent processus vaginalis, but, most common, they are idiopathic. Since the testicle is difficult to palpate through the hydrocele, a malignancy may be undetected until the hydrocele sac is opened. If the incision has been transscrotal, contamination not only of the hemiscrotum but also of the deep and superficial inguinal lymph nodes may result. This can best be avoided by inguinal exploration of all hydroceles in patients below the age of 50 when an underlying malignancy cannot be excluded.

Recurrence of a hydrocele is seen following procedures in which the hydrocele sac is merely plicated and not excised. The subsequent operative procedure should involve removal of the sac.

SPERMATOCELE

A spermatocele is a cystic mass containing spermatozoa located superior and posterior to the testicle. It is thought to arise from tubules connecting the rete testis with the epididymis. Although most are less than 1 cm in diameter, they occasionally become larger and then may be confused with a hydrocele of the cord. They are usually soft and cystic on palpation and will transilluminate. If they are firmer, differentiation from a tumor of the cord may be difficult. Most spermatoceles are small and asymptomatic and require no therapy. However, if they are unusually large or cannot be distinguished from a tumor, operative intervention may become necessary. There are no complications specific for spermatocelectomy, only the common complications of hemorrhage and wound infection.

VARICOCELE

A varicocele is a varicosity of the pampiniform plexus and internal spermatic vein. It presents clinically as a mass of dilated veins palpable along the spermatic cord in the scrotum and is almost always on the left side because that vein is longer and inserted into the renal vein rather than into the vena cava. Indications for operation are a large size or impaired spermatogenesis with infertility. Treatment is ligation of the internal spermatic vein at the level of the internal inguinal ring where the pampiniform plexus has become one or two large veins. Postoperative atrophy does not occur if only the vein has been ligated, since collateral venous drainage through the cremasteric and vasal veins is sufficient.

Complications specific to varicocelectomy include testicular atrophy when the internal spermatic artery is ligated and collateral arterial supply is insufficient and residual or recurrent varicocele, which may occur when all of the internal spermatic veins are not ligated.[4] Occasionally a varicocele may be due to occlusion of the left renal vein by a tumor embolus from a hypernephroma or to a circumaortic renal vein—the so-called left renal vein syndrome—and, because of this possibility, it has been suggested that intravenous urography or ultrasonography be part of the preoperative evaluation of all varicoceles of acute onset.[18]

TORSION OF THE SPERMATIC CORD

Torsion of the spermatic cord commonly but incorrectly referred to as "testicular torsion," is a dramatic event presenting as an acutely swollen and exquisitely painful testicle (Figs. 53-1 and 53-2). Conditions that may present as a similar picture include torsion of testicular appendage, epididymitis, epididymo-orchitis, and incarcerated inguinal hernia. Radioisotope and Doppler evaluation of testicular blood flow; the patient's age; and the presence or absence of fever, leukocytosis, and pyuria may help lead to the correct diagnosis; however, whenever any doubt exists, the best policy is to explore the scrotum in the operating room to make the definitive diagnosis and carry out the necessary operative procedure. It is far better to explore a case of epididymitis unnecessarily than to fail to operate on a torsion. If a twisted spermatic cord is found, it is untwisted

FIG. 53-1. Torsion of the spermatic cord. The left testicle is swollen and high in the scrotum on physical examination.

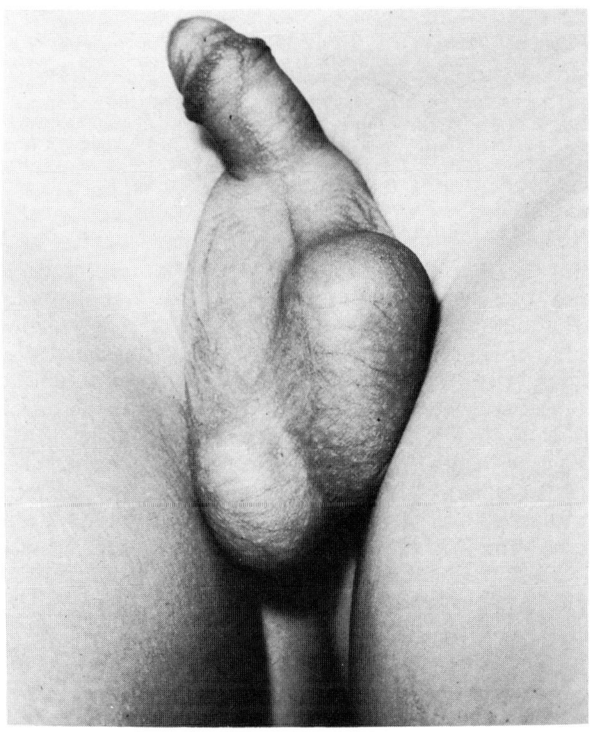

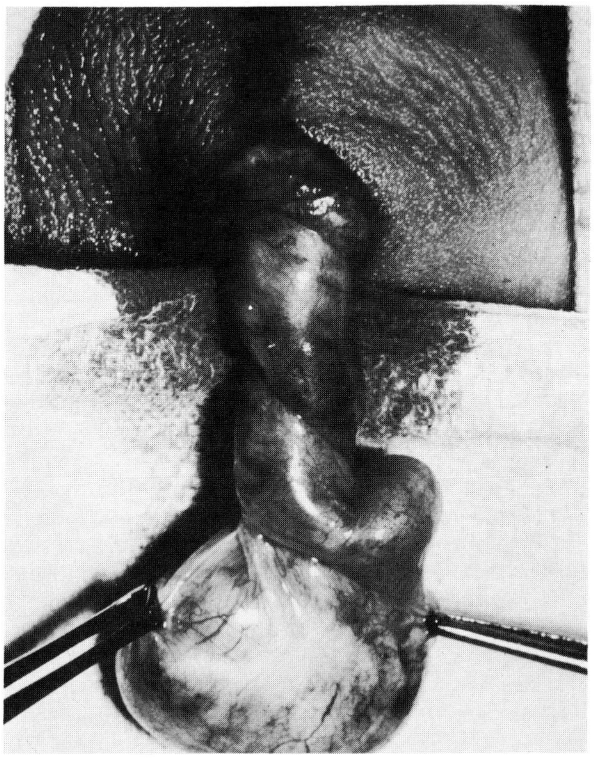

FIG. 53-2. Torsion of the spermatic cord. There is 360° torsion of the spermatic cord with an infarcted testicle.

and fixed by pexis with nonabsorbable sutures to the scrotal wall in two planes. The contralateral testicle is then also fixed by pexis in a similar fashion. It has been our policy to leave all but the most obviously nonviable testes in place, since Leydig cell function is quite resistant to ischemia.

There are two complications that may occur specifically with surgery for spermatic cord torsion: recurrent torsion and loss of exocrine and endocrine function. Recurrent torsion is rare, may be ipsilateral or contralateral, and is due to use of absorbable rather than nonabsorbable sutures to fix the testicle.[19] Preservation of function is directly related to the length of time between the torsion of the cord and successful detorsion. Generally, 4 hours is the length of time beyond which testicular function will be predictably and severely compromised.[3] Even with intervals of less than 4 hours, exocrine function may be irreversibly impaired, since the seminiferous tubules are much more sensitive to ischemia than are Leydig cells.

During any intrascrotal procedure, we remove the testicular appendages (appendix testis and appendix epididymis) so that torsion of these structures will not enter into the differential diagnosis of postoperative scrotal pain and swelling.

CRYPTORCHIDISM

Correct management of the undescended testis must take into account the age of the patient, the condition of the contralateral testis, and the location and gross anatomical appearance of the ipsilateral testis. Operative procedures range from orchiectomy to microvascular autotransplantation. However, most undescended testes are located distal to the internal inguinal ring, and the standard operative procedure involves division of the processus vaginalis and skeletization of the internal spermatic vessels and vas deferens to allow sufficient mobilization of the testicle to place it into the scrotum.[15] Between the ages of 1½ and 2½ years is the preferred time for orchidopexy, since spontaneous descent rarely occurs after the age of 1 year, and the earliest signs of seminiferous tubule damage occur by the age of 2 years.[12]

Complications specific to orchidopexy are testicular atrophy, damage to the vas deferens, retraction of the testicle, and peritoneal injury. Atrophy results from excessive traction on the spermatic artery with an intimal injury and thrombosis or inadvertent operative injury of the vessels. Recognition of the injury intraoperatively might allow successful microsurgical reanastomosis; however, most operating theaters and surgeons are not properly equipped or trained for this procedure. In most cases the surgeon can hope only that collateral circulation will be sufficient to prevent total loss of exocrine and endocrine function. Damage to the vas deferens, however, can be repaired successfully using only magnifying loops. Vasovasostomy utilizing sutures of 6-0 or 7-0 Prolene done with or without a stent has produced a high patency rate.[20] If the injury is not recognized intraoperatively, it generally produces no symptoms and will pass undetected. The testicle may retract back into the inguinal canal if the vascular pedicle is short and under considerable tension when the testicle is positioned in the scrotum. Management is by a second procedure 4 to 6 months later. Avoidance of this complication can be guaranteed by a staged orchidopexy, division of the spermatic vessels (Fowler–Stephens procedure), or autotransplantation.[6, 22]

Peritoneal injury occurs during division of the processus vaginalis and separation from the spermatic vessels. The peritoneum is filamentous at this level, and the edge can easily be lost or a tear extend up into the abdominal cavity. The peritoneum must be closed to prevent bowel herniation into the inguinal canal and possible strangulation or obstruction.

SCROTAL INFECTIONS

Scrotal infections require surgical intervention in two situations, abscess and synergistic gangrene (Fornier's gangrene). Both require prompt drainage and débridement. Fornier's gangrene, which is a necrotizing fasciitis originating in the scrotum, is a life-threatening emergency, since it can extend up the entire anterior abdominal wall in a matter of hours.[23]

The only complication of surgical management of scrotal infections arises from delayed drainage and inadequate débridement. The surgeon may be reluctant, with synergistic gangrene, to débride radically enough. This temptation must be resisted, and all tissue that does not actively bleed must be removed, even if that means débridement of all of the abdominal wall, perineum, and scrotum. These can later be covered with skin grafts. To do otherwise will lead to the patient's death (Fig. 53-3; see also Chap. 3).

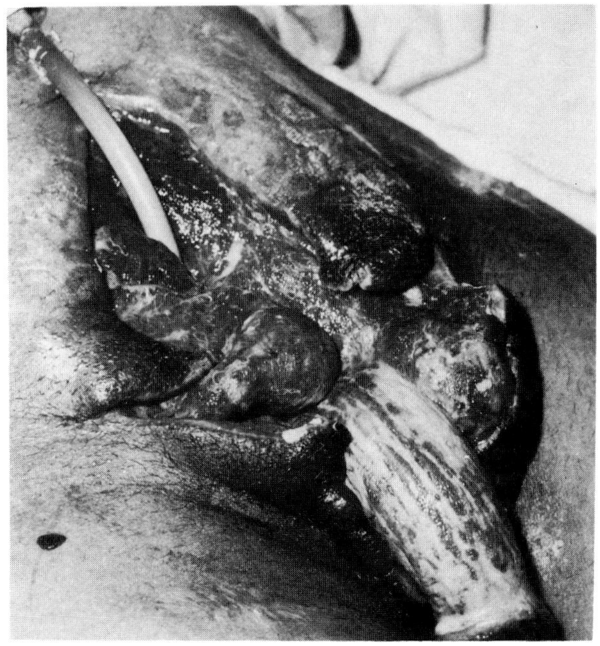

FIG. 53-3. Extensive débridement of the phallus, scrotum, and anterior abdominal wall in a patient with Fournier's gangrene.

TUMORS

The only complication specifically related to surgical management of testicular or spermatic cord tumors is scrotal contamination and potential spread of tumor to the inguinal lymphatics as a result of a scrotal rather than an inguinal incision.[13]

INFERTILITY

A number of procedures are used for evaluation and treatment of infertility, including testicular biopsy, vasography, and vasovasostomy. Vasectomy, a procedure to produce infertility, is included here. Testicular biopsy is associated with no specific complication. Vasography and vasovasostomy share the complication of leakage of semen and granulomatous formation in reaction to the sperm.[21] Local symptoms of tenderness and swelling over the vas deferens signal the presence of this complication. These symptoms will resolve spontaneously with time and require no specific treatment. More serious than the local complications has been the possible formation of antisperm antibodies as a result of the extravasation of semen.[1] It has been suggested that continued infertility following successful (*i.e.*, normal sperm count) vasovasostomy is due to the presence of these antibodies.[11] The issue is controversial and remains undecided.

Vasectomy is one of the most common surgical procedures performed in the world today. Complications include sperm granuloma and recanalization. Recanalization is rare, but presumably it results from re-epithelialization along the path created by extravasated semen. Avoidance of this complication can be ensured by excising a segment of the vas rather than merely dividing it, cauterizing the epithelium as well as ligating it, and leaving the two ends of the vas in separate tissue planes. Recently experimental animal data have implicated vasectomy as an accelerator of atherosclerosis.[2] The mechanism is thought to be endothelial injury by antisperm antibodies and other immunologic mediators. Clinical support of this in humans has not been forthcoming; however, until this controversy is resolved, it would seem prudent to avoid vasectomy in men with a strong family history of cardiovascular disease.

Scrotal Trauma

Traumatic scrotal injuries will most commonly present as part of the spectrum of pelvic trauma. The associated injuries to other genital and pelvic organs usually represent a much greater threat of morbidity and mortality than the scrotal trauma and are discussed in the various other chapters of this text. Injuries to the scrotum itself rarely present difficulties in management or serious complications. Injuries to the testicle represent a far more important aspect of scrotal trauma in management and morbidity.

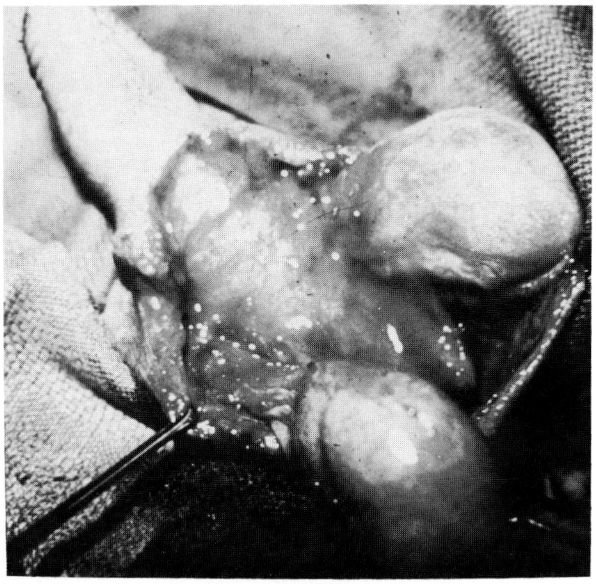

FIG. 53-4. Denuded testes following an avulsion injury of the scrotum.

TRAUMA TO THE SCROTUM ITSELF

Trauma of the scrotum may be classified as contusion, laceration, or avulsion. Contusions should be treated with ice packs and elevation and will heal with virtually no unfavorable sequelae. Lacerations, if not heavily contaminated, should be débrided, thoroughly cleansed, and closed with suture approximation. If the degree of contamination is thought to be significant and the chance of infection high, the wound should be thoroughly débrided and cleansed and packed open to allow healing by secondary intention. Avulsion injuries are treated in a similar manner (Fig. 53-4). Scrotal skin is so pliable that even with extensive loss of skin, the remaining portion will usually cover the scrotal contents and gradually expand during the ensuing months and years. Again, the degree of contamination dictates the decision as to whether to close the wound primarily or secondarily. If the scrotum has been totally avulsed but the testicles remain, they should be buried in the subcutaneous tissue of the medial thigh. At a later date a scrotal compartment can be constructed with skin grafts and pedicle flaps.

TESTICULAR TRAUMA

Testicular trauma also may be classified as a contusion, laceration or rupture, and avulsion. Contusion should be diagnosed only if the entire capsule remains intact on palpation of the gonad and there is no loss of the normal oval contour. This injury is managed by ice packs and elevation. Whether intratesticular scarring and altered spermatogenesis develop subsequently in some of these cases is unknown. A laceration or rupture should be suspected if the contour of the testicle is distorted or if a large scrotal hematoma precludes adequate examination of the testicle. Maximal preservation of testicular function is then achieved by scrotal exploration and suture repair of the injury.[9] Little can be done for avulsion injuries other than ligation of the spermatic vessels to control hemorrhage. The role of microvascular surgery in testicular salvage probably remains very limited. A prosthesis may be subsequently placed to correct the cosmetic deformity, but this is appropriate only as a delayed procedure and not at the time of the initial surgery.

COMPLICATIONS

The complications of scrotal and testicular trauma are hemorrhage and infection. Diagnosis and management of these problems is discussed previously. All traumatic scrotal wounds that are closed should be drained with a Penrose drain. If infection is a concern, it is best to pack the wound open and allow healing to occur secondarily. The cosmetic deformity from this type of closure is usually quite minimal. Broad-spectrum antibiotics are generally employed.

References

1. Alexander NJ: Autoimmune hypospermatogenesis in vasetomized guinea pigs. Contraception 8:147, 1973
2. Alexander NJ, Clarkson TB: Vasectomy increases the severity of diet-induced atherosclerosis in macaca fascicularis. Science 201:538, 1978
3. Bartsch G, Frank ST, Marberger H, Mikuz G: Testicular torsion: Late results with special regard to fertility and endocrine function. J Urol 124:375, 1980
4. Dubin L, Amelar R: Varicocele. Urol Clin North Am 5(3):563, 1978
5. Ewing L: Testis, Epididymis. The physiology of male reproduction. In Harrison JH, Gittes R, Perlmutter AD, Stamey TA, Walsh PC (eds): Campbell's Urology, vol 1, chap 5. Philadelphia, WB Saunders, 1979
6. Fowler R, Stephens FD: The role of testicular vascular anatomy in the salvage of high undescended testes. In Stephens FD (ed): Congenital Malformations of the Rectum and Anus and Genito-Urinary Tracts. Baltimore, Williams & Wilkins, 1963
7. Glover TD: The Epididymis. In Williams DI, Chisholm G, (eds): Scientific Foundations of Urology. London, William Heinemann, 1976
8. Gordon JA, Schwartz, BB: Delayed extrusion of testicular prosthesis. Urology 14:59, 1979
9. Gross M: Rupture of the testicle: The importance of early surgical treatment. J Urol 101:196, 1969
10. Gross RE, Replogle RL: Treatment of the undescended testis: Opinions gained from 1767 operations. Post Grad Med 34:266, 1963

11. Gupta I, Dhawan S, Goel SD, Saha K: Low fertility rate in vasovasostomized males and its possible immunologic mechanism. Int J Fertil 20:183, 1975
12. Hadziselimovic F, Herzog B, Seguchi H: Surgical correction of cryptorchidism at 2 years: Electron microscopic and morphometric investigations. J Pediatr Surg 10:19, 1974
13. Herr HW, Silber I, Martin DC: Management of inguinal lymph nodes in patients with testicular tumors following orchiopexy, inguinal, or scrotal operations. J Urol 110:223, 1973
14. Huggins CB, Entz FH: Absorption from normal tunica vaginalis testis, hydrocele, and spermatocele. J Urol 25:447, 1931
15. Kieswetter WB: Undescended testes: Surgery and its results. Am. Surg 37:201, 1971
16. Moosman DA, Oelrich TM: Prevention of accidental trauma to the ilioinguinal nerve during inguinal herniorrhaphy. Am J Surg 133:146, 1977
17. Nachtsheim DA, Gosink BB, Scheible WF, Schmidt JD: Ultrasonography of testis tumors. Presented at the 76th Annual Meeting of the American Urologic Association, Boston, May 10-14, 1981
18. Parker DS, Hicks T: Varicocele and renal tumor in the right side. Urology 5:530, 1975
19. Rabinovitch HH, McNellis DR: Repeat torsion of "Fixed" testis. Urology 16:476, 1980
20. Schmidt SS: Anastomosis of the vas deferens: An experimental study in the use of fine polyethylene tubing as a splint. J Urol 85:838, 1961
21. Schmidt SS, Morris RR: Spermatic granuloma: The complication of vasectomy. Fertil Steril 24:941, 1973
22. Silber SJ, Kelly J: Successful autotransplantation of an intra-abdominal testis to the scrotum by micro-vascular technique. J Urol 115:452, 1976
23. Tan RE: Fournier's gangrene of the scrotum and the penis. J Urol 92:508, 1964
24. Tobin CE, Benjamin JA: Anatomic and clinical re-evaluation of Camper's, Scarpa's and Colles' fasciae. Surg Gynecol Obstet 88:545, 1949

54 Complications of Bladder and Prostate Surgery and Trauma

John H. Texter, Jr.

OVERVIEW

Surgical injury or trauma to the urinary bladder is unique in that the bladder's vulnerability is dependent upon its state of fullness or distention at the time of injury. The empty bladder is less likely to be damaged, since its area of exposure to forces or cutting instruments is at a minimum and the thickness of the wall is maximal. Also, in the empty state, the bladder is situated well down inside the bony pelvis behind the symphysis pubis (Fig. 54-1). The exception to this anatomical arrangement is seen in children, in whom even the empty bladder occupies a much higher location and anatomically can be considered an intra-abdominal organ. The transition from childhood to adult configuration occurs gradually during the earlier and midteens.[10]

The full bladder, however, even in the adult, rises up out of the pelvis and may be subjected to trauma. Likewise, as the bladder fills, the wall becomes thinned and therefore more susceptible to penetration or rupture.

The presence of any preexisting disease increases the possibility of injury to the urinary bladder. This is seen very commonly in the older man who may have prostatic enlargement with urinary outflow obstruction. The enlarged prostate further pushes the bladder base up from the pelvis, and because of the obstruction large residual urine volumes may keep the bladder relatively full at all times. The presence of a tumor or an acute inflammatory disease is another cause that may weaken the bladder wall.

The health and state of the surrounding structures determines whether a given insult will produce bladder damage. A healthy muscular adult with powerful rectus muscles will be less likely to damage his bladder from blunt abdominal trauma than will a multiparous woman whose rectus muscles may be considerably weaker. Previous surgery with incisional changes to the fascia planes and points of adhesion may increase the stress and shearing during injury. Following hysterectomy, the bladder may be adherent to the pelvic wall and be less supported and protected posteriorly.

FIG. 54-1. As the urinary bladder fills, the area of exposure becomes greater and the wall becomes thinner. The protection from the bony pelvis decreases when the bladder is distended.

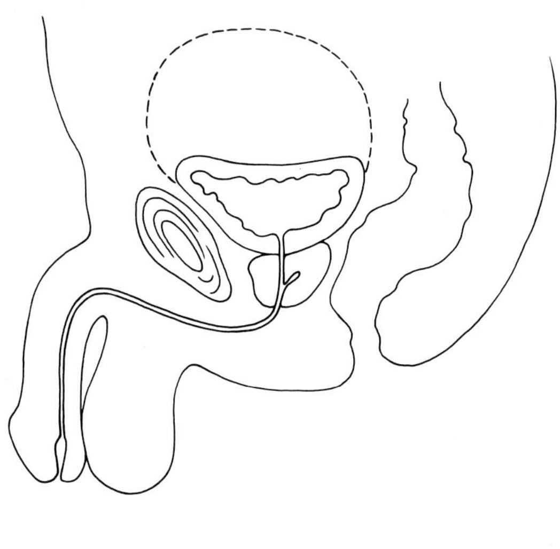

Blunt Trauma

Blunt trauma to the lower abdomen in a patient with a full or partially filled bladder will transmit the force directly to the bladder. Since the urine is a fluid, traumatic force or pressure impulses are transmitted equally throughout the bladder. The weakest point of the bladder surface will therefore be the point most likely to rupture. Since the bladder base is well supported and generally changes very little whether the bladder is full or empty, it is the area most resistant to traumatic rupture. As the bladder fills, however, the dome rises from the bony protection and becomes progressively thinner. In addition, other structures afford less protection, making the dome the most frequent point of rupture (Fig. 54-2). Only a thin layer of peritoneum covers the bladder dome and separates it from the abdominal cavity. As the bladder ruptures, the peritoneal lining is also disrupted, which allows free communication with abdominal contents (Fig. 54-3). This intraperitoneal extravasation is extremely dangerous, and it requires immediate surgical correction with provisions for urinary drainage.[1] If the urinary tract is infected at the time of injury, the condition is further complicated. The spillage of infected urine must be terminated as soon as possible, and adequate intravenous antibiotics are mandatory to prevent generalized peritonitis.

If the urine is sterile at the time of intraperitoneal bladder rupture, leakage of urine into the abdominal cavity may be initially well tolerated. Signs of peritonitis, shock, and hematuria may be absent, and it may even be possible to detect fairly normal bowel sounds for several hours following the injury, providing no other vital organ has been damaged. Usually, the patient will have little or no urine output, and eventually signs of chemical peritonitis will develop. Surgical repair, urinary drainage, and antibiotic coverage are necessary even if a urinary tract infection is not present.[8]

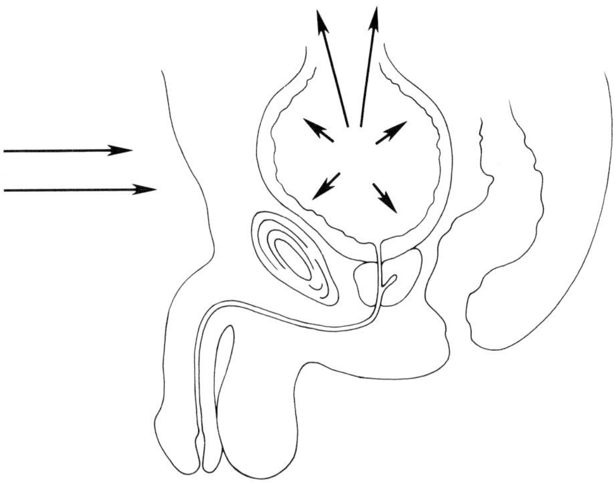

FIG. 54-2. Blunt trauma to the distended urinary bladder produces elevated intravesical pressure. If the pressure is great enough, the bladder will rupture through the dome, which is the weakest point.

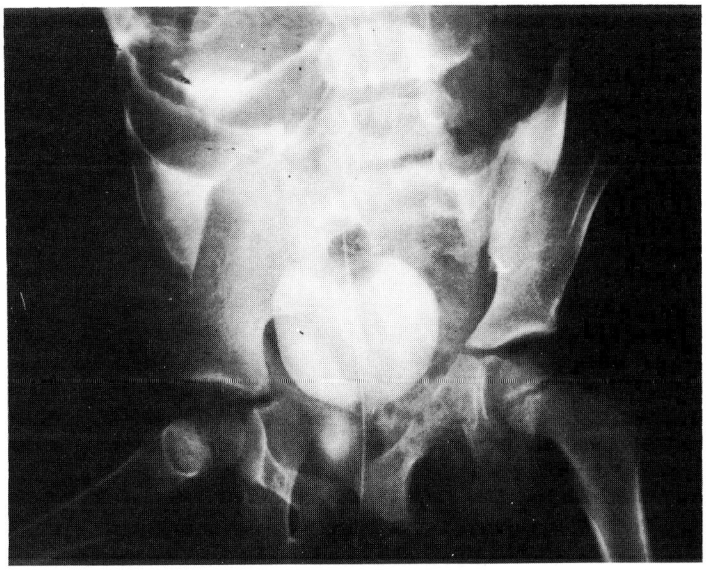

FIG. 54-3. A cystogram obtained on a youngster with fractured pelvis. The Foley-catheter balloon can be seen sitting outside the bladder through the ruptured dome. This intraperitoneal rupture allows contrast to flow into the abdominal cavity and outline loops of bowel.

EXTRAPERITONEAL EXTRAVASATION

If the bladder ruptures at some site other than the dome, such as along the side walls, or if the peritoneal covering is still intact, urine will leak into the perivesical tissues but will not gain access to the peritoneal cavity (Fig. 54-4). This extraperitoneal extravasation, although still a serious injury, is not generally as life threatening as is intraperitoneal injury. If the urine is infected, the area of extravasation must be drained and, if possible, the rupture site repaired and catheter drainage provided. If the urine is uninfected and the injury is genuinely extraperitoneal, there is some controversy over whether drainage and surgical repair are necessary.[5] This approach has been used in patients in whom other injuries such as major head trauma would make them unsuitable for any type of surgery. However, if other abdominal injuries are suspected and abdominal exploration is required, then the bladder should be repaired and drained. Also, if the urine is infected or the patient shows any signs of deterioration, exploration, drainage, and bladder repair are necessary. As with any type of bladder perforation, catheter drainage and antibiotic coverage are essential for successful recovery.[6]

FIG. 54-4. Extraperitoneal bladder rupture demonstrated on cystogram, which shows Foley balloon sitting at the bladder base. Contrast can be seen leaking into the left perivesicle space and into the left femoral canal.

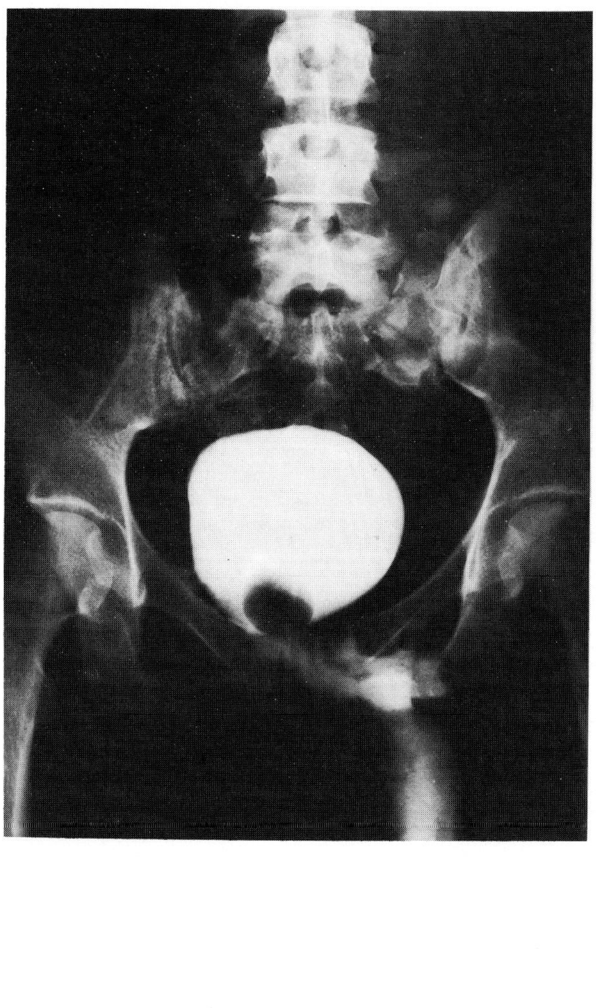

Penetrating Injuries

Penetrating injuries to the urinary bladder may come from any source such as a projectile or missile from a gun, penetration from a stab wound, or accidental incision at the time of other surgery. The bladder may be perforated during laparoscopy or at the time of peritoneal lavage, especially if the bladder was not emptied initially by catheter drainage prior to the procedure. During abdominal surgery, it is possible to enter the bladder inadvertently if there has been previous abdominal surgery and the bladder is adherent to the anterior abdominal wall. This is particularly troublesome if the patient has had suprapubic catheter drainage in the past. In this situation, the surgeon must cautiously dissect off the bladder to avoid accidental injury. Occasionally, when a large inguinal hernia is repaired, the bladder may be damaged because the bladder has prolapsed or been incorporated into the hernia sac contents (Fig. 54-5).

Occasionally a penetrating bladder injury may

FIG. 54-5. Cystourethrogram shows contrast in the urethra and bladder. The upper portion of the bladder is prolapsed off to the left side and is incorporated into the sac of a large left inguinal hernia. Damage or incision into the urinary bladder could easily occur during surgical repair of the hernia.

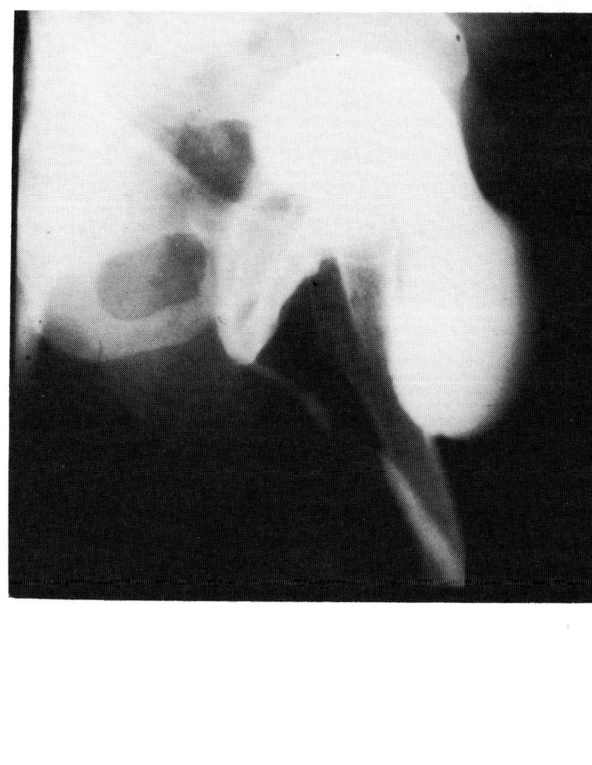

result from massive blunt trauma (e.g., extensive pelvic fractures). At the moment of impact when the pelvis is fractured, the sharp ends of the bone may penetrate the bladder wall. If the traumatic force is great enough, the broken bone fragments may become missiles and perforate the urinary bladder. Case reviews have indicated that approximately 10% of the patients with fractured pelvis will have an associated rupture of the bladder. Approximately 80% of these ruptures will be extraperitoneal.[3]

As with any type of penetrating injury from a high-speed projectile, the resulting damage is dependent not only upon the size of the missile, but also upon the speed with which it is driven through the tissue.[2] In a penetrating injury from an extremely high-speed projectile such as may be encountered from high-velocity firearms, there may be considerable surrounding tissue devitalization as a result of the dissipation of energy, even though the projectile itself may be quite small. It is therefore important to assess viability of the bladder wall to determine if débridement is necessary before simply oversewing the perforation site. Sometimes, this dissipated energy may damage the bladder even though the projectile has not directly penetrated the bladder surface. This energy may produce enough impact to injure the inside wall and produce a bladder wall contusion. Although gross hematuria may result, there should be no extravasation of urine. In such situations, it is wise to provide catheter drainage until the urine has completely cleared of blood and bladder filling will not subsequently perforate a thinned or partially ischemic section of the bladder wall.

Diagnosis

Any type of trauma to the lower abdomen should alert the clinician to possible bladder injury. Even though local pain, tenderness, and gross hematuria are usually encountered, occasionally the initial symptoms and findings may be minimal. It is helpful if the patient is awake to provide the time of the last urination, since it would give some estimate as to the state of filling at the time of injury.

The prompt appearance of clear urine when a catheter is passed into the bladder does not rule out bladder injury or perforation. Ruptured bladder should never be diagnosed on the basis of incomplete return of a known volume of irrigating solution. This antiquated technique can be extremely misleading. The use of an air cystogram should also be discouraged, since this adds little specific information and risks the possibility of air embolism.

If the urethra is intact and a catheter has been placed, it is simple to identify a bladder perforation by the use of contrast medium. This is the safest and surest technique for determining the integrity of the bladder. Not only should pictures be taken before the contrast has been introduced into the bladder, but also following drainage of the contrast from the bladder since an area of perforation may exist posterior to the bladder and not be evident when the bladder is completely filled with contrast medium. The medium should be nonirritating and nontoxic, since if extravasation is present the agent will come into contact with vital organs and may be absorbed into the general circulation. Intravenous pyelographic contrast agents that have been diluted with normal saline are quite safe and readily available in most emergency x-ray areas.

Bladder Injury During Pelvic Surgery

It is helpful to the surgeon to place a Foley catheter into the bladder per urethra at the start of the operation. This prevents inadvertent bladder injury in two ways. First, the catheter decompresses the bladder, making the entry into the lumen less likely. Second, the catheter balloon is usually palpable through the bladder wall and allows the surgeon to identify the bladder by palpation. If the surgeon suspects the bladder has been incised, it is usually quite easy to identify the smooth shining surface of the bladder mucosa. However, the diagnosis can easily be confirmed by the intravenous administration of the blue dye, indigo carmine. Providing that renal function and perfusion are normal, one ampule containing 5 ml of the dye will produce blue-stained urine in the bladder within a few minutes of injection. If renal function is not adequate, the presence of a bladder leak can be detected by irrigating the Foley catheter with saline or saline that contains a small amount of methylene blue. This is an excellent technique to use after the bladder has been repaired to ensure that a watertight closure has been accomplished.

During the repair of the bladder, only absorbable suture materials should be used for the closure. Nonabsorbable suture materials will lead to the development of stone deposits when they are exposed to urine for any length of time. A two-layer closure technique should be used with the inner suture line being continuous and incorporating the mucosa, submucosa, and superficial portions of the bladder muscle. This first layer should produce a watertight seal and is best done with a 3-0 chromic catgut. The outer second layer should be interrupted using 2-0 chromic catgut and incorporate the full thickness of the bladder wall. This layer provides strength to the repair. A catheter, either suprapubic or urethral Foley, is needed to divert the urine for 5 to 7 days so healing can occur. A cystogram obtained just before removing the catheter will assure that the healing is complete and that no extravasation will occur.

Complications of Surgery of the Prostate Gland—Complications of Transurethral Resection for Benign Disease

A special note of caution must be sounded about the use of the electrocautery unit during transurethral resection of the prostate.[7] Occasionally, intravesicle explosions, which can rupture the bladder, may occur. Thermal decomposition occurs as the tissue is resected, which produces flammable gases. The composition of this gas varies according to the intensity of the high-frequency current. Also, both hydrogen and oxygen are produced by electrolysis as a result of the electrode arc. This gas accumulates at the highest point of the bladder and may explode if it comes in contact with the activated loop.[9] This complication can be avoided by frequent emptying of the bladder during resection and allowing all the gas to escape each time. It is also important to keep the resectoscope loop immersed in the irrigating solution and away from the gas bubble.

FIG. 54-6. This patient had a perforation of the prostatic capsule during transurethral resection of the prostate. The extravasation is extraperitoneal and is clearly demonstrated by contrast in the periprostatic tissue on this drainage film taken after a cystourethrogram was performed.

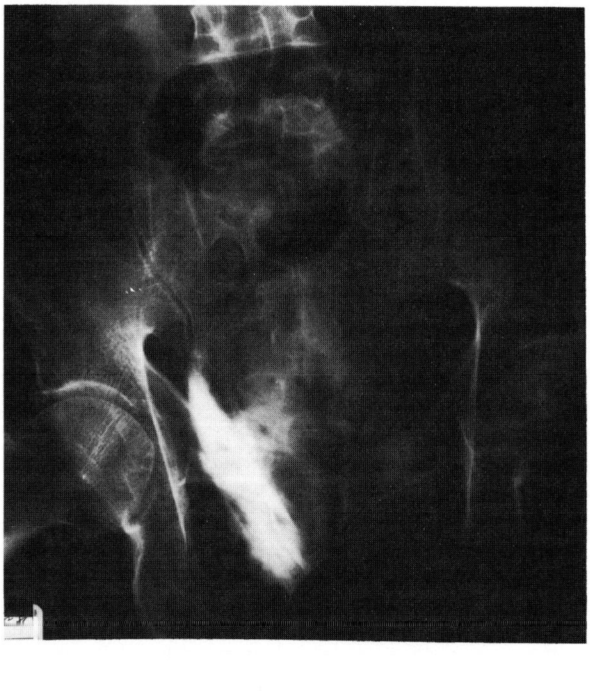

Massive amounts of irrigation solution may be absorbed during transurethral resection of the prostate, producing dilutional hyponatremia.[4] Distilled water is no longer used for irrigating solution, and therefore the problems of hemolysis and subsequent renal failure are no longer encountered. Some degree of hemorrhage is quite frequent during prostate surgery because of the extreme vascularity. Blood dyscrasias or hemorrhagic states may compound the bleeding. Hemorrhage from transurethral resections usually results from failure to identify specific bleeding points and to apply adequate direct electrocoagulation. With a vascular prostate gland, the surgeon may "fall behind" in obtaining adequate hemostasis by waiting until the end of the resection in order to provide coagulation. The bleeding by that time may be so profuse that the flow of irrigation fluid may not be adequate to keep the field of view unobscured. Additional flow and pressure of the irrigation solution may be required in order to enhance visualization of the prostatic fossa. This increases the likelihood of massive fluid absorption and dilutional hyponatremia. Hemorrhage from transurethral resections is best prevented by obtaining adequate hemostasis throughout the operation. The main blood supply from the prostatic arteries is located at the 5 and 7 o'clock positions, just at the junction of the prostate base with the bladder neck. However, capsular arteries may be encountered around the entire circumference and be the source of significant bleeding.

Usually, arterial bleeders can be readily identified by the jet or spurt of blood; however, sometimes the bleeding point may be hidden behind the irregularity of the floor of the partially resected prostate fossa. A particular artery may go into spasm and not actually be spurting at the time the operator inspects the fossa. At a later time, active bleeding may occur when the spasm is relieved and the vesicle lumen is again patent. To avoid such hemorrhagic problems, the operator should keep the surface of the resection as smooth as possible and electrocoagulate each bleeding point as it is encountered throughout the surgery.

Perforation of the prostatic capsule or the prostatovesical junction may occur. This is usually the result of manipulation or poor control of the beak of the resectoscope during the resection or of the operator's losing orientation of normal anatomical landmarks. Usually, these perforations will be extraperitoneal; however, there may be sudden changes in the vital signs such as fluctuation of the pulse or shock (Fig. 54-6). If the patient is under spinal anesthesia, there may be restlessness or sudden onset of pain, nausea, and vomiting. Shortly after the perforation, the abdomen may be quite tense and rigid, even in someone under general anesthesia.

If the operator suspects a perforation, it is mandatory that the surgery be terminated as soon as adequate hemostasis is obtained. A catheter should be placed into the bladder per urethra and a cystogram obtained. Baseline electrolytes should be drawn to determine any dilutional hyponatremia that may accompany the perforation. If there has been intraperitoneal extravasation and the perforation is limited to the prostatic capsule, adequate drainage can be obtained with a Foley urethral catheter. A continuous irrigating solution should not be utilized. Electrolyte abnormalities should be corrected and fluid overload managed with diuretics. These patients will also require appropriate antibacterial therapy.

If a perforation is intraperitoneal or if massive bleeding continues, open surgery will be required to repair the perforation, check the abdominal contents for possible injury, and provide suprapubic drainage. The bleeding from the prostatic fossa can be managed transvesically by placement of hemostatic sutures around the bladder neck. If hemostasis is not obtained with these measures, a gauze packing should be placed into the prostatic fossa around a Foley catheter. After the packing is complete, the Foley catheter balloon is then inflated to approximately 30 cm to 40 cm of water and traction is applied to the catheter. This traction compresses the Foley balloon down onto the packing and prevents any further bleeding by tamponade. The end of the packing is exited through the suprapubic wound and can be gradually withdrawn over the next several days. A suprapubic catheter should be left in place until the gauze packing has been removed and no further bleeding is encountered.

Open Prostatectomy

During open prostate surgery for enucleation of prostatic adenomas, complications from severe hemorrhage may be encountered. This may occur even in the absence of any blood dyscrasias or abnormalities of the coagulation components. Generally, the heaviest bleeding will be encountered at the level of the bladder neck or just inside the prostatic fossa. Bleeding may occur anywhere around the entire circumference of the bladder neck, although the main arterial supply enters the fossa just lateral to the midline on both the left and right sides. Even if active bleeding is not encountered, an arterial spasm may be present and hemorrhage may occur later. This situation accounts for the often-heard statement that the prostate fossa was completely dry at the time the surgical field was closed, but heavy bleeding began in the recovery room. Therefore, figure-of-eight sutures should be routinely placed at these locations even when no active bleeding is noted. Since these positions are very close to the ureteral orifices, it is mandatory to visualize the orifices for patency. If obstruction to the orifice with one of the hemostatic sutures is of concern, a single ampule of indigo carmine can be given intravenously. If there is normal function and perfusion of the kidney and the orifice is not obstructed, the blue dye should appear within a matter of a few minutes.

During surgical enucleation of the prostatic adenoma, difficulty may be encountered when attempting to define by blunt dissection the anatomical plane between the adenoma and the true prostatic capsule. This situation is most likely to occur posteriorly when there is preexisting inflammatory disease of the prostate or prostatic malignancy, which obliterates the normal tissue plane. If the surgeon uses any excessive force or loses his anatomical orientation, he may tear the prostatic capsule and even enter the rectal lumen. This latter complication is extremely serious and will lead to a rectal-prostatic fistula if the injury is not identified and corrective measures taken immediately.

If the rectal wall is intact and only the prostatic capsule has been torn, an attempt should be made to repair the prostatic capsule with absorbable sutures such as 2-0 or 3-0 chromic catgut. Urine drainage should be provided by means of a suprapubic catheter. During the first 10 to 14 days of the postoperative period, the patient should be kept on a low-residue diet and constipation prevented in order to protect the anterior rectal wall. Likewise, it is imperative that the patient not receive any rectal suppositories, have any rectal temperatures taken, or undergo any digital manipulation, which might jeopardize or perforate the rectal wall.

If the rectum has been damaged during the enucleation, the fecal stream must be diverted by a colostomy and the rectal tear repaired with a multiple-layer closure. Likewise, the defect in the prostatic capsule should be repaired with absorbable sutures. A suprapubic catheter will be required for urine drainage. No attempt should be made to remove the catheter or close the colostomy until complete healing has been demonstrated by both a cystourethrogram and a barium enema.

References

1. Cockett ATK: Urological trauma. Sym Contemp Surg 14:95-125, 1979
2. Henkel HB: The urologic battle injury in the Korean conflict. J Urol 70:637-647, 1953
3. Kessler R: Diagnosis and treatment of genitourinary emergencies. Urol Digest 15:12-28, 1976

4. Masoloff JI, Mitam JH, Bunts RC: Fluid and electrolyte changes associated with transurethral prostate resection. South Med J 59:1203-1208, 1966
5. Richardson JR Jr, Leadbetter GW Jr: Nonoperative treatment of the ruptured bladder. J Urol 114:213-216, 1975
6. Robards VL Jr, Haglund RV, Lubin EN, Leach JR: Treatment of rupture of the bladder. J Urol 116:178-179, 1976
7. Schellhammer PF: Electrosurgery: Principles, hazards and precautions. Urology 3:261-268, 1974
8. Smith DR: Injuries to the genitourinary tract. In General Urology, vol 16, pp 240–243. Los Altos, CA, Lange Medical Publications, 1978
9. Weyrauch HM: Transurethral prostatectomy. In Surgery of the Prostate, vol 13, pp 390–391. Philadelphia, WB Saunders, 1959
10. Wyker AW Jr: Trauma. In Wyker AW Jr, Gillenwater JV (eds): Method of Urology. Baltimore, Williams & Wilkins, 1975

55
Complications of Renal Surgery and Trauma

M. J. V. Smith

OVERVIEW

Complications are inherent in any surgical procedure, but certain complications are inherent and unique to the surgical approach to the kidney, and certain complications are associated with traumatic injuries to the kidney. The wise surgeon will be alert to a variety of possibilities and have an organized approach to their recognition and treatment. Such an approach will often mean that effective treatment, anticipation, and prevention will ameliorate if not completely avoid serious impairment of renal function. This chapter provides a broad overview of the various possible complications, reviews some of the possible evasive actions, and suggests effective methods to evaluate and care for complications when they occur.

It is wise also when reading a chapter of this nature to understand the credo of the author, which is to make every effort to save nephrons. Thus it should be apparent that the prophylactic "nephrectomy" is anathema to me.

Renal surgery has moved forward with such rapidity that a careful preoperative evaluation is of fundamental importance. The surgeon should be aware that the mortality from this surgery can be tripled in patients with infection, azotemia, or cancer.[8]

Pathophysiology

If the gross anatomy of the kidneys and their relationships to neighboring organs are clearly understood, many of the complications of renal surgery can be avoided. The posterior relationships of the kidneys are essentially similar, except that the right kidney, being lower, has a lesser relationship to the pleura. The renal bed is bounded medially by the psoas major and posteriorly by quadratus lumborum muscle, across which run three nerves (the subcostal, iliohypogastric, and ilioinguinal) and the subcostal vessels. Laterally lies the aponeurosis of transversus muscle and superiorly the diaphragm, which is attached to the inner aspect of the 12th and 11th ribs and separates the kidneys from these ribs and the pleura.

Anteriorly lies the peritoneum, which is in close apposition to the kidney. However, three structures on each side have no intervening peritoneum: on the right, the triangular adrenal overlies the upper pole of the kidney; just along the medial border lies the descending part of the duodenum; while the hepatic flexure overlies the lower pole. Unless great care is exercised during difficult dissections, these structures can be injured. Similarly, the left kidney has the adrenal, the tail of the pancreas, and the splenic flexure as direct anterior relationships.

Both kidneys have four coverings, the true capsule, the perirenal fat, Gerotas fascia, and the parirenal fat. Each plays an important role in protection and support of the kidney. The true capsule is a dense, fibrous structure that encloses the kidney substance. It can become extremely fibrotic and thickened. The surgeon must realize that this structure should always be closed if injured, because it is responsible for maintaining the integrity of the kidney by tamponade. Characteristically the true capsule will strip away from the kidney with great ease. Thus the discerning surgeon understands that if a difficult perirenal dissection suddenly becomes easy, "it must be subcapsular!"

The perirenal fat has a very characteristic firm, yellow consistency. It contains numerous interlacing fibrous strands. These act to form a functional support for the kidney and prevent it from tipping forward when a person assumes the upright position. These fibrous strands are particularly well-developed at the upper pole of the kidney. Surrounding this is the fascia of Gerota, which is a closed envelope open at its inferior end. It serves to form a barrier to the spread of blood or urine that extravasates into the space and also helps in tamponade of the kidney following trauma. Only in rare instances do the two sides connect across the midline. Gerota's fascia is firmly adherent to the adventitia of the major vessels. If at all possible, this layer should be reconstituted during surgical closure to prevent the kidney or ureter from becoming adherent to the underlying muscle, which interferes with their necessary mobility within the fatty layer.

The kidney is supplied by end-arteries and can be divided into five anatomical segments, each with its own segmental arterial supply. These were clearly described by Graves and are known as the apical, upper anterior, middle anterior, basilar, and posterior segments.[4] Various workers have tried to relate the arterial segments to the pyramidal distribution within the kidney.[14] These findings are very important and of considerable interest for those who plan intrarenal surgery. The original reviews should be consulted to delineate the arterial distribution to the various pyramids.[2, 14, 15] However, one constant finding is that the posterior segmental artery is the only supply to the posterior, middle third of the kidney. The junction of this arterial segment with the others lies in the plane of the anterior aspect of the posterior calyces. Thus an incision in this area will damage the blood supply to the smallest number of nephrons.[5]

There is considerable discussion of so-called aberrant arteries to the kidney. In the main, these are merely segmental vessels that find their origin from the main arterial trunk and represent the systems of the original segmental distribution.[4] There is an extensive collateral venous plexus within the kidney, and these vessels can usually be divided without fear of parenchymal damage. The major veins lie close to the bases of the infundibulum and along the outer border of the pelvis. The remaining veins form a series of longitudinal arcs, with one major group near the calices and the other in the juxtamedullary area.[12]

General Approaches to the Kidney

There are many approaches to the kidney, but regardless of the approach selected, a generous incision is necessary. The major complication of this type of surgery is massive hemorrhage, which is most difficult to control unless proper exposure has been obtained. The incision is usually influenced by the surgeon's preference, the patient's anatomy, and the nature of the operative problem. Thus, ectopic kidneys are often approached through unusual incisions, while in trauma or vascular surgery, it is easier to obtain control of the renal pedicle through an anterior approach.

The flank approach is the most commonly used incision by the urologic surgeon and is remarkably effective as long as the patient is correctly placed upon the table. If the patient is not correctly placed, then the malposition will prevent adequate exposure, and the procedure will become difficult and frustrating. Thus it should be a rule that in all flank approaches to the kidney, the patient be placed on the table by the operating surgeon. Particular attention must be paid during this placement to make sure that none of the restraining tapes or supporting structures cause damage. For example, the axilla should be protected with a soft support to prevent brachial plexus damage, and the area over the peroneal nerve should be protected.

It is well to remember that in the flank position, the vena cava can become obstructed by a renal mass. This can give rise to serious cardiovascular compromise, and the surgeon should check with the anesthesiologist concerning this possibility before proceeding with the surgery.

The most common complication following use of the flank approach to the kidney is inadvertent damage to the nerves that run between the transversus and internal oblique muscles. Care should always be taken to identify them so that they are not damaged. Injury to these nerves can lead to weakness of the abdominal wall or troublesome anesthesia. Some patients may develop a neuroma and continuing pain, and the neuroma will require excision by a neurosurgeon at a later date.

Many surgeons inject local anesthesia (*e.g.*, 0.5% bupivacaine) around these nerves during closure of the wound so that during the postoperative period there is a decrease in the use of analgesics and earlier patient ambulation. Lessening the need for analgesics is an important consideration, since narcotics may depress the cough reflex postoperatively, thus increasing the risk of pulmonary complications. It is essential that the physical signs and symptoms of acute atelectasis be checked and immediate action taken to correct this problem. Many patients develop the so-called down-lung syndrome during the first 4 hours postoperatively from aspiration of mucus into the most inferior lobe of the lung (usually the posterior lobe). Ipsilateral atelectasis occurs later and is due to poor respiratory excursion and depressed cough reflex.

Almost any incision that is used to expose the kidney will risk causing a pneumothorax. It is essential that this be recognized at the time of surgery and appropriate corrective action taken.

The flank approach is very good for the obese

patient, since the panniculus usually falls forward and away from the operative field. However, it is not a good approach in most children, since the space between the ilium and the costal margin is limited. This approach has the virtue of ready access to the upper portion of the kidney and its collecting system, effective retroperitoneal drainage postoperatively, and finally a very strong wound closure. The actual incision can be made subcostal, through the rib, or supracostal, each route having its proponents and indications.

If the main surgery is to involve the major vessels, then an anterior approach is chosen by many. Some will use a subcostal (chevron) incision, while others will use the midline incision. These incisions are much more useful where the space between the lower rib and the iliac crest is minimal, and they may be either transperitoneal or extraperitoneal, depending upon the preference of the surgeon.

Finally, there is the posterior lumbotomy, in which the incision is made parallel to paraspinus muscles from the angle of the rib to the anterior spine of the iliac crest so that the kidney is approached through the lumbodorsal fascia. This incision provides more limited access and is useful for operations in which direct access to the renal pelvis is the primary concern. Although access may be limited, the incidence of postoperative morbidity is reduced.

NEPHRECTOMY

It is important to mobilize the kidney out of its bed by means of blunt and sharp dissection. This is often facilitated by mobilizing the upper pole first so that the kidney does not disappear into the dome of the diaphragm. If this is not possible, it is wise to mobilize the ureter early, and after it has been transected, to use it for traction. If spillage of urine is of no concern, the traction can be improved further by passing a Foley catheter into the pelvis and inflating the balloon. Particular care should be taken when dissecting around the lower pole, since a polar artery may come directly from the aorta. A similar situation can occur at the upper pole. However, troublesome bleeding usually comes from the adrenal gland, which may be inadvertently injured. If this occurs, the bleeding is best controlled with a running suture.

Sometimes exposure of the renal hilus is hindered by a large cyst or hydronephrosis. The dissection may be facilitated by aspirating these structures.

The renal artery should be doubly ligated and divided first in order to prevent pooling of blood in the kidney. On the left side, it will be necessary to ligate the adrenal and gonadal veins as they enter the renal vein so that sufficient mobility is obtained and then to expose the other structures. Then the vein can be ligated safely. On both sides, particular attention should be paid to the posterior aspect of the renal vein, where it is not unusual for a lumbar vessel to drain directly. It should be noted that the old-fashioned concept of ligation en masse of the renal hilus is discouraged, since in a few cases such a maneuver gives rise to an arteriovenous fistula. If the dissection of the hilus proves difficult, then it is advisable to thin the pedicle mass as much as possible and then apply a large Satinsky-type vascular clamp. The kidney is then removed and each individual vessel identified and suture ligated.

Sometimes it may prove impossible to dissect the kidney out of the surrounding fibrotic tissue. In these cases it is sometimes necessary to carry out a subcapsular nephrectomy in which the capsule is opened and dissected away from the kidney. The vascular supply is then individually identified at the hilar lip and ligated. Again, it may be necessary to cross clamp the thinned pedicle.

Occasionally major hemorrhage can occur, and it must be controlled by direct compression of the renal pedicle against the lumbar vertebral bodies. Blind clamping in a pool of rising blood can only result in damage to neighboring structures (e.g., duodenum or colon). Once compression controls the bleeding, the patient's condition can be stabilized. After additional suction lines and vascular instruments are obtained, gradual release and point compression to the exact site of the bleeding can be obtained. The vessel is then dissected proximally and distally so that vascular clamps can be applied and the bleeding site repaired. The vena cava can be safely ligated as long as the most cephalad ligature is below the junction with the left renal vein. Complex problems in regard to the cava are discussed below (see under Radical Nephrectomy).

It is probably necessary only to drain the renal fossa if an infected kidney was removed. Very occasionally the area will have a persistent drainage due usually to nonabsorbable suture material that has become infected and that will have to be removed by surgical exploration.

A delayed retroperitoneal hemorrhage is usually manifested by the sudden development of ileus or acute gastric dilatation.

Not infrequently there is a temptation to allow patients who have undergone flank exploration to start taking nourishment by mouth very early. It is probably wise to wait at least 48 to 72 hours to avoid ileus.

Injuries to the tail of the pancreas and the spleen can occasionally occur on the left side. It is very important to recognize an injured pancreas so that it may be amputated and oversewn. Any persistent wound drainage should always be checked for amylase to exclude this rare injury.

Injury to the spleen can rarely be oversewn. Except in children, it is wise to perform a splenectomy. It is also advisable to leave the gastrosplenic vessels long, since postoperative gastric distension can push the ties off short vessels.

PARTIAL NEPHRECTOMY

Partial nephrectomy may be indicated for a variety of reasons. Whenever it is done, it is wise to remove the whole of the segment involved, if at all possible. It is also important to leave the covering capsule intact so that it may be closed over the defect. The collecting system should be closed watertight and all bleeding points suture-ligated with 4-0 chromic catgut. Sometimes it is necessary to use a peritoneal patch to cover the defect.

A drain should be brought out through a separate stab incision. Most patients will drain urine for awhile. If there are substantial amounts and no signs of the drainage diminishing, then an indwelling ureteral stent should be placed cystoscopically. If the drainage still does not stop, reexploration is indicated, because it is likely that a calix has been left open without connection to the main collecting system.

The question of whether partial nephrectomy should be done for a tumor in a solitary kidney has plagued surgeons for some time. It would seem that the results of a partial nephrectomy are comparable to those achieved by radical nephrectomy, but it is probable that these represent a very select group of people. Such an approach should never be taken unless dialysis is readily available, because all patients will have a period of azotemia of varying degree during the postoperative period.[8, 9]

RADICAL NEPHRECTOMY AND LYMPHADENECTOMY

The ready availability of CT scans and arteriography has made the diagnosis of renal mass lesions relatively simple. In addition, the use of preoperative infarction of tumors has become a recognized mode of therapy.[9] In selected cases, it is very helpful in controlling the vascularity of tumors. However, if coils are used, it is essential that surgeons account for all that were used. Otherwise they may migrate to other places (e.g., the opposite kidney or femoral artery).

It is essential in surgery for cancer that the artery and vein be tied before the tumor is manipulated. This means that the veins on both sides must be mobilized first so that the deeper artery can then be identified and ligated. Then the kidney within the envelope of Gerota's fascia is mobilized and excised.

Preoperative evaluation will have alerted the surgeon to the possibility of a tumor thrombus. This is often suggested by proteinuria or a prolonged arterial phase on the arteriograms. If this problem is suspected, an inferior venacavagram and sometimes a superior cavagram may be necessary to delineate the extent of the tumor, even though real-time sonography has shown that a tumor thrombus is present.

If there is a large thrombus, then the cava must be mobilized above and below so that occlusive clamps can be applied. The tumor thrombus can often be easily extracted from the vena cava once the ostium of the renal vein has been excised. Only rarely is there direct invasion of the wall of the vena cava. If the thrombus is more extensive, it may be necessary to milk the tumor thrombus out of the cava using a No. 14-French Foley catheter alongside the tumor by inflating the balloon and using it in the same manner as a Fogarty catheter. Care must be taken to maintain positive intrathoracic pressure to avoid embolism.

Rarely the thrombus may actually go into the right atrium, in which case extensive incisions and the use of cardiopulmonary bypass have been helpful.

In extensive left-sided tumors it is possible to excise the vena cava and either repair the remaining cava forming a tube from the right renal vein or occasionally anastomose the right renal vein into the portal vein. Sometimes the cava can be resected above the left renal vein when the tumor is on the right. The patient then relies upon collateral circulation, which may have developed through the gonadal, adrenal, lumbar, and azygos systems. Initially this may not be sufficiently developed to handle the venous return, and severe oliguria and azotemia may develop. Thus it is unwise to attempt such heroic surgery unless dialysis is readily available.

Most surgeons recommend that an ipsilateral lymphadenectomy from the level of the inferior mesenteric artery to the crus of the diaphragm should be done after the kidney and Gerota's fascial envelope have been removed. There are data only from retrospective studies to support this concept, but it is essential that the dissection be extensive and complete.[8] However, unless care is taken, the cisterna chyli may be injured. It should be formally identified and occluded, usually with a hemoclip. Similarly, the lumbar vessels should be identified and tied; otherwise they will retract into lumbar muscles and troublesome bleeding can occur.

A complication that is unique to radical nephrectomy is the development of acute bowel obstruction in the immediate postoperative period, due usually to failure to identify tears in the mesentery of the colon as it was reflected from Gerota's fascia. Unless these tears are closed, they present possible sites for internal herniation, resulting in the "localized loops" seen on roentgenography.[6]

NEPHROURETERECTOMY

Nephroureterectomy is indicated in patients with tumors of the collecting system or ureter. It requires that the kidney, ureter, and cuff of the bladder around the ureteral orifice be excised in continuity. This can be done through a single incision in a thin person, but usually it requires two incisions. Most surgeons will do the flank portion first and then push the specimen down into the wound and remove the specimen through a separate abdominal incision. Thus, except for the extensive surgery involved, no complications are unique to this type of surgery unless the surgeon decides to compromise the procedure by not removing the ureter and a cuff of bladder.

PYELOPLASTY

Many surgeons prefer the traditional approach to the kidney through the flank for pyeloplasty. This requires almost complete mobilization of the kidney. I prefer an anterior extraperitoneal approach, because minimal mobilization is necessary and the pyeloplasty is carried out with kidney in the position that it will be at the end of the operation. This avoids potential twisting of the repair and ensures that the drainage will be dependent.

Regardless of which type of repair is selected, it is essential that the ureter and pelvis be completely mobilized. Neither the ureter nor the pelvis should be handled with anything other than traction sutures (not with forceps or other crushing instruments). Any bleeding points must be handled with ligatures, *not* fulguration. "Marking sutures" should be used prior to opening the pelvis, because the pelvis collapses immediately upon release of pressure, producing distortion.

The repair should be precise and watertight. This should be checked by distending the pelvis. The pelvis should empty promptly when ureteral compression is released.

All pyeloplasties must be drained, preferably by a soft Penrose-type drain that is brought out through a separate stab incision. If copious urinary drainage ensues, the incision can be covered with an enterostomy collecting device to keep the patient dry. If no drainage occurs, the drain can be shortened and removed beginning on the fifth postoperative day. If, however, the drainage is copious, the drain should be advanced at 7 days in case the drain is exerting a wick effect at the repair site. If drainage continues, the patient should have an internal ureteral stent placed. It is most important that urinary leakage be kept to a minimum, since such leakage will often set up a dense, fibrous inflammatory response that will contribute to the failure of the repair.

Discussions of pyeloplasty always provoke comment on whether stents or nephrostomies should be employed. The lines of battle are usually clearly drawn.[8] On one hand, it is argued that stents or nephrostomies may cause bacteriuria or bleeding, while, on the other, it is pointed out that they provide drainage and prevent anastomotic leaks. The absolute indications for their use are fairly clear-cut: previous surgery or pyeloplasty on that kidney; significant inflammatory reaction in or around the proposed repair; and in repairs that are less than ideal, for example, incomplete suture closure, a reoperation, or when congenital anomalies exist.

It is important that the stents be placed *prior* to beginning the repair.

The stent can probably be removed at 7 to 10 days. A nephrostogram should always be performed first. This should show prompt passage of contrast material at low pressure. The nephrostomy tube should then be clamped for 24 hours. If there is no fever or flank pain, the nephrostomy may be removed after obtaining urine for culture.

NEPHROSTOMY

Nephrostomy drainage to provide temporary relief of obstruction or to protect the kidney is not an uncommon operation; but it is now only rarely used as a permanent method of urinary diversion, except in the elderly or poor-risk patient.

The type of tube used and its size are very much a matter of the preference of the surgeon. If the diversion is temporary, I prefer a Malecot catheter with two of the retaining wings removed. This provides a wide-bore tube that is not likely to cause intrapelvic obstruction, which can occur if a Foley catheter is used. Also the opening in the Malecot tube is the most dependent, while in the Foley catheter, the opening is beyond the retaining bag. Certainly it is easier to replace the Foley catheter nephrostomy, since a rigid instrument does not need to be used. This decreases the risk of renal damage.

At the time of placement of the tube, the complication of leakage around the tube can be avoided if the surgeon remembers that the nephrostomy tube should be brought out through the kidney. The first nephrotomy should be over the internally placed stone forceps, which pull a small red rubber catheter into the collecting system. This then brings the nephrostomy tube back. Thus the tubes that pass through the kidney are ever larger in size, thus causing tamponade at the site of egress.

Sometimes there will be poor drainage or bleeding after the tube is inserted. The commonest cause of this is that the tube lies in the intrarenal sinus rather than in the collecting system. The surgeon should always check for this complication *before* he closes.

It is extraordinarily important to pay close attention to the site at which the nephrostomy tube is brought out on to the skin. Those that exist posteriorly are liable to kinking, but, more important, the patient will be unable to sleep flat and unable to manage it should later circumstances require self-care.

The nephrostomy diversion may sometimes need to be permanent. If this is expected, then it is probably wise to insert a circle- or U-tube nephrostomy. Certainly this should be mandatory in children. This approach avoids dislodgement, allows excellent drainage, and is easy to change.

The complication of continued bleeding through a nephrostomy tube is best handled initially by obstructing the tube and allowing the clot to tamponade the bleeding. It is not necessary to remove the clot, since the urinary enzymes will lyse it satisfactorily.

A major drawback of the nephrostomy tube is that its presence will encourage urinary infection, which may result in rapid formation of urinary sand, sludge, and stones. This complication can be avoided to some extent by keeping the urine acid. Occasionally infections can be kept under control with local irrigations (see under Stone Surgery). Sometimes the walls of the tubing may be encrusted. These can be satisfactorily "reamed" using a cone-tipped ureteral catheter in much the same manner that a test-tube brush is used.

Nephrostomies should always be sewn in place at the skin using strong, nonabsorbable sutures. They should be carefully taped in place so that there is no danger of inadvertent removal of the tube.

Whenever a tube is changed, the proper positioning should always be checked by means of a nephrostogram.

The introduction of percutaneous nephrostomy under radiologic control has sparked a whole new armamentarium of instruments and exaggerated claims.[11] The field is developing at an extraordinary rate. It should be clear to all that this technique requires considerable expertise and should not be done by the uninitiated. Recently it has been claimed that up to 90% of nephrostomies can be done by this method.

These same techniques have also been adapted to the management of renal cysts and abscesses. These structures can be punctured and drained using percutaneous techniques. The problems are inadequate drainage, sepsis, and, finally, bleeding that may require open exploration.

PERINEPHRIC ABSCESS

The patient with a perinephric abscess is usually seriously ill; however, *NO* patient with this diagnosis is too sick to withstand incision and drainage. No patient has ever improved on conservative treatment alone; consequently, the sooner the abscess is drained, the more rapid the recovery.

It is wrong to believe that the incision should be very large. It is better to place numerous drains and utilize daily irrigation until the drainage ceases. Also, it is important that the skin and subcutaneous tissue be left open and a secondary closure planned for a week later. When this is not done and the skin is closed primarily, there is a high incidence of wound infections.[3]

It is not very wise to perform a nephrectomy at the time of the abscess drainage, because the danger of uncontrollable bleeding or injury to nearby structures is very high. It is not unusual for an apparently nonfunctioning kidney to resume activity after drainage of the abscess. The only time a nephrectomy *must* be done, regardless of the risk, is when emphysematous pyelonephritis has been diagnosed. Nephrectomy is then a life-saving operation more than 60% of the time.[3]

STONE SURGERY

In order to avoid the removal of a stone from the kidney representing just a surgical exercise, it is most important that every patient be evaluated metabolically prior to surgical excision. These patients should be approached with the concept that surgery is but one of the steps in their overall management. All too often a patient with a large stone has its presence blamed on infection. It is well to remember that patients who form struvite (infection) stones frequently have metabolic disorders.

Stones are bilateral in 15% to 20% of patients. Which stone should be operated upon first should signal a functional evaluation of each kidney to determine which kidney has the more compromised function. It has been clearly shown in experimental work that better results are achieved if the more compromised kidney is selected first.[10]

Recently a large number of adjunctive techniques have been developed that have decreased the morbidity associated with stone-removal procedures by decreasing parenchymal damage and ensuring complete removal. The aim of any surgery for stones is to remove all of the calcareous material, making certain that no foreign body is left behind to form the nidus for a recurrent stone. The major challenge in stone surgery is of course the staghorn, with its attendant dangers of sepsis and deteriorating renal function.

Occlusion of the renal artery and cooling of the kidney have improved surgeons' abilities to carry out prolonged operations upon the kidney with less blood loss and better preservation of renal function. Occlusion and cooling carry some complications. First, great care must be used in the application of the clamp or occlusive device to the renal artery. This instrument should have a wide blade and no sharp edges to prevent intimal tearing during subsequent renal manipulation. Prior to occlusion, it is wise to give 25 g of mannitol intravenously. This appears to protect against ischemic tubular injury.

It is unwise to occlude the circulation of the kidney for longer than 15 minutes unless the kidney is cooled to 15°C.

During hypothemia, it is important to use liquid, not ice, which will cause localized infarcts. It is also important to monitor the patient's temperature during hypothermic cooling of the kidney. All patients will experience a 1°C fall, and corrective devices such as a warming blanket should be available prior to surgery.

As mentioned above, stones that are left behind should be regarded as an operative failure, even though this occurs in some 20% of patients.[12] It is toward this problem that much of the present research is directed. Thus intraoperative organ roentgenograms are under study and modification. All the work is directed toward making these adjuncts readily available to all. The recent introduction of Polaroid TPX film shows great promise in locating small residual stones using simple techniques. Intraoperative real-time sonography has also proven extraordinarily successful in experienced hands. The more sophisticated nephroscopes with flexible tips and grasping forceps have shown great promise and are under continuing modification. Finally, a coagulum to entrap small stones has been used for a long time. Recently its use has been revived because it has been shown that instead of using bovine fibrin to make this coagulum, cryoprecipitate plasma (20 ml), thrombin (200 units), and calcium chloride (1 mg) could be used to form an excellent clot to extract small retained stones. Some fear has been expressed that thrombin could contribute to intravascular clotting. However, if the thrombin is not placed under pressure or is replaced with more calcium chloride, there is no problem.

Renal Trauma

If trauma to the kidneys is suspected, then it is mandatory that an excretory urogram be obtained. If the patient is the victim of multiple trauma, necessitating rapid transfer to the operating suite, the patient should still receive a bolus of contrast material during the resuscitative efforts so that once the patient's condition has been stabilized, at least one roentgenogram can be obtained that will establish the presence or absence of a kidney. The exploring hand can be easily misled.

A consideration that should always be kept in mind is that traumatic hematuria may be symptomatic of an underlying pathologic problem. This is particularly likely in children, in up to 30% of whom there may be severely diseased kidneys. The disease is revealed when minor trauma causes hematuria.[13]

The management of renal trauma is fairly straightforward and follows the usual surgical principles; that is to say, if there is contamination such as with injuries due to violence (gunshot or knife wounds), then exploration is usually necessary.[7] However, if the trauma is accidental, only deterioration of the patient's condition as manifested by a falling hematocrit or blood pressure mandates exploration.

The most important principle of the management of renal trauma is that the surgeon *must* obtain control of the renal pedicle *before* opening the retroperitoneum. If this principle is not observed, the surgeon will be forced into performing a nephrectomy, because once the retroperitoneum is opened and tamponade is removed, brisk and uncontrollable bleeding usually follows.

The renal pedicle is best approached transperitoneally by a longitudinal incision in the posterior parietal peritoneum over the aorta after the small bowel has been displaced out of the abdominal cavity. The duodenum should be in the upper portion of the wound and should be retracted upward to expose the renal veins. On the left, the gonadal vein must be divided to allow the necessary mobility to expose the artery, which lies posteriorly. This renal artery must be distinguished from the superior mesenteric and splenic vessels. The right renal artery is best exposed between the cava and the aorta.

If there is a major arterial injury and the facilities are available, the vessel can be occluded with an intra-arterial balloon preoperatively by the femoral route.

Once control of the artery has been established, the retroperitoneum can be opened along the paracolic gutter and the kidney dissected out and formally explored.

Complications are more common in the patient who has had violent trauma to the kidney, mainly because the surgeon may fail to appreciate the "blast" effect of the missile. Thus there may be persistent urinary drainage from the flank because necrosis of the renal pelvis or collecting system has occurred. If no nephrostomy drainage was established *a priori*, then the kidney will probably need to be reexplored.

Arteriovenous fistula or aneurysms are also more common following violent trauma and should be carefully excluded during the initial evaluation. However, it is not unusual for these to be late occurrences following trauma. It therefore behooves the physician to be aware of this problem and to reevaluate the patient should there be persistent hematuria, hypertension, or bruits.

All surgeons should be aware that there are certain injuries to the kidney that may not be associated with hematuria. Injury to the renal pedicle such as may occur during sudden vertical deceleration is rarely associated with hematuria. Tears of the renal parenchyma that do not disrupt the collecting system can give rise to brisk perirenal bleeding without hematuria. Finally, acute disruption of the ureteropelvic junction can occur. This will not be associated with hematuria but rather will only be diagnosed late when a flank mass becomes apparent. It is therefore a cardinal rule that excretory urograms must be done if renal trauma is suspected, even though the results of urinalysis are normal.

Patients who have extravasation of urine on early evaluation may need exploration. Only those in whom infected urine is present or a high-velocity missile injury has occurred require exploration. Most others will improve in the absence of distal obstruction, and conservative *close* observation and bed rest will take care of the problem.

Any patient with kidney trauma in whom the hematuria persists more than 2 weeks should be seriously considered for full reinvestigation. All patients should have a follow-up pyelogram at 6 months to delineate any damage that may have occurred so that whether continuing follow-up is necessary can be decided. Any patient who is going to develop posttraumatic hypertension will have manifested this problem by 6 months.

References

1. Boyce WH, Harrison LH: Complications in renal stone surgery. In Smith RB, Skinner DG (eds): Complications of Urologic Surgery. Philadelphia, WB Saunders, 1976
2. Boyce WH, Russell JM, Webb R: The management of the papillae during intrarenal surgery. Trans Am Assoc Genitourin Surg 71:76, 1979
3. Diaz R, Smith MJV: Air in the urinary system. J Urol (in press)
4. Graves FT: The Arterial Anatomy of the Kidney. Baltimore, Williams & Wilkins, 1971
5. Hodson J: The lobar structure of the kidney. Br J Urol 44:246, 1972
6. Humphrey RL: Renal complications. In Abeloff MD (ed): Complications of Cancer. Baltimore, Johns Hopkins University Press, 1979
7. Lucey DT, Smith MJV, Koontz WW Jr: A plea for conservative treatment of traumatic renal injuries. J Trauma 11:306, 1971
8. Lytton B: Renal surgery. Mon Urol 3:35, 1982
9. McDonald MW: Current therapy for renal cell carcinoma. J Urol 127:211, 1982
10. Miller JB, Marrion DW, Gillenwater JY: Patterns of recovery of renal function after surgical relief of chronic bilateral partial ureteral obstruction. Invest Urol 17:69, 1979
11. Smith AD: Symposium on endourology. Urol Clin North Am 9:1, 1982
12. Smith MJV: Anatrophic nephrolithotomy. In Roth RA, Finlayson B (eds): Stones: Clinical Management of Urolithiasis. Baltimore, Williams & Wilkins, 1983
13. Smith MJV, Bonacarti AF, Seidel RL: Accident trauma to the kidneys in children. J Urol 96:845, 1966
14. Sykes D: The correlation between renal vascularisation and lobulation of the kidney. Br J Urol 36:549, 1964
15. Vordermark JS II: Segmental anatomy of the kidney. Urology 17:521, 1981

56 Complications of Renal Transplantation

H. M. Lee | G. Mendez–Picon

Vascular Complications

ARTERIAL THROMBOSIS

Thrombosis of the renal artery following transplantation is one of the most devastating complications of renal transplantation. Fortunately, arterial thrombosis is a rare complication with an incidence reported from 0.5% to 2%.[43, 70, 101]

Thrombosis of the renal artery may be divided into two separate groups: early occlusion in the posttransplant period and late thrombosis (over 3 months posttransplant). The thrombosis that occurs early, from a few hours to 4 weeks posttransplantation, is usually related to technical factors: intimal tear of the donor artery during nephrectomy or during perfusion with subsequent intimal flap formation and thrombosis upon revascularization; if the hypogastric artery is used, failure to endarterectomize the arteriosclerotic plaque that is commonly present; if an end-to-side anastomosis is performed to the common iliac artery, a discrepancy in thickness between the iliac vessel and the renal artery, which can produce a faulty narrow anastomosis; multiple anastomoses needed because of the presence of multiple renal arteries; hypercoagulability state; hyperacute or acute accelerated rejection, which can produce renal artery thrombosis as the final event in the case of capillary and arterial thrombosis; a severe kinking of the artery following anastomosis, which can also produce thrombosis in the posttransplant period.[27, 104]

When the thrombosis occurs late (later than 3 months posttransplant), the cause is usually severe renal artery stenosis or low-flow states such as myocardial infarction and severe dehydration superimposed on moderate renal artery stenosis (Fig. 56-1).

The most important factors in management of posttransplant arterial thrombosis are prevention and early diagnosis. The lack of collateral circulation in the transplanted kidney adds to the urgency. Anuria in the posttransplant period is the most important sign. It is of greater significance if stable renal function has been present for a few hours to days prior to its development. The following steps should be taken: (1) irrigation of the catheter (if it is in the immediate posttransplant period) to rule out the presence of lower urinary tract obstruction secondary to bleeding; (2) if the anuria is not related to lower urinary tract obstruction postoperatively, the surgeon may immediately undertake operative ex-

FIG. 56-1. A renal artery thrombosis that occurred in the immediate posttransplant period.

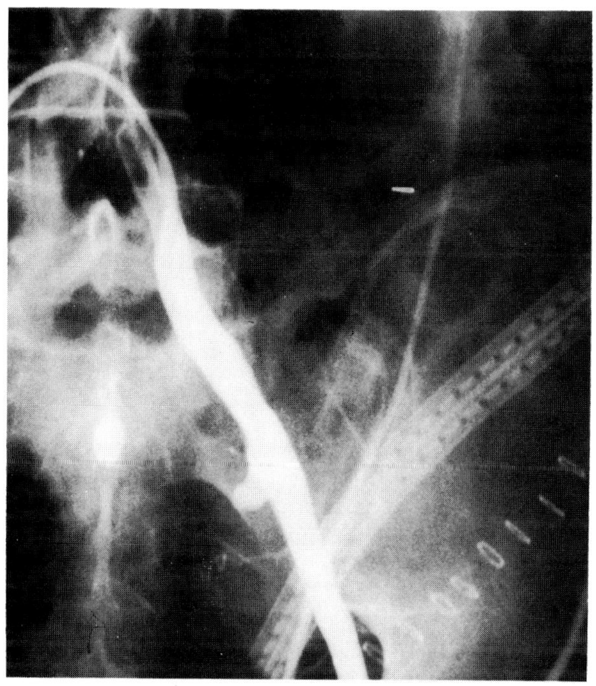

ploration without further diagnostic procedures; (3) if the surgeon is fairly confident in the integrity of anastomosis or if anuria occurs late, radionuclide scan (^{99m}Tc DPTA) can be obtained to assess the vascularity of the graft. Even though angiogram is the definitive confirmatory study, it is seldom necessary.

Usually a graft with an occluded renal artery is not salvageable, but there have been reports of thrombectomy performed 12, 24, and 48 hours after arterial occlusion.[44, 68, 95] In these reports renal function was preserved, in one instance with return of function to prethrombosis level.

We have experienced seven cases of renal thrombosis in 649 transplants (1%). Three of these thromboses occurred late in the course of the transplanted graft.[44] In all cases severe renal artery stenosis was present. Our experience suggests that repair of high-grade stenosis should be performed to avoid thrombosis.

Inspection of the renal artery prior to anastomosis as well as careful endarterectomy of the hypogastric artery is necessary.

In a few cases in our experience, arteriotomy in the common iliac artery, opposite the hypogastric, was performed to assess the intima after endarterectomy of the hypogastric vessel. If end-to-side anastomosis is contemplated without an aortic patch, it may be necessary to use a patch of vein in the common iliac artery to which the thin-walled renal artery or arteries can be anastomosed with more satisfactory results.

RENAL ARTERY STENOSIS

Transplant renal artery stenosis is a well-recognized complication, causing hypertension. Since hypertension and renal artery stenosis can cause deterioration of renal function, this complication presents important diagnostic and therapeutic problems to the transplant surgeon. The incidence has been variously reported as 1.5% up to 15.6%.[35, 36, 42, 70] Lacombe, based on his experience with routine angiograms in 100 patients showing a 23% incidence of renal artery stenosis, speculated that the actual incidence may be as high as 25%.[37]

Etiology

The exact cause of renal artery stenosis is unknown and probably multifactorial. The following causes have been said to contribute to the development of renal artery stenosis: (1) progressive atherosclerosis; (2) faulty surgical technique of anastomosis; (3) trauma from perfusion cannula or perfusion itself or vessel damage during the donor nephrectomy; (4) hemodynamic turbulence (Morris, reporting renal artery stenosis after an end-to-side anastomosis, suggested hemodynamic turbulence to be the major cause of renal artery stenosis.[62, 69] It also seemed to occur more often in multiartery grafts); (5) kinking, angling, and torsion of the renal artery anastomosis, probably due to excess lengths of the vessel and a rigid or poorly rotating iliac artery; (6) rejection process; and (7) excessive fibrosis around the vessel. Although the source of the donor kidney has been implicated, we have found the same incidence of stenosis with transplants from cadavers and living, related donors. The length of machine preservation prior to transplantation also has been suggested to influence the rate of development of renal artery stenosis. Our experience with 50 cases of renal artery stenosis in over 700 transplants does not support this theory. Histologic examination of resected specimens showed intimal hyperplasia, intimal fibrosis, typical atherosclerosis, and "rejection change," such as vascular lesions, granulation, and thrombosis at the anastomotic site. Rare, but isolated atherosclerotic lesions of the hypogastric arteries have also been described as "renal artery stenosis."

Diagnosis

Renal artery stenosis may become clinically significant anywhere from 1 month to 2 years posttransplantation, most often between 1 and 7 months posttransplantation. We have seen it as early as 1 month and as late as 6 years after the transplant. The indications for arteriography in all our patients have been newly developed hypertension with or without deterioration of renal function and the presence of a bruit over the graft. Some have reported the presence of bruit in 100% of the patients, but this has not been our experience, with bruit seen in 76% of the documented cases. Reduction in renal function is rather uncommon and usually occurs rather late; however, it has been reported to mimic acute rejection episodes and also to simulate chronic rejection.[67, 81, 87] Significant erythrocytosis has been found to be associated with this lesion. Selective angiography confirmed the diagnosis and required more than one plane, usually AP as well as oblique views.

Angiographically, three types of lesions can be seen in renal artery stenosis: (1) At the anastomotic site the lesion is usually short and sharp and is created by kinking, angling, torsion, or periarterial fibrosis (Fig. 56-2). This lesion is created quite often by excessive lengths of the hypogastric and renal arteries or discrepancy in size between the hypogastric and renal artery. Faulty technique creating intimal flap or enfolding has been also blamed. Rarely, it can be caused by extension of the atherosclerosis. (2 and 3) In most series, a lesion distal to the anastomosis is more common, as has been our experience.[42] Two types of lesions can be seen in this area: short and sharp, caused by fibrotic bands, atheroma, and kinking (Fig. 56-3); and long and smooth, usu-

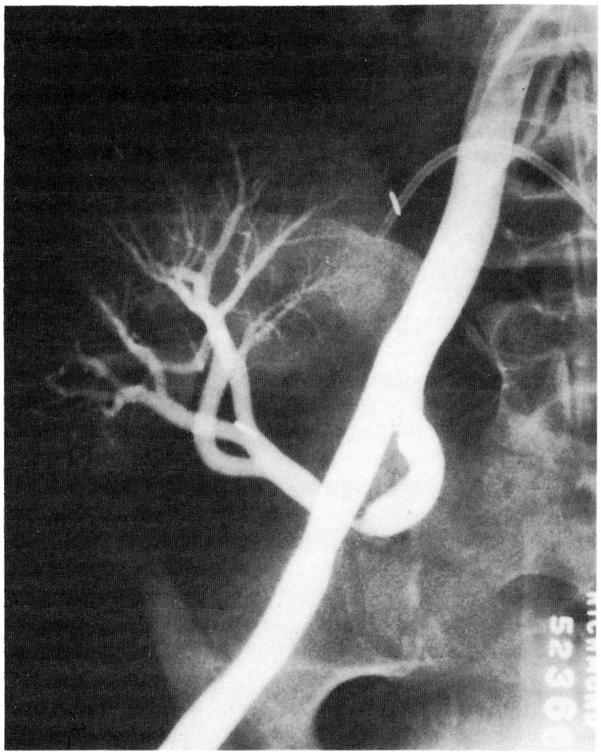

FIG. 56-2. Renal artery stenosis. The vessel is twisted and kinked just beyond the anastomosis.

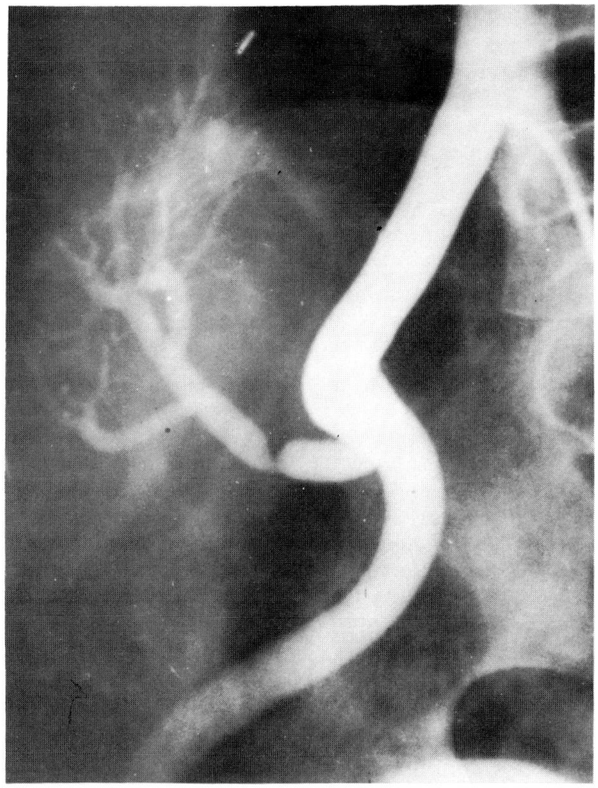

FIG. 56-3. Renal artery stenosis. Sharp, short stenosis is seen in the donor artery just beyond the anastomosis and is due to infolding or atherosclerosis.

FIG. 56-4. Renal artery stenosis. Segmental stenosis is seen in the donor artery.

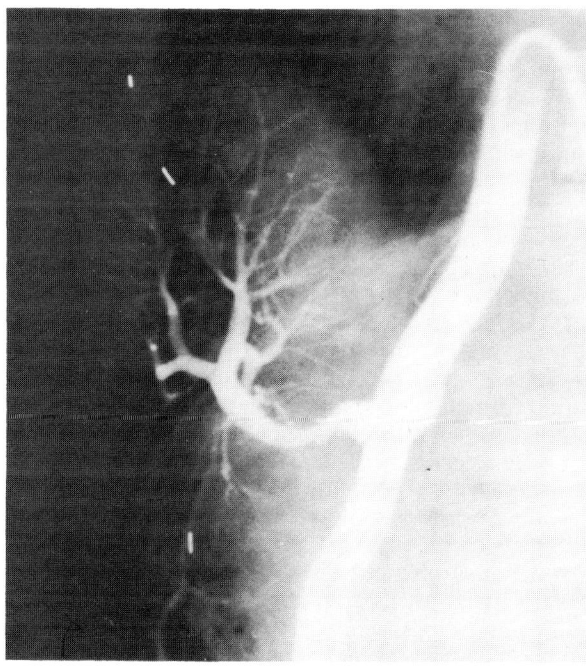

ally caused by fibrotic thickening of the vessel wall, presumably due to rejection damage or perfusion injury (Fig. 56-4).

Renal artery stenosis has been seen in normotensive patients, the reported incidence being from 5.3% to 13%.[37, 67, 105] Although some have noted that renal artery stenosis hypertension is generally more severe with higher renal vein and systemic plasma renin values, others have observed that the nature of hypertension is not predictive of the presence or degree of renal artery stenosis.[76, 105] Selective renin study has been recommended to define the source of hypertension in the patient who still has native kidneys. At times, in spite of the presence of renal artery stenosis, the actual source of renin may be from the native kidney.

Although the cause of the renal artery stenosis may be multifactorial, some preventive measures can be stressed.

1. Care in donor nephrectomy, with gentle handling of the renal vessels to avoid damage to the vasa vasorum
2. Avoidance of injury from perfusion jetstream by perfusing through the aorta, as well as avoidance of cannula injury by removing the portion of the vessel damaged by the cannula

3. Meticulous technique in the surgical anastomosis
4. Avoidance of excess lengths to prevent kinking or angling
5. Extreme care in handling the multiple artery graft, preferably using the aortic patch

Recently a few cases of spontaneous reversal of renal artery stenosis have been reported, including improvement of the hypertension.[75, 97, 100] The exact mechanism of spontaneous reversal is still unclear. The course of the renal artery stenosis is observed to be unpredictable, producing sudden unexpected hypertensive crisis.[32] We have also observed complete thrombosis of the renal artery in preexisting renal artery stenosis.

Treatment

In view of these observations including spontaneous reversal of the lesion and an unpredictable course along with possible complication of repair such as graft loss, the surgeon should be careful in deciding between medical and surgical treatment. Generally, surgical repair would be expected to produce poor results if renal function were poor with rejection in the hypertensive patient. The result would be better if renal function had not deteriorated and intrarenal arterial structures were normal. If surgical treatment is chosen, we prefer the transabdominal approach because of the ease of exposure of the blood vessel involved. Vein patch, resection and reanastomosis, vein bypass, and lysis of adhesions can be utilized.

Vein patch, when used on the long segment of the lesion in the donor artery, appears to be associated with a higher incidence of recurrence, either under or just beyond the patch. This may be because the vein patch does not extend quite beyond the pathologic lesion. Some state that this method should be used only at the anastomotic site. Resection and reanastomosis (reduction arterectomy) can be used effectively in the long artery with kinking.[31] In the majority of cases, vein bypass has produced quite satisfactory results. Lysis of periarterial adhesions has been least satisfactory; even after satisfactory loss of pressure gradient with this technique, recurrence is common, requiring additional surgery.[20] Recently, percutaneous angioplasty has been reported with good short-term results.[16, 89] Although there has been minimal morbidity, long-term follow-up has not been available. As an adjunct, Kauffman and colleagues have advocated the use of antiplatelet agents (dipyridamole) as a prophylactic agent, reporting satisfactory results from their experience.[35] Results of surgical repair have been reasonably good in the literature, with 74% overall satisfactory results, including secondary repair.[70] We have seen 88% immediate satisfactory results and 66% long-term.

ANASTOMOTIC LEAK AND SECONDARY MASSIVE HEMORRHAGE

Secondary massive hemorrhage from anastomotic leak or mycotic aneurysm in transplant patients is a most alarming and serious complication. Fortunately, the reported incidence is very low, ranging from 0.3% to 2.8%.[27, 70, 77] The mortality rate from this complication is reported to be high, ranging from 33% to 57%.[70, 99] Early massive hemorrhage is usually caused from an anastomotic leak due to faulty technique or a missed branch of the artery or vein, in either the recipient or the donor. Delayed appearance of massive hemorrhage is usually due to infection from perinephric abscess, urine leak, or development of a mycotic aneurysm from hematoma infection. At times the initial presentation of anastomotic leak might be a minor hemorrhage, but usually it is manifested by excrutiating pain at the graft site or back pain radiating to the flank and to the rectum, which is followed by a hematocrit drop or vascular collapse. Expeditious exploration and control of hemorrhage, with or without nephrectomy, are necessary to save the patient.

Resuturing of an anastomotic leak produced by infection is usually condemned to failure because of persistent infection in the arterial wall, although occasionally the salvage of graft by resuturing the leaking anastomosis has been reported.[47] If an end-to-side anastomosis to the common iliac artery leaks secondary to infection, it may be necessary to ligate the iliac system to prevent a repeat hemorrhage. Ischemic consequences of these ligations have been found to be very benign in most instances, and they do not necessitate urgent reconstructive procedures.[28]

With increases in cadaver donor transplantation and organ exchange, infection transmitted from the donor and contamination during organ perfusion as a source of transmission have become grave concerns.[90] Although contamination from *Staphylococcus epidermidis* may be of no grave consequence, contamination from gram-negative bacteria carries a high risk of graft loss and arterial hemorrhage.

Preventive measures should be stressed again, in view of the serious consequence of anastomotic leak, including careful dissection to reduce hematoma, lymphocele, and infection; careful technique in anastomosis; and strict sterile technique for donor nephrectomy and subsequent organ preservation, including culture of the perfusate as well as donor tissues. Prophylactic use of antibiotics has become standard practice in most transplant centers performing cadaver donor transplantation.

VENOUS THROMBOSIS

Renal vein thrombosis in renal transplants seems to be rather rare. Reported incidences range from 0.3% to 4%.[3, 70] One series reported 24 cases of renal vein thrombosis, an incidence of 9.8%; however, most of them were concomitant with arterial thrombosis and severe rejection found at the time of graft removal. Only four of these patients presented with a nephrotic syndrome, for an incidence of 1.5%. Some of the causative factors described in venous thrombosis are kinking of the anastomosis or iliac vein; extension of thrombosis from the iliac-venous system; and pressure on the iliac vein such as from lymphocele, uromas, hematomas, or silent left iliac vein compression syndrome. Severe rejection or arterial thrombosis were concomitant in some, as noted above, and result in venous thrombosis. A case of renal vein thrombosis occurring presumably as a part of the immune-complex-related nephrotic syndrome has been reported.[24]

Early thrombosis was reported in the immediate posttransplant period, and from the second day to the 18th day. Late appearance thrombosis was reported anywhere from 1 to 6 months. We have had a single case of renal vein thrombosis on the first postoperative day, manifested as sudden anuria. Immediate exploration with thrombectomy resulted in prompt return of renal function with diuresis. Acute manifestations include oliguria or anuria, reduction of renal function, graft swelling, and massive proteinuria or hematuria. At times, ipsilateral leg swelling can be seen from deep vein thrombosis. These features may mimic rejection episodes at times, necessitating a careful differential diagnosis.

The insidious delayed renal vein thrombosis may show only massive proteinuria with a very slight rise in the serum creatinine. The diagnosis can be entertained with a high index of suspicion, particularly in a case in which there was technical difficulty with the venous anastomosis. Delayed clearing of the perfusion scan may also suggest venous occlusion.

Selective venography would be the only confirmatory test of renal vein thrombosis in the immediate postoperative period. Prompt exploration may be undertaken with high index of suspicion to salvage the graft. Besides our experience in a single case, there have been five case reports of the success of surgical thrombectomy in the immediate postoperative period with return of normal function. Clarke reported a case of successful thrombectomy with return of function 15½ hours after the onset of symptoms.[12] Graft nephrectomy has been carried out in most other situations because of irreversible damage. The insidious type occurring later (1 month after transplant) may be treated with anticoagulation with stabilization of function.[3, 24, 70] If renal vein thrombosis is a consequence of progressive deep vein thrombosis and pulmonary embolism is present, vena cava interruption can be performed with the Greenfield filter without further jeopardizing renal function (Fig. 56-5).

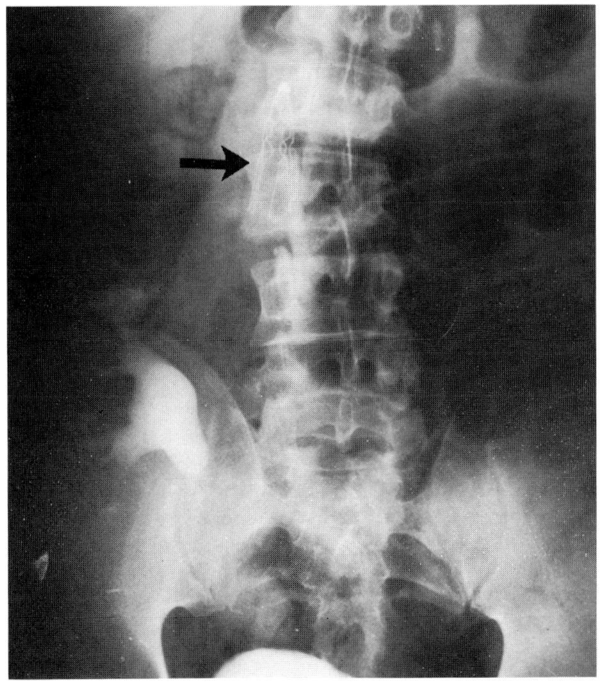

FIG. 56-5. Greenfield filter in the vena cava, placed for ileofemoral deep vein thrombosis with pulmonary embolism.

ARTERIOVENOUS FISTULA

Very few reports in the transplant literature concern arteriovenous (AV) fistula. Recently Debruyne reported two cases resulting from percutaneous needle biopsy of the transplanted kidney.[15] There are three other earlier reports in the literature. We had one small peripheral AV fistula, which was thought to result from biopsy at the time of transplantation. Two types have been noted: central (hilar), which is large and symptomatic, and peripheral, which is small and asymptomatic and may regress spontaneously. Small peripheral fistulae seem to be caused by percutaneous biopsy, while large central ones may be caused by surgical or technical factors or may be congenital in the donor kidney. They are manifested clinically by a bruit, which is continuous and high pitched. Some reduction in renal function as well as mild to severe hypertension, microangiopathic hemolytic anemia, and high-output cardiac failure have been noted. The diagnosis is confirmed by careful angiography.[7]

Treatment will be dictated by the location, size, and consequent physiologic change caused by the AV fistula. Small peripheral fistulae have very little clinical significance and reportedly often close spontaneously. If the fistula is fairly large and produces any of the above-mentioned problems, wedge resection or partial nephrectomy may be considered. In the central AV fistula, if technically feasible, ligation may be done as reported in the case of Bennett.[62] Successful ligation of the intrarenal AV fistula has been reported using an *ex vivo* surgical technique. If the central AV fistula is large and symptomatic and if mycotic infection is suspected, total nephrectomy may be necessary. Although some recommend open renal biopsy to avoid AV fistula, others suggest that needle biopsy is reasonably safe if there is tangential introduction of the needle.[15, 65] We have preferred open renal biopsy because of concern for both AV fistula creation and hemorrhagic complications.

LYMPHOCELE

Lymphocele, a collection of lymph around the graft in the retroperitoneum, has been described as a lymphatic complication of kidney transplantation. Although it is uncommon and relatively benign, lymphocele poses a problem to the transplant surgeon because of its effects: reduction in renal function mimicking rejection, which is caused by the mass effect compressing the ureter, and venous compression simulating deep vein thrombosis (Fig. 56-6).

The incidence of lymphocele has been reported to be from 0% to 22%.[29, 31, 47] As a perinephric collection of fluid, lymphocele appears somewhat later than the urine leak, which appears almost immediately after transplantation. However, there are reports of appearance as early as 1 week after transplant and as late as 5 years after transplantation.[9] The majority of lymphoceles develop clinically within the first 6 months after transplantation.[9, 46, 52, 83] The size of the lymphocele can vary from a 2-cm or 3-cm diameter collection, which is incidentally discovered during sonographic or radiologic investigation, to over 1000 cm, which presents as a large pelvic mass easily appreciated through the abdominal wall as well as during rectal or pelvic examination.

FIG. 56-6. Lymphocele compressing the iliac vein.

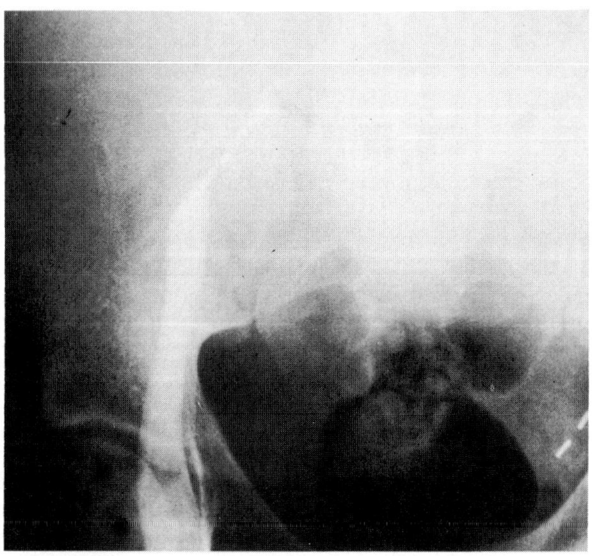

In about 70% of cases the first sign of a lymphocele is an increase in the serum level of creatinine, which can be confused with rejection.[11] Other common signs are suprapubic, abdominal, or ipsilateral leg edema and swelling over the graft. The remaining 30% of lymphoceles appear as a clear persistent drainage from the incision. Much less common forms of presentation include enlarged allograft, mild fever of unknown origin, iliofemoral thrombosis, urinary frequency, and urinary tract infection.

Occasionally the decreased urine volume can reach anuria, owing to compression of the kidney and ureter.[17, 32] Diastolic hypertension, presumably due to Goldblatt kidney effect, also has been reported in two of three patients in one series.[9]

Etiology

The source of these lymph leaks is an interrupted lymphatic chain along the iliac vessels.[37, 56, 103] Disruption of the lymphatic system of the donor kidney may also contribute.[9, 46] Some of the contributing factors in perpetuating a leak or increasing lymph flow have been said to include the use of steroids, diuretics, and anticoagulants; rejection episodes; ureteral obstruction; increased renal vein pressure; renal biopsy wound; radiation effect; postoperative hematomas; and active motion of the lower extremity. All of these may exist in the posttransplant period. There has been some suggestion that lymphocele occurs more often with cadaver kidney transplant and in female patients.

Diagnosis

The method of choice for the diagnosis of a perinephric collection in the posttransplant period is ultrasonography (Fig. 56-7). With increasingly sophisticated technique, the size and location of the collection can be determined exactly, and also effective differentiation can be made among lymphocele, abscess, and hematoma. CT scans have been used to complement ultrasonography findings.[45] If leg edema and swelling are the presenting symptoms, a venogram may be necessary to differentiate lymphocele from deep vein thrombosis. An intravenous pyelogram and cystogram would also diagnose a lymphocele by demonstrating mild hydronephrosis, ureteral displacement, and bladder compression.

Lymphoangiogram with radiographic dye or ^{99m}Tc sulfur colloid has been used in the past, but because of the morbidity associated with it and its invasive nature, it has been largely displaced by noninvasive techniques.[33]

The differential diagnosis between lymphocele and urinoma is difficult to make by ultrasound. If the intravenous pyelogram does not establish the diagnosis, aspiration of the fluid under sonographic control and analysis of the specimen for creatinine content can establish the diagnosis.[9, 45, 59, 91] If the fluid collection presents as an external leak, analysis of the fluid or injection of indigo carmine can establish the nature of the collection.

Treatment and Prevention

With the routine use of ultrasonography in the posttransplant period, the behavior of the lymphocele is better known.[13, 48, 72] Up to one third of lymphoceles are known to resolve spontaneously regardless of the size.[29, 61]

On the basis of that information, it is reasonable to establish an expectancy period if the lymphocele presents no clinical problems. If the symptomatology indicates compromised renal function or leg edema, percutaneous aspiration of the fluid under ultrasonographic guidance can be attempted. This maneuver should not be repeated if reaccumulation occurs, owing to the increased possibility of contamination.

Surgical intervention may be indicated because of pressure symptoms, including compression of the ureter and production of significant hydronephrosis and reduction of renal function attributable to venous compression. If surgery is undertaken, we prefer the abdominal approach for draining intra-abdominally by unroofing the wall of the lymphocele. Care should be taken to drain all of the collections completely in case of a multiloculated lymphocele. Recurrence with this approach is quite rare. Preventive measures include careful dissection of the perivascular tissue of the iliac vessels and ligation of the tissue containing the iliac lymphatic chain rather than the use of electrocautery.

RUPTURE

Spontaneous rupture of the transplanted kidney has been reported in increasing numbers in recent years. Reported incidence ranges from 0.8% to 10%.[19, 22, 93] Rupture is known to occur as early as 72 hours but as late as 5 months posttransplantation; however,

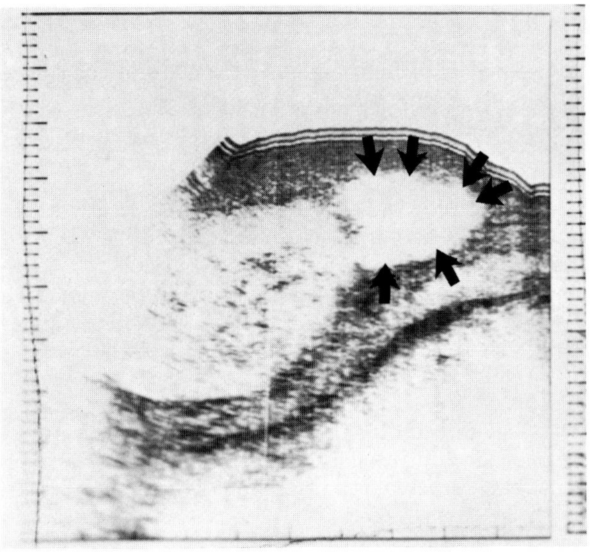

FIG. 56-7. Ultrasonogram shows a lymphocele (*arrows*).

the majority are known to occur within 2 weeks of transplantation.[10, 19, 50, 63] Clinically, rupture presents as painful swelling of the graft site, hypotension, and oliguria. At times the recipient may go into shock from rapid massive hemorrhage. In some reported cases massive exsanguination and death occurred before surgical repair could be attempted. Fever, hematuria, and an acute abdomen can also be part of the presenting syndrome. Interestingly, rupture can be asymptomatic in a rejected kidney and has been reported as an incidental finding at the time of nephrectomy.

The mechanism of rupture, although not clear, has been attributed to many factors. It should be noted that spontaneous rupture has been reported in the native kidneys in hydronephrosis, carcinoma, pregnancy, and in patients on anticoagulant therapy.[93]

In the transplant population, rupture has been attributed to acute rejection and edema of the graft, the renal biopsy site, ischemic damage, ureteral obstruction, trauma, capsulotomy, perfusion air embolism injury during machine preservation, cadaver graft, anticoagulation, and major graft vessel occlusions.[10, 19, 22, 26, 30, 51, 63, 74, 78, 98]

It is obvious that rupture of the graft is a multifactorial event, but the common finding is a swollen graft undergoing acute rejection or a nonfunctioning graft that requires the patient to undergo hemodialysis.

On the basis of poor second-graft survival in these patients, strong immunologic response has been suggested as one of the causative factors.

Review of the literature reveals that although

rupture occurs more often in cadaver kidney grafts than in living donor grafts, no correlation has been found between incidence of rupture and the length of the periods of warm and cold ischemia.

Treatment

The mortality rate from graft rupture has been reported to be from 9% to 16% with graft loss up to 74%; therefore rupture is obviously one of the more serious causes of graft loss.[39, 51] Although most ruptures of the graft result in nephrectomy and graft loss, control of hemorrhage and salvage of the graft have been reported also, with a salvage rate of 50% to 83%.[19, 22]

The salvage technique advocated has been closure of the rupture using horizontal mattress sutures of nonabsorbable material, reinforced if necessary with Teflon pledgets. Because of the possibility of rerupture, the patient should be watched very closely for the next 4 to 6 weeks.[51]

The strongest argument for immediate nephrectomy in all instances of kidney rupture is the high incidence of acute rejection in this group of patients and the relatively poor long-term survival of these grafts. The attempt at repair may also produce rerupture, sepsis, and possible death of the patient.

It seems logical that the plan of management should be individualized and that a decision to attempt to repair the kidney should be based on the general status of the patient, the kidney function before rupture, and the feasibility of obtaining hemostasis and repair at the time of surgery. It should be recognized, however, that in most cases the life of the patient is in jeopardy and that repair should be carried out only when the above criteria are most favorable.

Prevention

Whether capsulotomy of the graft can prevent rupture has been a controversial issue.[51] Although some cases of rupture have occurred in kidneys in which a capsulotomy had been performed, most of the reported ruptures have occurred in noncapsulotomized grafts.

In our experience with 700 kidney transplants, we have seen only one rupture, which occurred in a transplanted organ that had had total removal of the capsule during nephrectomy. The tear was shallow, 2 inches in length on the posterior surface of the kidney, and it was easily repaired.

We have routinely performed capsulotomies in all transplants, and our incidence of rupture is the lowest in published data, 0.14%.[43] We believe that routine, careful performance of capsulotomy is the best way to prevent this devastating complication.

Urologic Complications

Although a urologic complication demands special attention because of the great rates of morbidity and mortality, the incidence is fairly low. The incidence of urologic complications in general has been reported to range from a low of 0 to 10% to as high as 34%. Graft loss due to a urologic complication has been reported to be up to 22%. However, although some groups report a very low mortality of 0 to 0.6% (middle group ranging 10%–25%), others are as high as 47%, 68%, and 100%, mainly from sepsis. Urologic complications can be divided into two major categories: (1) urinary leak and (2) stenosis and obstruction.

URINARY LEAK

The incidence of urinary leak has been variously reported from less than 1% to 24%, the average ranging between 1% and 10%. We have had a 5% incidence of leak in our recent experience.

Ureteral Fistula

Urinary leak from ureteral extravasation has been reported recently to occur in from less than 1% to 10% of cases, the majority at the ureterovesical junction. Slough of the entire ureter as well as renal pelvis hemorrhage also has been noted. Usually ureteral fistulae occur within the first week after transplantation and most appear within 2 weeks. Clinically the fistula presents as a sudden reduction in urine volume, increase in wound drainage, fever, and, at times, swelling or palpable mass near the graft.

The major cause of the ureteral leak is poor vascularity. Graft rejection involving the ureter has also been implicated, while some question the importance of this factor in the clinical situation. Faulty technique also can be blamed. Some have reported a higher incidence of fistula with ureteropyelostomy, while others, more ureteral slough with ureteroneocystostomy. In most centers ureteroureterostomy has been abandoned owing to the high incidence of leak as well as stenosis. Renal pelvis rupture is known to follow ureteral obstruction, particularly in the high diuretic phase. Since such rupture can mimic rejection or a vascular complication, the differential diagnosis becomes extremely important. It also can pose such diagnostic problems as fever of unknown origin and perirenal fluid collection.

If reduction of the urine volume develops with deterioration of renal function or if there is sudden anuria, one must study the entire system. Diagnostic studies available include ultrasound, isotope scan, intravenous pyelogram, cystogram, and retrograde study. If wound drainage or fluid aspirate can be obtained, analysis of this fluid for creatinine, urea, and electrolytes (sodium and potassium) can be of diagnostic help. Intravenous injection of indigo carmine may help to differentiate urinary leak from other wound drainage. In recent years noninvasive techniques using ultrasound and radionuclide scans have improved greatly in facilitating early and prompt diagnosis of this grave complication.[79, 92, 96] Routine sequential ultrasound and radioisotope studies can detect perinephric collection as well as urine leak before they become symptomatic. In radionuclide scans, ^{131}I hippurate (excretion phase) remains the most reliable study, while ^{99m}Tc DPTA (perfusion phase) complements it to differentiate among other causes of reduction of renal function. Postvoid films should always be obtained, since they may be necessary to show early and small extravasation.[79, 96] The intravenous pyelogram is time consuming and may not show enough image with reduced renal function. Retrograde cytoscopy may become necessary to pinpoint the exact level of the ureteral leak. However, because of the possibility of infection and the invasive nature of instrumentation, this study is reserved for specific circumstances. As stated previously, analysis of the perinephric collection aspirate under ultrasound guidance can be of great help. Needless to say, this technique should be employed under strict sterile conditons.

Since the major cause of ureteral leak is poor vascularity, preventive measures should be directed toward the surgical technique of donor nephrectomy to preserve vascularity. Donor nephrectomy should be carried out without "undue haste" with en bloc removal. Hilar structures should be carefully preserved as well as periureteral tissue.[79] This should be done with sharp dissection rather than blunt dissection.[5] With multiple arteries in the donor kidney, the lower pole artery should be preserved carefully and revascularized since it serves as a major source of blood supply to the ureter. A small accessory upper polar artery can be ligated, but caliceal hemorrhage from segmental infarct of the renal parenchyma has been reported from this maneuver.[25] Ureteroneocystostomy is the preferred technique to reduce urinary leak.

Some advocate an "extravesical" technique of ureteroneocystostomy, reporting a lower incidence of urinary leak; others, however, report a higher incidence of leak with this technique.[21, 58] Careful cystostomy closure is necessary if the surgeon performs ureteroneocystostomy to reduce leak from this source. Some advocate a three-layer technique, while we have employed a two-layer technique without significant incidence of bladder leak.[41] Effective decompression of the bladder during the diuretic phase in the immediate postoperative period is extremely important. Most advocate leaving the indwelling catheter in place at least until the diuretic phase is over. The catheter should be more carefully handled and left in longer if the patient is diabetic and a neurogenic bladder is possible.

MANAGEMENT. Prompt diagnosis and aggressive management are necessary to save the graft and reduce the incidence of mortality by preventing sepsis. Recently some groups have reported success with conservative management.[58, 71] At times it may be difficult to decide between conservative and surgical management. The decision depends upon the severity of leak, its location (vesical or ureterovesical vs higher level of ureter), and the presence or absence of sepsis. Management should be individualized.

Small leaks have been managed successfully by continued urethral catheter drainage. Since most of the morbidity and mortality are due to sepsis, it is extremely important to prevent sepsis by early surgical management. If sepsis is present, wide drainage of the wound and urinary tract is important, and it may be necessary to remove the graft and stop immunosuppression. The differential diagnosis from a rejection episode is important to avoid unnecessary rejection treatment, thereby increasing the chance of sepsis. A variety of surgical techniques have been employed to reconstruct the urinary tract. The most commonly utilized and effective method has been ureteropyelostomy utilizing the recipient ureter. One modification of this technique is contralateral pyelocalicostomy.[57] Extravesical ureteroneocystostomy has been utilized to advantage when the ureter was short. To deal with the shorter ureter, psoas hitch, Boari flap, and pyelovesical anastomosis have been used.[88] Use of the rotational capsule flap has also been reported, and a segment of ileum has been used to replace the ureter.[14, 54] The usefulness of nephrostomy and ureteral catheter drainage of the urinary tract has been reemphasized recently. With an aggressive and individualized approach, a higher incidence of graft salvage with a reduced mortality rate has been reported in recent years. During the primary graft operation, the surgeon should avoid including the recipient ureteral orifice in the ureteral neocystostomy sutures so that the host ureter can be used in the future if the need arises.

Bladder Leak

The reported incidence of bladder leak ranges from less than 1% to 4%.[1, 5, 73] In contrast to ureteral leak, bladder leak is fairly benign. The usual cause of bladder leak is an improperly closed cystostomy wound and poor vascularity of the bladder from previous surgery. Some have reported perivesical hematoma to be the factor causing cystostomy wound disruption and leak. A higher incidence of bladder

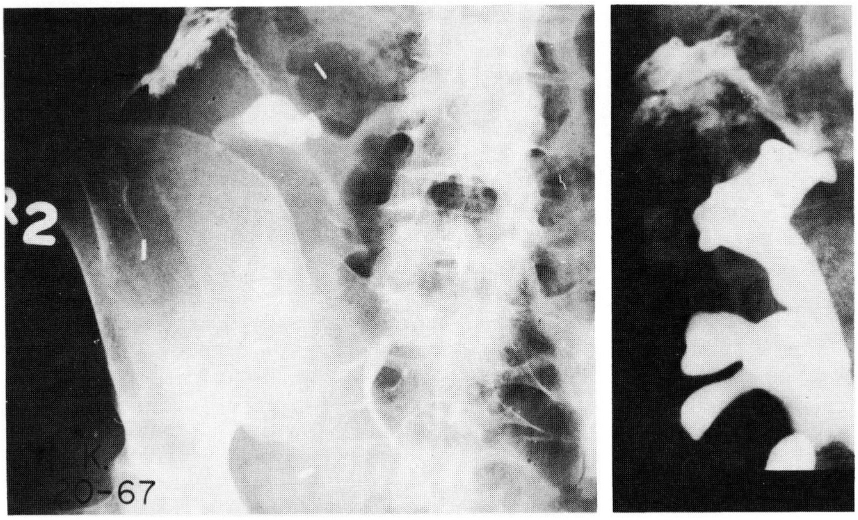

FIG. 56-8. Caliceal leak.

leak in the patient undergoing second or third transplant surgery has been well known. The need for cystostomy is one major disadvantage of the ureteroneocystostomy over the ureteropyelostomy.

To prevent bladder leak, meticulous and careful closure of the cystostomy wound is of upmost importance, as advocated by Belzer.[5] We have had no bladder leak in recent years using careful technique except one in a patient who underwent second transplant surgery on a bladder that had undergone multiple previous procedures to remedy lower urinary tract dysfunction. We leave transplant patients in the intensive-care area during the immediate postoperative period with careful monitoring of urinary output by indwelling catheter for 5 days unless they are diabetic patients. Longer decompression in diabetic neurogenic bladder patients has been stressed by others. At times, small bladder leaks can be managed conservatively by continuous drainage with an indwelling catheter if sepsis is not a component. In most cases, early surgical intervention is advisable with repair of the leak and, at times, redoing the ureteroneocystostomy. Some have advocated the use of an omental flap in repair of a bladder fistula.

Caliceal Leak

Caliceal leak is rather uncommon and, at times, difficult to diagnose. Reported incidences range from 0.8% to 2.2%—overall, 1.3%.[25, 80, 94] In one report the incidence was up to 2.6%, including the donor graft with multiple arteries. Contributing factors are reported to include difficult donor nephrectomies, multiple arteries, particularly polar or accessory arteries with a "low perfusion segment," segmental infarct due to nonvascularized polar artery or accessory artery, ureteral obstruction, and blunt trauma to the lower abdomen. Caliceal leaks usually occur within the first 3 months of the transplant. Since they occur rather late compared to a ureteral leak, the diagnosis can be difficult. In the late stage the patient may show swelling, fever, and tenderness in the flank. Caliceal leak with urinary extravasation in the retroperitoneal space can be suspected if the patient suffers repeated urinary tract infection. A high dose IVP may make the diagnosis, but most of the time retrograde study is necessary (Fig. 56-8).

Both graft loss and mortality rates are high in caliceal leak, ranging up to 87%, graft loss rate, and 50%, mortality rate. Perinephric sepsis and subsequent superinfection due to antibiotic treatment are the major problems. Early exploration is mandatory if one suspects or confirms the diagnosis of caliceal leak. If sepsis supervenes, prompt nephrectomy is the most definitive treatment to save the patient. Use of nephrostomy, partial nephrectomy, or repair of the leak with omental patch or muscle graft has been reported successful.

OBSTRUCTION AND STENOSIS

Ureteral Stenosis

The incidence of ureteral stenosis is very low, ranging from 1% to 10%; however, up to 20% ureteral stenosis has been reported in a small number of transplant patients.[18, 48, 58] Except for early obstruction from blood clot or edema during the immediate postoperative period, most ureteral obstruction appeared late, at 3 to 6 months.[58] Late appearance of ureteral obstruction, 5 to 6 years after transplant, has also been reported.[106]

Many causative factors in ureteral stenosis have been cited in the literature. In the immediate postoperative period, it is usually due to clots. Simply removing the clot without ureteral stent is sufficient.

Other factors include retroperitoneal or periureteral fibrosis, usually a late phenomenon (Fig. 56-9); intrinsic fibrosis of the ureter, presumably due to rejection; angling or kinking at the ureteroneocystostomy; kink with fibrosis; and compression by the spermatic cord.[18, 34, 82, 106] Fungus ball and renal calculus causing obstruction also have been reported. A case of the uterus of a pregnant woman leading to sudden anuria from ureteral obstruction has been reported.[55] Two cases of human polyoma virus infection causing ureteral stenosis in renal allograft recipients have also been reported.

Ureteral stenosis may mimic rejection by presentation as reduced urine volume and increased serum creatinine with mild fever. Late stenosis may show calicectasis and hydronephrosis in the follow-up routine IVP. The diagnosis can be made by radioisotope scan; sonogram, particularly in the early postoperative period; and IVP in late stenosis. Sequential radioisotope scan and sonogram have been quite useful in recent years in delineating ureteral compression due to perinephric fluid collection. It has been particularly useful in timing surgical intervention of lymphocele compression of the ureter. At times, cystoscopic retrograde study may be necessary to pinpoint the level of the stenosis.

Careful operative technique with gentle handling of the ureter is necessary to prevent early ureteral obstruction from mechanical angulation, faulty technique, or reactive edema. Some stent the ureter with a ureteral catheter to prevent early obstruction in the immediate postoperative period. We have found this unnecessary except in one case in our early experience. We, as well as others, find edema to be an extremely unusual cause of ureteral obstruction in the early postoperative period. It is important to provide a large bladder opening in creating ureteroneocystostomy to prevent future narrowing within the tunnel. Some speculate that late periureteric fibrosis is due to urine leak or hematoma and infection. Obviously, avoiding these complications by meticulous surgical technique is of importance in preventing future stenosis. The spermatic cord as a cause of ureteral obstruction has been implicated in one report in which the ureter was draping over the cord, and in another report in which there was compression of the ureter crossing under the cord.[18, 34] The author recommended division of the cord routinely to prevent this problem.[18] We have never divided the cord and have never had obstruction from this problem.

If ureteral obstruction occurs in the early postoperative period from blood clot, it may be necessary to explore promptly to remove the clot through the ureterotomy. In one case in our experience, temporary ureteral catheter drainage was sufficient to restore renal function. Late stenosis of ureter at the

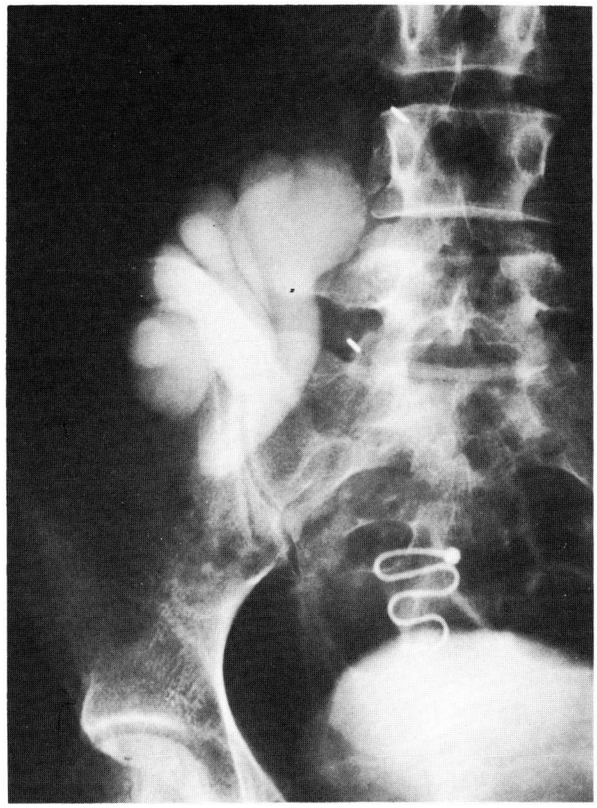

FIG. 56-9. Delayed ureteral stenosis due to ureteropelvic junction fibrosis. Repair was accomplished with ureteropyelostomy.

ureteroneocystostomy opening can be treated with transurethral meatotomy. However, in one report the meatotomy caused local abscess and eventually resulted in graft loss.[54] Ureteropyelostomy using the recipient ureter is a satisfactory method to bypass ureteral stenosis. At times, lysis of periureteric adhesions with ureteral catheter drainage may suffice, but we have found this not to be satisfactory because of recurrence. If stenosis of the midportion of the ureter due to compression by lymphocele is present, intraperitoneal drainage of the lymphocele relieves ureteral stenosis. Since the late-stage transplant ureter is often encased in dense fibrosis and has marginal vascularity, dissection of the ureter carries the risk of disintegration of the ureter. Ureteral stenosis rarely may be manifested by polyuric renal failure.[64] Although ureteral obstruction has less associated mortality as a urologic complication, it has a higher incidence of graft loss.

Bladder Neck Contracture and Urethral Stricture

A posttransplant incidence of 6.6% of urethral stricture has been reported and up to 10% in late follow-up.[49, 66] The usual cause is presumed to be instrumentation and the indwelling catheter used at the time of transplantation. The use of a large catheter (24 French) to ensure effective drainage of the bladder and purulent urethritis from long duration of the catheter may aggravate the urethral stricture. All patients with urethral stricture show obstructive voiding symptoms with some urinary retention. Transient hydronephrosis seen on the IVP has been reported. Urethral stricture may be seen within months, but most cases are found more than 1 year later. Bladder neck obstruction can be due to benign prostatic hypertrophy or the aftermath of previous transureteral resection of bladder neck obstruction. The incidence of bladder neck contracture has not been well documented, but in one series a 0.9% incidence was noted.[49]

As a preventive measure against urethral stricture, the surgeon should use the smallest possible catheter for adequate drainage or switch to a smaller catheter after the initial diuretic phase.[6] The catheter should be left indwelling for the shortest possible duration for the purpose. The medical team should be instructed to handle the indwelling catheter with aseptic technique, with frequent cleansing and use of antiseptic ointment.

Preoperative study of the lower urinary tract with cystoureterogram or cystometrogram is now part of the routine for preparation for transplantation. If lower urethral tract obstruction or bladder neck contracture is found, it is advisable to remedy this while the native kidney and urinary output are present. If the surgeon waits for the second transplant after primary graft failure, it is advisable to repeat the study of the lower urinary tract to ensure that it is adequate for another transplant.

Most urethral strictures can be managed with simple dilatation. Although this procedure is usually tolerated quite well, the urine should be checked for bacteria before instrumentation. If bacteria are present, the dilatation should be postponed until their identification allows the initiation of suitable antibiotic treatment. Prophylactic antibiotics should be started at least 12 hours before instrumentation.[49] Some have advocated use of the meatotomy, or first-stage Johanson urethroplasty, as the simplest and most expeditious method to overcome urethral stricture. We have not had any experience with this procedure in transplant patients.

If the bladder neck is contracted, transurethral resection can be performed. Ideally this should be done while the native kidney is still excreting urine to facilitate removal of blood clots. On some occasions, Y–V plasty can be performed at the time of transplant surgery to remove bladder neck contracture. In our early experience we performed Y–V plasty at the time of transplantation on a few occasions with satisfactory results. If bladder contracture develops while the patient is waiting for the second or third renal transplant, it should be repaired before the next transplant.

Acute Renal Failure

EARLY OLIGURIA OR EARLY ANURIA

The immediate concern upon completion of transplant surgery is the resumption of renal function. Ideally the grafted kidney resumes function immediately, usually with a diuretic phase when an adequate volume replacement and an osmotic load are provided. Acute renal failure with oliguria or anuria in kidney transplantation, as defined by a need for hemodialysis for the first week after transplantation, has been reported with an incidence ranging from 10% to 60% in cadaver donor transplantation. Some centers that rely on their own cadaver donor procurement network report a rate of acute renal failure of 10%. Other centers relying on national or regional networks for procurement of organs have reported up to 60% incidence of acute renal failure following transplantation. The Eurotransplant group reported 24.5% incidence of acute renal failure. The Southeastern Organ sharing group, surveying multicenter experience, reported an incidence of 36%, with the range being from 11% to 60%.[53]

Acute renal failure following transplantation can be due to extrinsic or intrinsic factors. In the former group, technical complications are the most prominent and include thrombosis of the artery or vein and compression of the kidney or its excretory system by lymphatic accumulation or hematoma (especially after hemodialysis). The intrinsic causes include factors that affect the kidney itself prior to and during organ harvesting or preservation as well as factors that may play a role during the implantation of the graft or in the environment of the graft.

During donor maintenance and harvesting, the age of the donor, oliguria of the donor, shock, the use of peripheral vasopressors, and prolonged warm ischemia time can contribute to delayed function of the graft.[53, 86] During preservation, the longer the period of ischemia, the higher the incidence of delayed function.

During implantation, several factors delay function of the graft, including prolonged periods of rewarming during anastomosis, multiple arteries, and careless handling of the kidney.[85]

Hypovolemia in the recipient can have a deleterious effect in a newly implanted kidney. Finally, hyperacute rejection, rare nowadays, can be a cause of anuria. Although most hyperacute rejections can be diagnosed immediately, sometimes delayed hyperacute rejection or acute accelerated rejection can cause acute renal failure a few hours posttransplant.

Diagnosis

It seems clear from our experience and that of others that acute renal failure following transplantation is a multifactorial phenomenon. Consequently the diagnosis is one of exclusion. Our practice has been to use a methodical approach in an effort to eliminate all correctable factors. Upon completion of the ureteral implantation, a kidney biopsy is performed to obtain a baseline of histology. At the same time, the diagnosis of hyperacute rejection can be ruled out. The patient is challenged in the immediate postoperative period by volume loading with blood and normal saline solution while the central venous pressure or the pulmonary wedge pressure is closely monitored. If the patient fails to respond, ultrasonography is used to rule out compression as the cause of the oliguria. Radionuclide scanning will demonstrate the patency of the vascular supply to the graft.

Acute renal failure with oliguria in the immediate postoperative period poses the problem of differentiating between acute tubular necrosis and ischemic damage and acute rejection superimposed on acute tubular necrosis. Recently many studies have reported increased use of radionuclide scan to differentiate "normal" acute tubular necrosis and acute rejection. Not only visual interpretation but also calculation of the activity–time graph or perfusion index, using the computer, have served to make this difficult diagnosis. Unfortunately, no definitive method can distinguish the damage of acute tubular necrosis from superimposed acute rejection. Because of the difficulty in diagnosing acute rejection superimposed on acute tubular necrosis, some have advocated routine use of antirejection treatment during the acute tubular necrosis period. However, the surgeon should keep the complication of overimmunosuppression in mind at all times.

The predictability of kidney function according to harvesting and perfusion parameters has not been accurate. Recently it has been confirmed in a multicenter prospective study that high diastolic and perfusion pressure (>20 torr) carry a high incidence of acute renal failure posttransplantation.[53] Ligandin in the perfusate (an intracellular organic anion-binding protein having transferase activity) has been reported to have a predictive value, as has renal blood flow 1 hour after transplant vascularization.[2, 23]

Earlier reports indicated that acute renal failure in the immediate postoperative period has no influence on eventual graft and patient survival. However, recent reports indicate poor long-term graft survival in a delayed-functioning kidney, while most reports indicate that patient survival has not suffered. McDonald and colleagues, reporting the Southeastern Organ Sharing group experience, stated that in the group poorly matched for histocompatibility and receiving transfusion, the adverse effect of early renal failure on graft survival was manifested in the first 12 months, while in the group well matched for histocompatibility with transfusion, the adverse effect appeared late (*i.e.*, 18–24 months posttransplant).[53] The European group has also reported that early acute renal failure affects eventual renal function as well as the incidence of late complications.

Acute renal failure from use of a living related donor is extremely rare and should immediately alert the surgeon to the possibility of hyperacute rejection or a technical disaster. Immediate reexploration is mandatory.

Wound Infections

Infection remains the major complication of renal transplantation. Wound infection requires particular attention because of serious rates of morbidity, mortality, and graft loss. The reported incidence of surgical wound infection in recent reports ranges from 1.9% to 34%.[4, 93] Wound infection of the uncomplicated or primary transplant wound has been reported to be fairly low, ranging from 0 to 1.7%; however, it is higher with a reopened wound, ranging from 3% to 18.5%.[4, 40, 52, 84] The incidence of deep wound infection or perinephric abscess remains high, with a reported overall incidence of 3.5% to 8.7%.[40, 93] The highest incidence of deep wound infection was reported after transplant nephrectomy, ranging from 17% to 34%.[38, 84] Earlier reports showed wound infection after transplant nephrectomy to be as high as 56%.[60]

Uremia, long-term nutritional depletion prior to renal transplant surgery, and immunosuppressive therapy after transplant surgery make these patients particularly vulnerable to infectious complications. Many contributing factors have been identified besides uremic conditions and immunosuppressive therapy, such as hematoma, reopening the wound, urinary fistula, urine infection, cadaver kidney transplant, use of a drain in the wound, diabetes, hemodialysis, and contaminated kidney.[8, 90, 102] Hematoma and urine leak are particularly serious causes of deep wound infection. The incidence of hematoma in the transplant wound has been reported from 7% to 9.5%.[13, 40, 84] Besides technical mishap at the time of surgery, such as missing a blood vessel in the cadaver donor kidney, a bleeding disorder with platelet dysfunction and the use of heparin in hemodialysis make these patients susceptible to bleeding. Schweizer found 60% of hematomas in the group of patients who underwent hemodialysis subsequent to transplant surgery.[84] The infection rate in hematoma patients is high, ranging from 43% to 46%. Use of a drain in the wound is also known to increase the incidence of infection, particularly with hematoma.

The bacterial agent involved in infection is usually a gram-negative rod (*E. coli*). A significant incidence of staphylococcus infection also is found. Other agents involved are enterococcus, candida albicans, pseudomonas, and klebsiella. Although the incidence of pseudomonas infection is fairly low, it is known to be the most virulent, up to 60% of them leading to septicemia with a high mortality rate. The overall mortality rate of wound infection ranges to 30%, becoming higher with septicemia, up to 50%.

Besides septicemia, which is known to occur in up to 62% of patients with deep wound infections, other serious consequences of wound infection are mycotic aneurysm and graft loss. Massive hemorrhage from rupture of a mycotic aneurysm or anastomotic leak is one of the most life-threatening complications of posttransplant wound infection. Mycotic aneurysms have been reported in as many as 37% of deep wound infections.[40] Diabetic patients appeared to be particularly vulnerable, with an incidence of mycotic aneurysm three times higher than that in nondiabetic patients.[40]

Wound infection is also the major cause of graft loss after rejection. Up to 75% of graft loss has been reported after deep wound infection. The altered clinical response in immunosuppressed patients, particularly in patients on steroids, makes the diagnosis of wound infection rather difficult at times. A high index of suspicion should be maintained and careful physical examination performed, including pelvic and rectal examinations. Routine ultrasonography supplemented by CT scans has become a useful diagnostic tool in recent years.[13,38] Frequently, however, surgical exploration is the only way to confirm the diagnosis. Gallium scan, intravenous pyelogram, and cystogram have not been useful for diagnosis in most hands.

It is obvious that the best way to counter the wound infection problem is to prevent it. Preventive measures should start prior to surgery. Preoperative measures include scrubbing of the operative field with antiseptic soap the day prior to surgery and shaving the field just before the operative procedure. At the time of surgery, measures should be taken to prevent hematoma by thorough hemostasis and meticulous surgical technique, including during the cadaver donor nephrectomy procedure. Lymph vessels should be ligated carefully to control lymph leak, and the surgical principle of obliteration of dead space should be practiced, including subcutaneous tissue.

Irrigating the wound at the time of surgery with topical antibiotic agents such as bacitracin, kanamycin, and neomycin has been reported by many to be effective in reducing wound infection. We routinely irrigate the wound with 1% neomycin solution during and at the termination of surgery. Many agree that the use of a Penrose drain should be avoided. If a drain is essential, a closed drainage system should be used for a very short period of time (*i.e.*, 12–48 hours).

Recently many authors have suggested short-term systemic prophylactic antibiotic therapy before, during, and after the transplant procedure, covering gram-negative as well as gram-positive agents. With increased use of exchanged organs with potential contamination, we use systemic prophylactic antibiotics routinely at the time of surgery. If a urinary infection exists, it should be treated with appropriate antibiotics, as should any other infection. To lessen the anticoagulant effect of hemodialysis just preceding and following transplant surgery, regional heparinization should be practiced and any anticoagulant effect neutralized before surgery. The bleeding diathesis of uremia may be lessened by frequent and effective hemodialysis. A prolonged period of careful follow-up is necessary for these patients because of the delayed appearance of an occult abscess. Routine sequential ultrasonography has been useful for this purpose.

Once infection is diagnosed, prompt and effective drainage should be employed, including irrigation with saline and antiseptic agents as well as a topical antibiotic solution at the time of surgery. At times it may be necessary to perform an early transplant nephrectomy to facilitate drainage and also to prevent an anastomotic leak. The importance of appropriate antibiotics with frequent culture and careful surveillance for superinfection is obvious.

Complications of Transplant Nephrectomy

Unfortunately transplant nephrectomy remains a fairly common operative procedure because of rejection and infection. The incidence of wound infection in transplant nephrectomy is high, as noted previously, from 17% to 34%. Also, massive hemorrhage from an anastomotic leak or mycotic aneurysm remains a life-threatening complication. Because of these complications use of this procedure has become more selective in recent years. Vascular and urologic problems are discussed in other sections. When the transplanted kidney becomes damaged irreversibly by hyperacute rejection at the time of transplantation surgery, the indication for immediate removal is obvious. However, when transplanted kidneys are damaged by irreversible acute rejection or progressive chronic rejection, it is not always necessary to remove them.

Selective indications justifying transplant nephrectomy include infection, hypertension originating from a transplant kidney, toxemia, and fever of unknown origin. If the surgeon elects to perform transplant nephrectomy, the ideal time is when the patient has reached optimal condition after cessation of immunosuppressive therapy and after an effective hemodialysis program with nutritional support has been started. Some technical aspects of transplant nephrectomy to lessen complications include prevention of hematoma and avoidance of the use of a Penrose drain, use of closed drainage for a short period, and use of a topical antibiotic solution and systemic prophylactic antibiotics. Although it is easy to remove the transplanted kidney *in toto* during the immediate postoperative period, it is not easy to remove the graft that has survived for a long period of time. Under these circumstances, it is preferable to remove the graft subcapsularly. The vascular pedicle can be mass clamped and at times mass ligated without undue risk. Wound closure should be simple, with single-layer closure utilizing synthetic monofilament material. If necessary because of gross contamination or obvious infection, secondary closure should be employed.

References

1. Anderson CB, Sicard GC, Haid SD, Etheredge EE: Cadaver kidney characteristics and immediate renal allograft function. Proc Clin Dial Transplant Forum 7:7, 1977
2. Anderson EE, Glenn JF, Seigler HF, Stickel DL: Urologic complications in renal transplantation. Trans Am Assoc Genitourin Surg 63:56, 1971
3. Arruda JAL, Jonasson O, Gutierrez LF et al: Renal vein thrombosis in kidney allografts. Lancet 2:585, 1973
4. Banowsky LH, Montie JE, Braun WE, Magnusson MO: Renal transplantation. III. Prevention of wound infections. Urology 4:656, 1974
5. Belzer FO: Technical complications after renal transplantation. In Morris PJ (ed): Kidney Transplantation, Principles and Practice. New York, Academic Press, Grune & Stratton, 1979
6. Belzer FO, Kountz SL, Najarian JS et al: Prevention of urological complications after renal allotransplantation. Arch Surg 101:449, 1970
7. Bennett WM, Strong D, Rosch J: Arteriovenous fistula complicating renal transplantation. Urol 8:254, 1976
8. Bore PJ, Basu PK, Rudge CJ, Sells RA: Contaminated renal allografts. Arch Surg 115:755, 1980
9. Braun WE, Banowsky LH, Straffon RA et al: Lymphoceles associated with renal transplantation. Am J Med 57:714, 1974
10. Brekke I, Flatmark A, Laane B, Mellbye O: Renal allograft rupture. Scand J Urol Nephrol 12:265, 1978
11. Brockis JG, Hulbert JC, Patel AS et al: The diagnosis and treatment of lymphoceles associated with renal transplantation. Br J Urol 50:307, 1978
12. Clarke SD, Kennedy JA, Hewitt JC et al: Successful removal of thrombus from renal vein after renal transplantation. Br Med J 1:154, 1970
13. Coyne SS, Walsh JW, Tisnado J et al: Surgically correctable renal transplant complications: An integrated clinical and radiologic approach. AJR 136:1113, 1981
14. Dabhoiwala NF, Ten Cate HW, Linschoten H et al: Conservative surgical management of urological complications after cadaveric renal transplantation. J Urol 120:290, 1978
15. Debruyne FMJ, Koene RAP, Moonen WA et al: Intrarenal arteriovenous fistula following renal allograft biopsy. Eur Urol 4:435, 1978
16. Diamond HG et al: Dilatation of critical transplant renal artery stenosis by percutaneous transluminal angioplasty. AJR Cec 133:1167, 1979
17. Diethelm AG: Anuria secondary to perirenal lymphocele: A complication to renal transplantation. South Med J 65(3):350, 1972
18. Donaldson RA, Jacobson JE, Pontin AR: Ureteric obstruction in renal allograft recipients. S Afr Med J 52:1077, 1977
19. Dostal G, Medrano J, Eigler FW: Die spontane nierentransplantruptur. Langenbecks Arch Chir 341:87, 1976
20. Doyle TJ, McGregor WR, Fox PS et al: Homotransplant renal artery stenosis. Surgery 77:53, 1975
21. Dreikorn K, Rohl L: Urological complications in renal transplantation. Eur Urol 1:170, 1975
22. Dryburgh P, Porter KA, Krom RAF et al: Should the ruptured renal allograft be removed? Arch Surg 114:850, 1979
23. Feinfeld DA, Levine RD, Levine SD, Fleischner G: Ligandin in perfusates from transplanted kidneys: A test for tubular necrosis. Nephrology 21:38, 1978
24. Golden J, Stone RA, Goldberger L: Immune-related renal vein thrombosis in a renal allograft. Ann Intern Med 85:612, 1976
25. Goldman MN, Burleson RL, Tilney NL et al: Calyceal-cutaneous fisulae in renal transplant patients. Ann Surg 184:679, 1976
26. Goldman MH, Leapman SB, Handy RD, Best DW: Renal allograft rupture with iliofemoral thrombosis. Arch Surg 113:204, 1978
27. Goldman MH, Tilney NL, Vineyard G et al: A twenty-year survey of arterial complications of renal transplantation. Surg Gynecol Obstet 141:758, 1975
28. Gorey TF, Bulkley GB, Spees EK, Sterioff S: Iliac artery ligation. The relative paucity of ischemic sequelae in renal transplant patients. Ann Surg 190:753, 1979
29. Griffiths AB, Fletcher EW, Morris PJ: Lymphocele after renal transplantation. Aust NZ J Surg 49(6):626, 1979
30. Homan WP, Cheigh JS, Kim SJ et al: Renal allograft fracture: Clinicopathological study of 21 cases. Ann Surg 186:700, 1977
31. Howard RJ, Simmons RL, Najarian JS: Prevention of lymphoceles following renal transplantation. Ann Surg 184:166, 1976
32. Hume DM: Kidney transplantation. In Rapaport FT (ed): Human Transplantation. New York, Grune & Stratton, 1968
33. Jackson FI, Lentle BC, Higgins MR et al: Lymphocutaneous fistula following renal transplantation. Clin Nucl Med 5:19, 1980
34. Karmi SA, Dagher FJ et al: Spermatic cord: Cause of ureteral obstruction in renal allograft recipients. Urology 11:380, 1978

35. Kauffman HM, Sampson D, Fox PS et al: Prevention of transplant renal artery stenosis. Surgery 81:161, 1977
36. Klarskov P et al: Renovascular hypertension after renal transplantation. Scand J Urol Nephrol 13:291, 1979
37. Koehler PR: Injuries and complications of the lymphatic system following renal transplantation. Lymphology 5:61, 1972
38. Kohlberg WI, Tellis VA, Bhat DJ et al: Wound infections after transplant nephrectomy. Arch Surg 115:645, 1980
39. Kootstra G, Meijer S, Elema JD: Spontaneous rupture of homografted kidneys. Arch Surg 108:107, 1974
40. Kyriakides GK, Simmons RL, Najarian JS: Wound infections in renal transplant wounds: Pathogenetic and prognostic factors. Ann Surg 182:770, 1975
41. Lacombe M: Arterial stenosis complicating renal allotransplantation in man: A study. Ann Surg 181:283, 1975
42. Lacombe M: Correction of renal transplant artery stenosis by transposing iliac arteries. Urology 13(1):21, 1979
43. Lee HM: Surgical technique of renal transplantation. In Morris PJ (ed): Kidney Transplantation Principles and Practice. New York, Academic Press, 1979
44. Lee HM et al: Renal artery occlusion in transplant recipients. Am Surg 43:186, 1977
45. Lerut T, Lerut P, Broos P et al: Lymphatic complications in renal transplantation. Proc Eur Dial Transplant Assoc 6:83, 1980
46. Lerut J, Lerut T, Gruwez JA, Michielsen P: An unusual case of lymphocele after renal transplantation. Lymphology 11:89, 1978
47. Lindstrom BL, Lindfors O, Eklund B, Ahonen J, Collan R et al: Surgical complications in 500 kidney transplantation. Proc Eur Dial Transplant Assoc 14:353, 1977
48. Lipshultz LI, Wein AJ, Arger PH et al: Post-transplantation lymphocyst: Use of ultrasound as adjunct in diagnosis. Urology 8(6):624, 1976
49. Loening SA, Banowsky LH et al: Bladder neck contracture and urethral stricture as complications of renal transplantation. J Urol 114:688, 1975
50. Lord RSA, Belzer FO, Kountz SL: Delayed spontaneous rupture of the allografted kidney. Arch Surg 100:607, 1970
51. Lord RSA, Effeney DJ, Hayes JM et al: Renal allograft rupture: Cause, clinical features and management. Ann Surg 177:268, 1973
52. Lorimer WS III, Glassford DM, Sarles HE et al: Lymphocele: A significant complication following renal transplantation. Lymphology 8:20, 1975
53. McDonald JC, Vaughn W, Filo RS et al: Cadaver donor renal transplantation by centers of the Southeastern Organ Procurement Foundation. Ann Surg 193:1, 1981
54. McLoughlin MG: Late ureteric obstruction in renal transplantation. Br J Urol 49:93, 1977
55. McLoughlin MG: Unusual cause of anuria in a transplant patient. J Urol 117:124, 1977
56. Madura JA, Dunbar JB, Cerilli GJ: Perirenal lymphocele as a complication of renal transplantation. Surgery 68:310, 1970
57. Martelli A, Reggiani A, Buli P: Post-transplantation ureteral stricture: Contralateral pyelocalicosty. Eur Urol 5:330, 1979
58. Mehta SN, Kennedy JA et al: Urological complications in 119 consecutive renal transplants. Br J Urol 51:184, 1979
59. Meyers AM, Levine E, Myburgh JA, Goudie E: Diagnosis and management of lymphoceles after renal transplantation. Urology 10:497, 1977
60. Moore TC, Hume DM: The period and nature of hazard in clinical renal transplantation: The hazard to patient survival. Ann Surg 170:1, 1969
61. Morley P, Barnett E, Bell PRF et al: Ultrasound in the diagnosis of fluid collections following renal transplantation. Clin Radiol 26:199, 1975
62. Morris PJ, Uadav RVS, Kincaid–Smith P et al: Renal artery stenosis in renal transplantation. Med J Aust 29:1255, 1971
63. Murray JE, Wilson RE, Tilney NL et al: Five years' experience in renal transplantation with immunosuppressive drugs. Ann Surg 168:416, 1968
64. Nagar D, Ferris FZ, Schacht RA: Obstructive polyuric renal failure following renal transplantation. Am J Med 60:702, 1976
65. Navani S, Athanasoulis CA, Monaco AP et al: Renal homotransplantation: Spectrum of angiographic findings of the kidney. AJR 113(3):433, 1971
66. Nerstrom B, Brix E, Clausen E, Lund FL: Late urological complications following human kidney transplantation. Acta Chir Scand (Suppl)433:113, 1973
67. Nerstrom B, Ladefoged J, Lund FL: Vascular complications in 155 consecutive kidney transplantations. Scand J Urol Nephrol 6:65, 1972A
68. Nicholson JD et al: Survival of a renal allograft after correction of a nearly total acute renal artery occlusion. Transplantation 26:131, 1978
69. Oakes DD, Spees EK et al: Arterial injury during perfusion preservation: A possible cause of post-transplantation renal artery stenosis. Surgery 89:210, 1981
70. Palleschi J, Novick AC, Braun WE, Magnusson MO: Vascular complications of renal transplantation. Urology 16(1):61, 1980
71. Pastershank SP, Ty M: Urologic complications in renal homotransplantation. J de L'Assoc Canad Radiol 29:34, 1978
72. Petrek J et al: Ultrasound in renal transplantation. Ann Surg 185:441, 1977
73. Pfeffermann R, Vidne B, Leapman S et al: Urological complications in renal primary and retransplantation. Experience with 202 consecutive transplants. Am J Surg 131:242, 1976
74. Prompt CA, Johnson WH, Ehrlich RM et al: Nontraumatic rupture of renal allografts. Urology 13:145, 1979
75. Raphael MK, Steiner RE, Shackman R, Ware RG: Postoperative angiography in renal homotransplantation. Br J Radiol 42:873, 1969
76. Ricotta JJ, Schaff HV, Williams GM et al: Renal artery stenosis following transplantation. Etiology, diagnosis and prevention. Surgery 84:595, 1978
77. Robson et al: Secondary hemorrhage from the arterial anastomosis of renal allografts. Br J Surg 59:890, 1972
78. Salaman JR, Calne RY, Pena J et al: Surgical aspects of clinical renal transplantation. Br J Surg 56:413, 1969
79. Salvatierra O Jr, Olcott C et al: Urological complications of renal transplantation can be prevented or controlled. J Urol 117(4):421, 1977
80. Schiff M, McGuire E, Webster J: Successful management of caliceal fistulas following renal transplantation. Arch Surg 110:1129, 1975
81. Schramek A, Adler O, Hashmonai M et al: Hypertensive crisis, erythrocytosis and uraemia due to renal artery stenosis of kidney transplants. Lancet 1:70, 1975
82. Schweizer RT, Bartus SA, Kahn CS: Fibrosis of a renal transplant ureter. J Urol 117:125, 1977
83. Schweizer RT, Cho S, Kountz SL: Lymphoceles following renal transplantation. Arch Surg 104:42, 1972
84. Schweizer RT, Kountz SL, Belzer FO: Wound complica-

tions in recipients of renal transplants. Ann Surg 177:58, 1973
85. Shimshak RR, Hattner RS, Tucker C, Salvatierra O: Segmental acute tubular necrosis in kidneys with multiple renal arteries transplanted from living-related donors. J Nucl Med 18(11):1074, 1977
86. Simmons RL: Kidney transplantation. In Najarian JS,Simmons RL (eds): Transplantation. Philadelphia, Lea & Febiger, 1972
87. Simmons RL, Tallent MB, Kjellstrand M, Najarian JS: Renal allograft rejection simulated by arterial stenosis. Surgery 68:800, 1970
88. Smith RB, Ehrlich RM: The surgical complications of renal transplantation. Urol Clin North Am 3:621, 1976
89. Sniderman KW et al: Percutaneous transluminal angioplasty in renal transplant arterial stenosis for relief of hypertension. Radiology 135:23, 1980
90. Spees EK, Williams GM et al: The consequence of microbial contamination of cadaver renal preservation media. II. A SEOPF prospective study, 1977–1981. Transplantation, 1981 (in press)
91. Spigos D, Capek V: Ultrasonically guided percutaneous aspiration of lymphoceles following renal transplantation. A diagnostic and therapeutic method. J Clin Ultrasound 4:45, 1976
92. Spigos DG, Tan W, Pavel DG et al: Diagnosis of urine extravasation after renal transplantation. AJR 129:409, 1977
93. Susan LP, Braun WE, Banowsky LH et al: Ruptured human renal allograft. Urology 11:53, 1978
94. Susan LP, Daughtry JD et al: Delayed calyceal cutaneous fistula after transplantation. Cleve Clin Q 45(3):287, 1978
95. Swanson DA, Sullivan MJ: Thromboendarterectomy for anuria 4½ years post-renal transplant: A case report. J Urol 116:799, 1976
96. Texter JH, Haden H: Scintiphotography in the early diagnosis of urine leakage following renal transplantation. Urology 116:547, 1976
97. Van Cangh PJ, Dautrebande J et al: Reversible renal artery stenosis in renal transplantation. Urology 13(5):529, 1979
98. Van Cangh PJ, Ehrlich RM, Smith RB: Renal rupture after transplantation. Urology 9:8, 1977
99. Vegeto A, Berardinelli L, Storelli G et al: Spontaneous rupture of the renal artery in kidney transplantation. Transplant Proc 11:1276, 1979
100. Vegter AJ et al: Spontaneous reversible renal artery stenosis after renal allotransplantation. Br Med J 1:1028, 1978
101. Vinde BA, Leapman SB, Butt KM, Kountz SA: Vascular complications in human renal transplantation. Surgery 79(1):77, 1976
102. Walter S, Poulsen LR, Friedberg M, Vejlsgaard R: The influence of drainage on the infection rate in kidney transplant patients. Br J Urol 50:160, 1978
103. Ward K: The origin of lymphoceles following renal transplantation. Transplantation 25:346, 1978
104. White RI, Najarian J, Loken M, Amplatz K: Arteriovenous complications associated with renal transplantation. Diagn Radiol 102:29, 1972
105. Woo KT et al: Transplant renal artery stenosis. Aust NZ J Surg 49:616, 1979
106. Zincke H, Woods JE, Hattery RR: Late ureteral obstruction mimicking rejection after renal transplantation. Urology 9(5):504, 1977

57
Complications of Gynecologic Surgery and Trauma

W. Glenn Hurt | Leo J. Dunn

OVERVIEW

In the female, the genital and urinary systems and, to a lesser extent, the lower bowel are closely related embryologically and anatomically. Congenital anomalies of one system are frequently associated with anomalies of another system. Gynecologic disease commonly involves all three systems, distorting anatomy and disturbing function. This is why gynecologic surgeons should acquire detailed knowledge of pelvic anatomy and become technically competent in both abdominal and vaginal surgery. They should be able to anticipate, recognize, and manage the common complications of pelvic surgery.

There are several characteristics of gynecologic surgery that may in themselves be sources of complications. Throughout life a woman may have more than one operation of a gynecologic nature. The prevalence of venereal disease and its sequelae; the desire to improve, retain, or terminate reproductive function; and the need for cesarean section are all causes for repetitive gynecologic surgery. Multiple entries into the peritoneal cavity and successive procedures on the same organs predispose the patient to incisional complications and adhesions.

The fact that the uterus, tubes, and ovaries are suspended within the pelvic cavity by ligaments and their accompanying vascular bundles encourages the surgeon to abandon careful dissection techniques and to crush bulky pedicles with multiple clamps and large sutures. When surgery is performed in this manner, it may injure adjacent organ systems. It also predisposes the patient to intraoperative and postoperative hemorrhage and leaves behind an excessive amount of traumatized tissue that may become a nidus for infection.

Gynecologic operations quite often require a combination of related surgical procedures as in the correction of pelvic relaxation or the removal of gynecologic neoplasms. There is reason to believe that multiple procedures increase the overall incidence of complications.

Gynecologic emergencies are infrequent; therefore most patients have time for thorough preoperative assessment. Cervical cytology should be routine. Anemias should be diagnosed and treated; infections should be cultured and eradicated; and electrolyte imbalances should be corrected. Preoperative electrocardiograms and chest roentgenograms should be performed when indicated. Pelvic ultrasonography, intravenous pyelography, cystoscopy, sigmoidoscopy, and barium enemas should be used liberally in evaluating pelvic masses and known or suspected gynecologic malignancies.

Prophylactic bowel preparation, antithromboembolic measures, and antibiotics are prescribed when specifically indicated. Preoperative bathing with special attention to the lower abdomen, vulva, and perineum; antiseptic vaginal douches; and cleansing enemas are recommended on the night before elective surgery.

Often major gynecologic surgery may be performed with equal facility using either general or regional anesthesia. The choice should be determined by prior consultation with the anesthesiologist and the patient.

After the patient has been brought to the operating room and anesthesia administered, the surgeon should check the position of the patient and supervise the preparation of the surgical site with special attention to the vagina and cervix. Bladder drainage should be effected using strict asepsis. When indwelling catheters are used, they should be connected to straight drainage and taped to prevent unnecessary trauma to the bladder and urethrovesical junction.

Endoscopy

LAPAROSCOPY

Laparoscopy is being used with increased frequency as a diagnostic and minisurgical technique. Contraindications to the procedure include severe cardiac disease, generalized acute peritonitis, intestinal obstruction, and massive intraperitoneal hemorrhage. The overall risk of laparoscopy is increased in the presence of significant cardiorespiratory disease, anticoagulant therapy, previous surgery likely to result in adhesions about the operative site, and diaphragmatic herniation.

Laparoscopy is performed using local, general, or regional anesthesia. Anesthetic complications are primarily those inherent to the technique.

The most common complications of laparoscopy include abdominal wall injuries, hemorrhage, gastrointestinal injury, uterine perforation, infection, and failure to effect sterilization. The abdominal wall may be injured by laceration of a blood vessel or by thermal burn. Bleeding from the abdominal wall is usually of little consequence and can be managed conservatively. Large hematomas require evacuation, ligation of bleeding vessels, and drainage. Electrosurgical burns must be widely excised and closed in layers.

Bleeding due to laceration of a mesosalpingeal blood vessel during sterilization procedures is usually controlled by cauterization or occlusion of the bleeding vessel by direct application of a sterilization device such as a ring or clip. If bleeding persists, laparotomy and ligation of the vessel may be indicated. Lacerations of major blood vessels require immediate laparotomy, transfusion, and repair of damaged vessels with vascular suture materials.

Gastrointestinal injury is most often the result of thermal burns or trocar lacerations. Burns are caused by defective instrumentation, electric arcing, contact with hot tissue or instruments, or the combustion of gas used to create the pneumoperitoneum. The most common sites of thermal injury are the terminal ileum and the rectosigmoid. Minor serosal burns may be managed conservatively by hospitalization and observation. However, since it is difficult to appreciate the extent of thermal injury, immediate laparotomy with resection of damaged small intestine or exteriorization of the damaged colon should be considered. Unrecognized thermal injuries may result in delayed bowel perforation and peritonitis. Trocar lacerations of the gastrointestinal tract require immediate laparotomy and repair. Gastric perforations are usually related to gastric distention from difficult general anesthetic inductions and can be prevented by gastric suctioning prior to the insertion of instruments into the abdominal cavity.

Uterine perforation may occur with the placement of the intrauterine probe, cannula, or curett. Direct observation during laparoscopy reveals the problem and determines treatment.

Wound infection is a rare complication of laparoscopic procedures and may be treated conservatively with hot compresses, drainage, and routine wound care. Suppurative salpingitis has been reported as a complication of laparoscopic sterilization in patients with an intrauterine device in place.[1] It is recommended that such devices be removed at least 2 weeks before laparoscopic sterilization.

The failure rate for laparoscopic sterilization, when corrected for luteal phase pregnancies and technical errors, is about two to three in 1000 cases. If laparoscopic sterilization is performed during pregnancy, it is associated with a significantly increased failure rate.[5] Inadequate cauterization, incorrect application of rings and clips, and inadvertent surgery on the round ligament and utero-ovarian ligament are all technical causes of "failure." Experience with the technique reduces these errors. Hysterosalpingography is not recommended as a routine postoperative test for tubal occlusion; if done, it is best to wait at least 3 months after the sterilization procedure, or it might contribute to recanalization. Sterilization failure may be an indication for abortion.

Abdominal Gynecologic Surgery

INCISIONS

The choice between a transverse or a vertical abdominal incision should be influenced by physical findings during the pelvic examination and by the preoperative diagnosis. An inadequate or inappropriately placed abdominal incision may complicate the entire procedure.

In repeating abdominal incisions, the relative advantage or disadvantage of entering through a previous incision must be considered. Removal of scars usually improves healing and appearance. New incisions in the vicinity of old scars often heal poorly and may result in incisional hernia.

Transverse lower abdominal incisions are frequently adequate for gynecologic surgery and cesarean sections. Advantages are a lower incidence of wound complications, including disruption and incisional hernia, and an improved cosmetic appearance. They are believed to cause less postoperative discomfort; this facilitates earlier ambulation. In comparison to vertical incisions, they require more time to perform and are associated with an increased loss of blood. The main disadvantage of transverse incisions is limited abdominal exposure.

If lateral retraction of the rectus muscles does not provide adequate exposure, the surgeon should consider cutting the tendinous insertions of the rectus muscles at the pubis or transversely cutting the muscles themselves. If either of these procedures is performed, reattachment of the muscles to the pubis or reapproximation of their cut edges and fascial coverings should be accomplished during closure.

Vertical midline incisions are rapidly performed and can be easily extended above the umbilicus to increase abdominal exposure. They facilitate exploration of the upper abdomen and should be used if the diagnosis is uncertain or upper abdominal procedures are anticipated. Since the incision is placed in a relatively avascular area, it is subject to more wound complications, including dehiscence and incisional herniation. Patients with vertical incisions who are at risk for poor wound healing may benefit by a primary Smead–Jones closure.[2]

Entry into the peritoneal cavity may be associated with bowel or bladder injury. To avoid injury, it is recommended that the point of entry be in the cephalad portion of the incision and clear of previous peritoneal incisions. Careful elevation and incision of a single fold of peritoneum will allow air to enter the peritoneal cavity and separate bowel from peritoneum. With the urachus as a guide, the translucent peritoneum may be incised to the dome of the bladder under direct vision.

RETRACTION AND PACKING

When self-retaining retractors are used, it is best to protect the walls of the incision with moist laparotomy pads. Excessive pressure tears blood vessels and causes tissue necrosis. The lower ends of the retractor's lateral blades should be visualized and palpated to be sure they are not in a position to compress or otherwise injure bowel, vessels, nerves, or the psoas mucles. Excessive pressure on the psoas muscle or compression of the external iliac artery, which diminishes or inhibits distal pulsations, implies femoral nerve compression and may be a cause of retraction-induced femoral neuropathy.[12]

Displacement of bowel into the upper abdomen with tight packing or compression by the superior blade of a self-retaining retractor may injure bowel or compress the inferior vena cava, causing systemic hypotension. Inferior blades or retractors should be carefully placed and constantly monitored to avoid bladder, vessel, and nerve injury.

UROLOGIC INJURY

The bladder, because of its anatomical location, is subject to direct and indirect injury during pelvic surgery. The most frequent sites of bladder injury are the dome, during entry of the peritoneal cavity; the fundus, during its dissection and displacement from the anterior surface of the uterus; its lateral margins, when clamping and suturing the cardinal ligaments; and the base or trigone, when excising the cervix and suturing the vaginal cuff. During reperitonealization of the pelvis, sutures may be placed in the bladder. Bladder injury can usually be prevented if traction is applied to the uterus and clean, sharp dissection is used to open anatomical planes. Prior cesarean sections, infections, endometriosis, or distortion by tumors complicates dissection and predisposes the patient to injury.

During abdominal gynecologic surgery, the bladder is often drained by an indwelling transurethral catheter. Hematuria is usually a sign of bladder mucosal trauma by the catheter or indirect bladder contusion secondary to retraction and dissection. Lacerations of the bladder may be demonstrated by allowing colored (methylene blue or indigo carmine) sterile water or saline solution to distend the bladder by means of the transurethral catheter and should be performed if injury is suspected. Some prefer to use sterile milk instead of colored solutions because it does not discolor the tissues about the laceration.

Partial-thickness bladder injuries should be reinforced by oversewing with absorbable suture. Full-thickness lacerations of the bladder require a two-layer closure with absorbable suture. When suturing near the trigone, it is important to avoid kinking or otherwise injuring the intramural ureter. Transvesical or transurethral catheterization of the ureter may be necessary to avoid this complication. Postoperatively, the lacerated bladder should be drained continuously for 7 to 10 days. Suprapubic or transurethral bladder catheters may be used. It is best to position the catheter so that it will not rest upon the suture line.

The ureter may be injured at any point along its course within the pelvis. Anatomically, it is closely related to the vascular bundles and ligaments of the uterus and ovaries. It is most frequently injured when clamping and ligating the cardinal ligament, the uterine artery, or the infundibulopelvic ligament and ovarian vessels (Fig. 57-1). Whenever ligatures are used to control pelvic hemorrhage, the risk of ureteral injury must be considered.

During surgery the ureters may be kinked, crushed, sutured, incised, divided, or devascularized. Suspected ureteric injury, in itself, is reason enough to dissect the pelvic course of the ureter. It may be further evaluated by unilateral intraureteral injection of dilute indigo carmine, intraoperative intravenous pyelography, or the insertion of ureteral catheters. Ureteral catheters may be inserted by linear ureterotomy, transvesically by cystotomy, or transurethrally by cystoscopy.

Kinking and suturing of the ureter requires removal of the suture and relief of obstruction. Crushed segments should be observed for viability. Minor crushing injuries may be treated with extraperitoneal drainage alone or, if more extensive, ureteral catheter stents. Significant crushing of the ureter requires excision of the segment and primary ureteroureterostomy or ureteroneocystostomy. Partial lacerations of the ureter may be sutured with interrupted extramucosal fine absorbable sutures. Complete division or the loss of a segment of ureter requires different management, depending upon the location of injury (Fig. 57-2). Injury to the distal 5 cm of the ureter is best treated by ureteroneocystostomy. Injury above that point may be treated by ureteroureterostomy, transureteroureterostomy, extraperitoneal ureteral catheter drainage, cutaneous ureterostomy, kidney transplantation, ligation of the ureter, and so on. The procedure to be used depends upon many factors: location and extent of injury, reason for surgery, condition of tissues, renal status, patient's prognosis, and surgeon's experience. All ureteric anastomosis should have extraperitoneal drainage by a closed suction technique. The tip of the drain should not be allowed to touch the anastomotic junction.

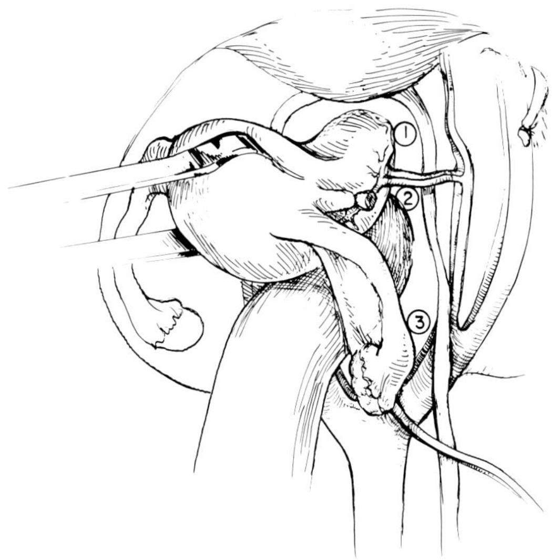

FIG. 57-1. The most frequent sites of ureteric injury associated with gynecologic surgery are at the level of (1) the cardinal ligaments, (2) the uterine arteries and veins, and (3) the infundibulopelvic ligaments.

INTESTINAL INJURY

Intestinal injury during abdominal gynecologic surgery is usually secondary to lysis of adhesions. Previous surgery may result in adhesions to the abdominal wall. Therefore, it is best not to enter the

FIG. 57-2. Surgical procedures recommended for segmental ureteric injury.

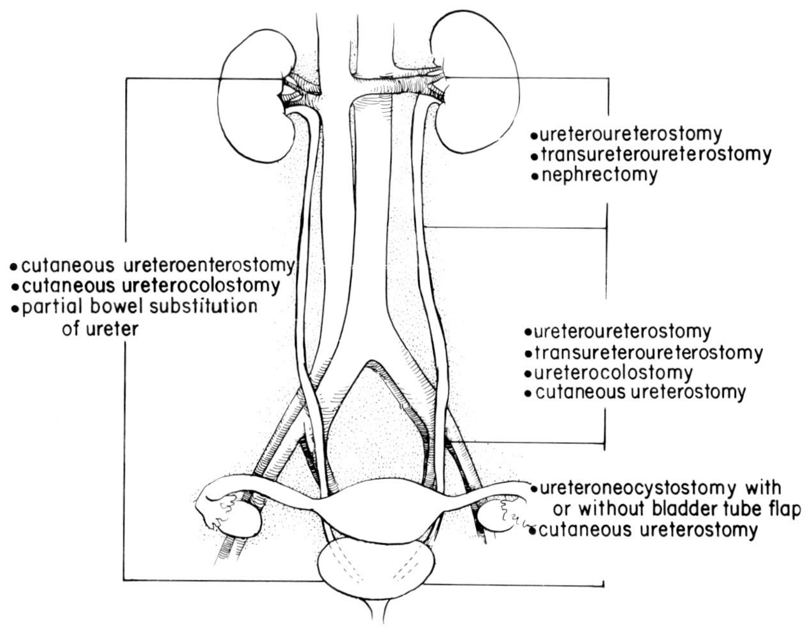

peritoneal cavity directly through the old peritoneal incision. Upon entry, the area about the old incision should be visualized, filmy adhesions lysed, and the more vascular adhesions clamped, incised, and ligated. Intraperitoneal "loops" created by omental adhesions or mesenteric defects should be sought and eliminated to prevent bowel strangulation.

Adhesions due to pelvic inflammatory disease and those due to endometriosis deserve special mention. Pelvic inflammatory disease tends to agglutinate serosal surfaces and to form an organ complex of tube, ovary, and bowel. Depending to some degree upon the interval since acute infection, it is often possible to identify the plane of agglutination and to separate the organs relatively easily with sharp and blunt dissection with very little risk of bleeding. The serosal surfaces maintain their integrity and are usually stronger than the adhesions that join them. Occasionally, vascular adhesions will require clamping and ligation. In endometriosis, the serosal surfaces do not maintain their integrity and the structures become "welded" together as a result of the invasive and destructive nature of the disease. Under these circumstances, blunt dissection may tear organs, and even sharp dissection may cause organ injury. If a difficult dissection is anticipated, it is best to prepare the bowel mechanically by diet and enemas and chemically by using antibiotics prior to surgery.

Injuries to the serosa and superficial muscularis of the small intestine are repaired by a single seromuscular layer of interrupted silk sutures. Minor lacerations of the small intestine should be closed in a transverse direction with one or more seromuscular layers of suture. If closure compromises the lumen of the small intestine or puts too much tension on the wall of the bowel, segmental resection and reanastomosis should be performed.

Superficial injury of the large intestine is also repaired by a single seromuscular layer of interrupted silk sutures. The lumen of the large intestine is not readily compromised. Management of lacerations of the large intestine varies with size, location, and bowel preparation. The laceration itself is closed in two layers; then the question is whether or not to perform a colostomy. In general, a proximal colostomy is indicated if the laceration is large, the blood supply to the damaged bowel is questionable, the closure is under tension, or the bowel is inadequately prepared. Copious peritoneal lavage, sump drainage, nasogastric suction, and antibiotic therapy also are indicated.

VASCULAR COMPLICATIONS

Blood loss is increased if the patient is pregnant or has pelvic inflammatory disease or endometriosis, a large tumor, or a coagulation defect. Certain medications, including birth control pills, may increase blood loss. Significant bleeding may come from the ovarian vessels, uterine arteries, vessels about the insertion of the cardinal ligament, or veins between the bladder and uterus. Skeletization of major vessels, clamping small bites of tissue, and double ligation of vascular pedicles will reduce blood loss. Venous ooze may be controlled by warm laparotomy pad compression. Hemoclips, absorable gelatin sponges, and occasionally the use of microfibrillar collagen hemostat may be useful. Intraoperative placement of suction drainage catheters will help prevent postoperative hematomas.

Uncontrolled pelvic bleeding may be treated by unilateral or bilateral hypogastric artery ligation, which reduces the pressure on the side of ligation.[4] Collateral circulation maintains viability of the pelvic organs. Hypogastric artery ligation should not be performed until the ureter, common iliac, and external iliac arteries and veins are identified. Then the hypogastric artery is dissected to demonstrate its posterior and anterior divisions. It is preferable to ligate the anterior division of the hypogastric artery just proximal to the uterine artery using one or two strands of heavy nonabsorbable suture material. Division of the artery is not necessary.

Injury to the major vessels during laparotomy for gynecologic disease is rare. Laceration of the common iliac or external iliac arteries requires repair by vascular techniques and suture material, preferably with the assistance of a vascular surgeon.

Postoperative thromboembolism is an important cause of mortality in gynecologic surgery. Abdominal hysterectomy appears to be associated with more risk of thromboembolism than is vaginal hysterectomy.[13] Recently the prophylactic perioperative use of support hose, intravenous low-molecular-weight dextran, and subcutaneous low-dose heparin has been advocated to reduce the incidence of venous thrombosis and embolism. However, the most important antithrombotic measures continue to be careful intraoperative positioning of the legs, postoperative leg elevation and movement, and early active ambulation.

Vaginal Surgery

DILATATION AND CURETTAGE

Contraindications to dilatation and curettage (D and C) are acute pelvic infection and pregnancy when abortion is not the intent. Complications of the procedure include uterine perforation, hemorrhage, infection, development of intrauterine synechiae, cervical stenosis, or an incompetent cervix.

The uterus may be perforated by dilators, sounds, curets, and forceps. Perforation is more likely to occur in patients with cervical stenosis, uterine malpositions, or uterine cancer. When perforation is the result of dilating the cervix or sounding the uterus, hemorrhage or injury to adjacent organs is rare. Uterine perforation by the sharp or suction curet or by forceps is more likely to cause bladder or bowel injury and hemorrhage. After perforating the uterus with these instruments, laparoscopy or laparotomy should be considered. Findings dictate therapy.

Hemorrhage as a result of gynecologic D and C is rare. Blood loss associated with obstetric D and C may be reduced by using the suction curet and the concomitant intravenous administration of dilute oxytocin. Hemorrhage may not be controlled until all of the products of conception have been removed from the uterine cavity. Postoperative ergotrate administration will assist in maintaining a contracted uterus and reducing blood loss.

Infection is more likely to complicate an obstetric D and C. Aseptic technique, removal of all products of conception, and a patent cervix reduce the incidence of infection. If infection develops, a pelvic examination should be performed and endometrial cultures obtained. Antibiotic therapy may be indicated.

Overzealous curettage, especially if associated with pregnancy and infection, may lead to the development of intrauterine synechiae (Asherman's syndrome), resulting in partial or complete obliteration of the uterine cavity and causing amenorrhea and infertility. The diagnosis may be confirmed by hysterosalpingography and hysteroscopy. Treatment consists of lysis of adhesions, temporary intrauterine placement of a device such as an IUD to separate the walls of the uterus, and the administration of estrogen to promote reepithelialization.

Traumatic cervical dilatation may cause the cervix to become either stenotic or incompetent. Gentle dilatation with Pratt or Hegar dilators reduces the incidence of these complications. Preoperative use of laminaria will make dilatation of the cervix for elective abortion less traumatic. Excessive dilatation should be avoided. Postoperative cervical stenosis requires repetitive dilatation to assure patency. An incompetent cervix may require cerclage during subsequent pregnancies.

CONIZATION OF CERVIX

Complications of cold knife conization of the cervix include laceration of the cervix, hemorrhage, infection, cervical stenosis, or an incompetent cervix.

Often the cervix that requires conization has old lacerations and is grossly irregular in contour or markedly stenotic. These conditions predispose the patient to laceration of the cervix and adjacent tissues. Hemostasis must be secured, and the laceration should be repaired with absorbable suture.

Immediate blood loss during conization may be reduced by prior injection of the cervix with dilute neosynephrine (1:2,000) or epinephrine (1:200,000) solution. Suturing the cervical branches of the uterine arteries with absorbable sutures is advisable. Additional sutures may be placed as needed. Sutures should not occlude or grossly distort the cervical canal. Early postoperative hemorrhage may require additional sutures or cervical packing. The patient should be told that delayed hemorrhage may occur when absorption of the suture material takes place. Resuturing of the bleeding points will be necessary and the need for supplemental iron therapy or blood transfusion will depend upon hemoglobin determination.

A low-grade cellulitis develops in the cervix after conization. If hysterectomy is to be performed, it is best to do it within 3 days or to delay it until the conization site is healed. Acute clinical infection requires pelvic examination, probing of the endocervical canal, culturing of the cervix, and usually antibiotic therapy.

The cervix is primarily fibrous tissue. Healing after conization can result in cervical stenosis. When the patient returns for her postoperative examination, she should be questioned about menstrual cramps and flow. If symptoms indicate cervical stenosis or if stenosis is apparent, the cervix should be dilated.

The incompetent cervix may require tracheloplasty or cerclage to help contain subsequent pregnancies.

VAGINAL HYSTERECTOMY

Contraindications to vaginal hysterectomy include active pelvic infection; large pelvic tumors; pelvic malignancies, other than occasional indication for a Schauta procedure; and the need for exploration of the upper abdomen. The risk of complications increases with dense pelvic adhesions secondary to previous operations, a history of pelvic infections, or endometriosis.

Technical competence in vaginal surgery and careful selection of patients for vaginal hysterectomy will do more than anything else to prevent complications. Complications of vaginal hysterectomy, with or without salpingo-oophorectomy, include hemorrhage, bladder and ureteral injury, intestinal injury, nerve injury, and infection.

Blood loss during vaginal hysterectomy appears to increase in a young patient. The injection of dilute neosynephrine (1:2,000) or epinephrine (1:200,000) solution about the cervix will reduce immediate blood loss. Since the ligatures on vascular pedicles tend to include more tissue and be less secure than those of abdominal hysterectomy, careful isolation, double ligation, and release of the pedicles is recommended. Avulsion of a pedicle may not result in immediate hemorrhage because of vascular spasm. To prevent delayed hemorrhage or hematoma formation, the pedicle should be reclamped and ligated. Although a continuous suture about the posterior vaginal cuff reduces access to the cul-de-sac, it will help control bleeding. Leaving an opening in the vaginal cuff helps prevent hematoma formation. The inability to control hemorrhage during vaginal hysterectomy may be an indication for laparotomy in order to gain hemostasis. Early or late postoperative hemorrhage is an indication for pelvic examination and an attempt at ligation of the bleeding point. Packing of the vagina is discouraged because it may conceal bleeding and contribute to hematoma formation.

The ureter may be injured when clamping or ligating the uterine artery. Because of its position alongside the uterus, the ureter is more prone to injury during surgery for uterovaginal prolapse. The ureter is also in jeopardy when clamping the infundibulopelvic ligament and vessels during vaginal salpingo-oophorectomy. If the ureter is crushed or ligated, urethral catheter drainage for up to 10 days should be considered. Division of the ureter is treated by transvaginal or transabdominal ureteroneocystostomy. Suspicion of partial or complete ureteral obstruction during the postoperative period is indication for intravenous pyelography, cystoscopy, and retrograde studies. Complete obstruction of the ureter may require percutaneous nephrostomy to preserve kidney function.

It is not uncommon to encounter adhesions between the uterus, bowel, and adnexal structures during vaginal hysterectomy. They may be lysed by sharp dissection. Occasionally bleeding points require ligation. If the small intestine is lacerated, a two-layer repair with absorbable suture and silk should be performed. Often this can be done through the vaginal port. If this is not technically feasible or if other injuries are suspected, the visible damage should be tagged for identification with sutures having long ends. Immediate laparotomy should be performed to repair damage. In general, the management of large intestinal injury is the same during vaginal hysterectomy as it is during abdominal hysterectomy.

Injury to the sciatic nerve is more common during vaginal hysterectomy than during abdominal hysterectomy.[9] This is primarily a result of placing the patient in variants of the lithotomy position. Padding pressure points helps to prevent damage to the anterior femoral cutaneous and lateral popliteal nerves. Since sciatic nerve injuries appear to be related to stretching, it is important not to overflex the thighs or overextend the legs. Nerve injury usually responds to physiotherapy. Recovery may be slow.

Postoperative infection of the vaginal cuff or adnexae is more frequently a complication of vaginal hysterectomy than of abdominal hysterectomy. Its incidence is greatest in patients of reproductive age. The onset of fever after the third postoperative day suggests vaginal cuff or adnexal cellulitis. It may progress to abscess formation if not diagnosed and treated. Postoperative fever is an indication for repeated pelvic examination to culture the vaginal cuff and to determine the probable cause of the fever. Probing the cuff will frequently provide drainage of a hematoma or an abscess. Large abscesses may require general anesthesia for vaginal drainage or laparotomy for the removal of infected adnexal tissues. Antibiotic therapy should provide coverage for anaerobic organisms.

Prophylactic antibiotics in gynecologic surgery appear to be of most value in reducing febrile morbidity when administered perioperatively to patients of reproductive age who are undergoing vaginal hysterectomy. Parenteral injections of cephalosporin before, during, and 6 hours after vaginal hysterectomy reduce the incidence of pelvic cellulitis.[7] When infection is the indication for surgery or when infection is encountered during surgery, a longer course of antibiotic therapy may be indicated.

Delayed complications of vaginal hysterectomy include enterocele and vaginal vault prolapse. It appears that removal of the uterus increases exposure of the cul-de-sac to changes in intra-abdominal pressure. Asymptomatic enteroceles may become symptomatic, and poorly supported vaginal vaults may become inverted. Suturing the cardinal and uterosacral ligaments to the vaginal cuff and prophylactic culdoplasty as advocated by McCall are generally accepted as important in the prevention of these complications.[8] An enterocele is usually corrected by dissection, ligation, and excision of the peritoneal sac; plication of the uterosacral ligaments; and posterior colporrhaphy. Occasionally enteroceles may be treated abdominally by excision or Moschcowitz closure using a series of purse-string sutures.[10] Many vaginal and abdominal procedures have been recommended for the suspension of a prolapsed vaginal vault. The selection of any one procedure should take into consideration the patient's age and desire for coital function. Two procedures to be considered are the vaginal sacrospinous ligament suspension as described by Randall and Nichols and the abdominal sacropexy as described by Birnbaum.[3, 11] In the elderly patient there is still the rare indication for partial or complete colpoclesis.

COLPORRHAPHY

Anterior and posterior colporrhaphy may be associated with excessive loss of blood. Submucosal injection of dilute neosynephrine (1:2000) or epinephrine (1:200,000) solution prior to incising the vaginal mucosa will assist hemostasis. Dissecting along anatomical planes and avoiding extensive lateral dissection will help control blood loss. Bleeding points should be ligated. Postoperative placement of a vaginal gauze pack will help obliterate submucosal spaces and prevent hematoma formation.

Anterior colporrhaphy may be complicated by urethral and bladder injury; urinary tract infections and voiding difficulties are not uncommon. Dissection of the distal urethra, which lies within the wall of the vagina, may result in meatal stenosis, requiring dilatation. Excessive mobilization and plication of the urethra damages its blood and nerve supply, contributes to fibrosis, and renders it a functionless conduit without sphincteric action. It is important not to overcorrect a cystocele. Marked elevation and fixation of the bladder base may abolish the posterior urethrovesical angle and result in stress urinary incontinence. Sutures that pass through the mucosa of the urethra or bladder should be avoided to prevent encrustations and possible fistulae. Lacerations must be identified in their full extent and closed with two layers of absorbable suture. Instillation of sterile dye solution or milk helps to identify lacerations and assures watertight closure.

Continuous postoperative bladder drainage is recommended after anterior colporrhaphy. If laceration occurs, catheterization should continue for 7 to 10 days. Bladder drainage may be by suprapubic, transurethral, or transvaginal cystotomy catheter. Catheters should not rest upon the site of laceration. Indwelling bladder catheters contribute to urinary tract infection. Prophylactic antibiotics will reduce the number of significant infections. Periodic urine cultures and sensitivity testing should be used to monitor the urinary tract and modify therapy.

Voiding difficulties and urinary retention are common after anterior colporrhaphy. They are usually due to overzealous surgery and partial obstruction of the bladder outlet. Most of these difficulties disappear with catheter drainage and healing; rarely will urethral dilatation be necessary.

Posterior colporrhaphy may be associated with injury to the rectum. Lacerations are closed primarily with two layers of absorbable suture prior to approximation of the edges of vaginal mucosa. Following repair of a laceration of the rectum, the anal sphincter should be dilated with two or three fingers immediately and for several days postoperatively to prevent gas collection and tension on the suture line. Such treatment is preferred over the use of a rectal tube. Lacerations of the small bowel at the time of posterior colporrhaphy are managed in the same manner as lacerations that occur during vaginal hysterectomy.

Late complications of colporrhaphy include vaginal strictures and dyspareunia. Most strictures respond to repeated dilatation. Rarely, vaginal Z-plasty or cutaneous pedicle grafts are required to increase the caliber of the vagina. Dyspareunia is usually the result of overzealous perineorrhaphy. The construction of a high perineum is of no advantage to the patient and is often the cause of dyspareunia.

Fistula

Emphasis has been placed on the intraoperative recognition and repair of urinary tract and intestinal injuries. A properly performed repair is successful in the majority of cases. When either primary repair was unsuccessful or injury was not recognized at the time of surgery, a fistula may form.

URINARY FISTULA

Most genitourinary fistulae are caused by gynecologic surgery. The fistulae usually open directly or indirectly into the vagina. A complaint of vaginal leakage of urine is highly suggestive of a urinary fistula and should be investigated. Visualization of all aspects of the vagina usually reveals the location of the fistula. The knee-chest position will assist visualization of the anterior vaginal wall. Gentle probing may reveal the origin of the fistula. The instillation of dye solutions into the bladder will usually reveal whether or not the origin of the fistula is the bladder. If the fistulous opening is difficult to locate, oral pyridium or intravenous indigo carmine may be administered, a tampon or four or more cotton balls placed in the vagina, and the patient told to walk for 20 to 30 minutes. Careful removal of the tampon or cotton balls, under direct visualization, will help locate the fistula along the vaginal axis.

Lower urinary tract fistulae are indications for urethroscopy and cystoscopy. The location and size of the defect must be documented, the condition of the tissues surrounding it evaluated, and its relationship to the ureters determined. Intravenous pyelograms and retrograde studies are useful in evaluating ureteric fistulae. It must be recognized that some fistulae are multiple and have complex tracts.

The first attempt at fistula repair is associated with the highest rate of successful closure and should be undertaken by an experienced surgeon. Timing of fistula repair depends upon many factors: the general condition of the patient and the lower urinary tract, the type of procedure resulting in fistula formation, previous attempts at repair, condition of tissues about the fistula, and the surgeon's experience. In general, delayed closures are more likely to succeed than are early closures.

The most common genitourinary fistula is the vesicovaginal fistula. Most are the result of total hysterectomy and are located just anterior to the vaginal apex. Smaller ones may close spontaneously with prolonged catheter drainage. Those that do not heal with catheter drainage may be repaired by the Latzko partial colpocleisis.[6] This procedure involves removal of vaginal mucosa about the fistula and a transverse two-layer watertight closure of the vaginal muscularis with absorbable suture. The edges of the vaginal mucosa are likewise approximated. The bladder need not be entered nor the fistulous tract excised.

Other types of vesicovaginal fistula and urethrovaginal fistulae can usually be repaired by the vaginal approach. The abdominal transvesical approach may be preferred for some cases of complicated vesicovaginal fistula. Whichever approach is used, the principles of repair are the same: mobilization of bladder or urethral wall, excision of fistulous tract, and multi-layered, extramucosal watertight closure with absorbable suture and no undue tension on the suture line. In all cases of vesicovaginal and urethral fistula, the bladder should be drained for 7 to 14 days postoperatively. Suprapubic drainage is recommended. Transurethral catheter or transvaginal cystotomy drainage may be substituted. An effort should be made to keep the catheter from the suture line.

Ureteral fistulae can be diagnosed by intravenous administration of indigo carmine and placement of vaginal cotton balls or tampons, once a vesicovaginal fistula has been ruled out. Intravenous pyelography, cystoscopy, and retrograde ureteral catheterization should be performed. Small ureteral fistulae may heal if the catheter can be passed beyond the fistulous opening and the urinary stream diverted. If this is not possible, the patient should be observed and managed conservatively until the time of surgical repair. If obstruction occurs and retrograde catheters cannot be passed, nephrostomy should be considered. The choice of operation for repair of ureteral fistulae varies according to the site of the fistula and the length of ureter that must be removed. Various types of operative procedures are suggested in Figure 57-2. Ureteroneocystostomy is recommended for fistulae below the bifurcation of the iliac arteries, especially in cases associated with previous pelvic irradiation or radical pelvic surgery.

INTESTINAL FISTULA

Intestinal fistulae following gynecologic surgery are most often associated with radical surgical procedures and radiation therapy. Manifestations depend upon location and size. High intestinal fistulae may have to be operated upon early because of the loss of electrolytes and irritating bowel contents. Hyperalimentation allows some latitude in this regard. Lower ileal and colonic fistulae may be treated conservatively. Careful injection of water-soluble radiopaque media into a bowel fistula under fluoroscopy and roentgenograms of the area help to locate the origin of the fistula. Dye solutions instilled into the rectum may be used to identify rectovaginal fistulae.

Large bowel fistulae may close unless they are complicated by distal obstruction, infection, or malignancy. In some cases, laparotomy with a two-layer intestinal closure or resection and reanastomosis may be necessary. Small rectovaginal fistulae should be excised and closed in two layers with absorbable suture. Fistulae near the external anal sphincter may be treated by proctotomy and an episiotomy-type closure. Larger and more complicated rectovaginal fistulae may require bowel preparation, temporary sigmoid colostomy, and delayed closure of the rectovaginal defect.

Complications of Cancer Therapy

Complications secondary to radiation therapy or radical surgery for the treatment of pelvic malignancies are more frequent and more serious than those for benign diseases. Since most of the patients who have been treated for malignancy are under the care of an oncologist, their management is not discussed in detail.

RADIATION THERAPY

Radiation damage requiring nonsurgical management includes radiation cystitis, radiation proctitis, and radiation enteritis. Cutaneous damage may still occur, but it less common since the advent of higher-energy radiation, which results in maximum ionization below rather than on the surface of the skin. Complications result from the inflammatory response of the tissues to the destructive effect of radiation. Inflammation of the affected organs may result in pain, diarrhea, and bleeding. Treatment includes reduction of the daily dose of ionizing radiation or temporary interruption of treatment if the severity of the symptoms warrant it. Interruption of therapy complicates the calculation of an appropriate tumor dose. Morphine derivatives may be used to slow intestinal motility, and steroids applied locally to the rectum as steroid enemas, suppositories, or foam are useful in the alleviation of symptoms.

The more serious complications of radiation therapy are due to an obliterative endarteritis. Resulting tissue hypoxia may produce necrosis sufficient to disrupt the wall of the affected organ. Ulceration, fistulization, or perforation of the intestine with subsequent peritonitis may result.

Lesser degrees of injury and scar formation may result in contraction of involved organs. The bladder capacity may be reduced; bowel may become stenotic and eventually obstructed. Surgical management of these complications involves a variety of procedures, which are not described in detail. However, it is important to recall the pathophysiology of these injuries, since surgery involves repair of heavily scarred tissues with a compromised blood supply. Repair of bladder and rectal fistulae following pelvic irradiation should employ a new source of healthy tissue with a good blood supply. Pedicle grafts utilizing the bulbocavernosus or a gracilis myocutaneous flap are currently in use.

Obstruction of the small bowel due to radiation stenosis poses difficult management. Currently bypass operations appear to have a higher success rate and lower morbidity rate than do resection and reanastomosis. Most often the area of stenosis is in the distal ileum and therefore ileoascending or ileotransverse side-to-side anastomosis to the colon is favored.

RADICAL SURGERY

Radical gynecologic procedures carry increased risks of hemorrhage, transfusion reactions, thromboembolism, infection, and fluid and electrolyte abnormalities.

Radical vulvectomy is associated with a high incidence of wound complications. Infection and necrosis of tissue about the wound are frequent problems. Suction drainage and utilization of skin flaps or grafts to avoid closure under tension can reduce this problem. Postoperative spontaneous rupture of the femoral artery has become rare since transplantation of the origin of the sartorius muscle over the vessel has been employed in radical vulvectomies with groin dissection. Late complications include urinary incontinence, which may be prevented by plication of the bladder neck at the time of the radical procedure. Contracture of the vaginal introitus, resulting in dyspareunia, may be avoided by making use of flaps of vaginal mucosa at the time of initial closure. Subsequent contractures may require Z-plasty or flaps.

Radical hysterectomy may be associated with immediate or late injury to surrounding organs. This is particularly likely when the procedure is undertaken because of recurrence of cancer after radiation therapy. Ureteral injury or tissue slough with resultant fistula formation has been reduced because suction drainage of the pelvis is commonly used and pelvic infections are more effectively treated with antibiotics. Also, greater care is given to avoidance of trauma and to the preservation of the blood supply of the ureters. Management of ureteral, bladder, and intestinal injuries is covered elsewhere.

Gynecologic Trauma

Traumatic injury of the female genitalia is relatively uncommon. Most often it consists of blunt trauma to the vulva or impalement of the vagina or rectum. In young girls it is usually associated with bike riding or fence climbing. Laceration of the pudendal or clitoral vessels and the pampiniform plexus may result in hematoma formation. It is most often treated conservatively. Rarely, exploration, drainage, and ligation of bleeding points will be required. Lacerations of the urethra, cul-de-sac, and rectum require immediate surgical exploration and repair.

References

1. Badra PL, Young JR, Laros RK Jr, Peterson EP: Suppurative salpingitis after laparoscopic tubal cauterization. Obstet Gynecol 42:511, 1973
2. Baggish MS, Lee WK: Abdominal wound disruption. Obstet Gynecol 46:530, 1975
3. Birnbaum SJ: Rational therapy for the prolapsed vagina. Am J Obstet Gynecol 115:411, 1973
4. Burchell C: Physiology of internal iliac artery ligation. Br J Obstet Gynaecol 75:642, 1968
5. Chi I-c, Mumford SD, Gardner SD: Pregnancy risk following laparoscopic sterilization in nongravid and gravid women. J Reprod Med 26:289, 1981
6. Latzko W: Postoperative vesicovaginal fistulas: Genesis and therapy. Am J Surg 58:211, 1942
7. Ledger WJ, Sweet RI, Headington JT: Prophylactic cephaloridine in the prevention of postoperative pelvic infections in perimenopausal women undergoing vaginal hysterectomy. Am J Obstet Gynecol 115:766, 1973
8. McCall ML: Posterial culdeplasty: Surgical correction of enterocele during vaginal hysterectomy, a preliminary report. Obstet Gynecol 10:595, 1957
9. McQuarrie HG, Harris JW, Ellsworth HS et al: Sciatic neuropathy complicating vaginal hysterectomy. Am J Obstet Gynecol 113:223, 1972
10. Moschcowitz AV: The pathogenesis, anatomy and cure of prolapse of the rectum. Surg Gynecol Obstet 15:7, 1942
11. Randall CL, Nichols DH: Surgical treatment of vaginal inversion. Obstet Gynecol 38:327, 1971
12. Sinclair RH, Pratt JH: Femoral neuropathy after pelvic operation. Am J Obstet Gynecol 112:404, 1972
13. Walsh JJ, Bonnar J, Wright FW: A study of pulmonary embolism and deep leg vein thrombosis after major gynecological surgery using labelled fibrinogen phlebography, and leg scanning. Br J Obstet Gynaecol 81:311, 1974

Part Nine

Complications of Musculoskeletal Surgery and Trauma

58
Complications of Multisystem Trauma Management

Kimball I. Maull

OVERVIEW—TRAUMA CARE SYSTEMS

Trauma is a sudden unanticipated interruption of life's routine. The trauma care system implies coordination of all essential resources necessary to facilitate care of the acutely injured patient from the time of injury until discharge from the hospital or completion of rehabilitation. With continued improvement in multisystem trauma management, the surgeon will more frequently be able to reply affirmatively to the trauma patient's lingering question: "Will I return to my routine?"

A trauma care system is an organized and coordinated approach to the acutely injured patient that provides personnel, facilities, and equipment for optimal trauma care in an appropriate geographical area under emergency conditions. A fully operational trauma care system requires (1) a communications capability to receive requests for help and to assure a prompt and appropriate response; (2) the capability for immediate on-site treatment and in-transit life support; and (3) the availability of suitable trauma treatment facilities prepared 24 hours, 7 days a week to receive injured patients from within the region.

Although full nationwide implementation of trauma care systems remains a challenge for the future, remarkable progress has taken place during the past 10 years. In 1966, the report of the National Academy of Sciences and National Research Council entitled "Accidental Death and Disability—The Neglected Disease of Modern Society" stimulated a critical examination of emergency care services in the United States and, together with the National Highway Safety Act of the same year, directly led to several important advances, of which the Emergency Medical Services System (EMSS) Act of 1973 was, by far, the most significant.[1,4] *Surgeons returning from Vietnam and accustomed to sophisticated battlefield intervention found relatively primitive emergency response systems. Ambulance attendants were given less formal training than were taxi drivers. The standard practice of "load and go" meant that helpless victims of highway accidents found themselves literally dumped in the back of ill-equipped vehicles that sped recklessly to the nearest, and often inappropriately staffed, hospital. The EMSS legislation was a necessary response to a national crisis in emergency health care.*

Phases of Trauma Care

There are certain factors regarding the trauma patient that, from the time the injury is incurred, act as determinants in final trauma outcome. These include, but are not limited to, the age of the patient, preexisting medical conditions, severity of injury, where the injury occurred, and, by implication, the time it takes from injury to definitive care. Unlike other types of emergencies, which often can be approached more casually, the characteristics of trauma require predetermined protocols in order to assure the most favorable outcome. Trauma care, therefore, exists as a continuum with four arbitrary but interdependent phases.[14]

PHASE I—PRETREATMENT

The pretreatment phase includes the incident and the processes of detection, notification of the emergency medical service (EMS) system, interpretation of the request for aid, dispatch of such aid, and transport of EMS resources to the incident site. Problems in the pretreatment phase relate primarily to delay in obtaining appropriate rescue, which may result from initial failure to detect the need for emer-

TABLE 58-1. LEVELS OF PREHOSPITAL PROVIDERS

Designation	Required Hours	Curriculum
Emergency Medical Technician—Ambulance (EMT-A)	81	Department of Transportation
Emergency Medical Technician—Shock-Trauma (EMT-ST)	EMT + 66	National Paramedic Training Program Modules I-III, V, VII-IX
Emergency Medical Technician—Cardiac (EMT-C)	EMT + 162	National Paramedic Training Program Modules I-VI, XV
Emergency Medical Technician—Paramedic (EMT-P)	EMT + 384	National Paramedic Training Program Modules I-XV

gency assistance, basically an unalterable circumstance. However, the ability of citizens to activate the EMS system is difficult in many parts of the United States. The reputedly universal 911 number for emergency police, fire, and medical assistance remains far from universal in practice. Thus, the citizen is often left to his own devices, resulting in life-saving time lost and inappropriate aid unless the correct resource is alerted. Even so, interpretation of requests for aid requires training and familiarity with both regional topography and relative risks and needs of illness or injury. The problems attending prompt dispatch of an advanced life support unit to the correct location is a phenomenon physicians rarely encounter. Yet, Adams, in a study of over 800 trauma victims injured in rural traffic accidents, showed that when assistance was provided within 15 minutes or less, 20% of the patients were already dead.[2] If 30 minutes had elapsed, 50% were already dead, and if 90 minutes had elapsed, 67% were already dead. Although this does not prove that earlier assistance would have saved those who died, improved survival rates with the rapid evacuation used in the Vietnam conflict would support such a conclusion. In certain types of trauma, therefore, it is more important to shorten the time it takes skilled rescuers to reach the scene than the time it takes to convey the victim to a trauma center, provided skilled resuscitation starts at the scene.

The emergency medical technician-ambulance (EMT-A) is the basic prehospital provider (Table 58-1). The EMT-A is trained in basic life support, oxygen administration, splinting, and other noninvasive skills. There are three recognized levels of advanced EMT training. The *EMT-shock trauma* (EMT-ST) is qualified to start intravenous infusions, apply the pneumatic antishock garment, and insert the esophageal obturator airway. The *EMT-cardiac* (EMT-C) has these same qualifications but receives additional instruction in EKG monitoring and telemetry, recognition of lethal cardiac rhythms, defibrillation, and drug therapy. The *EMT-paramedic* (EMT-P) is trained to perform at the most advanced level. The EMT-P receives a minimum of 167 hours of didactic instruction and 117 hours of clinical training and must serve 100 additional hours of field internship. This in-depth educational experience heightens the EMT-P's awareness of both medical and surgical emergencies and better enables the individual paramedic to establish appropriate treatment priorities.

PHASE II—PRELIMINARY CARE

The preliminary care phase includes on-site problem analysis and the sequential procedures of extrication (if needed), stabilization, treatment, loading, facility selection, and transport. Extrication, a vehicle crash rescue technique, requires scene assessment, hazard control, access, disentanglement, removal, and transfer.[7, 10, 15, 17] The difficulties encountered during vehicular extrication are unfamiliar to most surgeons, and it is this ignorance that commonly leads to misunderstanding delays that occur in the field. Additional delays in the field, however, are under the control of the emergency medical technician (EMT) and, by inference, the physician, in most advanced life support systems under direct medical control.

Before the development of EMS systems, trauma patients were often admitted to hospitals without any assessment of neurologic injury and without any attempt at stabilization. With improved training and communications, the level of prehospital expertise has steadily increased. The importance of early field trauma care is evident in several published postmortem studies demonstrating deaths from causes that need not have been fatal.[19, 21, 25] MacKay in a report on road accident postmortems suggested that 43% of riders or vehicle occupants fatally injured would have had a greater chance of survival if medical treatment were available at the scene of the accident within 10 minutes.[21] The World Health Organization estimated that 15% of early road deaths are caused by respiratory obstruction. Lauppi, in a series of 300 postmortem examinations performed on road accident casualties dying within 48 hours after injury, reported that respiratory obstruction was a sole cause of death in 15%.[19] He also noted victims dying from blood loss from injuries not in themselves incompatible with survival. These findings indicate that early skilled treatment may be able to reduce the mortality rate. Frey and colleagues estimated that about 20% of deaths at the scene of road accidents were needless if trained personnel could have been provided quickly.[11]

Trauma patients, particularly those in shock from major blood loss, offer the prehospital provider an opportunity to improve patient outcome. In reviewing a series of patients suffering from both penetrating and severe blunt trauma, Diamond reported that the establishment of intravenous lines raised the blood pressure and maintained the vital signs until definitive evaluation could be accomplished in the emergency unit.[9] Similar experiences accompany airway maintenance and the use of the pneumatic antishock garment.[6, 8, 20] Stabilization of trauma patients in the field, therefore, should include establishment and maintenance of an airway, ventilation, immobilization of the spine, intravenous volume replenishment, and application of pneumatic antishock garment and other splints as needed.

The airway is best established by the chin lift or jaw thrust maneuver with or without an oro- or nasopharyngeal tube, depending on the patient's level of consciousness. Careful suctioning is usually needed, and oxygen should be administered to all injured patients in shock. If the patient requires assistance with ventilation, a simple, safe, and effective method is the pocket mask using the rescuer's own lungs.[16] This method assures an open airway and adequate ventilatory volumes, and alignment of the cervical spine can be maintained (Fig. 58-1). Ventilation with a bag-valve-mask device is not recommended.

Whenever a trauma victim requires assisted ventilation without a definitive airway (*i.e.*, an intratracheal cuffed tube), vomiting and aspiration constitute an ever-present danger. Sudden turning of the head to the side to facilitate drainage may aggravate an unrecognized cervical spine injury and lead to permanent neurologic deficit. Provided the patient is unconscious, an esophageal obturator airway (EOA) may be a good compromise.[24, 26] This device is passed through the mouth into the esophagus, which is occluded by a balloon. Volume introduced by mask passes into the lungs, while gastric distention and regurgitation are prevented. The cervical spine may be maintained in a neutral position. Complications are uncommon but may be serious; they are listed below.[18]

- Pharyngeal or esophageal laceration
- Endotracheal intubation
- Bradycardia
- Driving blood or debris from pharynx into trachea
- Gastric distention
- Esophageal rupture
- Aspiration

The principal hazard attending field use of the EOA is unrecognized endotracheal intubation leading to acute gastric distention and asphyxia. This can be prevented by observing the rise and fall of the chest, listening for breath sounds, and searching for gastric borborygmi. If intratracheal placement is suspected, the tube should be removed and replaced. Improper removal of the EOA by the emergency physician is an additional hazard. If the patient is regaining consciousness and can protect his airway, the EOA may be carefully removed with suction at the ready. If the patient continues to require an airway, an endotracheal tube must be inserted prior to removal of the EOA.

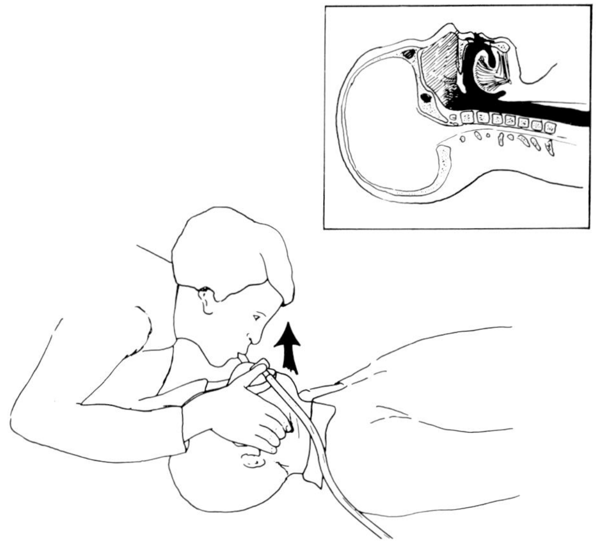

FIG. 58-1. Proper pocket mask ventilation assures adequate ventilatory volumes and maintenance of cervical alignment.

The pneumatic antishock garment, or military anti-shock trouser (MAST), is a three-chambered external counterpressure device applied circumferentially about both lower extremities and the abdomen, which has a salutory effect on circulatory hemodynamics. It functions by promoting central autotransfusion of a certain proportion of the intravascular volume while increasing the peripheral resistance and tamponading any bleeding points, both arterial and venous, which may lie underneath the garment. An added bonus is air-splinting of underlying fractures. Shock is the principal indication for the use of the device (see Chap. 26), and provided that cardiogenic shock with pulmonary edema has been ruled out, the MAST is safe and effective in the field.[3]

If the patient is in shock, intravenous access is indicated but may be difficult or impossible by usual percutaneous techniques. Often MAST application may result in adequate upper-torso venous engorgement, facilitating intravenous access. The decision to pursue intravenous administration in the field may be by protocol or by medical control, but inability to gain venous access should not be considered a stigma by prehospital personnel nor should patient transport be delayed.

Prior to movement of the patient, cervical stability should be assured. This is best accomplished by application of a rigid cervical collar and fastening the patient to a long spineboard.[3] The physician who receives a patient so immobilized is in no better position than is the EMT to determine the likelihood of cervical spine injury, and immobilization should be maintained until an unstable fracture is excluded by adequate roentgenograms.[23] Other splints should be placed wherever a fracture is suspected and treated in like manner by the receiving physician.

The measures cited can be performed quickly in the hands of skilled prehospital personnel and, under most circumstances, would be consistent with the primary rule governing emergency care, "Do no further harm." Taking a detailed medical history, further examinations, and other ill-advised maneuvers may adversely affect outcome when time to definitive care is so important. This confusion of priorities by prehospital personnel has led some to advocate a return to a "load and go" approach, and the experience in certain locales and with certain injuries would support such a concept.[13, 22] Enthusiasm for transport only has been superseded by a more realistic view that a small but significant number of patients should be managed in such a manner. Yet, the concept of prolonged stabilization in the field, although sometimes suitable for the cardiac victim, is ill suited for many trauma victims. The difficulties encountered in making some of these decisions point out the continued need for adequate communication and close medical direction.

One of the major problems in optimal trauma management during the preliminary care phase is that the full spectrum of anatomical and physiologic derangements may not be initially apparent. Both undertreatment and overtreatment may occur at the scene, and the patient may be misdirected to an inappropriate hospital where the entire clinical problem is not appreciated, is realized too late, or cannot be handled. Obviously, proper patient assessment, medical control, and successive assessment through the system either by protocol or by facility categorization will help to prevent these complications.

PHASE III—DEFINITIVE CARE

The definitive care phase begins with the transfer of patient care responsibility from the prehospital providers to the in-hospital medical personnel. This transfer includes the physical transfer of the patient but also the oral and written transfer of patient care information, which is almost always significant. Failure to review the "run sheet," lack of data about mechanism or time of injury, or poor communication in general may seriously impair trauma care at subsequent levels. The definitive care phase continues with rapid initial patient assessment and resuscitation, followed by establishment of patient care priorities, definitive diagnosis, and appropriate management.

Initial assessment is a brief 30-second look for airway adequacy and ability to ventilate, examination for pulses and signs of shock or external bleeding, and determination of level of consciousness. Patients must be disrobed prior to examination. Failure to do so may result in missing a significant injury. Life-threatening injuries require immediate treatment. The major pitfall in airway management relates to concern for a cervical spine injury. Based on a life-long cost for care exceeding $500,000 for a young paraplegic, it would appear that this attention is justified. Therefore, all comatose injured patients or patients with injuries above the clavicle should be considered at risk of cervical spine injury. Airway techniques that require little or no movement of the neck for establishment of ventilation are listed below.

Jaw thrust/chin lift
Pocket mask ventilation
Esophageal obturator airway
Nasotracheal intubation
Flexible bronchoscopic intubation
Cricothyroidotomy

An orotracheal tube may be inserted safely in certain instances of cervical spine injury, but the technique requires an assistant to provide in-line traction on the cervical spine. Deterioration following assisted ventilation suggests tension pneumothorax.

External bleeding is best controlled by direct pressure or by control of blood supply to the injured part. Tourniquets may be life saving but should not be employed unless the injured part is likely to be sacrificed since tourniquets crush underlying soft tissues and obstruct venous outflow.

Volume replenishment with lactated Ringer's solution from two large-bore catheters is indicated, and the MAST, if not previously applied, may be employed. Central venous lines are helpful, provided position and function of the line are confirmed by portable chest film. Pneumothorax, hydrothorax, and internal bleeding are the most immediate risks from central vein cannulation to the trauma patient. Urinary and gastric tubes should be inserted, provided that urethral and cribriform plate injuries are not suspected.

Following resuscitation and provided the patient has responded to initial therapy, a more detailed assessment is performed and is supplemented by suitable roentgenographic and laboratory tests. Missed injury is perhaps the surgeon's greatest concern. Use of diagnostic peritoneal lavage (DPL) has virtually assured finding significant intraperitoneal hemorrhage. Awareness of mechanisms of injury often suggests what injuries may be present (Fig. 58-2), and all inebriated patients warrant close observation and reevaluation in the hospital.[27]

An important factor in successful trauma management is the appointment of one surgeon as trauma team leader. This physician is responsible for patient management, sets patient care priorities, and guides the temporal aspects of specialty intervention. With this leadership, the timing and type of operative and intensive-care therapy can be established for the benefit of the patient.

PHASE IV—REHABILITATION

The rehabilitation phase begins after the patient has begun his initial recovery from the definitive care of his injuries. Rehabilitation often assumes a major early role in postinjury recovery and extends beyond the time of hospitalization to include the patient's transfer home or to an extended-care facility. Although it is certainly true that what happens in phases I to III often determines the ultimate outcome, the timely provision of rehabilitative services and the commitment of personnel to returning the patient to a productive status constitute a major influence in reducing long-term morbidity.

Special Problems in Multisystem Trauma Management

MULTIPLE CASUALTIES

In a disaster the number of injured patients exceeds what the trauma care system can optimally manage over a finite time period. This disproportion between the number of casualties and treatment resources requires that prioritization, a systematic approach to the individual patient that establishes the order of resuscitation and definitive care, yield to triage, a sorting procedure to determine which patients are treated first. To a small rural hospital with limited personnel and resources, a bad automobile crash with several critically injured victims may, indeed, qualify as a disaster. In an urban setting with multiple facilities capable of rendering emergency assistance, a coordinated disaster plan may disperse what would otherwise be a major disaster for any single hospital.

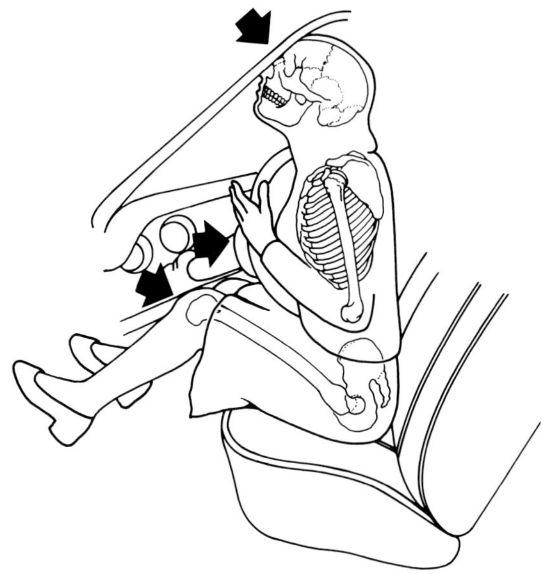

FIG. 58-2. The three levels of injury to the unrestrained driver demonstrate how knowing the mechanisms of injury can affect clinical management.

The major complications in multiple-casualty management relate to the sudden influx of injured persons who overwhelm available staff. If less severely injured and hysterical patients arrive first, the attention of staff may be diverted from the more seriously injured. Triage at the disaster scene can avoid this crisis and supports the concept of a mobile triage team to sort patients at the scene and select the appropriate receiving hospitals.[12] Others believe that specialized medical personnel perform best within the hospital environment and may actually impede efficiency at the disaster site.[17]

Triage at the hospital must be performed by the most experienced senior surgeon or clinician, one who can accept both the responsibility and the criticism for decisions reached under duress. Experience has confirmed the wisdom of identifying a triage area on the ground floor of the hospital separate from the emergency unit through which all casualties must pass. Irving considers clearing a single unit for care of all disaster victims the single most important factor in successful management of mass casualties.[17] This may not be practical in the United States where hospitals have designated intensive-care units and other less sophisticated general-care nursing areas.

More basic to the management of a multiple casualty incident is a workable disaster plan. Because junior staff usually have little knowledge of such contingencies and the few persons familiar with the plan may not always be available, the di-

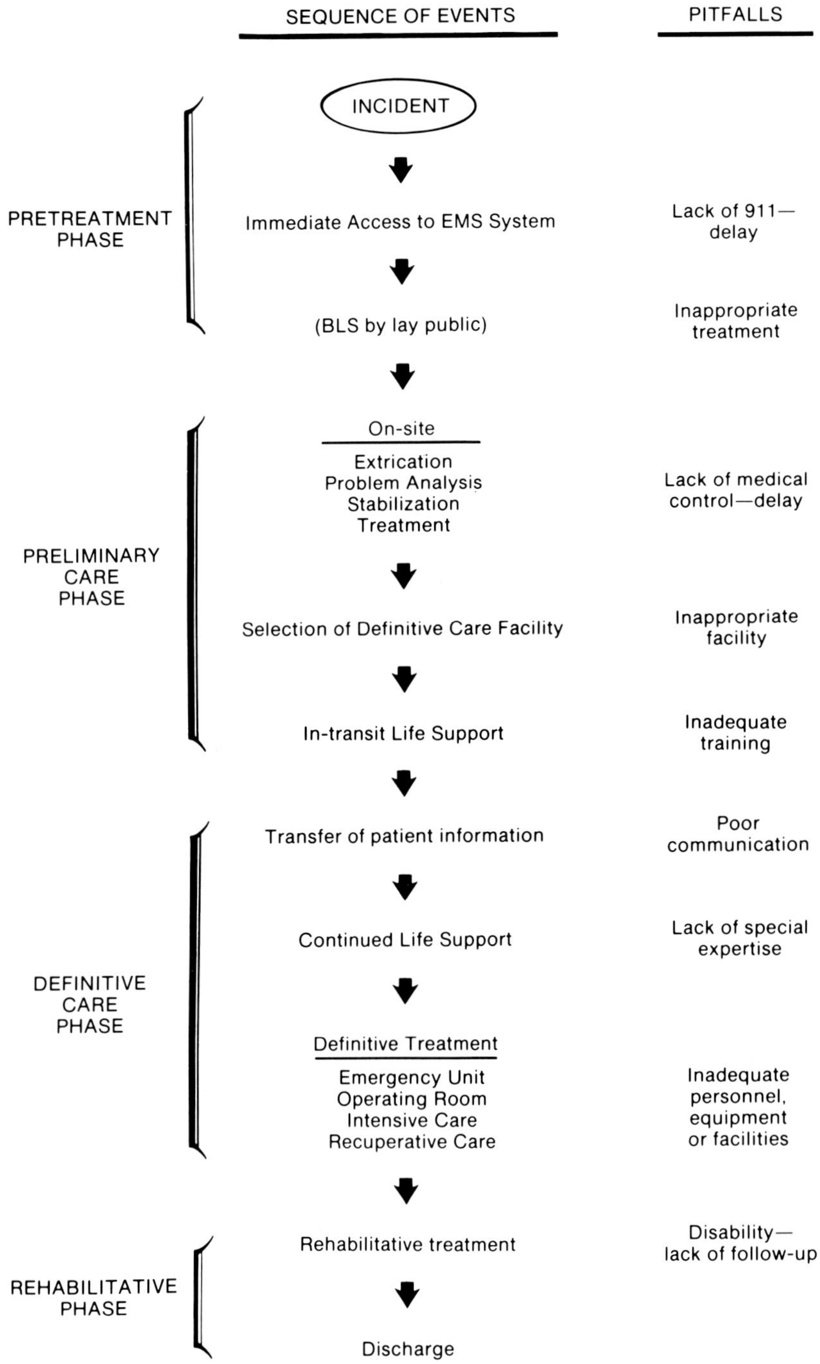

FIG. 58-3. Pitfalls in the optimal trauma-care system.

saster plan must be based on practical considerations and sound trauma care principles that fit both the institution and the area. No plan can be considered workable until it has been drilled, revised, and redrilled. The ultimate value of a disaster plan can be assessed only after its use in a disaster.

REGIONALIZATION OF TRAUMA CARE

Time/distance relationships are among the most critical factors affecting ultimate trauma outcome. In severe trauma, death will result if definitive care is not rendered within certain time constraints. Although over 80% of highway-related deaths occur in the spacious rural areas of the United States, it has been suggested that as many as 43% of these deaths could be prevented if adequate trauma care were available on a timely basis. Since trauma care is not a static phenomenon but a dynamic continuum with multiple interdependent phases, the lethality of an injury may be favorably affected by providing optimal but timely care at each of these phases (Fig. 58-3).[5] Although each phase is critical, in the final analysis it is often operative management and intensive postoperative care that are the final arbiters between life and death and between returning to a useful life and having a long-term disability. This concept has led to the evolution of regional trauma care systems, beginning with enlightened care at the scene; in-transit life support and resuscitation; and when possible, surgery at outlying hospitals or, when indicated, fast, safe transportation to advanced centers (trauma centers) for definitive management. This approach, when feasible in time and distance, offers the greatest chance for favorable outcome.[28]

Critically injured patients must be selectively triaged to centers with capabilities suited to the magnitude of the patient's injury. In urban areas this may not be the nearest hospital but a hospital the resources and capabilities of which are well known in the area. By contrast, in rural areas, the nearest hospital is often the only facility able to continue stabilization of the injured patient. In wilderness areas, the problem becomes even more difficult and may require the implementation of advanced systems of communication and transportation, including air medical evacuation.[5]

Regionalization of trauma care, therefore, seeks to address problems of limited personnel, both medical and technical, inadequate facilities and equipment, and the issues of priority of access. In order for regionalization to succeed, all phases must be operational.

PREHOSPITAL PATIENT TRIAGE

With a fully functional trauma care system, critical patient care needs can be assessed in the field and matched with the availability of local and regional expertise and facilities. The crucial issue is the question of bypassing the local hospital when rapid decay in physiologic status could be reversed at any emergency unit or inappropriately transporting a trauma victim to the local hospital when prompt sophisticated definitive care is the determinant of outcome. Prevention of these complications requires a sophisticated prehospital component with EMT paramedics, an intact and reliable communication network, and direct medical control of the EMS system (Fig. 58-4). With certain injuries, field stabilization and in-transit life support can afford the EMT-parmedic the capability to bypass the local hospital whereas with other injuries immediate transport to the closest facility is paramount.

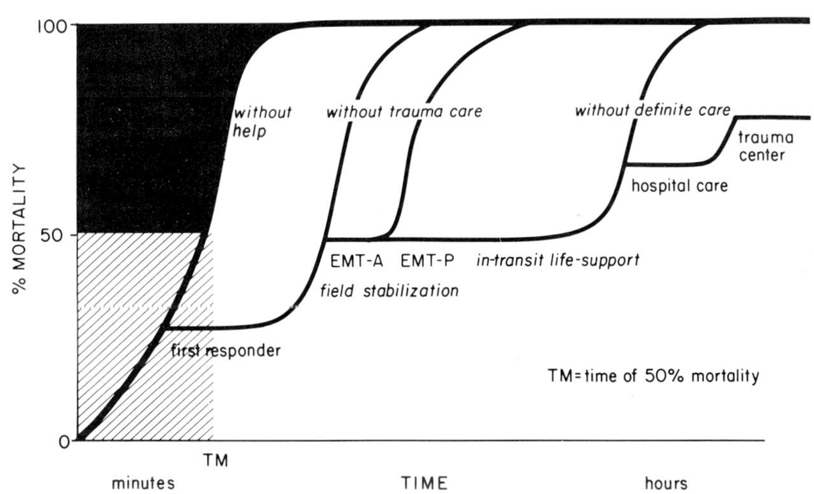

FIG. 58-4. Impact of appropriate prehospital and definitive care measures on trauma outcome. (Adapted from Boyd DR: Trauma: A controllable disease in the 1980s. J Trauma 20:16, 1980)

SAMPLE TRANSFER FORM

A. Patient's Name ____________________

Address ____________________

Age __________ Sex __________ Weight __________

Next of kin ____________________

Address ____________________

Phone ____________________

B. History of Injury
1. Pre-existing medical conditions
2. Previous medications

C. Condition on admission

Blood pressure _____/_____ Pulse _____ Temperature _____

D. Initial impressions

E. Diagnostic Studies
1. Laboratory
   a. Complete blood count
   b. Urinalysis
   c. Electrolytes
   d. Arterial blood gases
2. X-rays

F. Treatment rendered patient
1. Medications (amount and time)
2. Intravenous fluids (type and amount)
3. Other

G. Transfer Status

H. Management during transport

I. Name of physician transferring patient ____________________

Phone ____________________

J. Name of physician and hospital contacted ____________________

____

FIG. 58-5. Sample patient-transfer form.

MEDICOLEGAL PROBLEMS IN PREHOSPITAL CARE

With advances in the prehospital management of injured patients, the issue of accountability must be addressed. What happens if an untoward event occurs in the field and the patient suffers because of it? What happens if the patient succumbs en route to a trauma center after passing and not stopping at another hospital? These are questions that are frequently discussed, but the answers are incomplete. What is known is that prehospital providers functioning in a capacity consistent with their training are protected from liability by Good Samaritan laws in most states. Gross negligence, however, defines liability. In advanced life support systems with a designated medical director, the physician is responsible for events occurring in the field to the extent that mishaps result from faulty system design. Fortunately, such instances are rare. Close medical control of the system and documentation and review of each advanced life support (trauma) run are the best prevention.

INTERHOSPITAL TRANSFER OF TRAUMA PATIENTS

Nowhere in multisystem trauma management is the initial principle of trauma care "do no further harm" more applicable than in the transfer of the injured from one facility to another. Patients must not be allowed to die en route because of inadequate preparation.

Most injured patients will be able to receive total care of their injuries at the local hospital. Only a small number of injured patients require transfer to a facility with more advanced trauma care capabilities. It is crucial to patient outcome that the referring physician recognize this patient early and prepare for his orderly and safe transfer. This requires contact between the referring and receiving physician, initiated by the referring physician. The receiving doctor should define the criteria for the safe transfer and what information, what personnel, and what equipment should accompany the patient (Fig. 58-5). Certain injuries are best handled at a major trauma center, as listed below.[3]

Multisystem injuries
Open fractures
Uncontrolled bleeding
Severe maxillofacial injuries
Major head and spine injuries
Unstable chest injuries
Pelvic fractures
Blunt or penetrating abdominal trauma with hypotension

References

1. Accidental Death and Disability, Washington, DC, National Academy of Sciences—National Research Council, September, 1966
2. Adams AI: Death and injury on country roads: A study of 816 persons involved in rural traffic accidents. Med J Aust 2:799, 1967
3. Advanced Trauma Life Support—American College of Surgeons. Chicago, 1981
4. Boyd DR: Emergency medical services systems development: A national initiative, IEEE Transactions on Vehicular Technology 25:104, 1976
5. Boyd DR: Trauma—A controllable disease in the 1980's. J Trauma 20:14, 1980
6. Civetta JM, Nussenfield SR, Rowe TR et al: Prehospital use of the military anti-shock trouser (MAST). JACEP 5:581, 1976
7. Conrad MB: Principles of extrication. EMTJ 2:48, 1978
8. Cutler BS, Daggett WM: Application of the "G-suit" to the control of hemorrhage in massive trauma. Ann Surg 173:511, 1971
9. Diamond NJ, Schofferman J: Factors in successful resuscitation by paramedics. JACEP 6:42, 1977
10. Farrington JD: Extrication of victims—surgical principles. J Trauma 8:493, 1968
11. Frey CF, Huelke DF, Gikas PW: Resuscitation and survival in motor vehicle accidents. J Trauma 9:292, 1969
12. Gerace RV: Role of medical teams in a community disaster plan. Can Med Assoc J 120:923, 1979
13. Gervin AS, Fisher RP: The importance of prompt transport in the salvage of patients with penetrating heart wounds. J Trauma 22:443, 1982
14. Hanlon JJ: Emergency medical care as a comprehensive system. Health Services Reports 88:579, 1973
15. Harrison RR, Maull KI, Boyan CP: Vehicle crash rescue skills and residency training in emergency medicine. In Frey R, Safar P (eds): Emergency and Disaster Medicine. Sussex, England, John Wiley & Sons, Ltd (in press)
16. Harrison RR, Maull KI, Keenan RL, Boyan CP: Mouth-to-mask ventilation: A superior method of rescue breathing. Ann Emerg Med 11:74, 1982
17. Irving M: Major disaster: Hospital admission procedures. Br J Surg 63:731, 1976
18. Johnson KR, Genovesi MG, Lassar KH: Esophageal obturator airway: Use and complications. JACEP 5:36, 1976
19. Lauppi E: Traffic medicine. Therapeutische Umschau (Bern) 31:595, 1974
20. Lilja GP, Bataldan DJ, Adams BE et al: Value of the counterpressure suit (MAST) in pre-hospital care. Minn Med 58:540, 1975
21. MacKay GM: Some features of traffic accidents. Br Med J 4:799, 1969
22. McSwain GR, Garrison WB, Artz CP: Evaluation of resuscitation from cardiopulmonary arrest by paramedics. Ann Emerg Med 9:341, 1980
23. Maull KI, Sachatello CR: Avoiding a pitfall in resuscitation: The painless cervical fracture. South Med J 70:477, 1977
24. Meislin HW: Esophageal obturator airway: A study of respiratory effectiveness. Ann Emerg Med 9:54, 1980
25. Pacy H: Rural highway crashes—numbers of lives saved by treatment before transport. Med J Aust 2:780, 1974
26. Schofferman J, Dill P, Lewis AJ: Esophageal obturator airway: A clinical evaluation. Chest 69:67, 1976
27. Weisz GM, Schramek A, Barzilai A: Injury to the driver. J Trauma 14:212, 1974
28. West JG, Trunkey DD, Lim RC: Systems of trauma care. Arch Surg 114:455, 1979

59 Complications of Fractures

John A. Cardea

OVERVIEW

Fractures occur when excessive stress is applied to bone. Bone is a semirigid structure, and fractures from forces applied exceed first the bending point and subsequently the breaking point of the bone. Energy is accumulated in the bone, and the bone literally explodes at the breaking point. The ends of the fractured bone become secondary missiles and may lacerate, contuse, or stretch surrounding soft tissue. The amount of damage occurring to the soft tissue is directly proportional to the amount of initial trauma plus the secondary trauma created by the free bone ends and fragments (Fig. 59-1).

Fractures are produced by direct or indirect trauma.[7] An example of direct trauma is a fracture of the tibia that occurs when the tibia is struck directly by an automobile bumper. The forces directly applied to the tibia exceed the elastic limits of the bone, and fracture results. An indirect trauma occurs when a force is transmitted from the point of impact to create a fracture at a more distal point. An example of this type of fracture is a fall on the outstretched hand. The impact of the hand on the ground is transmitted through the forearm, elbow, arm, and shoulder to produce a fracture of the clavicle.

Indirect forces that result in fractures may be compressive, distractive, angulatory, or rotational, and each of these produces a distinct type of fracture.[7] A bursting fracture of a vertebral body represents a compression force. A patient falling from a height and landing on his feet creates a force directed vertically down the spine, producing a compression fracture of the vertebral body (Fig. 59-2). A basketball player jumping and landing on one leg produces a distraction force through the quadriceps

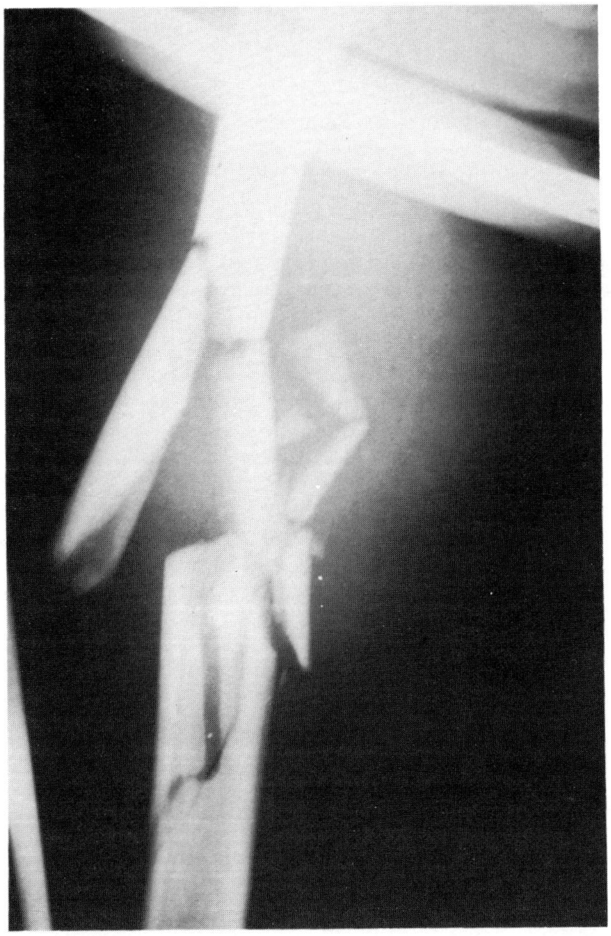

FIG. 59-1. Comminuted fracture of the femur with a high-energy injury secondary to a motorcycle accident. Multiple-bone fragments act as secondary missiles.

mechanism, resulting in an avulsion fracture of the patella (Fig. 59-3). A boot-top fracture of the tibia in a skier is an example of an angular force. The ski and boot stop abruptly and the skier continues forward, creating an angular force on the tibia at the top of the rigid ski boot (Fig. 59-4). An intertrochanteric fracture of the hip is another common example of an angular force that creates a fracture. The force created through the femoral head exerts an angular moment at the trochanteric area. If this force exceeds the elastic limits of bone, a fracture results (Fig. 59-5). Rotational forces occur when one end of the bone is held firmly, and a rotational torque is applied to the opposite end of the bone. This will produce a long spiral fracture (Fig. 59-6).

Fractures resulting from direct or indirect trauma may also be classified according to the configuration of the fracture. A common configuration classification is transverse fracture, short oblique fracture, long oblique fracture, spiral fracture, comminuted fracture, and comminuted fracture with a butterfly fragment (Fig. 59-7). The configuration of the fracture will determine the stability and must be considered in planning the treatment of the fracture.[5]

If the fracture fragments penetrate the skin, an open or compound fracture is created. This condi-

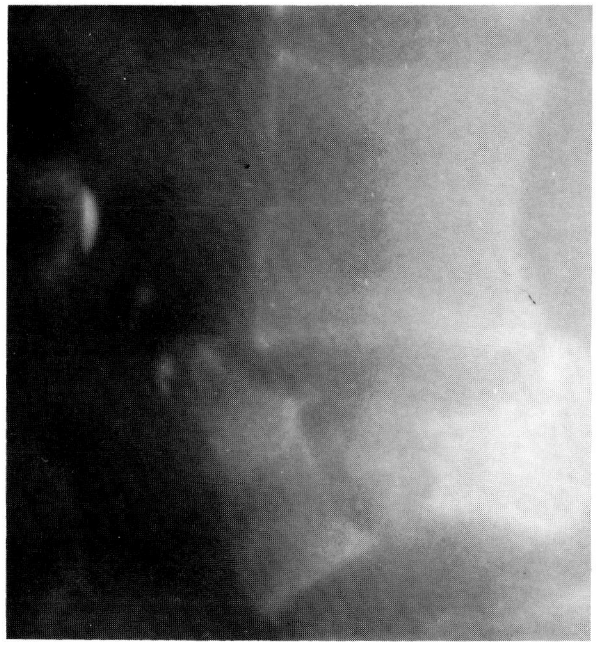

FIG. 59-2. A burst fracture of a vertebral body of the lumbar spine.

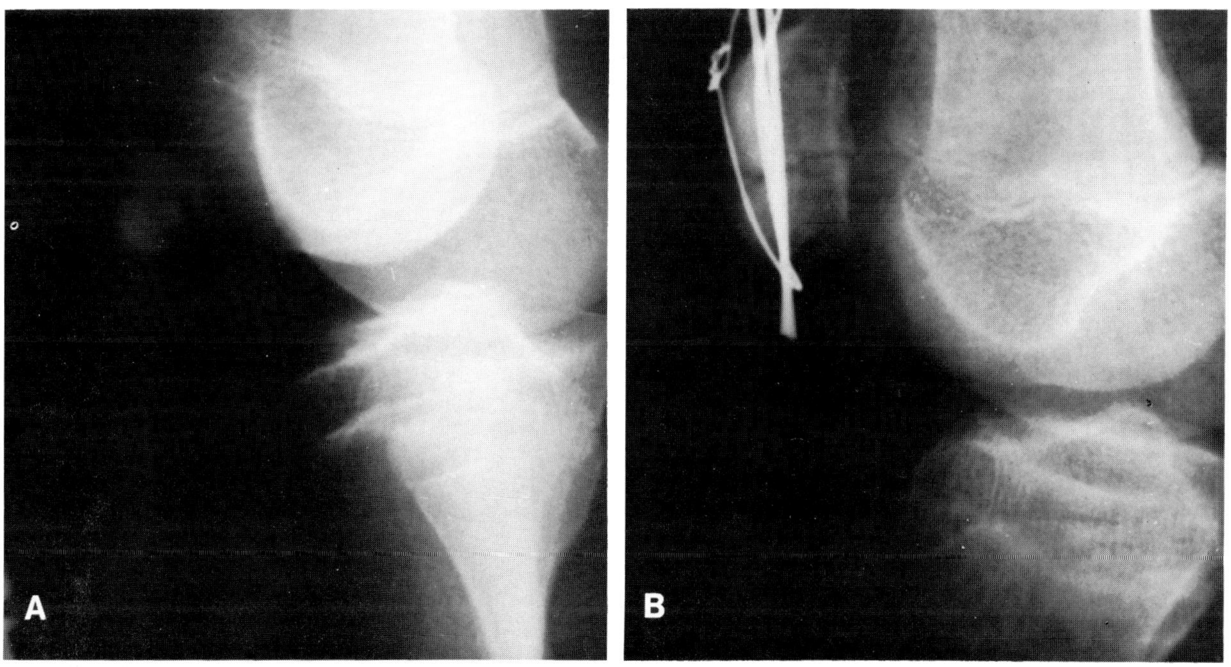

FIG. 59-3. (*A*) Traction fracture of the patella. Note the transverse fracture created by pulling the bone apart. (*B*) Fracture of the patella repaired by a tension band to resist the traction action of the quadriceps mechanism.

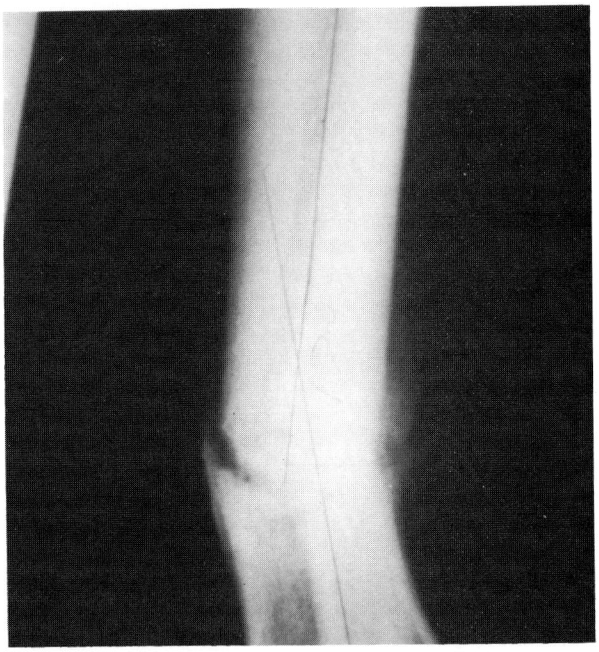

FIG. 59-4. Fracture of the tibia created by an angular force at the boot top of a skier.

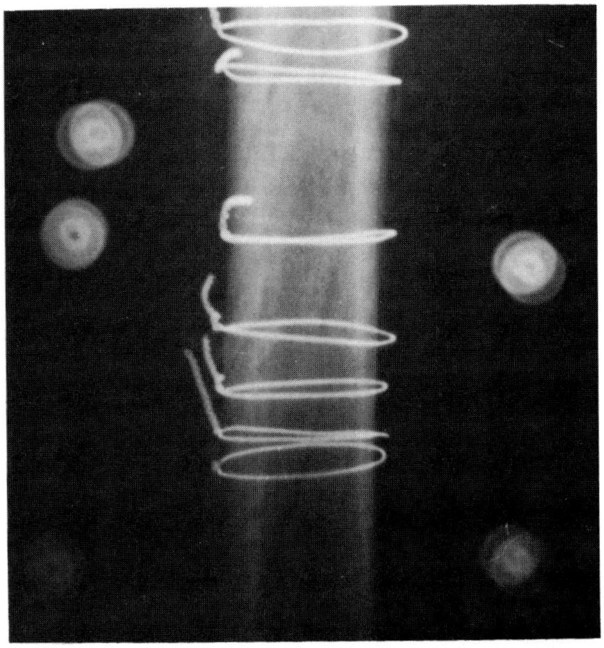

FIG. 59-6. Spiral fracture of the femur below a total hip femoral stem. The fracture has been stabilized with cerclage wires. Note the spiral nature of the fracture site. The fracture was created by excessive torque applied to the bone.

FIG. 59-5. Intertrochanteric fracture of the femur. The head and neck fragments act as a lever arm, transmitting excessive force to the intertrochanteric region.

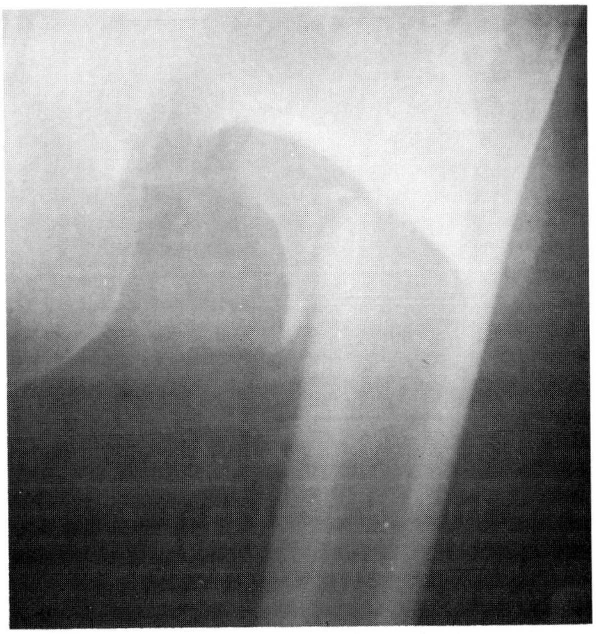

FIG. 59-7. Lateral view of a comminuted fracture of the proximal one third of the tibia with a butterfly fragment.

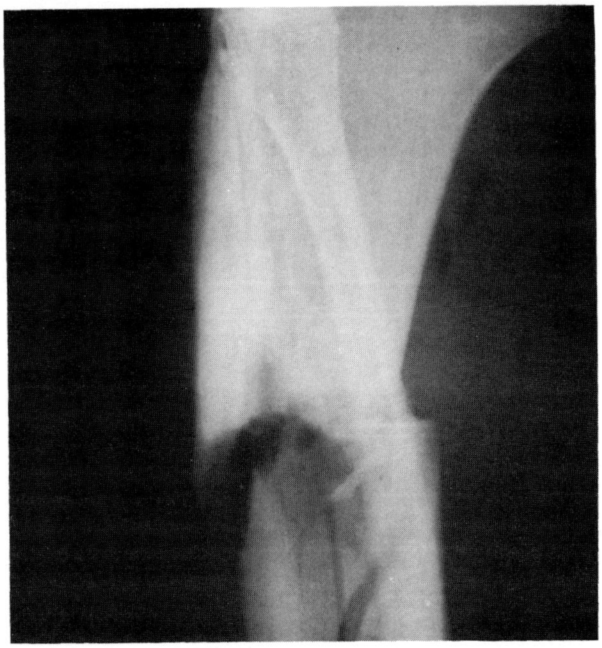

tion leads to bacterial contamination of the fracture and complicates fracture treatment to a much higher degree. The wound created by the fracture is classified according to the severity of the laceration and the severity of the soft tissue damage.[7] A minor puncture wound created from the end of a bone penetrating through the skin is classified as a type I wound. This classification proceeds to a type III wound, in which there is a laceration of greater than 2 inches in the skin with moderate to severe soft tissue damage.

Emergency treatment of fractures is extremely important and may decrease the complications associated with the injury. Proper immobilization will reduce the motion of the bone ends and minimize any further damage to the soft tissue. Application of pressure dressings will decrease hemorrhage of compound wounds, and elevation of the injured extremity will limit edema of the injured part and of the extremity distal to the fracture. Immobilization of a fracture will also decrease pain. The pain of a fracture is created by the periosteum and the soft tissue; there is no nerve fiber deep within the bone.

In the initial splinting of the fracture, the bone as well as the joint above and the joint below the fracture should be immobilized. Fractures of the lower extremity may be bound to the good extremity, and fractures of the upper extremity may be immobilized to the chest wall with sling and swath to provide emergency immobilization. Upon the patient's arrival in the emergency room, more conventional splints and traction methods may be employed to provide splinting and stabilization. Compression dressings should be applied directly over the bleeding points to control hemorrhage. The use of a tourniquet is contraindicated and may cause further ischemia or edema to the injured part and the extremity distal to the injured part.[6]

The complications of fractures are discussed individually rather than by anatomical area and are divided into acute and late complications. Acute complications result from the fracture and include problems that occur to the patient or the soft tissue. Late complications are related to the function of the bone or extremity. After discussing each complication, the most common bones involved and any peculiarities of those bones is discussed.

Acute Complications

SHOCK

In the management of any fracture the overall status of the patient should first be determined. Recognition and early treatment of shock is essential to prevent the complications of shock (see also Chap. 13). The clinical signs of shock include peripheral vascular collapse, low blood pressure, increase in pulse rate, and altered mental state of the patient. The circulation to an injured extremity may be difficult to assess in a patient in shock. A Doppler examination may be required to establish the presence or absence of a distal pulse in a patient with decreased peripheral circulation.

The most commonly fractured bones to produce hypovolemic shock are the pelvis and the femur.[7] The pelvic fracture causes bleeding directly from the large vascular flat bones, and the trauma that creates the pelvic fracture also may lacerate or avulse the pelvic veins and arteries. The resulting hypovolemic shock may require transfusion of as much as 20 units of blood to sustain the patient. The initial treatment is to stabilize the pelvic fracture. If a fracture dislocation of the pelvis is present, traction should be applied to the affected side through a distal femoral traction pin. This allows firm traction to be applied directly to the femur to reduce the displacement of the pelvic fracture. By decreasing the motion of the fragment, immobilizing the fracture, and reestablishing the normal tension, bleeding may be controlled. If further immobilization of the pelvis is necessary, an external fixator may be applied directly to the pelvis percutaneously.[4] Continued bleeding from the soft tissue arteries and veins must be controlled either by an external pressure suit or, under the guidance of localized arteriography, by injection of clotting material directly into the lacerated artery. If these techniques are used, it is seldom necessary to explore the pelvic vessels surgically.[6]

Fractures of the intertrochanteric region of the femur or fractures of the shaft of the femur also may precipitate shock. A blood loss of 2 to 6 units may accompany these fractures. The initial treatment is traction through the femur or tibia. In addition to stabilizing the bone ends, the traction causes the thick fascia of the thigh to exert a compression force on the injured muscle and bone, creating localized tamponade. This treatment does raise the intercompartmental pressure of the thigh, effectively decreasing the volume of that compartment; however, this assists in stopping the local hemorrhage and rarely creates problems with compartment syndrome in this large compartment.[8] In addition to its excellence as an emergency treatment, traction may also be used as the definitive treatment for fractures of the femoral shaft.[7]

Other bones that cause moderate hemorrhage when fractured are the humeral shaft and the tibial shaft. Pathologic fractures resulting from highly vascular metatastic lesions may also precipitate hemorrhage.

ARTERIAL INJURY

Arterial injury is a genuine surgical emergency. A laceration to a major artery of the extremity may result in permanent damage to nerves and muscles if the blood supply is not restored within 4 to 6 hours following injury. The initial evaluation of the extremity with a fracture should include the examination of distal pulses. If the pulse is not present to palpation, a Doppler examination is indicated. The pulses may be present but weak if the patient has any degree of shock secondary to peripheral vasoconstriction or if the vessels are under localized pressure applied by the fracture fragment or increased compartmental pressures.

Two types of arterial injury occur secondary to fracture. Complete laceration of a major artery produces profuse bleeding; however, the arterial ends contract owing to the elasticity in the vessel wall and usually clot as the mean blood pressure decreases. In partial lacerations, the artery remains intact and only the lacerated portion of the artery retracts, resulting in excessive hemorrhage. This type of injury may lead to more severe hemorrhage than if the artery were lacerated completely.

Excessive localized hemorrhage is the most important clinical sign in evaluating arterial lacerations. An arteriogram is diagnostic; however, direct exploration without arteriogram may be mandated by the circumstances; that is, there is no time for delay so that perhaps the study cannot be performed. Intramedullary fixation of the fracture prior to arterial repair is my recommended treatment of the fracture in civilian injuries. However, if the extremity is jeopardized because of delay in arterial repair, the arterial repair should be performed primarily as well as repair of any major venous injury (see also Chap. 27). The bone is then stabilized after the vascular repair or stabilized with traction by percutaneous external fixator.[4] If a surgical procedure on the bone is necessary, this should be delayed for 3 to 4 weeks until the arterial repair has healed.[6]

Common sites of arterial injury associated with fracture are as follows:

- Brachial artery at the proximal humeral shaft
- Brachial artery in the supracondylar area of the humerus
- Deep femoral artery at the subtrochanteric level of the femur
- Popliteal artery at the level of Hunter's canal in the supracondylar area of the femur
- Popliteal artery at the level of trifurcation adjacent to the metaphyseal area of the tibia
- Anterior tibial artery in the middle one third of the tibia

NERVE INJURY

Nerve injuries occur from direct contusion or laceration by the fracture fragment or by penetration of missiles (e.g., bullets or shotgun pellets). Nerves also may be stretched by excessive forces, producing fracture dislocation about the joint. Nerve injuries may be classified as

Neuropraxia
A transient denervation produced by a mild contusion of the nerve. The healing of this type of injury is usually complete by 8 weeks with some signs of nerve function return being present in a few days. An electromyographic study (EMG) shows no denervation potentials with this injury.

Axonotmesis
Complete physiologic denervation with intact nerve sheaths. This type of injury is called *severe contusion* or *stretch* of the nerve. The EMG will show reinnervation potentials at 2 to 3 months. The axon will regenerate through the intact nerve sheaths.

Neurotmesis
Complete denervation caused by complete laceration of the nerve including axons and sheaths. No reinnervation potentials on the EMG will return at any time, and this type must be identified and surgically repaired.

The nerve injury is identified by neurologic examination of the extremity distal to the fracture. As with pulses, the neurologic examination is mandatory on initial evaluation of the extremity, and reexamination is mandatory after manipulation or reduction of the fracture. The complications of nerve injury and nerve repair are discussed more fully in Chapter 48.

Common nerve injuries associated with bone injuries include

Axillary nerve injury with fracture and dislocation of the shoulder. This injury is identified by the motor loss of the deltoid muscle.

Radial nerve injury with fracture of the humerus at the distal one third of the humerus. Care should be taken to splint the hand and wrist properly following this injury. The wrist and MP joints should be splinted in extension, and the thumb should be splinted in extension and abduction. If the fracture requires open reduction and internal fixation, the nerve should be explored. If closed treatment is appropriate for the fracture, the nerve should be followed with serial EMG studies for up to 3 months along with specific physical examination for return of radial nerve function. If no return is present at all at 3 months, then surgical exploration and repair of the nerve are indicated.

Median nerve injury at the wrist with displaced radial fracture. This is a very common sequel of Colles' fracture or fracture of the distal radius with dorsal displacement and radial angulation, which creates a stretch as well as a direct contusion to the median nerve. The immediate treatment for this consists in accurate reduction of the fracture. If the neuropraxia does not respond to this treatment, a carpal tunnel release should be performed.

Sciatic nerve injury associated with fracture dislocation about the hip. Open reduction and internal fixation of the posterior acetabular wall is the treatment for this injury. In most instances the injury consists in a neuropraxia due to direct contusion of the nerve by the femoral head from the dislocation.

Peroneal nerve injury associated with fractures of the neck of the fibula. With peroneal nerve clinically or a peroneal portion of the sciatic nerve injury, clinically the result is a drop foot. This places the foot in its weakened position, and the prolonged plantar flexion may result in an equinus flexion contracture. This injury can be treated simply with physical therapy and a drop-foot brace, which maintains the foot in dorsiflexion and prevents inversion of the foot and ankle on ambulation.

FAT EMBOLISM

Fat embolism is a cause of the commonly diagnosed adult respiratory distress syndrome. It may follow the fracture of a single long bone or multiple trauma. It occurs from 6 to 24 hours after the injury and has a high correlation with shock in the postinjured patient.[7]

The clinical sign of fat embolism consists of tachycardia, dyspnea, mental confusion of any degree, and petechial hemorrhage. The hemorrhages occur in the axillary and pectoral areas of the chest as well as in the conjuctiva of the eye. The etiology of fat embolism may be from direct embolism of fat from the marrow of the long bones into the venous plexus; however, altered lipid stability can cause embolism of fat to the lungs, brain, and other parts of the body.[6]

There is no diagnostic test for fat embolism. Arterial blood gas with an oxygen tension of less than 50 torr is almost always present in the full clinical fat embolism syndrome. Increase in serum lipase and fat levels in the urine may be seen, but neither is pathognomonic for this condition. Thrombocythemia of less than 150,000 per ml^3 and precipitous drops in the hematocrit may also be present. A differential diagnosis of more severe pulmonary problems must be ruled out before treatment is initiated. These include posttraumatic shock lung syndrome, pulmonary contusion, and overhydration.

Fat embolism is a self-limiting entity if adequate ventilatory support and oxygenation are provided. Oxygen should first be given by mask and the oxygen tension monitored. An oxygen tension of greater than 70 torr should be maintained during this emergency treatment. If the mask ventilation is not adequate, the patient will require endotracheal intubation for adequate administration of oxygen. Intravenous high-dose steroids, alcohol, and heparin have all been used as adjunctive therapy; however, none of these has been definitively proved to be of benefit in the treatment of fat embolism.[6]

In a review of 53 consecutive cases of clinically proved fat embolism treated at the Medical College of Virginia with oxygen and various ventilatory supports, there were no deaths. When intubation was necessary, it was used for 3 days or less in all but one of the patients. No long-term measure of pulmonary compliance has been made in these patients. No case presented with marked hypoxia and coma. This presenting syndrome reportedly causes a higher mortality rate.[7]

COMPARTMENT SYNDROME

Compartment syndrome is a condition in which increased pressures in a closed space compromise the circulation to muscles and nerves of that compartment. The most common cause of compartment syndrome is fracture with bleeding from the bone into one or more compartments and contusion of the muscles within the compartment. Other causes include vascular injury, bleeding disorders, anticoagulation therapy, burns, intra-articular drug injection, snake bites, exercise, infiltrated infusion, and a tight cast or bandage.[8] Awareness of compartment syndrome must always be kept in mind when treating fractures. The resultant compartment pressures represent a combination of internal pressures from the fracture's bleeding and injury plus the external pressures created from casts or rigid dressings.[8] For a compartment syndrome to occur there must first be a compartment of a thick, unyielding envelope (fascia). There must then be an insult to increase the pressure either by increasing the content of the compartment (hemorrhage) or by applying external pressures effectively, thus decreasing the compartment (cast).

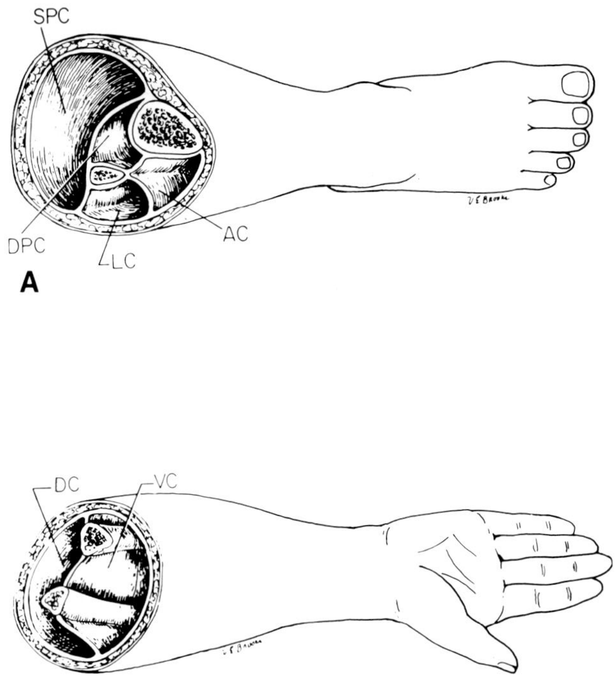

FIG. 59-8. (*A*) The four compartments of the leg: the anterior compartment (*AC*), the lateral compartment (*LC*), the superficial posterior compartment (*SPC*), and the deep posterior compartment (*DPC*). (*B*) The two compartments of the forearm: the volar compartment (*VC*) and the dorsal compartment (*DC*). (Matsen FA III: Compartmental Syndromes, p 82. New York, Grune & Stratton, 1980, by permission)

Common compartments involved in this syndrome include

In the leg, anterior, lateral, deep posterior, and superficial posterior compartments (Fig. 59-8*A*)
In the forearm, volar and dorsal compartments (Fig. 59-8*B*)

Less common compartments involved in compartment syndrome include

Hand (interosseous)
Thigh (quadriceps)
Arm (deltoid and biceps)
Buttock (gluteal)

The diagnosis is made by clinical signs and symptoms and by tissue pressure measurements.[9] These may be supplemented by direct nerve stimulation. The most important clinical finding is pain out of proportion to that expected for the injury. The pain is not relieved by narcotics after adequate splinting. Pain on passive stretch of the muscle is highly suggestive of ischemia, and also the muscles of the involved compartment may be weak on active extension or flexion. All of these findings may be present with bounding peripheral pulses. The presence of pulses must not be used to rule out compartment syndrome. The physician must always keep in mind that the microcirculation to the muscle and the ultimate delivery of oxygen to the muscle are cut off in the compartment syndrome. Hyperesthesia of nerves of the compartment may also be found as the compartment syndrome progresses.

In addition to the findings on active and passive motion and neurologic examination, the extremity itself must be examined. As the pressure increases, the compartment becomes extremely tense, owing to increased pressure pushing against the tight envelope of fascia. Palpation of this tense compartment will produce tenderness. Although the physical examination and clinical symptoms are highly reliable, direct tissue measurements may also be indicated. Continuous monitoring of compartment pressures may be mandatory in patients with multiple trauma, who are unconscious, or who have external pressure applied in the form of a MAST suit or cast.

Before the diagnosis of compartment syndrome is made, the physical findings as well as the compartment pressures must be taken into account. A tissue pressure of 45 to 60 torr will consistently give rise to compartment syndrome. Measurements of this magnitude with positive physical findings indicate the need for surgical decompression of the involved compartment.[8] Monitoring of the compartment and examinations must be repeated frequently. Compartments at risk may not attain the pressures or physical findings of a compartment syndrome immediately, and the pressures may continuously rise and require measurement for 72 hours. The newer techniques of compartment monitoring allow the introduction of catheters coupled to transducers, which allow continuous monitoring of one or more compartments.

The earliest of the diagnostic methods for tissue pressure measurement is by injection, which continues to be one of the most commonly used today because it is simple to perform and its results can be reproduced, if it is done properly.[9] This method is also inexpensive. It requires a mercury manometer and disposable needles and tubing. In this method, a needle is placed through the fascia into the muscle. The needle is connected to a mercury manometer through a three-way stopcock, on the third arm of which a syringe filled with air is applied. Pressure is then exerted very slowly through the syringe, and the mercury manometer and meniscus are observed simultaneously.[9] As the air–fluid meniscus begins to move, the measurement is directly read from the mercury manometer (Fig. 59-9). The examination is performed with all of the systems in a horizontal plane at heart level. More sophisticated continuous monitoring systems that are more expensive and more complicated have been developed, but they offer no substantial difference in the technical results. The principle of these methods is basically the same: a needle, catheter, or wick is inserted through the fascia and into the muscle of the compartment and connected to a solid column of heparinized saline, which is connected to a transducer monitor from which readings in millimeters of mercury are made.

Once the compartment syndrome has been diagnosed, the compartment or compartments should be surgically released. The four compartments of the leg are most commonly involved, with the anterior and peroneal compartments the most common followed by the deep posterior and superficial posterior compartments. It has been our practice to release only the compartment or compartments involved with elevated pressures, and in 8 years no patient has had to have a second operation for releasing additional compartments. Therefore, I do not recommend that a four-compartment release always be done when a compartment syndrome is present.

If a four-compartment release is needed, there are two methods currently used. The first is an incision from 2 inches above the lateral malleolus to 2 inches below the fibular neck centered over the fibula. The dissection is then carried down through the subcutaneous tissue to the fascia, with care being taken to identify the superficial branch of the peroneal nerve. The fibula should not be exposed subperiosteally, but there should be an extraperiosteal dissection around the fibula. This will open all four compartments laterally, and the fibula need not be resected. The other method of four-compartment release is a linear incision over the junction of the anterior and lateral compartments. The dissection is carried down to the intramuscular septum, and subcutaneously the fascia over the anterior compartment is identified and divided, as is the fascia over the lateral compartment. A second incision is made 1 cm posterior to the medial tibial crest from 2 inches above the medial malleolus to the flare of the tibia, and the fascia over deep and superficial posterior compartments is released through this medial incision. Both of these procedures give adequate exposure and adequate decompression of the compartments.[8] The two-incision technique requires slightly less dissection than a perifibular technique; however, it does require two incisions. The wound should then be dressed open and some splinting for the fracture utilized.

If multiple compartments are involved, internal or external fixation of the bone may be indicated. The compartment pressures can be measured individually on the operating table with the injection technique and the decreased to zero pressures noted. The patient can then be returned to the operating room in 3 to 5 days for delayed primary closure. If the swelling requires 7 to 10 days to subside, skin grafting will be necessary (Fig. 59-10). Muscle need not be resected at the time of decompression unless there is obviously dead muscle. The regenerative power of muscle is good, and only muscle that is obviously necrotic need be removed at the initial operation. If the patient develops fever within 24 hours, reexploration of the wound is indicated if there is no obvious pulmonary cause for this fever. Early temperature elevation is an indication of ischemic muscle.

FIG. 59-9. Injection technique. The pressure in the system is slowly increased by depressing the plunger of the syringe while observing the manometer and the air–water meniscus. The pressure at which the meniscus first moves toward the limb reflects the tissue pressure. (Matsen FA III: Compartmental Syndromes, p 12. New York, Grune & Stratton, 1980, by permission)

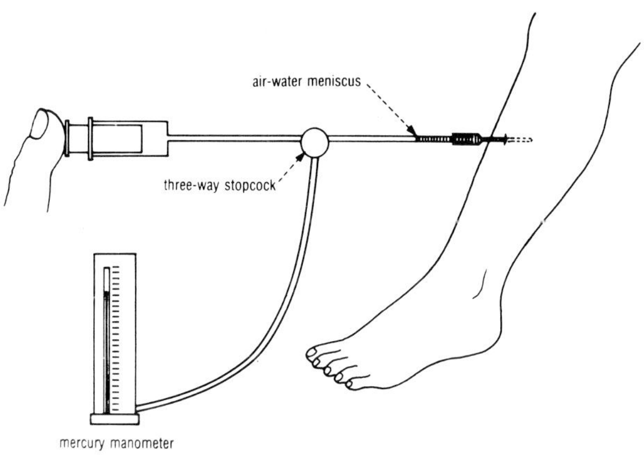

FIG. 59-10. Split-thickness skin-graft coverage of a defect created by compartment release.

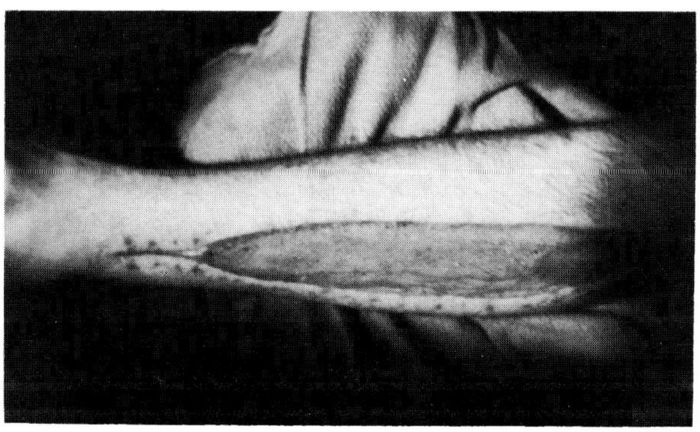

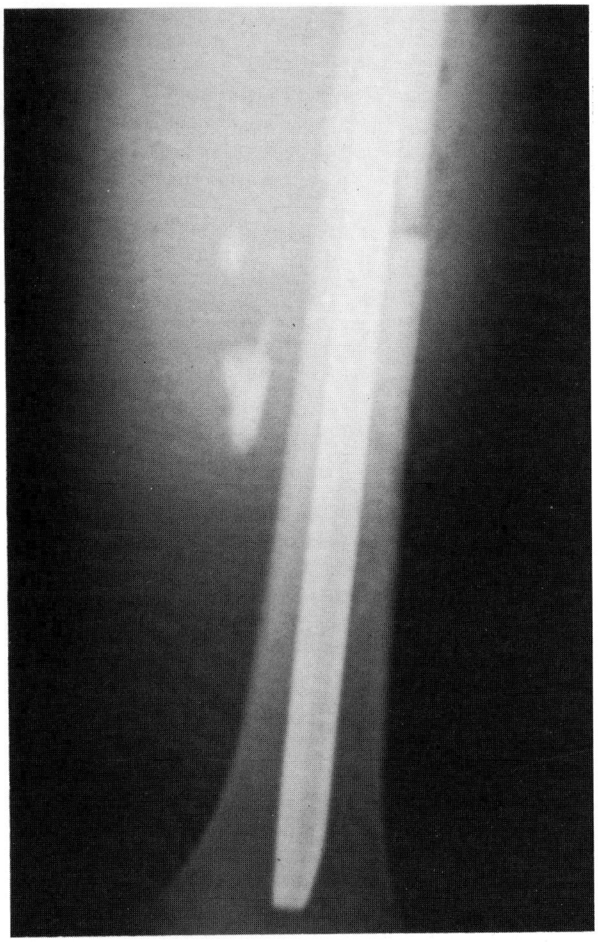

FIG. 59-11. Internal fixation of a femur fracture using a Küntscher intramedullary nail.

OPEN FRACTURES

An open wound with exposed bone is a complication of the fracture. This type of injury implies laceration of muscle, fascia, subcutaneous tissue, and skin. The bones as well as the wound have been contaminated. These are the most serious types of injury, and the prognosis is guarded. Many open injuries are caused by gunshot or shotgun wounds; however, the majority of open fractures are caused by laceration of the soft tissues by bone from within out. This type of injury not only creates a compound wound but also causes marked internal damage and stripping of tissues from the bone.

The fracture should be splinted and the wound dressed with clean gauze. A pressure dressing should be applied to all brisk bleeding. After x-ray evaluation of the fracture, the wound should be explored and débrided in the operating room. Included in the emergency treatment is the administration of prophylactic antibiotics. A wide-spectrum antibiotic is recommended because 75% of contaminated wounds have mixed flora with both gram-positive and gram-negative organisms.[6]

Antibiotics are no substitute for thorough surgical débridement of the wound, and this surgical débridement must be given the highest priority. The wound should not be probed or partially débrided in the emergency room. In the surgical suite, thorough preparation of the wound should be performed and each level of tissue damage thoroughly débrided. All dead or severely damaged tissue must be excised and the wound cleansed gently with saline lavage. The fracture should be maintained in proper alignment and be splinted or stabilized. Stabilization of the fracture may be obtained with cast or by internal or external fixation (Fig. 59-11). The application of a cast to stabilize the fracture may be used for extremities with small or moderate compound wounds. A rigid cast material may add external pressure to the compartments as the soft tissues swell, in which case the cast must be partially removed or windowed to attend to the wounds. This may jeopardize fracture stabilization. In more extensive soft tissue injuries, cast or plaster splints are not the most effective means of stabilization for the wound management. The surgeon must keep in mind that the first priority is soft tissue wound care.

Internal fixation of fractures may be utilized to stabilize the bone under ideal circumstances. If the wound is tidy and excised properly and if the internal fixation material is completely covered by soft tissue, plates and screws or intramedullary rods or pins may be safely used. The preferred internal fixation devices are intramedullary rods or pins. These devices may be introduced through small holes at the end of long bone and are confined to the medullary canal and therefore completely covered. Devices that require no intramedullary reaming are preferred to those that require intramedullary reaming, provided stability can be obtained. Plates and screws may be used; however, they require much more surgical exploration and soft tissue stripping of the bone than do intramedullary devices. If used, plates should be placed under available local soft tissues, preferably muscle. The plate should never be exposed because this will lead to bacterial contamination and local wound infection.

External fixation devices are ideal for stabilizing fractures and allowing easy access to soft tissue wounds (Fig. 59-12).[1] Pins are placed through the bone at a distance from the fracture site and are coupled to each other and to a rigid external frame.[4] The fracture is stabilized because the pins are rigidly fixed to the frame. Extreme caution in pin placement must be used. The pins should be applied with no tension to the soft tissues. There should be minimal binding of muscle tendon units and no perforation of arteries, nerves, or veins.[4]

The goal of treatment of compound fractures is to provide coverage and healing of the soft tissue as soon as possible. Only after this has been accomplished can the definitive fracture care be undertaken. The systematic plan of wound débridement and local wound care should be followed by a systematic plan of wound closure. In many cases of types I and II open wounds, a delayed primary closure may be accomplished from 5 to 7 days following the injury. If primary closure cannot be accomplished, split-thickness skin grafting should be performed as soon as the proper bed of granulating tissue has formed (see also Chap. 4). A mesh skin graft of 0.015 to 0.017 inches has yielded uniformly good results in our treatment of compound injuries. Delayed primary closure or skin grafting is facilitated by the ability to close the muscles over the bone. Bone that has circumferential muscle coverage—that is, the humerus, femur, and radius—is easily treated in this manner. The tibia, which is the most common bone to sustain a compound fracture, presents special problems. The tibia has one third of its circumference subcutaneous, and this area is almost always involved in the compound wound. Large areas of tibia may be left with no material available for primary coverage. The use of muscle pedicle flaps from the gastrocnemius, the soleus, and the flexor muscles of the foot to cover areas of exposed tibia is now widespread.[6] These muscle pedicle flaps should be used as a delayed procedure unless the surgeon is very experienced in treating open wounds of the tibia. If a flap is used for primary coverage and there is further necrosis of the wound, the entire flap may be lost. My recommendation for treating large denuded areas of the tibia is first débridement and stabilization of the bone, followed by reevaluation of the wound in the surgical suite 3 to 5 days later. If the necrosis progresses no further or if no major débridement is necessary at that time, coverage is obtained by the use of the muscle pedicle flap. The surgeon should strive to have the open wound closed and healed within 3 weeks. This will allow the fracture to be treated properly (Fig. 59-13).

FIG. 59-12. External fixator used to stabilize the bone in a type III compound fracture of the tibia.

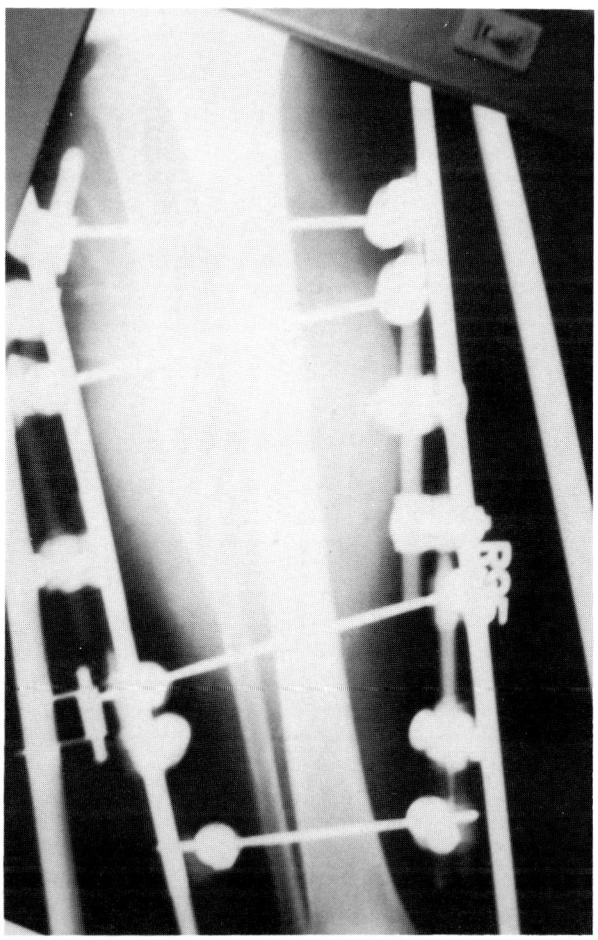

FIG. 59-13. External fixator device used to stabilize a severely comminuted fracture about the knee with extensive soft tissue loss. While in the external fixator, wound débridement, muscle pedicle flap, and skin grafting of the wound were accomplished.

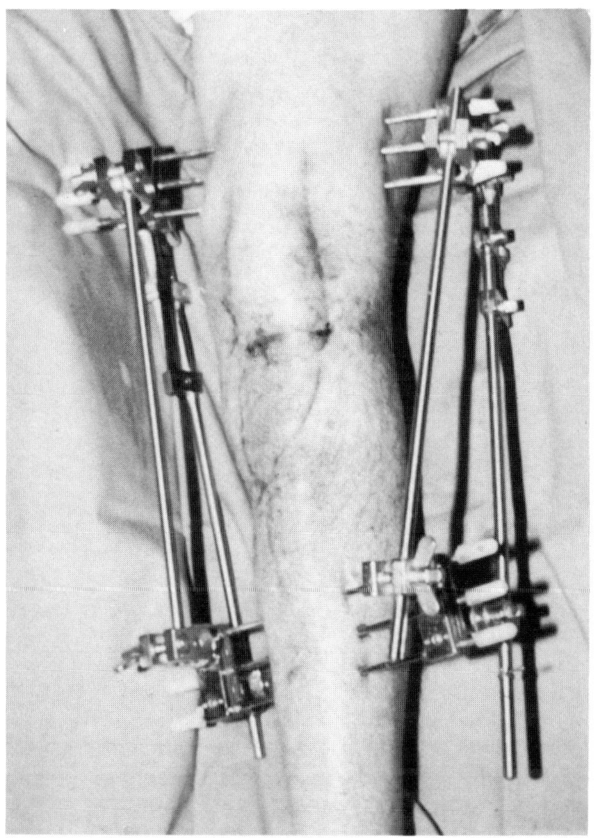

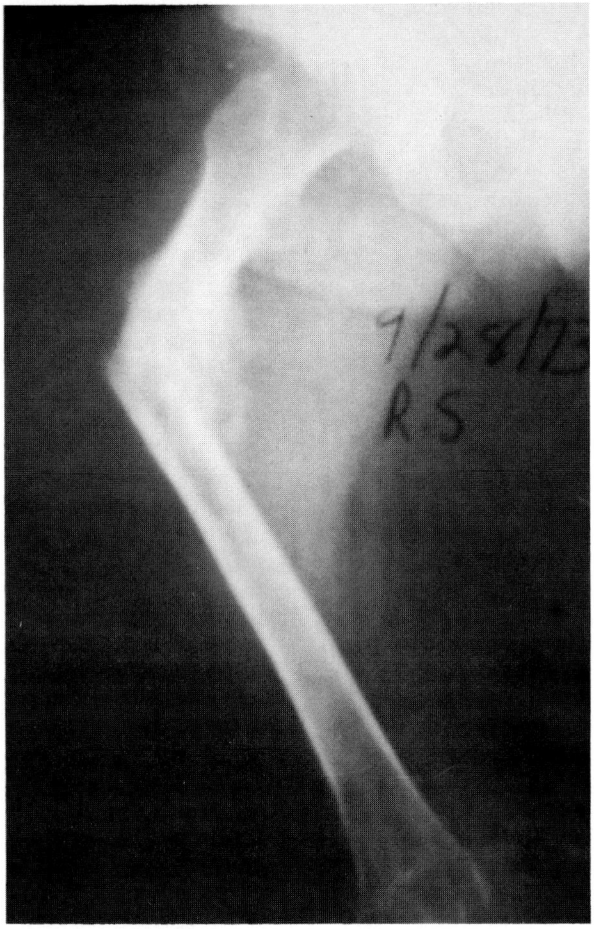

FIG. 59-14. Malunion of a pathologic fracture of the femur with 50° of angulation.

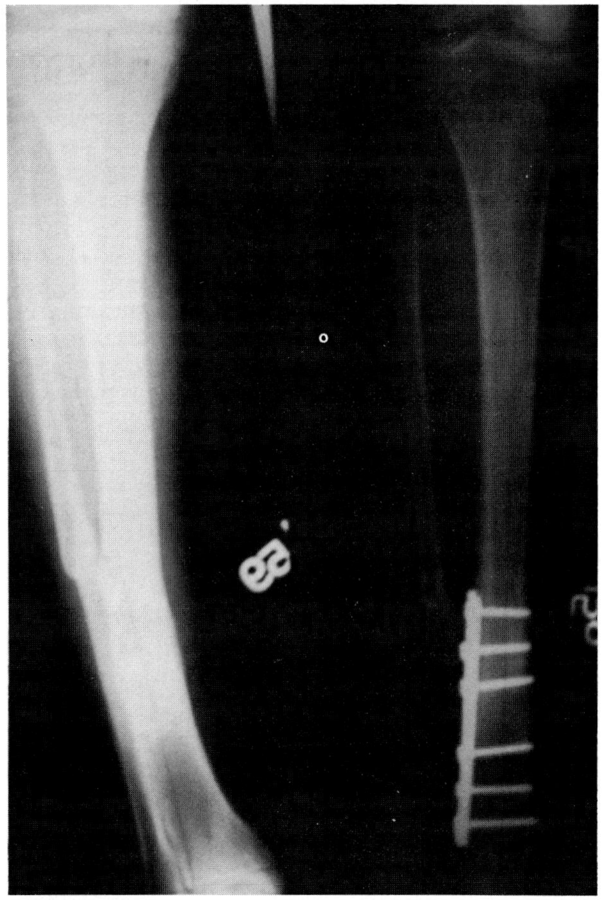

FIG. 59-15. Malunion of the tibia treated with corrective osteotomy and plate fixation.

THROMBOEMBOLIC DISEASE

Thromboembolic disease is a frequent complication of fractures. It is most commonly associated with fractures of the pelvis, hip, and femoral shaft and is uncommon in upper extremity fractures. Prophylactic treatment may be used in patients at high risk who have pelvic and femoral fractures. High-risk patients include those with a history of thromboembolic disease, obesity, on prolonged bedrest, and young women on birth-control pills. The form of prophylactic treatment must be weighed against the problems of hemorrhage secondary to the interference with the clotting mechanism. Coumadin, aspirin, and low-molecular-weight dextran are the most common medications used in prophylactic treatment of fracture patients. The management of thromboembolic disease is discussed in Chapter 30.

Late Complications

Late complications are problems with healing of the fracture and function of the extremity.

MALUNION

Malunion is defined as a fracture that has healed with the fragments in an abnormal position (Fig. 59-14). The deformity may result in shortening, angulation, or rotation of the bone. Malunion occurs from inadequate reduction or improper immobilization during the healing process.[5] Malunion that interferes with the function of the extremity should be treated by corrective osteotomy (Fig. 59-15). Rotational or angular deformities in the weight-bearing bones may cause abnormal stress upon the joints and lead to arthritis (Fig. 59-16). In the upper extremity, malunion may lead to improper function of the limb and is not associated with arthritis. Malunion of an intra-articular fracture will lead to traumatic arthritis of the joint.

Before surgical correction of the malunion, the patient should undergo intensive physical therapy to regain full range of motion of the joints and as much rehabilitation of the muscle–tendon unit as possible. This therapy will counteract the atrophy and decreased range of motion that resulted from appropriate immobilization to treat the malunion. After full function of the extremity is restored, surgical correction may be undertaken.

Angular and rotational deformities may be corrected by osteotomy and repositioning of the fragments. It is best to correct these deformities at the original fracture site, if possible. Stable internal fixation is required as well as bone grafting in the healing of the osteotomy (Fig. 59-17*A* and *B*).

Shortening of a bone by 1 inch or greater causes major disability. In children or young adults, lengthening of the affected bone may be possible. The lengthening of a bone requires a special external fixation device specifically for this purpose.[6] This device is calibrated or motor-driven to lengthen the gap between the bone fragments 1 mm every 24 hours after its application. It is applied to the bone by percutaneous pins in the same fashion as previously described external fixation devices. After the desired length of the bone has been achieved, bone grafting of the defect must be performed. The vascular and nerve supply to the extremity must be continuously monitored because these structures are stretched during the lengthening process. Tendon

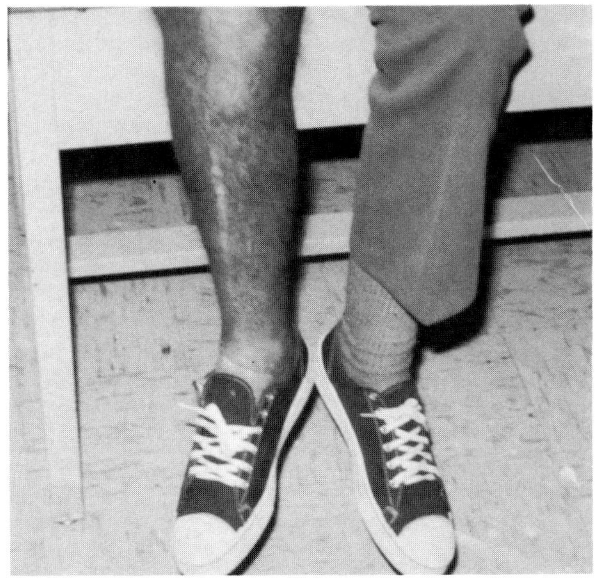

FIG. 59-16. Malunion of the right tibia resulting in 15° of external rotation. The patient had pain in his ankle and difficulty in walking.

FIG. 59-17. (*A*) AP x-ray film of a malunion of the distal tibia. (*B*) Rigid compression plate fixation and bone graft of the malunion.

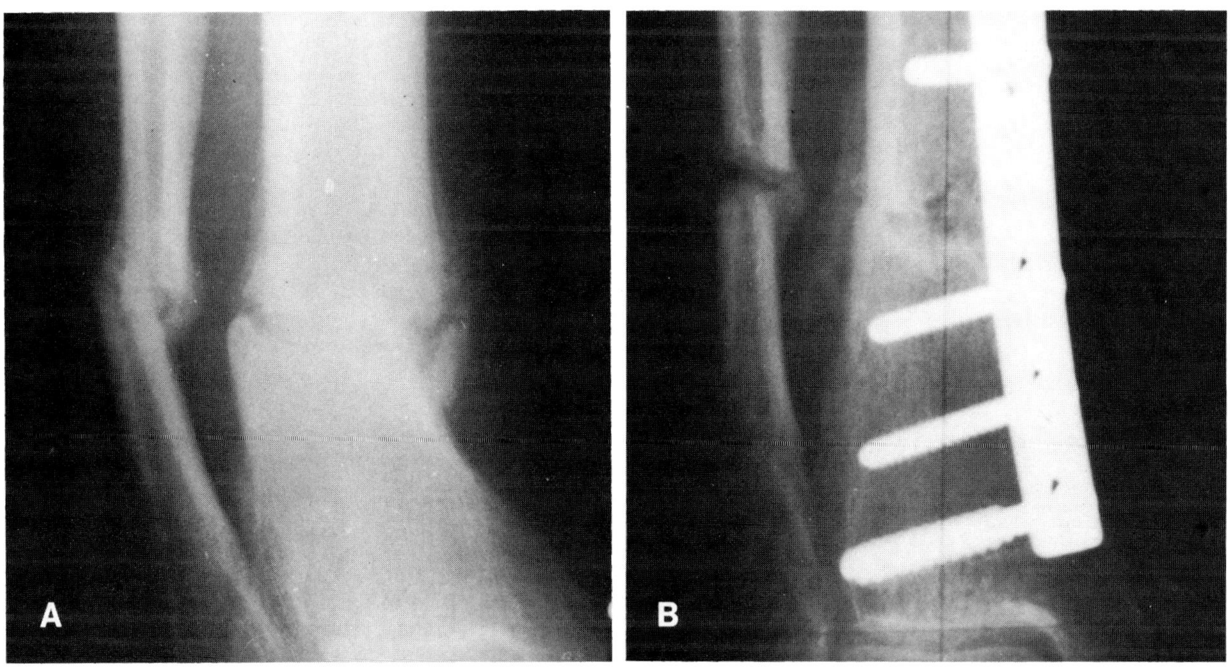

lengthenings may be necessary if the muscle–tendon unit does not stretch adequately. This is most common in the tibia. Lengthening procedures are used in the long weight-bearing bones to provide equal leg length for proper ambulation. The procedure is rarely indicated in the upper extremity. Thirty percent to 50% of lengthening procedures in adults require a second or third bone grafting to achieve final union of the long bone.

An alternative to lengthening of the affected bone is to shorten the opposite normal bone. In a growing child, a epiphysiodesis of the affected bone may be performed at a properly planned time.[5] By stopping the growth of the normal bone, the shortened bone continues to grow and catches up to a normal bone. If growth of the bone has completed, a segment of the normal bone may be removed. This procedure may require internal fixation and bone grafting to ensure proper alignment and healing.

FIG. 59-18. Avascular nonunion 7 months after fracture. Note almost no healing process at the fracture site.

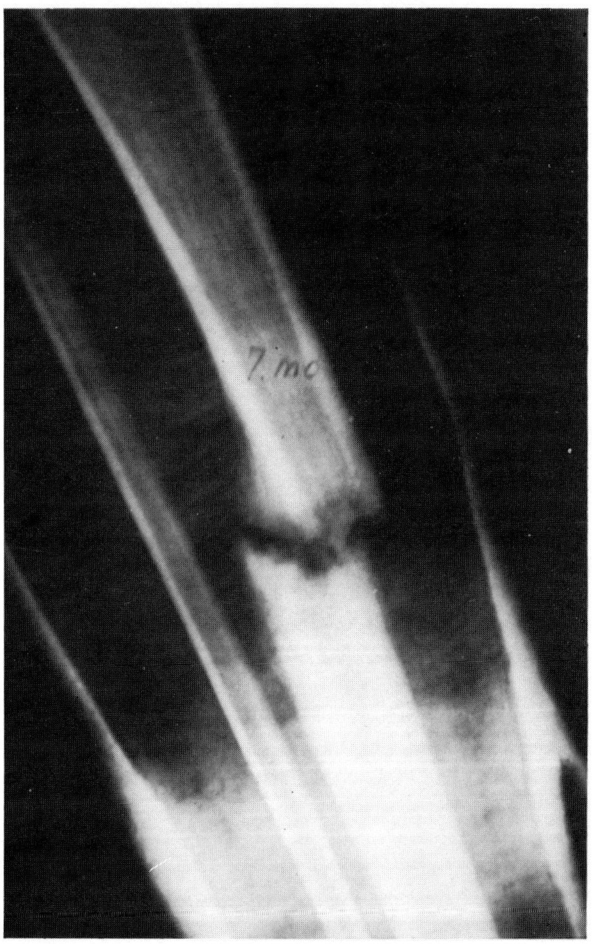

Intra-articular malunion of greater than 2 mm may lead to traumatic arthritis of that joint. In the weight-bearing bones, corrective osteotomy may be used to redirect the forces across the joint, thus delaying or preventing severe arthritis of the joint. If severe arthritis does occur, reconstructive surgery of the joint is the treatment of choice.

NONUNION

Nonunion is defined as a fracture that has not united within a prescribed period of time. The amount of time required for a fracture to unite is directly proportional to the amount of injury imparted to the extremity. A simple fracture of a long bone requires approximately 4 months to heal. A more significant injury will require additional time. A fracture that has not healed in 6 months may be declared a delayed union, and fractures that have not healed in 8 to 9 months are defined as a nonunion. If continued motion occurs at the fracture site, a pseudocapsule with a true synovial lining will form, and this is defined as a *pseudoarthrosis*.

There are two types of nonunion, hypervascular and avascular. An avascular nonunion has a marked decrease in blood supply to the fracture site (Fig. 59-18). A hypervascular nonunion has an abundant blood supply at the fracture site. The diagnosis may be made by a technetium-99 bone scan. The scan will be cold (decreased uptake) for the avascular type and hot (increased uptake) for the hypertrophic type.

Factors that lead to an increased incidence of nonunion are wound infection, severity of trauma, distraction of fracture fragments, excessive motion at the fracture site, poor immobilization during the healing phase, segmental fracture, and open reduction using plates and screws with insecure fixation.

The treatment for nonunion of a long bone must be individualized for each fracture. If the nonunion is stable without malalignment and it is of a hypervascular type by bone scan, a simple bone grafting procedure with functional bracing is all that is required (Fig. 59-19*A* and *B*). Compression plating or intramedullary fixation with or without bone grafting is acceptable treatment for a hypervascular nonunion (Fig. 59-20). If malalignment is present, open reduction and internal fixation are required. For avascular nonunion, a bone graft is mandatory. The bone graft is used as a stimulus for osteogenesis. The same principles of internal fixation and correction of malalignment must be followed, as previously discussed.

Electrical stimulation of the bone has been shown to be an effective method in treating nonunion.[2, 3] Electrical current produces osteogenesis at the cathode when properly applied to bone. An elec-

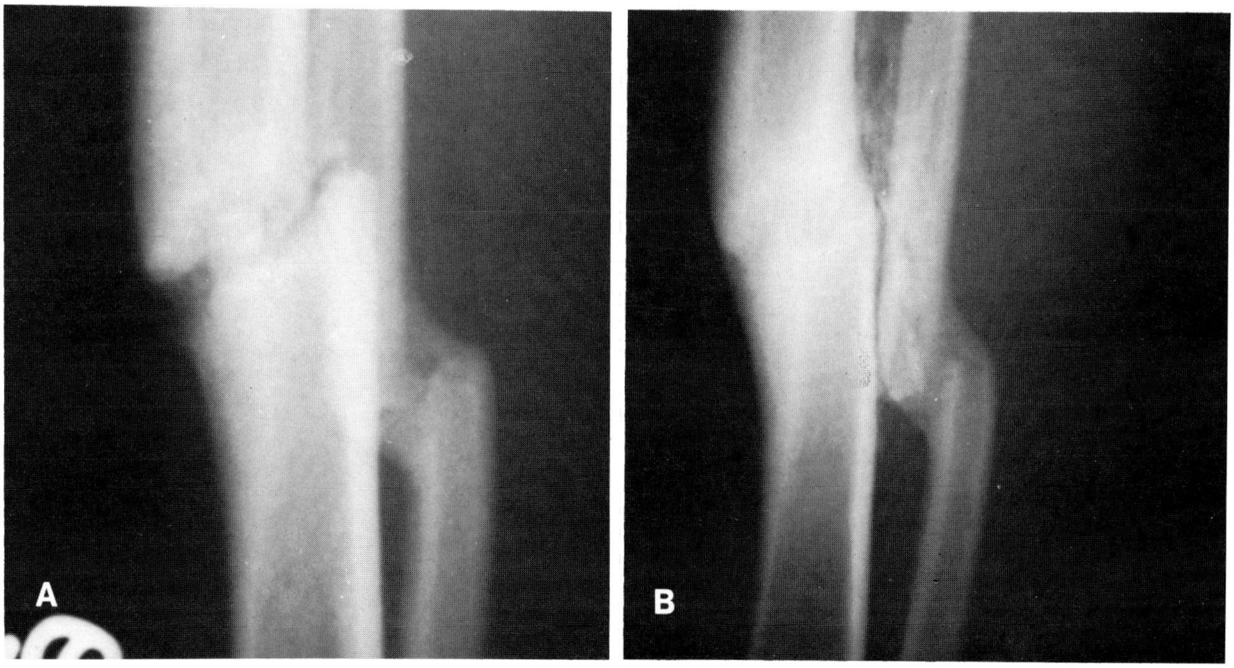

FIG. 59-19. (*A*) Stable nonunion of the tibia 8 months after the fracture with a hot bone scan. (*B*) Healed nonunion following a posterior onlay bone graft and treatment with functional cast bracing.

trical current of 20 μamp will induce osteogenesis in bone. There are three types of electrical stimulation of bone.

A percutaneous introduction of electrodes into the fracture site may be performed using image intensification to guide the position of the electrodes. With this type, the power source for the electricity is external to the bone and the electrodes must pass through the skin and into the fracture site.

A second method is to implant the electrode directly into the fracture site and also to implant the power source in the soft tissues of the extremity. This system totally implants the electrical stimulating apparatus, and it is necessary for an additional operation to be performed to remove the battery pack from the extremity after the fracture has healed.

A third application of electricity is through an electromagnetic field using coils placed externally on either side of the fracture site. This requires precise placement of the electromagnetic coils, and the fracture must be completely immobilized. This method is totally noninvasive.

An 85% success rate has been reported with the use of electrical stimulation of bone for nonunion.[3] Open bone grafting with or without internal fixation has a success rate of 85% to 92% but may require one or two additional operations to achieve the higher percentage.[5] The exact role of the treatment of nonunion by electrical stimulation will evolve over the next few years.

INFECTED NONUNION

Infected nonunion is the most serious complication of a fracture. Not only has the bone failed to unite, but also there is chronic infection (Fig. 59-21). The tibia is the most common bone affected by infected nonunion. This followed in frequency by the femur, both bones of the forearm, and the humerus.

The basic principles of treating infection and nonunion must be followed in infected nonunions. The fracture must be evaluated to determine the presence or absence of sequestered bone. Any dead bone fragments must be removed to improve chances of healing the chronic osteomyelitis. The amount of blood supply to the fracture site must also be determined. This is best determined by the use of a technetium-99 bone scan. The evaluation of the bone for sequestrum is best made by polytomography.

A débridement of the infected nonunion is the first step in treatment. The débridement should include removal of all infected material and of fully

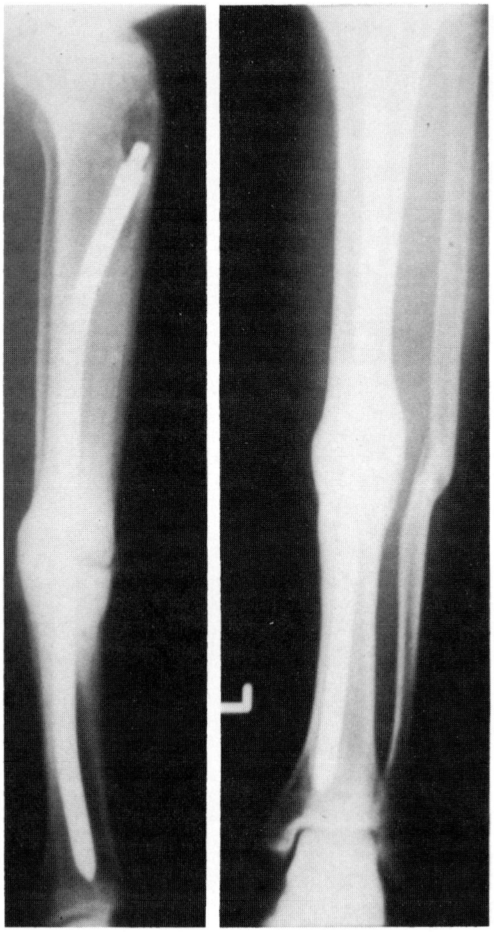

FIG. 59-20. AP and lateral x-ray films of a healed nonunion of the tibia treated with intramedullary fixation, posterior bone grafting, and functional bracing.

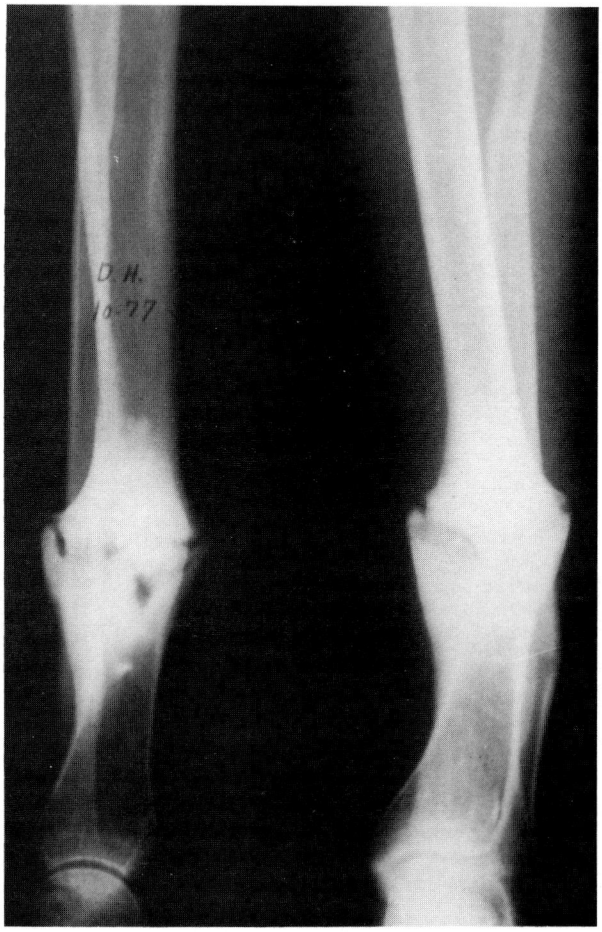

FIG. 59-21. AP and lateral x-ray films of an infected nonunion of the tibia.

devascularized scar tissue about the fracture site. The bone ends must be immobilized and the appropriate antibiotic therapy begun. Immobilization may necessitate the use of an external fixator to ensure complete immobilization of the bony fragments. If the débridement requires removal of large amounts of tissue covering the bone, a muscle pedicle flap may be required to close the wound. Such a flap will also enhance the delivery of local blood supply to the bone fragment. Creation of the flap should be done as a secondary procedure and not during the initial débridement of the acute infection.

After the infection has been brought under control, the second phase of treatment of the nonunion is carried out. The fracture is bone grafted, and on occasion internal fixation may be necessary. Since the débridement is done through the anterior part of the wound and the bone grafting through a posterior lateral incision, the anterior compartment containing the infection is not entered during bone grafting. The bone graft consists of massive onlay calleous bone graft on a roughened subperiosteal bony surface.

Using the above principles in treating 30 consecutive infected nonunions of the tibia at the Medical College of Virginia, the infection was brought under control in 29 patients, and union was successfully attained with posterior onlay bone graft and no internal fixation in 28 patients (Fig. 59-22*A* and *B*). Seven of the patients required two bone grafting procedures, and three required two or more surgical débridements of the fracture.

AVASCULAR NECROSIS

Avascular necrosis is a specific entity in which a portion of bone is rendered avascular secondary to fracture and interruption of blood supply. This is

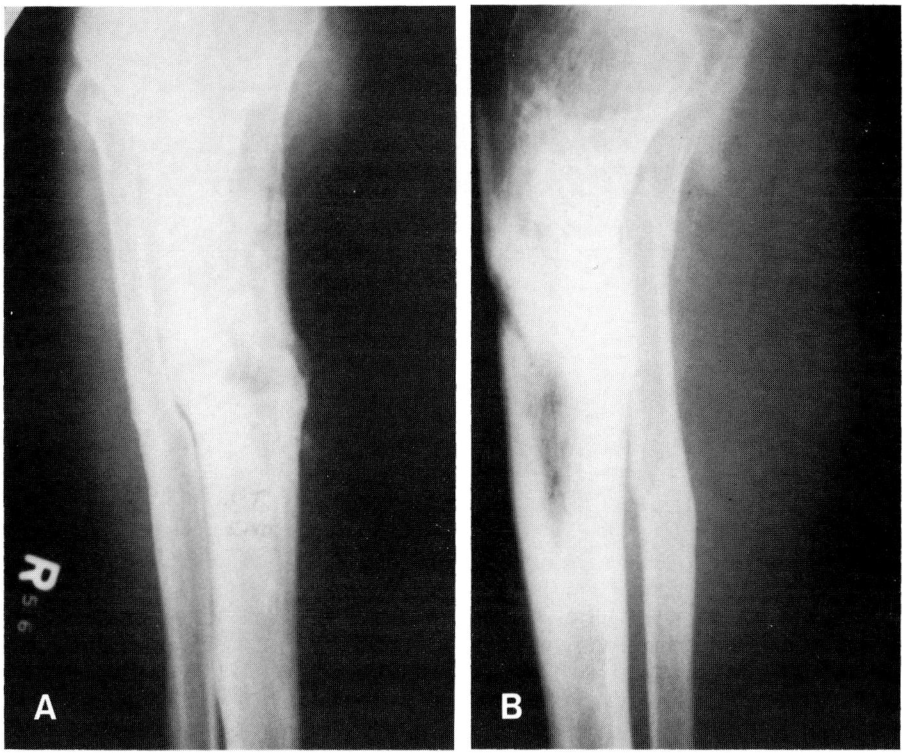

FIG. 59-22. AP (*A*) and lateral (*B*) x-ray films of a healed infected nonunion of the proximal tibia treated with débridement and a posterior bone graft. Note the defect in the anterior portion of the bone from débridement of the sequestrum and the healed posterior cortex from the onlay bone graft.

most commonly seen in intracapsular fracture of the femoral neck, fracture of the proximal pole of the navicular, and in the body of the talus secondary to displaced vertical fractures of the talar neck. The early management of these specific fractures is anatomical reduction and rigid immobilization. If avascular necrosis is recognized early, it may be treated by bone grafting procedures. If initial treatment fails and avascular necrosis persists, it may lead to traumatic arthritis, which will require replacement arthroplasty or surgical fusion of the joint.

MYOSITIS OSSIFICANS

Myositis ossificans is heterotrophic bone formation, and it may occur in muscle, ligament, and tendinous tissue of an injected extremity. If myositis ossificans is recognized early, the extremity must be placed at rest and treated with passive range of motion. Rarely, following trauma, is there bone formation significant enough to interfere with function; however, if it does occur and the joint motion is obstructed, the bone may be surgically removed after it has become mature nonreactive bone. This requires 1 to 2 years, and the activity of the bone should be followed with technitium-99 bone scan. Only when the bone scan is cold should the bone be excised. If myositis ossificans occurs in a major muscle mass (*i.e.*, the quadriceps with a direct injury), the appropriate treatment is rest followed by gentle exercise and progressing to full range of motion once the pain has subsided. There is rarely an indication to excise the ectopic bone forming in a muscle mass. After adequate conservative therapy, range of motion will usually return.

References

1. Behrens F, Jones RE III, Fisher DA, Mears DC: External skeletal fixation. Instr Course Lect 30:112, 1981
2. Brighton CT: Nonunions: The treatment with electricity. J Bone Joint Surg 63A:847, 1981
3. Brighton CT, Black J, Friedenberg ZB et al: Nonunion: The treatment with constant direct current, a multi center study. J Bone Joint Surg 63A:2, 1981
4. Brooker AF, Edwards C: External Fixation: The Current State of the Art. Baltimore, Williams & Wilkins, 1979
5. Edmonson AS, Crenshaw AH: Campbell's Operative Orthopaedics, 6th ed. St Louis, CV Mosby, 1980
6. Epps C: Complications of Orthopaedic Surgery. Philadelphia, JB Lippincott, 1978
7. Rockwood CA Jr, Green DP: Fractures. Philadelphia, JB Lippincott, 1975
8. Matsen FA III: Compartmental Syndromes. New York, Grune & Stratton, 1980
9. Whiteside TE, Harada H, Morimoto K: Compartment syndromes and the role of fasciotomy, its parameters and techniques. Instr Course Lect 26:179, 1977

60 Complications of Dislocations

Robert S. Adelaar

OVERVIEW—ANATOMY

In considering the complications associated with traumatic joint dislocations, the surgeon must appreciate the basic architecture of all moving joints, typified by the knee joint (Fig. 60-1A).[8] *Joints contain cartilage surfaces of varying configurations sliding over each other in a distinct biomechanical pathway determined by the center of the arc of joint motion. The center of the arc of motion of each joint determines the type of motion possible between the cartilaginous surfaces (Fig. 60-1B). Most joints have a structure similar to that of the knee joint: a meniscuslike structure and internal and external ligaments provide a constraint to motion and a shock-absorbing quality that protects the articular surface from direct injury. The surrounding muscular envelope provides the force that initiates joint motion and also restricts abnormal force and motion. Traumatic dislocations can alter these anatomical restraints and joint functions.*

Every dislocation offers a potential for alteration of joint mechanics, which results in asymmetrical loading and increased force, leading to eventual articular damage.

The cartilage receives its nutrition from synovial fluid lubrication. If the joint mechanics are altered, lubrication and cellular nutrition will also be affected.

FIG. 60-1. (*A*) The basic architecture of moving joints is typified by the knee joint. All joints have constraints such as the menisci, cruciate ligaments, and external ligaments. (*B*) The center of motion of the knee joint is located in the posterior femoral condyles.

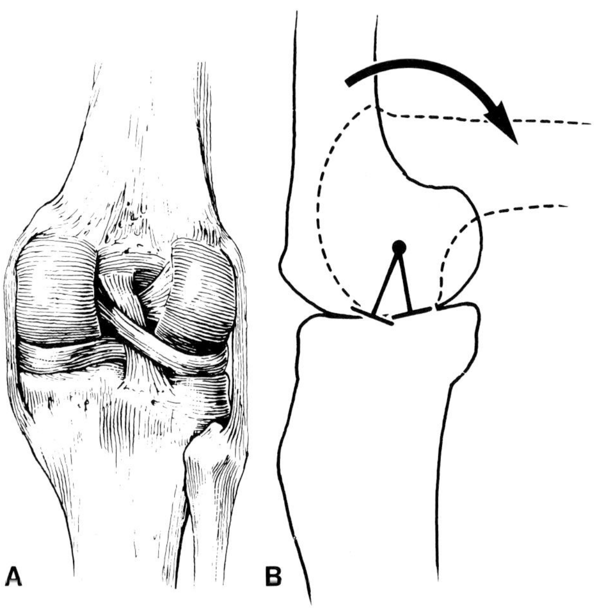

Pathophysiology

The most common mechanism of action that causes a dislocation involves a force transmitted down the axis of one of the articulating members. For example, when the knee strikes a dashboard with the hip in a flexed position, a force is transmitted down the axis of the femur to the hip joint (Fig. 60-2). Depending on the position of the hip joint, force transmitted, and the capsular and muscular restraints, a dislocation may result. The force is distributed to the articular surface; the fibrocartilage restraint (*i.e.*, meniscus, the capsule, and ligaments); and the muscular envelope. Any one of these restraints may be injured, and the postdislocation function will depend upon the ability of all the injured tissues to return to their original anatomical positions and functions. A second common mechanism that causes joint dislocations is a direct force to the joint as, for example, an acromioclavicular dislocation caused by a fall in which the shoulder strikes the ground (Fig. 60-3).

Acute Complications

PROGNOSTIC FACTORS

The immediate dislocation complications depend on many factors, including the applied force, muscle conditioning, arthrosis or preexisting joint injury, the degree of bone mineralization, and capsule and static ligamentous constraints.[4, 16]

Applied Force

The amount of transmitted force and the angle and point of application will determine whether the constraining tissue can prevent a dislocation. If the joint-restraining structures are not able to contain these forces, a dislocation will result. The resultant injury will also depend on the velocity of the force and the joint position at the time of injury.

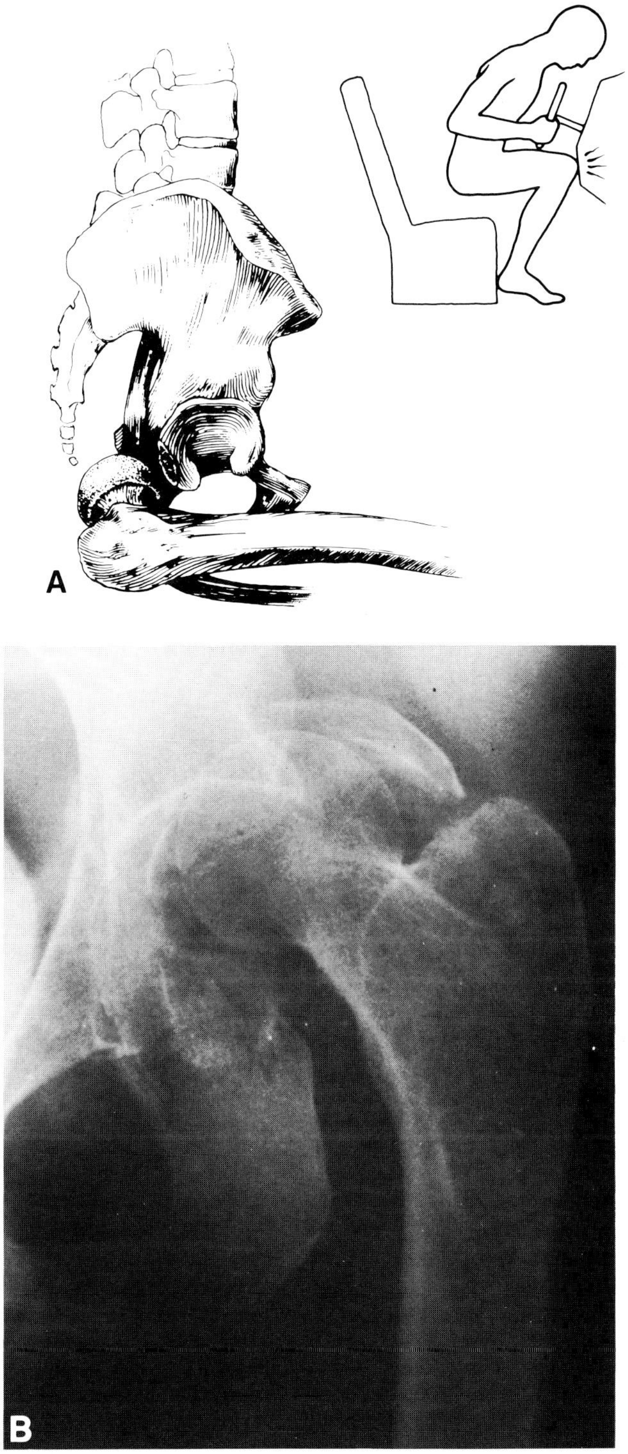

FIG. 60-2. (*A*) A posterior hip fracture dislocation will occur if a flexed hip and knee strike a dashboard, producing a large axial force. (*B*) A comminuted posterior hip fracture dislocation in a 70-year-old woman who was injured in an automobile accident.

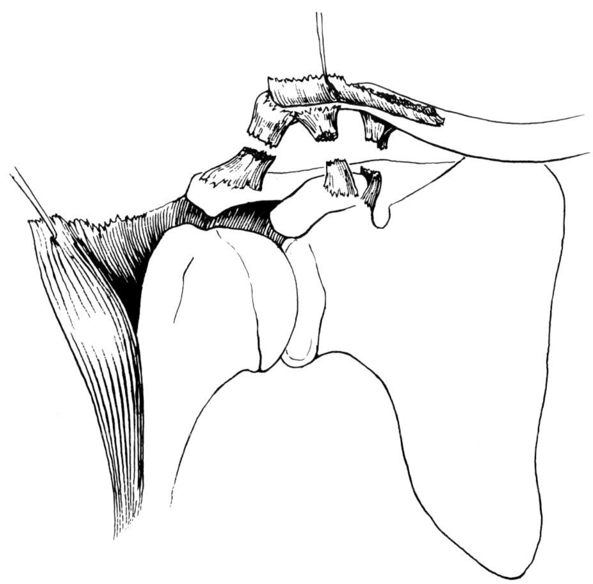

FIG. 60-3. A complete acromioclavicular dislocation with rupture of the acromioclavicular capsule, coracoclavicular ligaments, and the deltoid and trapezius muscle.

Muscle Conditioning

The muscles that control joint motion also protect the joint from applied force. If the muscle is well conditioned, its contraction at the time of injury can result in a decrease in the applied force. For example, a well-conditioned quadricep muscle can prevent the knee from undergoing damage to its static ligamentous constraints. Preexisting neurologic disorders that affect muscular function can cause greater unopposed joint forces.

Arthrosis or Preexisting Joint Injury

Conditions that cause joint destruction or incongruity will predispose the patient's joint to more damage for a given applied force. Cartilage defects will cause localization of stress. Arthritic disorders will also alter joint mechanics and lubrication.

Degree of Bone Mineralization

Conditions that cause a reduction in the structural integrity of subchondral bone may cause increased cartilage damage for a given force. Articular cartilage is supported by subchondral bone; therefore, when bone structure is weakened, less cartilage support is provided. Medications, such as steroids, which decrease the collagen linkage and mineralization of bone, also increase the susceptibility to injury.

Capsule and Static Ligamentous Constraints

Weakness in the supporting structures secondary to preexisting injury will render a joint more prone to injury. Alteration of static ligamentous constraints, such as the knee cruciate ligaments, can cause further stretching of normal ligament constraints to the knee by the fatigue failure of cyclic loading.

INJURY-RELATED COMPLICATIONS

In a dislocation complications directly relate to the injury and relate to treatment. The injury-related complications can be categorized as soft tissue and muscular injury; capsule, ligament, or meniscus injury; articular cartilage injury; associated fractures; neurovascular and visceral structure injury; compound injuries; and structural interposition.

Soft Tissue and Muscular Injury

Direct injury to soft tissue and muscles occurs with every dislocation. Hemorrhage into the surrounding joint tissue occurs with all dislocations. The healing process can cause fibrosis and alteration of the function of the muscular component as well as of the pericapsular tissue. Numerous sensory fibers exist in these tissues and are responsible for some of the acute pain that occurs at the time of dislocation.

Capsule, Ligament, Meniscus Injury

Injuries occurring to the static restraining structures are notoriously difficult to heal. All joints should be treated with adequate immobilization in order to attempt healing the static restraining structures in their original anatomical positions. Instability of these structures will cause immediate problems, that is, instability directly related to the ligament injured or chronic problems related to increased stress on the remaining normal ligamentous structures.

Articular Cartilage Injury

Articular cartilage has multiple layers, and the surface or the deeper structures may be damaged, depending on the force applied. Due to the decreased blood supply and slow metabolic rate, healing will be slow. The articular hyaline cartilage will be replaced with a fibrous-type cartilage, which has inferior biomechanical properties.

Associated Fractures

Fractures can occur to either portion of the articulating components. They are often associated with hemorrhage and can create articular loose bodies. Damage to the articular surface is greater, and the traumatic arthrosis rate increases with fractures.

Neurovascular and Visceral Structure Injury

A dislocation can cause a direct injury to surrounding neurovascular tissue. Each neurovascular bundle consists of an artery, nerve, and usually a vein. Several joints have visceral structures, such as the lung and bladder, in close proximity. Care should be taken to evaluate whether these structures have been injured at the time of the dislocation; there may be injuries to the genitourinary tract with pelvic dislocations. The injury edema and hemorrhage can exert pressure on the joint neurovascular structures or viscera, resulting in dysfunction. Venous or lymphatic obstruction at the site of injury can lead to stasis and thrombosis.

Compound Injuries

Compound joint dislocations can cause infection, resulting in articular and soft tissue damage. Care should be taken with compound injuries to ensure thorough débridement, good drainage, and appropriate antibiotic management. Compound injuries are usually the result of greater forces and involve more extensive injury to surrounding, restraining structures, and articular surfaces.

Structural Interposition

With each dislocation, joint structures such as tendons and articular loose bodies can be trapped and block concentric reduction. Adjacent tendons, such as the biceps tendon in the shoulder and posterior tibial tendon in the ankle, can cause irreducible dislocations. Entrapment should be considered with asymmetrical reductions.

COMPLICATIONS IN THE TREATMENT OF ACUTE DISLOCATIONS

The reduction of a dislocation can result in injury to adjacent structures. Reduction should be gentle and performed with good muscular relaxation. Adequate anesthesia should be used employing local, regional, or endotracheal general techniques. The reduction should be checked for congruity in order to avoid entrapment of adjacent structures. Forceful reductions can result in fractures, articular damage, ligament disruption, and neurovascular injury.

Late Complications

A dislocation is a significant injury to all surrounding joint structures. The integrity of the joint and its adjacent structures may not be restored to normal after reduction. The following are some of the problems that can be seen after a dislocation and its acute treatment.

JOINT STABILITY

Subluxation and recurrent dislocations can occur if the capsule, ligaments, or surrounding muscular tissues have been injured. Recurrent dislocations or subluxations further distort the supporting tissue and make it easier for the next dislocation to occur. After repeated dislocations or subluxations, surgical procedures are often indicated to stabilize the joint.

HETEROTOPIC OSSIFICATION AND MYOSITIS OSSIFICANS

Injury to the joint and supporting structures may be associated with calcification as part of the healing tissue. Heterotopic ossification occurs primarily in the capsular and pericapsular tissue. It can be painful and actually obstruct joint motion. The capsules about the elbow and the hip are particularly prone to this problem. Diphosphonates have been used in an attempt to decrease calcification. Myositis ossificans is a pseudotumor that occurs in injured muscle. It contains all grades of fibrous tissue elements as well as osteoid, and its immature state can be mistaken for a malignant process. Myositis ossificans should be allowed to mature prior to any surgical attempt at removal.

LOSS OF RANGE OF MOTION

Injury to the capsular and pericapsular tissue will lead to fibrous proliferation. It is important to immobilize all joints so that the ligaments will heal at their anatomical length. Motion should be started early to prevent pericapsular fibrous restriction.

MALUNION AND NONUNION JOINT FRACTURES

Failure to unite or malposition of intra-articular fractures will cause distortion of cartilage and formation of stress risers with associated pain and arthritic involvement. Malunited fractures will also alter the joint mechanics.

NEUROVASCULAR DAMAGE

Muscle damage from neurologic injury will alter joint mechanics and cause loss of power. Injury to the deep venous system may result in venous stasis and thrombosis. Arterial injuries may result in chronic vascular insufficiency with claudication.

REFLEX SYMPATHETIC DYSTROPHY

Injury to soft tissue or major nerve trunks can damage the accompanying sympathetic fibers. This will result in a physiologic alteration of the autonomic nervous system with resultant causalgia and poor vascular regulation. The ultimate outcome of this disorder can be chronic fibrosis with loss of motion and hypersensitivity. Treatment usually involves psychological counseling, biofeedback, temperature deregulation, sympathetic blocks, and physical therapy.

Common Dislocations

The preceding discussion presented the general complications of any dislocation. The following is a discussion of the common dislocations and their specific regional complications.

DISLOCATIONS OF THE WRIST

In order for humans to evolve into bipedal organisms, the wrist evolved to give the hand increased mobility and dexterity for complex tasks. This occurred by phylogenetic recession of the ulna in the quadriped, causing the wrist to be unstable.[2] Dislocation of the wrist occurs with dorsiflexion past 90° and causes rupture of the important volar and ulnar ligamentous complexes (Fig. 60-4).[20] If these ligaments do not heal, they cause characteristic instability patterns (Figs. 60-5 and 60-6).[2, 11]

An injury only to the radioscaphoid ligament will cause type I or scapholunate instability, and as the forces continue and the tears progress, a complete lunate dislocation can develop. The postinjury result depends upon accurate anatomical reduction with supplemental pin fixation and rehabilitative efforts to gain wrist motion and strength. Acute complications associated with carpal injury are discussed below.

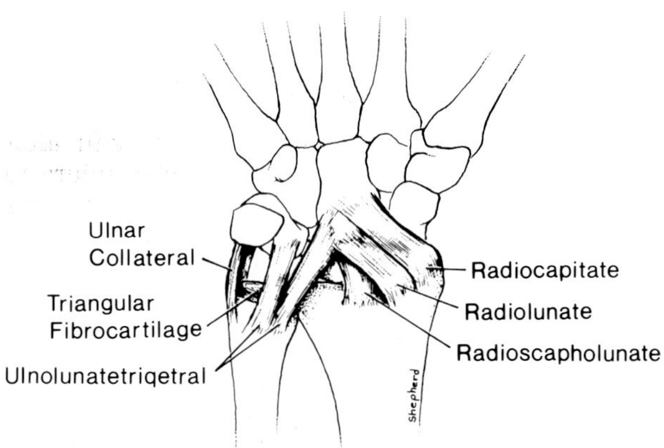

FIG. 60-4. The important wrist-stabilizing ligaments are the deep volar and ulnar ligament complexes.

Median Nerve Injuries

The median nerve within its carpal tunnel is placed under pressure by the dorsiflexion mechanism or by direct pressure from the dislocated lunate. The majority of the acute median nerve symptoms are transient and improve significantly with early anatomical reduction and elevation. If median nerve deficit does not improve or increases, the carpal tunnel should be decompressed.

Carpal Fractures

Fractures of the midportion of the carpal scaphoid are common, since it is the articulating link between the proximal and distal carpal row (Fig. 60-7). The scaphoid is prone to avascular necrosis of the proximal pole owing to the disruption of the common distal blood supply from the radial artery (Fig. 60-8).[6] Malunions and nonunions of the scaphoid are related to fracture location, amount of displacement, and the degree of fixation obtained.[1] The scaphoid is a vital link to carpal motion and requires secure anatomical fixation at the time of surgery. Fractures of the capitate and hamate have also been reported.

Carpal Instability

The worst complication that can occur from these injuries is instability of the carpal bones with pain, clicking, and loss of grip strength. An accurate diagnosis can be made by evaluating the anteroposterior stress x-ray films in search of an increased sca-

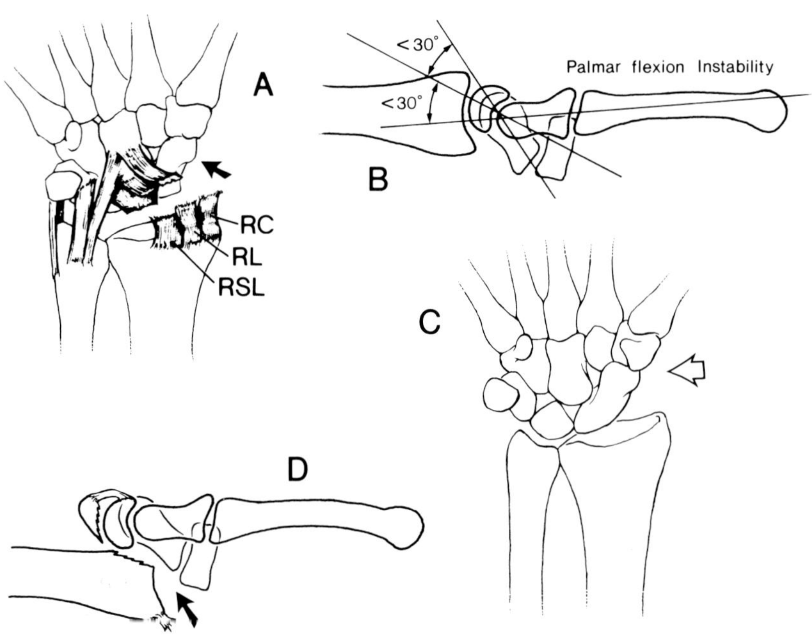

FIG. 60-5. The patterns of wrist instability. (*A*) Dorsiflexion instability, which is common in trauma. (*B*) Palmar-flexion instability, which is common in rheumatoid arthritis. (*C*) Ulnar translocation, which is common in trauma and congenital ligament laxity. (*D*) Dorsoradial instability, which occurs with trauma. *RC*, radiocapitate; *RL*, radiolunate; *RSL*, radioscapholunate.

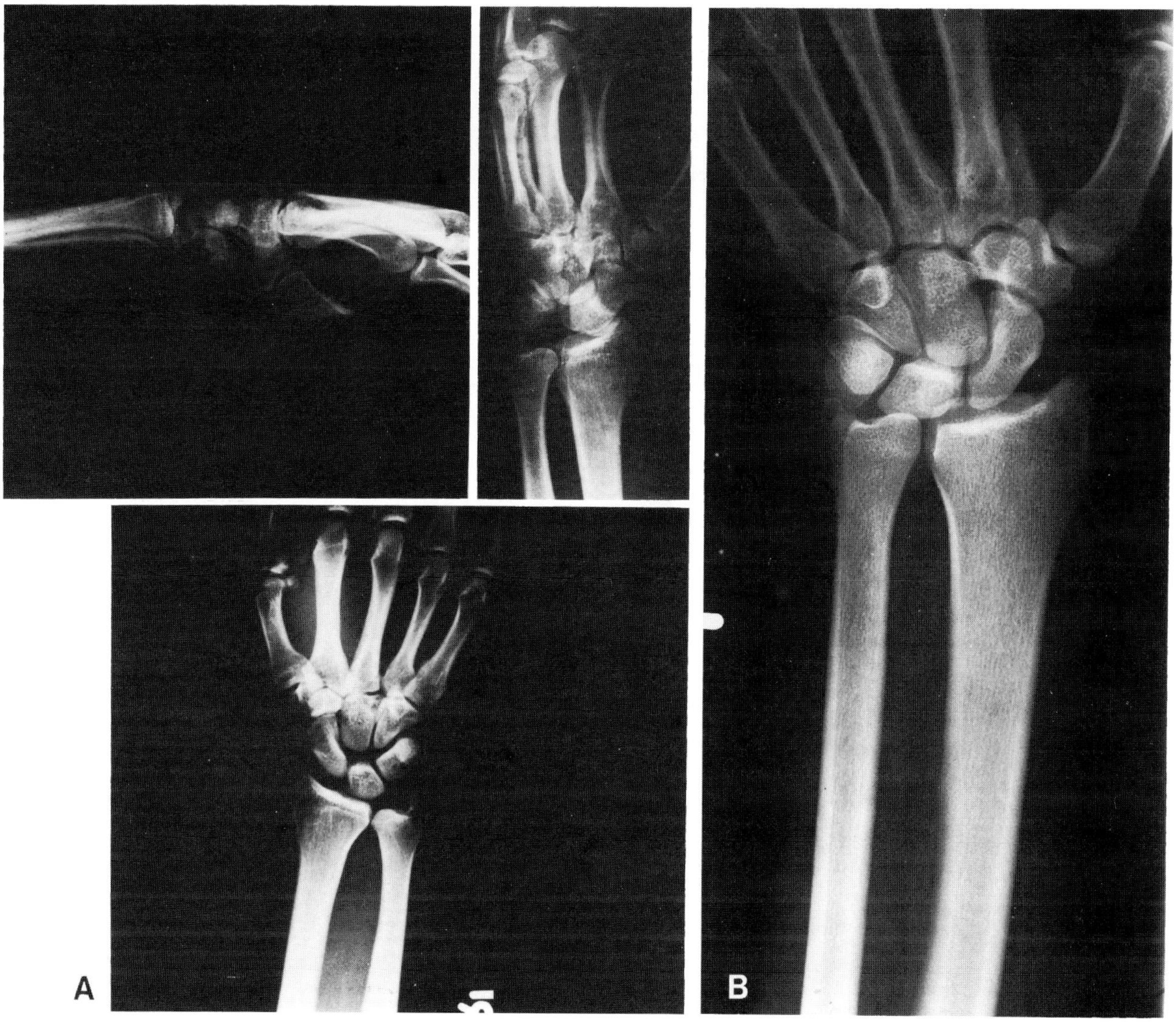

FIG. 60-6. (*A*) Perilunate instability is demonstrated in this lunate dislocation. The lower x-ray film shows the instability in traction. (*B*) A traumatic ulnar translocation of the entire carpus.

pholunate gap. The lateral x-ray film will reveal a more vertical orientation of the navicular and a dorsiflexed position of the lunate (see Fig. 60-6*B*). Chronic instability is due to inaccuracy of the initial diagnosis and failure to obtain anatomical reduction.

DISTAL RADIAL–ULNAR DISLOCATION

Injuries of the radial–ulnar joint are usually undetected owing to the attention paid to the carpal or radius injury. The ulnar complex (see Fig. 60-4) is an important stabilizing element, consisting of the triangular fibrocartilage, meniscus, and ulnar lunocapitate ligament. This complex can be injured in dorsal dislocations of the ulna (Fig. 60-9). Future painless wrist motion depends upon the anatomical position and type of acute treatment at the time of injury. Often these dislocations occur with distal radial fractures, and attention to the distal ulna is an important part of treatment.

Failure to treat this injury will result in pain with gripping and motion in the ulnar and radial direction. The distal ulna is also important in supination and pronation. With a distal ulnar subluxation, supination is limited, and pronation contracture of the forearm occurs. The other problem

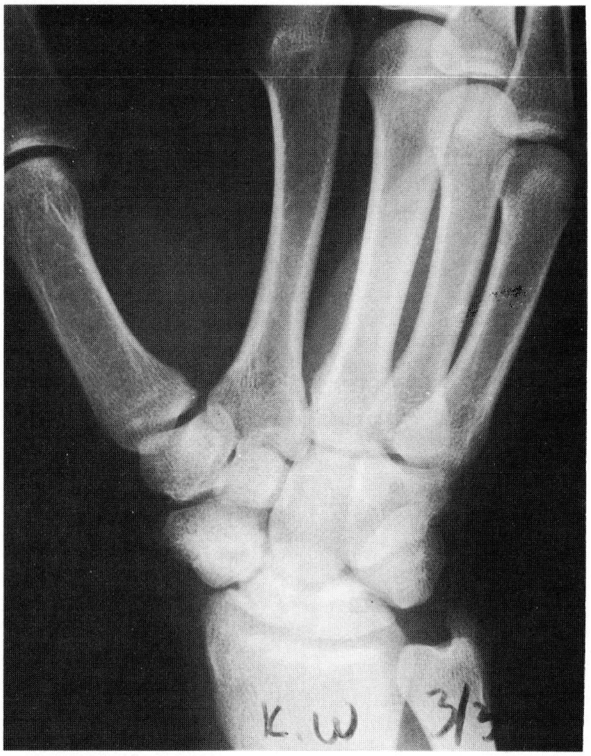

FIG. 60-7. A fracture of the midpole of the scaphoid.

associated with distal ulnar dislocation is subluxation of the extensor carpi ulnaris secondary to rupture of the retinaculum.

RADIAL HEAD DISLOCATION

Radial head dislocation can occur as an isolated injury or in combination with elbow dislocation and fractures about the elbow and forearm. A Monteggia's fracture is a fracture of the ulna associated with a radial head dislocation (Fig. 60-10). Subluxation of the radial head can occur in young children who have been hyperextended and pronated, as in the characteristic nursemaid's deformity, in which the annular ligament snaps around the radial head.[16] It is important to demonstrate the normal alignment of radial head–capitellum axis in a good lateral elbow x-ray film.

With more severe trauma, the radial head can be dislocated in an anterior, posterior, or lateral direction and associated with fractures of the ulna (see Fig. 60-10).[15, 16] The mechanisms of injury usually involve a fall on a flexed elbow with a pronated forearm. Recognition of radial head dislocation is key since, if unreduced in growing children, growth abnormalities occur at the elbow and also at the distal radial ulnar joint. The posterior interosseous nerve, which passes below the radial head, can be injured. Posterior interosseous nerve injuries can be detected by loss of motor function in the extensor pollicis longus, extensor indicis proprius, abductor pollicis longus, and extensor pollicis brevis muscles. Occult radial head fractures can occur with dislocations and should be treated by open reduction if significant incongruity occurs. Radial humeral arthrosis postinjury is associated with incongruity of reduction and articular surface damage.

ELBOW DISLOCATIONS

Dislocations of the radius and ulna can occur in many directions. The posterior dislocation is the most common, but anterior, medial, lateral, and divergent dislocations do occur.[10] The usual mechanism is a fall on an outstretched arm with hyperextension and abduction forces. In the common posterior dislocation, the coronoid slips below the distal humerus, and the humerus can cause significant damage to the anterior capsule and its sur-

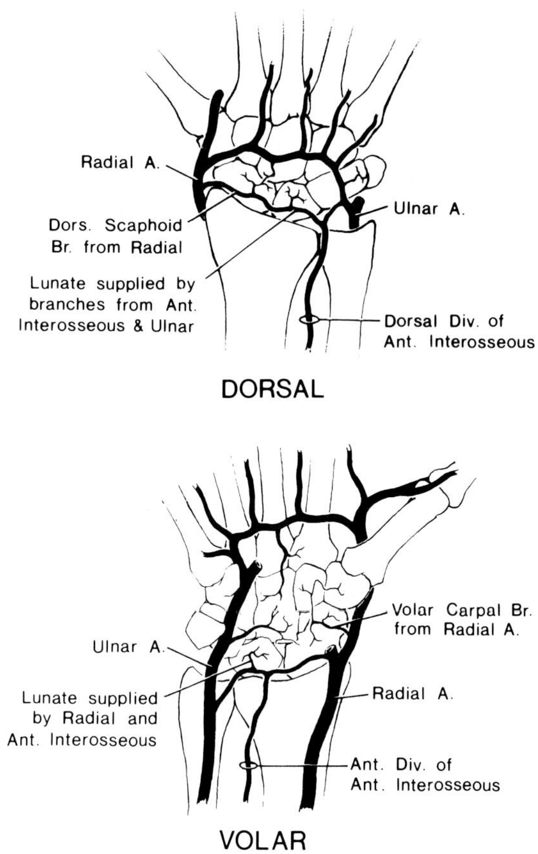

FIG. 60-8. The vascular supply of the lunate and scaphoid (Gelberman).

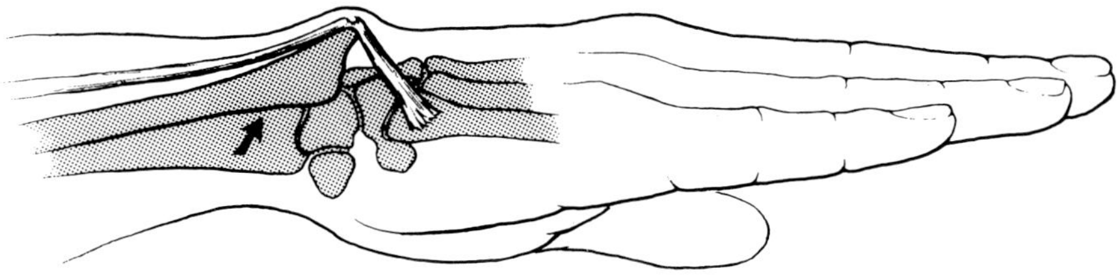

FIG. 60-9. Dorsal dislocation of the ulna may occur with dorsiflexion injuries to the wrist. The extensor carpi ulnaris tendon is often involved with distal ulnar injuries.

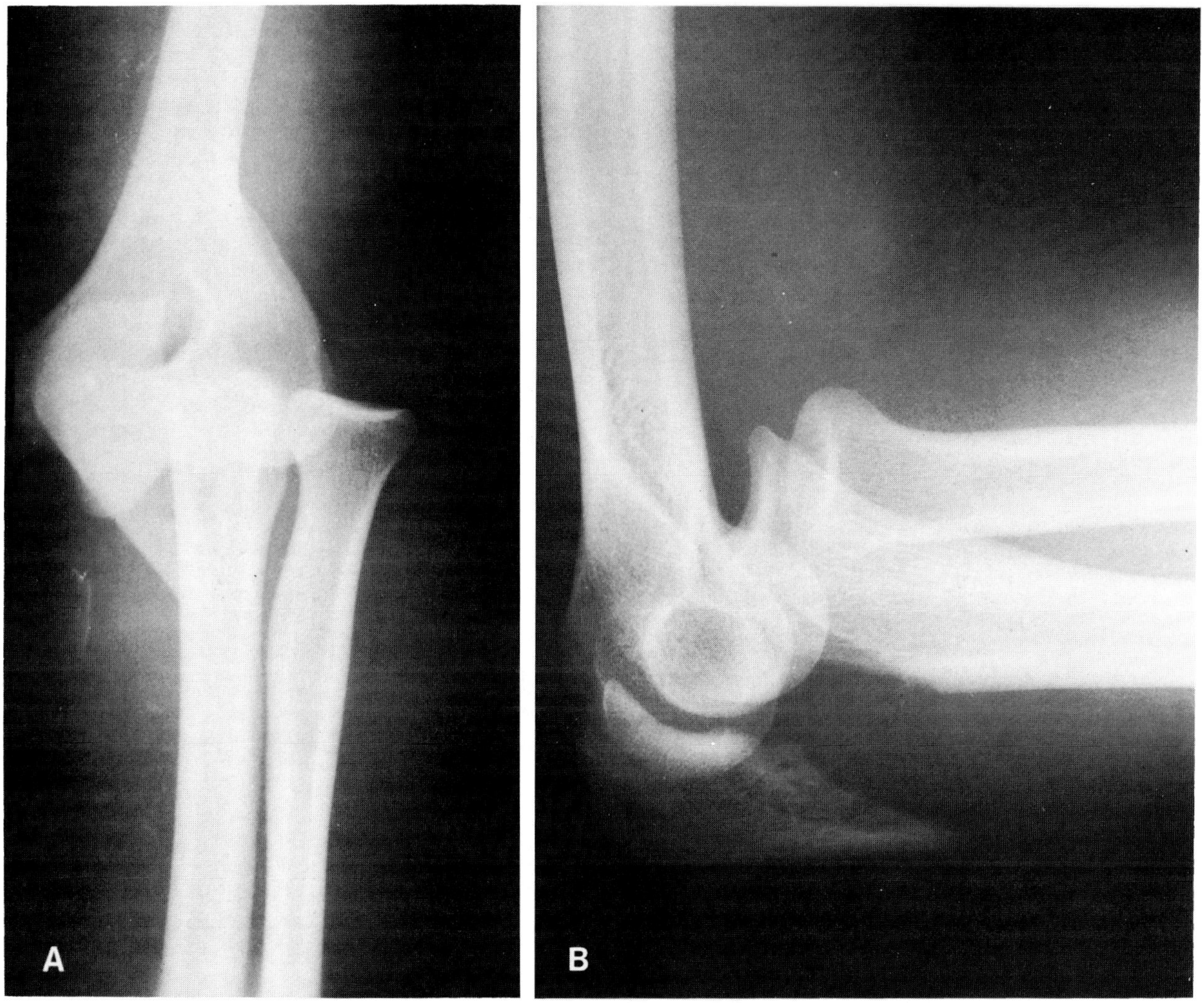

FIG. 60-10. (*A*) A Monteggia fracture is a dislocation of the radial head with a fracture of the ulna. (*B*) A lateral view of a Monteggia fracture.

rounding anatomical structures (Fig. 60-11). The complications that follow depend upon the injury to the soft tissue and neurovascular structures.

Acute complications involve damage to the surrounding structures and reduction. The following are the most common acute complications:

Irreducibility

Most acute posterior dislocations will reduce with adequate muscle relaxation. Entrapment of tendons and possible fracture fragments can occur and block reduction, necessitating open reduction.

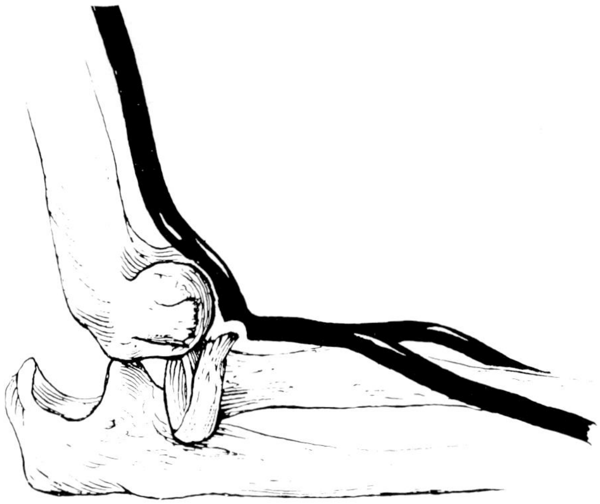

FIG. 60-11. Dislocations of the elbow are associated with anterior elbow capsule and vascular injuries.

Fractures

Fractures to the coronoid and epicondyles can occur. They are uncommon but should be watched for since they are difficult to detect, particularly in children.[16, 19] These fractures can block reduction if they are intra-articular and may require an arthrotomy for excision. Nonunion of a coronoid fracture can cause instability since it tends to block the mechanism of a posterior dislocation.

Nerve Injury

The ulnar nerve is exposed at the medial condyle and tethered at the cubital tunnel and lateral intermuscular septum of the tricep; therefore, it is vulnerable to injury with elbow dislocations (Fig. 60-12). These injuries usually result in a temporary neuropraxia of the ulnar nerve, and treatment of the ulnar nerve should be delayed until this loss of func-

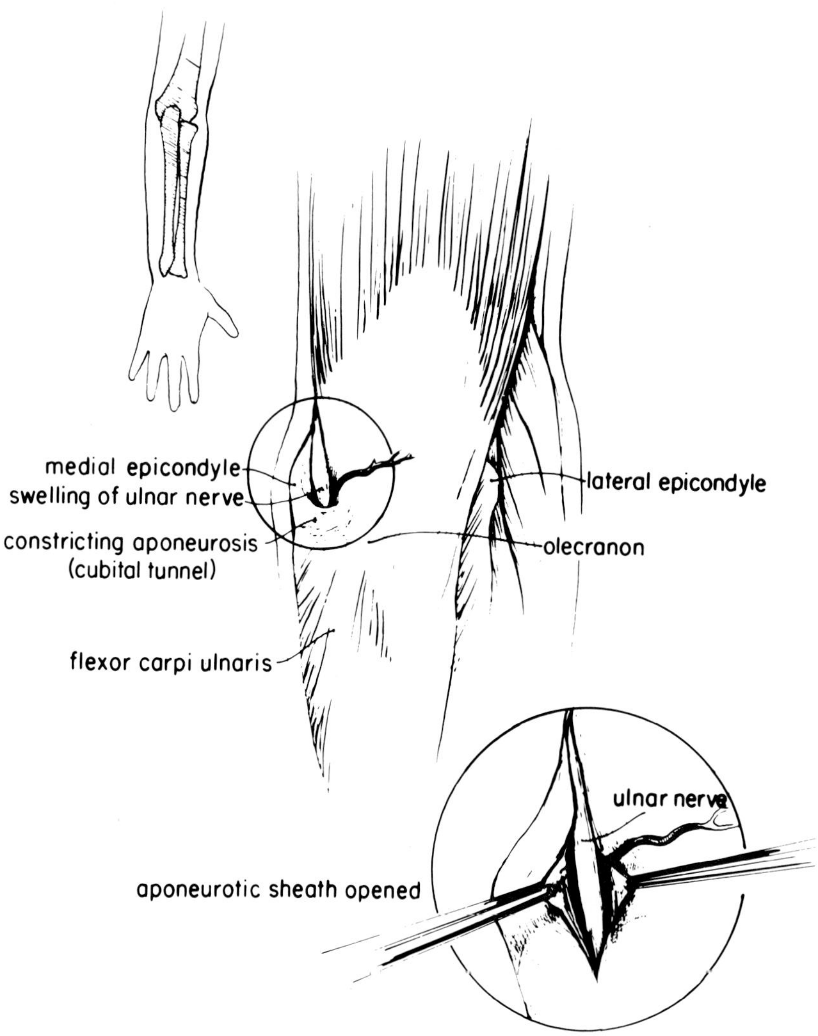

FIG. 60-12. The ulnar nerve in the cubital tunnel formed by the two heads of the flexor carpi ulnaris is vulnerable to injury.

tion can be documented with serial electromyograms. Injuries to the median and radial nerves also occur, but less frequently.

Compartment and Vascular Injury Syndromes

Injuries to the soft tissue, large veins, and brachial arteries can occur. Major arterial lesions should be diagnosed by arteriogram and treated appropriately. Because of a good collateral blood supply around the elbow, repair of the brachial artery is not absolutely necessary in all cases. Hemorrhaging into the deep volar compartments can result in an ischemic process by increasing the venous pressure, which first blocks venous return causing further increases in pressure, thus resulting in blockage of capillary flow and, finally, arterial compromise.[3, 7] Elevated compartment pressures can occur in the face of good distal arterial pulses. The compartment should be palpated for firmness; extension of flexor tendons causes severe pain, and loss of anterior interosseous medial nerve function to the index proprius muscle can occur. Compartment pressure measurements should be done, and if elevation is close to the diastolic pressure, then surgical fasciotomy is recommended.[21] The end result of an undiagnosed compartment syndrome is a Volkmann's ischemic paralysis with ischemic contracture of the muscles of the forearm.[3]

Chronic complications usually are related to loss of motion and capsular calcification. Hemorrhage and damage to the soft tissue capsule usually result in fibrosis and loss of extension. These elbows are usually placed in a flexed position for a short time, and motion is started when the elbow is stable.

Pathologic Calcification

Heterotopic calcification of the capsule and ligaments can be associated with loss of motion. Myositis ossificans occurs in the brachialis muscle and is usually related to the amount of soft tissue injury or the manipulation of the tissue postinjury. It should be allowed to mature prior to any revision.

Instability

Recurrent dislocation of the elbow is rare and usually occurs in sports-related injuries because of inappropriate care of coronoid fractures. A long delay in reduction may cause tightness of the ligaments and inability to obtain a full reduction.

Intra-articular fractures can result in loose bodies, which block motion and reduction. These can occur in the coronoid process but also in the humeral condyles. In children they are often difficult to see because of the lack of ossification; therefore, comparison views are mandatory.

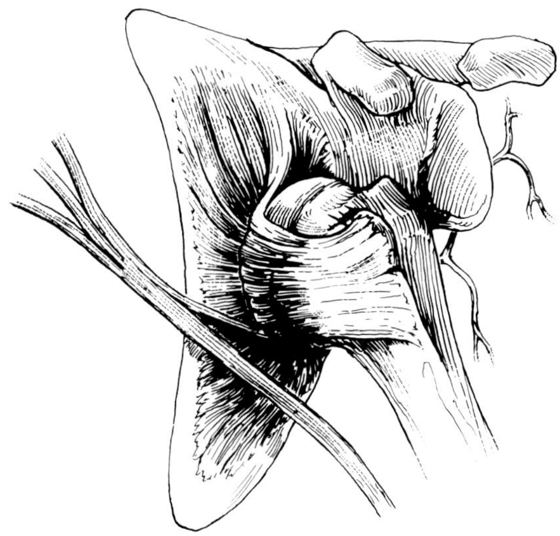

FIG. 60-13. The anterior shoulder dislocation is the most common and can cause injury to the axillary nerve.

SHOULDER DISLOCATIONS

Dislocations of the shoulder can occur in an anterior, posterior, subglenoid, subclavicular, or intrathoracic direction.[16] The anterior dislocation (Fig. 60-13) is the most common and usually occurs because of a fall on the posterior lateral aspect of the shoulder or a force pushing the shoulder into abduction and external rotation. Posterior dislocations are unusual and are associated with seizure disorders and electroconvulsive treatments. The younger the patient, the higher the forces of the initial dislocation, and the greater the chance for recurrent instability and future dislocations. The acute complications are related to the mechanisms of injury, the forces of injury, and the treatment of the injury. Forceful manipulation without adequate muscle relaxation can cause neural problems, fractures, or rotator cuff tears.

Fractures

Fractures of the glenoid or humeral head are not uncommon. The glenoid fracture usually involves an avulsion fracture of the long head of the tricep. Fractures of the greater tuberosity with its rotator cuff attachment often do not reduce anatomically and require an open reduction. The bicep tendon can also slip out of the groove and block reduction of the greater tuberosity fracture. The stability of the reduction may be affected when there is an accompanying fracture, and if the fracture is large enough, as of the glenoid, fixation of the fracture is necessary for a stable reduction. Cartilage lesions can also occur and develop into osteochondral loose bodies.

Rotator cuff tears, with or without associated fractures, do occur, although they are not very common.

Neural Injuries

Neural injuries to the axillary, radial, musculocutaneous, and ulnar nerves have been reported with injury to the axillary nerve being the most common.[4, 16] Axillary nerve injuries usually occur with first dislocations since they are the most forceful and are not very common with recurrent dislocations.

Malreduction

Failure to obtain a symmetrical reduction will cause contractures about the joint, which will make future reduction difficult. The chance of asymmetrical reduction is increased the longer a complete dislocation persists or a malreduction is present. If the dislocation has been present for more than 3 months and is not painful, it is sometimes best to leave the shoulder dislocated.

Vascular Injury

Vascular injuries to the axillary artery and vein can occur, and the surgeon should be alert for expanding hematomas. The collateral circulation about the shoulder is excellent, and there is often no loss of brachial pulsation. An arteriogram should be done when axillary artery injury is suspected.

Recurrent Dislocations

In anterior dislocations, stretching of the anterior capsule and attenuation of the subscapularis muscle occur. This will predispose the patient's shoulder to recurrent subluxation and dislocations. There also can be damage to the glenoid labrum with tears or detachment, causing instability. The age of the patient is related to the incidence of recurring dislocation, with the older patient being much less prone to recurrent problems.

FIG. 60-14. Posterior dislocation of the sternoclavicular joint can involve important vascular structures.

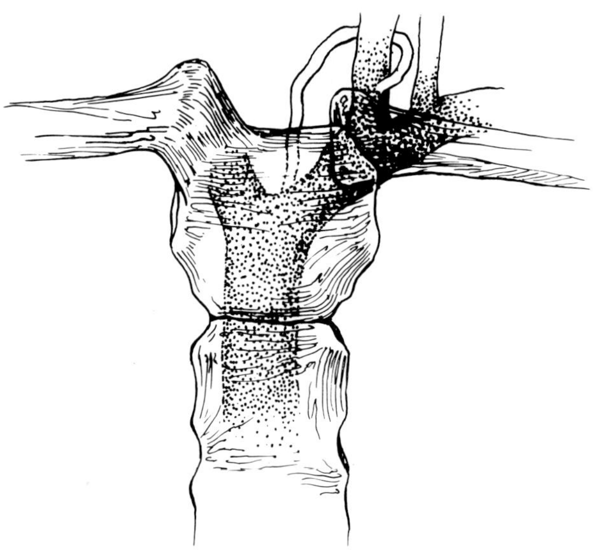

ACROMIOCLAVICULAR DISLOCATIONS

The acromioclavicular joint plays an integral part in scapulothoracic motion by allowing clavicle rotation and stability. The clavicle is stabilized to the acromion by the acromioclavicular capsule, to the coracoid by the coracoclavicular ligaments and also by the deltoid origin and trapezius insertion. In order for a dislocation to be unstable, disruption of the acromioclavicular capsule, coracoclavicular ligaments, and the deltoid and trapezius attachments must occur (see Fig. 60-3). Dislocations occur because of force conducted through the outstretched arm by a fall and also by direct trauma to the posterior acromion. Complications are arthrosis, instability with lack of reduction, and cosmetic deformity.

Malreduction

Damage to the intra-articular meniscus of the acromioclavicular joint occurs. The meniscus is torn and displaced, and an arthrosis develops with pain on clavicular rotation. A complete dislocation is not at all painful since no arthrosis between the clavicle and acromion can occur. Dislocations with the muscular envelope still intact and with no significant cosmetic problems should be left alone.

Cosmetic Problems

Complete subluxation with loss of muscular envelope can cause cosmetic deformity. Unfortunately, it is difficult to obtain a stable reduction with internal fixation in a long-standing problem. Soft tissue repairs in the chronic dislocation are not helpful. The incision should be in the skin lines in order to avoid the unsightly scar that develops because of tension on the wound.

Pin Migration

Fixation pins cannot be left indefinitely. Pins have been reported to migrate through the thorax, heart, and mediastinum.[4, 16] Therefore, any fixation device should be secured externally and removed when appropriate soft tissue stability is obtained.

STERNOCLAVICULAR DISLOCATIONS

Dislocations of the sternoclavicular joint (Fig. 60-14) are uncommon. The anterior dislocation is more frequent, easier to diagnose and reduce, and should be reduced in the acute situation, if possible. If the

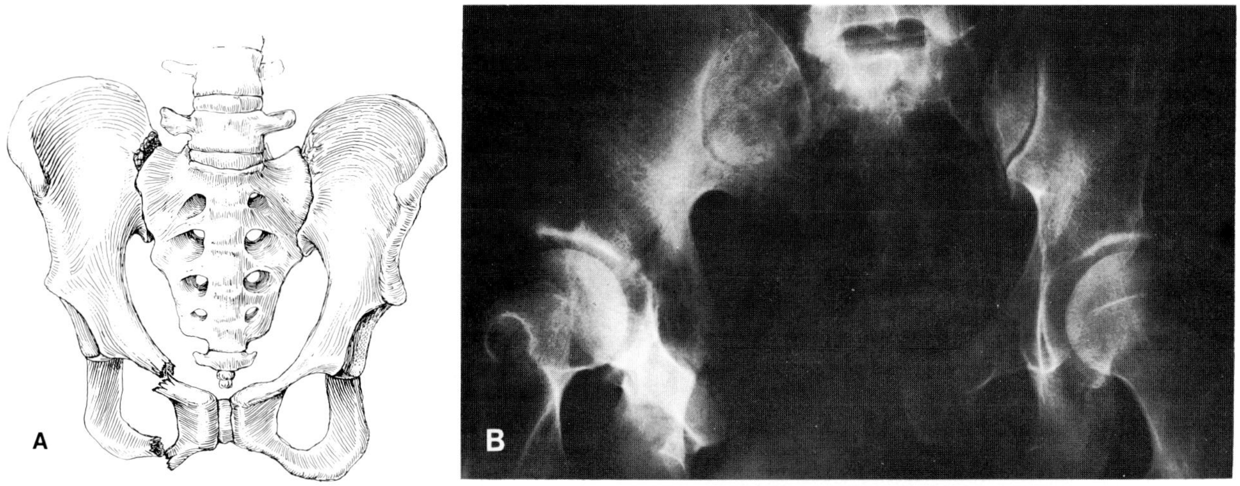

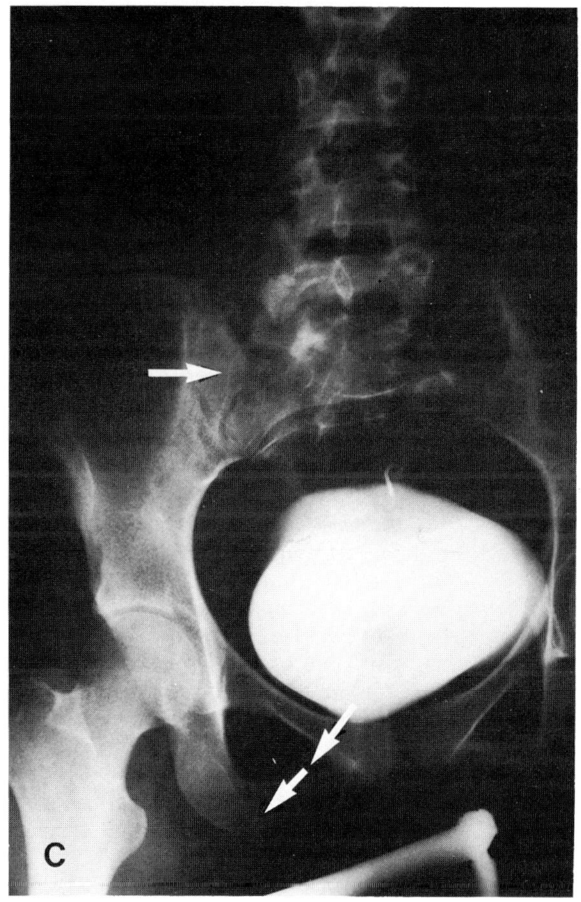

FIG. 60-15. (*A*) A Malgaigne's fracture dislocation of the pelvis has two or more fractures of the pelvic ring and a sacroiliac fracture or dislocation. (*B*) A complete dislocation of the pubic symphysis and disruption of the anterior sacroiliac joints. In this injury, the pelvis opens like a book with intact posterior sacroiliac ligaments. (*C*) A Malgaigne fracture dislocation of the pelvis with fractures in the lower pelvic ring and sacrum (*arrows*).

dislocation is old or reduction is difficult, then it can be left unreduced since this produces few cosmetic or functional problems. Often the cosmetic and potential complications of the fixation devices are much greater than the problems that follow an unreduced anterior dislocation.

A posterior dislocation requires reduction because of potential problems for the surrounding important organs (see Fig. 60-14). Pressure on the subclavian artery, vein, or thoracic duct can occur. Closed or open reduction should be attempted to obtain a permanent and stable reduction. Fixation devices should be used with caution.

DISLOCATIONS OF THE PELVIS (MALGAIGNE'S FRACTURES)

Disruption of the sacroiliac joint with an associated pubic diastasis or unilateral pelvic ring fracture has many potential complications (Fig. 60-15). Due to the great force associated with this injury, hemorrhage and genitourinary problems can be significant.

Vascular Injury

Major arterial injury occurs in approximately 1% of the fractures of the pelvis.[4] The internal iliac artery is firmly bound and is most susceptible to disruption. Angiography should be used to make the diagnosis, and treatment should consist of flushing with thrombotic agents or autologous blood clot. A gravity suit can be used for massive hemorrhage, but this can also cause arterial compromise. Vascular injuries are often associated with posterior lateral fractures of the pelvis, owing to the violent force involved.

Genitourinary Injury

There is a 15% incidence of genitourinary tract involvement with pelvic fractures (see Fig. 60-15*B*). The male posterior and prostatic urethras are most commonly injured. Hematuria or gross urethral bleeding is the presenting symptom, and an intravenous pyelogram and cystometrogram should be performed. Bladder ruptures occur less frequently, most commonly extraperitoneal. If a pelvic fracture and signs of peritoneal irritation are present, contrast urethral and bladder studies should be done.

Neural Injuries

Neural injuries are uncommon with pelvic dislocations or fractures. These usually occur with severe injury to the pelvis or when fractures involve the sacrum. Sciatic nerve injury, particularly the peroneal component, is most frequent.

Malunions or Nonunions

A pelvic nonunion is unusual and hard to diagnose; it can be painful and sometimes a fusion is indicated. A malunion will alter the pelvic gait mechanics and also may cause skin problems in spinal cord patients with unequal ischial tuberosity pressure. Sacroiliac arthrosis can develop, which sometimes needs to be treated with fusion.

Thrombosis of the pelvic veins is common after severe pelvic injury. There is an incidence of pulmonary embolism from deep venous involvement in this area, and anticoagulation should be used when fear of hemorrhage is past. Gynecologic, abdominal, or testicular injury can accompany pelvic injury.

POSTERIOR HIP DISLOCATIONS

Dislocation of the hip requires violent force and results in considerable injury to surrounding structures. Posterior dislocations are the most common and usually occur from force directed axially up the femur with the hip held in flexion and adduction. The position of the hip and amount of force involved determine the type of complication (see Fig. 60-2).

Avascular Necrosis

The important posterior lateral vessels can be injured with capsular injury. Vascular problems of the hip can take up to 2 years to appear and x-ray follow-up should be done. The extent of initial injury, length of time the hip is dislocated, and the difficulty of reduction are all related to the incidence of vascular death.

Associated Fractures

When the hip is abducted and flexed, there is a 15% incidence of posterior acetabular fractures. Stability of the hip must be determined after reduction, and if the hip is unstable, the fracture must be repaired. A CT scan and tomography are used to look for intra-articular fragments. The treatment of these fractures is controversial; Epstein believes that they should all be fixed while others believe that surgery increases the rate of avascular necrosis.[5, 18] Fractures of the femoral head are uncommon, but if they are large and in a weight-bearing area, they should be repaired. These usually have satisfactory capsular blood supply, and avascular necrosis of the fragment is not common.

Neural Injury

There is a 15% incidence of sciatic nerve injuries. The peroneal component of the sciatic nerve is the most vulnerable.[4, 16] The rate of recovery is related to the amount of neural injury and the length of time that the dislocation persists. The overall prognosis is good for return of the sciatic component, and patients should be splinted to prevent deformities during the acute phases of recovery. An electromyogram can be used after 3 weeks to evaluate potential neural recovery.

ANTERIOR HIP DISLOCATIONS

Anterior dislocations are less common than are posterior dislocations and are classified according to the location of the femoral head, obturator, iliac, and pubis. The type of dislocation depends upon the degree of hip flexion at the time of injury. The mechanism usually involves a forceful abduction and is associated with falls from heights, force on the back while in a squatting position, and automobile accidents.[16] Femoral head fractures are associated with these anterior dislocations, and avascular necrosis can also occur.

CENTRAL ACETABULAR DISLOCATIONS

Acetabular fracture dislocations usually occur from violent lateral force on the greater trochanter (Fig. 60-16). The prognosis depends upon the amount of femoral head weight-bearing dome remaining, the comminution of the fractured acetabulum, and any associated femoral head fracture.[17] Significant pelvic protrusion may be associated with hemorrhage and genitourinary problems, as seen in severe pelvic fractures.

Posttraumatic arthrosis, thrombosis, and heterotopic ossification are other complications characteristic of central acetabular fracture dislocations. It is important in the treatment of these injuries to obtain a symmetrical reduction as soon as possible. Failure to obtain reduction by traction requires early

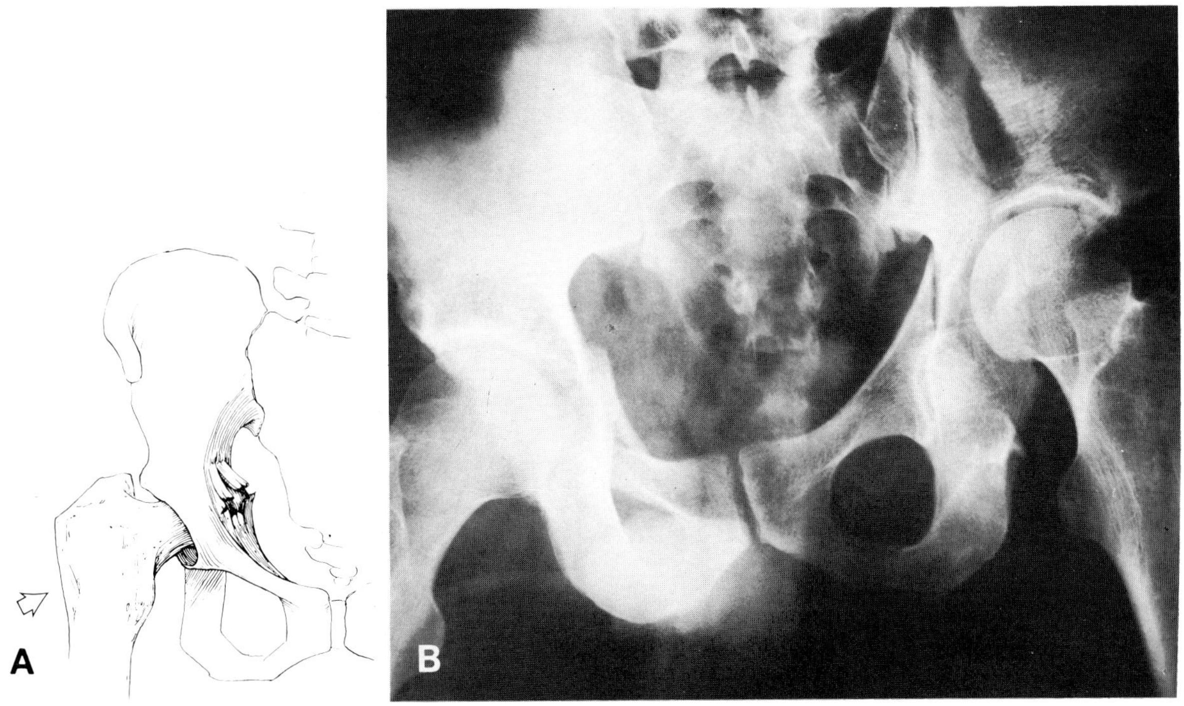

FIG. 60-16. (*A*) Fracture of the acetabulum with protrusion of the femoral head. These fractures are associated with posttraumatic arthritis. (*B*) Bilateral central acetabular fracture dislocations in a 40-year-old man who was in a motorcycle accident.

operative intervention, and infection and significant operative hemorrhage are associated with extreme difficulty in obtaining adequate fixation of acetabular fractures. The CT scan has been helpful in determining the operative approach. Fractures of the anterior and posterior pelvic pillars of support usually require internal fixation.

PATELLA DISLOCATIONS

Traumatic dislocations of the patella are an uncommon injury and usually are associated with sudden changes in direction, an external rotation and valgus force upon the knee, or a direct force that drives the patella laterally (Fig. 60-17). There are certain predisposing factors such as a high riding patella, valgus knee alignment, atrophy of the lateral femoral condyle, deficiency of the patellar facets, weakness of the vastus medialis, internal femoral rotation, and generalized hyperextension laxity of the knee.[16] The injury can cause weakness and fibrosis of the vastus medialis, osteochondral fractures of the patella and lateral femoral condyle, and chondromalacia. Patients with predisposing etiologic fractures are more likely to develop recurrent problems with subluxation and dislocation after a traumatic dislocation. Chondromalacia of the patella can lead to long-term patellar femoral arthrosis. These injuries should be treated by reduction and immobilization until soft tissue healing occurs and then rehabilitation to redevelop the vastus medialis musculature.

KNEE DISLOCATIONS

Dislocations of the knee represent a genuine surgical emergency because of the potential of vascular compromise (Fig. 60-18). The dislocations are often reduced upon the patient's arrival in the trauma unit; a high index of suspicion is required with any severe knee injury. There are several types of dislocations, each with its own potential complications. Treatment of all knee dislocations, or suspected knee dislocations, should involve Doppler examination of the arterial and venous systems and an arteriogram with good venous study. The diagnosis and appropriate treatment should be performed within the first 6 hours of injury to prevent any problems from vascular compromise. The anatomy of the popliteal artery with proximal fixation to the adductor magnus hiatus and distal tibial fixation by the soleus muscle makes it prone to injury with any dislocation of the knee (see Fig. 60-18).[9]

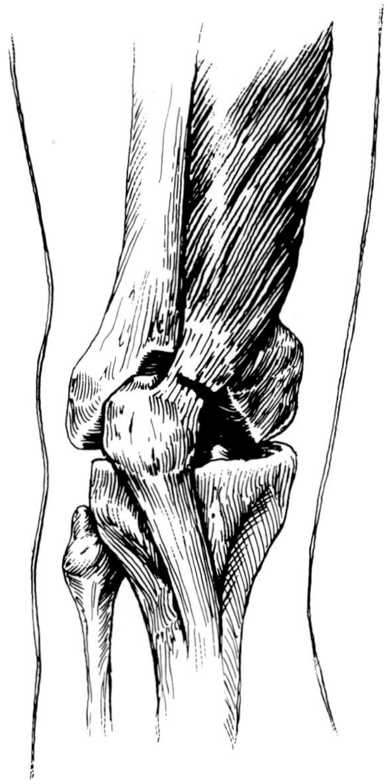

FIG. 60-17. Traumatic patella dislocations occur in a lateral direction and usually involve injury to the vastus medialis.

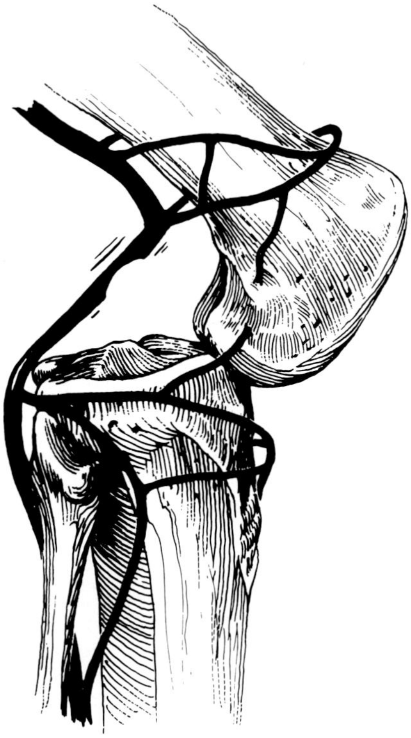

FIG. 60-18. Posterior dislocation of the knee may cause injury to the popliteal vessels and peroneal nerve.

Other complications that can occur are neural injury, osteochondral fractures, traumatic arthrosis, and generalized joint stiffness in addition to ligamentous laxity. There are five basic types of dislocations: anterior, posterior, medial, lateral, and rotatory.[4, 9, 12, 16]

Anterior Dislocations

Anterior dislocations are the most common and are usually associated with hyperextension forces or severe abduction and medial rotation on a flexed knee.[9, 16] The anterior dislocations have a high rate of vascular problems due to stretching of the popliteal artery; the posterior capsule is usually injured, in addition to a high incidence of cruciate ligament avulsions. Hyperextension laxity is a common physical finding. The peroneal nerve can also be stretched over the posterior femoral condyle.

Posterior Dislocations

Posterior dislocations (see Fig. 60-18) occur with crushing injuries and can be associated with patellar tendon avulsions. Vascular injury can involve double tears in the popliteal artery from its proximal and distal fixation.[9, 16] Care should be taken to examine both areas of likely injury at the time of surgery or angiography.

Posterior Lateral Dislocations

Posterior lateral dislocations can be associated peroneal nerve injuries with stretching of the peroneal nerve over the posterior femoral condyle.

The amount of recovery is dependent upon the initial amount of stretch injury and rate of reduction. Posterior lateral dislocations can be associated with difficult reduction if the medial femoral condyle is button-holed through the medial femoral capsule.[4, 12]

Ligament Injuries

Ligament injuries can occur with any of the dislocations. Superior results have been reported from primary surgical repair.[12] Instability should be diagnosed at the time of injury under appropriate anesthesia. The ligamentous injury should certainly be repaired if there is an exploration for arterial damage. Injury to the ligaments is also accompanied by periarticular injury, and there can be problems with joint stiffness and future arthrosis.

PROXIMAL TIBIAL/FIBULAR JOINT DISLOCATIONS

Proximal tibial/fibular joint dislocation is a rare injury that usually occurs with falls from heights, such as skydiving, or by a direct blow to the fibula. This joint is constrained by an anterior and posterior ligament. The peroneal nerve is posterior and is prone to injury, particularly in the posterior dislocation. The anterior dislocation is the most common. Superior dislocations are accompanied by tears of the interosseous membrane and dislocation of the lateral malleolus.[13] The major problem with this injury is in diagnosis; it should be considered when this area is tender and in accidents that carry a high incidence of these dislocations.

ANKLE DISLOCATIONS

The ankle region is one of the few that has very little muscular coverage. The skin is very susceptible to hypoxic damage secondary to trauma.[4] The objective in treating injuries in this area is to reduce the dislocation and stabilize the joint as soon as possible with provision for adequate drainage of soft tissue hemorrhage. Dislocations of the ankle are uncommon and usually occur in an anterior or posterior direction (Fig. 60-19).

Ligament–Capsular Damage

Significant force is involved in ankle dislocations with the ligaments, capsule, retinaculum, and tendons suffering significant injury. After ankle dislocations, problems occur with subluxation of extrinsic tendons such as the peroneal and posterior tibial, since their retinaculum may have been injured. This damage usually occurs in the peroneal and posterior tibial tendon structures. Also, there is usually significant pericapsular fibrosis with traumatic arthritis, capsular calcification, and stiffness after ankle dislocations.

Associated Fractures

Osteochondral fractures of the anterior or posterior dome of the tibia and talus are associated with ankle dislocations. Talar fractures are a greater problem because of the poor vascularity in the body of the talus. Care should be taken to remove all intra-articular fragments. The presence of these osteochondral fractures increases the likelihood of arthritic problems in the future.

FIG. 60-19. In anterior dislocations of the talus there may be ligament and neurovascular damage.

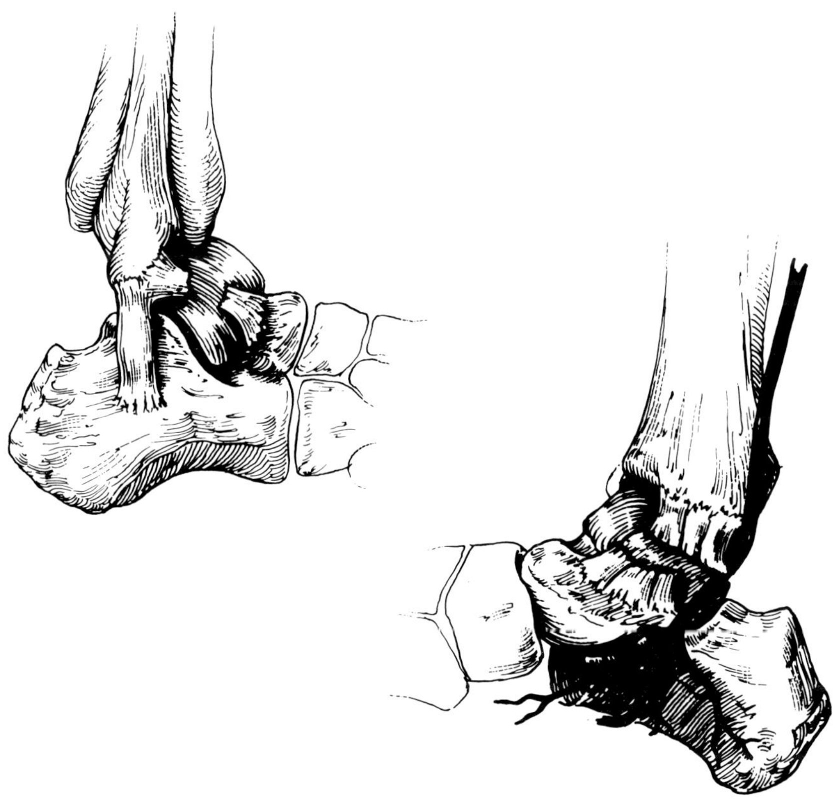

Sudeck's Atrophy

Sudeck's atrophy is a disorder of the sympathetic nervous system that is relatively frequent about the ankle and foot. This disorder is a sympathetic malfunction with patchy osteoporosis, inappropriate pain to pressure, and vasomotor instability. In the active phase of this disorder, there is significant pain and loss of motion. Treatment should include temperature biofeedback, sympathetic blocks, and physical therapy.

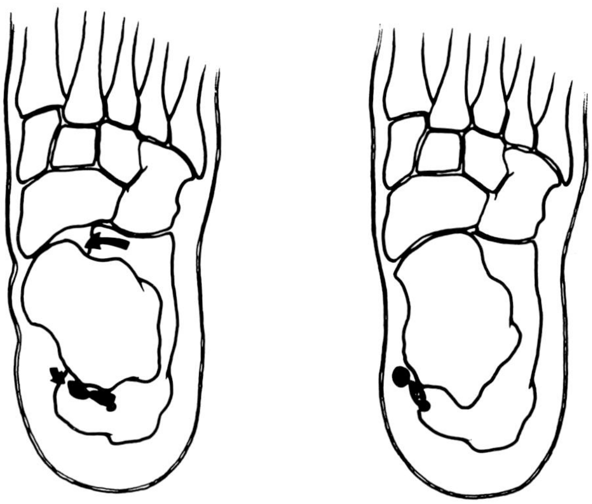

FIG. 60-20. Subtalar dislocations require large forces, but the morbidity following injury is very low with timely reduction.

FIG. 60-21. Tarsometatarsal dislocation involves rupture of the base of the second metatarsal–cuneiform complex, which is a rigid support for the foot.

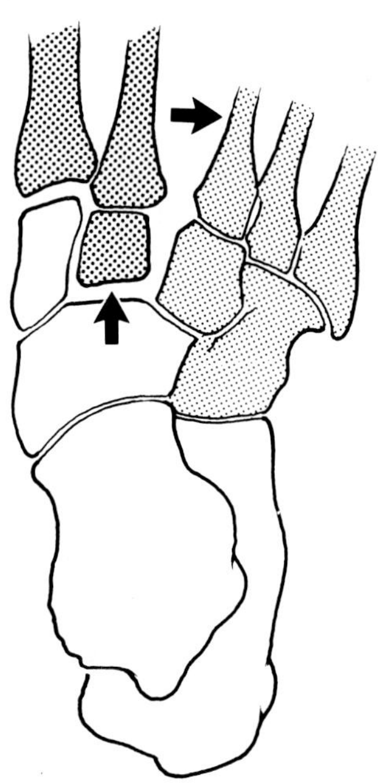

Neurovascular Injuries

Vascular compromise to anterior tibial, posterior tibial, or peroneal arteries can occur with ankle dislocations. Patients with preexisting vascular disorders should be watched carefully for posttraumatic swelling. A compartment syndrome can also occur with bleeding extending into the anterior, peroneal, and deep posterior compartments.[21] Neural injury usually involves direct neuropraxic damage to the superficial peroneal, deep peroneal, sural, or saphenous nerve.

TALAR DISLOCATIONS

Dislocations of the talus without associated fractures are rare and usually occur in severe flexion injuries with complete rupture of the anterior, medial, and lateral capsular restraint.[14, 16] The force involved in these injuries is great; therefore, there is a high incidence of compound wounds. Severe skin hypoxia occurs with all talus dislocations, and rapid reduction with measures to increase the vascular blood supply and adequate drainage should be taken. Avascular necrosis is an inevitable complication of this type of dislocation.

SUBTALAR DISLOCATIONS

Subtalar dislocations account for 15% of all talar injuries and usually are associated with fractures of the talus. Fortunately, with a timely reduction, there is a low incidence of avascular necrosis; the major complication is loss of subtalar motion secondary to the pericapsular swelling and ligamentous disruption (Fig. 60-20).[14, 16]

TARSOMETATARSAL DISLOCATIONS

The key to stability of the metatarsal cuneiform complex is the second metatarsal (Fig. 60-21). Rupture of this articulation occurs from a longitudinal force with the foot in extreme plantar flexion. The injury is associated with dislocation of the other tarsometatarsal joints as well as fractures of the second, third, fourth, and fifth metatarsal heads. Vascular compromise of the forefoot is the major, immediate complication and should be treated by early reduction, drainage, and stability. Failure to achieve an anatomical reduction may lead to chronic foot pain and loss of motion.

Conclusions

In treating dislocations of the musculoskeletal system, the surgeon should be aware of potential regional complications. Knowledge of the anatomy of the joint and adjacent structures is the key to treatment. All reductions should be performed in a timely and gentle manner with anesthesia, if needed. The postreduction x-ray film should be checked in multiple views. There is a high rate of complications associated with dislocations because of the forces involved; therefore, complete pre- and postreduction neurovascular examinations should be documented. No dislocation can occur without injury to cartilage and supporting structures, and a postinjury rehabilitation program is mandatory.

References

1. Cooney WP, Dobyns JH: Nonunion of scaphoid: Analytical results for bone grafting. J Hand Surg 5:343, 1980
2. Dobyns JH, Linscheid RL et al: Traumatic instability of the wrist. AAOS Instructional Course Lectures 182:199, 1975
3. Eaton RG, Green WT: Volkmann's ischaemia. Clin Orthop 50:219, 1973
4. Epps CH (ed): Complications in Orthopaedic Surgery. Philadelphia, JB Lippincott, 1978
5. Epstein HC: Posterior fracture dislocation of the hip. J Bone Joint Surg 56A:1103, 1974
6. Gelberman RH et al: Vascularity of scaphoid bone. J Hand Surg 5:508, 1980
7. Griffith PC: The management of acute circulatory failure in an injured limb. J Bone Joint Surg 30B:280, 1948
8. Hollinshead WH: Anatomy for Surgeons, The Back and Limbs, vol 3. Hagerstown, Harper & Row, 1964
9. Kennedy JC: Complete dislocation of the knee joint. J Bone Joint Surg 45A:889, 1963
10. Linscheid RL, Wheeler DK: Elbow dislocation. JAMA 194:1171, 1965
11. Mayfield JK, Johnson RP: Carpal dislocation: Pathomechanics and progress in perilunar instability. J Hand Surg 5:226, 1980
12. Myers MH, Harvey JP: Traumatic dislocation of the knee joint. J Bone Joint Surg 53A:16, 1971
13. Ogden JA: Subluxation and dislocation of the proximal tibia-fibula. J Bone Joint Surg 56A:145, 1974
14. Pennal GF: Fractures of the talus. Clin Orthop 30:53, 1963
15. Penrose JH: The monteggia fracture with posterior dislocation of radial head. J Bone Joint Surg 33B:69, 1951
16. Rockwood CA, Green DP (eds): Fractures. Philadelphia, JB Lippincott, 1975
17. Rowe CR, Lowell JD: Progress of fractures of the acetabulum. J Bone Joint Surg 43A:30, 1981
18. Stewart MJ, McCarroll HR: Fracture dislocation of the hip. J Bone Joint Surg 52B:773, 1970
19. Tachdjian MO (ed): Fractures and dislocation. Pediatric Orthopedics, vol 2, chap 8, pp 1532–1738. Philadelphia, WB Saunders, 1972
20. Toleisnik J: The ligament of the wrist. J Hand Surg 1:110, 1976
21. Whitesides TE et al: Tissue pressure measurements as a determinant for need of fasciotomy. Clin Orthop 50:219, 1973

61 Complications of Amputations

Robert S. Adelaar

OVERVIEW

Amputations are one of the most ancient of surgical procedures. The incidence of lower extremity amputation in men over 60 is 129 per 100,000.[4] *The most common etiology of amputations in the older male population is peripheral vascular disease, resulting in a 70% incidence of amputation, while 22% of amputations are secondary to trauma.*[3] *Other common etiologies of amputations are neurotrophic disorders such as myelomeningocele and diabetes mellitus, infection, tumors, and congenital disorders such as leg length inequality.*

Problems Associated With Amputation

Each time an amputation is performed, the potential problems of prosthetic wear for the area involved and the increased patient energy requirements for the type of amputation must be considered, as well as the medical condition of the patient.

INCREASED ENERGY REQUIREMENT

A patient with severe cardiopulmonary problems may not be able to handle the increased energy requirements that prosthetic usage requires. For example, with an amputation above the elbow, the opposite shoulder must be used as the initiating mechanism, which requires a great deal of power and energy consumption. The lower the level of amputation, the less the cost in energy consumption.[13] Therefore, in cardiopulmonary patients the lowest level amputation possible would be the most suitable.

PROSTHETIC FITTING PROBLEMS

Difficult prosthetic fitting problems occur with short stumps, knee disarticulation, and hindfoot amputations. A Boyd amputation, in which the calcaneus and heel pad remain, is a difficult prosthesis to fit. A Syme's amputation can be accommodated in the normal patient, but large and neurotrophic stumps present prosthetic problems. Amputations that are too close to a joint also present prosthetic wear and fitting problems. A below-knee amputation, which is too short, is as difficult as a knee disarticulation or a long above-knee amputation. The elbow, shoulder, and hip are other areas where a stump that is too short is of no mechanical advantage for prosthetic management. The space required for a prosthetic joint, such as the knee, should also be accounted for in the ideal stump length.

JOINT CONTRACTURES

Contracture of a joint or anatomical variation should be considered in potential prosthetic wear. Flexion contractures of the hip, knee, or elbow make prosthetic fitting difficult. Full passive range of motion is ideal for joints around the amputation site.

SKIN COVERAGE

Each particular prosthesis has its own areas for increased stump pressure. For example, in the normal amputee a patellar-tendon-bearing below-knee prosthesis has increased pressure in the distal lateral tibial, proximal medial tibial, and patellar tendon areas. These areas should be covered with sensitive tissue that can resist pressure. Areas of poor sensa tion and skin coverage will lead to skin breakdown and prosthetic failure.

Amputation Level

The ideal functional levels for amputations are demonstrated in Figure 61-1. In the foot and hindfoot, it is important to leave adequate dorsiflexors and plantar-flexors with the heel pad to prevent equinus contractures. The hindfoot is usually not used in the vascular or neurotrophic amputation because of the pressure on the heel pad. The below-knee level should be at least 4 to 5 inches below the tibial tubercle for ideal patellar tendon-bearing prosthetic fitting. The patellar tendon-bearing prosthesis is the best type of prosthesis to use for below-knee amputation. In the above-knee and the upper extremity amputation, the lower the amputation, the less the morbidity and the easier the prosthetic fitting. A space should be left to accommodate the knee mechanism.

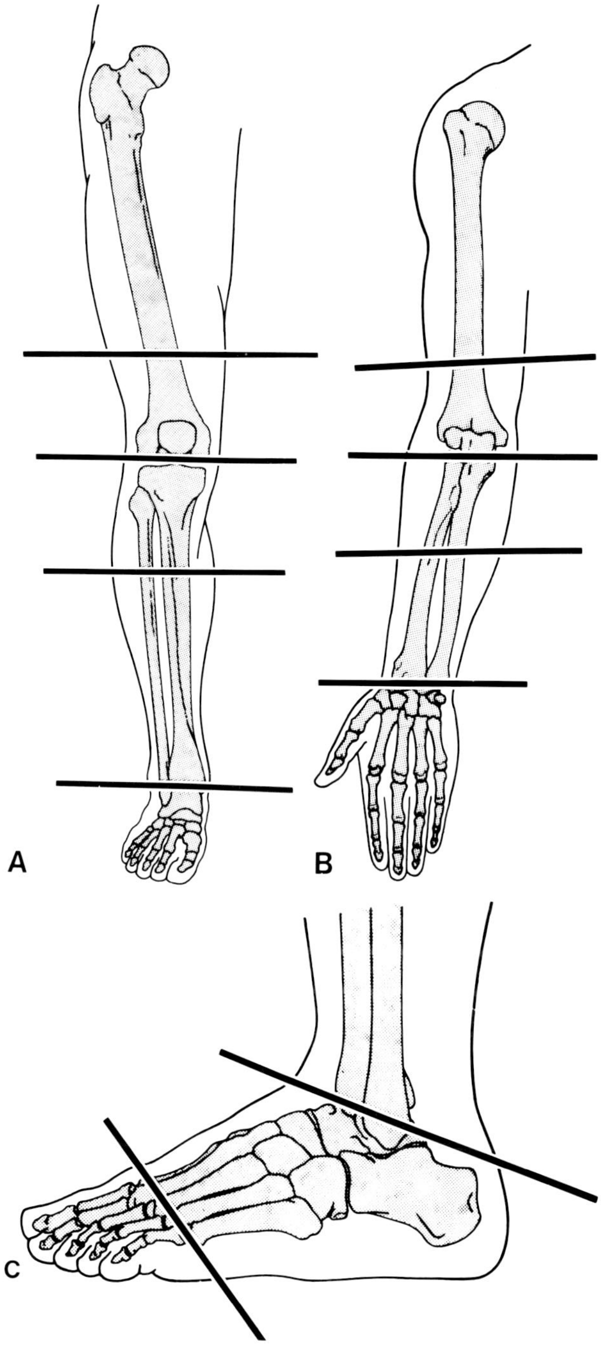

FIG. 61-1. (*A*) Ideal levels of amputation for the lower extremity. (*B*) Ideal levels of amputation for the upper extremity. (*C*) Ideal levels of amputation for the foot and ankle.

Surgical Technique

Well-designed skin and muscle flaps should be used. Skin flaps with the highest blood supply and innervation, such as the posterior calf skin in a below-knee amputation, are ideal. The suture line should be placed away from areas of prosthetic pressure. For example, below-knee amputation suture lines should be anterior where there will be little prosthetic pressure (Fig. 61-2).

The end of the bone should be cut short enough so that there will be no pressure at the end of the stump, and it should be smoothed as well. Each stump passes through a 6-month period of soft tissue shrinkage after amputation; however, the level of the bone during this time remains the same.

The end of the stump should not be left bulky. Nonviable muscle should be débrided for firm closure. In heavy patients, adipose tissue should be defatted to avoid problems with poor blood supply and fat necrosis.

CIRCULATORY CARE

Major arterial and venous channels should be ligated. Extra precautions should be taken in patients with hypertensive and arteriosclerotic vascular disease. The tourniquet should be released prior to closure of these amputation stumps to facilitate complete hemostasis. Any skin flap that has poor capillary filling should be débrided and the stump shortened.

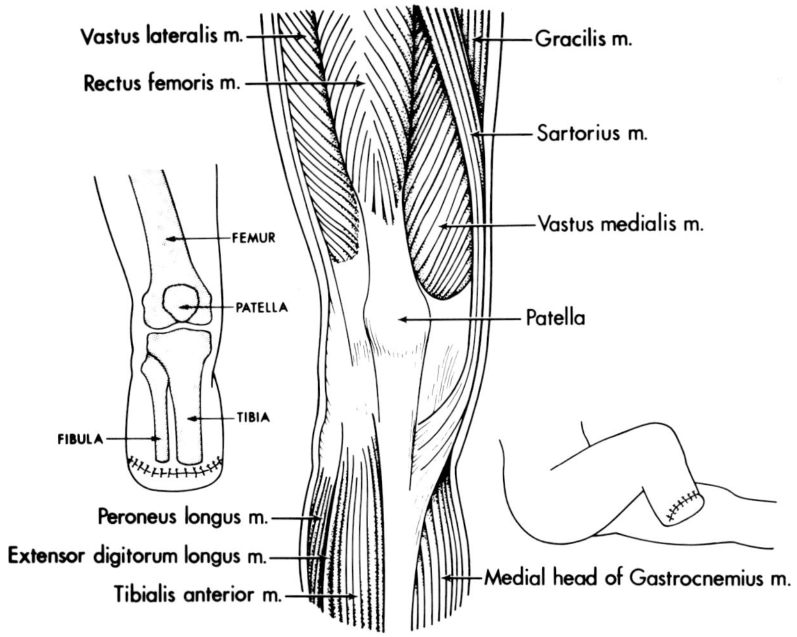

FIG. 61-2. The ideal below-knee amputation stump. There is a well-placed incision and a good muscular pad.

NERVE MANAGEMENT

Neuromas can be a difficult postoperative problem but can be prevented with good operative techniques. Neural tissue should be handled carefully, and no significant tension should be applied. Nerves should be cut sharply so that they retract into areas with good soft tissue coverage that will not be sites of future prosthetic pressure. Damaged nerves should be sacrificed, since they have been implicated in some postamputation pain problems.

Etiology

JUVENILE AMPUTATION

Amputations in juvenile patients particularly with open growth centers pose problems with bone overgrowth. The amount of overgrowth depends on how much skeletal growth remains. The stump should be adjusted to accommodate for this, and multiple revisions may be necessary.

TRAUMATIC AMPUTATION

Amputations performed for trauma should be conservative. All devitalized tissue should be removed. The amputation should be left open and closed secondarily. Determination of how much skin or muscle will survive is often difficult. Agents such as low-molecular-weight dextran have been used to increase the capillary perfusion of traumatized tissue. Adequate débridement, irrigation, and antibiotics, if appropriate for contaminated open wounds, should always be used. Care should also be taken to eliminate any possibility of anaerobic or clostridial infection prior to closure. If fractures accompany the trauma, they should be repaired so that early mobilization can be attained. An appropriate level of amputation should be chosen for optimal prosthetic fitting and wear.

NEUROTROPHIC AMPUTATION

Patients with myelomeningocele and diabetes mellitus have stumps with poor sensation, which are not ideal for prosthetic wear. The diabetic also has poor arterial supply, and most amputations in diabetics are done because of infection.[11] The stump should be left open, and the level of amputation chosen will depend on the availability of viable skin and muscle flaps. Care should be taken to prevent infection, edema, and hematomas in these stumps, since they are vulnerable to infection. The energy consumption of the diabetic patient who also has cardiopulmonary problems should be considered.[13]

The level of amputation in patients with diabetes mellitus is still controversial. Amputations of the foot and hindfoot have been advocated as a method of preserving ambulatory status. However, the morbidity and revision rates are very high when multiple foot amputations are done in the presence of poorly vascularized infected tissue. There are also problems in prosthetic fitting for Syme's and distal foot amputations, and equinus contractures can develop with foot amputations because of insufficient dorsiflexion muscle power. In light of these factors, it is often preferable to amputate immediately below the knee.

TUMOR AMPUTATION

Primary sarcomas of the musculoskeletal system require precise amputation in order to minimize the chance of metastatic spread and improve the chance of survival. Each tumor has certain defined surgical margins, which can be determined by CT scan, tomography, bone scanning, and angiography. The surgical plane will give the margins of safety for the location and aggressiveness of each particular tumor. If a sarcoma is localized to bone and is not violating the integrity of the periosteum, treatment should consist of a radical *en bloc* resection of the tumor. The chance of secondary local spread decreases the more proximal the area is from the bone lesion. The decision, then, involves the potential for local spread *versus* a longer stump for better prosthetic wear. For example, a fibrosarcoma confined to the bone in the distal femur has a good chance for stump metastasis when a proximal femoral amputation is performed instead of a hip disarticulation. Hip disarticulation would theoretically give the best tumor-free interval. The problem becomes one of quality of life because the above-the-knee prosthesis is much more functional than the hip disarticulation prosthesis. For proximal femoral amputations, hip disarticulations, and hemipelvectomies, a hip disarticulation type of prosthesis must be used, which is cumbersome and difficult to use and has high energy consumption.

In soft tissue sarcomas, the planes of the tumor must be well defined. For example, if a low-grade fibrosarcoma is confined to the midsoleus region, then removal of the deep and superficial posterior compartment with the posterior tibial artery and gastroc attachment should be performed. Limb-saving procedures should always be considered for central axis sarcomas, such as a chondrosarcoma of the scapula, which rarely metastasize distally to the extremities.

Care should be taken to avoid spreading the tumor to a new place when performing the initial biopsy. The biopsy incision should be removed with a wide local margin at the time of the definitive amputation. Ideally, the pathologist and surgeon decide at the time the initial frozen section and the definitive amputation are done to decrease possible secondary spread of tumor from the biopsy procedure.

Complications that are characteristic of tumor amputations are wound breakdown and secondary seeding to the stump. The use of radiation and chemotherapy in the immediate postoperative period can delay collagen bonding and cause wound dehiscence. An amputation stump that develops wound complications after radiation is difficult to heal.

PERIPHERAL VASCULAR DISEASE AMPUTATION

Peripheral vascular disease is the most common etiology of adult amputations. Good surgical techniques should be followed, since edema, hematoma, and infection, in combination with poorly oxygenated tissue, will result in failure. Preoperative assessment of arterial and venous supply is mandatory. Doppler examination, thermography, and fluorescein injection can all be utilized. The key determinant of success, however, is the actual bleeding at the time of the operation. A tourniquet should not be used because of the problems with postoperative thrombosis. The posterior skin flap has a better blood supply for a below-knee amputation and should be left longer than the anterior flap (see Fig. 61-2). Muscle that has poor contractility and blood supply should be débrided. Muscle atrophy occurs postoperatively, and it is not important, therefore, to leave muscle bulk behind.

Operative Mortality

Vascular amputees usually have multisystem disease with generalized arteriosclerotic vascular disease. There are reports of up to 30% mortality in below-knee amputations. The lower the amputation, the lower the mortality rate.[5, 7] Pneumonia, cerebrovascular accidents, myocardial infarction, and pulmonary embolism are the major postoperative medical problems.[5, 10] The use of anticoagulation therapy reduces thromboembolic complications, and spinal anesthesia has been shown to reduce the mortality rate more than general anesthesia does.[10, 12]

Local Complications

Local complications are common to all types of amputations but are critical in vascular amputations since they involve stump failure and high revision rates.

INCISIONAL PROBLEMS

The use of a vascularized skin flap, good drainage, lack of contamination, and no tension will decrease incisional problems. Major incisional problems are skin necrosis, wound dehiscence, and dry gangrene (which usually occurs because of thrombosis of the stump vessels). It is imperative to use meticulous skin handling and good drainage to avoid thrombosis, and anticoagulation is recommended for the first 5-day period. Collagens in poorly vascularized skin take longer to bond; therefore, nonreactive sutures such as wires should be left for 2 to 3 weeks. Care should be taken in the use of electrical coagulation near the skin edges, and as many veins as possible should be preserved. A uniform external compression dressing should be used, and it should not be applied so tightly that the external pressure becomes greater than the already diminished arterial pulse pressure.

HEMATOMA

A tourniquet should not be used in vascular amputations. Instead, meticulous hemostasis and special care in using electrical coagulation should be utilized. Ligatures should be used around large vessels. The soft tissue, fascia, and muscle should be closed in order to avoid any dead space. It is important to remember that the bone end has a good medullary blood supply, and agents such as Avitene or bone wax are recommended to stop bleeding. Adequate drainage is recommended for 24 to 48 hours. A closed suction irrigation system is used in combination with a rigid external dressing. If a hematoma does develop, it is important that it be evacuated and the skin closed in the operating room.

INFECTION

Infection of the stump is usually secondary to necrosis of the skin edges and deep muscle tissue or hematoma formation. The stump is poorly vascularized, and systemic antibiotic tissue levels are low. It is best to approach a deep infection by adequate surgical débridement and secondary closure. Hospital contamination from resistant organisms sometimes occurs. Appropriate antibiotic management is difficult, and anaerobic infections can be severe because of the low oxygen level. These anaerobic infections should be handled by aggressive débridement.[5] Clostridial infections should be débrided back to viable tissue and hyperbaric oxygenation used if available. Use of prophylactic antibiotics is encouraged, but it should be remembered that antibiotic levels at the stump will be low.

Most infections of the stump are superficial and secondary to skin necrosis. These should be handled by local débridement of devitalized tissue and wound care to stimulate granulation. The use of a skin graft is not recommended in areas of prosthetic pressure.

EDEMA

Edema can result in proximal vessel necrosis in vascular amputations. The stump should be closed and a rigid compression dressing applied.[1, 9] Unless severe pain occurs, this dressing should be left in place for at least 10 days and then changed with a similar rigid dressing. It is not necessary to inspect the wound daily. Immediate prosthetic fitting is controversial. Some believe that the immediate use of a prosthetic device will decrease the amount of postoperative complications, increase prosthetic efficiency, and decrease the period of hospitalization.[3] Management consists of the use of rigid dressings for 3 weeks followed by appropriate stump wrapping and prosthetic fitting after the acute atrophy of the stump has occurred.

PAIN

Pain in the immediate postoperative period is normal. The normal postoperative pain is usually felt over the entire stump and subsides over a 4- to 5-day period. Pain that is severe, unresponsive to analgesics and limb elevation, and localized to certain areas should be investigated since it may be due to localized pressure. Failure to investigate this type of pain may result in pressure necrosis and may abort the beneficial effects of a rigid postoperative dressing.The immediate use of the rigid dressing is thought to decrease the amount of postoperative pain by decreasing the amount of edema.

Long-Term Complications

The long-term complications of amputations are prosthetic adaptation, stump problems, pain syndromes, and the psychological aspects of amputations.

STUMP PROBLEMS

During prosthetic adaptation, a non-weight-bearing portion of the body must handle excessive pressure. Increased local pressure can result in pressure necrosis and stump breakdown with long delays in prosthetic wear for healing. Abnormal stump and prosthetic stress risers must be handled with revision of both the stump and the prosthesis. Chronic skin problems may develop because of the increased pressure and the damp stump environment. Some common chronic problems are folliculitis, which is usually caused by staphylococcus infection, epidermoid cysts with keratinc plugging of the hair follicles, contact dermatitis, and eczema.[2, 5]

The stump will usually atrophy for the first 6 months after amputation, and permanent prosthetic fitting should be delayed until the stump size has stabilized. This is more of a problem in below-knee amputations than in other areas. A redundant stump, usually caused by bulky muscle flaps, will cause problems because of pressure and local skin irritation. These redundant skin folds should be revised. Weight increase will cause the stump to become too large for the prosthesis and result in excessive pressure. Extensive scarring, which is common with traumatic amputations, will cause problems with local pressure areas and desensitized skin.

Contracture of the stump should be avoided, since this can cause problems with the prosthetic fitting and increased pressure areas. Contractures occur when the stump is short, as in the elbow, hip, and knee. Equinus contractures are a particular problem with forefoot and hindfoot amputations, owing to the unopposed action of the gastroc complex. Physical therapy modes should be used to prevent and treat these contractures. When a contracture becomes too severe, it precludes use of the prosthesis, and a revision must be brought to the next higher joint.

Bursitis occurs where there is increased pressure or friction in the moving parts. Bursitis should initially be treated with revision of the prosthesis in order to recess the areas of increased pressure. If pressure continues, revision of the stump or a new prosthesis may be required.

PAIN SYNDROMES

Phantom limb pain occurs frequently with amputations (see also Chap. 49). It becomes a pathologic disorder in approximately 10% of amputations. Pathologic phantom limb pain is more common in upper extremity amputations, patients with abnormal personality profiles, and patients who have had chronic pain prior to amputation. The personality profile most likely to develop pathologic phantom limb pain is that of the compulsive, hard-working type.[2, 5, 6, 8] Phantom limb pain can be classified into three types: postural, with cramping characteristics; burning; and sharp nerve root irritation. The burning and nerve root types can lead to chronic pain.[5] The effective treatment of phantom limb pain is difficult and involves the use of psychotherapy, transcutaneous stimulation, and neurosurgical procedures.

A neuroma develops each time a nerve is transected. It can become a pathologic source of pain when it is in an area of increased pressure. The neuroma will usually require a tension-free resection and movement into an area of low stress with good soft tissue coverage. Recurrent neuromas are significant problems, and the therapeutic modalities used have not been able to control them effectively.

PSYCHOLOGICAL PROBLEMS

The loss of a limb can bring out pathologic personality disorders. It is natural to have a period of depression with loss of limb. The psychological adaptation is influenced by the premorbid personality, type of amputation, medical condition, and the success of the prosthetic program. Patients who are rapidly rehabilitated and become good prosthetic users have a low percentage of chronic psychological problems. Psychological and psychiatric counseling is always useful for patients such as young, traumatic, or tumor amputees. We know that these patients have problems accepting their amputations, and psychiatric counseling should be an early part of rehabilitation.

References

1. Burgess EM, Romano RL: The management of lower extremity amputees using immediate post-surgical prosthesis. Clin Orthop 57:137, 1968
2. Edmonson AS, Crenshaw AH (eds): Campbell's Operative Orthopedics, vol 1, chap 8, pp 821–873. St. Louis, CV Mosby, 1980
3. Hanssone J: The leg amputee: A clinical follow-up study. Acta Scand (Suppl 1) 69, 1964
4. Kay H, Newman JD: Relative incidences of new amputations. Orthotics and Prosthetics 29:3, 1975
5. McCollough RJ III: Complications of amputation surgery. In Epps CH Jr (ed): Complications of Orthopaedic Surgery, vol 2, chap 40, pp 1159–1189. Philadelphia, JB Lippincott, 1978
6. Melzau R: Phantom limb pain. Anesthesiology 35:409, 1971
7. Otteman MG, Stahlgren LH: Evaluation of factors which influence mortality and morbidity following major lower extremity amputation for arteriosclerosis. Surg Gynecol Obstet 120:1217, 1965
8. Parkes CM: Factors determining the persistence of phantom pain in amputees. J Psychosom Res 17:197, 1973
9. Sarmento A et al: Immediate post-surgical prosthetic fitting. Clin Orthop 68:22, 1970
10. Sarmento A, Warren WD: A re-evaluation of lower extremity amputations. Surg Gynecol Obstet 129:799, 1969
11. Silbert S: Amputation of lower extremity in diabetes mellitus: Follow-up of 294 cases. Diabetes 1:297, 1952
12. Thompson RC Jr, Delblanco TL, McAllister FF: Complication following lower extremity amputation. Surg Gynecol Obstet 120:301, 1965
13. Waters RL et al: Energy cost for walking of amputees. J Bone Joint Surg 58A:42, 1976

62
Complications of Hand Surgery and Trauma

Wyndell H. Merritt

OVERVIEW

Surgical conditions of the hand are far more common than most physicians realize. Indeed, hand injury alone causes 16 million Americans annually to seek medical aid. Labor Department statistics show that one fourth of disabling work injuries are to hands and one half million of these victims receive compensation.[34]

Because of the magnitude of this problem, most of the initial treatment must be by surgical personnel at general emergency facilities rather than by hand surgeons. However, in a busy emergency room, hand injuries or infections may seem of minor importance to both surgeon and patient. Unfortunately, major morbidity may then result from incorrect appraisal or inadequate initial treatment. The final result following any surgical condition of the hand will be directly proportional to the accuracy of evaluation and the efficiency of initial treatment.

Certainly, most preventable complications stem from acute hand injuries. Primary care physicians need to recognize that the hand is an organ; injury to any part biologically influences the entire organ. By developing such respect for hand injury, much can be done to protect function in the uninjured portion as well as to repair obvious damage.

Biologic Consequences of Hand Trauma

BIOLOGIC BASIS OF THE STIFF HAND

The most frequent and most frustrating complication of hand injury is the stiff hand. Basically, in the stiff hand the dense connective tissue has remodeled. In general, the degree of inflammation will predict the amount of remodeling and stiffness to be anticipated, although other variables such as age, immobilization, and individual motivation play vital roles. For example, a patient with severe crushing injury to the hand will invariably experience permanently limited motion in spite of intact skin, bone, tendon, nerve, and other structures because of the predictable severe inflammation. Although dense connective tissue such as fascia, ligament, and tendon is not recognized to be highly reactive, wounded fascia will actually show far greater collagen synthesis than will comparable skin wounds.[52] Furthermore, the increased turnover of collagen in dense connective tissue appears to persist far longer than collagen turnover in simple skin wounds.[53] Thus, the mobility of an injured hand may be modified long after skin wounds have completely healed. The areolar covering of ligaments, joint capsule, and fascia appears to respond to simple wounding with intense collagen proliferation, even greater in extent than within the dense connective structure itself.[48] This thickened coat of new collagen (Fig. 62-1) acts almost as an external cast over the mobile structures, and collagen cross-linking then fixes these structures in a limited position. It is therefore important to immobilize patients in positions from which they can recover the maximal degree of useful function (Fig. 62-2).

Much evidence now implicates inflammatory cells, especially the macrophage, as the major stimulus for altering collagen metabolism. Indeed, tissue culture studies show this cell capable of stimulating fibroblast proliferation, increasing collagen deposition, and also increasing collagen degradation.[15, 76] Two very important clinical consequences should be recognized. First, when there is increased collagen turnover, there is increased remodeling, so that the natural balance between the mobility and stability of ligaments and other dense connective tissue can be lost. Because of inflammation, there is proliferation of "young" or uncross-linked collagen, which is capable of slippage of subunits in response

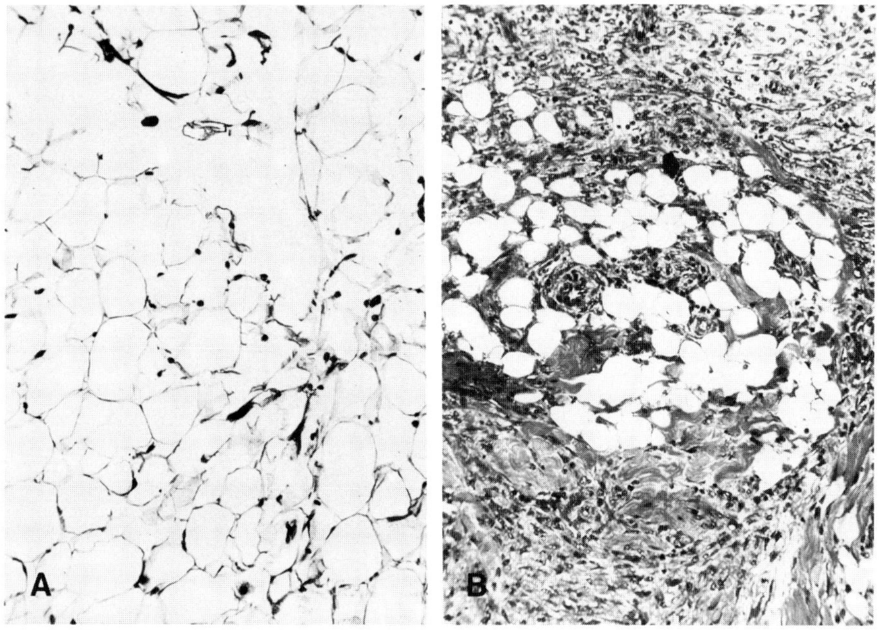

FIG. 62-1. Photomicrographs of collagen in the areolar covering of canine fascia lata stained with Masson's trichrome reagent. (*A*) at the time of injury; (*B*) 5 days following skin and adjacent fascia laceration, showing 20 times greater collagen synthesis on biochemical analysis.

to tension.[3] Therefore, to avoid stiffness, the inflamed hands should be moved, but only within the range that will not further increase inflammation and accelerate collagen turnover. Second, if the macrophage accelerates connective tissue turnover, it will do so whether the adjacent ligament is injured or not. When there is severe injury, such as a crushed fingertip, the inflammatory response is not confined to the precise site of injury but will also adversely influence adjacent normal hand structures. Therefore, an important first consideration is preservation of adjacent uninjured structures, which can easily be lost due to the inflammatory response. The "position to protect function" may be valuable in these situations. For example, one unfortunate and frequent complication is loss of metacarpophalangeal (MP) joint flexion due to tongue-blade splinting of finger fractures. Because tongue blades are so ubiquitous, they provide an irresistible and inexpensive splinting device. However, when a distal or middle phalangeal fracture is splinted for crush injury, the inflammatory response will certainly extend to the MP joint where the collateral ligaments are normally lax in extension and tight in flexion (Fig. 62-3). If the tongue blade extends into the palm, this ligament is allowed to remodel in extension, and the patient becomes incapable of flexing the MP joint. After 3 weeks, the surgeon may rejoice that the fracture is stable but will regret that the remodeled collateral ligament now prevents MP joint flexion. This is avoided by immobilizing the MP joints in flexion, one of the principles of the position to protect function (see Fig. 62-2).

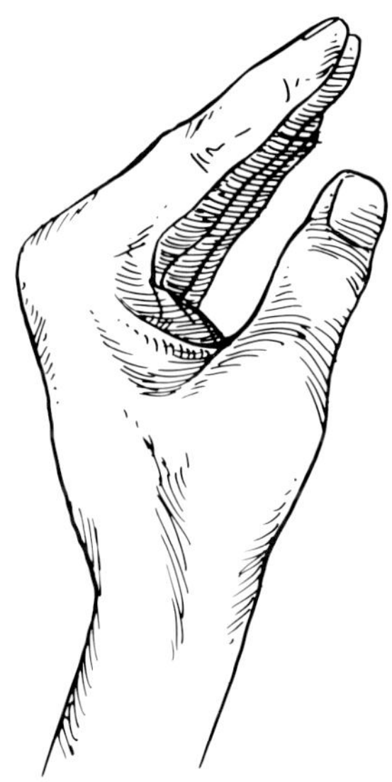

FIG. 62-2. Position to protect function: wrist extension, MP flexion, IP extension, thumb abduction, and opposition.

WOUND COVERAGE AND CONTRACTURES: SKIN GRAFTS OR FLAPS

A profound stimulus for the inflammatory response occurs with loss of protective coverage of the hand. The bacterial contamination and inflammation of skin loss not only may cause wound contraction but also may influence remodeling of the deeper connective tissue structures. The debate whether to skin graft a wound primarily or let it heal by secondary

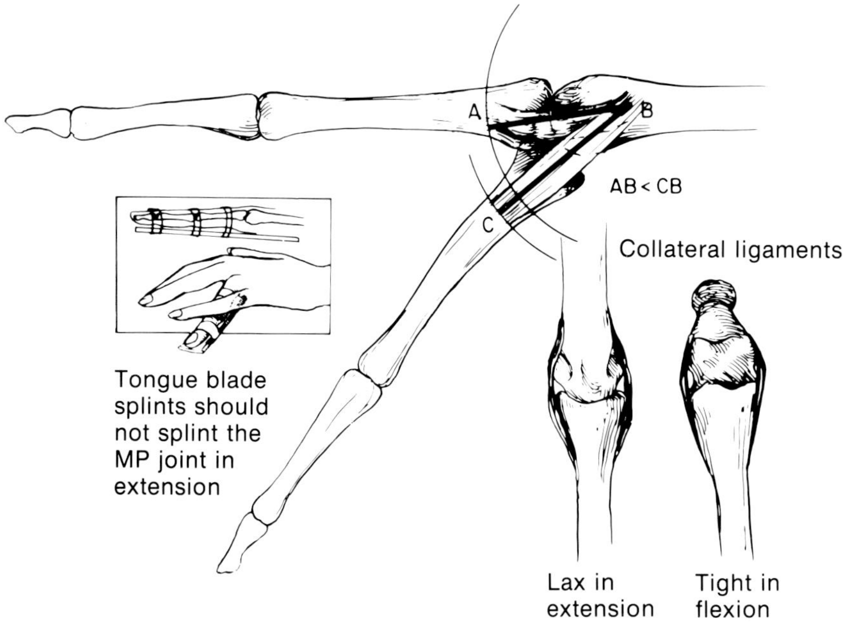

FIG. 62-3. Metacarpophalangeal joints should be splinted in flexion because the collateral ligament is lax in extension and tight in flexion. If collateral ligaments remodel in extension, they prohibit later MP joint flexion.

intention should be influenced by two important factors. One is whether the depth of injury and size of defect will cause contraction that interferes with function. Second is whether the amount of prolonged inflammation during secondary healing will cause adverse remodeling and stiffness. In many patients primary skin grafts may be done to provide healing more quickly, which will reduce inflammation and permit earlier mobilization. Early excision and split-thickness grafting of deep partial-thickness loss of skin in the hand is an acceptable approach and may be indicated for many patients.[56] Certainly, when the burned hand is managed with topical antibiotic therapy, it is important to maintain mobilization so that the inflamed dense connective tissues will not remodel in a fixed functionless position.

When the thin and highly vascular areolar covering of extensor tendons or other dense connective tissue is lost, skin grafts should not be expected to become vascularized and survive. When an injury exposes the raw collagen of these dense connective tissue structures, it is necessary to mobilize adjacent areolar tissue or skin for coverage. When this is not possible, a skin flap is necessary. In the hand, tissue for skin flaps is limited, although many innovative local flap methods have been designed. When injury is severe, such as loss of the entire dorsal surface of the hand, distant flaps become necessary. These may be from an axial flap with a known vessel supply, such as the groin flap, or may be a random flap as can be designed from the chest or abdominal wall. The groin flap supplied by the superficial circumflex iliac vessels has gained popularity because it is relatively thin and easily tolerated. It should be remembered that skin flaps do not contract the way skin grafts do. Furthermore, full-thickness skin grafts, if completely vascularized, will contract less than will split-thickness skin grafts. Generally, the thinner the skin graft the greater the contraction, and this should be considered when choosing grafts and flaps. Rarely, microvascular "free flaps" may be attached to hand vessels to provide neurovascular function.

THE POSITION TO PROTECT FUNCTION

The hurt hand automatically assumes a functionless posture with wrist flexion, MP extension, interphalangeal flexion, and thumb adduction (see Fig. 62-2). Although the original injury may be only to the wrist or skin, when remodeling occurs in this posture, the whole hand is rendered functionless (Fig. 62-4). Fifty years ago, Kanavel described a "position of function" for infected hands in which even a small amount of motion could be functional after the ravages of bacterial inflammation.[31]

When analyzing how to position hands to protect function best, the surgeon should recognize four important anatomical considerations. First, the amplitude of the flexor profundi and sublimi require wrist extension to achieve strong power grip. Therefore, the wrist should be immobilized in extension when the injury permits. Indeed, wrist extension may be regarded as the key to hand function. Second, the MP joint is a "cam" joint in that the dense portion of the collateral ligament is so arranged that it is lax in extension and tight in flexion. Furthermore, in flexion this ligament must pass over the condyles of the metacarpal head, an additional factor tightening the joint (see Fig. 62-3). This makes it possible to "waggle" the finger in extension but allows less "waggle" and greater stability in flexion. If this ligament remodels in extension, flexion of the MP joint is no longer possible unless the ligament is ruptured or divided. Therefore, the MP joint should be immobilized in flexion to preserve the length of the collateral ligament. Third, the most important anatomical consideration preserving interphalangeal joint function is the relative strength of the powerful flexors of these joints compared to the weaker intrinsic muscles that provide extension. If an interphalangeal joint is held in flexion, the volar plate remodels in a shortened position. It becomes difficult to overcome this change with the weak intrinsic extensor mechanism, and usually serial casting or splints become necessary. When immobilized in extension the remodeled, shortened dorsal capsule of these joints is far more capable of being stretched by the powerful flexors of the interphalangeal joint than the remodeled volar plate is by the weak intrinsic extensors. Therefore, the interphalangeal joints should be held in extension. Finally, the thumb web is a highly specialized structure that has the unique capacity to collapse on itself in an accordianlike fashion. This is possible because of the special quality of its thin mobile skin. Unfortunately, this skin also has a remarkable ability to remodel rapidly and disappear if the thumb is held in an adducted position in the inflamed hand. Furthermore, the adductor pollicis fascia may remodel in a shortened position to limit additionally efforts to correct thumb adduction contractures. None of the web-plasty procedures restores the original elegant quality of thumb web skin, so it is important to preserve this special structure by maintaining the thumb in an abducted position opposed to the fingertips. This is perhaps the most frequent oversight, leading to a serious preventable complication when hands are immobilized.

To avoid unnecessary loss of function, all four anatomical features should be considered any time the injured hand is placed at rest. Of the four, interphalangeal joint extension is the most difficult to recover and wrist extension the easiest.

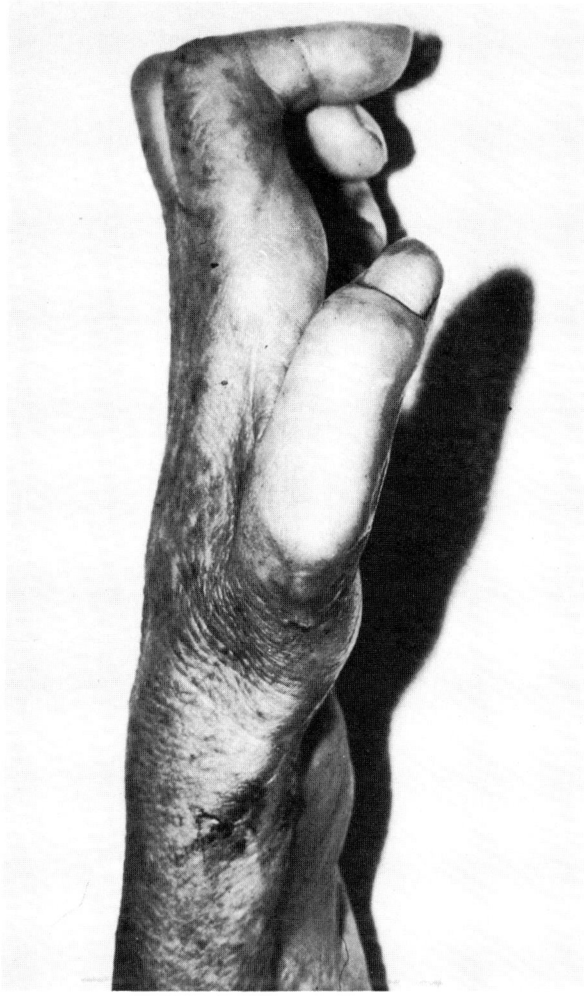

FIG. 62-4. The hurt hand characteristically assumes IP flexion, MP hyperextension, thumb adduction, and wrist flexion as in this patient with wrist electrical injury.

WHEN AND HOW TO IMMOBILIZE HANDS

Hands should be immobilized any time acute injury or inflammation is present. Acute inflammatory changes will be aggravated and increased by motion, and the patient will choose to place his hand in a functionless posture. Hand pain, edema, or inflammatory signs dictate the need for protective immobilization, which will not only protect function but will also afford much symptomatic relief. One popular method of hand immobilization was described by Peacock.[57, 58] This technique creates a conformer effect by placing several layers of gauze over the wound and between the fingers (without cotton in the interstices). Sponges and a bolus of cotton waste or similar material is carded into a loose arrangement and placed on top of the sponges. A loosely woven roll of gauze can then be used to wrap the bolus of cotton waste in position. A finely woven, nonyielding cotton gauze roll may then be used to tighten the dressing into final size and shape, making the entire structure compact and relatively solid. A plaster splint or a few tongue blades can be added to maintain wrist extension. Finally, adhesive tape may be added to provide a degree of permanent stability. Tips of the digits should always be left exposed so that sensation and circulation can be monitored.

After proper immobilization, it is equally important to initiate an active program of mobilization as soon as the acute inflammatory process subsides or injured structures are adequately healed. Many times it is advantageous to place the hand at rest in a position to protect function at night and to work actively on mobilization during the day until scars from the injury have matured.

ROLE OF EDEMA FOLLOWING HAND TRAUMA

There are no data documenting the precise biologic mechanism whereby edema causes hands to become stiff, although empirical observation has led to this popular belief. Indeed, many surgeons and therapists are sufficiently enamored of this concept that treatment of edema becomes a primary therapeutic objective without much regard for its origin. Hand edema should be regarded as a symptom of inflammatory changes following trauma. These inflammatory changes lead to collagen remodeling and hand stiffness, not the edema itself. This explains why hand edema from renal or congestive heart failure does not have a high fibrin content and does not generally cause stiffness. It is more important to focus initial therapeutic goals on the cause and control of inflammation rather than on the resultant edema. Control of edema becomes important once acute inflammation subsides and mobilization is initiated. The edematous hand maintains MP extension, some interphalangeal flexion, and thumb adduction, all opposed to positions that will protect function. Indeed, edema basically immobilizes the hand in a poor functional position at a critical time of rapid dense connective tissue remodeling. Successful mobilization programs must therefore use measures to control edema, including elevation, elastic stockings, elastic wrappings, periodic immobilization, and whatever splinting is needed to recover a functional amplitude of motion. This may be necessary for many months following severe trauma.[8]

Evaluation and Treatment of Acute Hand Injury

EVALUATION

Perhaps the most unjustified violation of wounds occurs following acute hand injury. All too frequently, emergency room personnel attempt assessment by widely opening wounds and inspecting them to see if any important looking structures are divided. This not only leads to inadequate appreciation of injuries, such as a flexor tendon laceration, which may be 7 cm from the skin wound, but also increases bacterial inoculation and stimulates additional hemorrhage, inflammation, and harm. Wounds of the hand should be gently protected by a moist sterile dressing while the hand itself is examined, not the wound. To do so the surgeon must have some fundamental understanding of hand functional anatomy.

Accurate Brief Hand Examination

SENSORY AND FLEXOR TENDON EXAMINATIONS. Examination following acute hand injury is usually brief but must include an accurate history as well as accurate

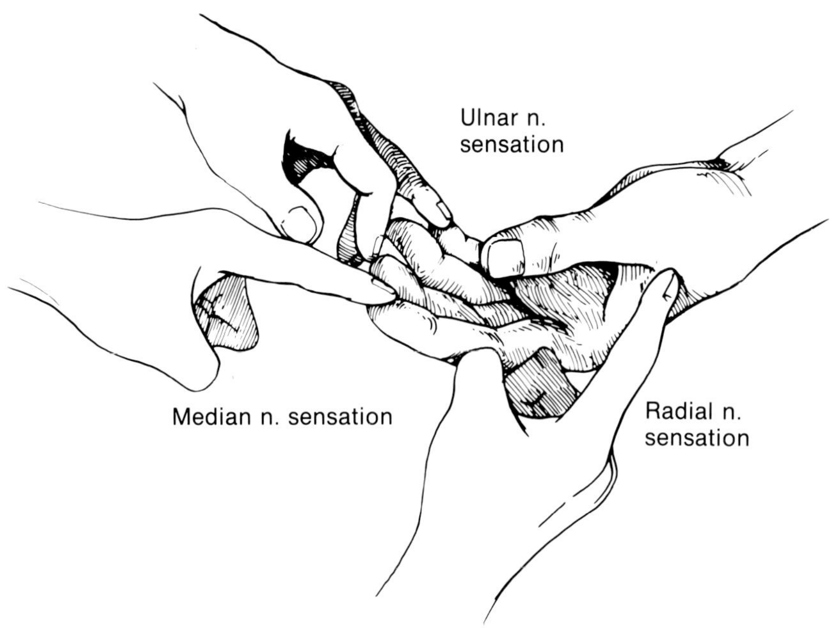

FIG. 62-5. Fingertip examination for sensation can be performed with the index finger for median, fifth finger for ulnar, and dorsum of thumb web for radial. The patient's eyes must be averted during examination.

sensory and motor assessments. X-ray films are also included when structural injury is suspected. It is important to assess sensation while the patient keeps his eyes closed or looks somewhere other than at the injured hand. As surely as one may "see" with fingertips, searching a pocket for the right key, one can also "feel" with eyesight, anticipating touch or pin prick. Therefore, the patient's eyes must be averted to examine sensation accurately. On initial examination, if the very soft touch of the surgeon's index digit pulp is perceived by the patient while he looks elsewhere, other tests of sensation are unnecessary. However, care must be taken not to move the interphalangeal joints in this examination because joint receptors may be activated and confuse the clinical picture. When severe injury is present, there may be an overall dampening of soft touch, and gentle movement on the skin may be needed to activate touch receptors even when the nerve supply is intact. When no soft touch seems present, pain testing with pin prick will immediately determine whether there is complete anesthesia, as when the nerve has been divided.

Median nerve sensation may be evaluated using the index digital pulp region, ulnar nerve by use of the fifth digit pulp, and the radial nerve by examination of an area on the dorsum of the thumb web (Fig. 62-5).

One common error in hand injury assessment is failure to appreciate flexor sublimis tendon laceration. This actually is the most likely flexor tendon laceration because of its superficial location in the palm and proximal finger. Digital flexor tendon function can be determined by remembering two anatomical facts: the profundus flexes the DIP joint, and the sublimi are independent while the profundi are not. Sublimis function is tested by holding the other digits in full extension and observing PIP joint flexion (Fig. 62-6). Profundus function is established by curling the DIP joints as in making a fist. It should be remembered that the intrinsic muscles will still flex the MP joints in complete lacerations of both tendons, but the finger interphalangeal joints will be extended. There is a 10% incidence of absent sublimis tendons in the fifth digit and approximately the same percentage of patients may be so fortunate as to have an independent profundus to the index digit, making repair of the sublimis in such a circumstance unnecessary.[32] Flexor pollicis longus function of the thumb is easily assessed by thumb interphalangeal joint flexion.

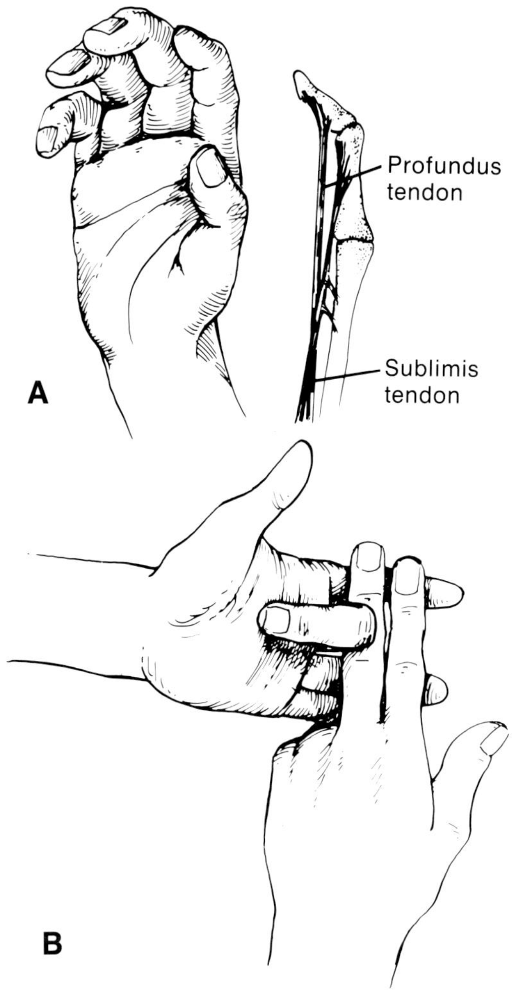

FIG. 62-6. Profundus tendon function is determined by distal joint flexion. Sublimis tendon function is identified by holding adjacent distal interphalangeal joints in extension, permitting sublimis flexion of the proximal interphalangeal joint.

INTRINSIC MUSCLE EXAMINATION. Function of the small muscles that arise and insert in the hand can be assessed as well by direct palpation as by observation of function. The usual reason for examination is to determine motor nerve continuity, which can be quickly ascertained by palpating contracting muscles. The ulnar nerve can be tested by abducting the fifth digit against resistance while simultaneously palpating the abductor digiti quinti (Fig. 62-7). This should be the first intrinsic muscle innervated by the motor division of the ulnar nerve. On the radial side of the hand, the first dorsal interosseous is easily palpated during index and thumb pinch to confirm the integrity of the ulnar motor branch all the way across the palm (see Fig. 62-7). The motor branch of the median is in a vulnerable location in the superficial fascia of the thenar eminence, where it is frequently injured. It is important to recognize laceration of this small nerve if primary repair is to be considered. The distal end of this match-sized

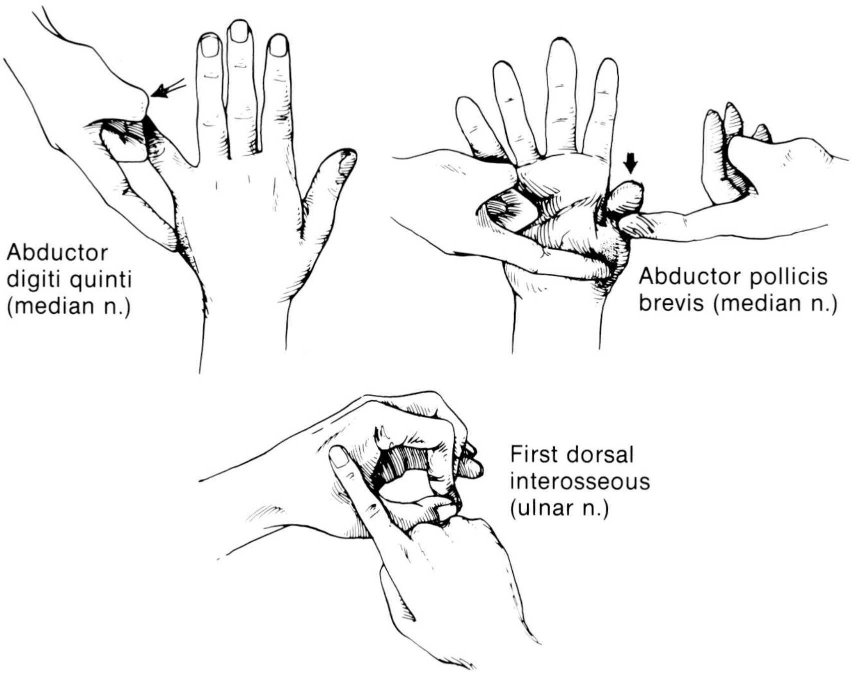

FIG. 62-7. Intrinsic muscle function is checked by palpation of the first dorsal interosseous and the abductor digiti quinti muscles for ulnar nerve function and the abductor pollicis brevis muscle for median-nerve motor-branch function.

nerve will rarely be found after it has undergone wallerian degeneration, so primary repair soon after injury is necessary. The abductor pollicis brevis is the best thenar muscle to test for integrity of the median motor branch. This is done by having the patient abduct his thumb against resistance while the abductor pollicis brevis is palpated (see Fig. 62-7). Following late injury, the defect from the atrophied muscle is apparent, but it is too late to repair, and tendon transfer becomes necessary to restore function. Therefore, it is important to identify paralysis in this muscle after an acute injury while repair can still be accomplished. Circumduction can also be tested using the standard pencil test, but the examiner must remember there is a 12% incidence of anomalous ulnar cross innervation, which may obscure motor median nerve laceration (Fig. 62-8).[39] Because the abductor pollicis brevis is the most likely palpable muscle to be paralyzed, this should always be tested when nerve laceration is suspected. Although this common injury may appear to be a minor laceration, it can lead to major morbidity, requiring tendon transfers if not recognized.

EXTENSOR EXAMINATIONS. Single long extensor tendon lacerations to the fingers are common and are commonly missed. Because of the oblique anatomical attachments between the tendons of the extensor digitorum communis, complete laceration on the back of the hand will produce extensor lag rather than complete inability to extend the MP joint (Fig. 62-9). Although the patient can still extend the finger by means of the juncturae tendinae attachment to the adjacent tendons, he will complain bitterly that "it doesn't feel right." The wise examiner will appreciate the significance of this 15° to 30° "lag" and schedule the patient for tendon repair and possible dynamic splinting of the digit (Fig. 62-10). It is not uncommon for all of the common extensor tendons to be lacerated on the dorsum of the wrist. This permits only the independent index and fifth function so that these two fingers extend even though all of the common extensors are divided.

Disruption of the extensor tendon hood over the PIP joint causes boutonnière deformity. It is important that this be anticipated. Very often, laceration or partial rupture of this structure will not cause any apparent abnormality until the lateral bands migrate downward and the scar over the extensor hood attenuates. Thus, the patient seems normal on initial examination, then the deformity gradually increases days or even weeks following injury (Fig. 62-11). When this injury is suspected, either careful follow-up to diagnose early failure of complete PIP extension or prophylactic extension splinting is mandatory.

Disruption of the extensor lateral bands crossing the DIP joint causes mallet deformity (Fig. 62-12). Similar to late boutonnière, late mallet deformity can occur with injury over the DIP joint. When there is partial laceration of these small thin tendons or an inflammatory process in the skin above them, spontaneous rupture can occur as the patient pulls with his strong flexor profundus tendon. The examiner should anticipate this possibility when there is a deep laceration or inflammation above the DIP joint and prophylactically splint this joint in full extension. When there is definite disruption, the DIP joint should be splinted in some hyperextension, or a lag is likely after healing.

EXAMINATION OF CHILDREN. Although most adults are quickly and easily examined for hand disorders, children require special attention and patience, and the examiner must gain their confidence. Giving them an object or task will often permit adequate observation to make a diagnosis. (The multiply injured patient can also prove difficult to evaluate, especially when there is significant head injury.) If surgery is necessary for other reasons and there is a high index of suspicion, exploration of the hand is warranted to rule out significant injury.

Appreciation of the Most Important Features

NATURE OF THE INJURY. Proper appraisal of an acute hand injury requires an understanding of the nature of the injury. Injuries from a sharp cutting force may produce lacerations in which the damage is confined to a narrow path, whereas injuries with a crushing or tearing force can cause tissue damage that is far more widespread. Knowing the nature of the injury will modify management. For example, repair of a median nerve laceration caused by a sharp knife could be done immediately but that caused by a chainsaw should be delayed. Other important factors associated with the nature of the injury are the degree of bacterial contamination and the degree of devascularization. The management of a blast wound of the hand may require delayed primary closure to assess the degree of muscle devasculari-

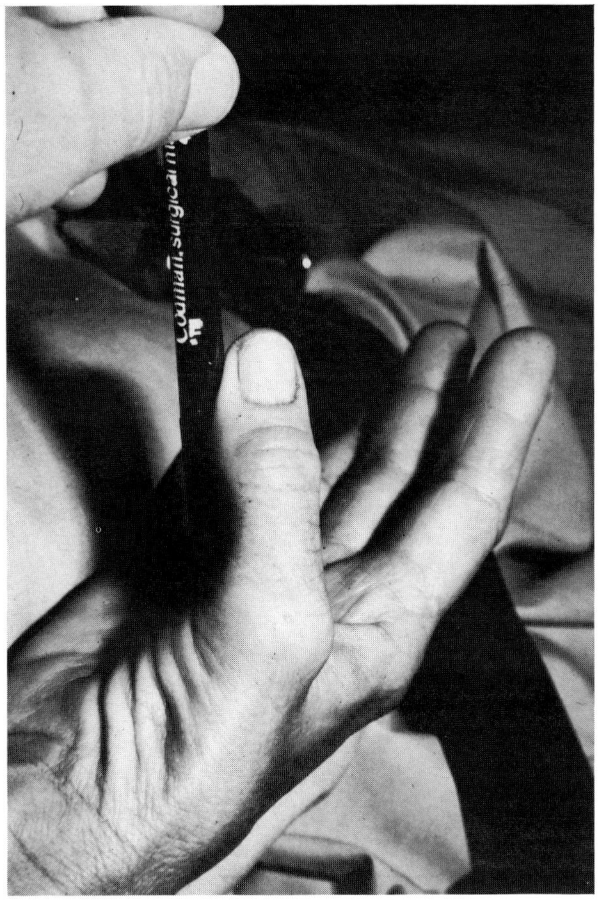

FIG. 62-8. The pencil test for median motor-branch function is misleading if there is anomalous ulnar-nerve crossover as in this patient who performs the test but has paralysis and atrophy of the abductor pollicis brevis muscle.

FIG. 62-9. Only extensor lag occurs with complete laceration of a common extensor tendon on the dorsum because of adjacent pull by the junctura tendinum.

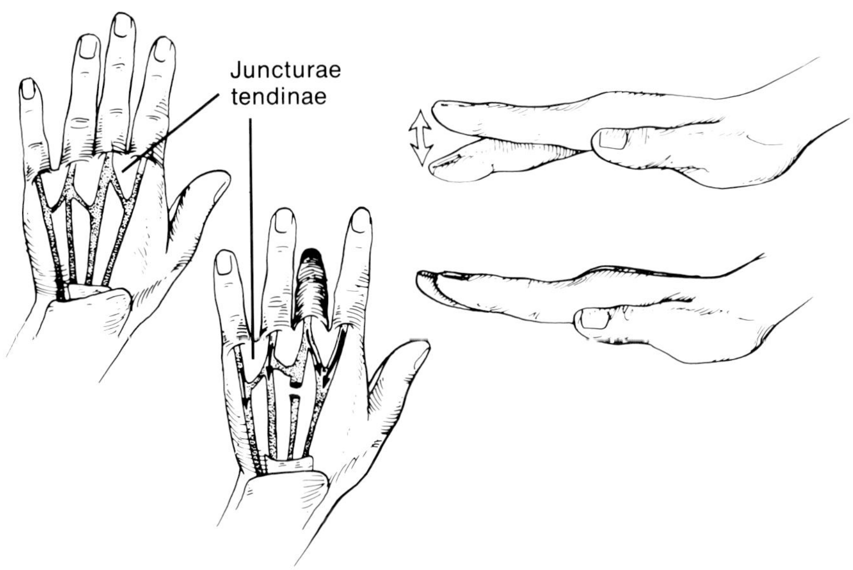

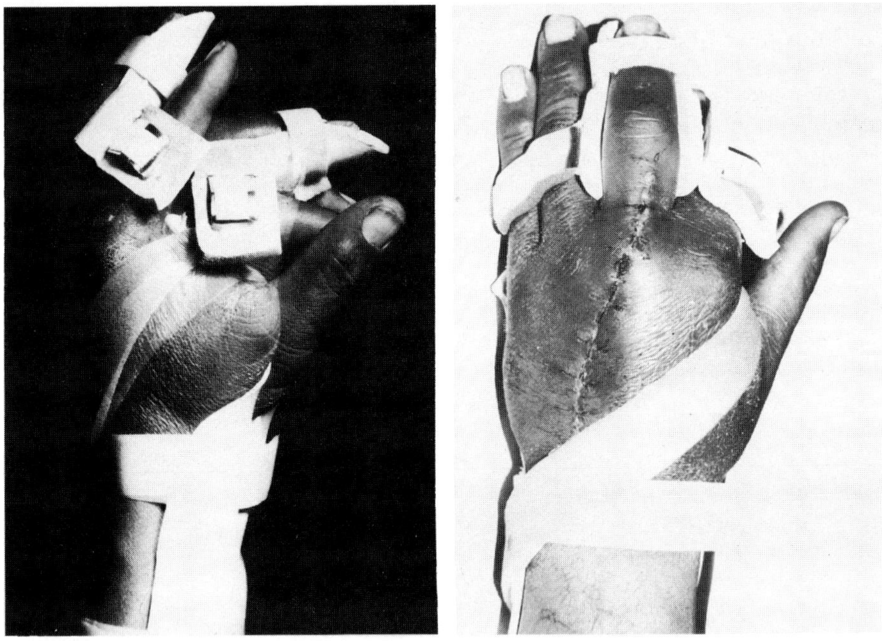

FIG. 62-10. Following repair of a common extensor tendon on the dorsum, motion can be allowed by dynamically splinting that digit in greater extension than adjacent digits and stabilizing the wrist in extension.

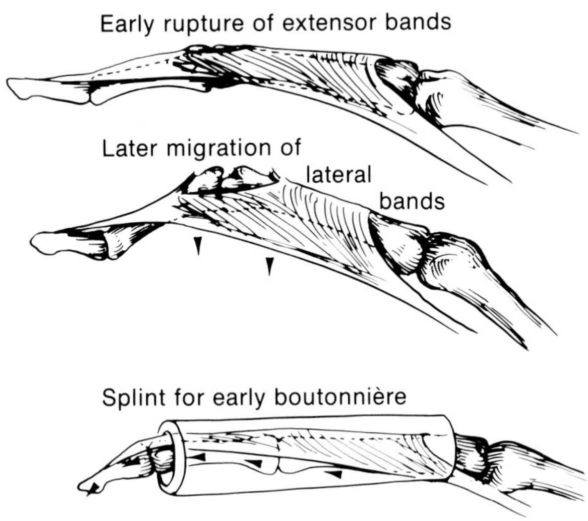

FIG. 62-11. Early boutonnière can be deceptive by delay in the volar migration of the lateral bands. Splinting for boutonnière should permit distal joint flexion to encourage dorsal return of the lateral bands from the resulting tension.

zation accurately, whereas a clean laceration may permit repair of all structures, even in replantation.

TIDY AND UNTIDY WOUNDS. Rank and Wakefield divided open wounds into two classifications, *tidy* and *untidy*.[62] Although most domestic injuries are tidy, it must be remembered that the history may suggest a foreign body buried in the depth of the wounds and that the appearance of the surface wound may have no bearing on the extent of involvement of the deeper structures. The problem in tidy wounds, therefore, is to be suspicious of important deeper injuries. Untidy wounds in which tissues are torn, crushed, or avulsed require the utmost judgment. Because of widespread damage, the surgeon must resist attempting extensive anatomical reconstruction with severely damaged tissues, destined to necrosis. However, the temptation to ablate all damaged tissues must be restrained, recognizing that potential function may be removed. A course midway between these extremes should be charted, neither to carry out extensive reparative surgery with questionable tissue nor needlessly to sacrifice structures solely for the purpose of quick healing. In the severely mutilated hand, there often is advantage in initial débridement of all clearly devitalized and unsalvageable tissues, leaving the wound open and inspecting the tissues of questionable status 5 days later. This management method provides more certainty at the time of delayed wound closure.

INDIVIDUAL NEEDS OF THE PATIENT. Finally, initial appraisal of the most important features of acute hand injury may include the needs of the specific patient. Many times a manual laborer will be best served by amputation of a digit, while a computer operator or fashion model would prefer preservation even though it requires multiple operations with minimal function. It is important to consider an individual's

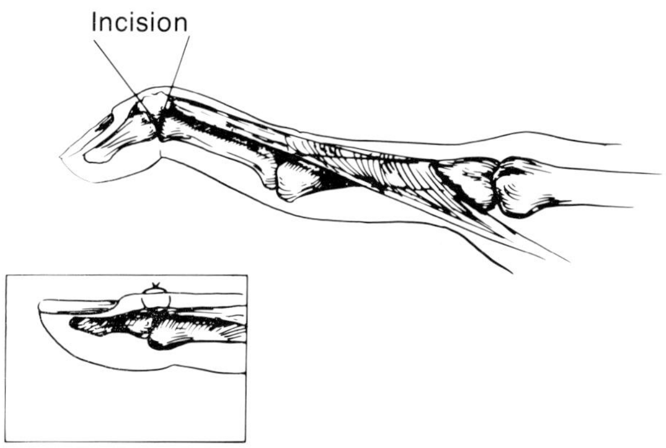

FIG. 62-12. Mallet deformity occurs with the rupture of the lateral bands over the distal interphalangeal joints. Late deformity correction by the Iselin "dermotenodesis" simply excises a tissue wedge above the joint, suturing through the skin and underlying tendon.

hobbies as well as occupation and age in making such judgments. Perhaps the most frequent error is a failure to include the patient in the individual decision. This requires honest communication, explaining limitations. For example, the public is well informed about the possibility of replantation surgery but unaware of the very poor functional results. Once informed of the morbidity rate of salvage procedures, most patients can assist with rational surgical judgment, rather than later express concern about the choices that were made. It is the surgeon's responsibility to offer individual patients any possible choices.

WOUND CARE OF HAND INJURY

Following an accurate examination and appraisal of traumatic hand injury, the wound should be immobilized in a comfortable position and protected by a moist sterile saline dressing until the primary surgical procedure. "Atraumatic technique," a term popularized by Sterling Bunnell, should be employed regardless of whether the injury is handled as an outpatient emergency room procedure or requires major surgery. Meticulous handling of tissue is the essence of hand surgery and will do much to prevent wound infection and avoid unnecessary injury to the delicate anatomical structures. To do so, it is essential to know how to use a tourniquet properly, to manipulate small instruments, and to utilize nonirritating materials for repair of deep structures.

Priorities

When the surgeon confronts a complex injury of the hand, it is necessary to recognize which aspects of repair take precedence and determine the scope of the primary procedure, considering all aspects including both the patient and the procedure.

Vascular Considerations

In acute injury, vascular supply becomes the most important consideration, and when the whole hand or digit is at risk, this cannot be delayed. If the vascular status is clearly embarrassed, it is naive to observe in hopes of improvement. Usually, the injury will lead to edema, further blood supply compromise, and thrombosis. Injuries with a vasospastic component, such as drug injection injuries, often benefit from prolonged sympathetic blocks with long-acting anesthetics; however, acute traumatic injuries with evidence of compromise in the major hand vessels should be explored or at least investigated by Doppler or angiographic study. A delay-and-observe approach will disenfranchise the patient of opportunity for microvascular revascularization because the small vessels will occlude and microvascular reconstruction of common volar or digital arteries will then be of no avail. Where microsurgical facilities are not available and major vascular compromise is suspected, the primary physician should immediately refer the patient. This is true even of massive crush injuries because these can many times be salvaged by multiple long vein grafts to the distal vessels. However, when only skin flaps are of questionable viability and the major vessels of the hand are intact, a wait-and-see approach may be appropriate with delayed débridement; coverage is then possible 3 to 5 days following injury, depending upon viability of the tissues.

Skeletal Stabilization

The next important consideration is stabilization of the skeletal structures of the hand. This may be by internal or external methods. If unstable structures are left unattended, motion may cause vascular or nerve injury and will further increase damage and inflammation. When replantation is done, stabilization is usually accomplished prior to revascularization.

Soft Tissue Coverage

Once the vascular supply is assured and skeletal structures stabilized, attention must be directed to soft tissue coverage. When the viability of muscle or skin flaps is questionable, the surgeon may choose to keep a moist sterile dressing on the defect for a few days before definitive closure.

TENDON AND NERVE REPAIR

Repair of tendons and nerves can be safely delayed beyond the time of injury, provided the wound is cleaned and the skin closed. Indeed, in the untidy questionable injury, secondary repair is usually preferable. In most cases, delayed tendon repair should be accomplished within approximately 10 days.[40] When there has been avulsion or an irregular type injury, such as might be seen with a chainsaw laceration, secondary nerve repair is recommended.[11] A 10-day or longer interval provides opportunity to assess viability of the nerve and to trim the ends accurately before repair. Primary repair of badly contused nerve endings leads to a fibrotic repair site, which may form a barrier to regeneration and lead to a poor result.[9] Indeed, a case can be made for delayed nerve repair in all but the cleanest and sharpest of lacerations. All severed nerves undergo a variable amount of retrograde wallerian degeneration, and in the case of blunt, crushing or avulsion injuries, there is greater proximal degeneration.[18] The amount of time before nerve regeneration reaches the site of nerve repair is also reported to produce an adverse effect on nerve regeneration, probably due to collagen cross linking, which may interfere with axoplasmic growth across the repair site.[53] Therefore, in an avulsion or crushing-type nerve laceration, a better result might be anticipated if regeneration is permitted at the injury site before definitive repair, limiting the amount of time the scar matures at the repair site before axoplasmic growth crosses it. Nerve repair may be delayed many weeks or months without significant problem except that motor recovery will decrease proportionally to the length of time before reinnervation. No muscle function should be expected after 2 years, owing to fibrosis at the motor end plates.[65, 78] However, sensory return may follow nerve repair many years after the injury. When the surgeon anticipates a long interval before regeneration can reach the muscle, early tendon transfers may be worthwhile. At minimum, the patient should be splinted in a functional position.

OPERATIVE PRINCIPLES OF HAND INJURY

Need for Hospitalization and Observation

Hippocrates advocated inspecting injured hands many hours after dressings and immobilization.[59] This principle is still true today. Observation is necessary whenever the injury requires a compressive dressing, because swelling may render this too tight. Usually, this is best accomplished in a hospital where frequent examination, appropriate sedation, constant elevation, and protective inactivity are possible. Nerve injury requires particular attention because the patient is no longer able to recognize the pain and paresthesias of vascular compromise. The classic signs of Volkmann's ischemic contracture should be a major concern when the upper arm or forearm is immobilized in cast or other compressive dressing.[55] These include the "five Ps": paresthesia, pallor, pulselessness, pain with finger extension, and paralysis.[5] This indicates immediate need for release of dressings, better stabilization of fractures, escharotomy, or whatever it takes to correct the vascular compromise. Certainly, this complication is more easily prevented than treated. It is indeed tragic to see a simple injury such as a Colles' fracture render a hand completely useless with no motor or sensory function. Widespread neurolysis and repositioning of median and ulnar nerves in the forearm are recommended for early forearm Volkmann's ischemic contracture.[57] There is no satisfactory late treatment, but free microvascular muscle flap reconstruction has been used to afford flexor replacement.[45]

Volkmann's ischemic contracture of the intrinsic muscles is not as easily recognized and may occur in injuries confined to the hand. The early manifestations include intrinsic tightness and pain when the "intrinsic test" is performed. This consists of placing the MP joint in extension and assessing whether tight intrinsic tendons now cause the IP joints to remain extended or to resist flexion (Fig. 62-13). The surgeon must consider this possibility, or the diagnosis will be overlooked until late contraction and swan neck deformity occur. Early ischemic intrinsic contraction is best handled by intrinsic muscle fasciotomy.[69] Later established ischemic contracture requires intrinsic muscle release (Fig. 62-14). Available data suggest that this ischemia induces myofibroblast formation, activity and contraction in the intrinsic muscle fascia.[44]

Anesthesia

Obviously hands are so sensitive they can replace sight for the blind and talk for the mute. Anesthesia for such a highly sensitive organ must be excellent as surely as if the eye or vocal cord were to be repaired. Acceptable anesthesia may include local nerve blocks, brachial plexus nerve blocks, intravenous Bier blocks, or general anesthesia, depending on the nature of the injury and general medical condition of the patient.

For digital nerve block, it is an error to include epinephrine in combination with a local anesthetic agent because the vasoconstriction may cause thrombosis of the digital arteries and complete loss of a digit. This anesthetic might be useful in proximal nerve blocks because it will prolong the anesthetic effect, but it is contraindicated at levels where distal small arteries are susceptible or damaged tissue can be lost.

Nerve blocks at any level distal to the elbow region can be used satisfactorily in selected cases, and regional infiltration may be sufficient for lacerations or injuries that are confined in the hand. If too much of a local anesthetic agent is injected

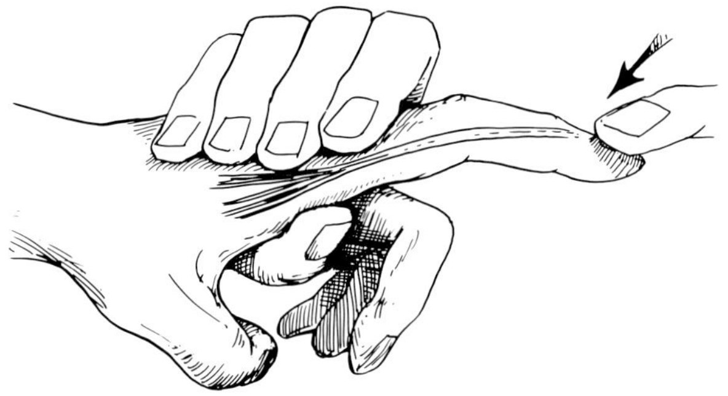

FIG. 62-13. Early intrinsic contracture tested by the intrinsic tightness test extends the MP joint, then tests resistance to IP passive flexion. This is compared to the resistance with the MP joint flexed, relaxing the intrinsic mechanism.

around the proximal phalanx, the vascular supply to a finger may be impaired. It is a safer technique to block the digital nerve in the palm at the level of the distal flexion crease. To do so, the needle is inserted through the soft tissue on the dorsum of the web space and then directed proximally and volarward to the level of the digital nerve. If the surgeon chooses to place the anesthesia in the digital space, he should be careful not to use a large quantity but rather a higher concentration of anesthetic.

The Bier intravenous block may be a highly useful anesthetic when surgery will be of a brief duration and does not require assessment of the viability of tissues.[1] This method involves the use of two tourniquets, the more proximal of which is inflated after exsanguination of the venous blood using an Ace or Esmark bandage, then placing an appropriate quantity of half percent Xylocaine intravenously in the extremity. Although many anesthesiologists prefer to place the intravenous needle distally in the hand, the anesthetic is equally well administered with an intracath in the antecubital fossa, where it may remain during surgery to avoid extravasation of anesthetic from the puncture site, but well away from the operative field. The amount of anesthetic is determined by the patient's weight. Once anesthesia has been achieved, the lower tourniquet, which is in the anesthetized region, can be elevated and will keep the patient from developing tourniquet pain. Care should be taken to wait at least 15 or 20 minutes after anesthesia before releasing these tourniquets, regardless of how rapidly the surgery has been performed. After a quick procedure, such as a dislocated digit, tourniquet release too soon can cause seizures and respiratory arrest. The surgeon must wait until the anesthetic becomes fixed in the extremity. This may also be true when a concentration higher than half a percent of anesthetic is used. Intravenous anesthesia is not recommended for severe open injuries of the hand because it interferes with assessment of viability and also loads the tissues with anesthetic, which will extrude from the lacerations. It is an excellent anesthetic for infections of the hand; however, the hand should be only elevated and not exsanguinated before inflating the tourniquet, and the intravenous needle should be placed well away from the site of infection. Exsanguination in the infected hand will cause the patient undue pain and could force infection into uninvolved adjacent areas.

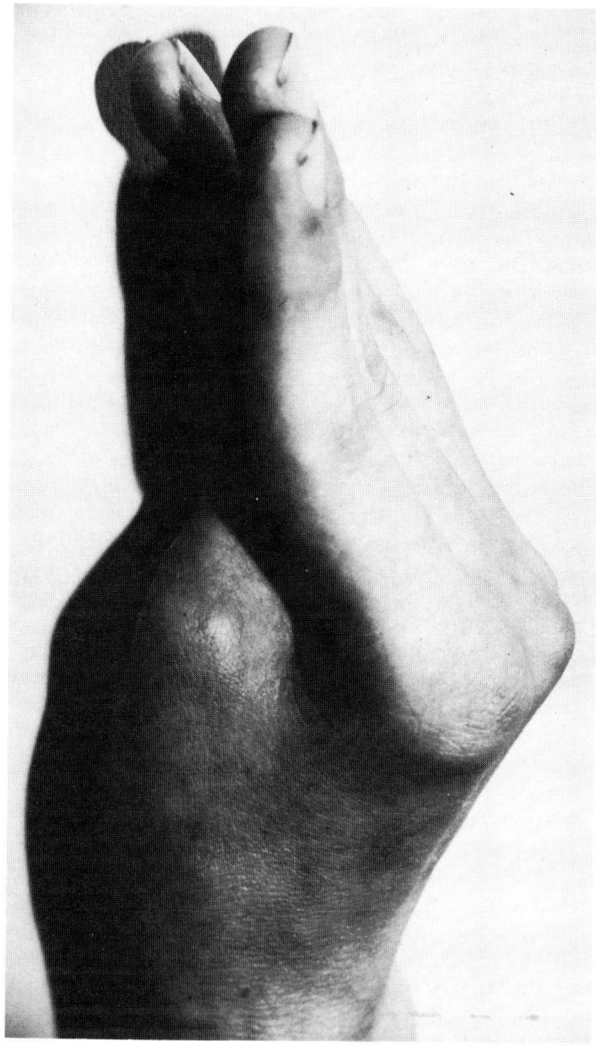

FIG. 62-14. Fixed swan neck deformity from late Volkmann's intrinsic ischemic contracture in a patient with radial artery drug-injection injury.

The Bier block is usually not employed for procedures that take longer than 1 hour. Recently, some surgeons have used long-acting anesthetic agents intravenously, but for most operations of a greater duration, a brachial plexus block or general anesthetic will be preferred.

General anesthesia or brachial plexus block, by either the supraclavicular or axillary method, is generally chosen for the treatment of extensive hand injuries. General anesthesia is usually mandatory if the injury requires a skin graft or pedicle flap from another part of the body. The patient's general welfare is the major consideration in choosing between these two methods. It should be remembered that the anxious patient with questionable cardiorespiratory status is not always best served by an anesthetic method that may increase anxiety during the operation. Sedation of such elderly patients may be associated with profound decrease in arterial oxygenation; therefore, careful anesthesiology monitoring is as necessary when brachial plexus block is employed as when a general anesthetic is used in the high-risk patient. When a prolonged operation is anticipated, the use of long-acting local anesthetic agents for brachial plexus block will not only offer adequate anesthesia but will also afford postoperative pain relief for many hours.

Bloodless Field

When asked why he used a tourniquet, Bunnell quipped, "Would a watchmaker repair a watch in an inkwell?"[12] For the majority of hand operations, a bloodless field is a prerequisite. This not only permits accurate identification of delicate structures with minimal trauma but also obviates the need for repeated irritating sponging in the wound. Most surgeons prefer to use a special pneumatic apparatus, although an ordinary blood pressure cuff or an Esmarch bandage can be used. However, there is a special danger in using the Esmarch because it can deliver pressures as high as 500 torr, and the surgeon has no way accurately to monitor the pressure he applies with this bandage. For that reason, the Esmarch bandage tourniquet should be utilized only when no better apparatus is available. Tourniquet paralysis is reported more frequently from too much pressure than from too great a duration.

Use of any tourniquet can be dangerous unless the surgeon takes a few simple precautions. First, he should be familiar with his tourniquet and confident of its accuracy. It is well known that as rubber components age and become more brittle, errors will occur in the pressure gauge reading. It is a simple matter to check the accuracy of the system against the blood pressure monitor of the anesthesiology cart; many surgeons recommend this be done every 2 weeks, recording the date and error on the cuff so the next surgeon will use it with accuracy. During the operation, many surgeons suggest a reading between 250 torr to 300 torr pressure for adults, 200 to 250 torr for children, and 150 torr for infants. We have preferred simply to use a reading that is 90 torr to 100 torr greater than the patient's systolic pressure, once a steady blood pressure has been achieved. This will afford adequate hemostasis, often at a much lower pressure, and will lessen the tissue injury at the tourniquet site. This is especially useful in patients with capillary fragility, such as those with connective tissue diseases. Tissue damage is also lessened by one or two turns of sheet wadding on the arm beneath the tourniquet. Care must be taken to avoid wrinkling this wadding, or the underlying skin will blister. Although suitable cuffs in smaller sizes are available for children, these narrower cuffs should not be used for adults because they may produce injury. For the adult, the cuff width should not be less than 3 inches. Most surgeons limit tourniquet time to 2 hours. Even with that limit, marked anoxic changes are present and when additional time is needed, the tourniquet should be released for no less than 20 minutes.[77] Thereafter, it should be released every hour.

Troublesome "tourniquet ooze" is a frequent complaint when tedious dissection is needed, as in microsurgery (Fig. 62-15). This occurs due to blood flow through the humerus, which obviously is not collapsed by the tourniquet. Tourniquet ooze can be completely controlled by the Furlow maneuver, which is a simple venous tourniquet applied at the elbow where the ooze must pass out of the humerus at no greater than venous pressure. When tedious dissection is anticipated, tourniquet ooze is prevented by use of this elbow venous tourniquet in association with the upper arm arterial tourniquet.[26]

When only a block in the hand is used, tourniquet pain may become a problem. Most adults will tolerate up to 20 minutes of tourniquet pressure, especially with sedation. If a longer interval is anticipated, local infiltration beneath the skin at the tourniquet site will permit longer use.

Most surgeons use the Esmarch or an Ace bandage to wrap and exsanguinate venous blood before inflating the tourniquet. However, when there is infection, severe injury, or unstable fractures, it is a safer and more humane method simply to elevate the arm for 2 minutes rather than wrapping it before tourniquet inflation.

When injury is severe, such as a crushing avulsion wound, the use of a tourniquet will be variable. A tourniquet may be employed to facilitate identification and repair of deep and delicate structures but must be released to assess the viability of skin and muscle for débridement and repair.

Preparation of the Wound

The temptation to scrub any significant hand injury or infection vigorously and roughly should be resisted and replaced by gentle mechanical cleansing,

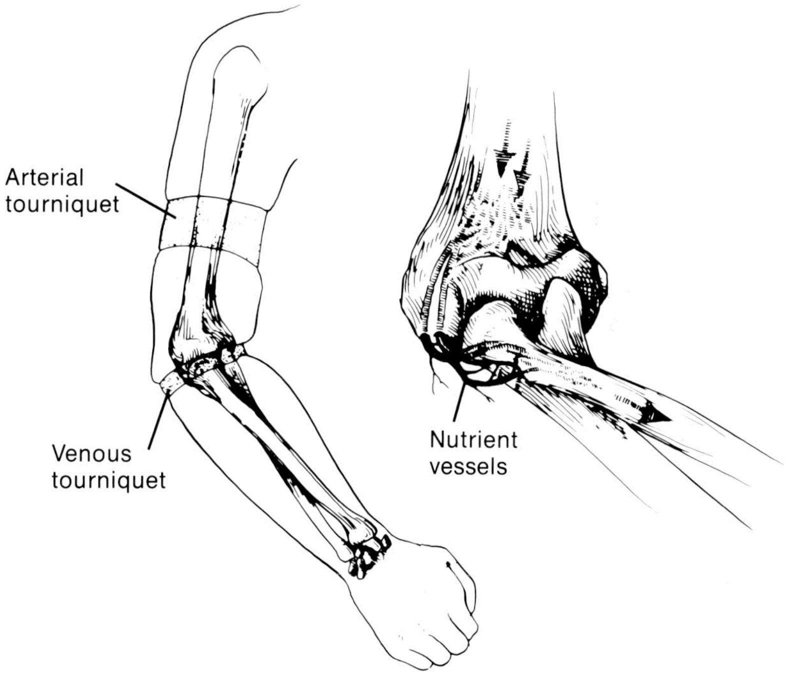

FIG. 62-15. Tourniquet ooze is caused by blood flow through the humerus. This is blocked by the Furlow method of venous tourniquet at the elbow, occluding flow through nutrient vessels.

under sterile conditions, with soap and water. Generous saline irrigations are preferable to use of any antiseptic agent in a wound, and thorough irrigation and preparation of a hand injury usually require adequate anesthesia.

Choice of Incision for Additional Exposure

Thoughtless hand incision, when incisions are erroneously placed across flexion creases or in the highly sensitive digital pulp, may easily convert a simple problem into a complicated contracture or painful scar. The two major principles are never to cross a finger flexion crease inside the "neutral line" and not to place incisions in the most sensitive sites when this can be avoided. The zigzag incision used to expose the finger flexor apparatus has gained recent popularity. Unfortunately, most descriptions of this technique include incision diagonally across the fingertip pulp.[10] This creates an unnecessarily painful scar, and when this incision is used, we recommend a midlateral continuation at its most distal point to avoid this complication (Fig. 62-16). To do so, it is necessary to identify and protect the digital nerve. Whether a Brunner-type zigzag incision or a midlateral linear incision is used in the digit, care should be taken to place the lateral most points near the end of the flexion creases to avoid some degree of scar contracture (see Fig. 62-16). Incisions that cross the wrist should do so in a curved or angled fashion to avoid contracture at that site and, when possible, should be placed on the ulnar side of the median nerve level to avoid injury to the superficially located palmar sensory branch of the median nerve. Incisions at the base of the thumb should take into consideration the very superficial location of the motor branch of the median nerve, and when incisions are placed over the dorsum of the wrist, as frequently needed for ganglionectomy, the location of the superficial branch of the radial nerve must be considered. This nerve probably produces the most frequent and troublesome painful neuroma in the hand and often is needlessly injured during elective minor surgery.

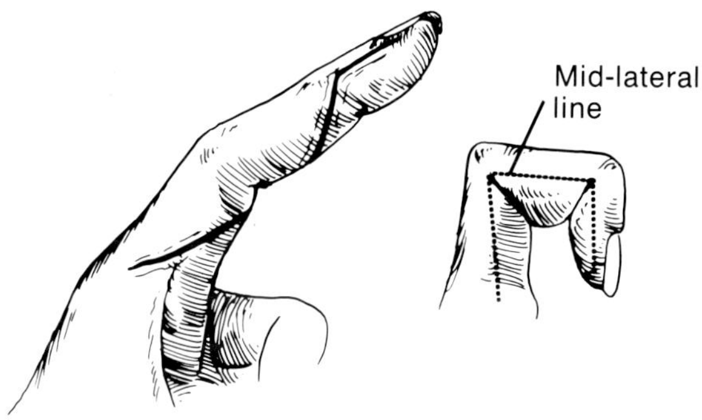

FIG. 62-16. The zig-zag incision can be extended midlaterally in the distal digit to avoid scarring the sensitive pulp. The midlateral line is along the ends of the digital flexion creases, dorsal to neurovascular bundles.

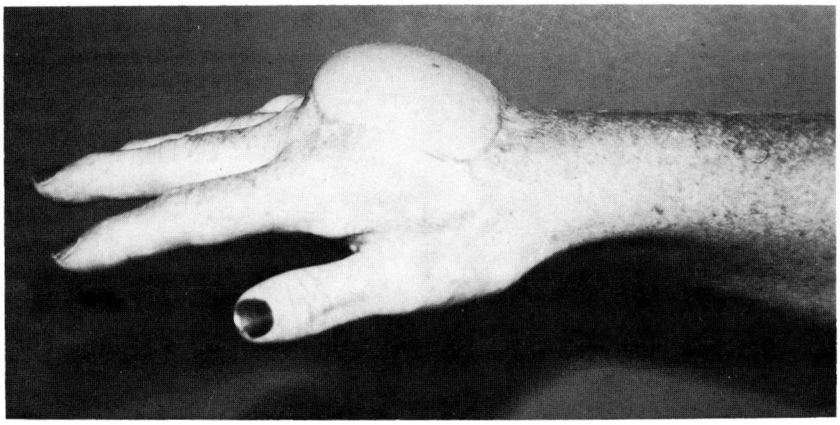

FIG. 62-17. The groin flap on the hand retains the abdominal tendency for fat accumulation, even when it is thinned at surgery.

Débridement

Although removal of devitalized tissue is as important in the hand as in injuries elsewhere, here there must be greater effort to preserve marginal tissue that may be functionally important. Muscle and skin can be assessed with the tourniquet deflated and preserved when their edges bleed. Tendon, ligament, joint capsule, and nerve are not so easily assessed and can usually survive on minimal blood supply; therefore, they should be minimally débrided unless they are clearly damaged beyond recognition or are contaminated. Bone fragments are left in place if they have any soft tissue attachment, since these may later be molded back into proper position.

Wound Closure Techniques

The volar surface of the hand is firmly attached to the bony framework by a fascial network that gives stability with grasp. This also obviates the need for deep sutures when the skin is closed and a single layer of 4-0 or 5-0 nylon or wire suture is all that is required for most skin lacerations. Steristrips are rarely, if ever, indicated for hand lacerations. The combination of sweating and motion will surely cause these strips to depart from the laceration, leaving the wound to heal by secondary intention. When a skin graft is used, it is important to place the hand in a position that produces the maximum-sized recipient site. For example, if the dorsum of the hand is grafted, the MP joint should be placed in maximum flexion. Otherwise, the graft may limit motion after it has healed.

When a skin flap is used, it should be thinned and defatted as much as can be done safely. It is well to remember that these flaps will always maintain the characteristics of the donor site and will never adopt the thin, mobile features of the hand itself. Thus, an abdominal flap will fatten and resemble a "dough ball" if the patient gains weight, unlike the rest of the hand (Fig. 62-17). Many of these fat flaps will require excision of all but the deepest layer with skin grafting of this layer to achieve a satisfactory late cosmetic result. Following closure, the hand should be placed in the position to protect function for hand injury of any consequence (see Fig. 62-2).

Complications of Common Hand Infections

Hand infection no longer poses the major threat to life it did in the preantibiotic days of Kanaval; however, infection still causes major morbidity with hand stiffness the predominant complication. Unfortunately, an undue reliance is now placed on antibiotics, ignoring many of the early principles of hand infection management. Indeed, an attitude may prevail suggesting "wait until it points, then drain it." This leads to greater delay in drainage, prolonged inflammation, and ultimately greater fibrosis, stiffness, and loss of function than is necessary.

MANAGEMENT

The first important principle in hand infection is to make a diagnosis more specific than "hand infection." The management of cellulitis, suppurative tenosynovitis, and thenar web space abscess are all quite different, and only accurate diagnosis will lead to selection of proper management. Second, all patients with hand infection should be placed at rest with the hand immobilized except in streptococcal cellulitis. To allow patients to continue to move interferes with the inflammatory effort to wall off and localize the infection and increases the number of delicate hand structures involved with infection and inflammation. Much morbidity could be eliminated by simply placing the infected hand at rest in the position to protect function (see Fig. 62-2). Third, the surgeon who diagnoses hand infection should immediately place the patient on antibiotics that will cover penicillin-resistant staphylococci and penicillin-sensitive streptococci because these two organisms are responsible for 78% of hand infections.[20] After drainage, specific cultures may lead to an even better selection of antibiotics. Fourth, immediate drainage of abscesses should be planned, and the hand should be placed at complete rest, both before and after drainage. If the anatomical location of the infection is unclear, it is reasonable to place the patient at rest on antibiotics until further localization allows a more specific diagnosis. This is best done in the hospital with frequent examination of the hand in order to drain it at the earliest possible time. Finally, once a hand infection has been well drained and the postoperative inflammation and edema have subsided, usually in 3 to 5 days, all attention should be directed to active and passive mobilization before the newly synthesized collagen induced by inflammation can cross link and cause permanent stiffness. A good hand therapist can be invaluable at this time.

CELLULITIS

Most hands carry a bacterial flora with a colony count of approximately 10^3 streptococcal and staphylococcal organisms, and this may become the inoculum when there is puncture wound of the hand. However, serum aliquot studies show greater natural serum resistance to staphylococci than streptococci. Indeed, it appears that the fatty acid layer of the skin is the major barrier to streptococcal infection, explaining why small puncture wounds of the hand often lead to the characteristic red streaking of streptococcal lymphangitis rather than to abscess formation from staphylococcal infection. When streptococcal lymphangitis is diagnosed, only penicillin and reassurance are needed. However, the surgeon must be wary of the possibility of a primary staphylococcal or coliform abscess with secondary streptococcal lymphangitis. For that reason, it is necessary to examine the patient diagnosed with streptococcal lymphangitis a day or two after penicillin therapy has been initiated. If there has been no significant improvement, immobilization and close observation are indicated to be certain the lymphangitis is not secondary to an occult abscess from another organism.

COLLAR BUTTON ABSCESS

Laborers who use tools and military personnel who carry weapons are frequent victims of collar button abscess at the site of a palmar callus. On examination, this can be deceptive because the palmar fascia is unyielding and there is dorsal swelling from the lymphatic drainage. The unwary surgeon may misinterpret these findings as a dorsal abscess and drain the wrong site when on careful palpation the patient will pinpoint the right location on the palm (Fig. 62-18). The popular management method of placing the patient on antibiotics and waiting for the abscess to "point" to the surface is to be condemned. Should the infection find easier access to the midpalmar space than through the dense fascial layers of the palmar surface, it may erode along the lumbrical canals and destroy the finger web skin, as in the patient illustrated in Figure 62-19. The proper management of collar button abscess is immediate drainage and débridement of necrotic material from the abscess and callus.[17] Staphylococci are almost always present, and the wound can be left open to heal by secondary intention. This surgery must be done under tourniquet control to ensure preservation of the digital nerves and vessels as this necrotic

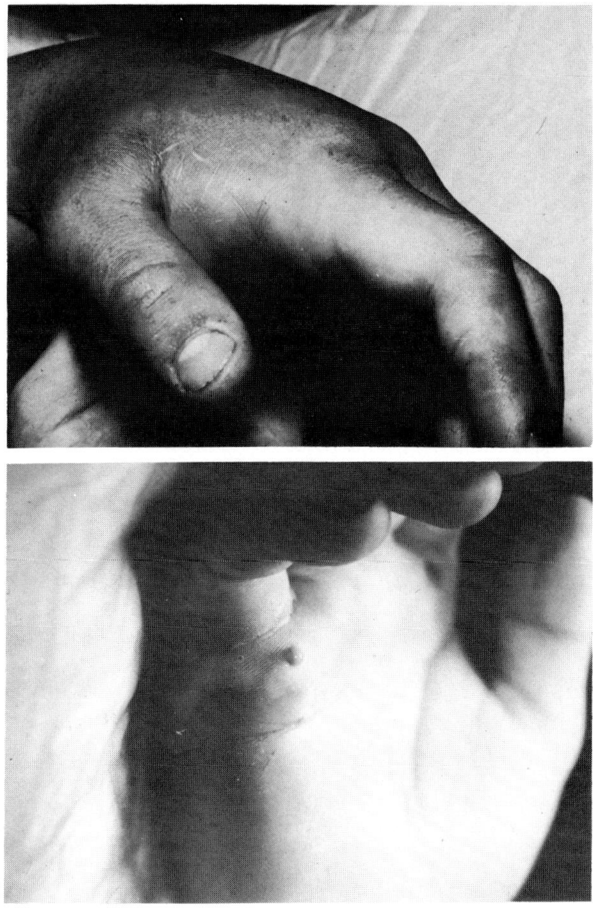

FIG. 62-18. Collar-button abscess causes predominantly dorsal hand swelling.

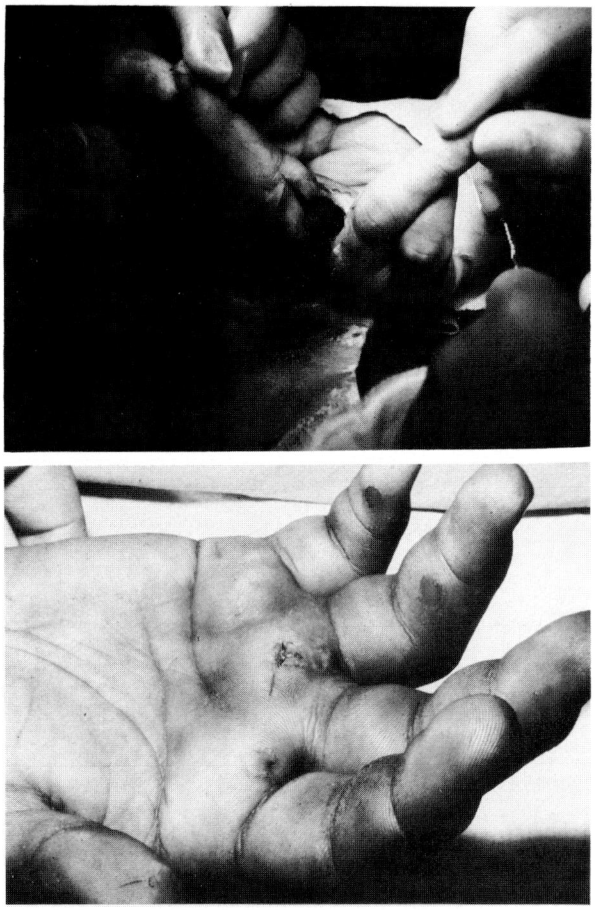

FIG. 62-19. Collar-button abscess that eroded into the midpalmar, then lumbrical spaces, causing finger-web loss. The patient had been on only antibiotic therapy.

material is débrided. The hand should be placed at rest immediately afterward.

MIDPALMAR SPACE INFECTION

Most midpalmar space infections occur from a deep puncture wound or an extension of a collar button abscess. If not drained, they will likely lead to lumbrical canal involvement and may cause loss of finger web tissue (Fig. 62-19). Drainage should be parallel to a palmar crease, and any necrotic material should be débrided.

THENAR SPACE INFECTION

Most thenar space infections also occur from inoculation of the potential space by direct puncture wounds. Drainage over the thenar surface may lead to a painful scar or injury to the motor branch of the median nerve. Therefore, it is better to place the incision on the dorsal aspect of the thumb web, then to enter the thenar space through the adductor fascia. The thenar space can be adequately drained by this approach without danger of injury to the motor branch of the median nerve and avoiding a painful scar over the important sensitive thenar eminence. However, when the abscess has already advanced through the palmar fascia to the thenar skin, careful direct drainage and débridement may as well be instituted (Fig. 62-20).

DIGITAL SPACE INFECTION

Puncture wounds and calluses over the proximal and middle phalangeal areas of the fingers are the usual cause of digital space infection. Although the finger may become quite tense over the space involved, these infections do not usually enter the flexor tendon sheath and are distinguishable from suppurative tenosynovitis by the absence of tenderness along the flexor tendon sheath proximal or distal to the involved digital space. Extension of the digit, however, may be quite painful when involvement is severe, and the diagnosis can be confused

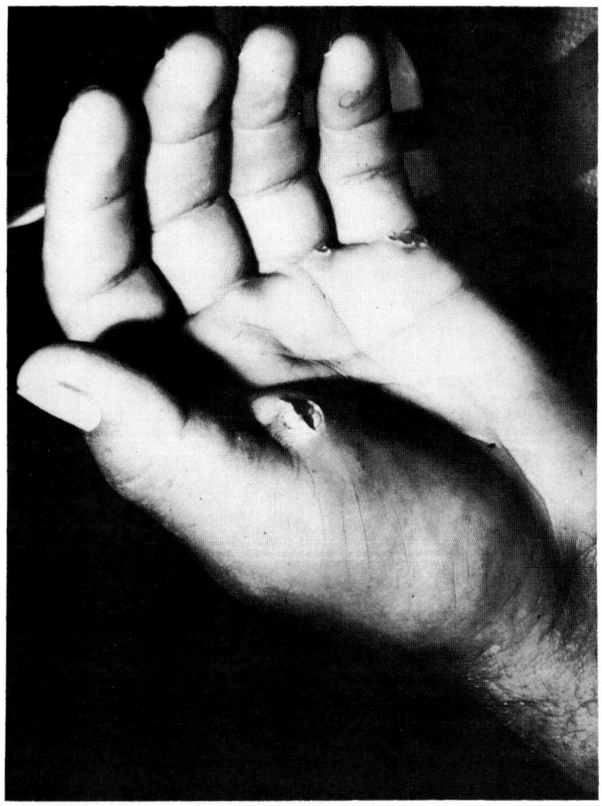

FIG. 62-20. Thenar-space abscess from a puncture wound.

with suppurative tenosynovitis if the flexor tendon sheath region is not palpated. It is important to avoid entering the uninvolved tendon sheath in these patients; the infection will not usually invade this barrier even though it may be so extensive as to cause major skin loss, occlusion of the digital vessels, and anesthesia of the digital nerves (Fig. 62-21). In patients with digital space infection, the tendency to treat this with antibiotics and observation alone leads to occlusion of the vessels in this closed space. Early drainage is of great importance in these infections. When there is severe digital space infection, as may be seen with a fish fin injury, there may be anesthesia distal to the site of infection. This anesthesia indicates that the outcome for useful function is questionable even with immediate drainage and débridement. It should be regarded as an ominous finding.

Felon

Digital space infection of the finger pulp in the region of the distal phalanx deserves special consideration. Because the skin of the finger pulp is densely adherent to the distal phalanx by means of fibrous septa, infection from a puncture wound in this highly vulnerable region will not produce noticeable swelling, and the seriousness of the condition may not be appreciated (Fig. 62-22). However, patients will complain bitterly, the most characteristic lament being that they cannot sleep because of throbbing severe pain. The fingertip itself will be highly tender, and this history and finding should lead the surgeon to drain the digital pulp immediately and place the patient on antibiotics. If it is left untreated or treated only by antibiotics, one of three serious complications will likely occur. The least serious of these is spontaneous rupture and drainage through the pulp surface (Fig. 62-23). Although this affords relief, the site of spontaneous drainage is likely to be on an opposing surface and leave a large painful scar. The patient is better served with either a laterally placed incision or drainage at the site of maximal tenderness (see Fig. 62-22). Second, avascular necrosis of the distal phalanx occurs if there is no spontaneous rupture through the surface because as the pressure increases in the enclosed pulp space, the blood supply to the distal phalanx becomes compromised. This will not be so bad if secondary osteomyelitis of the phalanx does not occur.

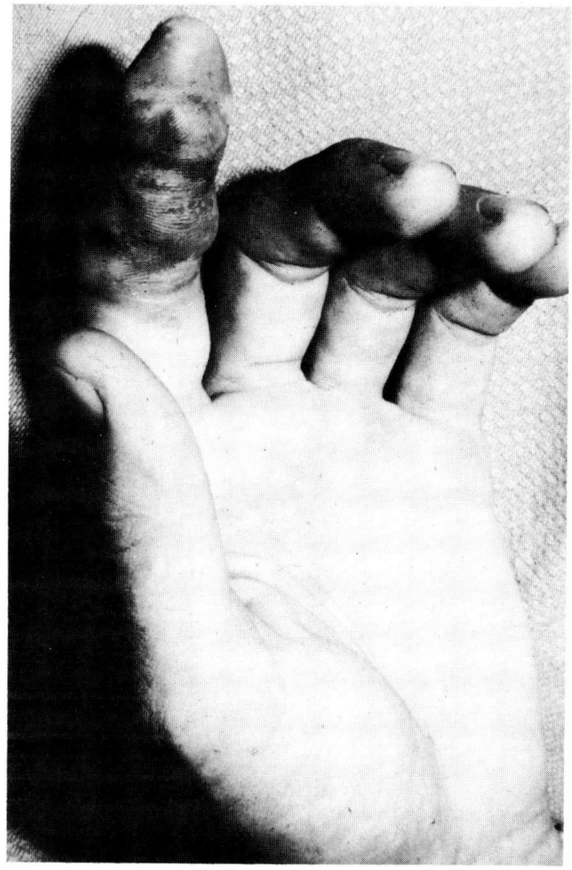

FIG. 62-21. Late digital space infection.

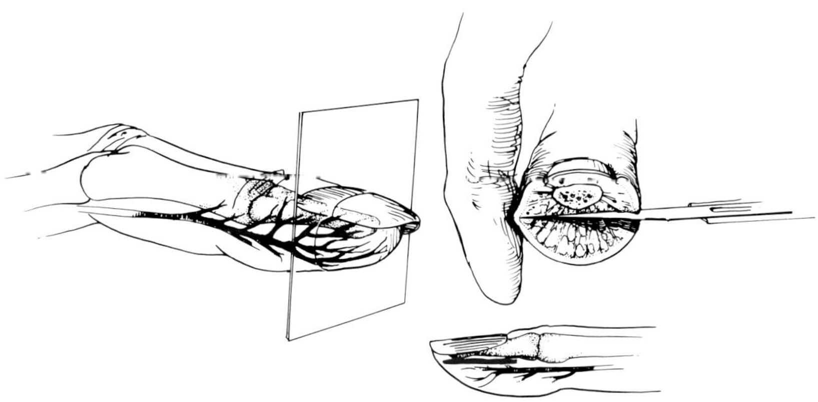

FIG. 62-22. Felons have minimal swelling and maximal pain owing to the fibrous attachments between skin and bone. Incisions should cross the attachments but remain dorsal to the neurovascular branches.

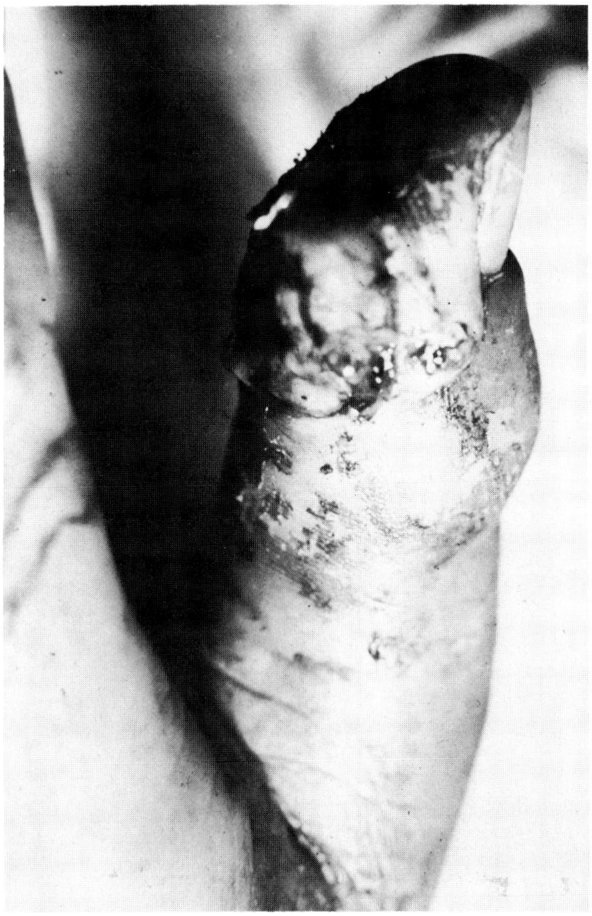

FIG. 62-23. Spontaneous rupture of a felon.

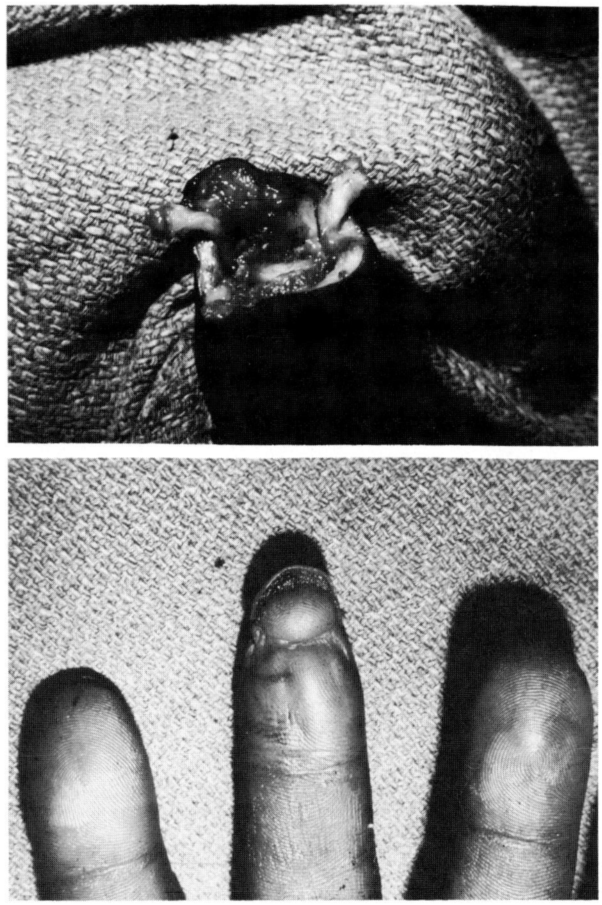

FIG. 62-24. Painful digital neuromas from a felon fish-mouth incision. The neuromas were resected and the nerve ends repositioned dorsally using chromic sutures.

Indeed, it is well shown that revascularization and reossification often occur in late treated felon.[66] However, if the devascularized bone develops osteomyelitis, then it becomes necessary to débride all bone that is infected. Certainly, this complication is far more easily prevented than treated. Finally, when osteomyelitis of the distal phalanx becomes established, suppurative tenosynovitis may occur owing to involvement of the flexor profundus insertion on the distal phalanx. This necessitates wide débridement of all infected distal phalanx and thorough drainage along the entire flexor tendon sheath.

There is current literature supporting a "conservative" felon management of waiting until the abscess has eroded to the surface to drain it where it presents.[66] This management should be condemned. For humanitarian reasons alone, early drainage should be performed to give relief, as well as to prevent all three possible complications. Morbidity from early diagnosis and drainage is minimal. Simple felon drainage should be an emergency room outpatient procedure under digital block anesthesia. The old fish mouth incision across the fingertip creates significant morbidity and has little or no justification (Fig. 62-24). There are two preferred incisions. One is midlateral along the pulp, not crossing the fingertip and not passing the knife through the opposite side but dividing all of the fibrous septa. This can be accomplished by palpating the blade tip through the intact skin of the other side (see Fig. 62-22). With this incision, care must also be taken to avoid a proximal sweep of the knife along the base of the phalanx, or the flexor profundus tendon insertion might be cut. Other surgeons advocate early incision at the site of maximal tenderness to minimize nerve and septa damage.[36] Postoperatively, a small drain may be left in place a few days, and the patient may be sent home on antibiotics and analgesics. Follow-up is necessary to be certain osteomyelitis did not occur, although most patients will return only to praise the dramatic relief of pain.

DIGITAL SUPPURATIVE TENOSYNOVITIS

The four signs of Kanaval offer the best diagnostic criteria for digital suppurative tenosynovitis, an uncommon but very important surgical emergency.[31] These include diffuse swelling along the finger, which may be minimal; inability to extend the digit completely, owing to pain; tenderness along the entire flexor tendon sheath from its insertion at the distal phalanx to the cul-de-sac in the distal palmar crease over the MP joints; and, finally, maintenance of a rigid semiflexed position. Perhaps the mesotenon of the tendon sheath should be thought of as the peritoneum of the flexor tendon cavity. Mesotendonitis is like peritonitis, causing tenderness to palpation, diffuse distention along its entire surface, and rigidity. Like peritonitis, another striking finding may be chills and fever in some patients. Even with early diagnosis and surgical treatment, suppurative tenosynovitis still has significant morbidity owing to the development of hand stiffness. When the surgeon considers the tendon's fragile blood supply through the vincula within this fibrocartilagenous tube, it is easy to see how the pressure of infection can cause loss of this delicate blood supply, leading to fibrosis and adhesion formation.

Most patients with digital suppurative tenosynovitis are inoculated through a puncture wound over the finger flexion crease. Skin at this location is directly over the sheath and even a small, innocent-seeming wound may penetrate directly into this synovial cavity. The patient may not even be aware of injury, but when findings lead to this diagnosis, immediate drainage is indicated. This procedure should be performed in a major surgical facility with excellent anesthesia and tourniquet control. The degree of involvement will determine whether the procedure will consist of a simple midline incision and drainage of the puncture site of the sheath or whether the entire flexor sheath is exposed and constant flow irrigation catheters placed. Suppurative tenosynovitis is a condition requiring the utmost judgment by an experienced hand surgeon. Even then, the results are often disappointing, especially if diagnosis has been delayed.

HUMAN BITE INFECTION

As many as 50% of hand injuries from human tooth wounds may have significant complications.[24] These consist of osteomyelitis, septic joints, and amputation. It is well shown that the length of time before institution of therapy has the highest correlation of any factor with development of significant complications. In light of the usual mechanism of injury, an intoxicated fist into teeth, it is easy to see how a sobering delay may occur. The mouth flora include anaerobic streptococci and bacteroides. These, along with the staphylococcal inoculum from the skin, can cause a synergistic infection that is difficult to control. Furthermore, the skin wound of the fist is removed from the inoculum into adjacent dense connective tissue of the joint capsule or tendon once the fist is opened, setting up an ideal environment for anaerobic organisms from the mouth. Most patients with human bites should be hospitalized, their wounds thoroughly débrided and irrigated, and intravenous antibiotics administered because of the rate of morbidity associated with these injuries.

PARONYCHIA

Paronychia, small staphylococcal infections beneath the fingernail cuticle, are common and usually easily handled by opening the involved region and permitting exit of the small pocket of staphylococci. Antibiotics and warm soaks may also speed recovery. Left untreated or treated only by antibiotics, the entire nail matrix may become involved, lead to erosion into the pulp space and felon formation, and finally advance to osteomyelitis of the phalanx and possible suppurative tenosynovitis of the finger. Certainly, there should be no reluctance to open the small area between the cuticle and the nail and avoid these possible sequelae. The surgeon should try to identify *Herpes zoster* of the finger, which may present as either paronychia or felon. Herpes will usually have characteristic small vesicles and more diffuse skin involvement, and often a history will help the diagnosis. It is common among intensive-care personnel who have handled tracheostomy sites.

Complications of Tendon Injuries

FLEXOR TENDON LACERATIONS

The most frequent complication of flexor tendon lacerations in the finger is a poor amplitude of motion. Under the best of surgical care, an adult with flexor tendon lacerations in the "no man's land" region of the tendon sheath should not expect to regain completely normal amplitude of flexion. The inability to restore normal gliding to this important structure is primarily a biologic, not technical, problem. However, technique does play an important role in obtaining the best possible result, and the inexperienced hand surgeon should carefully cleanse and close the skin wound, immobilize the hand, and refer the patient to someone who can perform definitive repair within 7 to 10 days. Failure to immobilize the hand can lead to pull on the delicate vincula of the proximal lacerated tendon, which may tear this blood supply, causing the tendon end to retract to the palm. This increases the amount of resultant inflammation and the length of incision needed to find the tendon and further devascularizes the repair site.

Current research on tendon healing clearly shows that chicken flexor tendons can heal from their intrinsic blood supply, synovial nutrition alone, or by adhesion formation with blood supply through the adhesions.[42, 46, 61] Indeed, chicken and human tendons isolated in tissue culture show a basic intrinsic capacity to heal even in the absence of blood supply, synovial fluid, or adhesions.[4] No one knows just how human tendons will heal when lacerated. All these different mechanisms may exist simultaneously, and each may predominate variously. However, the hand surgeon should expect human tendons to heal predominantly by adhesion formation and should adopt measures to encourage "favorable scar" in these adhesions. These measures include very delicate handling of the mesotenon surface of the tendon, use of suture techniques that do not strangulate the tendon, careful approximation of the tendon ends so that "raw" cut tendon surface is not exposed, and delay in repair if the digit is greatly contaminated or widely damaged. When a compound fracture or contused and contaminated tissue are present, "unfavorable" adhesions should be anticipated, and repair or later tendon grafting should be delayed. Favorable tendon adhesions are capable of remodeling with hand therapy, permitting a functional degree of gliding for the patient's needs. The concept of "breaking adhesions" should be condemned because this causes increased inflammatory response and can increase new adhesion formation. Surgical tenolysis should be used when adhesions cannot remodel adequately after 3 months of well-conducted hand therapy. This will benefit patients fortunate enough to have an isolated area of unfavorable adhesion formation, as though the tendon were "spot welded" at one site. Patients with dense adhesions along much of the tendon surface will reform adhesions after tenolysis in spite of excellent amplitude in the operating room and excellent therapy following tenolysis. These may later require two-staged tendon grafting with use of a Silastic tendon rod.

When digital nerve injury is associated with tendon laceration, both can be repaired and immobilized for 3 weeks. If only one digital nerve is involved, there will be no unfavorable effect on the outcome; however, if both nerves are lacerated, it is more difficult for the patient to mobilize the insensible digit, and the final range of motion will be somewhat compromised.[6]

One of the most frequent preventable complications from flexor tendon repair is the inability to extend the interphalangeal joints fully. The delicate intrinsic extensor hood mechanism is weaker than the repaired flexor profundus and cannot overcome remodeled and shortened volar plates on the flexor side of the finger. Wrist extension is far more easily recovered than is finger interphalangeal extension, and the MP joints benefit from immobilization in flexion. Therefore, the proper position for hands with repaired flexor tendons in the finger is with the MP joints in almost 90° of flexion, the interphalangeal joints in almost full extension, and the wrist in adequate flexion to remove tension from the repair site. Most patients remain in this position for 3 weeks following repair.

EXTENSOR TENDON INJURIES

Whereas the major problem in flexor tendon injury is inadequate gliding caused by adherence, extensor tendon injury complications are usually from incomplete restoration of motion caused by attenuation and elongation. These problems can often be prevented merely by early diagnosis and appropriate protection of the patient, but function can be extremely complex to restore once the deformity is established.

Extensor Hood Laceration: Boutonnière Deformity

One of the most treacherous extensor injuries is laceration or rupture of the extensor hood mechanism. The initial appearance is deceptive. The patient may have minimal or no obvious problem until the lateral bands slide further to the volar side of the PIP joint, giving the characteristic flexion deformity of the proximal interphalangeal joint and hyperextension of the distal interphalangeal joint, called *boutonnière* or buttonhole deformity (see Fig. 62-11). When the hood has been repaired or when rupture or attenuation is suspected, it is imperative to immobilize the PIP joint completely in full extension and maintain this position 4 to 6 weeks. It is advantageous to leave the distal joint free to flex in this splint because, with flexion of the distal joint, the pull on the lateral bands will encourage a more dorsal position at the proximal interphalangeal joint (see Fig. 62-11). It is not necessary to immobilize the MP joint with this splint. Whenever the surgeon suspects injury to the extensor hood, this splint should be used, or at minimum the patient should be reexamined in a few days to be certain that normal extension of the proximal interphalangeal joint has been maintained. Extensor hood attenuation leading to boutonnière deformity can occur from infection of the skin over the proximal interphalangeal joint or from a deep second-degree burn in this region. The inflammatory response alone can cause remodeling of this delicate adjacent structure, the thoughtful surgeon will anticipate this possibility and protect the extensor hood, thereby preventing this difficult complication. Once established, boutonnière deformity is among the most difficult of hand conditions to treat successfully. Whether the patient will be best served by the Fowler procedure, dividing the lateral bands over the middle phalanx to release the distal joint hyperextension, exploration and late repair of the hood itself to reposition the lateral bands, tendon grafting of the hood mechanism, or acceptance of the deformity is a highly individual decision to be reached according to the degree of deformity and the particular patient's functional problems.[21, 25] Certainly, early proper management is easier than making difficult judgments once this deformity becomes established.

MALLET DEFORMITY

Rupture of the weak lateral bands as they cross the distal interphalangeal joint is common in injuries in which direct force is exerted against the extended fingertip, such as a "baseball injury." The deceptive feature in this injury is the possibility of a perfectly normal range of motion immediately afterward because the bands are only 98% ruptured or their insertion on a distal phalanx fracture fragment is not yet displaced. Later, the patient may finish rupturing the tendons or may displace a fracture fragment to develop progressive mallet deformity (see Fig. 62-12). As in boutonnière deformity, inflammatory conditions such as severe paronychia or laceration over the distal joint may lead to attenuation of these lateral bands; this should be anticipated by the attending surgeon. Late mallet deformity is associated with progressive uncomfortable hyperextension of the proximal interphalangeal joint. The late deformity is most easily and successfully repaired by the Iselin "tenodermodesis" technique, which simply reestablishes the original injury by resecting skin and scar and repairing the skin and tendon defects with a single layer of sutures.[29] The patient should be immobilized in slight DIP hypertension as for an acute injury.

COMMON EXTENSOR TENDON LACERATIONS

Failure to diagnose isolated laceration of long extensor tendons is common because of their unique anatomical arrangement on the back of the hand. The junctura tendinae attachments between adjacent long extensor tendons permit some deceptive digital extension even though the tendon is completely divided proximal to these attachments (see Fig. 62-9). However, these attachments do not permit full extension, and the small amount of extensor "lag" in the lacerated digit should alert the surgeon. When a suspicious laceration of the hand is associated with a 15° to 30° lack of extension, complete laceration of the extensor digitorum communis to that digit should be expected and surgical repair initiated.

The two most common complications following extensor tendon repair are lack of full extension due to lengthening at the repair site and loss of MP flexion from remodeled collateral ligaments. Both can be minimized by proper management. Attenuation and lengthening of the extensor tendon repair site are fairly common, causing persistent extensor "lag." This is usually due to inadequate immobilization so that the powerful flexor tendons can exert their full force on the weak extensor repair site before collagen cross linking permits sufficient tensile strength to resist slippage of subunits and lengthening of the scar. Some type of protection from the full flexor force should be used for up to 6 weeks after extensor tendon repair to prevent this complication. However, prolonged immobilization of the MP joints in extension is likely to permit remodeling of the lax collateral ligaments of the joint and lead to a loss of flexion. One conservative method to manage this injury is to use wrist and limited MP joint extension immobilization 3 or 4 weeks after repair and then only wrist extension splinting for an additional 2 to 3 weeks while full MP joint motion is recovered. During this initial immobilization, interphalangeal joint flexion contracture must be avoided.

At the Medical College of Virginia, we have used dynamic splinting with immediate motion in reliable patients following isolated extensor tendon repair. This method takes advantage of the single motor system of the extensor digitorum communis by placing the injured digit in approximately 25° more extension than the adjacent normal digits, creating less tension on the repaired tendon than on its intact neighbor. By maintaining this relationship, the MP joints may pass through a normal range of motion except that the injured digit is always held in 25° more extension. The wrist is also protected in extension for a month to reduce tension, and the splint is maintained for 6 weeks (see Fig. 62-10). Our early results using this method are encouraging, avoiding both complications of attenuation of the repair site and remodeling of the collateral ligament.

WRIST EXTENSOR LACERATIONS

Wrist extension has been termed the "key to hand function." Indeed, loss of wrist extension causes wrist flexion with attempted power grip, rendering the hand relatively useless unless it is stabilized with a splint. Although wrist extensors are amazingly powerful muscles, they have a relatively short amplitude of motion.[35] Therefore, when these important tendons are divided, repair should be done as soon as safely possible to avoid remodeling of the muscle fascia in a contracted position. Such remodeling will cause loss of tone and amplitude in these important muscles. The technique of repair is less important provided it is secure and the wrist is protected in extension for 3 or 4 weeks. When a laceration of wrist extensors is badly contused, avulsed, or infected, repair may not be safe. Under these circumstances, the cut ends of the wrist extensor tendons may be sutured to adjacent dense connective tissue or to bone in such a way that muscle tone can be preserved for later definitive repair or tendon grafting.[51]

Complications of Common Hand Fractures

Stiff digits are probably the most common complication following treatment of simple hand fractures. Much of this problem could be avoided by simply adhering to the concept of immobilization in the position-to-protect function to the extent the specific fracture allows (see Fig. 62-2). When a patient presents with only a broken bone, an unfortunate result would be shortened volar plates, causing loss of interphalangeal extension, and tight collateral ligaments, causing loss of MP flexion.

A frequent misconception, which leads to prolonged immobilization and stiffness, is that x-ray evidence of callus formation is needed before mobilizing the hand. Simple fractures of phalanges and metacarpals are stable at 3 weeks following injury if they have been properly immobilized. Although x-ray films will not show union, it is safe to mobilize these patients, while protecting them from severe stresses at the fracture site for another week or so. Unnecessarily long immobilization of these fractures produces unnecessarily stiff finger joints.

Additional less frequent hand fracture complications include malunion, nonunion, joint instability, and traumatic arthritis.

PHALANGEAL FRACTURES

When "crush" injuries cause a fractured tuft of the distal phalanx, management is to rest the digit and advise the patient that this will be very tender for a prolonged period of time. However, if the dorsal area of the interphalangeal joint is involved, special attention should be directed toward immobilization in distal interphalangeal hyperextension to avoid the complication of late mallet formation from displacement of the fracture fragment or from the inflammatory process causing attenuation of the lateral bands. This is especially likely if a fracture involves the dorsal edge of the distal phalanx where the lateral bands insert. Three weeks' immobilization is usually adequate for union of the fracture site. Maintaining patients with distal phalangeal fractures in extension will afford greater comfort as well as protect the lateral bands and the length of the volar plate. Flexion of the DIP joint is far more easily recovered by the powerful flexor profundus tendon than extension is by the weak lateral bands. Therefore, the position of distal interphalangeal joint extension is preferred for almost all fingertip injuries.

Most phalangeal fractures will heal with simple splinting unless there has been tissue loss or unstable comminution, whereupon Kirschner wire fixation may be required. The most likely complication, stiffness of adjacent joints, is usually a flexion contracture of the proximal interphalangeal joint due to volar plate shortening. Whenever fractures cannot be properly reduced and aligned without markedly flexing this joint, it is far better to use Kirschner wires or miniplate fixation to avoid a prolonged position in flexion.

Fracture dislocation of the proximal interphalangeal joint poses a very special problem with frequent complications. Management of this difficult injury requires careful judgment about the degree of injury and sometimes the specific needs of the patient. The inexperienced hand surgeon should consult in dealing with this difficult injury rather than using a standard "splint 3 weeks" approach. The likely problems include failure to correct the dislocation, instability at the site of injury, stiffness, and late traumatic arthritis. To minimize these complications, the surgeon should reduce the dislocation under a local anesthetic and then have the patient attempt range of motion against gravity to verify the degree of stability. When the fracture dislocation cannot be reduced or held in position or when greater than one third of the joint surface is involved, open reduction and internal fixation are indicated. In many of these patients, a volar plate advancement technique will stabilize the joint and decrease the likelihood of late traumatic arthritis. Surgery on these joints always causes some stiffness, and a vigorous postoperative hand therapy program will be necessary. When the joint can be adequately reduced but is unstable as the patient actively flexes or extends, it should be immobilized for 3 weeks in the reduced position. Afterward, stiffness should be anticipated, and vigorous hand therapy is again required. When the patient is fortunate enough to have a stable joint following reduction, early motion with protective splinting will achieve the best possible range of motion (Fig. 62-25). This is usually done by a "figure-of-eight' splint to protect the patient from hyperextension, and there may be slight loss of extension. Flexion is well preserved by this method. Nonunion of the small fracture fragment attached to the volar plate is of no consequence if good flexion

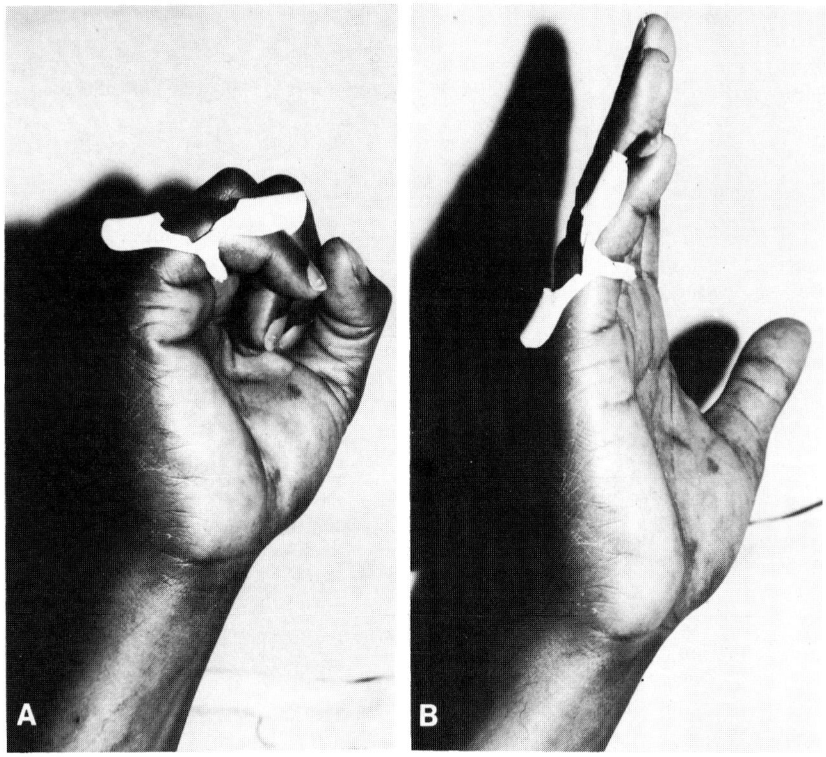

FIG. 62-25. A figure-of-eight splint prevents hyperextension (*B*) but permits full flexion (*A*) after stable closed reduction of a PIP-fracture dislocation.

and extension are maintained with a stable joint. The stiffness that occurs with complete immobilization is therefore avoided.

Late PIP subluxed fracture dislocation or late traumatic arthritis is a very difficult problem with options including fusion, replacement arthroplasty, volar plate advancement, and even perichondrial-cartilage homografting.[23] We have been pleased with the use of interpositional hyaline cartilage grafts from the nasal septum in selected young patients, but they have been followed for less than 5 years. Certainly, adequate primary treatment results are far better.

METACARPAL FRACTURES

Rotation deformity of the fingers is one of the most frustrating and frequent complications of metacarpal fractures. A simple transverse metacarpal fracture can appear deceptively aligned on x-ray and physical examination when the digits are held in extension (Fig. 62-26). However, only 2° to 3° rotation deformity at the fracture site may be amplified in the arc of finger flexion.[38] The unwary surgeon may accept apparently reduced fractures that will cause "scissoring." This complication can be prevented by being certain the flexed fingers point toward the tuberosity of the scaphoid and that the nails of the digits are lying parallel. Therefore, when immobilization is undertaken, the fingers should be carefully checked in flexion following reduction to avoid impingement of the digit against others when they are flexed. Late deformity is correctable by rotational osteotomy.

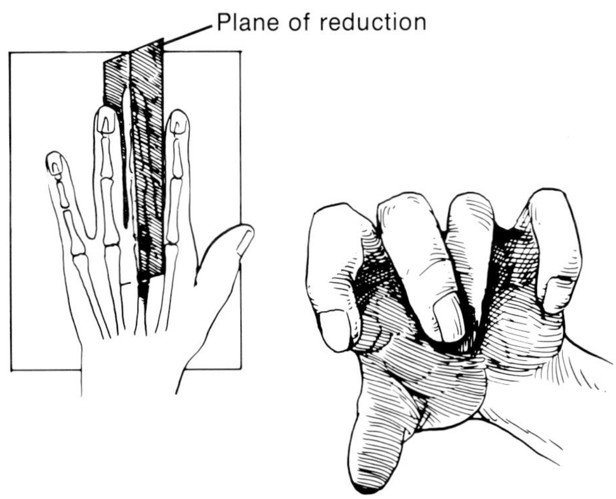

FIG. 62-26. Rotation malunion of metacarpal fractures causes scissoring in digital flexion although they may appear normal in extension.

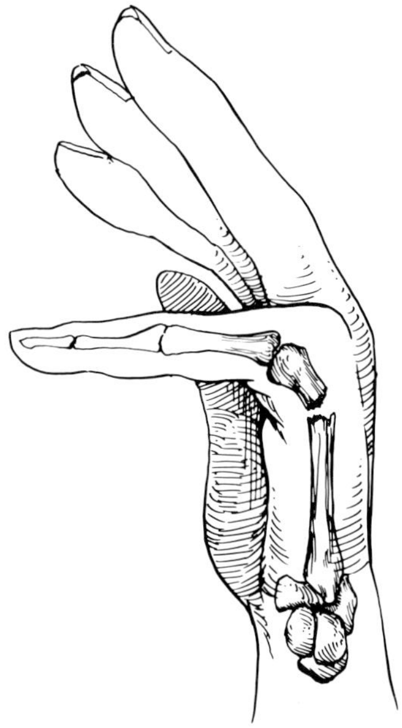

FIG. 62-27. Boxer fractures in the fifth metacarpal do not usually require reduction with less than 30° angulation. When reduced and immobilized, the IP joints should be held in extension to avoid unnecessary flexion contractures.

Boxer and Other Metacarpal Neck Fractures

By far the most common metacarpal fracture occurs at the neck of the fifth metacarpal, usually from a blow with a clenched fist. There is characteristic angulation volarward. When reduction is attempted, it usually is done with the fifth digit fully flexed, applying pressure against the proximal phalanx (Fig. 62-27). There has been an unfortunate tendency for surgeons then to immobilize this digit in full flexion, causing the previously undamaged interphalangeal joints to remodel into flexion contractures. This is unnecessary, since fracture angulation of 25° or even 30° is acceptable and seldom causes any permanent deformity or functional deficiency. Indeed, many surgeons believe that immobilization of this fracture is not necessary. However, in the middle three metacarpals, this degree of angulation is not acceptable because it will cause a prominence in the palm, which is painful on gripping.[38] Fractures in the metacarpal neck of these middle digits must be reduced and immobilized.

Bennett's Fracture

Fracture of the base of the thumb metacarpal is usually unstable, owing to the unopposed pull of the abductor pollicis longus. As a consequence, the temptation to control this fracture with closed reduction and cast should be resisted. Failure to maintain reduction of this intra-articular fracture leads to late, very troublesome traumatic arthritis at the base of the thumb (Fig. 62-28). Most surgeons prefer to secure this fracture by a percutaneous Kirschner wire, fixing the first metacarpal shaft to the adjacent second metacarpal or into the carpus to prevent late slippage.

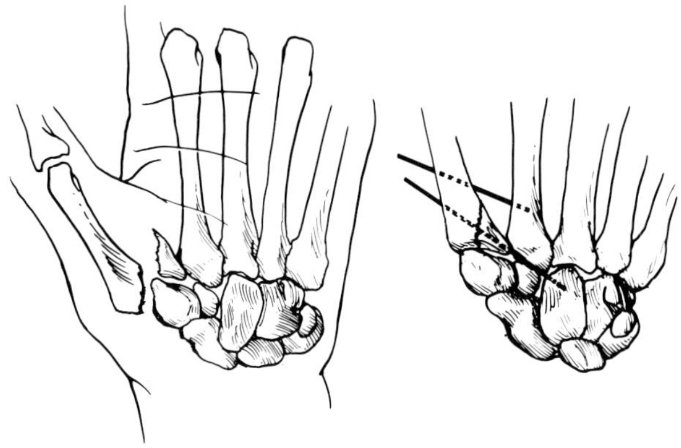

FIG. 62-28. Bennett's fracture is usually unstable unless percutaneously pinned.

Fracture at the base of the fifth metacarpal may be unstable, similar to Bennett's fracture, with tendency for the metacarpal to slip proximally from the hamate. Percutaneous fixation to the fourth metacarpal shaft following reduction will secure this and avoid late traumatic arthritis.[19]

NAVICULAR FRACTURE

Whenever a patient complains of wrist sprain and has tenderness in the snuff box region of the wrist, the presumptive diagnosis should be navicular fracture, regardless of x-ray findings. A simple thumb spica short-arm cast can be applied for 2 weeks. It will provide excellent treatment for wrist sprain if x-ray films at that time show no fracture on navicular view. Sufficient resorption at the fracture site will make a previously inapparent navicular fracture easily visible on x-ray film 2 weeks following injury. Failure to immobilize early navicular fracture may lead to vascular damage and avascular necrosis.

Major Pain Syndromes Following Minor Hand Trauma

HYPERSENSITIVITY SYNDROMES: PAINFUL AMPUTATION NEUROMATA

Certain hand injuries are likely to produce hypersensitivity, best characterized by inability to use the hand due to pain. These include crush injury; fingertip laceration; amputation; frostbite; thermal, chemical, and electrical partial-thickness burns; and most severe avulsion-type injuries. Prolonged edema, cold intolerance, and disuse changes usually accompany these injuries, and the patient may develop a disuse pattern that greatly amplifies restrictions of use. For example, Seddon reports as many as 60% of fingertip amputations develop complications of painful neuromata that interfere with function.[65]

The very best treatment for hypersensitivity syndromes is prevention of the disuse pattern before it becomes established. To do so, the surgeon must anticipate this possibility and engage the patient in a vigorous hand therapy regimen during early postoperative management. For example, the patient with a car-door laceration of the fingertip should be told, "after this heals it will surprise you how much and long it hurts when you use it, possibly many months, but it is best to use it because although it may hurt you, you won't hurt it, and you will tolerate use much sooner." Often, such patients return, proud of their ability to overcome this discomfort, rather than surprised, disappointed, and suspicious over the degree of discomfort.

Once a pain pattern becomes established, it may be further complicated by secondary gain, such as from the local workmen's compensation agency where the patient is told he must be "completely" recovered before returning to work. The patient will always experience some discomfort when he first engages in work. Direct communication with his employer will often do much to break this cycle.

When hypersensitivity has become well established, we recommend instituting a system of desensitization organized on the basis of objective measurements and a series of objective goals for the patient. It is essential to have an empathetic and supportive therapist or physician working closely with the patient to achieve this. The program starts with tuning-fork stimulation and ends with simulated work activity. The series of objectives is outlined in Figure 62-29, and it has been surprising how well many patients with a prolonged disability will quickly take pride in achieving these objectives and returning to healthy functional use. In our series of 16 patients, the average length of time out of work before desensitization therapy was 5 months; once this therapy was instituted, the average length of time before returning to gainful employment was 2 months.[28] Although the results of this desensitization regimen seem promising, it is far better to avoid

FIG. 62-29. The Medical College of Virginia desensitization protocol.

Table of Desensitization Treatment Program

Time	Level 1	Level 2	Level 3	Level 4	Level 5
Week 1	Tuning-fork paraffin massage				
		Vibration—battery operated Friction massage Constant touch/pressure			
↓			Vibration—electric Textures Splints Activities		
				Vibration—electric Object identification	
Discharge					Work and activities simulation

the hypersensitivity syndrome by preventing establishment of the pain pattern.

In certain patients, such as those with a painful amputation neuroma, surgical procedures may be of benefit. However, we believe most patients should engage in desensitization before surgery to assist their recovery. The literature describes treatments of amputation neuroma consisting of cauterization, ligation, resection, and capping. None of these methods has proved altogether satisfactory, and consequently desensitization should be the initial mode of treatment.[72] Many patients who are improved but continue to have some discomfort will then do far better after the neuroma is resected and the end of the nerve repositioned in a less sensitive location away from the fingertip (see Fig. 62-24).

MAJOR CAUSALGIA

During the American Civil War, Dr. Wier Mitchell described a Yankee who received a musket wound in his upper arm and developed severe pain that was exaggerated by temperature change, loud noise, and emotional stress.[74] We now recognize this as major causalgia, the symptoms of which can be dramatically reduced by sympathectomy. Unfortunately, the term *causalgia* now has wide usage. It should probably be confined to that complication associated with proximal nerve injury, temperature intolerance, relief from sympathectomy, and severe pain that prohibits function. Sympathetic block will confirm the diagnosis. Doups' theory suggests a biologic mechanism involving crossover of sympathetic fibers into pain tracts at the site of injury; however, Sunderland regards the problem to be at the central nervous system level in the "internuncial pool."[16, 71] Major causalgia is an uncommon but distinctive condition that should not be confused with shoulder–hand syndrome, Sudeck's atrophy, reflex sympathetic dystrophy, or other less well defined pain syndromes.

REFLEX SYMPATHETIC DYSTROPHY

Whereas major causalgia appears to have specific findings associated with a precise anatomical injury, reflex sympathetic dystrophy belongs to a vague group of disorders best described as *psychophysiologic pain syndromes*. There are some 37 different diagnoses variously used to describe these ill-defined disorders including minor causalgia, osteodystrophy, shoulder–hand syndrome, and so forth. The most distinguishing feature is significant autonomic dysfunction and pain for what would not seem a severe injury or operation, such as a phalangeal fracture, an elective carpal tunnel release, or ganglionectomy. In 1937, Bunnell expressed his opinion that these patients were emotionally unstable, but this was not convincingly studied until recent work by Maureen Hardy, R.P.T., M.S., at the Medical College of Virginia. To investigate this problem, she established objective criteria for the diagnosis of reflex sympathetic dystrophy including temperature differences of 4° or more in the uninjured hand. She then tested these patients psychologically for comparison with a control group of hand injured patients who did not meet her criteria. Her data showed significant differences in the psychological profile of reflex sympathetic dystrophy patients, particularly in areas of anxiety, depression, and self-image. Furthermore, these patients had sustained lesser injuries than had the control group. However, pain measurement, using the linear analogue scale and the ischemic ratio test, showed no difference between the two groups so that the lack of function and resistance to improvement did not appear related to the degree of pain. A small number of these patients treated with temperature biofeedback therapy developed voluntary control of their temperature and reported improvement or relief of their pain.[49, 50] Serial sympathetic blocks, intravenous reserpine therapy, and transcutaneous electroneurostimulation have all been reported as successful methods of treating these patients. However, these reports do not provide their criteria for diagnosis and have no control groups. It may very well be that the psychological support offered by those who render any of these treatments is the major therapeutic value. Certainly, the patient who has had a less severe injury or operation and who is anxious and depressed and complains of disproportionate pain should immediately be treated by compassionate, intensive hand therapy to obviate development of this very difficult complication. The worst possible approach is to try to minimize the patient's plea for support by appearing nonchalant and classifying him as a "crock." These patients feel rejected, become hostile, and will prove that the physician is wrong by developing a severe disability that is far more easily prevented than treated.

SUDECK'S ATROPHY AND OSTEOPOROSIS

In 1900, Sudeck described a dramatic condition in which minimal injury resulted in a severe pain syndrome characterized by muscle atrophy, intolerance of soft touch and cold, progressive osteoporosis, thinning of the skin, and eventual contracture and ankylosis of the fingers (Fig. 62-30).[70] The most astonishing early feature is the disproportionate degree of pain and functional disability for what appears to be a relatively minor injury or operation. The patient holds the hand in a protected position and avoids even light touch. The surgeon should immediately recognize this as a dangerous finding and engage the patient in a comprehensive hand therapy program with strong emotional support. Most patients with Sudeck's atrophy give a history that includes hostility over the rejection they felt when their early symptoms and findings were diagnosed as a minor pain syndrome. If these patients have pending litigation, they should be encouraged to resolve it as quickly as possible and to expect only gradual improvement with prolonged therapy, usually not to a normal level. Transcutaneous neuroelectric stimulation, temperature biofeedback therapy, desensitization therapy, and psychotherapy may all be used to treat these patients. In spite of the anatomical changes, many patients with Sudeck's atrophy can be improved by prolonged intensive hand therapy. However, all surgical efforts should be postponed until after the patient is able to control pain and tolerate use of the hand; otherwise the syndrome may recur.

Complications of Finger Amputations

Today, the public is far better informed about the possibility for replantation of amputated digits than it is about the probability of a poor functional result. The amount of inflammation following successful replantation causes ankylosis of the small joints and dense fibrosis along the tendon and its sheath. For that reason, single digit replantation attempts are not recommended for most patients. Replantation is justified only when multiple digits or the thumb is lost. It is important for the referring physician to cool the tissue to be replaced; however, in the absence of circulation, frostbite will develop if it is placed directly on ice. Therefore, the amputated tissue should be suspended in a saline-filled basin or wrapped in sterile moist towels before placing on ice. The amputation stump should be treated with a pressure dressing in most instances. If control of vessels is necessary, this should be with vascular clamps to avoid damage.

Preventable technical errors are responsible for two important complications after elective finger amputations. One of these occurs from the irresistible temptation to use the flexor profundus tendon as a buffer over the raw end of the amputated phalanx. This is done by suturing the cut end of the profundus to the cut end of the extensor mechanism. If the profundus is then under greater tension than the adjacent profundi of the remaining fingers, flexion of these normal digits will be functionally restricted because the single muscle for these tendons is now under tension and cannot contract normally. Late correction of this complication is by division of the profundus. However, this may be difficult owing to adherence along the tendon sheath, and it may require incision in the palm. Painful amputation neuroma at the stump is another frequent complication of digital amputations, with an incidence reported as high as 60%.[65] This is often due to the technical error of allowing the digital nerve cut ends to remain at the site of skin closure. When the nerve is dissected during amputation, enough length should be maintained to attach an absorbable suture and direct the cut end of the nerve in a proximal dorsal direction, well away from the tip of the amputation stump. Revision for painful amputation neuromas can be done in this fashion, but a desensitization therapy regimen may first be tried (Fig. 62-29).

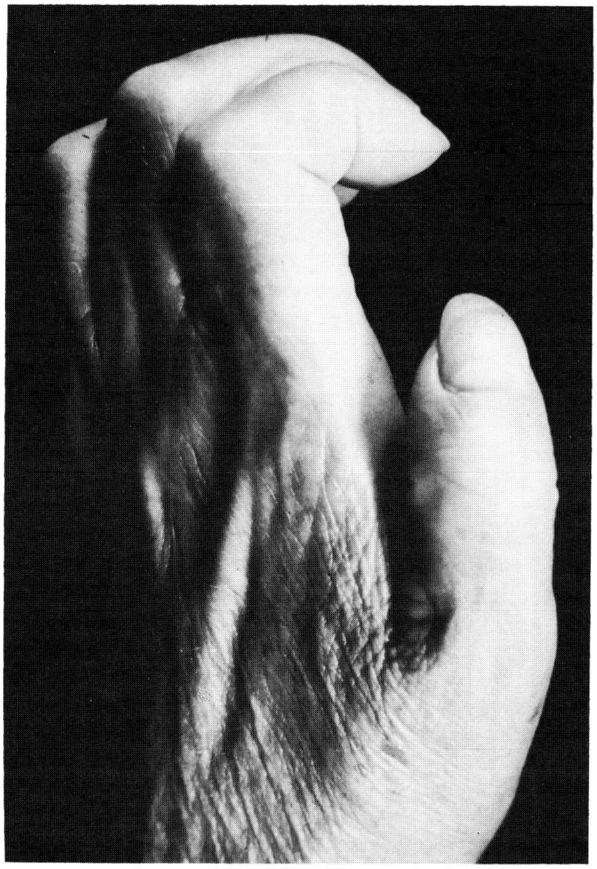

FIG. 62-30. Sudeck's atrophy and osteoporosis from a painful Colles' wrist fracture.

Injection Injuries of the Hand

Two types of injection injuries are particularly prone to serious complications if initially improperly managed. These are drug injection injury and high velocity "paint gun" or "grease gun" injuries.

Arterial injection of illegal drugs may often cause widespread vasospasm, thrombosis, and sometimes embolism. Amputation or Volkmann's ischemic contracture may result from this injury (see Fig. 62-14). The initial management should include prolonged sympathetic block using either a long-acting agent such as bupivacaine (Marcaine) or an indwelling catheter by the axillary nerve to permit frequent xylocaine injections. If arteriography is done, consideration should be given to use of streptokinase or similar fibrinolytic agents in an attempted dissolution of thrombosis. This has been successful in a few reported cases and our own experience.[33] It has been necessary to maintain streptokinase for a few days to prevent recurrent thrombosis.

Paint spray gun or grease gun injection injuries are indications for emergency exploration if the digit is swollen or the patient knows material was actually injected into the digit. Far more injected material will be found than the inexperienced surgeon expects, and it usually extends well beyond the site of injection, sometimes from the fingertip into the palm. Surgical removal of all the material that can reasonably be removed should be accomplished for the best result.[63] A troublesome inflammatory response will occur even after the best surgical effort, and early vigorous hand therapy is needed to restore function.

Complications Associated with Common Elective Surgical Conditions

CARPAL TUNNEL SYNDROME

The surgical treatment of carpal tunnel syndrome is widely regarded as "safe, simple, and successful."[60] Unfortunately, careful review of complications in carpal tunnel surgery reveals significant difficulty in 12% of postoperative patients.[14] These surprising figures probably reflect a lack of careful postoperative follow-up by most surgeons, many of whom regard this operation as a minor office procedure. The complications arise from three categories: diagnostic problems, technical problems, and management problems both preoperative and postoperative. Most are easily prevented if they are considered before surgery.

Diagnostic Problems

Incorrect diagnosis is commonly responsible for the lack of relief or limited relief from carpal tunnel syndrome surgery. A major cause of this complication arises from undue reliance on nerve conduction studies. It is well known that there are instances of both false-positive and false-negative results, and it is necessary to review the clinical signs and symptoms in relation to nerve conduction and EMG studies.[64] In a prospective study of 20 patients diagnosed with carpal tunnel syndrome at the Medical College of Virginia, the most common clinical finding was night pain causing the patient to awaken (80%); next was a positive Phalen's sign with the wrist flexed 2 minutes (68%); and next was a positive Tinel's sign in 50%.[54, 75] When these clinical signs are present, they are sufficient to warrant surgical correction, even if the nerve conduction study does not confirm a delay at the wrist. Raynaud's phenomenon may appear to be a part of carpal tunnel syndrome but will not be relieved by median neurolysis. Hypothyroidism causes carpal tunnel syndrome but is corrected by medical therapy alone. Amyloidosis frequently has carpal tunnel syndrome as an early symptom, and syringomyelia may easily mimic median nerve compression. Pregnancy is associated with carpal tunnel syndrome in as high as 50% of patients, but the syndrome will rarely persist following delivery, and therefore splinting alone is recommended.[27] Steroid wrist injections are contraindicated in pregnancy because of the possibility of congenital anomalies. Some believe that the carpal tunnel syndrome associated with oral contraceptives and with pregnancy may be due to vitamin B_6 deficiency. Although the data for this explanation are controversial, a trial of pyridoxine therapy, 100 mg per day, may safely be attempted.[22, 67]

Diabetic patients have a higher incidence of carpal tunnel syndrome than does the normal population, but distinguishing the findings of diabetic polyneuropathy from those of nerve compression may be quite difficult. Although nerve conduction studies may show delayed conduction at the wrist, the surgeon cannot determine if this is polyneuropathy at the wrist or nerve compression. Surgeons should be pessimistic about improvement if the patient does not have the characteristic night pain or a positive Tinel's or Phalen's sign. I believe in performing an internal neurolysis in these patients so that another surgeon will not have cause to justify a return to surgery if there is persistent postoperative difficulty.

"Double-crush" syndrome is responsible for incomplete recovery after carpal tunnel release in many patients. When the proximal nerve is compressed, as may occur from cervical compression, the nerve becomes more susceptible to carpal tunnel compression at the wrist with typical signs and symptoms of carpal tunnel syndrome. The clinician should be suspicious of this entity if the patient also complains of neck pain, has cervical osteoarthritis, or has a Tinel's sign of the ulnar nerve at the elbow as well as the median nerve at the wrist. It is recommended that both proximal and distal levels of nerve compression be treated to relieve these patients' symptoms completely.[47, 73]

Technical Problems

Improper technique has proved to be an unfortunately common cause of complications in patients treated for carpal tunnel syndrome. Most of these complications arise from using local anesthesia without a tourniquet, a transverse incision across the volar wrist crease, and "blind" division of the volar carpal ligament in an attempt to follow the ulnar side of the median nerve. This method of carpal tunnel release leads to neuroma of the median palmar sensory branch, division of the median motor branch, laceration of the superficial palmar vascular arch, and incomplete release. The transverse incision, as well as the popular S-shaped incision, is likely to divide the palmar sensory branch of the median nerve. Although most patients will find this to be only an annoying loss of feeling in a dime-sized area of their palm, others will develop a painful neuroma at the incision site. In a small number this appears to precipitate reflex sympathetic dystrophy. This problem is avoided by recognizing and protecting this sensory branch. The palmar sensory branch usually exits from the median nerve proximal to the volar carpal ligament and runs superficially above the radial border of the nerve. Incisions over the radial side of the median nerve will divide this sensory nerve. When this has occurred, desensitization therapy may help, and the patient should be reassured that this problem is not progressive. Of far greater significance, this blind technique endangers the important motor branch of the median nerve to the thumb thenar muscles. Although blind passage of scissors along the ulnar edge of the median nerve is safe in most patients, 12% have some anatomical variation in the location of this branch.[39] In the few whose motor branch exits from the ulnar side, this important nerve will likely be divided by this technique. If this division is unrecognized, later correction will require tendon transfers, such as the extensor indicis proprius, to restore circumduction of the thumb. Incomplete release of the distal end of the volar carpal ligament is more common with the transverse wrist incision technique as is division of the superficial palmar vascular arch. Because this vascular arch is located at the distal end of the volar carpal ligament, the timid surgeon may blindly stop before adequately releasing the ligament, and the bold surgeon may divide the vascular arch as well as the ligament. Proper technique for carpal tunnel release requires a bloodless field, block or general anesthesia, and an incision that protects the palmar sensory branch and permits direct observation of the median nerve and superficial palmar arch (Fig. 62-31). If the incision crosses the volar wrist crease, it should be angled to avoid a flexion contracture or hypertrophic scar at this site. When only the median nerve is to be released, I prefer to use a blunt fasciotomy method of dividing the proximal transverse carpal ligament without making an incision across the wrist crease at all. In so doing, care must be taken to remain on the ulnar side of the median nerve to protect the palmar sensory branch. When the ulnar nerve is also to be released from Guyon's canal, extension across the wrist by an ulnar-angled incision facilitates dissection.

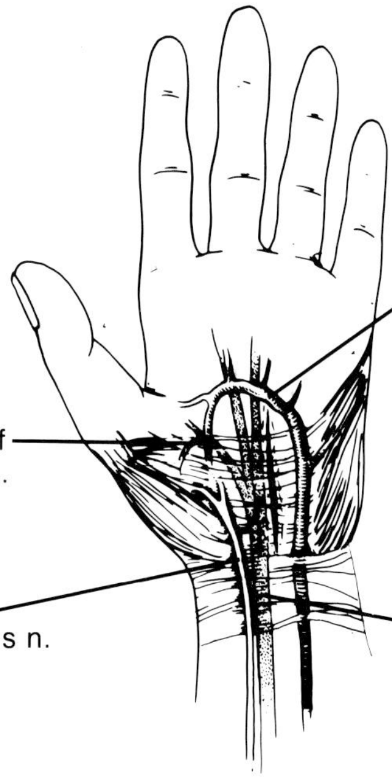

FIG. 62-31. The design of the carpal tunnel incision for median neurolysis may enable it to avoid the median palmar sensory and motor branches. Scar hypertrophy at the wrist crease is avoided by proximal fasciotomy of the volar ligament, but the incision should be angled across the wrist if ulnar neurolysis is also done.

When rheumatoid synovitis is the cause of carpal tunnel compression, it is wise to release both median and ulnar nerves even though only one may be symptomatic. This prophylactic release avoids the need for later surgery in the other canal when additional proliferative synovitis occurs. Consideration should also be given to a limited tenosynovectomy while the surgeon has exposure of the proximal palm and wrist. However, this additional procedure requires more intense postoperative management to ensure a satisfactory return of motion.

"Internal neurolysis" is indicated when severe carpal tunnel compression has been prolonged so that the epineurium of the median nerve has thickened and remodeled in a constricted position. Mere release of the volar carpal ligament alone will not afford relief to these patients. Direct inspection of the nerve will help the surgeon recognize the need for further release, which should be performed under magnification. Although this is called *internal neurolysis*, in many patients only an epineurotomy is required to permit visualization of healthy fascicular groups so that the tubular structure is again recognizable as a nerve rather than as a tendon. Unnecessary invasion of the nerve may lead to progressive intraneural fibrosis or reflex sympathetic dystrophy. Once healthy fascicular groups are freed, further dissection is unnecessary and unwarranted.

Management Problems

Routine steroid injection is popular as initial management for carpal tunnel syndrome. Few physicians recognize how devastating this can be if there is direct penetration into intraneural tissue. The findings in clinical cases show severe intraneural fibrosis. Experimentally, there is complete necrosis of the nerve from any of the steroid agents studied when the injection is into the perineural tissue. Injection outside the epineurium or even just beneath the epineurium caused no change.[43] Any time a patient complains of paresthetic pain during steroid injection beneath the carpal ligament, the needle should be withdrawn immediately. Indeed, it may be safer to confine steroid injections only to patients in whom an inflammatory condition is thought to cause the nerve compression, justifying the risk.

Flexor tendon "bowstringing" at the wrist due to loss of the volar carpal ligament is an unusual complication that occurs in active athletic patients who forcibly tighten their long flexor tendons early after surgery with the wrist flexed. This atypical position is likely to occur in pipe fitters or athletes who lift weights or use a horizontal bar. If the surgeon suspects that these postoperative activities are likely, the problem is avoided by splinting the patient's wrist in neutral position for 3 weeks following surgery.[41]

Many patients will become concerned because of the prolonged tenderness and discomfort at the palm scar site following carpal tunnel release. They should be reassured that this discomfort is common and will subside, usually within 6 to 8 weeks.[30] Because of the discomfort, most manual laborers will need to rest 3 weeks before resuming their work.

GANGLIONECTOMY

The three most common complications associated with ganglionectomy are recurrent ganglion, painful neuroma of the dorsal sensory branch of the radial nerve, and error in diagnosis. Electron micrographic and histologic studies suggest that ganglions arise from a one-way valve system through a defect in the dorsal wrist capsule.[2] Others believe that they develop from mucinous degeneration of the joint capsule or other dense connective tissue.[14, 68] With either of these hypotheses, resection requires removal of the base of the ganglion to reduce the chance for recurrence. This base is usually the dorsal joint capsule itself. Wrist ganglionectomy cannot be performed easily under local anesthesia or without a tourniquet. Recurrence rates as high as 40% have been described, likely owing to failure to remove the base of the ganglion at the wrist capsule.[2] With proper technique under adequate anesthesia in a bloodless field, a recurrence rate of 5% should be expected. I believe it is also helpful to immobilize the wrist in a splint for 3 weeks following surgery to allow adequate collagen cross linking across the scar that replaces the joint capsule. However, no data document the value of wrist immobilization. With this method, normal hand activity is permitted while the wrist is splinted.

Painful neuroma of the dorsal sensory branch of the radial nerve is one of the most troublesome and difficult complications to manage. Unfortunately, the most common location of dorsal wrist ganglions is directly adjacent to this nerve over the dorsoradial border of the wrist.[2] Laceration of the nerve causes loss of sensation over the radial side of the back of the hand, which is usually of no functional significance. However, laceration also causes a painful neuroma at the scar site. Under local anesthesia and without a tourniquet, identifying this nerve is difficult. If the divided nerve ends are identified, immediate repair with 8-0 nylon suture should be performed. In late injury, the best initial treatment may be desensitization therapy, which will be adequate for many patients. Other patients will have functional difficulty owing to painful neuroma at the proximal divided end. This has been so troublesome that many surgical techniques have been described, none of which seems to work in certain patients. The most popular method of surgical management is to resect the neuroma and implant the proximal end in bone or muscle. I prefer to try to repair the nerve, regardless of how long it has been since injury. However, with an old injury, the distal end may be difficult to identify because of wallerian degeneration. Furthermore, remodeling of the cut ends may make reanastomosis impossible without tension, and nerve grafting is not indicated because of the donor sacrifice. Therefore, one provocative method suggested by Snyder is to implant the proximal end into an adjacent dorsal vein, providing tubularization for irregular growth along this vein rather than formation of another painful neuroma. This appears successful in our limited experience.

Inclusion cysts, xanthomata, and other benign tumors may be incorrectly diagnosed as ganglions;

however, the correct diagnosis becomes evident at surgery, and the operation can be modified properly. More important, extensor tenosynovitis from undiagnosed rheumatoid arthritis can easily be misdiagnosed as a dorsal ganglion. Because medical rather than surgical treatment is initially indicated, it is important to make the correct diagnosis preoperatively. This is done by having the patient flex and extend his fingers; a "dimple" or "tuck" sign will appear in the skin just distal to the tumor as the fingers are fully extended. This occurs because the tenosynovitis moves with the tendon whereas the usual ganglion remains at the same site, arising much deeper from the joint capsule.

Aspiration of ganglions is not harmful if sterile technique is used, but it is generally ineffective, and the patient should be counseled to expect recurrence. Physicians should not encourage patients to attempt to rupture ganglions by hitting them with a book unless they are willing to be held liable for carpal dislocations.

DE QUERVAIN'S DISEASE

The most frequent complications following release of the first dorsal compartment for the stenosing tenosynovitis of De Quervain are inadequate release, injury to the radial nerve dorsal sensory branch, and "snapping" of the released tendons as they move in and out of the former compartment.

Inadequate release for De Quervain's disease usually occurs owing to separate anomalous slips of the abductor pollicis longus in separate isolated portions of the first compartment so that complete release is not accomplished. This is prevented by good visualization, using an incision parallel to the compartment and a bloodless field to be sure any divisions in the first dorsal compartment have been released. Similarly, a bloodless field and vertical incision should prevent injury to the adjacent sensory branch of the radial nerve. Local anesthesia is adequate for this procedure in most patients. Occasionally, the tendons will snap postoperatively as they slide into and out of the released compartment. This is corrected by splinting the patient for 3 weeks with the tendons at rest in the compartment. The scar at the site of release will gain sufficient tensile strength to maintain them there.

RELEASE OF "TRIGGER FINGER"

"Triggering" usually is caused by a flexor tendon nodule passing through the first tendon sheath pulley in the palm, although the condition is described as *stenosing tenosynovitis*. This "locking" may also be due to the trapping of a profundus nodule at the division of the sublimis tendons in the fingers. The first pulley mechanism in the palm should therefore be released under local anesthesia so that the patient can continue to perform and the surgeon will know when release has been adequate. When the locking is at the sublimis level, the patient continues to experience it after the entire first pulley has been divided. A new incision should then be made at the proximal interphalangeal joint level and one slip of the sublimis tendon divided. In so doing, it is important to preserve the A_2 pulley now that the A_1 has been sacrificed. Otherwise, bowstringing of the flexor tendons may occur. The surgeon cannot always locate the level of the locking until the patient performs, and local anesthesia provides the opportunity to confirm the correction.

A tourniquet should also be used for this procedure to visualize and protect the neurovascular bundles lying adjacent to the flexor tendon sheath in the palm. Digital nerve neuropraxia is not uncommon following this operation, but digital nerve laceration should not occur.

WARTS OF THE HAND

Verruca vulgaris of the hand is a common condition with a wide spectrum of management techniques. It has long been suspected that a positive attitude on the part of those who render treatment bears the highest correlation with success.[13] Surgical excision may be indicated, but it should be considered only after all the conventional or folk remedies have failed. Incomplete excision of a single lesion may be followed by a series of warts all along the scar, the virus having been implanted into the site. To avoid this complication, excision must include a normal rim of tissue as though skin cancer were being removed. Sometimes this will require a skin graft to close the defect, especially in the volar portions of the digits. I have frequently been successful with ultrasonic therapy for warts, explaining with enthusiastic confidence how "ultrasonic waves fracture the viral walls." Spontaneous regression is far preferable to surgical excision because of the hazard of recurrence along the incision and the possibility of a tender scar in the hand. Trimming the warts while conducting conservative efforts may be beneficial.

Cryotherapy for warts on the fingers has caused late degenerative changes in adult interphalangeal joints and growth disturbances in children's digits. Therefore, cryotherapy for warts is contraindicated over the small joints of the fingers.[7, 37]

FOREIGN BODIES IN THE HAND

Hands are particularly susceptible to penetration by glass, metal, wood, and other foreign bodies. It is a mistake for surgeons to embark on an adventuresome exploration of the hand for these foreign bodies unless they cause a functional problem. Furthermore, foreign bodies to be removed because of chronic inflammation, nerve compression, or pain should be localized preoperatively to minimize the exploration. Metallic and leaded glass can be seen on routine x-ray film. Nonmetallic objects may be identified on xeroradiography of the hand, which can be indispensable for locating glass or other particles. However, wood slivers can usually be seen on xeroradiography only early after penetration. Later absorption of water will often cause similar density as the surrounding tissue, and therefore the absence of wood foreign body on xeroradiography does not rule it out. Exploration under these conditions must rely on the suspicion of the surgeon.

References

1. Adams J, Dealy E, Kenmore P: Intravenous regional anesthesia in hand surgery. J Bone Joint Surg 46A:4, 1964
2. Angelides AC, Wallace PF: The dorsal ganglion of the wrist: Its pathogenesis, gross and microscopic anatomy, and surgical treatment. J Hand Surg 1(4):228-235, 1976
3. Arem AJ, Madden JW: Effects of stress on healing wounds: I. Intermittent noncyclical tension. J Surg Res 20:93-102, 1976
4. Becker H, Grahm MF, Cohen IK, Diegelmann RF: Intrinsic tendon cell proliferation in tissue culture. J Hand Surg 6(6):616-619, 1981
5. Boyes JH: Bunnell's Surgery of the Hand, 5th ed. Philadelphia, JB Lippincott, 1970
6. Boyes JH, Stark HW: Flexor-tendon grafts in the fingers and thumb. J Bone Joint Surg 53-A:1332-1342, 1971
7. Brown FE, Spiegel PK, Boyle WE: Digital dysplasia: An effect of frostbite in children. Presented at the American Association for Hand Surgery Annual Meeting, Maui, Hawaii, October 8, 1982
8. Brown M: Management of edema. In Hunter JM (ed): Rehabilitation of the Hand. St. Louis, CV Mosby, 1978
9. Brown PW: Factors influencing the success of the surgical repair of peripheral nerves. Surg Clin North Am 52(5):1137-1155, 1972
10. Bruner JM: The zig-zag volar-digital incision for flexor tendon surgery. Plast Reconstr Surg 40:571, 1967
11. Buncke HJ Jr: Digital nerve repairs. Surg Clin North Am 52(5):1267-1285, 1972
12. Bunnell S: Surgery of the Hand, 2nd ed. Philadelphia, JB Lippincott, 1949
13. Cannon B, Constable JD: Reconstructive plastic surgery of the lower extremity. In Converse JM (ed): Reconstructive Plastic Surgery. Philadelphia, WB Saunders, 1974
14. Carp L, Stout AP: A study of ganglion with special reference to treatment. Surg Gynecol Obstet 47:460, 1928
15. Diegelmann RF, Cohen IK, Kaplan AM: Effect of macrophages on fibroblast DNA synthesis and proliferation. Proc Soc Exp Biol Med 169:445-451, 1982
16. Doupe J: Post-traumatic pain and the causalgic syndrome. J Neurol Neurosurg Psychiatry 7:33, 1944
17. Dubos RJ: Bacterial and Mycotic Infections of Man, 3rd ed. Philadelphia, JB Lippincott, 1958
18. Ducker TB: Metabolic factors in surgery of peripheral nerves. Surg Clin North Am 52(5):1109-1122, 1972
19. Eaton RG: Joint Injuries of the Hand. Springfield, IL, Charles C Thomas, 1971
20. Eaton RG, Butsch DP: Antibiotic guidelines for hand infections. Surg Gynecol Obstet 130(1):119-122, 1978
21. Elliott RA Jr: Boutonniere deformity. In Cramer LM, Chase RA (eds): Symposium on the Hand. St. Louis, CV Mosby, 1971
22. Ellis J, Folkers K, Watanabe T et al: Clinical results of a cross-over treatment with pyridoxine and placebo of the carpal tunnel syndrome. Am J Clin Nutr 32:2040-2046, 1979
23. Engkvist O, Johannson SH: Perichondrial arthroplasty. A clinical study in 26 patients. Scand J Plast Reconstr Surg 14:71, 1980
24. Farmer CB, Mann RJ: Human bite infections of the hand. South Med J 59(1):515-518, 1966
25. Fowler SB: Extensor apparatus of the digits. J Bone Joint Surg 31B:477, 1949
26. Furlow LT Jr: Cause and prevention of tourniquet ooze. Surg Gynecol Obstet 132:1069-1072, 1971
27. Gould J: Carpal tunnel syndrome in pregnancy. South Med J 71(2):144-145, 1978
28. Hardy MA, Moran CA, Merritt WH; Desensitization of the traumatized hand. Va Med J 109:134–137, 1982
29. Iselin F, Levanne J, Godoy J: A simplified technique for treating mallet fingers: Tenodermodesis. J Hand Surg 2(2):118-121, 1977
30. Jabaley ME: Personal observations on the role of the lumbrical muscles in carpal tunnel syndrome. J Hand Surg 3(1):82, 1978
31. Kanavel AB: Infections of the Hand. A Guide to the Surgical Treatment of Acute and Chronic Suppurative Processes in the Fingers, 7th ed. Philadelphia, Lea & Febiger, 1939
32. Kaplan EB: Functional and Surgical Anatomy of the Hand, 2nd ed. Philadelphia, JB Lippincott, 1965
33. Kartchner WWC: Thrombolysis of palmar and digital artery thrombosis by intra-arterial thrombolysin. J Hand Surg 1:67-74, 1976
34. Kelsey JL, Pastides H, Kreiger N et al: Upper Extremity Disorders: A Survey of Their Frequency and Cost in the United States, St Louis, CV Mosby, 1980
35. Ketchum LD, Brand PW, Thompson D, Pocock GS: The determination of moments for extension of the wrist generated by muscles of the forearm. J Hand Surg 3:205, 1978
36. Kilgore ES, Brown LG, Newmeyer WL et al: Treatment of felons. Am J Surg 130:194, 1975
37. Kuylenstierna R, Annike M, Lundquist P, Nathanson A: Experimental cryosurgery on bone: A light and electron microscopical investigation. Cryobiology 17:563-570, 1980
38. Lamb DW, Kuczynski KMB: The Practice of Hand Surgery. Boston, Scientific Publications, 1981
39. Lanz U: Anatomical variations of the median nerve in the carpal tunnel. J Hand Surg 2(1):44-53, 1977
40. Leddy JP, Packer JW: Avulsion of the profundus tendon insertion in athletes. J Hand Surg 2(1):66-69, 1977
41. MacDonald RI, Litchtman DM, Hanlon JJ: Complications of surgical release for carpal tunnel syndrome. J Hand Surg 3(1):70-76, 1978

42. McDowell CL, Snyder DM: Tendon healing: An experimental model in the dog. J Hand Surg 2(2):122-126, 1977
43. Mackinnon JE, Hudson AR, Gentile F et al: Peripheral nerve injection injury with steroid agents. Plast Reconstr Surg 69:482-489, 1982
44. Madden JW, Carlson EC, Hines J: Presence of modified fibroblasts in ischemic contracture of the intrinsic musculature of the hand. Surg Gynecol Obstet 140(4):509-516, 1975
45. Manktelow RT, McKee NH: Free muscle transplantation to provide active finger flexion. J Hand Surg 3:416-426, 1976
46. Manske PR, Lesker PA: Nutrient pathways of flexor tendons in primates. J Hand Surg 7(5):436-444, 1982
47. Massey EW, Riley TI, Fleet A–B: Coexistent carpal tunnel syndrome and cervical radiculopathy (double crush syndrome). South Med J 74:957-959, 1981
48. Merritt WH; Studies of the biological response of fascia to injury. Presented at the Plastic Surgery Research Council, Downey, California, April 18, 1977
49. Merritt WH, Hardy MA: A model to study sympathetic dystrophy: Psychological testing and biofeedback results. American Society for Surgery of the Hand Annual Meeting, New Orleans, Louisiana, January 18-20, 1983
50. Merritt WH, Hardy MA, Acharya G: Treatment for Raynaud's: Preliminary results of temperature biofeedback therapy and digital artery sympathectomy. Orthopaedic Transactions (abstr), vol 4, September 1980
51. Merritt WH, Peacock EE Jr, Chvapil M: Comparative biology of fascial autografts and allografts. Surg Forum 25:524, 1974
52. Merritt WH, Peacock EE Jr, Chvapil M: Studies on the inductive capacity of canine fascia lata. Surg Forum 26:553, 1975
53. Merritt WH, Szumski AJ, Clamann HP, Ely JF: Influence of Scar Maturation in Nerve Grafts. Transactions of the 7th International Congress of Plastic and Reconstructive Surgery, pp 743–745. Sociedade Brasileira De Cirurgia Plastica, Sao Paulo, Brazil, 1980
54. Moran CA, Merritt WH, Personius WJ: Comparison of sensory testing methods using carpal tunnel syndrome patients. Presented at the American Society of Hand Therapists' Meeting, New Orleans, Louisiana, January, 1982
55. Newmeyer WL, Kilgore ES: Volkmann's ischemic contracture due to soft tissue injury alone. J Hand Surg 1:221-227, 1976
56. Peacock EE: Management of the burned hand. South Med J 56:1094, 1963
57. Peacock EE, Van Winkle W Jr: Surgery and Biology of Wound Repair. Philadelphia, WB Saunders, 1970
58. Peacock EE, Van Winkle W Jr: Wound Repair, 2nd ed. Philadelphia, WB Saunders, 1976
59. Peterson WF: Hippocratic Wisdom: For Him Who Wishes to Pursue Properly the Science of Medicine, p 97. Springfield, IL, Charles C Thomas, 1946
60. Phalen S: The carpal tunnel syndrome. Seventeen years' experience in diagnosis and treatment of six-hundred fifty-four hands. J Bone Joint Surg 48A:211-228, 1966
61. Potenza AD: Tendon healing within the flexor digital sheath in the dog. J Bone Joint Surg 44-A:49-64, 1962
62. Rank BK, Wakefield AR: Surgery of Repair as Applied to Hand Injuries, 2nd ed. Baltimore, Williams & Wilkins, 1961
63. Ramos H, Posch JL, Lie KK: High-pressure injection injuries of the hand. Plast Reconstr Surg 45:221-226, 1970
64. Schwartz MS, Gordon JA, Swash M: Slowed nerve conduction with wrist flexion in carpal tunnel syndrome. Ann Neurol 8:69-71, 1979
65. Sedden SH; Surgical Disorders of the Peripheral Nerves. Edinburgh, Churchill Livingstone, 1972
66. Seddon J: Infections of the Hand. London, E & S Livingstone, 1970
67. Shizukuishi S, Nishii S, Ellis J, Folkers K: The carpal tunnel syndrome as a probable primary deficiency of vitamin B6 rather than a deficiency of a dependency state. Biochem Biophys Res Commun 95:1126-1130, 1980
68. Soren A: Pathogenesis and treatment of ganglion. Clin Orthop 48:173, 1966
69. Spinner M, Aiache A, Silver L, Barsky AJ: Impending ischemic contracture of the hand: Early diagnosis and management. Plast Reconstr Surg 50:341, 1972
70. Sudek P: Uber die akut entzundlicke Knochenatrophie. Arch Klin Chir 62:147, 1900
71. Sunderland SM: Nerves and Nerve Injuries. Edinburgh, Churchill Livingstone, 1978
72. Tupper JW, Booth DM: Treatment of painful neuromas of sensory nerves in the hand: A comparison of traditional and newer methods. J Hand Surg 1:144-151, 1976
73. Upton ARM, McComas AJ: The double crush in nerve entrapment syndromes. Lancet 3:359-361, 1973
74. Weir Mitchell MS: Injuries of Nerves and Their Consequences. London, Smith, Eldor, 1872
75. Wein P: Significance of Tinel's sign. Acta Neurochir (Wein) 49(3-4):255-258, 1979
76. Werb Z, Gordon S: Secretion of a specific collagenase by stimulated macrophages. J Exp Med 142:346, 1975
77. Wilgis EFS: Tourniquet ischemia, muscle anoxia and operative edema. In Littler JW, Cramer LM, Smith JW (eds): Symposium on Reconstructive Hand Surgery, vol 9. St Louis, CV Mosby, 1974
78. Woodhall B (ed): Peripheral Nerve Regeneration. A Follow-Up Study of 3,656 World War II Injuries. Veterans' Administration Medical Monograph. Washington, DC, Supt of Documents, 1956

Part Ten

Prevalence of Complications

63
A Synopsis of Surgical Complications

George A. Parker

OVERVIEW

Both the patient and physician sectors of society have placed greater and greater demands upon the medical profession to be accountable for its performance. No longer are patients satisfied with "just making it through an operation"; they desire firm evidence that optimal therapy has been rendered at all times. As advocates for the patient, third-party insurance carriers have stepped into the discussion, not only to insure that patient care is above reproach, but also to attempt to control costs. In addition, physicians have always desired to be certain that the care they give is optimal and that their results are comparable to those achieved by other physicians under similar circumstances. The aspirations and expectations of these three separate groups must be kept in mind when evaluating the current approach to medical auditing.

In its simplest terms, an audit is an attempt to document the reasons for hospitalization and the results of therapies, as well as the performance of physicians during the administering of therapy. Heavy reliance is placed upon the written medical record as the sole source of documentation.

The mainstay of any type of audit is the establishment of standards of care that are recognized as acceptable norms. Nonphysician data collectors then are able to scan charts for evidence of such standards in the written medical record. Before discussing the establishment of standards, it is important to consider the different types of audits that can be applied to hospitalization.

The first is the input-type audit, which is retrospective and is an attempt to determine if acceptable standards are being met for justifying hospitalizations of patients for any variety of disease processes or operative procedures. Obviously, one of the main thrusts behind such an audit is the continuing desire to decrease the cost of hospitalization by decreasing utilization of hospitals for administration of care.

The second type of audit, utilization review, likewise is an attempt to decrease the amount of monies spent on hospitalization. Such a review is basically an ongoing, in-house review to ascertain whether certain standards, which are prearranged and accepted ahead of time by a physician review panel, are being met continually to justify the hospitalization of patients. Such a review often is viewed as unnecessary meddling in the doctor–patient relationship, but it is a very powerful tool for assessing performance and providing impetus for continued updating of practice activities.

The third type of audit is most familiar to physicians in general, since it very closely resembles the process used at most hospital death and complications conferences, although it performs such a function on a much more rigid and standardized format. The medical audit is a retrospective analysis of the charts of patients admitted with a given disease or subjected to a certain surgical procedure to document adherence to agreed upon standards of care.

It is important to realize that the reason for the audit will lead to different goals. Patients and, specifically, the third-party insurance carriers, look upon such an audit as a method of quality control and cost containment in a very pragmatic way. Physicians, in contrast, look upon it as a method to obtain information that might lead to improvement in patient care, either in the treatment of a given disease per se or in the performance of a given physician.

The performance of a medical audit usually takes the form of a retrospective chart review. Either a disease process listed as an admission or discharge diagnosis or an operative procedure is chosen for review. Preestablished standards of care need to be delineated clearly so that the nonphysician reviewers may be able to find the information in a chart sufficient to establish whether or not the standards were present or followed. It is obvious, even to the most inexperienced, that all possible standards cannot be delineated for any given procedure or for establishment of any given diagnosis. Therefore, exceptions must be delineated clearly on a case-by-case basis, and it is in this area that a great degree of debate over what are acceptable exceptions for the establishment of diagnoses or performance of procedures arises. The reason for this is that in any hospital situation, the patient population being treated is not necessarily comparable to that of any other hospital; for example, the patients seen at a large urban tertiary-care center are not comparable necessarily to patients seen at a small community hospital in a rural setting.

With a medical audit on a surgical service, the two areas of interest, most of the time, are either disease processes and their treatments or operative procedures and the attendant complications. In either case, the events of importance to the surgeon, and to his patients, are the operative mortality rate associated with the treatment for a given disease and the complications attendant upon such treatment. The long-term outcome of treatment, such as survival following a resection of a malignancy, do not lend themselves well to auditing procedures because of the time lag involved in such analysis.

It is important to emphasize that the medical audit does differ from the standard death and complications conference. The purpose of an audit is to document presently achieved results and to outline clearly areas for improvement. These areas might be in the performance of a given physician, the treatment of a given disease at that particular hospital in general, or the like. The important difference is a standardized approach to improve results.

As mentioned previously, the standards that are applied to the evaluation of a given event need to be agreed upon ahead of time. As also mentioned, it is difficult to apply the same standards to every single hospital or practice situation. Accordingly, it would be helpful to have representative data on the reported outcomes of treatments of various diseases to use as guidelines for the establishment of acceptable standards of therapy in any given institution. Obviously, standards acceptable 30 years ago are no longer applicable to the level of care achievable today. In order to provide such background information, the literature for the past 10 years has been reviewed, and the reported mortalities and complications encountered in the treatment of various disease processes commonly seen by a general surgeon have been recorded.

In Section A, disease processes and complications are organized on the basis of the affected organ system. For purposes of comparison, the commonly encountered complications of various operations categorized by operation, with subheadings according to disease being treated, are tabulated in Section B. It must be emphasized, however, that the data given are merely guidelines as to what seem to be acceptable morbidity and mortality rates for commonly performed operative procedures.

Section A

Commonly performed operative procedures and their attendant complications (listed alphabetically by involved organ system)

ABDOMINAL WALL

Pathologic Condition	Therapy	Mortality (%)	Morbidity	Percent
Gastroschisis and omphalocele[1, 90, 135]	Primary or skin flap closure	3.3	Skin necrosis	10
	Silastic silo	22	Infarcted or perforated bowel	12
Inguinal hernia[103, 234]	Inguinal herniorrhaphy	0.01	Wound infection	0.5
			Recurrence	0.8

ADRENAL GLAND

Pathologic Condition	Therapy	Mortality (%)	Morbidity	Percent
Hyperaldosteronism[16, 130, 137]	Transabdominal adrenalectomy	8.1	Lacerated spleen	8.1
			Venous bleeding	4.1
			Wound infection	4.1
	Adrenalectomy (posterior approach)	0	Wound infection	2.9
			Wound hematoma	4.1
Cushing's syndrome[72, 122]	Transabdominal adrenalectomy*	15.6	Lacerated spleen	3
			Venous bleeding	0
			Wound infection	3
	Adrenalectomy (posterior approach)	0	Wound infection	0
			Wound hematoma	0
Pheochromocytoma[229, 246]	Transabdominal adrenalectomy	3	Wound infection	3

*Includes several cases from before 1970, during which the mortality rate was excessive

APPENDIX

Pathologic Condition	Therapy	Mortality (%)	Morbidity	Percent
Acute appendicitis[163, 168]	Appendectomy	0	Wound infection	6.8
			Abdominal abscess	1
Perforative appendicitis[163, 168]	Appendectomy	1.9	Wound infection	17.1
			Abdominal abscess	13.3

BILE DUCTS

Pathologic Condition	Therapy	Mortality (%)	Morbidity	Percent
Biliary atresia[50, 169]	Hepaticoportoenterostomy	5.9	Wound infection	0
			Abdominal abscess	5.9
			Gastrointestinal hemorrhage	5.9
Carcinoma of bile ducts at hilus of liver[8, 14, 48, 162]	Resection	16.7	Wound infection	2.6
			Abdominal abscess	13.2
	Decompression	16.9		
Carcinoma of bile ducts (middle portion)[86]	Resection	8.3	Wound infection	8.3
			Abdominal abscess	16.7
			Bile leak (transient)	41.7
Benign stricture[34, 49, 68, 126, 161, 172]	Hepaticojejunostomy	3.9	Abdominal abscess	13.2
			Gastrointestinal hemorrhage	9.1

(continued)

BILE DUCTS (*continued*)

Pathologic Condition	Therapy	Mortality (%)	Morbidity	Percent
Choledochal cyst[158, 166, 302]	Excision	0		
	Bypass	6.3	Abdominal abscess	1.1
Stricture or stenosis at sphincter of Oddi[71, 95, 118, 150, 190, 267]	Choledochoduodenostomy	2.2	Wound infection	7.3
			Biliocutaneous fistula	3.3
			Pancreatitis	0.8
	Sphincteroplasty	1.1	Wound infection	4.5
			Biliocutaneous fistula	1.1
			Pancreatitis	2.3
Choledocholithiasis[105, 289]	Common bile duct exploration	4.9		
Primary common bile duct stone[235]	Common bile duct exploration	0		

BREAST

Pathologic Condition	Therapy	Mortality (%)	Morbidity	Percent
Carcinoma[173, 179]	Radical and modified radical mastectomy (excluding extended radical mastectomy)	0	Skin necrosis	4.3
			Seroma	4.7
Metastatic breast carcinoma[38, 253]	Adrenalectomy (transabdominal approach)	4.2	Wound infection	7.1
			Hemorrhage	3.6
			Splenic laceration	12.1
	Adrenalectomy (posterior approach)	2.6	Wound infection	15.4
			Hemorrhage	2.6
	Oophorectomy[167, 219]	4.1		

COLON

Pathologic Condition	Therapy	Mortality (%)	Morbidity	Percent
Carcinoma of intra-abdominal colon*[291]	Resection and primary anastomosis	3.3	Wound infection	6.3
			Anastomotic leak	9.0
			Abdominal abscess	2.7
Carcinoma of ascending colon and cecum[273]	Right colectomy	7.9		
Carcinoma of transverse colon[18, 291]	Transverse colectomy	2.7	Wound infection	2.7
			Abdominal abscess	2.7
Carcinoma of descending and sigmoid colon[9, 27, 46, 193, 297]	Left colectomy	6.3	Wound infection	18.8
			Anastomotic leak	6.3
	Anterior resection	1.7	Anastomotic leak	6.6
	Low anterior resection	1.9	Anastomotic leak	9.8

* Summary figures reflecting all intra-abdominal sites

COLON (*continued*)

Pathologic Condition	Therapy	Mortality (%)	Morbidity	Percent
Carcinoma of the rectum[88, 210]	Abdominoperineal resection	7.8	Wound infection	15.5
			Abdominal or pelvic abscess	3.2
			Wound dehiscence	5.9
	Fulguration[178, 236]	0	Hemorrhage	15
			Abscess	6.7
			Perforation	2.7
Perforative colon carcinoma[293]	Colostomy	35.5	Wound infection	11
	Primary resection	21.1	Abdominal abscess	5.9
	Staged resection	26.1		
Obstructing colon carcinoma[292]	Colostomy	46.7		
	Primary resection	16.1		
	Colostomy followed by resection	3.8		
Crohn's colitis[108, 113]	Resection	5.3	Wound infection	10.4
			Abdominal abscess	3.9
			Anastomotic leak	3
			Wound dehiscence	1.3
Diverticular hemorrhage[24, 79]	Abdominal colectomy (urgent)	11.1	Wound infection	10
			Anastomotic leak	3.3
Diverticulitis (perforated)[57, 85, 196]	Colostomy ± drainage	10.9	Wound infection	14.7
	Colostomy + resection	5.6	Wound infection	22.2
			Abdominal abscess	5.6
	Resection + anastomosis	0	Wound infection	3.5
			Abdominal abscess	2.8
Colostomy[4, 23]	Colostomy closure (end to end)	0	Wound infection	3.9
			Anastomotic leak	3.9
			Abdominal abscess	5.3
	Colostomy closure (simple)	0	Wound infection	13.8
			Anastomotic leak	2.9
Hirschsprung's disease[238, 258, 269, 271]	Duhamel procedure	2.1	Wound infection	8.5
			Anastomotic leak	4.3
	Soave procedure	0	Wound infection	13.3
			Anastomotic leak	20
	Swenson procedure	3.1	Wound infection	4.7
			Anastomotic leak	5.5
			Abscess	4.6
Trauma (penetrating)[99, 128, 264]	Closure + proximal colostomy	10.6	Wound infection	51.1
			Abdominal abscess	28.7
	Primary closure*	1.9	Wound infection	28.4
			Abdominal abscess	10.3
			Colocutaneous fistula	3.9
	Exteriorized primary closure[203]	4.2	Wound infection	2.1
			Abdominal abscess	2.1
			Conversion to colostomy	41.7
Ulcerative colitis[5, 109, 247]	Urgent proctocolectomy	8.3	Wound infection	23.4
			Abdominal abscess	10.6
	Urgent colectomy	7	Wound infection	20.9
	Elective abdominal colectomy	2.9	Abdominal abscess	18.6
Volvulus of cecum[15, 156, 205, 257]	Right colectomy	17.6	Wound infection	21.4
	Cecopexy	10.1	Wound infection	10
	Cecostomy	26.7	Wound infection	16.7
Volvulus of sigmoid[15, 156]	Urgent colectomy	40.6		
	Elective colectomy	10.4		

* Applied to selected cases

DIAPHRAGM

Pathologic Condition	Therapy	Mortality (%)	Morbidity	Percent
Congenital hernia[115, 120, 188, 225, 251]	Repair	32.7	Contralateral pneumothorax	9.5
			Ipsilateral pneumothorax	19.6
			Pneumonia	49
Traumatic hernia[25, 114, 157, 200]	Repair	21.9	Aspiration ± pneumonia	22.6
			Empyema	12.5

DUODENUM

Pathologic Condition	Therapy	Mortality (%)	Morbidity	Percent
Mural hematoma secondary to trauma[144, 298]	Nasogastric suction	7.7		
	Bypass	0		
			Wound infection	38.7
Perforation secondary to trauma[59, 74, 89]	Bypass or closure	23.5	Duodenal fistula	16.7
			Abdominal abscess	20.8

ESOPHAGUS

Pathologic Condition	Therapy	Mortality (%)	Morbidity	Percent
Achalasia[26, 42, 300]	Heller myotomy	0	Gastroesophageal reflux	20.8
			Pneumonia	8.3
			Empyema	4.2
	Pneumatic dilatation	0	Gastroesophageal reflux	6.3
			Aspiration	4.2
	Bougienage	0	Esophageal perforation	6.3
Boerhaave's syndrome[31, 270]	Drainage and repair	20	Wound infection	22.2
			Recurrent leak	6.7
			Mediastinal abscess ± empyema	33.3
Carcinoma of the thoracic esophagus[84, 117, 215]	Esophagogastrectomy	13.4		
	Colon transplant	24.1	Cervical fistula	28.4
			Mediastinitis	8
			Pneumonia	10.7
			Necrosis of colon	7.8
Carcinoma of the cervical esophagus[7]	Extrathoracic esophagectomy and gastric pull-through	5.9	Anastomotic leak	4
Carcinoma of the cardia[52, 129, 248, 265]	Esophagogastrectomy	14.3	Anastomotic leak	10
			Wound infection	5.7
			Pneumonia	8
			Abdominal abscess	2.3
Reflux esophagitis[19, 28, 45, 77, 232, 252]	Nissen procedure	1.2	Splenectomy	16.8
			Wound infection	6
			Subphrenic abscess	1.3
	Belsey procedure	0.5	Splenectomy	7.3
			Wound infection	4.7
			Perforation	2.3
	Hill procedure	4.3	Splenectomy	8.7

GALLBLADDER

Pathologic Condition	Therapy	Mortality (%)	Morbidity	Percent
Chronic cholecystitis or cholelithiasis[145, 278, 286]	Elective cholecystectomy	0.3	Wound infection	1.6
			Pneumonia	0.4
			Abscess	0.4
Acute cholecystitis[105, 181, 191]	Urgent cholecystectomy	0.8	Wound infection	2.3
			Abscess	0.4
			Wound dehiscence	1
			Pneumonia	0.6
	Cholecystostomy[104]	11.7		

LIVER

Pathologic Condition	Therapy	Mortality (%)	Morbidity	Percent
Abscess (pyogenic)[222, 240, 284]	Drainage	25.4	Recurrent abscess	7.1
			Abdominal abscess	3
			Hemorrhage	7.1
Carcinoma—primary liver[20, 65, 147, 170, 259]	Resection	14.2	Wound infection	9.6
			Abdominal abscess	6.4
			Bile leak	5.3
			Hemorrhage	1.2
Carcinoma—metastatic to liver[6, 92, 119]	Lobectomy	8.9	Wound infection	18.2
	Wedge and segmental resections	2.6		
Portal hypertension[110, 143, 206, 226, 231, 256, 274]	Portacaval shunt	29.2	Occluded shunt	7.8
	Distal splenorenal shunt	11.5	Occluded shunt	7.7
	Mesocaval shunt	13.2	Occluded shunt	19.6
Trauma, simple laceration[10, 208]	Suture ± drainage	7	Wound infection	4.2
			Abdominal abscess	2.3
Trauma, complex laceration[10, 208]	Débridement or resection + drainage	14.3	Wound infection	5.9
			Abdominal abscess	8.9

LUNG

Pathologic Condition	Therapy	Mortality (%)	Morbidity	Percent
Carcinoma of the lung[78, 106, 148, 216, 250, 279]	Mediastinoscopy	0.1	Hemorrhage	0.8
			Pneumothorax	0.6
			Wound infection	0.3
			Chylothorax	0.2
	Anterior mediastinotomy	0	Pneumothorax	4.8
Carcinoma of the lung[63, 76, 124, 290]	Pneumonectomy	16	Pneumothorax	11.2
			Pneumonia	8
			Bronchopleural fistula	8
			Hemorrhage	6.4
			Wound infection	5.9
			Empyema	5.9
	Lobectomy	9.5		
	Exploratory thoracotomy	9.3		
Cancer metastatic to lung[136, 138, 139, 285]	Resections	0		
Mesothelioma[288]	Resection or biopsy	1.9	Hemorrhage	13
			Trapped lung	3.7
Diffuse pulmonary disease[171, 223]	Open lung biopsy	4.8	Pneumothorax*	5.8
			Pleural effusion*	24.4
			Hemothorax	0.5
			Wound infection	0.9
Bronchial carcinoid[43, 202, 281]	Resection	10.3		
Respiratory insufficiency[123]	Tracheostomy	1.6	Hemorrhage	3.7
			Infection	3.3
			Obstruction	2.7
			Displaced tube	1.5
			Pneumothorax	0.9
Trauma—flail chest[64, 249, 280]	Ventilator	16.3	Tracheoesophageal fistula	10.5
			Pneumonia	50
			Hemorrhage	5.3
	Conservative management of pulmonary contusion	0	Pneumonia	10

* Majority of cases closed without thoracostomy tube initially

LYMPHATICS

Pathologic Condition	Therapy	Mortality (%)	Morbidity	Percent
Hodgkin's disease[237, 255, 261, 282]	Staging laparotomy	0	Wound infection	3.3
			Abdominal abscess	0.9
			Hemorrhage	0.4
			Pancreatitis	0.6
			Wound dehiscence	0.8
Metastatic cancer	Axillary lymph node dissection[55]	0		
	Radical groin dissection[125, 287*]	0	Wound necrosis	28.2
			Seroma	20.3
			Wound infection	9
			Hemorrhage	3.7
	Superficial groin dissection†	0	Wound necrosis	38.1
			Seroma	7.9
			Wound infection	20.6
			Hemorrhage	1.6

* Chretien PB: Unpublished data

† Parker GA: Unpublished data

OBESITY

Pathologic Condition	Therapy	Mortality (%)	Morbidity	Percent
Obesity	Gastric bypass or partitioning[40, 185, 207, 211]	1.4	Perforation or leak	3.6
			Splenectomy	4
			Wound infection	3.1
			Dehiscence	0.5
			Abscess	2.7
	Jejunoileal bypass[17, 87, 146, 245]	2.3	Anastomotic leak	0.5
			Wound infection	12.7
			Wound dehiscence	0.9
			Abdominal abscess	0

PANCREAS

Pathologic Condition	Therapy	Mortality (%)	Morbidity	Percent
Abscess[47, 187]	Drainage	23.5	Recurrent abscess	32.6
			Wound infection	26.1
			Wound dehiscence	5.2
			Diabetes	17.6
			Pancreatic cutaneous fistula	30.7
Carcinoma[30, 62, 82, 91, 199, 230]	Resection	21.1	Abdominal abscess	5.6
			Pancreatic leak	11.3
			Biliary leak	4.8
			Gastric leak	2.4
			Hemorrhage	9.7
			Wound dehiscence	0.8
	Biliary bypass	18.4	Abdominal abscess	7.1
			Recurrent biliary obstruction	11.9
			Subsequent duodenal obstruction	28.2
	Biliary and gastric bypass	22.8	Abdominal abscess	2
			Recurrent biliary obstruction	5.9
Pseudocyst[97, 127, 184, 283]	Cystgastrostomy	6.5	Hemorrhage	4.3
			Recurrence	18.3
			Pancreatic fistula	5.6
	Cystjejunostomy	3.6	Hemorrhage	4.1
			Recurrence	8.2
	External drainage	11.5	Recurrence	25.6
			Hemorrhage	7.7
			Pancreatic fistula	10.9
			Dehiscence	2.1
			Abscess	11.9
Trauma[12, 149, 155, 260, 299]	Drainage	14.2	Pancreatic fistula	7.3
			Pseudocyst	3
			Pancreatitis	16.7
			Hemorrhage	8
			Sepsis*	10.8
	Resection	15.8	Pancreatic fistula	11.4
			Pseudocyst	0
			Pancreatitis	10.5
			Hemorrhage	4.7
			Sepsis*	25.9

* Wound, abdominal, and pelvic infections

PARATHYROID

Pathologic Condition	Therapy	Mortality (%)	Morbidity	Percent
Primary hyperparathyroidism[58, 81, 294]	Subtotal parathyroidectomy	0	Hypoparathyroidism	20
			Recurrent hyperparathyroidism	10
	Excision of enlarged glands	0	Hypoparathyroidism	3
			Recurrent hyperparathyroidism	0.4
Recurrent hyperparathyroidism[22, 36]	Reexploration and resection	4.8	Persistent hyperparathyroidism	19.4
			Hypoparathyroidism	30.6
			Vocal cord paresis	8.1

PULMONARY EMBOLUS

Pathologic Condition	Therapy	Mortality (%)	Morbidity	Percent
Pulmonary embolus[2, 60, 112, 165, 189, 195]	Inferior vena cava filter	1.7	Recurrent embolus	2.3
			Misplaced	18.4
			Edema	11.8
	Inferior vena cava ligation	16.8	Recurrent embolus	4.4
	Inferior vena cava clip	13.8	Recurrent embolus	5.2

RECTUM

Pathologic Condition	Therapy	Mortality (%)	Morbidity	Percent
Abscess (perirectal)[29, 177]	Incision and drainage	6.5	Recurrent abscess	9.8
	Primary fistulectomy	0	Recurrent abscess	2.1
			Hemorrhage	0.4
Squamous cell carcinoma of anus[21, 107]	Abdominoperineal resection	3.5	Wound infection	7.4
			Hemorrhage	5.3
			Abscess	1.1
Squamous cell carcinoma of perianal skin[107]	Wide local excision	0		

SMALL BOWEL

Pathologic Condition	Therapy	Mortality (%)	Morbidity	Percent
Atresia[73, 272]	Resection and anastomosis	35.5	Anastomotic leak	23.5
Crohn's disease[121, 134, 212]	Resection	1.2	Wound infection	0
			Anastomotic leak	3.8
			Abdominal abscess	2.6
			Wound dehiscence	0.9
	Bypass	0	Wound infection	2.2
			Anastomotic leak	2.2

SPLEEN

Pathologic Condition	Therapy	Mortality (%)	Morbidity	Percent
Abscess[98, 164, 214]	Splenectomy	0	Abdominal abscess	14.3
Cyst[159, 233, 254]	Splenectomy	0	Wound infection	0
			Abdominal abscess	0
Trauma[32, 44, 180, 186, 266]	Splenectomy	1.5	Abdominal abscess	2.2
			Wound dehiscence	1.1
	Splenorrhaphy	0		
Iatrogenic injury[56, 67, 204]	Splenectomy	10.1	Wound infection	9.4
			Abdominal abscess	4.3
			Hemorrhage	0.9
			Wound dehiscence	0.3

STOMACH

Pathologic Condition	Therapy	Mortality (%)	Morbidity	Percent
Carcinoma[3, 80, 133, 142, 160, 295]	Distal or subtotal gastrectomy	10.4	Wound infection	6.5
	Total or proximal gastrectomy	12.8	Enterocutaneous fistula	5.4
	Exploration or bypass	16		
Congenital hypertrophic pyloric obstruction[102]	Pyloromyotomy	0	Wound infection	0.8
			Perforation	0.8
Peptic ulcer disease[11, 152, 176, 209, 217 239]	Vagotomy and drainage	3	Wound infection	9.8
			Wound dehiscence	3
			Splenectomy	3.2
			Esophageal perforation	0.8
	Vagotomy and antrectomy	2.3	Wound infection	2
			Wound dehiscence	0.7
			Duodenal leak	1.8
	Parietal cell vagotomy	0	Wound infection	6.6
			Wound dehiscence	2.2
			Abdominal abscess	0.7
	Vagotomy*	0.4	Splenectomy	4.9
			Esophageal perforation	0.7
Perforated ulcer[61, 151, 242, 243]	Plication and parietal cell vagotomy	4	Wound infection	10
			Abdominal abscess	10.3
	Plication	9.8	Wound infection	25.2
			Abdominal abscess	7.6
Massive hemorrhage[39, 263]	Resection	10.6	Duodenal leak	6.9
			Abdominal abscess	3.4
	Vagotomy and drainage	7.1		

*Analysis of complication related to the technical aspects of performing a vagotomy, regardless of the accompanying procedure

THYROID

Pathologic Condition	Therapy	Mortality (%)	Morbidity	Percent
Carcinoma[41, 94, 277]	Thyroid lobectomy	1.4	Hypoparathyroidism	1.4
			Vocal cord paralysis	0.7
			Hemorrhage	0.3
	Total thyroidectomy	0.8	Hypoparathyroidism	8.2
			Vocal cord paralysis	3.1
			Hemorrhage	1.3
Hyperthyroidism[35, 94, 213, 244]	Subtotal thyroidectomy	0.3	Hypoparathyroidism	3.7
			Vocal cord paralysis	0.6
			Hemorrhage	1.9
	Total thyroidectomy	0.6	Hypoparathyroidism	5.1
			Vocal cord paralysis	2.7
			Hemorrhage	2.1
Thyroglossal duct*[70, 116]	Excision	0.6	Hematoma	4.4
			Wound infection	2.7

* Both studies from same institution, but not inclusive

VASCULAR CONDITIONS

Pathologic Condition	Therapy	Mortality (%)	Morbidity	Percent
End-stage distal lower extremity ischemia[192]	Below-the-knee amputation	7.4	Failure to heal*	17.6
			Wound infection	7.4
			Hematoma	1.9
Aneurysm—abdominal aortic[131, 262, 275, 301]	Grafting of abdominal aortic aneurysm	8.3	Myocardial infarction	7.7
			Renal failure	5.3
			Distal ischemia	5.4
			Wound infection	0.4
			Wound dehiscence	0.8
			Infected graft	1.7
Aneurysm—ruptured abdominal aortic[53, 131, 132, 220]	Grafting of abdominal aortic aneurysm	42	Myocardial infarction	16.1
			Renal failure	16.1
			Distal ischemia	8.4
			Infected graft	5.4
Aneurysm—popliteal artery[33, 54, 141]	Grafting of popliteal artery aneurysm	0.6	Distal ischemia	4.3
Aortoiliac occlusive disease	Aortofemoral bypass graft[37, 93, 100, 182]	2.6	Distal ischemia	1.1
			Infected graft	0.6
			False aneurysm†	2.5
	Aortoiliac endarterectomy[37, 100, 140]	5	Distal ischemia	4.1
			Wound infection	1
			Hemorrhage	0.5
	Axillofemoral bypass graft[175, 224]	6.5	Acute graft failure	5.6
			Wound infection	1.9
			False aneurysm†	1.9
	Femorofemoral bypass graft[69, 75, 101, 181]	3.8	Acute graft failure	9.9
			Wound infection	2.1
			False aneurysm†	0.8
Carotid artery stenosis or ulceration[51, 218, 268, 276, 296]	Carotid endarterectomy	1.8	Stroke	3.1
			Myocardial infarction	0.9
			Hemorrhage	0.9
			Wound infection	0.9
Embolus[96, 111, 241]	Fogarty catheter embolectomy	28.4	Subsequent amputation	16.4
			Wound infection	3.3
			Hematoma	4.1
Subclavian steal syndrome	Axilloaxillary bypass graft[194]	0	Wound infection	0
Superficial femoral artery occlusion	Femoropopliteal bypass graft[66, 154, 174, 197, 198, 221, 228]	2	Acute graft failure	11.7
			Wound infection	2.7
			Hemorrhage	2.7
	Femorotibial or femoroperoneal bypass graft[83, 153, 201, 227]	3.7	Acute graft failure	11.3

* Requiring higher level of amputation

† Late complication

Section B

Complications for each disease process treated by a given operation (listed alphabetically)

Operation	Indication	Mortality (%)	Complications (%)		
			Wound Infection	*Abdominal Abscess*	*Wound Dehiscence*
Abdominoperineal resection	Carcinoma of the rectum[88, 210]	7.8	15.5	3.2	5.9
	Ulcerative colitis (fulminant)[5, 109, 247]	8.3	23.4	18.6	*
	Squamous cell carcinoma of anus[21, 107]	3.5	7.4	1.1	

* Data not available

Operation	Indication	Mortality (%)	Complications (%)			
			Wound Infection	*Wound Hematoma*	*Lacerated Spleen*	*Venous Hemorrhage*
Adrenalectomy (transabdominal approach)	Hyperaldosteronism[16, 137]	8.1	4.1		8.1	4.1
	Cushing's syndrome[72, 122]	15.6	3		3	0
	Pheochromocytoma[229, 246]	3	3			
	Metastatic breast carcinoma[38, 253]	4.2	7.1		12.1	3.6
Adrenalectomy (posterior approach)	Hyperaldosteronism[16, 130, 137]	0	2.9	4.1	0	0
	Cushing's syndrome[72]	0	0	0		
	Metastatic breast carcinoma[38]	2.6	15.4			2.6

Operation	Indication	Mortality (%)	Complications (%)					
			Wound Infection	*Infected Graft*	*Wound Dehiscence*	*Distal Ischemia*	*Renal Failure*	*Myocardial Infarction*
Aortic graft	Abdominal aortic aneurysm[131, 262, 275, 301]	8.3	0.4	1.7	0.8	5.4	5.3	7.7
	Ruptured abdominal aortic aneurysm[55, 131, 132, 220]	42		5.4		8.4	16.1	16.1
	Aortoiliac occlusive disease[37, 100, 182]	2.6		0.6		1.1		

Operation	Indication	Mortality (%)	Complications (%)		
			Wound Infection	*Abdominal Abscess*	*Wound Dehiscence*
Cholecystectomy	Cholelithiasis[145, 279, 286]	0.3	1.6	0.4	
	Acute cholecystitis[105, 191]	0.8	2.3	0.4	1

Operation	Indication	Mortality (%)	Complications (%)		
			Wound Infection	*Biliary Fistula*	*Pancreatitis*
Choledochoduodenostomy[71, 95, 267]	Bile duct stricture	2.2	7.3	3.3	0.8

Operation	Indication	Mortality (%)	Complications (%)			
			Wound Infection	*Abdominal Abscess*	*Anastomotic Leak*	*Wound Dehiscence*
Colectomy and primary anastomosis	Carcinoma[291]	3.3	6.3	2.7	9	
	Perforative carcinoma[293]	21.1	5.9	11		
	Obstructing carcinoma[292]	16.1				
	Crohn's colitis[108, 113]	5.3	10.4	3.9	3	1.3
	Diverticular hemorrhage[24, 79]	11.1	10		3.3	
	Perforated diverticulum*[85, 196]	0	3.5	2.8		
	Volvulus of sigmoid (emergency procedure)[156]	40.6				
	Volvulus of sigmoid (elective procedure)[156]	10.4				

* Selected cases

Operation	Indication	Mortality (%)	Complications (%)		
			Pneumonia	*Empyema*	*Pneumothorax*
Diaphragmatic hernia repair	Congenital hernia[115, 120, 182, 225, 251]	32.7	49		29.1
	Traumatic hernia[25, 114, 157, 200]	21.9	22.6	12.5	

Operation	Indication	Mortality (%)	Complications (%)		
			Wound Infection	*Anastomotic Leak*	*Abdominal Abscess*
Esophagogastrectomy	Carcinoma of the esophagus[84, 117, 215]	13.4			
	Carcinoma of the gastric cardia[52, 129, 248, 265]	14.3	5.7	10	2.3

Operation	Indication	Mortality (%)	Complications (%)		
			Wound Infection	*Enterocutaneous Fistula*	*Wound Dehiscence*
Gastrectomy (distal)	Cancer[3, 80, 133, 142, 295]	10.4	6.5	5.4	
	Ulcer[152, 209, 217]	2.3	2	1.8	0.7

Operation	Indication	Mortality (%)	Complications (%)			
			Wound Infection	*Abdominal Abscess*	*Bile Leak*	*Hemorrhage*
Hepatic lobectomy	Primary liver carcinoma[20, 65, 147, 170, 259]	14.2	9.6	6.4	5.3	1.2
	Metastatic carcinoma in the liver[6, 92, 119]	8.9	18.2			
	Trauma[10, 208]	14.3	5.9	8.9		

Operation	Indication	Mortality (%)	Complications (%)			
			Wound Infection	*Abdominal Abscess*	*Gastrointestinal Hemorrhage*	*Bile Leak*
Hepaticojejunostomy	Biliary atresia[50, 169]	5.9	0	5.9	5.9	
	Carcinoma of hepatic hilar bile ducts[8, 14, 48, 162]	16.7	2.6	13.2		
	Benign stricture of bile duct[34, 49, 68, 161, 172]	3.9		13.2	9.1	

Operation	Indication	Mortality (%)	Complications (%)	
			Skin Necrosis	*Seroma*
Mastectomy (radical and modified radical)[173, 179]	Carcinoma of the breast	0	4.3	4.7

Operation	Indication	Mortality (%)	Complications (%)					
			Abdominal Abscess	*Pancreatic Leak*	*Biliary Leak*	*Gastric Leak*	*Hemorrhage*	*Wound Dehiscence*
Pancreatic resection	Carcinoma[62, 82, 91, 199, 230]	21.1	5.6	11.3	4.8	2.4	9.7	0.8
	Trauma[12, 149, 155, 299]	15.8	*	11.4	*	*	4.7	

* Total of these plus wound infection = 25.9%

Operation	Indication	Mortality (%)	Complications (%)		
			Wound Infection	*Abdominal Abscess*	*Wound Dehiscence*
Splenectomy	Splenic abscess[98, 164, 214]	0		14.3	
	Trauma[32, 44, 180, 186, 266]	1.5		2.2	1.1
	Iatrogenic injury[56, 67, 204]	10.1	9.4	4.3	0.3

Operation	Indication	Mortality (%)	Complications (%)		
			Hypoparathyroidism	*Vocal Cord Paralysis*	*Hemorrhage*
Total thyroidectomy	Cancer[41, 94, 277]	0.8	8.2	3.1	1.3
	Hyperthyroidism[35, 94]	0.6	5.1	2.7	2.1
Thyroid lobectomy	Cancer[41, 94]	1.4	1.4	0.7	0.3
Subtotal thyroidectomy	Hyperthyroidism[94, 213, 244]	0.3	3.7	0.6	1.9

References

1. Aaronson IA, Eckstein HB: The role of the Silastic prosthesis in the management of gastroschisis. Arch Surg 112:297-302, 1977
2. Adams JT, Feingold BE, DeWeese JA: Comparative evaluation of ligation and partial interruption of the inferior vena cava. Arch Surg 103:272-276, 1971
3. Adashek K, Sanger J, Longmire WP: Cancer of the stomach: Review of consecutive ten-year intervals. Ann Surg 189:6-10, 1979
4. Adeyemo A, Gaillard WE et al: Colostomy: Intraperitoneal or extraperitoneal closure? Am J Surg 130:273-274, 1975
5. Adson MA, Cooperman AM, Farrow GM: Ileorectostomy for ulcerative disease of the colon. Arch Surg 104:424-428, 1972
6. Adson MA, Van Heerden JA: Major hepatic resections for metastatic colorectal cancer. Ann Surg 191:576-583, 1980
7. Akiyama H, Hiyama M, Miyazono H: Total esophageal reconstruction after extraction of the esophagus. Ann Surg 182:547-552, 1975
8. Akwari OE, Kelly KA: Surgical treatment of adenocarcinoma. Location: Junction of the right, left, and common hepatic biliary ducts. Arch Surg 114:22-25, 1979
9. Akwari OE, Kelly KA: Anterior resection for adenocarcinoma of the distal large bowel. Am J Surg 139:88-94, 1980
10. Aldrete JS, Halpern NB, Ward S, Wright JO: Factors determining the mortality and morbidity in hepatic injuries. Ann Surg 189:466-474, 1979
11. Amdrup E, Jensen HE et al: Clinical results of parietal cell vagotomy (highly selective vagotomy) two to four years after operation. Ann Surg 180:279-284, 1974
12. Anane–Sefah J, Norton LW, Eiseman B: Operative choice and technique following pancreatic injury. Arch Surg 110:161-166, 1975
13. Andersson A, Bergdahl L, van der Linden W: Volvulus of the cecum. Ann Surg 181:876-880, 1975

14. Andersson A, Bergdahl L, van der Linden W: Malignant tumors of the extrahepatic bile ducts. Surgery 81:198-202, 1977
15. Arnold GJ, Nance FC: Volvulus of the sigmoid colon. Ann Surg 177:527-533, 1973
16. Auda SP, Brennan MF, Gill JR: Evolution of the surgical management of primary aldosteronism. Ann Surg 191:1-7, 1980
17. Baber JC, Hayden WF, Thompson BW: Intestinal bypass operations for obesity. Am J Surg 126:769-772, 1973
18. Bacon HE, Gennaro AR: Carcinoma of the transverse colon and the splenic flexure. Surg Gynecol Obstet 127:523-527, 1968
19. Bahadorzadeh K, Jordan PH: Evaluation of the Nissen fundoplication for treatment of hiatal hernia: Use of parietal cell vagotomy without drainage as an adjunctive procedure. Ann Surg 181:402-408, 1975
20. Balasegaram M: Complete hepatic dearterialization for primary carcinoma of the liver. Am J Surg 124:340-345, 1972
21. Beahrs OH, Wilson SM: Carcinoma of the anus. Ann Surg 184:422-428, 1976
22. Beazley RM, Costa J, Ketcham AS: Reoperative parathyroid surgery. Am J Surg 130:427-429, 1975
23. Beck PH, Conklin HB: Closure of colostomy. Ann Surg 181:795-798, 1975
24. Behringer GE, Albright NL: Diverticular disease of the colon: A frequent cause of massive rectal bleeding. Am J Surg 125:419-423, 1973
25. Bekassy SM, Dave KS, Wooler GH, Ionescu MI: "Spontaneous" and traumatic rupture of the diaphragm: Long-term results. Ann Surg 177:320-324, 1973
26. Benjamin B, Cohen D, Glasson M: Tracheomalacia in association with congenital tracheoesophageal fistula. Surgery 79:504-508, 1976
27. Berne CJ, Caneday RH, Rosoff L: Acute septic complications of anterior resection for carcinoma of the rectum. Surg Gynecol Obstet 134:767-770, 1972
28. Berry WB: Surgical correction of refractory reflux esophagitis using the standard unmodified Belsey Mark IV technique. Ann Thorac Surg 26:102-106, 1978
29. Bevans DW, Westbrook KC, Thompson BW, Caldwell FT: Perirectal abscess: A potentially fatal illness. Am J Surg 126:765-768, 1973
30. Blievernicht SW, Neifeld JP, Terz JJ, Lawrence W: The role of prophylactic gastrojejunostomy for unresectable periampullary carcinoma. Surg Gynecol Obstet 151:794-796, 1980
31. Bolooki H, Anderson I, Garcia–Rivera C, Jude JR: Spontaneous rupture of the esophagus: Boerhaave's syndrome. Ann Surg 174:319-324, 1971
32. Bostrom PD, Page HG: Splenectomy. Arch Surg 98:167-170, 1969
33. Bouhoutsos J, Martin P: Popliteal aneurysm: A review of 116 cases. Br J Surg 61:469-475, 1974
34. Braasch JW, Warren KW, Blevins PK: Progress in biliary stricture repair. Am J Surg 129:34-37, 1975
35. Bradley EL, DiGirolamo M, Tarcan Y: Modified subtotal thyroidectomy in the management of Graves' disease. Surgery 87:623-629, 1980
36. Brennan MF, Doppman JL et al: Reoperative parathyroid surgery for persistent hyperparathyroidism. Surgery 83:669-676, 1978
37. Brewster DC, Darling RC: Optimal methods of aortoiliac reconstruction. Surgery 84:739-748, 1978
38. Brown PW, Terz JJ, King R, Lawrence W: Bilateral adrenalectomy for metastatic breast carcinoma. Arch Surg 110:77-81, 1975
39. Buckingham JM, ReMine WH: Results of emergency surgical management of hemorrhagic duodenal ulcer. Mayo Clin Proc 50:223-226, 1975
40. Buckwalter JA, Herbst CA: Complications of gastric bypass for morbid obesity. Am J Surg 139:55-60, 1980
41. Buckwalter JA, Thomas CG: Selection of surgical treatment for well differentiated thyroid carcinomas. Ann Surg 176:565-578, 1972
42. Buker RH, Cox WA, Pauling FW, Seitter G: Complications of congenital tracheo-esophageal fistula. Am J Surg 124:705-710, 1972
43. Burcharth F, Axelsson C: Bronchial adenomas. Thorax 27:442-449, 1972
44. Burrington JD: Surgical repair of a ruptured spleen in children. Arch Surg 112:417-419, 1977
45. Bushkin FL, Neustein CL, Parker TH, Woodward ER: Nissen fundoplication for reflux peptic esophagitis. Ann Surg 185:672-677, 1977
46. Busuttil RW, Foglia RP, Longmire WP: Treatment of carcinoma of the sigmoid colon and upper rectum: A comparison of local segmental resection and left hemicolectomy. Arch Surg 112:920-923, 1977
47. Camer SJ, Tan EGC, Warren KW, Braasch JW: Pancreatic abscess: A critical analysis of 113 cases. Am J Surg 129:426-431, 1975
48. Cameron JL, Gaylor BW, Zuidema GD: The use of Silastic transhepatic stents in benign and malignant biliary strictures. Ann Surg 188:552-561, 1978
49. Cameron JL, Skinner DB, Zuidema GD: Long-term transhepatic intubation for hilar hepatic duct strictures. Ann Surg 183:488-495, 1976
50. Campbell DP, Smith EI et al: Hepatic portoenterostomy: An assessment of its value in the treatment of biliary atresia. Ann Surg 181:591-595, 1975
51. Carmichael JD: Carotid surgery in the community hospital. Arch Surg 15:937-939, 1980
52. Chassin JL: Esophagogastrectomy: Data favoring end-to-side anastomosis. Ann Surg 188:22-27, 1978
53. Chiariello L, Reul GJ et al: Ruptured abdominal aortic aneurysm: Treatment and review of eighty-seven patients. Am J Surg 128:735-738, 1974
54. Chitwood WR, Stocks LH, Wolfe WG: Popliteal artery aneurysms: Past and present. Arch Surg 113:1078-1082, 1978
55. Chretien PB, Ketcham AS, Hoye RC, Sample WF: Axillary dissection with preservation of the pectoralis major muscle. Ann Surg 173:554-560, 1971
56. Cioffiro W, Schein CJ, Gliedman ML: Splenic injury during abdominal surgery. Arch Surg 111:167-171, 1976
57. Classen JN, Bonardi R et al: Surgical treatment of acute diverticulitis by staged procedures. Ann Surg 184:582-586, 1976
58. Coffey RJ, Lee TC, Canary JJ: The surgical treatment of primary hyperparathyroidism: A 20-year experience. Ann Surg 185:518-523, 1977
59. Corley RD, Norcross WJ, Shoemaker WC: Traumatic injuries to the duodenum: A report of 98 patients. Ann Surg 181:92-98, 1975
60. Couch NP, Baldwin SS, Crane C: Mortality and morbidity rates after inferior vena caval clipping. Surgery 77:106-112, 1975
61. Coutsoftides T, Himal HS: Perforated gastroduodenal ulcers: Factors affecting morbidity and mortality and the role of definitive surgery. Am J Surg 132:575-576, 1976

62. Coutsoftides T, MacDonald J, Shibata HR: Carcinoma of the pancreas and periampullary region: A 41-year experience. Ann Surg 186:730-733, 1977
63. Cromartie RS, Parker EF et al: Carcinoma of the lung: A clinical review. Ann Thorac Surg 30:30-35, 1980
64. Cullen P, Modell JH et al: Treatment of flail chest: Use of intermittent mandatory ventilation and positive end-expiratory pressure. Arch Surg 110:1099-1103, 1975
65. Curutchet HP, Terz JJ, Kay S, Lawrence W: Primary liver cancer. Surgery 70:467-479, 1971
66. Cutler BS, Thompson JE, Kleinsasser LJ, Hempel GK: Autologous saphenous vein femoropopliteal bypass: Analysis of 298 cases. Surgery 79:325-331, 1976
67. Danforth DN, Thorbjarnarson B: Incidental splenectomy: A review of the literature and the New York Hospital experience. Ann Surg 183:124-129, 1976
68. Daugherty M, Ernst CB, Sachatello CR, Griffen WO: Proximal hepatic duct reconstruction: Repair using sutureless mucosal graft hepaticojejunostomy. Arch Surg 113:490-495, 1978
69. Davis RC, O'Hara ET et al: Broadened indications for femorofemoral grafts. Surgery 72:990-994, 1972
70. Deane SA, Telander RL: Surgery for thyroglossal duct and branchial cleft anomalies. Am J Surg 136:348-353, 1978
71. Degenshein GA: Choledochoduodenostomy: An 18-year study of 175 consecutive cases. Surgery 76:319-324, 1974
72. Delaney JP, Solomkin JS, Jacobson ME, Doe RP: Surgical management of Cushing's syndrome. Surgery 84:465-470, 1978
73. deLorimier AA, Fonkalsrud EW, Hays DM: Congenital atresia and stenosis of the jejunum and ileum. Surgery 65:819-827, 1969
74. DeMars JJ, Bubrick MP, Hitchcock CR: Duodenal perforation in blunt abdominal trauma. Surgery 86:632-638, 1979
75. Dick LS, Brief DK et al: A 12-year experience with femorofemoral crossover grafts. Arch Surg 115:1359-1365, 1980
76. Didolkar MS, Moore RH, Takita H: Evaluation of the risk in pulmonary resection for bronchogenic carcinoma. Am J Surg 127:700-703, 1974
77. Dilling EW, Peyton MD et al: Comparison of Nissen fundoplication and Belsey Mark IV in the management of gastroesophageal reflux. Am J Surg 134:730-733, 1977
78. Doctor AH: Mediastinoscopy: A critical evaluation of 220 cases. Ann Surg 174:965-968, 1971
79. Drapanas T, Pennington DG, Kappelman M, Lindsey ES: Emergency subtotal colectomy: Preferred approach to management of massively bleeding diverticular disease. Ann Surg 177:519-526, 1973
80. Dupont JB, Lee JR, Burton GR, Cohn I: Adenocarcinoma of the stomach: Review of 1,497 cases. Cancer 41:941-947, 1978
81. Edis AJ, Beahrs OH, van Heerden JA, Akwari OE: "Conservative" versus "liberal" approach to parathyroid neck exploration. Surgery 82:466-473, 1977
82. Edis AJ, Kiernan PD, Taylor WF: Attempted curative resection of ductal carcinoma of the pancreas. Mayo Clin Proc 55:531-536, 1980
83. Edwards WH, Wright RS: Tibial and peroneal bypass in severe occlusive disease of the lower extremities. Ann Surg 183:710-718, 1976
84. El–Domeiri A, Martini N, Beattie EJ: Esophageal reconstruction by colon interposition. Arch Surg 100:358-362, 1970
85. Eng K, Ranson JHC, Localio SA: Resection of the perforated segment: A significant advance in treatment of diverticulitis with free perforation or abscess. Am J Surg 133:67-72, 1977
86. Evander A, Fredlund P et al: Evaluation of aggressive surgery for carcinoma of the extrahepatic bile ducts. Ann Surg 191:23-29, 1980
87. Fikri E, Cassella RR: Jejunoileal bypass for massive obesity: Results and complications in fifty-two patients. Ann Surg 179:460-464, 1974
88. Fitzgibbons RJ, Harkrider WW, Cohn I: Review of abdominoperineal resections for cancer. Am J Surg 134:624-629, 1977
89. Flint LM, McCoy M, Richardson JD, Polk HC: Duodenal injury: Analysis of common misconceptions in diagnosis and treatment. Ann Surg 191:697-702, 1980
90. Fonkalsrud EW: Selective repair of neonatal gastroschisis based on degree of visceroabdominal disproportion. Ann Surg 191:139-144, 1980
91. Forrest JF, Longmire WP: Carcinoma of the pancreas and periampullary region: A study of 279 patients. Ann Surg 189:129-138, 1979
92. Foster JH: Survival after liver resection for secondary tumors. Am J Surg 135:389-394, 1978
93. Foster JH, Dean RH, Pinkerton JA, Rhamy RK: Ten years experience with the surgical management of renovascular hypertension. Ann Surg 177:755-766, 1973
94. Foster RS: Morbidity and mortality after thyroidectomy. Surg Gynecol Obstet 146:423-429, 1978
95. Freund H, Charuzi I et al: Choledochoduodenostomy in the treatment of benign biliary tract disease. Arch Surg 112:1032-1034, 1977
96. Freund U, Romanoff H, Floman Y: Mortality rate following lower limb arterial embolectomy: Causative factors. Surgery 77:201-207, 1975
97. Frey CF: Pancreatic pseudocyst—Operative strategy. Ann Surg 188:652-662, 1978
98. Fry DE, Richardson JD, Flint LM: Occult splenic abscess: An unrecognized complication of heroin abuse. Surgery 84:650-654, 1978
99. Garfinkle SE, Cohen SE et al: Civilian colonic injuries: Changing concepts of management. Arch Surg 109:402-404, 1974
100. Gaspard DJ, Cohen JL, Gaspar MR: Aortoiliofemoral thromboendarterectomy versus bypass graft: A randomized study. Arch Surg 105:898-901, 1972
101. Gazzola LM, Hirsch SA, Kaufer GI: Femorofemoral bypass. Surgery 76:841-844, 1974
102. Gibbs MK, van Heerden JA, Lynn HB: Congenital hypertrophic pyloric stenosis: Surgical experience. Mayo Clin Proc 50:312-316, 1975
103. Glassow F: Inguinal hernia repair: A comparison of the Shouldice and Cooper ligament repair of the posterior inguinal wall. Am J Surg 131:306-311, 1976
104. Glenn F: Cholecystostomy in the high risk patient with biliary tract disease. Ann Surg 185:185-191, 1977
105. Glenn F, Beil AR: Choledocholithiasis demonstrated at 586 operations. Surg Gynecol Obstet 118:499-506, 1964
106. Goldberg EM, Shapiro CM, Glicksman AS: Mediastinoscopy for assessing mediastinal spread in clinical staging of lung carcinoma. Semin Oncol 1:205-215, 1974
107. Golden GT, Horsley JS: Surgical management of epidermoid carcinoma of the anus. Am J Surg 131:275-280, 1976
108. Goligher JC: The outcome of excisional operations for

primary and recurrent Crohn's disease of the large intestine. Surg Gynecol Obstet 148:1-8, 1979
109. Goligher JC, Hoffman DC, de Dombal FT: Surgical treatment of severe attacks of ulcerative colitis, with special reference to the advantages of early operation. Br Med J 4:703-706, 1970
110. Graziano JL, Sullivan HJ: Portal decompression: Clinical experience with the "H" graft. Ann Surg 178:209-214, 1973
111. Green RM, DeWeese JA, Rob CG: Arterial embolectomy before and after the Fogarty catheter. Surgery 77:24-33, 1975
112. Greenfield LJ, Zocco J et al: Clinical experience with the Kim-Ray Greenfield vena caval filter. Ann Surg 185:692-698, 1977
113. Greenstein AJ, Meyers S et al: Surgery and its sequelae in Crohn's colitis and ileocolitis. Arch Surg 116:285-288, 1981
114. Griswold FW, Warden HE, Gardner RJ: Acute diaphragmatic rupture caused by blunt trauma. Am J Surg 124:359-362, 1972
115. Grmoljez PF, Lewis JE: Congenital diaphragmatic hernia: Bochdalek type. Am J Surg 132:744-746, 1976
116. Guimaraes SB, Uceda JE, Lynn HB: Thyroglossal duct remnants in infants and children. Mayo Clin Proc 47:117-120, 1972
117. Gunnlaugsson GH, Wychulis AR, Roland C, Ellis FH: Analysis of the records of 1,657 patients with carcinoma of the esophagus and cardia of the stomach. Surg Gynecol Obstet 130:997-1005, 1970
118. Haff RC, Torma MJ: Oddi sphincteroplasty in the management of complicated biliary and pancreatic disease. Am J Surg 129:509-512, 1975
119. Hanks JB, Meyers WC et al: Surgical resection for benign and malignant liver disease. Ann Surg 191:584-592, 1980
120. Harberg FJ, Meagher D, Wetchler S, Harris F: Congenital anomalies of the diaphragm: Personal experience with thirty-five consecutive cases. Am J Surg 132:747-748, 1976
121. Hardin CA, Friesen RH: Surgical treatment of regional enteritis. Am J Surg 125:595-600, 1973
122. Hardy JD: Surgical management of Cushing's syndrome with emphasis on adrenal autotransplantation. Ann Surg 188:290-307, 1978
123. Hardy KL: Tracheostomy: Indications, technics, and tubes. Am J Surg 126:300-310, 1973
124. Harmon H, Fergus S, Cole FH: Pneumonectomy: Review of 351 cases. Ann Surg 183:719-722, 1976
125. Harris MN, Gumport SL, Berman IR, Bernard RW: Ilioinguinal lymph node dissection for melanoma. Surg Gynecol Obstet 136:33-39, 1973
126. Hart MJ, White TT: Central hepatic resection and anastomosis for stricture or carcinoma at the hepatic bifurcation. Ann Surg 192:299-305, 1980
127. Hastings PR, Nance FC, Becker WF: Changing patterns in the management of pancreatic pseudocysts. Ann Surg 181:546-551, 1975
128. Haygood FD, Polk HC: Gunshot wounds of the colon: A review of 100 consecutive patients, with emphasis on complications and their causes. Am J Surg 131:213-218, 1976
129. Hermreck AS, Crawford DG: The esophageal anastomotic leak. Am J Surg 132:794-798, 1976
130. Herwig KR: Primary aldosteronism: Experience with thirty-eight patients. Surgery 86:470-474, 1979
131. Hicks GL, Eastland MW et al: Survival improvement following aortic aneurysm resection. Ann Surg 181:863-869, 1975
132. Hildebrand HD, Fry PD: Ruptured abdominal aortic aneurysm. Surgery 77:540-544, 1975
133. Hoerr SO: Prognosis for carcinoma of the stomach. Surg Gynecol Obstet 137:205-209, 1973
134. Homan WP, Dineen P: Comparison of the results of resection, bypass, and bypass with exclusion for ileocecal Crohn's disease. Ann Surg 187:530-535, 1978
135. Hrabovsky EE, Boyd JB, Savrin RA, Boles ET: Advances in the management of gastroschisis. Ann Surg 192:244-248, 1980
136. Huang MN, Edgerton F et al: Lung resection for metastatic sarcoma. Am J Surg 135:804-806, 1978
137. Hunt TK, Schambelan M, Biglieri EG: Selection of patients and operative approach in primary aldosteronism. Ann Surg 182:353-361, 1975
138. Hutchison DE, Deaner RM: Resection of pulmonary secondary tumors. Am J Surg 124:732-737, 1972
139. Huth JF, Holmes EC et al: Pulmonary resection for metastatic sarcoma. Am J Surg 140:9-16, 1980
140. Inahara T: Eversion endarterectomy for aortoiliofemoral occlusive disease: A 16-year experience. Am J Surg 138:196-204, 1979
141. Inahara T, Toledo AC: Complications and treatment of popliteal aneurysms. Surgery 84:775-783, 1978
142. Inberg MV, Heinonen R, Rantakokko V, Viikari SJ: Surgical treatment of gastric carcinoma: A regional study of 2,590 patients over a 27-year period. Arch Surg 110:703-707, 1975
143. Jackson FC, Perrin EB, Felix WR, Smith AG: A clinical investigation of the portacaval shunt: V. Survival analysis of the therapeutic operation. Ann Surg 174:672-701, 1971
144. Janson KL, Stockinger F: Duodenal hematoma: Critical analysis of recent treatment technics. Am J Surg 129:304-308, 1975
145. Jarvinen HJ, Hastbacka J: Early cholecystectomy for acute cholecystitis: A prospective, randomized study. Ann Surg 191:501-505, 1980
146. Jewell WR, Hermreck AS, Hardin CA: Complications of jejunoileal bypass for morbid obesity. Arch Surg 110:1039-1042, 1975
147. Joishy SK, Balasegaram M: Hepatic resection for malignant tumors of the liver: Essentials for a unified surgical approach. Am J Surg 139:360-369, 1980
148. Jolly PC, Li W, Anderson RP: Anterior and cervical mediastinoscopy for determining operability and predicting resectability in lung cancer. J Thorac Cardiovasc Surg 79:366-371, 1980
149. Jones RC: Management of pancreatic trauma. Ann Surg 187:555-564, 1978
150. Jones SA, Smith LL: A reappraisal of sphincteroplasty (not sphincterotomy). Surgery 71:565-575, 1972
151. Jordan GL, DeBakey ME, Duncan JM: Surgical management of perforated peptic ulcer. Ann Surg 179:628-633, 1974
152. Jordan PH: A prospective study of parietal cell vagotomy and selective vagotomy-antrectomy for treatment of duodenal ulcer. Ann Surg 183:619-628, 1976
153. Kahn SP, Lindenauer SM et al: Femorotibial vein bypass. Arch Surg 107:309-312, 1973
154. Kaminski DL, Barner HB et al: Femoropopliteal bypass with reversed autogenous vein. Ann Surg 177:232-236, 1973
155. Karl HW, Chandler JG: Mortality and morbidity of pancreatic injury. Am J Surg 134:549-554, 1977

156. Kerry RL, Ransom HK: Volvulus of the colon: Etiology, diagnosis, and treatment. Arch Surg 99:215-222, 1969
157. Kessler E, Stein A: Diaphragmatic hernia as a long-term complication of stab wounds of the chest. Am J Surg 132:34-39, 1976
158. Kimura K, Tsugawa C et al: Choledochal cyst. Arch Surg 113:159-163, 1978
159. King MC, Glick BW, Freed A: The diagnosis of splenic cysts. Surg Gynecol Obstet 127:509-512, 1968
160. Koga S, Kishimoto H et al: Results of total gastrectomy for gastric cancer. Am J Surg 140:636-638, 1980
161. Lane CE, Sawyers JL, Riddell DH, Scott HW: Long-term results of Roux-en-Y hepatocholangiojejunostomy. Ann Surg 177:714-722, 1973
162. Launois B, Campion JP, Brissot P, Gosselin M: Carcinoma of the hepatic hilus. Ann Surg 190:151-157, 1979
163. Law D, Law R, Eiseman B: The continuing challenge of acute and perforated appendicitis. Am J Surg 131:533-535, 1976
164. Lawhorne TW, Zuidema GD: Splenic abscess. Surgery 79:686-689, 1976
165. Leather RP, Clark WR et al: Five-year experience with the Moretz vena caval clip in 62 patients. Arch Surg 97:357-364, 1968
166. Lee SS, Min PC, Kim GS, Hong PW: Choledochal cyst. Arch Surg 99:19-28, 1969
167. Lee YN: Therapeutic castration for advanced breast cancer. Am J Surg 122:42-49, 1971
168. Lewis FR, Holcroft JW, Boey J, Dunphy JE: Appendicitis. Arch Surg 110:677-684, 1975
169. Lilly JR, Altman RP: Hepatic portoenterostomy (the Kasai operation) for biliary atresia. Surgery 78:76-86, 1975
170. Lin T: Results in 107 hepatic lobectomies with a preliminary report on the use of a clamp to reduce blood loss. Ann Surg 177:413-421, 1973
171. Lincoln CP, Grover FL, Trinkle JK: Open versus needle biopsy of the lung. J Thorac Cardiovasc Surg 69:507-509, 1975
172. Lindenauer SM: Surgical treatment of bile duct strictures. Surgery 73:875-880, 1973
173. Livingston SF, Arlen M: The extended extrapleural radical mastectomy: Its role in the treatment of carcinoma of the breast. Ann Surg 179:260-265, 1974
174. LoGerfo FW, Corson JD, Mannick JA: Improved results with femoropopliteal vein grafts for limb salvage. Arch Surg 112:567-570, 1977
175. LoGerfo FW, Johnson WC et al: A comparison of the late patency rates of axillobilateral femoral and axillounilateral femoral grafts. Surgery 81:33-40, 1977
176. McDonald GO, Abtahi H: Critical appraisal of vagotomy and pyloroplasty: Treatment of peptic ulcer. Arch Surg 100:414-420, 1970
177. McElwain JW, MacLean MD et al: Anorectal problems: Experience with primary fistulectomy for anorectal abscess, a report of 1,000 cases. Dis Colon Rectum 18:646-649, 1975
178. Madden JL, Kandalaft S: Clinical evaluation of electrocoagulation in the treatment of cancer of the rectum. Am J Surg 122:347-352, 1971
179. Madden JL, Kandalaft S, Bourque RA: Modified radical mastectomy. Ann Surg 175:624-646, 1972
180. Magee RB, D'Luzansky JJ: Acute blunt traumatic rupture of the spleen. Arch Surg 99:121-122, 1969
181. Malmstrom P, Olsson AM: Cholecystostomy for acute cholecystitis. Am J Surg 127:397-402, 1973
182. Malone JM, Moore WS, Goldstone J: Life expectancy following aortofemoral arterial grafting. Surgery 81:551-555, 1977
183. Mannick JA, Maini BS: Femorofemoral grafting: Indications and late results. Am J Surg 136:190-192, 1978
184. Martin EW, Catalano P et al: Surgical decision-making in the treatment of pancreatic pseudocysts: Internal versus external drainage. Am J Surg 138:821-824, 1979
185. Mason EE, Printen KJ et al: Risk reduction in gastric operations for obesity. Ann Surg 190:158-165, 1979
186. Miller DW, Kelley DL: Splenic trauma: Surgical management in children. Arch Surg 105:561-563, 1972
187. Miller TA, Lindenauer SM, Frey CF, Stanley JC: Pancreatic abscess. Arch Surg 108:545-551, 1974
188. Mishalany HG, Nakada K, Woolley MM: Congenital diaphragmatic hernias: Eleven years' experience. Arch Surg 114:1118-1123, 1979
189. Mobin–Uddin K, Callard GM et al: Transvenous caval interruption with umbrella filter. N Engl J Med 286:55-58, 1972
190. Moody FG, Berenson MM, McCloskey D: Transampullary septectomy for postcholecystectomy pain. Ann Surg 186:415-423, 1977
191. Moore EE, Kelly GL, Driver T, Eiseman B: Reassessment of simple cholecystostomy. Arch Surg 114:515-518, 1979
192. Moore WS, Hall AD, Lim RC: Below the knee amputation for ischemic gangrene: Comparative results of conventional operation and immediate postoperative fitting technique. Am J Surg 124:127-134, 1972
193. Morgenstern L, Yamakawa T, Ben–Shoshan M, Lippman H: Anastomotic leakage after low colonic anastomosis: Clinical and experimental aspects. Am J Surg 123:104-108, 1972
194. Myers WO, Lawton BR et al: Axillo-axillary bypass for subclavian steal syndrome. Arch Surg 114:394-399, 1979
195. Nabseth DC, Moran JM: Reassessment of the role of inferior-vena-cava ligation in venous thromboembolism. N Engl J Med 273:1250-1253, 1965
196. Nahrwold DL, Demuth WE: Diverticulitis with perforation into the peritoneal cavity. Ann Surg 185:80-83, 1977
197. Naji A, Barker CF et al: Femoropopliteal vein grafts for claudication: Analysis of 100 consecutive cases. Ann Surg 188:79-82, 1978
198. Naji A, Chu J et al: Results of 100 consecutive femoropopliteal vein grafts for limb salvage. Ann Surg 188:162-165, 1978
199. Nakase A, Matsumoto Y, Uchida K, Honjo I: Surgical treatment of cancer of the pancreas and the periampullary region. Ann Surg 185:52-57, 1977
200. Nano M, DeiPoli M, Mossetti C, Maggi G: Traumatic diaphragmatic hernias. Surg Gynecol Obstet 151:191-192, 1980
201. Nicholas GG, Barker CF, Berkowitz HD, Roberts B: Reconstructive surgery distal to the popliteal trifurcation: Effect on the history of arterial occlusive disease. Arch Surg 107:652-656, 1973
202. O'Grady WP, McDivitt RW, Holman CW, Moore SW: Bronchial adenomas. Arch Surg 101:558-561, 1970
203. Okies JE, Bricker DL et al: Exteriorized primary repair of colon injuries. Am J Surg 124:807-810, 1972
204. Olsen WR, Beaudoin DE: Surgical injury to the spleen. Surg Gynecol Obstet 131:57-62, 1970
205. O'Mara CS, Wilson TH, Stonesifer GL, Cameron JL: Cecal volvulus: Analysis of 50 patients with long-term follow-up. Ann Surg 189:724-731, 1979
206. Orloff MJ, Bell RH, Hyde PV, Skivolocki WP: Long-term results of emergency portacaval shunt for bleeding esophageal varices in unselected patients with alcoholic cirrhosis. Ann Surg 192:325-340, 1980

207. Pace WG, Martin EW et al: Gastric partitioning for morbid obesity. Ann Surg 190:392-400, 1979
208. Pachter HL, Spencer FC: Recent concepts in the treatment of hepatic trauma: Facts and fallacies. Ann Surg 190:423-429, 1979
209. Palumbo LT, Sharpe WS: Distal antrectomy with vagectomy for duodenal ulcer. Ann Surg 182:610-616, 1975
210. Patel SC, Tovee EB, Langer B: Twenty-five years of experience with radical surgical treatment of carcinoma of the extraperitoneal rectum. Surgery 82:460-465, 1977
211. Peltier G, Hermreck AS et al: Complications following gastric bypass procedures for morbid obesity. Surgery 86:648-654, 1979
212. Pennington L, Hamilton SR, Bayless TM, Cameron JL: Surgical management of Crohn's disease: Influence of disease at margin of resection. Ann Surg 192:311-318, 1980
213. Perzick SL: Total thyroidectomy in the management of Grave's disease. Am J Surg 131:284-287, 1976
214. Pickleman JR, Paloyan E, Block GE: The surgical significance of splenic abscess. Surgery 68:287-293, 1970
215. Postlethwait RW, Sealy WC, Dillon ML, Young WG: Colon interposition for esophageal substitution. Ann Thorac Surg 12:89-107, 1971
216. Preciado MC, Duvall AJ, Koop SH: Mediastinoscopy: A review of 450 cases. Laryngoscope 83:1300-1310, 1973
217. Price WE, Grizzle JE et al: Results of operation for duodenal ulcer. Surg Gynecol Obstet 131:233-244, 1970
218. Prioleau WH, Aiken AF, Hairston P: Carotid endarterectomy: Neurologic complications as related to surgical techniques. Ann Surg 185:678-683, 1977
219. Puga FJ, Welch JS, Bisel HF: Therapeutic oophorectomy in disseminated carcinoma of the breast. Arch Surg 111:877-880, 1976
220. Rainer WG, Sadler TR, Guillen J: Ruptured abdominal aortic aneurysm. Am J Surg 126:794-797, 1973
221. Ramsburgh SR, Lindenauer SM et al: Femoropopliteal bypass for limb salvage. Surgery 81:453-458, 1977
222. Ranson JHC, Madayag MA, Localio SA, Spencer FC: New diagnostic and therapeutic techniques in the management of pyogenic liver abscesses. Ann Surg 181:508-518, 1975
223. Ray JF, Lawton BR et al: Open pulmonary biopsy: Nineteen-year experience with 416 consecutive operations. Chest 69:43-47, 1976
224. Ray LI, O'Connor JB et al: Axillofemoral bypass: A critical reappraisal of its role in the management of aortoiliac occlusive disease. Am J Surg 138:117-128, 1979
225. Rees JR, Redo SF, Tanner DW: Bochdalek's hernia: A review of twenty-one cases. Am J Surg 129:259-261, 1975
226. Reichle FA, Fahmy WF, Golsorkhi M: Prospective comparative clinical trial with distal splenorenal and mesocaval shunts. Am J Surg 137:13-21, 1979
227. Reichle FA, Martinson MW, Rankin KP: Infrapopliteal arterial reconstruction in the severely ischemic lower extremity. Ann Surg 191:59-65, 1980
228. Reichle FA, Rankin KP et al: Long-term results of 474 arterial reconstructions for severely ischemic limbs: A fourteen year follow-up. Surgery 85:93-100, 1979
229. Remine WH, Chong GC et al: Current management of pheochromocytoma. Ann Surg 179:740-748, 1974
230. Richards AB, Sosin H: Cancer of the pancreas: The value of radical and palliative surgery. Ann Surg 177:325-331, 1973
231. Rikkers LF, Rudman D et al: A randomized, controlled trial of the distal splenorenal shunt. Ann Surg 188:271-282, 1978
232. Rogers DM, Herrington JL, Morton C: Incidental splenectomy associated with Nissen fundoplication. Ann Surg 191:153-156, 1980
233. Ross ME, Ellwood R, Yang SS, Lucas RJ: Epidermoid splenic cysts. Arch Surg 112:596-599, 1977
234. Rutledge RH: Cooper's ligament repair for adult groin hernias. Surgery 87:601-610, 1980
235. Saharia PC, Zuidema GD, Cameron JL: Primary common duct stones. Ann Surg 185:598-604, 1977
236. Salvati EP, Rubin RJ: Electrocoagulation as primary therapy for rectal carcinoma. Am J Surg 132:583-586, 1976
237. Sandusky WR, Jones RCW et al: Staging laparotomy in Hodgkin's disease. Ann Surg 187:485-489, 1978
238. SanFilippo JA, Allen JE, Jewett TC: Definitive surgical management of Hirschsprung's disease. Arch Surg 105:245-248, 1972
239. Santos GH, Nordberg RE, Stamford WP, Efron G: Operative complications of abdominal vagotomy. Am J Surg 133:662-664, 1977
240. Satiani B, Davidson ED: Hepatic abscesses: Improvement in mortality with early diagnosis and treatment. Am J Surg 135:647-650, 1978
241. Satiani B, Gross WS, Evans WE: Improved limb salvage after arterial embolectomy. Ann Surg 188:153-157, 1978
242. Sawyers JL, Herrington JL: Perforated duodenal ulcer managed by proximal gastric vagotomy and suture plication. Ann Surg 185:656-660, 1977
243. Sawyers JL, Herrington JL et al: Acute perforated duodenal ulcer: An evaluation of surgical management. Arch Surg 110:527-530, 1975
244. Sawyers JL, Martin CE, Byrd BF, Rosenfeld L: Thyroidectomy for hyperthyroidism. Ann Surg 175:939-945, 1972
245. Scott HW, Dean R et al: New considerations in use of jejunoileal bypass in patients with morbid obesity. Ann Surg 177:723-735, 1973
246. Scott HW, Oates JA et al: Pheochromocytoma: Present diagnosis and management. Ann Surg 183:587-593, 1976
247. Scott HW, Sawyers JL et al: Surgical management of toxic dilatation of the colon in ulcerative colitis. Ann Surg 179:647-656, 1974
248. Sefton GK, Cooper DJ, Grech P, Giddings AEB: Assessment and resection of carcinoma at the gastroesophageal junction. Surg Gynecol Obstet 144:563-566, 1977
249. Shackford SR, Smith DE et al: The management of flail chest: A comparison of ventilatory and nonventilatory treatment. Am J Surg 132:759-762, 1976
250. Shah HH, Lambert CJ et al: Cervical mediastinal lymph node exploration for diagnosis and determination of operability. Ann Thorac Surg 5:15-22, 1968
251. Shochat SJ, Naeye RL et al: Congenital diaphragmatic hernia: New concept in management. Ann Surg 190:332-341, 1979
252. Sillin LF, Condon RE, Wilson SD, Worman LW: Effective surgical therapy of esophagitis: Experience with Belsey, Hill, and Nissen operations. Arch Surg 114:536-541, 1979
253. Silverstein MJ, Byron RL et al: Bilateral adrenalectomy for advanced breast cancer: A 21 year experience. Surgery 77:825-832, 1975
254. Sirinek KR, Evans WE: Nonparasitic splenic cysts. Am J Surg 126:8-13, 1973
255. Slavin R, Nelsen TS: Complications from staging laparotomy for Hodgkin's disease. Natl Cancer Inst Monogr 36:457-459, 1973
256. Smith RB, Warren WD et al: Dacron interposition shunts for portal hypertension. Ann Surg 192:9-16, 1980

257. Smith WR, Goodwin JN: Cecal volvulus. Am J Surg 126:215-222, 1973
258. Soper RT, Figueroa PR: Hirschsprung's disease: Pitfalls in diagnosis and surgical management. Arch Surg 104:429-433, 1972
259. Sorensen TIA, Aronsen KF et al: Results of hepatic lobectomy for primary epithelial cancer in 31 adults. Am J Surg 138:407-410, 1979
260. Steele M, Sheldon GF, Blaisdell FW: Pancreatic injuries: Methods of management. Arch Surg 106:544-549, 1973
261. Sterchi JM, Myers RT: Staging laparotomy in Hodgkin's disease. Ann Surg 191:570-575, 1980
262. Stokes J, Butcher HR: Abdominal aortic aneurysms. Arch Surg 107:297-302, 1973
263. Stone AM, Stein T, McCarthy K, Wise L: Surgery for bleeding duodenal ulcer. Am J Surg 136:306-308, 1978
264. Stone HH, Fabian TC: Management of perforating colon trauma: Randomization between primary closure and exteriorization. Ann Surg 190:430-436, 1979
265. Stone R, Rangel DM, Gordon HE, Wilson SE: Carcinoma of the gastroesophageal junction: A ten year experience with esophagogastrectomy. Am J Surg 134:70-76, 1977
266. Strauch GO: Preservation of splenic function in adults and children with injured spleens. Am J Surg 137:478-483, 1979
267. Stuart M, Hoerr SO: Late results of side to side choledochoduodenostomy and of transduodenal sphincterotomy for benign disorders: A twenty year comparative study. Am J Surg 123:67-72, 1972
268. Sundt TM, Sandok BA, Whisnant JP: Carotid endarterectomy: Complications and preoperative assessment of risk. Mayo Clin Proc 50:301-306, 1975
269. Swenson O, Sherman JO, Fisher JH, Cohen E: The treatment and postoperative complications of congenital megacolon: A 25 year follow-up. Ann Surg 182:266-273, 1975
270. Symbas PN, Hatcher CR, Harlaftis N: Spontaneous rupture of the esophagus. Ann Surg 187:634-640, 1978
271. Talbert JL, Seashore JH, Ravitch MM: Evaluation of a modified Duhamel operation for correction of Hirschsprung's disease. Ann Surg 179:671-675, 1974
272. Thomas CG, Carter JM: Small intestinal atresia: The critical role of a functioning anastomosis. Ann Surg 179:663-670, 1974
273. Thomas WH, Larson RA, Wright HK, Cleveland JC: An analysis of patients with carcinoma of the right colon. Surg Gynecol Obstet 127:313-318, 1968
274. Thompson BW, Casali RE, Read RC, Campbell GS: Results of interposition "H" grafts for portal hypertension. Ann Surg 187:515-522, 1978
275. Thompson JE, Hollier LH, Patman RD, Persson AV: Surgical management of abdominal aortic aneurysms. Ann Surg 181:654-661, 1975
276. Thompson JE, Talkington CM: Carotid endarterectomy. Ann Surg 184:1-14, 1976
277. Thompson NW, Harness JK: Complications of total thyroidectomy for carcinoma. Surg Gynecol Obstet 131:861-868, 1970
278. Todd GJ, Reemtsma K: Cholecystectomy with drainage: Factors influencing wound infection in 1,000 elective cases. Am J Surg 135:662-623, 1978
279. Trinkle JK, Bryant LR, Hiller AJ, Playforth RH; Mediastinoscopy—Experience with 300 consecutive cases. J Thorac Cardiovasc Surg 60:297-300, 1970
280. Trinkle JK, Richardson JD et al: Management of flail chest without mechanical ventilation. Ann Thorac Surg 19:355-363, 1975
281. Turnbull AD, Huvos AG, Goodner JT, Beattie EJ: The malignant potential of bronchial adenoma. Ann Thorac Surg 14:453-464, 1972
282. Urlaub BJ, Mack E: Evaluation and complications of 107 staging laparotomies for Hodgkin's disease. Ann Surg 190:45-47, 1979
283. VanHeerden JA, ReMine WH: Pseudocysts of the pancreas. Arch Surg 110:500-505, 1975
284. Verlenden WL, Frey CF: Management of liver abscess. Am J Surg 140:53-59, 1980
285. Vidne BA, Richter S, Levy MJ: Surgical treatment of solitary pulmonary metastasis. Cancer 38:2561-2563, 1976
286. Uori EE: Treatment of cholecystitis: Cholecystostomy or cholecystectomy? Am J Surg 132:75-80, 1976
287. Wagner DE, Rochlin DB, Weber AP: A new approach to radical retroperitoneal iliac and femoral node dissection. Arch Surg 103:681-683, 1971
288. Wanebo HJ, Martini N et al: Pleural mesothelioma. Cancer 38:2481-2488, 1976
289. Way LW, Admirand WH, Dunphy JE: Management of choledocholithiasis. Ann Surg 176:347-359, 1972
290. Weiss W: Operative mortality and five-year survival rates in men with bronchogenic carcinoma. Chest 66:483-487, 1974
291. Welch JP, Donaldson GA: Recent experience in the management of cancer of the colon and rectum. Am J Surg 127:258-266, 1974
292. Welch JP, Donaldson GA: Management of severe obstruction of the large bowel due to malignant disease. Am J Surg 127:492-499, 1974
293. Welch JP, Donaldson GA: Perforative carcinoma of colon and rectum. Ann Surg 180:734-740, 1974
294. Wells SA, Farndon JR et al: Long-term evaluation of patients with primary parathyroid hyperplasia managed by total parathyroidectomy and heterotopic autotransplantation. Ann Surg 192:451-458, 1980
295. White RR, Mackie JA, Fitts WT: An analysis of twenty years' experience with operations for carcinoma of the stomach. Ann Surg 181:611-615, 1975
296. Whitney DG, Kahn EM, Estes JW, Jones CE: Carotid artery surgery without a temporary indwelling shunt. Arch Surg 115:1393-1399, 1980
297. Wilson SM, Beahrs OH: The curative treatment of carcinoma of the sigmoid, rectosigmoid, and rectum. Ann Surg 183:556-565, 1976
298. Woolley MM, Mahour GH, Sloan T: Duodenal hematoma in infancy and childhood. Am J Surg 136:8-14, 1978
299. Yellin AE, Vecchione TR, Donovan AJ: Distal pancreatectomy for pancreatic trauma. Am J Surg 124:135-142, 1972
300. Yon J, Christensen J: An uncontrolled comparison of treatments for achalasia. Ann Surg 182:672-676, 1975
301. Young AE, Sandberg GW, Couch NP: The reduction of mortality of abdominal aortic aneurysm resection. Am J Surg 134:585-590, 1977
302. Yue PCK: Choledochal cysts: A review of 18 cases. Br J Surg 61:896-900, 1974

Suggested Reading

Kelman S: Improving Doctor Performance. New York, Human Sciences Press, 1980

Index

Index